Muir's Textbook of Pathology

Muir's Textbook of Pathology

Eleventh Edition

Edited by J. R. Anderson

C.B.E., B.Sc., M.D., F.R.C.P.(Glas.), F.R.C.P.(Lond.), F.R.C.Path., F.R.S.(Edin.)
Professor of Pathology, University of Glasgow

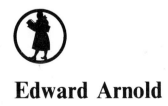

Edward Arnold

© J. R. Anderson, 1980

First published 1924
by Edward Arnold (Publishers) Ltd.
41 Bedford Square, London WC1B 3DQ

Reprinted, 1924, 1926, 1927
Second edition, 1929
Reprinted, 1930, 1932
Third edition, 1933
Fourth edition, 1936
Fifth edition, 1941
Reprinted, 1944, 1946
Sixth edition, 1951
Reprinted, 1956
Seventh edition, 1958
Eighth edition, 1964
Reprinted, 1968
Ninth edition, 1971
Reprinted, 1972, 1973, 1975
Tenth edition, 1976
Revised reprint, 1978
Reprinted, 1979
Eleventh edition, 1980
Reprinted, 1981

ELBS edition of Eighth edition first published 1964
Reprinted, 1967, 1968, 1969
ELBS edition of Ninth edition, 1971
Reprinted, 1974, 1975
ELBS edition of Tenth edition, 1976
Reprinted, 1979
ELBS edition of Eleventh edition, 1980

Italian Edition—Casa Editrice Universo
Portuguese edition—Editorial Espaxs
Spanish edition—Editorial Espaxs

Filmset in 'Monophoto' Times 10 on 11 pt. by
Richard Clay (The Chaucer Press), Ltd., Bungay, Suffolk
and printed in Great Britain by
Butler & Tanner Ltd., Frome and London

British Library Cataloguing in Publication Data

Muir, *Sir* Robert
  Muir's textbook of pathology.
  1. Pathology
  I. Anderson, John Russell
  II. Textbook of pathology
  616.07   RB111

  ISBN 0–7131–4357–6

Preface

It has long been appreciated that the undergraduate course in medicine cannot do more than lay the basis for further training, and that the newly-qualified doctor must undergo a further period of general training, followed by the appropriate specialist or vocational training, before commencing independent practice. There are, however, wide differences of opinion on what the undergraduate student should be expected to know, and this is nowhere better illustrated than by the variations in the time allocated to pathology in the curricula of medical schools. Clearly the authors of textbooks of pathology are faced with a problem, both in the selection of topics to be included and in the depth of treatment of each topic. The purpose of this book is to provide a text suitable for both undergraduate students and for doctors training or practising in various specialties, including junior trainees in pathology. It contains more than will be assimilated by most undergraduate students during their formal course in pathology, and students using it should receive guidance from their teachers on which topics deserve their closest attention. I hope it will continue to be of use throughout the clinically-oriented part of the curriculum and during subsequent training.

A brief introductory chapter defines pathology, explains its central position in medical education, and describes its importance in patient care and in the advancement of medical knowledge. The remainder of the book is divided into two main sections—'general' and 'systematic' pathology.

The twelve chapters on 'general' pathology describe pathological processes of fundamental importance—mechanisms and effects of cell injury, the inflammatory response to injury, healing and repair, the physiology of the immune response and its beneficial and harmful consequences, infection and host–parasite relationships, local and general disturbances of blood flow, and the causation, types and behaviour of tumours. It is in some of these basic processes that advance has been most rapid, and indeed this has necessitated production of this edition

earlier than had been intended. The accounts of the cellular basis of immune responses and of the causation of tumours have been very largely rewritten and most of the other chapters have been changed considerably. These basic processes are applicable to a wide range of species and although they are, where possible, illustrated by human material, much of the text is based on the results of experimental work. The size of the general chapters has been determined not just by the clinical importance of the physiological and pathological processes they describe, but also by the amount of firm information that can usefully be imparted to students and trainee doctors. For example, the mediators of the inflammatory reaction and the basis of neoplasia are both subjects of considerable practical importance, but knowledge on them is still very limited and larger accounts would, I believe, be more likely to confuse than help the student. By contrast, the immunity system and its abnormalities are still relatively unimportant as the basis of primary illness in man, and yet they merit detailed consideration because they continue to be the subject of rapid scientific advance. In spite of our efforts at brevity, it has not been possible to avoid some increase in the length of the general section, which I hope will be of use to medical students and to biological scientists in general.

The 'systematic' section consists of fourteen chapters, each devoted to the more important diseases of man which affect a particular organ or system—the heart, lungs, blood and haemopoietic tissues, alimentary system, etc. Emphasis has been placed on the aetiology of those diseases, and their structural changes and effects on function, together with brief clinico-pathological correlations. Every effort has been made to update these chapters. A section has been added on dental and related oral pathology, while the disorders of the male and female reproductive systems have been rewritten as separate chapters with a brief account of sexually-transmitted diseases placed appropriately between them. Multi-authorship has been of particular value in the systematic chapters, for the expert who is also an experienced teacher knows how much emphasis to place on particular topics and, most important, what may be omitted. Although the number of illustrations has been increased and now includes approximately 1200 photographs and diagrams, some reduction in the text has been achieved in this section, the total length of which is virtually unchanged.

Bibliography (now given at the end of each chapter) is confined mainly to reviews and larger texts. We have included some references to classical work, and to original papers representing important advances, but in general have avoided the temptation to append long lists of references to recent, often unconfirmed reports. I believe that it is the duty of the teacher to guide the student in his search for further information.

A final point relates to the value of cross-references, which are numerous in this text. They are useful in saving repetition, but they can, of course, be ignored by those readers who find them a distraction.

Acknowledgements

I am grateful to all my fellow authors, not only for their contributions but also for granting me wide editorial licence. I have used this in order to achieve uniformity of style and nomenclature, to avoid unnecessary repetition, and hopefully to provide a balanced account. I accept responsibility for errors of fact and judgement.

In addition to named contributors, I have received help with the accounts of certain topics from a number of colleagues. They include Drs J. J. Brown, A. F. Lever and J. I. S. Robertson of the MRC Hypertension Research Unit (the renin-angiotensin system, the aetiology of hypertension and Conn's syndrome), Professor J. Hume Adams (diseases of muscle) and Dr C. D. Forbes (haemostasis, clotting and fibrinolysis). I am grateful also, for their helpful discussion and advice to Dr J. Douglas Briggs (renal diseases), Dr J. W. Kerr (atopic hypersensitivity) and Professor I. A. Ledingham (shock).

My thanks are due also to colleagues who have contributed to previous editions, parts of whose contributions may still be embodied in the text. They include Professors Sir Douglas Black, M. J. Davies, W. A. Harland and N. Woolf and Drs E. L. Murray and J. M. Vetters. The contributions of the late Drs R. F. Macadam and H. E. Hutchison are also gratefully acknowledged.

In addition to those who have contributed directly to the text, all my colleagues in this Department have been most helpful in making useful suggestions, providing illustrations and participating in the correction of proofs. Illustrations provided by former colleagues and others outwith the Department are acknowledged in the legends.

I wish to thank Mr Robin Callander, FFPA, MMAA, for his skilful preparation of diagrams and Mr David McSeveney, FIMLT and his colleagues for their willing co-operation and skill in providing histological preparations and electron micrographs of the highest quality. Mr Peter Kerrigan has once again contributed an enormous amount of skilful and painstaking work in the preparation of photographs and he and Dr A. T. Sandison are largely responsible for the improved standard of many of the illustrations.

The revision has involved much secretarial work, for which I am particularly grateful to Miss Helen Scott who has dealt successfully with a large amount of correspondence and a considerable amount of typing, often from scarcely legible manuscripts. In the latter, she has been ably assisted by Mrs Pat Bonnar, Miss Margaret Brough, Mrs Pat Johnson, Mrs Jean Lyall and Mrs Maureen Ralston.

It is a pleasure once more to thank Messrs Edward Arnold, and particularly Miss Barbara Koster and Miss Jane Church for their enthusiastic co-operation and determination to overcome delays in publication.

Many readers have sent me useful comments and criticisms on the previous edition. This is most helpful and I hope it will continue.

For all this help, I offer my grateful thanks.

Finally, I wish to thank my wife for many things. Not only has she advised me on bacteriological topics and helped with proof reading, but she and our family have been unfailing in their support in spite of my pre-occupation and irritability during the preparation of this edition.
                                        J. R. ANDERSON
Glasgow, July, 1980

Reprinted 11th Edition. I am grateful to the many readers, and particularly to Dr. J. F. Boyd, for helping with the corrections and minor changes which have been made in the reprinted edition.

Contents

viii   *Contents*

1

Introduction

What is pathology?

Pathology is the study of disease by scientific methods. Disease may, in turn, be defined as an abnormal variation in the structure or function of any part of the body. There must be an explanation of such variations from the normal—in other words, diseases have causes, and pathology includes not only observation of the structural and functional changes throughout the course of a disease, but also elucidation of the factors which cause it. It is only by establishing the cause (*aetiology*) of a disease that logical methods can be devised for its prevention or cure. **Pathology may thus be described as the scientific study of the causes and effects of disease.**

Methods used in pathology

These include (*a*) **histology** and **cytology**, in which the structural changes in diseased tissues are examined by naked-eye inspection, or by light and electron microscopy of tissue sections or smears; (*b*) **biochemistry**, in which the metabolic disturbances of disease are investigated by assay of various normal and abnormal compounds in the blood, urine, etc.; (*c*) **microbiology**, in which body fluids, mucosal surfaces, excised tissues, etc., are examined by microscopical, cultural and serological techniques to detect and identify the micro-organisms responsible for many diseases.

These methods may be applied to the study of individuals suffering from a disease, and to animals in which a model of the disease occurs naturally or has been induced experimentally. The development of special techniques to investigate some types of disease has led to further specialisation in pathology. For example, the diagnosis of disorders of the blood involves various quantitative tests on, and morphologi-

cal examination of, the cells of the blood and haemopoietic tissue, assay of the factors involved in clotting, investigation of the metabolism of iron, vitamin B_{12}, etc., the detection of abnormal antibodies to cells of the blood and blood group serology. The many techniques involved have required the establishment of **haematology** laboratories: application of techniques to determine chromosome anomalies has led to the establishment of **cytogenetics** laboratories, and microbiology has divided into **bacteriology** and **virology**. Finally, **immunology**, a subject of enormous interest in biology and of increasing clinical significance, now requires special laboratory facilities. It will be apparent that pathology covers a wide spectrum of techniques, both in the diagnosis of patients and in research into the causes of various diseases. The relative importance of the several branches of pathology varies for different types of disease. In some instances, for example in diabetes mellitus, biochemical investigations provide the best means of diagnosis and are of the greatest value in the control of therapy. By contrast, recognition of the nature of many diseases, for example tumours, and so the choice of the most appropriate therapy, depend very largely on examination of the gross and microscopic features. For most diseases, diagnosis is based on a combination of pathological investigations. To give an example, biochemical tests may indicate that a patient is suffering from impairment of renal function, but the nature of the renal disease responsible for this commonly requires removal of a piece of renal tissue for histological examination (*renal biopsy*). Another example is provided by the condition of anaemia, which may have many causes. The changes in the cells of the blood and the bone marrow may suggest deficiency of a factor essential for erythropoiesis, and biochemical and physiological tests are then indicated to con-

1

firm the deficiency, e.g. of vitamin B_{12} or folic acid. Alternatively, anaemia may result from blood loss and this may be due to a structural lesion of the gastro-intestinal tract or of the endometrium, diagnosis of which may require histological examination.

The hospital pathologist is becoming much more clinically orientated. He must co-operate closely with clinicians, not only in diagnosis, but also by applying his skills to assessment of the effects of treatment, e.g. by examination of multiple biopsies of cancers and other lesions, removed serially during the course of treatment. He must also monitor patients for unwanted effects of treatment, e.g. the harmful effects of some drugs on the cells of the liver, kidney or haemopoietic tissue.

Finally, it is important to emphasise the continuing value of the clinical necropsy. In the past, when diagnostic procedures were relatively limited and primitive, a high proportion of diagnoses were made in the post-mortem room. In many cases, the more sophisticated diagnostic procedures now available have not diminished the value of necropsy, even in hospitals providing a very high standard of patient care (Cameron, 1978). The important role of post-mortem examination in elucidating the natural history of disease processes is well illustrated by the extensive studies of Willis (1973) on the spread of tumours within the body. This role of the necropsy is still important, for it is revealing the changes in the patterns of many diseases, and also new and unwanted effects, resulting from use of the ever-increasing number and variety of powerful drugs and therapeutic procedures available to the clinician.

Why learn pathology?

Most medical students are not going to become pathologists. It is nevertheless essential that the medical school curriculum should include a course of pathology which provides a clear account of the causes, where these are known, and of the pathological changes, of the more important diseases. Most disease processes bring about structural changes and these usually provide a logical explanation for the symptoms and signs and commonly also for the biochemical changes. A basic knowledge of the pathological processes of disease thus aids the

doctor in the correct interpretation of the clinical features of the patient's illness. This applies not only to the clinical diagnostician but also to the surgeon who must recognise the nature of the structural changes exposed at operation and act accordingly, and to the radiologist who must be familiar with the structural changes of diseases in order to interpret the shadows they cast on an x-ray film. To the research worker, histopathology and electron microscopy are superb techniques; both can be adapted to enzymic and other chemical investigations (**histochemistry**), including immunohistological techniques which make use of the exquisite specificity of antigen–antibody reactions to detect tissue and cell constituents and abnormal substances (see Fig. 22.20, p. 820 and Fig. 26.1, p. 1005).

Accordingly, pathology is of central importance to the medical student, regardless of the branch of medicine he intends to pursue.

How to learn pathology

Pathology is no exception to the general rule that learning is dependent mainly on the student's own effort. Most medical schools provide lectures and/or small-group tutorials, demonstrations and practical classes in pathology, but self-education by reading, preferably supplemented by audio-visual aids, is essential. The student should also take full advantage of opportunities to compare the clinical features of patients' illnesses with the underlying pathology. Clinico-pathological conferences on selected cases, held for teaching purposes, are helpful but one of the best places to see pathology and to compare the clinical features of disease with the pathological changes is the post-mortem room. A well-conducted necropsy, presented jointly by a clinician who cared for the patient and the pathologist performing the necropsy, is still unsurpassed as a teaching method. Students should also gain experience by following the progress of the patients they examine, noting the results of laboratory investigations and where possible examining the lesions removed surgically or revealed at necropsy.

Pathology in the medical curriculum

There is a logical sequence in the pattern of teaching of most medical schools. After courses in the basic sciences—chemistry, physics, biology—often provided before starting at medical school, the student is introduced to normal human structure (anatomy and histology) and function (physiology and biochemistry), followed by courses in pathology (the causes, features and effects of diseases) and pharmacology, and finally concentrates on the clinical subjects, i.e. the diagnosis and treatment of patients. Classically, the subjects are dealt with on a broad front. For example, the courses in anatomy, etc. deal with the whole of the body. In many medical schools, this policy has been replaced by what is variously termed 'integrated', 'topic' or 'systems' teaching, in which each of the body's major systems (cardiovascular, alimentary, respiratory, etc.) is the subject of a teaching course provided by a multidisciplinary team. Thus the course on, say, the alimentary system will include its anatomy, physiology, biochemistry, pathology, pharma-

cology and clinical aspects. Each method has its advantages, but it has become abundantly clear that the second method requires considerable organisation, and good co-operation between departments in the preparation and delivery of the course on each system. At present, there is a tendency to revert to the classical type of curriculum, or to compromise between the two.

One of the great advantages of a course in pathology, spanning the gap between the preclinical and clinical subjects, is that it provides the student, in the early part of his hospital experience, with a basic knowledge of the diseases he is likely to encounter most often in the wards and clinics. By contrast, the integrated course must either be brief and intensive or must extend over much of the curriculum, with the result that some systems come very late, leaving little time for their personal clinical study by the student.

Pathological processes

It was first pointed out by Virchow that all disturbances of function and structure in disease are due to cellular abnormalities and that the phenomena of a particular disease are brought about by a series of cellular changes. Pathological processes are of a dual nature, consisting firstly of **the changes of the injury** induced by the causal agent, and secondly of **reactive changes** which are often closely similar to physiological processes. If death is rapid, as for example in cyanide poisoning, there may be little or no structural changes of either type. Cyanide inhibits the cytochrome-oxidase systems of the cells and thus halts cellular respiration before histological changes can become prominent. Similarly, blockage of a coronary artery cuts off the blood supply to part of the myocardium and death may result immediately from cardiac arrest or ventricular fibrillation. When this happens, no structural changes are observed in the myocardium. If, however, the patient survives for some hours or more, the affected myocardium shows changes which occur subsequent to cell death and the lesion becomes readily visible both macroscopically (Fig. 15.9, p. 404) and microscopically (Fig. 2.5, p. 11).

Reactive changes may be exemplified by enlargement of the myocardium in the patient with high blood pressure (Fig. 4.31, p. 100). In this condition, there is an increase in the resistance to blood flow through the arterioles and consequently the normal rate of circulation can be maintained only by a rise in blood pressure. Reflex stimulation of the heart results in more forcible contractions of the left ventricle, and in accordance with the general principle that increased functional demand stimulates enlargement (**hypertrophy**) and/or proliferation (**hyperplasia**) of the cells concerned, the myocardial cells of the left ventricle increase in size. Although part of a disease state, the reactive hypertrophy of the myocardium in hypertension is closely similar to the physiological hypertrophy of the skeletal muscles in the trained athlete. To give another example, the invasion of the body by micro-organisms, in addition to causing injury, stimulates reactive changes in the lymphoid tissues, with the development of immunity. The distinction between the changes due to injury and those due to reaction are not usually so well defined as in the above examples. In many instances where cell injury persists without killing the cells, the cytological changes are complex and those due to injury often cannot be distinguished from those due to reaction. Some examples of the various types of cell injury and reaction are provided in Chapter 2.

In order to facilitate the understanding of pathological processes, it is helpful to group together those which have common causal factors and as a consequence exhibit similarities in their structural changes. For example, bacterial infections have certain features in common, and may with advantage be further sub-divided into acute and chronic infections. The features and behaviour of neoplasms (tumours) are sufficiently similar to classify most tumours into two categories, benign and malignant, and to provide a general account of each group. The changes resulting from a deficient blood supply are similar for all tissues. Accordingly, the next twelve chapters of this book are of a general nature and deal with the commoner pathological processes. The remaining chapters are systematic and go on to describe the special features of disease processes as they affect the various organs and systems.

The causes of disease

Causal factors in disease may be genetic or acquired. **Genetically-determined disease** is due to some abnormality of base sequence in the DNA of the fertilised ovum and the cells derived from it, or to reduplication, loss or misplacement of a whole or part of a chromosome. Such abnormalities are often inherited from one or both parents. **Acquired disease** is due to effects of some environmental factor, e.g. malnutrition or micro-organisms. Most diseases are acquired, but very often there is more than one causal factor and there may be many. Genetic variations may influence the susceptibility of an individual to environmental factors. Even in the case of infections, there is considerable individual variation in the severity of the disease. Of the many individuals who become infected with poliovirus, most develop immunity without becoming ill; some have a mild illness and a few become paralysed from involvement of the central nervous system (Fig. 21.44, p. 759). This illustrates the importance of **host factors** as well as causal agents. Spread of tuberculosis is favoured by poor personal

and domestic hygiene, by overcrowding, malnutrition and by various other diseases. Accordingly, disease results not only from exposure to the major causal agent but also from the existence of **predisposing** or **contributory factors**.

Congenital disease. Diseases may also be classified into those which develop during fetal life (congenital) and those which arise at any time thereafter during post-natal life. Genetically-determined diseases are commonly congenital, although some present many years after birth, a good example being adenomatosis (polyposis) coli, which is due to a dominant abnormal gene (see below) and consists of multiple tumours of the colonic mucosa, appearing in adolescence or adult life (Fig. 19.79, p.652). Congenital diseases may also be acquired, an important example being provided by transmission of the virus of rubella (German measles) from mother to fetus during the first trimester of pregnancy. Depending on the stage of fetal development at which infection occurs, it may result in fetal death, or involvement of various tissues leading to mental deficiency, blindness, deafness or structural abnormalities of the heart. The mother may also transmit to the fetus various other infections, including syphilis and toxoplasmosis, with consequent congenital disease. Ingestion of various chemicals by the mother, as in the thalidomide disaster, may induce severe disorders of fetal development and growth. Another cause of acquired congenital disease is maternal–fetal incompatibility. Fetal red cells exhibiting surface antigens inherited from the father may enter the maternal circulation and stimulate antibody production: the maternal antibody may pass through the placenta and react with the fetal red cells, causing a haemolytic anaemia.

Genetically-determined disease

As already mentioned, this results from abnormalities in the DNA which forms the genome. In some instances the abnormality consists of gain or loss of a whole chromosome or of part of a chromosome. Such gross abnormalities can now be detected by cell culture techniques. Most of them probably arise by non-disjunction of chromosomes in the meiosis which precedes germ-cell formation, and only a few appear to be compatible with life, e.g. an additional chromosome 21, which is the usual cause of Down's syndrome (mongolism).

A very large number of diseases result from the inheritance of an abnormal (mutant) gene, or combination of genes, from one or both parents. The development of abnormal genes (**mutation**) can be provoked by irradiation, mutagenic chemicals and probably by viruses, but in most instances the cause of mutations in man remains unknown. Examples of the many conditions resulting from an abnormal gene are colour blindness, albinism, haemophilia, sickle-cell anaemia, dystrophia myotonica and polyposis coli. The abnormal gene may be dominant, i.e. may induce an abnormality in spite of the presence of a normal corresponding gene from the other parent, or it may be recessive, i.e. causing disease only in the absence of a corresponding normal gene. The latter circumstance arises most usually in abnormalities of genes on the X chromosome, males being thus affected (Fig. 17.50, p. 555), or from the presence of two abnormal corresponding genes, one from each parent, the likelihood of which is enhanced by inbreeding.

In addition to those diseases due to mutations or recognisable chromosomal anomalies, there are many which show a **familial tendency**, but in which the mode of inheritance has not been elucidated. Examples include diabetes mellitus, chronic thyroiditis (see (**6**) below) and some of the commoner cancers, e.g. of the breast and of the bronchus. It is likely that both genetic and environmental factors are of causal importance in these conditions.

Acquired disease

The major causal factors may be classified as follows:

(1) **Deficiency diseases.** Inadequate diet still accounts for poor health in many parts of the world. It may take the form of deficiency either of major classes of food, usually high-grade protein, or of vitamins or elements essential for specific metabolic processes, e.g. iron for haemoglobin production. Often the deficiencies are multiple and complex. Disturbances of nutrition are by no means restricted to deficiencies, for in the more affluent countries obesity, due to overeating, has become increasingly common, with its attendant dangers of high blood pressure and heart disease.

(2) **Physical agents.** These include mechanical injury, heat, cold, electricity, irradiation and rapid changes in environmental pressure. In all instances, injury is caused by a high rate of transmission of particular forms of energy (kinetic, radiant, etc.) to or from the body. Important examples in this country are mechanical injury, particularly in road accidents, and burns. Exposure to ionising radiations cannot be regarded as entirely safe in any dosage. While radiation is used with benefit in various diagnostic and therapeutic procedures, any pollution of the environment with radioactive material is potentially harmful to those exposed to it and probably to subsequent generations.

(3) **Chemicals.** With the use of an ever increasing number of chemical agents as drugs, in industrial processes, and in the home, chemically-induced injury has become very common. The effects vary. At one extreme are those substances which have a general effect on cells, such as cyanide (see above) which causes death almost instantaneously, with little or no structural changes. Many other chemicals, such as strong acids and alkalis, cause local injury accompanied by an inflammatory reaction in the tissues exposed to them. A third large group of substances produces a more or less selective injury to a particular organ or cell type. Because of their important and complex metabolic activities, hepatocytes are injured by many chemical substances, including paracetamol and alcohol in high dosage. Many toxic chemicals or their metabolites are excreted by the kidneys, and because of their concentrating function the renal tubular epithelial cells are exposed to high levels of such substances. Accordingly toxic hepatic and renal tubular cell death are common. Fortunately both types of cell have a high regenerative capacity. Specific effects of chemicals are illustrated also by injury of neurones by overdosage of barbiturates and lung injury by paraquat (Fig. 16.37, p. 486).

(4) **Parasitic micro-organisms.** These include bacteria, protozoa, lower fungi and viruses. In spite of the advances in immunisation procedures and the extensive use now made of antibiotics, many important diseases still result from infection by micro-organisms, and the danger of widespread epidemics, e.g. of influenza and cholera, has been enhanced by air travel. The

disease-producing capacity of micro-organisms depends on their ability to invade and multiply within the host, and on the possibility of their transmission to other hosts. The features of the disease produced by infection depend on the specific properties of the causal organism. Bacteria bring about harmful effects mainly by the production of chemical compounds termed **toxins**, and the biological effects of these, together with the response of the host, determine the features of the disease. Viruses colonise host cells, and have a direct cytopathic effect: features of virus disease depend largely on which cells are colonised, the rate of viral replication, the nature of the cytopathic effect, and the response of the host. Of the protozoa, the malaria parasite is of enormous importance as a cause of chronic ill health in whole populations.

(5) Metazoan parasites are also an important cause of disease in many parts of the world. Hookworm infestation of the intestine and schistosomiasis are causes of ill health prevalent in many tropical countries.

(6) Immunological factors. The development of immunity is essential for protection against microbes and parasites. Harmful effects, both local and more widespread, can, however, result from the reaction of antibodies and lymphocytes with parasites, microbes and their toxic products. Also, the immunity system does not distinguish between harmful and harmless foreign antigenic materials, and injury may result from immune reactions to either. Such **hypersensitivity reactions** are numerous and complex. Local examples include hay fever, asthma and some forms of dermatitis, while hypersensitivity to many foreign materials, including penicillin and other drugs, sometimes causes fatal generalised reactions. Hypersensitivity reactions may also result from the development of **auto-immunity** in which antibodies and lymphocytes develop which react with and injure normal cells and tissues: examples include chronic thyroiditis, commonly progressing to myxoedema, and the excessive destruction of red cells in auto-immune haemolytic anaemia.

In another group of disorders, the immunity system is deficient, and the patient lacks defence against micro-organisms: this may result from abnormalities of fetal development, as an effect of various acquired diseases, or may be induced by immuno-suppressive therapy.

(7) Psychogenic factors. The mental stresses imposed by conditions of life, particularly in technologically advanced communities, are probably largely responsible for three important and overlapping groups of diseases. First, acquired mental diseases such as schizophrenia and depression, for which no specific structural or biochemical basis has yet been found. Second, diseases of addiction, particularly to alcohol, various drugs and tobacco: these result in their own complications, for example alcohol predisposes to liver damage (Fig. 20.27, p. 682) and causes various neurological and mental disturbances, while cigarette smoking is the major cause of lung cancer (Fig. 16.45, p. 498) and chronic bronchitis, and is concerned also in peptic ulceration and coronary artery disease. The third group of diseases is heterogeneous, and includes peptic ulcer (Fig. 19.28, p. 609), high blood pressure and coronary artery disease (Fig. 15.12, p. 406). In these three important conditions, anxiety, overwork and frustration appear to be causal factors, although their modes of action are obscure.

References

Cameron, H. M. (1978). The autopsy: its role in modern hospital practice. *Investigative Cell Pathology*, 1, 297–300.

Willis, R. A. (1973). *The spread of tumours in the human body*, 3rd edn., pp. 400. Butterworths, Sevenoaks and London.

2

Cell Damage

All metabolic activities of the body are carried out and regulated by the cells of the tissues, and since the time of Virchow cell injury has been recognised as the central problem in pathology. It is clearly important to know what factors cause cell damage and how these lead to the cellular disorders which result in the states we recognise as diseases. Our knowledge of this large and important subject has been slow to develop due to the extremely complex interrelationship of biological activities within the cell. Recently, however, there have been rapid advances, partly due to greatly improved techniques of biochemical analysis, fractionation of subcellular organelles and microscopy, and partly to the use of homogeneous experimental systems such as cultures of clones of genetically identical cells (bacterial or mammalian). Equally important has been the strategic use of cellular disorders in which the initial damage affects only one molecular constituent of the cell, thereby providing information about the normal and abnormal function of that constituent and its relationship to other activities of the cell. For this reason the most instructive forms of cellular damage are those due to abnormality of a single gene or to the effects of a selective poison.

Single gene defects. In at least one disease, sickle-cell anaemia, we probably know the entire sequence of events leading to cellular destruction. The sickle-cell abnormality is an inherited defect characterised clinically by rapid destruction of red blood cells. Apparently an error has occurred in copying one base in the sequence of 146 base triplets in the DNA constituting the gene for the beta polypeptide chain of haemoglobin. This error, transcribed through messenger RNA, results in the insertion of the amino acid valine instead of glutamic acid in position 6 from the N terminal end of the beta polypeptide chain and the shape of that end of the chain is altered. This abnormality does not matter when haemoglobin is oxygenated, but as the haemoglobin molecule gives up oxygen it expands and the abnormal parts of the two beta chains come to project from the surface of the molecule and unite with alpha chains of adjacent molecules. Masses of long helical fibres of polymerised deoxygenated haemoglobin form and these impart to the red cells abnormal rigidity and a characteristic sickle shape which make them unduly prone to mechanical injury and subsequent phagocytosis within the spleen. It should be noted that, compared with most cells, red cells have a very simple structure and are easily obtained for study. Also, haemoglobin is one of the few proteins whose molecular configuration and amino acid sequences are known in detail, so that the substitution of a single amino acid is detectable and indicates, in turn, a single error in the DNA base sequence.

Many other defects of single genes result in clearly defined primary lesions. There may be absence of a particular enzyme with predictable effects such as accumulation of substrate and deficiency of the product of the missing enzyme, but these effects often lead to secondary, more complex abnormalities which may result also from various other primary defects. Genetic disorders are further considered on p. 14.

Experimental poisoning. Many genetic defects are incompatible with cell survival and so cannot readily be investigated. Accordingly, toxic chemicals have been widely used to investigate more severe forms of cell injury, for example the impairment of oxidative phosphorylation by fluoroacetate or cyanide (p. 9). Much information has been obtained by use of drugs known to have a specific effect on particular cellular functions: examples include actinomycin D which inhibits transcription of

7

DNA to mRNA, and colchicine which interferes with microtubular function. Various bacterial and other biological toxins have specific effects, for example cholera toxin disturbs the sodium pump and α-bungarotoxin from snake venom blocks acetylcholine receptors. It is possible, however, that such substances have additional effects on other cellular mechanisms. The action of some other poisons is indirect and less specific. Thus the classical experimental poison carbon tetrachloride is toxic to liver cells because it is metabolised by the microsomal enzyme P450 to produce free CCl_3^+ and Cl^- radicals which lead to peroxidation of mRNA and of unsaturated fatty acids in cell membranes, and also to secondary disturbances of protein, fat and carbohydrate metabolism: electron microscopy shows damage to rough endoplasmic reticulum and later to other cellular organelles. Several other poisons cause similar effects on liver cells and, as in genetic abnormalities, it is evident that various different injuries cause trains of common secondary events, some of which lead to cell death.

In the following account only a few examples of cellular damage have been selected. The topic arises frequently in later chapters and our superficial treatment of this important subject is merely a reflection of our present basic ignorance.

It is convenient to consider the effects of cellular injury under two main headings: **(1) cell death** or *necrosis*, in which irreversible changes take place in the cell so that no further integrated function such as respiration or maintenance of selective membrane permeability is possible: **(2) lesser forms of damage** (sometimes described as degenerations) in which functions important for the economy of the cell or body are diminished or lost but in which integrated vital functions such as respiration and selective membrane permeability remain possible. Many lesser forms of cellular damage are reversible when the cause is withdrawn, for example the injury to neurones by therapeutic doses of anaesthetic drugs. Others, not resulting in cell death, are irreversible, e.g. radiation damage to chromosomes resulting in non-lethal genetic mutation.

Necrosis

Necrosis means the death of cells or groups of cells. It may occur suddenly, for example when cells are exposed to heat or toxic chemicals, or may be preceded by gradual and potentially reversible damage in which case the term **necrobiosis** is occasionally used.

Causes of necrosis

(a) **Marked impairment of blood supply,** usually due to obstruction of an end-artery (that is, one without adequate collaterals) is a common and important cause of necrosis, the necrotic area being known as an **infarct** (p. 246). Different cells can withstand the anoxia which results from ischaemia (impaired blood flow) for different periods, nerve cells, for example, die after only a few minutes, while fibrocytes survive much longer periods of anoxia.

(b) **Toxins.** Certain bacteria, plants, and animals such as snakes and scorpions, produce toxic organic compounds which even in very

small quantities can cause cell damage amounting to necrosis. Some toxins have identifiable enzyme activity; for example, the causal organism of gas gangrene, *Clostridium welchii*, forms a lecithinase which digests the lipoprotein of cell membranes. Diphtheria toxin appears to inhibit cellular protein synthesis by indirect interference with the transfer of aminoacyl–tRNA to ribosomes. Certain bacterial toxins, including those mentioned above, exert their effects not only locally, but are distributed via the bloodstream and other routes and so injure the cells of organs remote from the infection. The necrosis accompanying bacterial infection may be partly due to interference with the circulation brought about by toxic injury to the vascular endothelium with inflammation and sometimes thrombosis.

(c) **Immunological injury.** As will be described in Chapter 6, cell injury results in various ways from immune reactions. This is a feature of many infections, including tuberculosis in which tuberculoprotein, a nontoxic product of the tubercle bacillus, evokes an immune reaction which, though protective in function, paradoxically leads also to necrosis of cells in the neighbourhood of the organism.

(d) Infection of cells. In certain infections, notably by viruses, the infecting agent proliferates within cells. Many viruses kill infected cells in tissue culture (cytopathic effect) and this is probably the cause of necrosis *in vivo* of the anterior horn cells of the spinal cord in poliomyelitis.

(e) Chemical poisons. Many chemicals in high concentration cause necrosis by non-selective denaturation of the cellular proteins (e.g. strong acids, strong alkalis, carbolic acid, mercuric chloride). Cyanide and fluoroacetate are much more selective poisons and in low concentrations quickly cause cell death by interfering with oxidative production of energy from glucose, fatty acids and amino acids. As shown in Fig. 2.1 cyanide inhibits the enzyme cytochrome oxidase, thereby preventing the use of oxygen, while fluoroacetate forms a powerful competitive inhibitor of the enzyme aconitase which normally converts citrate to isocitrate in the Krebs citric acid cycle. Necrosis of liver or other specialised cells results from the effects of poisoning, but in many instances the mode of interaction between poison and cell is obscure.

(f) Physical agents. Cells are very sensitive to heat and, depending on the type of cell, they die after variable periods of exposure to a temperature of 45°C. Cold is much less injurious and, provided certain precautions are taken, cell suspensions and even small animals can be frozen without being killed. Necrosis after frostbite is due to damage to capillaries, resulting in thrombosis which may even extend to the arteries. Radiation damage, also a cause of necrosis, is considered on p. 32. Mechanical trauma such as crushing may cause direct disruption of cells. Certain disorders of the nervous system are sometimes accompanied by necrotic lesions in the limbs; these 'trophic' lesions were previously attributed to an ill-defined effect of denervation on tissue nutrition but are now thought to result from mechanical trauma which occurs unnoticed because of sensory loss.

The recognition of necrosis

As a rule it is not possible to determine exactly when a particular cell becomes necrotic—i.e. when the disintegration of its vital functions has reached an irreversible stage. Many of the changes by which necrosis is recognised occur *after* cell death and are due to the secondary release of lytic enzymes normally sequestered within the cell, e.g. in the lysosomes; this process of **autolysis** is described below.

Necrosis of cell suspensions in tissue culture can be studied conveniently by observing changes of permeability of cell membranes to dyes such as neutral red or trypan blue. These dyes are normally excluded from the nucleus but when cells die, the nuclei become stained due to increased permeability of the membranes of the cell (Fig. 2.2). Alternatively, membranous components of the living cells may be labelled with radioisotopes such as ^{51}Cr or ^{32}P; subsequent severe injury to the cell, probably lethal, is recognised by release of the radio-active label from the cells into the culture medium.

In organised tissues such as liver or kidney,

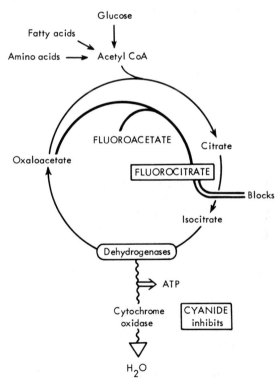

Fig. 2.1 The effects of fluoroacetate and of cyanide on cellular metabolism. Note that fluoroacetate is converted to fluorocitrate which inhibits conversion of citrate to isocitrate by aconitase.

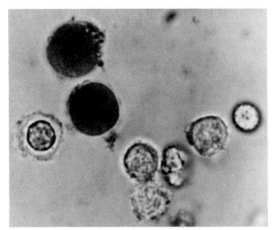

Fig 2.2 A suspension of lymphocytes treated with cytotoxic iso-antibody and complement. Some of the cells have been killed, and have become stained by trypan blue dye present in the suspending fluid: other cells have survived and are unstained. × 1250.

necrosis is usually recognised by secondary changes seen on histological examination. In preparations stained with haematoxylin and eosin, the nuclei may gradually lose their characteristic staining with haematoxylin so that the whole cell stains uniformly with eosin (Fig. 2.3), although the nuclear outline may persist; this change, the result of hydrolysis of chromatin within the cell after its death, is called **karyolysis**. Sometimes the chromatin of necrotic cells, especially those with already dense chromatin such as polymorphonuclear leukocytes, forms dense haematoxylinophilic masses (**pyknosis**) and these may break up (**karyorrhexis**) to form granules inside the nuclear membrane or throughout the cytoplasm (Fig. 2.4). In many necrotic lesions the outlines of swollen necrotic cells can be recognised but the cytoplasm is abnormally homogeneous or granular and frequently takes up more eosin than normal. In other tissues, e.g. the central nervous system, necrotic cells absorb water and then disintegrate, leaving no indication of the architecture of the original tissue; the lipids derived from myelin etc. persist in the debris of the necrotic tissue. The activities of certain enzymes, e.g. succinic acid dehydrogenase, diminish rapidly after cell death and appropriate tests provide useful indicators of recent tissue necrosis.

Electron microscopy of cells which have undergone necrosis shows severe disorganisa-

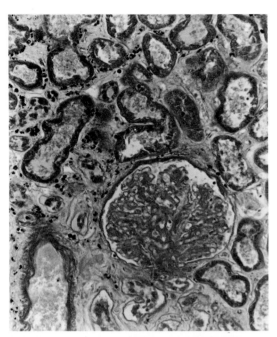

Fig. 2.3 Part of an infarct of kidney, showing coagulative necrosis. A glomerulus and tubules are seen, but the nuclei have disappeared and the structural details are lost. × 172.

tion of structure. Gaps are seen in the various membranes and abnormal polymorphic inclusions, presumably derived from membranes, lie in the ground substance. Fragmentation and vacuolation of endoplasmic reticulum and mitochondrial membranes precede the disap-

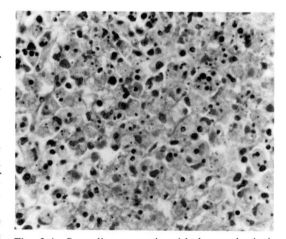

Fig. 2.4 Spreading necrosis with karyorrhexis in lymph node in typhoid fever. Note destruction of nuclei and numerous deeply-stained granules of chromatin. × 412.

pearance of these structures. Curious lamellar structures with concentric whorling form from the cell membrane, especially where there have been microvilli. Ribosomes and Golgi apparatus are unrecognisable from an early stage. There is loss of density of the nucleoplasm and large chromatin granules accumulate just inside the nuclear membrane before it disappears.

Less severe injury affecting single cells sometimes leads to **shrinkage necrosis**, a gradual process in which water is lost from the cell so that the nucleus becomes condensed and the cytoplasm appears strongly eosinophilic due to the closely packed organelles. Later the cell breaks into rounded fragments with preservation of ultrastructure and some functional activities which persist until the fragments are phagocytosed and digested by neighbouring parenchymal cells or macrophages. The circula Councilman bodies formed from hepatocytes are examples of this form of necrosis which can be an expression of normal cell turnover in the parenchyma of tissues like liver and adrenal cortex. The term **apoptosis** ('dropping off') has also been used in this context.

Necrosis can often be recognised macroscopically when large groups of cells die. The necrotic area may become swollen, firm, dull and lustreless, and is yellowish unless it contains much blood. This appearance is often found in kidney, spleen and myocardium. Histologically the outlines of the dead cells are usually visible (Figs. 2.3 and 2.5) and the firmness of the

tissue may be due to the action of tissue thromboplastins on fibrinogen which together with other plasma proteins has been shown to diffuse through the damaged membranes of necrotic cells. This type of necrosis is appropriately described as **coagulative necrosis**. By contrast, necrotic brain tissue, which has a large fluid component, becomes 'softened' and ultimately turns into a turbid fluid (**colliquative necrosis**) with profound loss of the previous histological architecture.

Certain necrotic lesions develop a firm cheese-like appearance to the naked eye and microscopy shows amorphous granular eosinophilic material lacking in cell outlines; a varying amount of finely divided fat is present and there may be minute granules of chromatin. Because of its gross appearance this lesion is described as 'caseation'. It is very common in tuberculosis but essentially similar changes are occasionally seen in infarcts, necrotic tumours and in inspissated collections of pus.

Necrotic lesions affecting skin or mucosal surfaces are frequently infected by organisms which cause putrefaction, i.e. the production of foul-smelling gas and brown, green or black discoloration of the tissue due to alteration of haemoglobin. Necrosis with putrefaction is called **gangrene** (Fig. 2.6). It may be primarily due to vascular occlusion, e.g. in the limbs or bowel where the necrotic tissue is exposed to putrefactive bacteria, but it may also result from infection with certain bacteria, namely the clostridia which cause gas gangrene (p. 203) or fusiform bacilli which result in **noma** (p. 205).

The special features of **fat necrosis** are described on pages 717 and 972.

Autolysis

The structural disintegration of cells as a result of digestion by their own enzymes is largely responsible for the softening of necrotic tissues and the associated loss of histological structure. In the intact cell, the enzymes concerned do not have general access to the protoplasm. For example, various hydrolytic enzymes are associated with endoplasmic reticulum, mitochondria and lysosomes. The hydrolases confined within the lysosomal membranes include proteases which are most effective at low pH, a state which prevails in necrotic cells due to acid production from anaerobic glycolysis and the

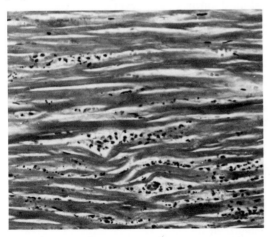

Fig. 2.5 Coagulative necrosis in infarction of heart muscle. The dead fibres are hyaline and structureless; remains of leukocytes, which have migrated from the venules, are present between them. × 125.

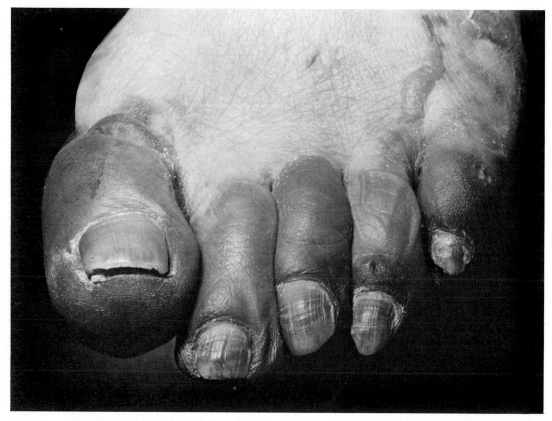

Fig. 2.6   Gangrene of toes.

action of phosphatases and proteolytic enzymes. The small molecules produced by hydrolysis of macromolecules lead to osmotic swelling of the necrotic cells and their organelles provided that the membranes are sufficiently intact.

It should be noted that when many polymorphonuclear leukocytes are present in necrotic tissue the enzymes from their abundant lysosomes may contribute to the hydrolysis of other cells. This is an important factor in the liquefaction of pus and in the softening seen in infected organs at necropsy.

If tissue is killed by heating, e.g. to 55°C, or by immersion in fixative such as formalin, the enzymes and other proteins are denatured and the histological features of necrosis attributable to autolysis do not develop. By contrast, if a piece of tissue is deprived of its blood supply by removal from the living body and kept at 37°C the development of autolysis can be observed, with marked osmotic swelling of membrane-bounded structures.

Two points of practical importance in the recognition of necrosis deserve emphasis. First, morphological signs of necrosis are not apparent until autolysis has developed in the necrotic tissue, and this takes 12–24 hours. Second, following death of the individual (somatic death), all cells of the body will in time die due to lack of blood supply and post-mortem autolysis will gradually take place. This is particularly marked in the parenchymal cells of the liver and kidney tubules and when seen at necropsy it may be mistaken for true necrosis, i.e. cell death occurring while the individual was still alive. This problem is of great importance in electron microscopy which shows fine structural evidence of necrosis and of post-mortem autolysis within a very short time.

Somatic death

Though not strictly related to cell necrosis, the interesting subject of somatic death (death of the individual) deserves some consideration.

Until recently, somatic death has been defined as complete and persistent cessation of respiration and circulation. For legal purposes the persistence of the state is arbitrarily taken as five or more minutes, by which time irreversible anoxic damage will have developed in the neurones of the vital centres. However, it is now possible to restore the circulatory and respiratory functions of heart and lungs in many cases of somatic death as defined above, and integrated function both of cells and of organs (excluding those of the central nervous system) can then continue for prolonged periods with the aid of special equipment. This fact is of great importance in obtaining organs for transplantation from cadaveric donors and a legal redefinition of somatic death in terms of extensive and irreversible brain damage is now necessary.

Effects of necrosis

By definition, necrotic cells are functionless. The effect of cell necrosis on the general well-being of the body accordingly depends on the functional importance of the tissue involved, the extent of the necrosis, the functional reserve of the tissue, and on the capacity of surviving cells to proliferate and replace those which have become necrotic. For example, splenectomy is compatible with good health in man (although it increases the risk of certain infections) and extensive splenic necrosis is apparently of little importance. By contrast, extensive necrosis of renal tubular epithelium results in the serious clinical condition of renal failure which is likely to be fatal unless the patient is kept alive (e.g. by haemodialysis) until there is regeneration of tubules by proliferation of surviving cells. Necrosis of a relatively small number of motor nerve cells may produce severe paralysis which persists because nerve cells cannot proliferate to replace those lost. Since myocardial cells have not only a contractile but also a conducting function, quite small necrotic lesions may result in striking alterations in the electrical activity of the heart.

The breakdown of necrotic cells results in escape of their contents. Enzymes such as aminotransferases released into the plasma from necrotic liver or myocardial cells form the basis of clinical tests for necrosis in these tissues. It should be emphasised, however, that abnormal enzyme release occurs from cells with damage short of necrosis (e.g. in muscular dystrophy). In poisoning by alloxan, which kills the β cells of the pancreatic islets, discharge of stored insulin from the necrotic cells results in hypoglycaemia which may be fatal: those animals which survive develop diabetes from lack of insulin.

Reactions to necrosis

Neutrophil polymorphs frequently accumulate in small numbers around necrotic cells (Fig. 2.5). Occasionally infarcts and caseous lesions are invaded by large numbers of these cells and this leads to softening as already described. Such softening is a notable feature in a small proportion of myocardial infarcts (which usually show coagulative necrosis) and may lead to rupture of the heart; it is also common in tuberculosis of the lumbar vertebrae where the caseous material liquefies and tracks down beneath the psoas fascia to form a 'cold abscess' in the groin.

Individual cells killed by toxins rapidly undergo autolysis and are absorbed, especially when the circulation is maintained. They may be quickly replaced by proliferation of adjacent surviving cells. When a large mass of tissue undergoes necrosis, e.g. in an infarct, the necrotic material may be gradually replaced by ingrowth of capillaries and fibroblasts from the surrounding viable tissue so that a fibrous scar results. If this process is incomplete the necrotic mass becomes enclosed in a fibrous capsule, may persist for a long time, and may become calcified. Areas of necrotic softening in the brain are usually invaded by macrophages and eventually become cyst-like spaces containing clear liquid and surrounded by proliferated astroglia.

Old caseous lesions and necrotic fat have a marked affinity for calcium and frequently become heavily calcified.

Cell Damage Short of Necrosis

Many forms of injury may cause cellular abnormalities short of necrosis, which may seriously affect health. Such cellular abnormalities may be detected by impairment of a physiological activity such as conduction of a nerve impulse, by chemical or histochemical means (diminished or excessive enzyme activity or storage or depletion of a chemical substance), by structural abnormality revealed by microscopy of one kind or another, or by a combination of these methods. Some of these forms of cellular injury lend themselves to scientific study because they can be accurately, if arbitrarily, defined.

The following discussion deals with very heterogeneous topics. First we consider damage to the nucleus, membranes and organelles of the cell, then give examples of damage resulting in abnormal storage of metabolites. Next, the important problem of irradiation damage, both to single cells and cell populations, is discussed and finally, shrinkage of cells (**atrophy**) and alteration of cell structure to a form more resistant to injury (**metaplasia**).

Nuclear damage

The importance of nuclear damage depends on the fact that the cell nucleus contains the genetic information upon which all the vital activities of the cell ultimately depend. Indeed, as already explained, severe nuclear damage indicated by pyknosis and karyolysis are customarily taken as evidence of cell necrosis. It should be remembered, however, that red blood cells, although devoid of a nucleus, maintain selective membrane permeability, produce energy by anaerobic glycolysis and perform their vital specialised function of oxygen transport in the blood for over 100 days in man. Protozoa such as *Amoeba proteus* survive at least for several days following microsurgical removal of their nucleus: motility and phagocytic activity are arrested but these return, together with the ability to reproduce, when the nucleus from another amoeba is introduced. It is therefore clear that cells can survive despite total cessation of nuclear function; their metabolic versatility will, however, be greatly reduced and their ability to multiply lost.

Gene mutation

Perhaps the best understood form of nuclear damage is that due to irradiation or to mutagenic chemicals such as nitrogen mustards. These and other unidentified factors may result in errors in the sequence of purine and pyrimidine bases in DNA molecules. If the damage is sufficiently localised, e.g. affecting only one base, it is most unlikely to lead to an alteration in the nucleus demonstrable by available chemical or morphological techniques. Its presence may be inferred if there is a familial disease which can be shown to be due to genetic rather than purely environmental factors. Such diseases are essentially mediated by an abnormal gene resulting in incorporation of a 'wrong' amino acid at a functionally important part of a protein molecule, or by deletion of a gene with consequent absence of the protein. In most known examples, the affected proteins are enzymes, as in phenylketonuric oligophrenia which affects 1 in 10 000 of the population. It is due to deficiency in the liver cells of phenylalanine hydroxylase, which normally converts phenylalanine to tyrosine, and brain damage apparently results from raised blood and cerebrospinal fluid levels of phenylalanine and its metabolites. There are also many genetic abnormalities of haemoglobin (haemoglobinopathies p. 522), the sickle cell abnormality (p. 7) being a good example. Other carrier proteins, for example transferrin which binds iron, may also be defective. Genetic abnormalities of cell surface receptors, e.g. for low density lipoproteins (p. 30) have been described and there are probably errors in genes coding for the polypeptide chains of structural proteins such as collagen and also for proteins which regulate the activity of other genes. Many of the so-called inborn errors of metabolism are inherited as a recessive trait—i.e. are apparent only in the homozygous individual, although sometimes the symptomless heterozygote can be identified by demonstrating subnormal activity of the gene product. It should be noted that similar but not identical genetic diseases may result from mutations affecting different genes concerned in a particular function, for example the various factors involved in blood coagulation, or by different mutations affecting a single gene and causing various degrees of functional impairment of the gene product. The influence of environmental factors in causing lesions may result in variations among individuals with an identical genetic abnormality, for example the severity of brain damage in phenylketonuric oligophrenia (see above) is influenced by the amount of phenylalanine in the diet.

Some genetic disorders are evident at birth (i.e. are **congenital**), particularly those resulting in abnormalities of physical development. Fig. 2.7 shows the masculinising effect of an excess of the androgenic steroid 17 α-hydroxyprogesterone on the development of the external genitalia of a female child. This is due to genetic deficiency of the adrenocortical enzyme which normally converts that substrate to a non-androgenic steroid in the biosynthesis of cortisol. Other genetic disorders become apparent when the demands of an independent existence after birth reveal a disorder of function such as renal failure, increased susceptibility to infection, or mental deficiency. Some genetic diseases are first recognised later in childhood or even in adult life because of the existence of metabolic pathways or functions peculiar to later periods of life or to the cumulative effects of factors which injure the genetically abnormal cells. The number of genetic disorders of metabolism is increasing rapidly, although the biochemical basis of many has not yet been elucidated. In recent years it has become possible to diagnose certain genetic abnormalities by investigation of fetal cells obtained in aspirated amniotic fluid and this has sometimes provided the opportunity to terminate pregnancy before the fetus is viable.

In the above examples the mutation has occurred in a germ cell and is transmitted to the descendents of the affected individual, resulting in a familial pattern of disease. Mutation can also occur in cells other than germ cells—**somatic mutation**—but this is likely to be apparent only when the genetically altered cell proliferates abnormally to form a large family or clone of similar cells, e.g. when a tumour forms (pp. 319, 551).

An interesting abnormality encountered in many types of tumour is the synthesis of substances normally restricted to fetal life, e.g. α-fetoprotein (normally produced by fetal hepatocytes) by liver cell cancer in the adult. Some tumours produce compounds characteristic of other tissues, e.g. parathyroid hormone by cells of tumours arising in the bronchus. The mechanism of the underlying disorder of genetic control in such tumours is unknown.

Chromosomal abnormalities

Damage to the genetic apparatus more gross than that described above can sometimes be seen when the chromosomes of dividing cells are examined microscopically. An extra chromosome may be found, e.g. three instead of the normal pair of No. 21 chromosomes are commonly present in cases of Down's syndrome, (Fig. 2.8), but it is not understood how the chromosome abnormality leads to the physical and mental defects found in this condition. Total absence of one chromosome from all body cells is almost invariably incompatible with survival, with the notable exception of the Y sex chromosome, present in males (XY) but not in normal females (XX). Individuals with one X and no Y chromosome are phenotypically female but have a group of physical abnormalities including dwarfism and failure of ovarian development known as Turner's syndrome. Structural abnormality of chromosomes in the form of deleted portions

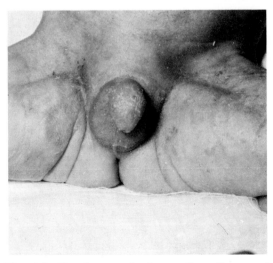

Fig. 2.7 Developmental abnormality of external genitalia of newborn female child due to an inborn error of metabolism, androgen being synthesised in the adrenal cortex instead of cortisol. (Adrenogenital syndrome due to 21 hydroxylase deficiency.) (Professor M. A. Ferguson-Smith.)

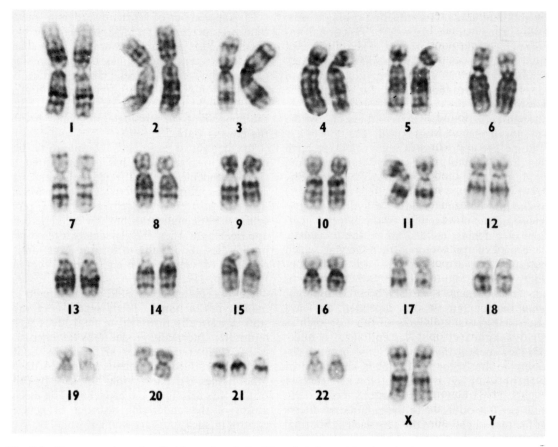

Fig. 2.8 Karyotype (trypsin – Leishman banded) of female infant with trisomic Down's syndrome. Three 21 chromosomes instead of the normal two. (Professor M. A. Ferguson-Smith.)

or added pieces derived from other chromosomes, or unusual shapes such as rings, are sometimes found and may be associated with characteristic clinical syndromes (Fig. 2.9). In a familial variety of Down's syndrome the two No. 21 chromosomes are normal but there is an abnormal No. 13 chromosome with an attached extra piece derived from a No. 21. This arises from a reciprocal exchange of fragments between two chromosomes during meiosis.

As would be expected, the gross chromosomal abnormalities described above, affecting all the cells of the body, lead to complex abnormalities since many genes must be involved. They arise during meiotic division of germ cells, the presence of an extra chromosome or absence of a chromosome being due to failure of separation of a pair of homologous chromosomes (**non-disjunction**); one of the resulting gametes will have an extra chromosome and

the other will be correspondingly defective. Structural chromosomal abnormality is due to chromosome breakage with re-arrangement of

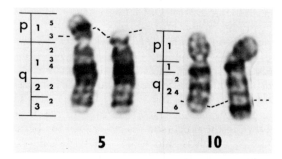

Fig. 2.9 Inherited structural chromosome abnormality in phenotypically normal individual. There is translocation of part of the short arm of a chromosome 5 to the long arm of chromosome 10 as shown by the banding pattern. (Professor M. A. Ferguson-Smith.)

fragments during repair. The reciprocal exchange of unequal fragments between non-homologous chromosomes (**translocation**) accounts for the occurrence of abnormally large or small chromosomes.

Abnormal chromosome numbers (**aneuploidy**) and structural chromosomal aberrations are invariably found in the cells of malignant tumours. The best known example of a consistent structural chromosomal aberration is the 'Philadelphia' chromosome, present in white and red blood cell precursors in the marrow in chronic myeloid leukaemia (a neoplastic proliferation of leukocytes). Radiation damage is known to cause chromosomal abnormalities in somatic cells and the frequency of chromosomal breakage has been used to assess exposure to radiation. Aneuploidy and structural abnormalities in individual chromosomes are also found in other circumstances, e.g. in thyroid epithelial cells which have proliferated following stimulation by pituitary thyrotrophic hormone, and in cells damaged by viruses.

Staining techniques which demonstrate structural transverse banding patterns are revealing less gross abnormalities and variations in chromosomes and are proving valuable in relating normal and abnormal genes to particular sites on individual chromosomes (**gene mapping**).

Nutritional nuclear damage

An interesting and clinically important form of nuclear damage is encountered in patients deficient in vitamin B_{12} or folic acid. The nuclei are larger than normal but contain less than optimal amounts of DNA for cell division. The chromatin of the large nuclei is arranged in a fine threadlike fashion (Fig. 17.2, p. 505) compared with the condensed masses seen normally (Fig. 17.1, p. 505), and when mitosis occurs the chromosomes in affected individuals are longer and less tightly coiled than normal. These changes occur in many tissues but are best known in the precursors of red cells in the bone marrow which is said to exhibit **megaloblastic erythropoiesis**. In addition to nuclear enlargement in megaloblasts there is increased amount

of cytoplasm, cytoplasmic basophilia due to excessive RNA and premature haemoglobinisation as judged by the immature state of the nucleus.

The mechanism of these changes is incompletely understood. Folate plays an essential role in the synthesis of purine bases and thymine, and deficiency of these substances presumably impairs nucleic acid synthesis, especially DNA which, unlike RNA, contains thymine. This could explain the delay of DNA synthesis prior to cell division together with excessive cytoplasmic growth and premature haemoglobinisation. Vitamin B_{12} is thought to influence nuclear structure by affecting folate metabolism (see Chanarin, 1979). Methyl folate is inactive in purine and thymine biosynthesis and one of the main functions of vitamin B_{12} is the transfer of methyl groups from methyl folate for the synthesis of choline. Accordingly, when there is severe vitamin B_{12} deficiency as in pernicious anaemia (p. 535), megaloblastic change occurs due to accumulation of methyl folate, and is reversed temporarily by the administration of folic acid, and permanently by life-long administration of vitamin B_{12}.

Toxic nuclear damage

Many drugs used in the treatment of cancer impair DNA replication either by combining directly with DNA (e.g. the alkylating agents nitrogen mustard and cyclophosphamide and certain antibiotics such as Actinomycin and Adriamycin) or by acting as analogues of normal metabolites and blocking the enzymes involved in nucleic acid synthesis. These include purine antagonists (mercaptopurine and its derivatives), pyrimidine antagonists (fluorouracil, cytarabine) and folic acid antagonists (methotrexate). The periwinkle alkaloid Vincristine damages the mitotic spindle. Amanitine (a toxic peptide from the mushroom *Amanita phalloides*) and D-galactosamine interfere with RNA synthesis in different ways and result respectively in fragmentation of nucleoli and in their disorganisation and replacement by small fibrillar bodies.

Damage to membranes and organelles

Electron microscopy reveals membranous structures which form the boundary wall around the cell and various compartments (organelles) within. The membranes are composed of lipoprotein or of phosphoglyceride bilayers containing enzymes, etc., and have the general properties of semipermeable membranes. The important definition of cellular compartments depends to a large extent on this property since soluble proteins of different types can thereby be sequestered within the cell; for example, hydrolases, potentially harmful to the cell, are confined within the lysosomes. As a result of the semipermeability of the membrane, the cell and its organelles tend to be subject to swelling and shrinkage depending on the relative osmotic pressures of the solutions in their various compartments and in the extracellular fluid. The membranes are not, however, inert but actively regulate the transport of crystalloids, including electrolytes, by enzymatic action which constantly modifies the chemical structure of the membrane and requires the provision of energy from ATP. Thus although K^+ and to a smaller extent Na^+ can passively diffuse through cell membranes, the intracellular concentration of K^+ is much higher, and of Na^+ lower, than that of the extracellular fluid; these differences are due to the outward 'pumping' of sodium by the cell membrane.

An additional important function of the membranes of the cell is that they form a cytoskeleton. This influences the shape of the cell and provides supporting structures for arrays of enzymes which form sequential functional units, such as those involved in the citric acid cycle and the flavoprotein and cytochrome systems of the cristae of the mitochondria.

Cell membranes

It has been shown by microsurgery that cells can survive incision of the surface membrane, and presumably self-sealing gaps develop in membranes when particulate material (e.g. nuclear fragments from normoblasts) is extruded from cells. However, most forms of reversible injury to surface membranes are not associated with demonstrable structural lesions. When antibody reacts with antigen associated with the cell surface, complement may be activated (p.143) with formation of complexes which bind to and injure the cell membrane, producing blebs and holes in it (Fig. 2.10): cell death results from osmotic disturbances.

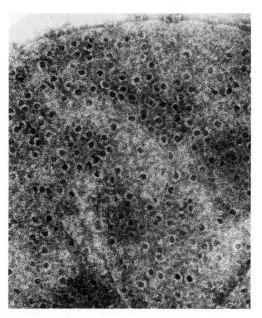

Fig. 2.10   Electron micrograph of part of the cell membrane of *Esch. coli* treated with antibody and complement, followed by treatment with trypsin. Activation of complement at the sites of antigen–antibody reaction has resulted in lesions—apparently holes—in the cell membrane, and these are accentuated by trypsin. × 140 000. (Dr. R. Dourmashkin.)

An indication of surface membrane dysfunction frequently encountered following anoxia and certain poisons is osmotic swelling of the cell with accumulation of water in the cytoplasm and resulting separation of organelles (Fig. 2.11 and 2.12). Such intracellular oedema, when reversible, may be the result of increased permeability of the surface membrane to sodium, or due to failure to remove sodium from the cell consequent upon diminished supply of ATP, or to poisoning of the enzymes involved in the sodium pump, e.g. by the drug ouabain. Increased cell volume leaves less room for extracellular fluid and this may impair the transport of metabolites between cells and the

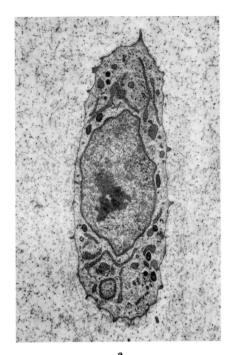

a

Fig. 2.11 Electron micrographs of chicken cartilage cells **a** before and **b** after injury by glutamylaminoacetonitrile. The damaged cell is swollen due to accumulation of water. × 6000. (Dr. Morag McCallum.)

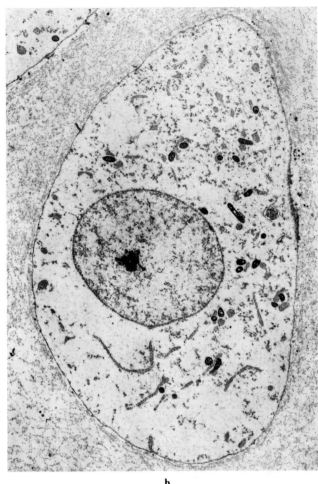

b

circulation, with further cell injury. When sodium is taken up by large numbers of cells, for example around extensive burns, there may be severe hyponatraemia (**sick cell syndrome**) which should not be treated by administering sodium.

The cell membrane controls the passage not only of water and inorganic ions, but also of organic molecules, into the cell cytoplasm. An inherited disorder characterised by failure of membrane transport of diamino acids, including lysine and ornithine, results in their presence in the urine because the renal tubular epithelium cannot re-absorb them: there is also a raised blood level of ammonia which is not converted to urea because ornithine does not enter hepatocytes in amounts adequate for the urea cycle.

The cell membrane also has an important role in receiving information from the environment of the cell through specialised surface receptor molecules which can combine specifically with polypeptide hormones, antigens, etc. Diminished numbers of surface receptors, leading to altered cellular responses, may result from genetic abnormality (e.g. in hyperbeta-lipoproteinaemia, p. 30), blocking by poison (e.g. the acetylcholine receptor on skeletal muscle by curare) or from prolonged overstimulation (e.g. of the insulin receptor by chronic hyperinsulinaemia).

Damage to **desmosomes** (the adhesion points of cell membranes which bind epithelial cells together), apparently caused by antibody and complement acting on adjacent intercellular material, is seen in the skin disease pemphigus. The desmosomes of the stratified squamous epithelium of the skin and mucous membranes

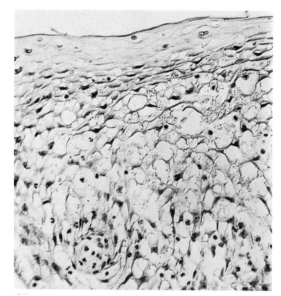

Fig. 2.12   Ballooning of epithelial cells due to bacterial toxic injury in acute laryngitis. × 250.

(the 'prickles' of the prickle cell layer) disappear and the resulting loss of cellular adhesion (acantholysis) is expressed in the formation of large intra-epidermal blisters (bullae) containing viable disaggregated prickle cells.

Endoplasmic reticulum

Loss of parallel arrays of endoplasmic reticulum and vacuolation due to accumulation of water within the membrane-lined spaces are frequently encountered as reversible lesions in anoxia and various poisonings, again presumably due to alterations in membrane permeability (Fig. 2.13). The swelling may be so severe in carbon tetrachloride poisoning as to give the cells a ballooned appearance. A marked increase of smooth endoplasmic reticulum bearing the mixed-function oxidases, e.g. cytochrome P450, is seen following the administration of certain drugs, notably phenobarbitone. This change is of special importance in

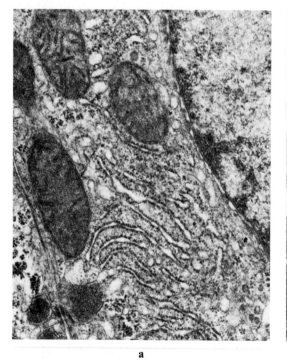

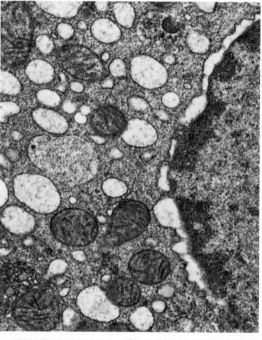

a   b

Fig. 2.13   Effect of carbon tetrachloride on the liver cells. **a** Part of normal mouse liver cell: note the regular parallel plates of granular endoplasmic reticulum and discrete clusters of ribosomes. **b** Part of a mouse liver cell 4 hours after oral administration of carbon tetrachloride. The plates of granular endoplasmic reticulum appear to have segregated into smaller oval vesicles from which many of the ribosomes have become detached and are dispersed singly in the cytoplasmic matrix. Mitochondria show no abnormality. × 23 000.

the study of cellular damage since these enzymes are responsible for the initial stages in
the metabolism of many drugs, some of which
are detoxicated and rendered less effective
while the oxidation products of others are more
toxic than the parent substances.

Disaggregation of polyribosomes, presumably associated with decreased production
of mRNA, has been noted in ischaemic cell
damage and with certain poisons, some of
which also cause loss of ribosomal particles
from the rough endoplasmic reticulum. The
resulting failure of protein synthesis has been
corrected in experimental situations by the
provision of a synthetic mRNA, but when the
outlines of the ribosomal particles (as seen by
electron microscopy) become indistinct, there is
irreversible failure of protein synthesis.

Mitochondria

Diminished oxygen supply quickly interferes
with the important mitochondrial function of
oxidative phosphorylation—the production of
high energy phosphate bonds in ATP by combination of oxygen with hydrogen through the
flavoprotein-cytochrome enzyme systems. One
minute of ischaemia causes a ten-fold decrease
in the ATP:ADP ratio. Mitochondrial function
can be restored by a return of adequate oxygenation even after lethal changes have occurred elsewhere in the cell.

Anoxia and many poisons cause reversible
osmotic swelling of mitochondria which gives
the cell cytoplasm a swollen, cloudy and granular appearance in light microscopy (Fig. 2.14).
This change, long known as 'cloudy swelling',
is seen especially in metabolically active tissues
such as liver, kidney and myocardium, and is
exactly the same as that which develops within
a few minutes of cessation of the circulation
after death of the body or excision of the tissue.
For this reason, pathological significance can
be attached to its finding only if pieces of tissue
small enough to be permeated rapidly are
promptly placed in fixative. Isolated mitochondria can be made to swell and contract *in vitro*
by adding calcium ions and ATP respectively
to the medium in which the mitochondria are
suspended.

Electron microscopy of injured mitochondria, in addition to showing in detail the site
of swelling, reveals other abnormalities. A very
early indication of anoxic damage is the dis-

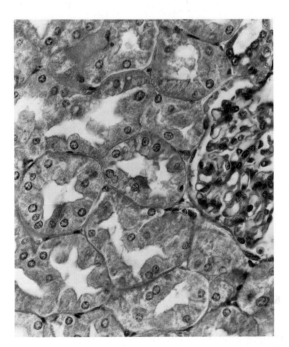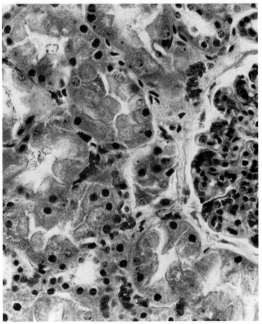

Fig. 2.14 *Left*, normal kidney. *Right*, cloudy swelling of renal tubular epithelium, showing cytoplasmic granularity. × 300.

appearance of the dense granules occasionally seen in the matrix of normal mitochondria. These bodies are thought to represent lipid-bound calcium which accumulates under the influence of respiration and ATP. A later structural change, characteristic of mitochondrial damage following various types of cell injury, is development in the matrix of dense poorly defined aggregations of unknown composition. A second type of abnormal mitochondrial inclusion apparently composed of calcium (sometimes as hydroxyapatite) is found in very varied circumstances, e.g. in renal tubular epithelium when there is excessive calcium in the urine due to vitamin D poisoning or to hyperparathyroidism, and in myocardial mitochondria in

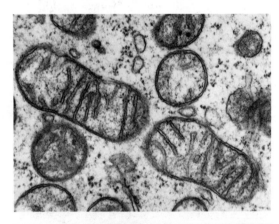

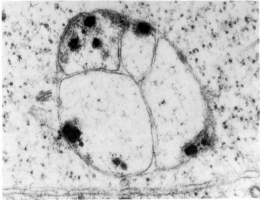

Fig. 2.15 Electron micrographs of human erythroblasts. *Above*, mitochondria of normal erythroblast. *Below*, mitochondrion of erythroblast from a patient with sideroblastic anaemia. The mitochondrion is swollen and has an electron-lucent matrix in which lie electron-dense masses of iron-containing material. × 37 400. (Dr. A. M. Mackay.)

magnesium deficiency. Dense mitochondrial inclusions (Fig. 2.15) containing iron are found in the red cell precursors in sideroblastic anaemia in which there is impairment of iron utilisation (p. 540).

Lysosomes

These are cytoplasmic organelles limited by a single membrane. They contain various hydrolases which digest proteins, fats, carbohydrates, etc. Under the electron microscope they present very varied appearances and can be recognised with certainty only by histochemical demonstration of their acid hydrolase activity. The enzymes have a low pH optimum and become active when the membrane of the **primary lysosome** is altered, e.g. by fusion with a phagocytic vacuole to form a **secondary lysosome (phagosome, or phagolysosome)**.

Lysosomal hydrolases seriously impair the biochemical function and structure of subcellular particles *in vitro* and there has been much speculation on the importance of lysosomal damage in cell injury *in vivo* (see Dingle and Fell, 1973). Damage to the lysosomal membrane leading to release of lysomal enzymes into the cytoplasm of living cells results in various degrees of cell damage up to necrosis. This happens in certain bacterial infections, e.g. by streptococci, and appears to result from the action of bacterial toxins. It is also encountered in hypervitaminosis A where it is attributed to the surfactant effect of the vitamin on the lysosomal membranes. Another example is the necrosis of macrophages which have ingested silica particles; some of the silica of the particles within phagolysosomes is converted to silicic acid and this forms hydrogen bonds with the phospholipids of the lysosomal membrane which then ruptures and releases the enzymes into the cytoplasm. Phagocytosis of monosodium urate crystals by neutrophil polymorphs in patients with gout is said to increase lysosomal permeability with resultant cell injury. Some photosensitivity reactions are due to lysosomal membrane damage when certain pigments, e.g. porphyrin, taken up by lysosomes, release energy on exposure to light of appropriate wavelength. Cortisol and chloroquine, drugs known to stabilise lysosomal membranes, diminish cell damage in vitamin A poisoning and some photosensitivity reactions. In many forms of cellular injury, however, the 'suicidal' release of lysosomal enzymes into the cytoplasm does not seem to be an important factor. For example, autolysis by lysosomal enzymes in cells injured by hypoxia, carbon tetrachloride and many other poisons occurs only after the cells have become necrotic.

Phagosomes containing membranous structures (e.g. damaged mitochondria) are commonly encountered in cells with focal cytoplasmic damage such as follows irradiation (Fig. 2.16), during starvation, in tumour cells, etc. The damaged parts of the cell are taken into an autophagic vacuole which coalesces with a primary lysosome to form a phagosome, and the activated hydrolases digest the contents of the vacuole. This process is accelerated by glucagon which acts via adenyl cyclase and cyclic AMP. Material resistant to digestion sometimes remains within a phagosome and forms one variety of **residual body** seen on electron microscopy. Lipofuscin pigment (p. 285) seems to originate from undigested lipid-rich material in this way. The hydrolysis of effete membranous structures and the re-utilisation of the products of digestion are probably of considerable importance in cellular economy.

Many inborn errors of lysosomal function have been described. Most of these involve deficiency of an enzyme and are characterised by progressive accumulation of the appropriate substrate within greatly swollen lysosomes. Some examples of the resulting 'storage diseases' are given on p. 28 and p. 32. Marked accumulation of metabolites in lysosomes with normal enzymes also occurs as a result of excessive production of substrate, e.g. α-chains of

haemoglobin in red cell precursors in β thalassaemia (p. 523) and lipids in macrophages in certain hyperlipoproteinaemias (p. 566). Storage of heavy metals, e.g. iron in the form of ferritin and haemosiderin and copper, occurs in lysosomes when cells are overloaded with these substances.

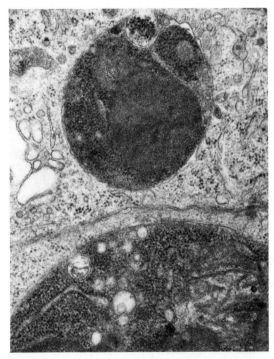

Fig. 2.16 Electron micrograph showing two autophagic vacuoles in adjacent cells of intestinal mucosa of mouse following radiation injury. Mitochondria and glycogen granules can be identified in the large, electron-dense vacuoles. × 57 000.

Abnormal storage of triglyceride fat

Triglycerides (or neutral fats) are glycerol esters of long-chain fatty acids and their storage in excess is a common and conspicuous feature of cell damage. Historically one of the first recognised features of sublethal cellular injury, its mode of development has been a centre of interest for many years. It is important to distinguish between an abnormal increase in the cells of adipose tissue (**pathological obesity**—or, when the condition is localised, **pathological adiposity**) and the accumulation of fat in other types of cell (**fatty change**). The two processes are quite distinct although in pathological obesity fat also commonly accumulates in the liver cells.

Fat metabolism

Before outlining the main features of fat metabolism, it is important to appreciate that water-insoluble lipids are transported in the plasma mainly as complexes of triglyceride fats, cholesterol and its esters, phospholipid and carrier protein (apoprotein). There are four major classes of such complexes in the plasma, namely chylomicrons and α, β and pre-β lipoproteins. These complexes differ in molecular size and in the proportion of their constituents, and so in density.

The apoproteins are essential for the aqueous solubility of the lipoproteins: the three main ones are called *apoprotein* (or *apo-*) A, B and C, and are synthesised mainly in the liver.

Over 95 per cent of the triglyceride in the diet is normally absorbed in the small intestine: much of it is hydrolysed in the gut into free fatty acids and monoglycerides, but these are re-esterified in the jejunal mucosal cells, and incorporated into large (up to 100 nm diam.) particles, the **chylomicrons**, which contain apo-B and -C. The chylomicrons pass via the gut lymphatics to the plasma, and are mainly responsible for its turbidity after a fatty meal. They consist of 90 per cent triglyceride fats, which are carried in the plasma mainly in this form. Reduction in size of the chylomicrons, and hydrolysis of fat, is effected by lipoprotein-lipase in the plasma, and the resulting glycerol and fatty acids are taken up by the cells of various tissues, including the liver. Some of the fatty acid is oxidised to provide energy, but much of it is re-esterified to triglyceride which is incorporated into **pre-β** or **very low density lipoproteins**: these are then secreted into the plasma and provide a means of transporting triglycerides in water-soluble form. The pre-β-lipoproteins, which make use of apo-B and apo-C, re-cycle through the liver, but are also taken up by the cells of the fat depots and other tissues, where the triglyceride is either used for energy or stored.

Triglyceride stored in adipose tissue is continuously being hydrolysed, and the fatty acids are secreted into the plasma where they are complexed with albumin. These so-called **free fatty acids** are taken up by muscle and other cells of high metabolic activity for the production of energy: that taken up by the liver cells is either oxidised or re-esterified to form triglyceride.

The α or **high density lipoproteins** of the plasma are assembled in the liver, and make use of apoprotein A. Their function is uncertain but they seem to be of importance in the transport of cholesterol (see α-lipoprotein deficiency, p. 29). The β or **low density lipoproteins**, which contain apoprotein-B, transport cholesterol from the various tissues which synthesise it (especially the intestinal mucosa) to the liver, where it is added to that synthesised by the liver cells: much of it is then secreted into the bile.

The control of these major metabolic processes is influenced by food intake and also by various hormonal and emotional factors: insulin stimulates the deposition of triglyceride in the adipose tissue depots; adrenal hormones (probably catecholamines and corticosteroids acting together) stimulate hydrolysis in the depots and release of fatty acids into the plasma, as does growth hormone and also thyroxine. The rate of uptake of triglyceride and fatty acids by various other tissues, particularly the liver, is dependent on their concentrations in the plasma. Starvation results in release of fatty acids from the depots, and this is suppressed after a fatty meal. In addition to that provided by the diet, triglyceride is synthesised within the body, particularly in the liver and adipose tissues, from glucose, amino acids and fatty acids, and enters the metabolic pathways outlined above.

Fatty change

This is the accumulation of fat in cells other than adipose tissue cells, and was previously subdivided into fatty infiltration and fatty degeneration. It is due to imbalance between fat and fatty acids entering the cell and the rate of utilisation or release of fat by the cell. Probably all parenchymal cells which accumulate an abnormal amount of fat are injured. Even the gross fatty change seen in the liver in obesity (p. 667) can be regarded as a form of injury to the liver cells due to the disturbed fat metabolism resulting from overeating.

Because of its major role in fat metabolism, the liver requires special consideration in fatty change. However, fatty change is seen not only in the liver cells, which are usually most seriously affected, but also in various other organs and tissues. The cells most prone to undergo fatty change are the parenchymal cells of the various organs, and skeletal and heart muscle cells, i.e. the cells which because of their specialised functions have a high metabolic activity. Part of their energy is normally supplied by the oxidation of fatty acids, provided largely by uptake from the plasma of free fatty acids released from the fat depots, and lipoproteins secreted mainly by the liver.

Microscopic appearances

In fatty change of most organs, small droplets, consisting mainly of triglyceride, appear in the cytoplasm of the affected cells. Even in an advanced stage the droplets remain small and discrete, and do not greatly enlarge the cell (Fig. 2.17). In the liver, however, they may fuse to form much larger droplets (Fig. 2.18) and the liver cells may be greatly distended. In most instances, the centrilobular cells* are affected first and most severely, but in phosphorus poisoning the change may be very severe and yet confined to the cells in the outer part of the lobules. The distribution of these lesions has not been fully explained.

Electron microscopy shows the fat globules to lie free in the cytoplasmic matrix, without a limiting membrane.

Causes of fatty change

The four major causes of fatty change are (*a*) hypoxia, (*b*) starvation and wasting diseases, (*c*) metabolic disorders, and (*d*) numerous chemicals and bacterial toxins.

(a) Hypoxia. The hypoxia resulting from chronic anaemia is a common cause of fatty change in the various organs and tissues. In the liver it occurs especially in the central zone of lobules, which receives the poorest supply of oxygenated blood, while in the heart it is more marked in parts farthest from the arterioles, that is, it is pararterial in distribution. In the heart, the change may be seen through the endocardium as a fine mottled pallor ('thrush breast') of the myocardium of the left ventricle and papillary muscles.

The fatty change commonly present in the cells of rapidly growing tumours is probably of the same nature, although in this instance there is inadequate blood supply or flow, and not just hypoxia.

(b) Starvation and wasting diseases. Fatty change is observed in the liver and to a smaller extent in the myocardium and elsewhere in

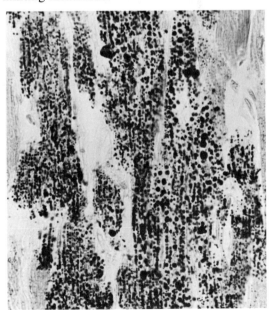

Fig. 2.17a Fatty change of heart muscle, stained with osmic acid. Note the very numerous minute intracellular droplets arranged in rows. × 380.

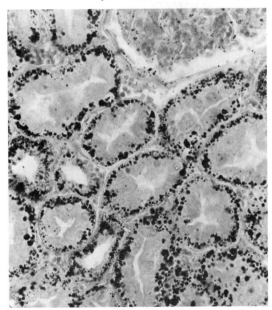

Fig. 2.17b Fatty change of tubules of kidney, stained with osmic acid. × 325.

* The lobule, centred on a hepatic venule, is still widely used, as above, to describe the location of changes in the hepatic parenchyma. However, it now seems more logical to consider the functional unit as the acinus centred on a portal tract, as explained on p. 661.

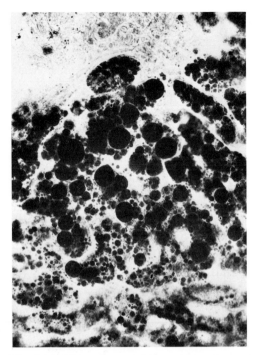

Fig. 2.18 Fatty change of liver. The cells are filled with large globules of fat. (Stained with Sudan IV.) × 190.

some patients who, previously well nourished, have died of a wasting disease such as gastric carcinoma or pulmonary tuberculosis. In other instances of equally or even more severe wasting, fatty change is not found. This was explained by Dible and his co-workers in 1941 who demonstrated experimentally that fat accumulates in the cells of the liver and other tissues under conditions of near-starvation so long as some adipose tissue remains. Once the fat depots are depleted, the fatty change disappears. The low food intake in wasting diseases leads to excessive lipolysis in the depots and release of fatty acids into the blood: these are taken up in increased amounts by the cells of various tissues and converted to triglyceride. Failure of carbohydrate metabolism resulting from the low caloric intake may also be of importance by interfering with intracellular oxidative breakdown of fatty acids, particularly in the liver.

Where a wasting disease is attributable to a toxic condition or complicated by severe infection, this may further impair hepatic fat metabolism, as explained below: a good example is provided by infantile gastro-enteritis due to certain strains of *Esch. coli*, in which dietary intake is severely impaired by anorexia, vomiting and diarrhoea, and the liver is subjected to toxins absorbed from the infected gut. The liver usually shows gross fatty change in fatal cases.

(c) Metabolic disorders. The fatty change in uncontrolled **diabetes mellitus** is attributable mainly to excessive release of fatty acids from the fat depots and impaired carbohydrate metabolism, both of which are a consequence of deficiency of insulin. The situation is thus similar to that in starvation, and in both conditions oxidation of fatty acids in the liver is incomplete and partial breakdown products, acetoacetic and hydroxybutyric acids, escape into the blood, resulting in ketosis. The subject is discussed more fully on p. 1031.

Fatty change is common in the liver in various inborn errors of carbohydrate metabolism including some types of glycogen storage disease (p. 30), galactosaemia, and also in disorders of amino-acid metabolism.

(d) Chemical and bacterial toxins. Of the many simple chemicals which can cause fatty change, phosphorus, carbon tetrachloride and puromycin are well-known examples. As in fatty change from other causes, the liver is usually most severely affected, but the changes are widespread, and may involve not only parenchymal cells, but also vascular endothelium and connective tissue cells. Fatty change is also a feature of severe infections, e.g. typhoid, smallpox and septicaemias.

Two factors are involved in the production of fatty change by chemicals and toxins. Firstly, they directly injure the cells; secondly, they produce anorexia and often vomiting, and the low calorie intake results, as described above, in increased mobilisation of fatty acids from the depots. The nature of the cell injuries by many chemicals and toxins and the way these cause fatty change is by no means fully understood.

As a result of recent experimental investigations, it has been established that fatty change in the liver is attributable largely to reduced production of lipoprotein. The triglyceride which would normally have been released as lipoprotein thus accumulates in the liver cells. This applies to fatty change induced in rats by administration of chlorinated hydrocarbons, ethionine, phosphorus, puromycin, orotic acid or a diet deficient in choline, each of which interfere with lipoprotein synthesis in different ways. There is some evidence that choline deficiency impairs the production of phospholipids, which are an essential constituent of lipoproteins.

It still remains unexplained how the various chemicals and toxins which cause fatty change in the liver affect also the cells of various other tissues. With the exception of the intestinal mucosa, which shares with the liver the property of converting fat to lipoprotein, tissue cells in general expend fat mainly by oxidative breakdown. It therefore seems likely that the various chemicals and toxins which produce widespread fatty change interfere in some way with this latter process.

Effects of fatty change

Fatty change results from cell injury, but varies in degree in different types of cell injury. For example, liver cell necrosis in viral hepatitis is not preceded or accompanied by any significant degree of fatty change, but there is severe fatty change associated with liver cell necrosis in phosphorus poisoning. Also the gross fatty change in the liver which may accompany obesity or alcoholism is not itself usually accompanied by severely impaired hepatic function.

Fat accumulates less rapidly in the other organs than in the liver but, as in the liver, the important factor is the severity of the cell injury, which is not reflected by the degree of the fatty change.

Fatty change in the heart may indicate severe myocardial injury, from which heart failure may result. For example, in severe anaemia attributable to a lesion requiring surgical intervention, such as recurrent haemorrhage from a peptic ulcer, it is important that, when practicable, the anaemia should be treated and time allowed for the myocardium to return to normal before any major operation is undertaken. The administration of a large volume of blood or packed red cells over a short period carries a risk of overloading the impaired myocardium, especially if followed immediately by major surgery.

Pathological obesity

Obesity, the accumulation of excessive amounts of adipose tissue, is a subject in which it is dif-ficult, if not impossible, to draw a sharp dividing line between physiological and pathological states. However, there is no doubt that gross obesity is harmful, and must be regarded as pathological.

Causes. Basically, obesity is very simply explained, being due to a dietary intake of calories in excess of those expended to provide energy for the body's metabolism. It is thus attributable to overeating, particularly of carbohydrates and fats, often combined with lack of exercise. Attempts to demonstrate metabolic differences between fat and thin people, e.g. in efficiency of intestinal absorption or in basal metabolic rate have, in general, been unsuccessful and the main problem of obesity appears to be the cause of overeating, a subject involving psychological factors which will not be discussed here. Some individuals, however, seem to be predisposed to obesity more than others, and genetic factors may be involved, as in some inbred strains of animals. It has been observed that when healthy young adults are given a high calorie diet and kept at rest in bed, those who are overweight gain more weight than the thinner subjects. The activity of the thyroid gland, by influencing the rate of general metabolism, has an important influence on energy expenditure, and the pituitary, adrenals and gonads all influence the amount of fat deposited. Damage to the hypothalamus with deficiency of pituitary secretion in early life leads to adiposity along with failure of sexual development, and there is evidence that some forms of obesity in the adult are of similar causation. Extreme degrees of adiposity can be induced in rats by small precisely placed experimental lesions in the tuber cinereum, the mode of action of which appears to be the development of a voracious appetite.

Gross abnormalities of the hypothalamus or of endocrine function have not been demonstrated in the great majority of obese subjects investigated, but it may be that more subtle variations in the functioning of these organs are of importance.

Structural changes. Apart from the increase in size of the normal depots, e.g. the subcutaneous tissue, the omentum, retroperitoneal tissues and epicardium, adipose tissue in obesity may extend to sites where it is normally absent. For example, in pathological adiposity of the heart, adipose tissue extends along the lines of con-

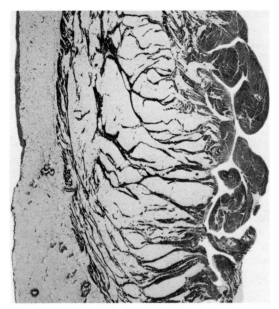

Fig. 2.19 Pathological adiposity of heart. The whole thickness of the wall of the right ventricle is infiltrated with adipose tissue extending from the epicardial layer between the muscle fibres which are

consequently atrophied. Even the columnae carneae are involved. × 6.

nective tissue through the heart wall (Fig. 2.19), and leads to atrophy of the muscle fibres and consequent weakening of the wall to such an extent that the right ventricle may rupture. A similar accumulation of stromal fat is seen occasionally in the pancreas.

In obese individuals, the liver may be grossly enlarged by accumulation of large droplets of fat in the liver cells. This is discussed on p. 667.

Effects. Apart from the limitations imposed on physical activity by obesity, it has long been recognised, and notably by life insurance companies, that obesity is associated with a reduced expectation of life attributable to an increased incidence of high blood pressure, coronary artery disease, heart failure, chronic bronchitis and respiratory infections, and late-onset diabetes.

The high and increasing incidence of obesity in affluent societies poses a major health problem.

Abnormal storage of other lipids

The lipids of the body other than triglyceride are chemically very heterogeneous and include sterols (cholesterol and its esters), phospholipids and complex lipids (e.g. glycolipids). These substances are frequently united with proteins to form lipoproteins, some of which constitute the insoluble membranes of cells, while others are soluble and play an important part in the transport of triglyceride in suspension in the plasma. Many diseases are known in which one or more of these substances accumulate in cells in abnormal amounts. By far the most important is **atheroma**, a poorly understood disorder in which various lipids, including sterols, phospholipids and triglyceride, accumulate in the intima of arteries and cause narrowing or occlusion of the lumen with consequent impairment of blood flow.

Most of the other disorders are much less common but illustrate interesting principles. Pathological accumulation of lipids other than triglycerides within cells may develop in the following ways.

Inherited deficiency of lysosomal enzymes

Cells may accumulate lipids derived from the normal turnover of the membrane material bounding the cell surface and organelles. This occurs in individuals lacking an enzyme necessary for the catabolism of membrane-derived lipids, and the accumulation of lipid is often especially prominent in macrophages because of their phagocytic function. A good example is Gaucher's disease in which there is a genetic deficiency of a lysosomal β-glucosidase. Normally, old worn-out red cells are phagocytosed and digested by macrophages, mainly in the spleen. In Gaucher's disease the glucocerebrosides of the red cell membrane accumulate in phagosomes in the macrophages, which consequently become greatly enlarged and develop a characteristic appearance (Fig. 18.3, p. 567) and are termed Gaucher cells. Their accumulation causes gross splenomegaly, hepatomegaly, and anaemia due to replacement of the haemopoietic tissue by Gaucher cells. Another form of Gaucher's disease affects the cerebral neurones (p. 567).

In marked contrast to Gaucher's disease, the lesions of Krabbe's disease are confined to the central and peripheral nervous systems because galactocerebroside, the substrate of the deficient enzyme galactocerebroside β-galactosidase, is a major component only of myelin. This recessive lysosomal enzyme defect causes, in infancy, severe central and peripheral nervous dysfunction due to unexplained demyelination of axons. Krabbe's disease is also known as 'globoid leukodystrophy' since the white matter of the brain is particularly affected and the lesions contain macrophages: these are globoid in shape because they are distended with PAS-positive galactocerebroside which has characteristic electron-microscopic appearances. Gaucher's disease and Krabbe's disease illustrate the great differences between lesions due to inherited deficiency of enzymes responsible for intracellular breakdown of lipids and demonstrate some of the reasons for these differences.

Disordered plasma lipid transport

Several inherited abnormalities of plasma lipoproteins are known which lead to massive accumulation of lipid in macrophages. These cells become spherical and enlarged due to the presence of numerous lipid vacuoles which give the cytoplasm a foamy appearance (Fig. 2.20). The predominant lipids stored are cholesterol esters

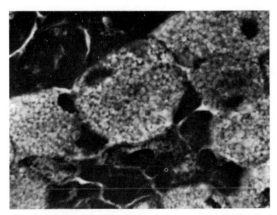

Fig. 2.20 Macrophages distended with multiple fine droplets of doubly-refractile lipid. Photographed through crossed polarising prisms. × 500.

which are seen to be doubly refractile when viewed under the microscope with polarised light (Fig. 2.21). Large accumulations of these cells (often accompanied by extracellular lipid deposits) may form nodules, called **xanthomas** because of their yellow and tumour-like appearance.

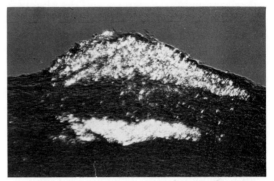

Fig. 2.21 Deposition of doubly-refractile lipid in early atheroma of aorta, photographed by polarised light.

The rare **familial α-lipoprotein deficiency** (Tangier disease) is due to absence of apoprotein A. There is a moderate increase in the plasma level of triglyceride which is associated with β-lipoproteins as unstable complexes. These are phagocytosed by macrophages in the spleen, liver, tonsils and lymph nodes, all of which organs become enlarged due to accumulation of cholesterol esters, presumably derived from the β-lipoprotein. Great enlargement of the tonsils, orange in colour due to the stored lipid, is a unique finding in this disease.

Familial hyperchylomicronaemia, apparently due to inherited deficiency of serum lipoprotein lipase, is characterised by a milky appearance of the serum, even after overnight fasting, due to chylomicrons which are not cleared from the plasma at the normal rate. There is lipid storage in macrophages in the enlarged liver and spleen, and xanthomas may be found in the dermis. It is of interest that in both of the above diseases the stored lipid is predominantly cholesterol ester, although the main elevation in serum lipid affects the triglycerides in the chylomicrons. Presumably the latter are broken down following phagocytosis by the macrophages, leaving a steadily increasing residue of less digestible esters of cholesterol. The steroid nucleus cannot readily be broken down and is mainly disposed of by excretion.

Familial hyperbetalipoproteinaemia is a relatively common disorder, inherited as a Mendelian dominant, in which the plasma β-lipoprotein is greatly increased. Cholesterol, an important integral part of the lipoprotein molecule, is correspondingly raised, hence the old name 'familial hypercholesterolaemia'. There is little elevation in triglycerides and the plasma is not milky. Atheroma, fatal even in childhood in rare homozygous individuals, and in many cases xanthomas affecting skin and tendon sheaths, increase with time and parallel in severity the plasma lipoprotein abnormality.

Many kinds of cells, including fibroblasts and aortic smooth muscle cells (but not liver or intestinal epithelium), have surface receptors for the apoprotein of β-lipoproteins. High lipoprotein concentrations in plasma and interstitial fluid saturate these receptors and this leads to diminished production of the rate-limiting enzyme for cholesterol synthesis in these cells (i.e. there is a negative feed-back control). In individuals homozygous for hyperbetalipoproteinaemia, the receptors are absent and cholesterol synthesis is greatly increased. Heterozygotes have half the normal number of receptor sites and this is compensated by raised levels of β-lipoproteins.

These and other inherited lipoprotein disorders illustrate the varied metabolic abnormalities underlying excessive storage of cholesterol esters in foam cells in different parts of the body. Hyperlipoproteinaemia also develops secondary to other diseases; for example, transitory hyperchylomicronaemia is encountered sometimes when severe diabetes mellitus is inadequately controlled and secondary hyperbetalipoproteinaemia, reversible by thyroxine therapy, is seen in hypothyroidism. These and other disorders (e.g. obstructive jaundice, pancreatitis, alcoholism and nephrotic syndrome) may be associated with various forms of hyperlipoproteinaemia.

Other lipid depositions

Submucosal aggregates of foam cells are often found in the gallbladder giving it a 'strawberry' appearance (Fig. 20.64, p. 710); presumably this results from intracellular storage of part of the cholesterol that is normally reabsorbed from the bile.

The important subject of atheroma will be considered later (p. 362). Suffice it to say here that pressure filtration of lipoprotein from the plasma into the intimal layer of the arteries leads to a difficult problem in disposing of the associated cholesterol by the local population of modified smooth muscle cells. At first the filtered lipid is found within these cells but these are quickly overwhelmed and most of the accumulated lipid eventually lies in an extracellular position. As already indicated, atheroma is particularly prone to develop in individuals with certain of the inherited lipoprotein abnormalities; it seems to result also from modern western dietary habits which lead to alterations in serum lipoproteins and lipids.

Abnormal storage of glycogen

The normal human body contains approximately 500 grams of glycogen, present mainly in muscle and liver cells, but also found in small amounts in the other tissues. Glycogen is a water-soluble branched polymer, composed exclusively of glucose units, and is broken down by enzymes (glycogenolysis) to provide glucose needed to meet increased energy requirements, e.g. during muscular exercise. The depolymerisation is effected mainly by phosphorylase enzymes which liberate glucose 1-phosphate, and this in turn is converted into glucose 6-phosphate which can be used for the intrinsic metabolic needs of the cell. For the maintenance of blood glucose levels during fasting and exercise, glucose 6-phosphate must be converted to glucose before release from the cell, and this happens almost exclusively in the liver, but also in the kidney, both of which contain the necessary enzyme, glucose 6-phosphatase.

Largely as a result of the brilliant biochemical studies of G. E. Cori, a number of distinct inherited **glycogen storage diseases** have been recognised, each associated with a different single enzyme deficiency. In several forms of the disease, the affected organs are enlarged due to an increased content of glycogen. Histological examination of sections stained by haematoxylin and eosin reveals clear unstained material distending the affected cells (Fig. 2.22); histochemical confirmation of the nature of the material is given by Best's carmine, or the periodic acid Schiff (PAS) stain (with and without prior hydrolysis of the section with diastase), and this is most satisfactorily obtained with tissue fixed promptly in alcohol in which glycogen is insoluble. Glycogen also has a characteristic appearance on electron microscopy, occurring as dense particles larger than

ribosomes; these sometimes form rosette-like clusters (Fig. 2.23).

In **von Gierke's disease** (Cori Type 1) there is deficiency of glucose 6-phosphatase, an enzyme which is associated with the endoplasmic reticulum. The resulting failure to convert glucose 6-phosphate to glucose for release into the circulation leads to hypoglycaemia and a tendency to increased glycogen storage in liver and kidney, the organs which normally contain glucose 6-phosphatase. As a consequence of the excessive glycogen storage, these organs become enormously enlarged. The disordered carbohydrate metabolism leads to increased lipogenesis and raised serum levels of triglyceride (as the very low density pre- β-lipoprotein), xanthomatosis, obesity, fatty change in the liver and ketoacidosis. The affected children also show retarded growth.

Pompe's disease (Cori Type 2) has recently been shown to result from an inherited deficiency of the lysosomal enzyme acid α-glucosidase which is normally present in all tissues and presumably hydrolyses the small amount of glycogen present in phagosomes as a result of

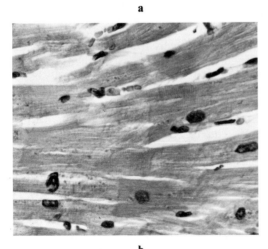

Fig. 2.22 Myocardium in Pompe's disease **a**, compared with normal myocardium. **b**. The affected muscle fibres are distended with glycogen and appear vacuolated. × 460.

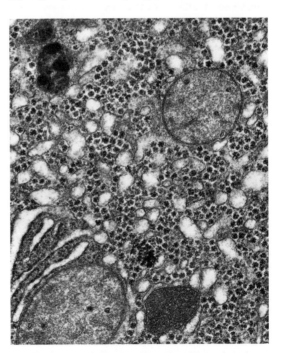

Fig. 2.23 Electron micrograph of normal liver showing the characteristic small, dense, round particles of glycogen. The large dense organelle at the top of the field is a residual body. × 30 000.

autophagy. In Pompe's disease, the glycogen in autophagosomes persists and accumulates, being inaccessible to the general cytoplasm with its normal complement of phosphorylase and other enzymes in the major glycogenolytic pathway. Accordingly much of the stored glycogen is seen by electron microscopy to be within greatly enlarged lysosomes, and it seems likely that the serious cellular dysfunction encountered in Pompe's disease is the result of lysosomal rupture and spilling of harmful hydrolases into the general cytoplasm of the cell. This explains most of the features of Pompe's disease, namely generalised glycogen storage—e.g. in myocardium, skeletal muscle, nervous and lymphoid tissue, and peripheral blood leukocytes—enlargement of organs, cardiac failure, mental deficiency, severe muscle weakness and absence of hypoglycaemia.

Other extremely rare forms of glycogen storage disease include deficiency of muscle phosphorylase (**McArdle's syndrome**) which results in abnormal accumulation of glycogen in skeletal muscle and rapid muscle fatigue without hypoglycaemia, and deficiency of liver phosphorylase which causes hepatomegaly and hypoglycaemia.

Another interesting disorder is the deficiency of the enzyme responsible for the branching of the tree-like glycogen molecule during its synthesis: in this condition the stored glycogen has an abnormal fibrillary structure seen by electron microscopy and is resistant to breakdown by phosphorylase.

In contrast to the rare disorders described above in which deficiency of a particular enzyme satisfactorily explains most of the observed pathological findings, increased glycogen storage is found in many other disorders but the mechanisms involved are usually obscure. In diabetes mellitus utilisation of glucose is seriously impaired and excess of glycogen is deposited in cardiac muscle, in Henle's tubules in the kidney, in liver cell nuclei, in polymorphonuclear leukocytes and in the hydropic β-cells of the pancreatic islets seen in early Type I diabetes (p. 1032). The glycogen content of skeletal muscle is, however, reduced. More glycogen than normal is found in polymorphs in acute inflammation, in recently formed pus and in the peripheral blood when there is a leukocytosis. Glycogen is abundant in embryonic tissues and in some malignant tumours arising from cells normally rich in glycogen, e.g. liver and renal tubular epithelium. It is particularly constant in clear cell carcinoma of kidney.

Cell damage due to ionising radiation

Because of the widespread use of radiation and radioactive materials in industry and medicine the study of their effects on living matter is now of great importance. Of all the branches o radiation biology—molecular, sub-cellular, cellular, organ and whole animal—cellular radiation biology is the most instructive in the present state of knowledge. This is firstly because the measurement of its effects on proliferation of cells in culture makes quantitation fairly easy. Secondly, it is mainly by the study and analysis of cellular effects that information can be obtained on molecular and sub-cellular processes in the development and repair of radiation damage. Thirdly, it appears that effects on whole organs or whole animals can often, to a first approximation at least, be described or explained on the basis of cellular injury. This third principle will be illustrated below in terms of the impaired ability of sub-lethally irradiated cells to divide, although it must be emphasised that the effects of radiation on the individual cannot easily be explained fully by its effects on his component cells.

Radiation causes its effects by transferring energy to the substance through which it passes. This energy can produce two changes, excitation or ionisation. Excitation is a change in the energy state of some electrons or charged parts of molecules. Radiations which, like ultraviolet light, produce excitations only, are of very low penetrating power and are not discussed in this section. Other radiations produce mixtures of ionisations and excitations.

Measurement of radiation

No widely useful and accurate biological method of measuring radiation dose has so far been developed. This is because the ultimate biological effects produced are very complex. The standard methods of measuring radiation dose are purely physical. The first is based on the application of a voltage to an air-filled chamber through which the ionising radiation passes. This voltage has the effect of separating the positive and negative electric charges produced by the ionisations. The flow of these charges under the influence of the applied voltage constitutes a small electric current which can be measured with great sensitivity and accuracy. The unit of *exposure* measured by this method is thus based on the electric charge per mass of air (coulomb/kilogram) and was called the *röntgen* (R). This method ignores the excitations produced by the radiation, but *exposure* expressed in R agrees roughly with the absorbed dose (see below) measured in rads.

The second method of measuring radiation dose is based on the measurement of the total energy absorbed from a beam of radiation by a solid material. The material must be one in which no radiation-produced chemical energy can be stored, all of it being transformed into heat which can be measured by sensitive calorimetry. The unit of absorbed dose is the *gray* (Gy), called after the British scientist who did fundamental work on the oxygen effect described below. Absorbed dose used to be expressed in units called *rads*. The new unit, Gy, equals 100 rads.

Much research has been done on the effects of radiation on aqueous solutions; these are mediated primarily through the decomposition products of the water, and probably reflect the initial damage produced in living biological material. However, this initial damage has never been directly observed. The effects which are observed are the result of an interaction, between the disruptive effects on the complex of normal biochemical processes arising from the initial molecular damage, and the response of the cell or organism in trying to overcome the disruption. From an analysis of these effects much has been learned about the nature of the disruption and repair, but very much more still remains unknown.

Types of ionising radiation

Ionising radiations fall into three categories; electromagnetic radiation, charged particles and uncharged particles. The ionisation is caused by the charged particles—electrons, protons or heavy nuclei: electromagnetic radiation and uncharged particles produce charged particles.

All of these radiations can be administered to animals and human beings externally or internally. External sources include x-ray machines, electron or other charged particle accelerators, high activity radiation γ-ray sources, neutron generators, nuclear reactors and atomic bombs. Internal irradiation arises from the ingestion of any of the hundreds of known radionuclides (radioactive isotopes) many of which are used for medical diagnostic or therapeutic purposes, for commercial non-destructive testing and for irradiating materials for industrial purposes; they are produced in nuclear reactors. The dosage has, in the past, been expressed as *curies* (Ci), but the modern unit is the *becquerel* (Bq) after the French scientist who discovered radioactivity. One Ci equals 3.7×10^{10} Bq. The best known severe radiation damage from accidental ingestion of radioactive material is that produced by radium which was once used extensively in luminising paints. Some sufferers from radium poisoning have been under medical supervision for up to fifty years and the effects are well documented. Today, in spite of strict regulations and control, occasional accidents occur in nuclear reactors, industry and hospitals, which result in significant radiation of personnel. Ionising radiation for diagnosis and therapy, however, has a secure and important place in modern medicine and has been essential for many research purposes.

Cellular radiation effects

Measurement of cellular radiation effects is based on the survival curve, i.e. on the ability of cells to multiply in appropriate environmental conditions. One of the most marked effects of radiation is the destruction of this ability. The number of cells in which the ability survives can be readily measured by counting the number of clones in cultures of the irradiated cells.

The percentage 'survival', that is, the percentage of cells which still retain the ability to produce clones after irradiation, is plotted on a logarithmic scale and the radiation dose is plotted on a linear scale (Fig. 2.24). Since log

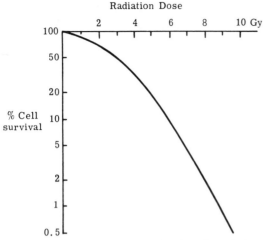

Fig. 2.24 Radiation injury, showing the relationship between percentage cell survival and dose of ionising radiation.

percentage survival decreases continuously with increasing dosage, the origin is placed in the top left corner of the figure. The resultant curve usually approximates to a straight line after an initial shoulder. This shoulder shows that an accumulation of sub-lethal damage is necessary before an observable effect is produced. After sufficient dose has been given to reach the straight portion of the survival curve, no further accumulation of sub-lethal damage occurs. If, however, the cells are allowed to recover for some hours, it is found that once again a considerable accumulation of sub-lethal damage is necessary before the radiation effects are produced with maximum efficiency. It appears that the shoulder therefore represents the repair process by which the cells can overcome some of the damage.

The slope of the portion of the survival curve which is almost straight on the log-linear plot of Fig. 2.24—the exponential part—represents the rate at which additional lethal damage is produced as additional dose is administered. The fact that this portion of the curve is almost straight means that, irrespective of the damage already created, a given amount of irradiation always reduces the survival by the same fraction. This kind of relationship, in which increasing dosage decreases proportionately the fraction of surviving cells, is indicative of an effect controlled by probability. In this case it is usually regarded as the probability of the track of ionisations, produced by charged particles, causing damage to small discrete targets in individual cells.

The available evidence suggests that, for each type of radiation, no great differences exist in the slopes of survival curves for various types of mammalian cells, unless they are hypoxic when irradiated. The magnitude of the shoulder, however, is dependent on the history, the environment, and the biochemical condition of the cells.

Linear energy transfer effect. Survival curves referring to different types of radiation have different shapes. The reason for this is that although, for equal doses of different radiations, the total number of ionisations are equal, the geometrical distribution of these ionisations in the cell can vary greatly. These large variations in distribution have a considerable effect on the mean number of ionisations necessary to produce the kind of biological damage which, after complex development, results in a cell losing its ability to continue to divide.

Heavy charged particles moving relatively slowly produce dense columns of ionisations, while electrons produce sparse lines of ionisations with occasional small clumps (Fig. 2.25).

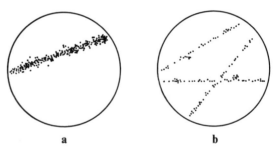

Fig. 2.25 The distribution of ionisations for high LET radiation (**a**) and low LET radiation (**b**).

The average amount of energy deposited per micron of track of a particle or photon is called the linear energy transfer (LET) and can be used to characterise the quality of the radiation. A number of ionisations grouped closely together are more likely to initiate a lethal chain of biological events than the same number of ionisations widely separated. The dense group of ionisations also prevents the cellular repair mechanisms from acting effectively. Thus the survival curves for high LET radiation such as α-particles show no shoulder, and have a steeper slope than those for low LET radiation such as x-rays or electrons (Fig.

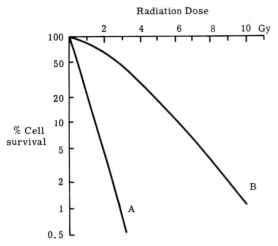

Fig. 2.26 The comparative cytotoxic effects of α-particles (A) and electrons (B).

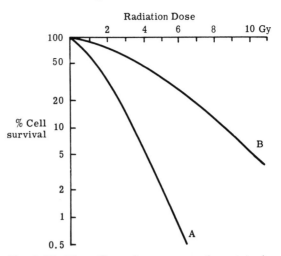

Fig. 2.27 The effect of oxygen on the cytotoxic effect of x-irradiation. A, high oxygen tension; B, low oxygen tension.

2.26). For both these reasons a dose of high LET radiation produces far more biological damage than an equal dose of low LET radiation.

Effect of oxygen. Another factor which has a striking effect on survival curves is the presence or absence of oxygen. Oxygen has the ability to combine with freshly severed ends of molecular structures thus preventing them from rejoining, which they commonly do if the opportunity presents itself. Oxygen thus interferes with a natural recovery process —a different one from that which produces the shoulder—and causes a given dose of radiation to be much more damaging than it would be in hypoxic or anoxic conditions. The ratio of the doses required to reduce the survival to the same level in anoxic and normal conditions is called the **oxygen enhancement ratio** (OER) (Fig. 2.27).

There are many other radio-sensitisers and radio-protectors which affect different levels of recovery and repair processes. Estimation of the biological damage produced by a given dose of radiation must therefore take into account both the type of radiation, the environment in which it is administered and the time allowed for repair and recovery.

Tissue radiation effects

The effect of radiation in destroying the ability of cells to continue dividing has been discussed above in relation to individual cells. It is important because it plays a major part in causing tissue effects. Cell function which is not related to mitosis and division is relatively insensitive to radiation. Much higher doses of radiation are required to produce gross changes in such function than are required to inhibit cell division. Hence the typical radiation effect on tissues arises from an inhibition of division.

Tissues whose cells are undergoing continuous controlled division, and whose integrity requires a continual flow of new cells, are therefore the first tissues to show the effects of radiation. The most obvious are the skin, the intestinal tract, the bone marrow and the immunity system. Similar considerations apply to the therapeutic use of radiation for malignant tumours, in which there is excessive division of cells. The initial effect upon a tissue is a reduction in cell numbers as the supply of new cells falls below the normal rate. The drop in cell numbers leads via homoeostatic feedback mechanisms to a build up of the population of viable stem-cells from which new cells are produced, and to an increase in the rate of cell division. If this compensation is successful, then in due course enhanced production of cells not only restores the depleted population but commonly results in a temporary hyperplasia or overshoot before the cell numbers return to normal (Fig. 2.28). The inflammatory response to trauma follows injury by irradiation and commonly results in permanent structural changes, e.g. fibrosis (see p. 38).

The fall, rise, overshoot and return to

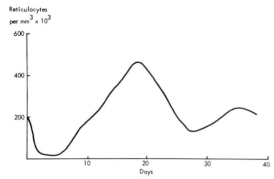

Fig. 2.28 Changes in the numbers of reticulocytes in the blood following 2 Gy whole-body irradiation.

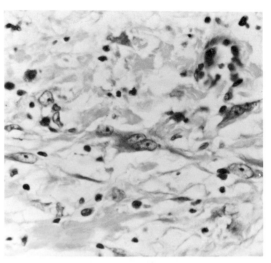

Fig. 2.29 Changes in the sub-epithelial connective tissue of the tongue following irradiation therapy for an epithelial tumour six years ago. Note the abnormally large connective tissue cells, one of which is binucleate. × 340.

normal of the cell populations exhibiting such behaviour after irradiation can be understood and explained in cellular terms if the appropriate homoeostatic feedback mechanisms are known. The normal cell turnover controls the rate at which the cell population falls following irradiation. The extent of the fall depends on the percentage of surviving cells and the rate at which they can divide.

If the cell population of a tissue falls below a critical value the tissue can lose its functional effectiveness. In the cases of the intestinal tract and the bone marrow the result is death of the individual. A rapidly administered x-ray dose of about 8 Gy to the bone marrow and 12 Gy to the intestinal tract reduces the number of surviving cells to such low levels that the delay before an adequate production of cells can be re-established is long enough to allow the cell population to fall below the critical value.

The cells whose reproductive ability has been destroyed by the irradiation often remain in the tissue for some time. Their abortive attempts to divide or prepare to divide can produce gross abnormalities in cytological appearance (Fig. 2.29). Toxic products of cell disintegration can increase the damage. However, the damaged cells are no longer directly relevant to the course of events leading to permanent damage or repair. This course is determined by the number of surviving cells still capable of division and by the kinetics of proliferation in the tissue. Ultimately, however, if a large enough dose is given (about 18 Gy in a single exposure) a tissue condition described as the **limit of tolerance** is reached. Although the nature of this is not understood, it is the determining factor for

radiotherapy, and represents an accumulation of permanent, irreparable damage.

Tissues whose cells are long-lived and therefore are not normally dividing show very little effect after doses of several grays. Damage has been done, however, and becomes apparent if the cells are stimulated to divide, even after long intervals of time (Fig. 2.30). Examples of such tissue are the adult liver, adult thyroid and long-lived lymphocytes. Again the major effect is that many of the cells are unable to divide successfully when called upon to do so.

Radiation damage to the gonads may lead to infertility due to impairment of germ cell division. Errors also occur in copying the base sequence of DNA in the germ cells, the number of errors—mutations—being related to the radiation dosage as shown in Fig. 2.31. A given dose of radiation insufficient to cause infertility gives rise to the same total number of mutations irrespective of the number of individuals among whom it is distributed. As a corollary there is no 'safe' level of background radiation. It is known that radiation induces the development of malignant tumours, (p. 301) possibly by causing mutations in somatic cells (p. 319).

Microscopic appearances. Following a substantial dose of radiation there is a latent interval of hours or days before histological evidence of tissue injury is seen. As already explained, the

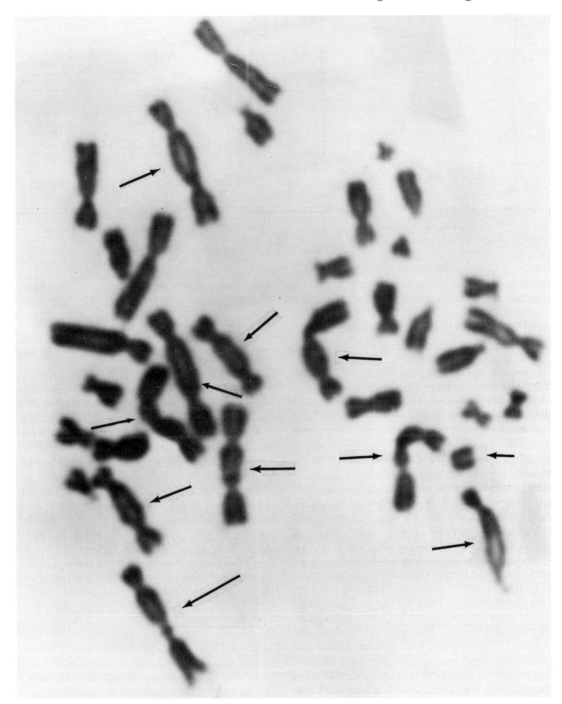

Fig. 2.30 Dividing lymphocyte in peripheral blood culture from a patient with bronchial carcinoma and spinal metastases, treated by five 5 Gy of ^{60}Co radiation to the lumbar spine. This cell shows the result of extensive chromosome breakage followed by random fusion of broken ends due to radiation. There are nine dicentric chromosomes, one possible tricentric, one acentric fragment and at least three other abnormal chromosomes. 44 centromeres can be counted, indicating elimination of two chromosomes. Aceto-orcein stain. $\times 2000$. (Professor M. A. Ferguson Smith.)

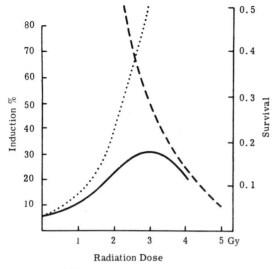

Fig. 2.31 The effect of dosage of radiation on mutation rate in mice. As the dose is increased, the mutation rate rises (dotted line), but the survival rate diminishes (interrupted line). The incidence of mutation-dependent abnormality, in this case leukaemia, is dependent on mutation and survival rates, and is shown by the continuous line.

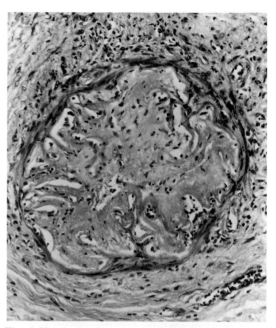

Fig. 2.32 A small artery occluded by hyaline fibrous tissue following radiotherapy. (Same case as in Fig. 2.29.) × 126.

damage depends on the dose and type of radiation, on the interval following exposure and on the tissue exposed. Early changes in the skin include dilatation of blood vessels and other signs of acute inflammation and these reflect acute tissue injury. With a single dose of 15 Gy mitotic activity of the basal cells is arrested, with subsequent loss of the epidermis and epilation. The walls of the dermal vessels are infiltrated with fibrin; later a characteristic concentric proliferation of intimal fibrous tissue is seen (endarteritis obliterans), followed by replacement with dense homogeneous (hyaline) collagen (Fig. 2.32). Large bizarre fibrocytic nuclei are present in the dermal connective tissue (Fig. 2.29). With repeated exposure to radiation the dermal collagen becomes very dense and there is a tendency for the dermal fibrous tissue to become necrotic even years after exposure; persistent melanin pigmentation and vascular dilatation are also noted. Comparable changes found in other tissues following irradiation are described later in the appropriate chapters; the detailed findings depend, of course, upon the radio-sensitivity of the various types of tissue present, their turnover of cells and potential for cell multiplication, and the architectural features of the tissue.

Atrophy

By atrophy is meant diminution in size of a cell or reduction in the essential tissue of an organ due to decrease in the size or numbers of its specialised cells. Pathological atrophy has its prototype in the physiological atrophy of old age, which affects all the tissues, and notably the bones, lymphoid tissue and the sexual organs; and although some of the changes occurring in old age are the result of atrophy of the gonads, this atrophy in its turn cannot be explained. The cause of **senile atrophy** is of course merely part of the larger question of what limits the duration of life. Atrophic specialised epithelial cells tend to lose their special features and to become de-differentiated, as may be seen in local atrophic changes in the liver and kidneys. Senile atrophy is commonly accompanied by accumulation of the yellowish-brown pigment lipofuscin and the term *brown atrophy* is then applied. As already indicated (p. 23) lipofuscin represents indigestable lipid which forms residual bodies and is often the product of cellular autophagia.

An organ may be undersized as the result of imperfect development, and the term **hypoplasia** is then applied; for example, the hypoplasia of the genital glands which results from deficiency of the pituitary secretion in early life.

Causes of atrophy

1. Defective nutrition. This may be produced locally by arterial disease interfering with the blood supply to a part, when the reduction is not so severe as to cause necrosis. The functioning parenchymatous elements of the tissue then undergo atrophy, and sometimes there is also a concomitant overgrowth of fibrous tissue. This is often seen in the myocardium (Fig. 15.5, p. 402) and in the kidneys, in which small atrophic depressions result from narrowing of the lumina of the small arteries. **General atrophy** is seen in cases of starvation; emaciation depends chiefly upon utilisation of the fat of the adipose tissue but there is also a general wasting of the tissues. The various organs may thus diminish in weight, the liver and spleen are markedly affected, the kidneys and heart to a less though distinct degree, whilst the central nervous system is only slightly affected. In most cases of wasting disease, however, such as malignant tumours of the alimentary tract, chronic tuberculosis or suppuration, other ill-defined factors appear to contribute to the wasting. Various other forms of cellular damage and diminished cell production may thus come to be associated with atrophy; secondary anaemia, for example, is present, although slight or absent in wasting due to starvation alone. The term **cachexia** is often applied to a combination of wasting, anaemia and weakness.

2. Diminished functional activity. It is a general law that diminution in the catabolic processes leads to reduced anabolism and thus to diminution in the size of cells. When the function of a part is in abeyance the blood supply also diminishes. **Disuse atrophy**, as it is sometimes called, is seen when a gland, for example,

the pancreas, has its duct obstructed; its functional activity is thus stopped and the exocrine glandular tissue undergoes atrophy. The muscles responsible for operating a joint which has been immobile for some time undergo marked atrophy and the bones also are affected. Unless such atrophy has become extreme it is reversible and full functional activity may be restored.

3. Interference with the nerve supply. This form of atrophy is seen where there is any destructive lesion of the lower motor neutrons or their axons. In this type, **neuropathic atrophy**, there is not only a simple wasting, but also more active shrinkage of the muscle tissue (Fig. 23.68, p.935). For at least a few weeks after nerve section, during which the muscle fibre mass may be reduced by half, anabolic processes take place at a normal rate: catabolism due to increased lysosome numbers and activity is

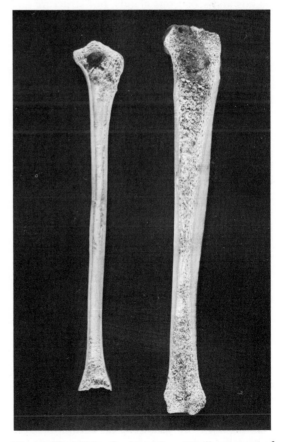

Fig. 2.33 Tibia from a longstanding case of poliomyelitis, showing marked atrophy (*left*). Normal tibia for comparison (*right*). × 0·3.

greatly accelerated. That this form is different in nature from disuse atrophy is shown by the electrical 'reactions of degeneration' which are given by the muscles and indicate that a complete return to normal is no longer possible. Sometimes marked atrophy occurs also in the bones of paralysed limbs; for example, in cases of poliomyelitis the bones of the limb may become thin and light, and this appears to be due simply to inactivity (Fig. 2.33). In some forms of inherited muscular atrophy, however, no nerve lesion is present and the terms *primary myopathy* or *muscular dystrophy* are often applied (p. 933).

4. Deficiency of endocrine glands. Atrophy of thyroid, gonads and adrenal cortex are seen when destruction of the pituitary results in diminished secretion of trophic hormones. In hypothyroidism there occurs marked atrophy of the structures of the skin, hair follicles, sweat glands and sebaceous glands, but structure and function may be restored by oral administration of thyroid hormone.

5. Fever. A good example of atrophy is provided by wasting of the muscles in fevers. No doubt inactivity and loss of appetite play a part, but the wasting is probably due mainly to utilisation of proteins, as is indicated by the increased excretion of nitrogen. This increased protein catabolism is characteristic not only of fever but also follows severe trauma such as fractures or major surgical operations. Other tissues may suffer atrophy in a corresponding way, but in the parenchymatous organs other expressions of cellular injury are more common.

6. Pressure atrophy is also described. The pressure acts mainly by interfering with the blood supply and also with the functions of a tissue. Thus atrophy of the organs may be brought about by the pressure of benign tumours and cysts. When bone is subjected to pressure there is active absorption by osteoclasts.

Examples of atrophy are provided in the later chapters on diseases of the different systems.

Metaplasia

An interesting cellular response to injury is the phenomenon of metaplasia—the transformation of one type of differentiated tissue into another. An example is provided by the surface epithelium of the bronchi which commonly changes from the normal ciliated pseudostratified columnar type to squamous (Fig. 2.34). In this example it appears that chronic injury or irritation, often due to cigarette smoke, results in adaptive changes in the surface epithelium to a type likely to be more resistant to the cause of the irritation. Similarly stratified squamous epithelium may form as a result of chronic irritation in the mucous membrane of the nose, salivary ducts, gallbladder, renal pelvis and urinary bladder. In some cases the injurious stimulus is apparent, e.g. when there is a stone in the renal pelvis or in cases of extroversion of the urinary bladder, while in others the cause is obscure. In vitamin A deficiency, in addition to xerophthalmia, stratified squamous epithelium may replace the transitional and columnar epithelia of nose, bronchi, urinary tract, and the specialised secre-tory epithelia of the lacrimal and salivary glands. In auto-immune chronic gastritis, in which there is an immunological attack on the mucosa of the fundus of the patient's own stomach, the specialised surface-lining cells and chief and parietal cells of the gastric glands are often replaced by tall columnar cells with striated borders, goblet cells and Paneth cells, i.e. metaplasia to an intestinal type of mucosa.

In the connective tissues, metaplasia occurs between fibrous tissue, myxoid tissue, bone and cartilage. Bone formation occasionally follows the deposition of calcium salts in such tissues as arterial walls (Fig. 2.35), bronchial cartilage and the uveal tract of the eye. In healing fractures cartilaginous metaplasia may occur especially when there is undue mobility. The flattened serosal endothelium of the rabbit pleural cavity becomes cubical, columnar, transitional or even squamous following injection of the dye Sudan III with sodium cholate in olive oil and the lining of adjacent alveoli also becomes cubical or columnar. Similar changes, which

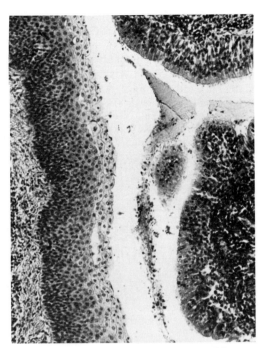

Fig. 2.34 Metaplasia of bronchial epithelium to stratified squamous type is seen on the left side, persistence of columnar ciliated epithelium on the right. × 200.

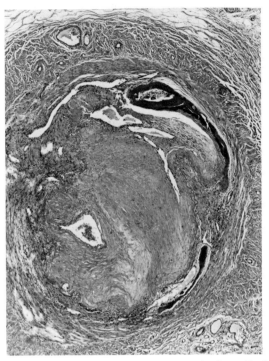

Fig. 2.35 Metaplastic bone formation in the wall of a largely obliterated artery. × 50.

are rapidly reversible, follow the injection of strontium chloride.

Metaplasia is to be distinguished from a mere loss of the special characters of cells, for example the dedifferentiation which is encountered when there is interference with the function of glands. Developmental epithelial abnormalities, e.g. squamous epithelium within the thyroid, arising from the thyroglossal duct, do not constitute metaplasia, nor does encroachment of one tissue upon another. Thus the fatty marrow of the long bones is replaced in certain types of anaemia by red haemopoietic marrow: in this case the haemopoietic tissue has spread by proliferation of haemopoietic stem cells and not by metaplasia of the adipose tissue cells originally present.

It is believed that all nucleated cells carry a complete list of the genetic information required for bodily development, including all types of cellular differentiation and function, but little is yet known about the factors which determine the differentiation of cells in an orderly manner to form the various tissues. The way in which the many different stimuli producing metaplasia act within the cell is correspondingly obscure. It seems likely that a change in gene repression and activation takes place in serosal endothelium when it undergoes metaplasia to squamous epithelium. By contrast, in surfaces lined by columnar epithelium, metaplasia may result from gradual atrophy of the columnar cells and proliferation and maturation of the less well differentiated basal or reserve cells to form squamous epithelium. It is noteworthy that many stimuli which bring about metaplasia are also capable of inducing neoplasia, and indeed tumour formation is relatively common in some metaplastic epithelia; conversely metaplasia is frequently encountered in malignant tumours. Indeed metaplasia may represent a cellular change in response to injury intermediate between the kind we have been considering earlier in this chapter and that which underlies the development of tumours.

Further Reading

Chanarin, I. (1979). *The Megaloblastic Anaemias*, 2nd edn., pp. 1100. Blackwell Scientific Publications, Oxford.

Cori, G. T. (1952–3). Glycogen Structure and Enzyme Deficiency Glycogen Storage Disease. *Harvey Lecture* **Vol. 48**, p. 145.

Dingle, J. T. and Fell, Dame Honor (1973 and 1975). *Lysosomes in Biology and Pathology*, 4 vols. North Holland Publishing Co., Amsterdam.

Emery, A. E. H. (1979). *Elements of Medical Genetics*, 5th edn., pp. 243. Churchill Livingstone, Edinburgh and London.

Popper, H. and Schaffner, F. (Eds.) (1976). *Progress in Liver Diseases*, **Vol. V**, Chapters 4 and 14. Grune and Stratton, New York.

Stanbury, J. B., Wyngaarden, J. B. and Fredrickson, D. S. (1975). *The Metabolic Basis of Inherited Disease*, 3rd edn., pp. 1778. McGraw Hill, New York and London.

3

Inflammation

Definition and nature of inflammation

Inflammation may be defined as *a series of changes which take place in living tissue following injury*. While commendably brief, this definition is useless without qualification. We have seen in Chapter 2 how tissue cells may be injured, i.e. rendered abnormal, in many ways, and how the effects may range from pathological storage of metabolites to neoplasia. These are not examples of inflammation, and so it is necessary to qualify both the type of injury and the nature of the changes resulting from it.

The injury which causes inflammation may be brought about by: (1) **physical agents,** such as excessive heating or cooling, mechanical trauma, ultraviolet or ionising radiations; (2) a wide variety of **chemical agents,** both inorganic and organic, and including the **toxins** of various bacteria; (3) the intracellular replication of **viruses;** (4) **hypersensitivity reactions,** i.e. the reaction of antibody or sensitised lymphocytes with antigenic material such as invasive bacteria or inhaled organic dusts; and (5) **necrosis of tissue,** which induces inflammation in the surrounding tissue.

A very important cause of inflammation is **microbial infection.** As indicated above, bacteria produce harmful toxins, viruses injure the host cells which they colonise, and all types of micro-organisms may induce hypersensitivity reactions by the host.

The main features of inflammation. When an appropriate injury, such as excessive heat, is applied to living tissue, an **acute inflammatory reaction** develops. The small vessels in the vicinity of the injury become engorged with blood which at first flows rapidly but gradually slows down. Protein-rich fluid and red cells and subsequently leukocytes escape from the engorged vessels into the tissue spaces. This reaction is due to changes in the small vessels and, because it includes the escape of blood constituents into the tissues, it is commonly termed **exudative.** When the tissue injury has been slight and brief, the exudative inflammatory reaction is correspondingly mild and soon subsides. However, if the injury persists, the exudative inflammatory reaction can continue for months or even years, as in some persistent bacterial infections, and it is therefore wrong to equate it solely with acute lesions, i.e. those having a short course.

A second type of inflammatory response, sometimes called **productive** or **formative** (to distinguish it from exudative) inflammation, is characterised by proliferation of fibroblasts and production of new fibrous tissue. This occurs particularly in prolonged tissue injury and so is seen especially in **chronic inflammation.** In some instances, both exudative and productive reactions are conspicuous, but in prolonged low-grade injury, fibrous tissue formation is often the more prominent. At first, the young fibrous tissue is highly vascular, soft and gelatinous, and is known as *granulation tissue.* As it ages, it becomes less vascular, progressively more collagenous, and is thus gradually converted to pale, dense *scar tissue.*

The present account follows tradition in using the terms 'acute inflammation' and 'acute inflammatory reaction' for the exudative process, and 'chronic inflammation' for persistent inflammatory lesions, in which fibrous tissue formation is a prominent feature. It must, however, be emphasised that the two types of reaction commonly occur together.

Leukocytes migrate from the blood vessels into the tissues in both acute and chronic inflammation: in the former neutrophil polymorphs usually predominate, while in the latter lymphocytes, plasma cells and monocytes are often more conspicuous.

The inflammatory nature of a lesion is usually indicated by the use of the suffix **-itis.** Thus inflammation of the appendix is appendicitis, inflammation of the meninges, meningitis, and so on.

Inflammation is usually beneficial. It is essential in combating various infections and in limiting the harmful effects of toxic compounds. Like other beneficial processes, it is not without disadvantages: for example, in acute bacterial infection of the larynx there may be sufficient inflammatory swelling to obstruct the airway and even to cause death from asphyxia, and inflammatory reactions caused by hypersensitivity to harmless substances, as in hay fever,

appear entirely disadvantageous to the host. Fibrous tissue formed in chronic inflammation may help to wall off bacteria or harmful compounds such as silica particles, but it may also cause disability by distorting and compressing important structures. Inflammatory fibrosis of a hollow viscus, such as the intestine, may cause narrowing of the lumen, and fibrosis occurring in any tissue can constrict blood vessels, nerves, ducts, etc.

This chapter deals with the acute inflammatory reaction, the mechanisms involved in its production and its effects, the special features of chronic inflammation, and the types of cell involved in inflammatory reactions.

The Acute Inflammatory Reaction

Acute inflammation has been recognised since the earliest days of medicine. Celsus (30 B.C. to A.D. 38) gave as its cardinal signs **heat, redness, swelling** and **pain,** to which may be added **limitation of movement,** e.g. of an inflamed limb. The explanation of these features has been provided by microscopic studies, which have revealed that the inflammatory reaction is composed of a number of phenomena, all of which involve the small blood vessels in the inflamed tissue. These phenomena were described by Cohnheim (1889) who observed microscopically the changes in the living transparent tissue of the frog's tongue and foot-web during inflammation caused by mechanical injury or chemical irritation. His superb account is a model of accurate observation and the changes he described have since been confirmed by others in mammalian tissues following thermal or chemical injury. They are as follows.

(a) Active hyperaemia. Immediately after thermal or chemical injury there is a transient blanching of the tissue due to arteriolar contraction. This effect, which is not of practical importance, is followed within a few minutes by relaxation of the arterioles in and around the injured tissue, so that the capillary network and post-capillary venules become engorged (Fig. 3.1) with rapidly flowing blood (*active hyperaemia*). This accounts for the redness (*erythema*) of the inflamed tissue, and when the normally cool skin is involved the increased

flow of blood warms it up and so explains the **heat** of inflammation.

(b) Exudation. Following the onset of active hyperaemia, protein-rich fluid (the **inflammatory exudate**) escapes from the blood vessels into the surrounding tissues and is largely responsible for the **swelling (inflammatory oedema).**

The **pain** of acute inflammation is due partly to the rise in tissue pressure resulting from inflammatory oedema; this accounts also for the **relative immobility**, for the oedema increases the rigidity of the tissues and movement further increases the pressure and thus aggravates the pain. Palpation has a similar effect and this explains why inflamed tissues are often exquisitely tender. The original injury (heat, chemicals, etc.) may also be directly painful and, as described later, a number of pain-inducing endogenous compounds (histamine, kinins, prostaglandins, etc.) are released in acute inflammation.

(c) Slowing of the blood flow. The microcirculation remains engorged but the blood flow, at first rapid, becomes progressively slower, with even momentary arrests in some of the small vessels.

(d) Emigration of leukocytes. Phagocytic leukocytes, at first neutrophil polymorphs and later monocytes, adhere to the endothelium of venules and migrate through the vessel walls into the tissue spaces (Fig. 3.1).

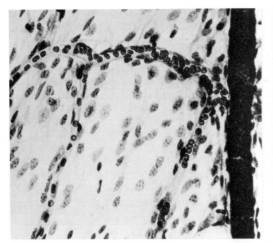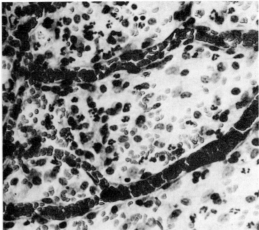

Fig. 3.1 Surface view of stained preparations of guinea-pig omentum showing the normal appearances (*left*) and acute inflammation (*right*). Note engorgement of the small vessels with blood and infiltration of the tissue with neutrophil polymorphs. × 300.

The time of onset, intensity and duration of each of these phenomena vary considerably depending on the type and severity of their causal injury. The reaction to thermal burns and many irritating chemicals is almost immediate: as sunbathers learn to their cost, inflammation of the skin due to excessive ultraviolet irradiation is delayed for several hours, while with ionising radiations, e.g. x-ray, acute inflammation may develop up to a week later.

The features of the inflammatory reaction to microbial infections vary greatly depending on the properties of the microbes and on the host–parasite relationships.

The major phenomena of acute inflammation will now be described in more detail, not only because of their fundamental importance, but also because elucidation of their mechanisms is essential to the advancement of rational therapy.

Active hyperaemia

Normal microcirculatory control

The flow of blood through a tissue is controlled mainly by changes in the tone of the circular smooth muscle of its arterioles. This is regulated in part by the autonomic nervous system, and especially by the sympathetic adrenergic vasoconstrictor nerves, which maintain arteriolar tone and are largely responsible for controlling the blood pressure, the cardiac output, and to some extent the distribution of blood flow among the various tissues. Superimposed on this overall control are local factors determined by the conditions in individual tissues. Thus when an organ or tissue is in a resting state of low metabolic activity, many of its arterioles are contracted and blood flow is diminished. When local metabolism increases, for example in the gastric mucosa after a meal, or in an exercising muscle, accumulated metabolites act directly on the arterioles, causing them to relax and the consequent rise in pressure of blood reaching the capillaries causes them and their draining venules to become engorged with rapidly flowing blood. This engorgement or congestion, due to the rise in pressure of blood entering the capillaries, is termed **active hyperaemia** to distinguish it from the congestion due to a rise in venous pressure (passive hyperaemia) which occurs in other conditions and is not accompanied by an increase in blood flow.

Although the arterioles and venules are greatly dilated in active hyperaemia, the size of capillaries is restricted by their basement membrane: their diameter is approximately 5–8 μm and in active hyperaemia they become conspicuous not so much by dilatation but because they are filled with whole blood, whereas in the resting tissue state most of them contain slowly flowing plasma with few cells.

In most tissues, the capillaries form an anastomosing network providing routes of various lengths between arterioles and venules. The individual entrances to the network are the *terminal arterioles,* which do not anastomose, and which are the smallest vessels controlled by smooth muscle cells: they function as pre-capillary sphincters and determine the flow of blood through individual capillaries. It is probable that, in resting tissues, the pre-capillary sphincters are so adjusted that blood flows mainly through the shortest capillary routes—the so-called thoroughfare channels—in accordance with the needs of general circulatory control: the pre-capillary sphincters guarding the longer capillary routes are contracted, and most of the capillaries contain only plasma.

The engorgement and rapid flow of active hyperaemia are brought about mainly by relaxation of the arterioles, including most of the pre-capillary sphincters. The capillaries themselves are not contractile and so the amount of blood passing through them depends on the state of the arterioles.

The active hyperaemia of acute inflammation

This is a local phenomenon and is due to predominance of local factors over the general system of arteriolar control. As in physiological activity (see above), the arterioles relax and active hyperaemia results. The mechanism of the arteriolar relaxation is unknown and is difficult to investigate. Either endogenous mediators or neural factors must be involved, for the active hyperaemia extends beyond the immediate site of injury.

In his classical experiments, Lewis (1927) provided evidence for both chemical endogenous mediators and neural factors. He induced mild inflammation in the skin of the human forearm by firm stroking with a blunt point or by mild thermal injury and observed three components in the inflammatory response, namely a *flush* (erythema at the site of injury), a *flare* (erythema of the surrounding skin) and a *weal* (swelling due to inflammatory oedema). Lewis showed that the flush was prolonged by applying a tourniquet to the arm and considered that it was due to capillary dilatation induced by a chemical endogenous mediator, removal of which was dependent on

blood flow. He showed that the erythema caused by a local injection of histamine was prolonged by a tourniquet and called his hypothetical mediator 'H' substance. In subjects with nerve injuries, Lewis showed that the flare could be elicited for up to ten days after severance of the sensory nerve to the part, but not later. Accordingly he postulated that the inflammatory stimulus (firm stroking or thermal injury) triggered off an axon reflex which induced the flare by causing relaxation of the arterioles in the surrounding skin (Fig. 3.2).

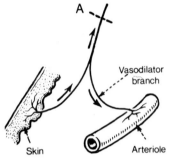

Fig. 3.2 Diagram of peripheral end of sensory nerve fibre with vasodilator axon branch. Stimulation of sensory nerve ending in the skin results in an anti-dromic reflex along the vasodilator branch, with resulting arteriolar dilatation. Section of the nerve fibre at A does not abolish this reflex until the fibre distal to A has degenerated.

It is now known that acute inflammation occurring in long-denervated tissues presents all the usual features and so neural factors clearly play no essential role: it is thus likely that Lewis's postulated axon reflex is not of much practical importance. His work did, however, stimulate considerable interest in the role of endogenous chemical mediators in the acute inflammatory reaction, and an ever-increasing number of endogenous compounds capable of inducing one or more features of acute inflammation has since been detected in inflammatory lesions. The list of possible endogenous chemical mediators of inflammatory hyperaemia includes histamine, 5-hydroxy-tryptamine, kinins, prostaglandins, products of activation of the complement system, fibrin degradation products and various other polypeptides. These and other vaso-active agents can all induce hyperaemia: what is in doubt is their relative importance in the natural process. To complicate matters further, most of them are capable also of inducing exudation (escape of protein-rich fluid from the small blood vessels) and yet the hyperaemia and exudation of inflammation do not closely parallel one another either in their timing or in their degree. In inflammation produced in the skin by sunburn, for example, exudation may only occur during a short part of the period of hyperaemia.

Changes in blood flow

The rapid blood flow of active hyperaemia is readily explained by the increased hydrostatic pressure of blood in the microcirculation resulting from arteriolar relaxation.

Slowing of the blood flow. This supervenes gradually until, in some vessels, there may be temporary stasis of blood. In severe inflammation, stasis may be prolonged and clotting may occur. Several factors contribute towards the slowing of the blood flow through inflamed tissues (Fig. 3.3). Firstly, active hyperaemia results in *loss of fluid from the blood* in capillaries and post-capillary venules, and the concentration of cells in the blood is thus increased. Secondly, although the exudate is rich in protein, loss of fluid is so great that there is an *increase in the local concentration of the plasma proteins.* Both of these changes increase the viscosity of the blood locally. Thirdly, the increased protein concentration of the plasma and slowing of blood flow result in *aggregation of the red cells in rouleaux,* with so-called sludging of the blood, and this further increases viscosity. A fourth factor which impairs the blood flow is the *adhesion of leukocytes to the walls of post-capillary venules.* Not only do the leuko-

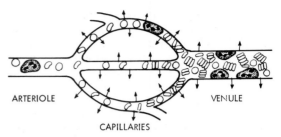

Fig. 3.3 The causes of slowing of the blood flow in acute inflammation. Loss of intravascular fluid (arrows) results in haemoconcentration, with consequent increase in blood viscosity. Increase in plasma protein concentration promotes rouleaux formation by the red cells, further increasing blood viscosity, while pavementing of polymorphs in the venules, together with rouleaux formation, partially blocks the venules. (Modified after Dr Roe Wells; *see* Zweifach, 1973–4.)

cytes adhere to the endothelium but also to one another, and considerable reduction in the effective lumen of venules may result.

Slowing of the blood flow will tend to impair the supply of oxygen, glucose, etc., to the tissues, and also the removal of metabolites, but these effects are diminished by the increased flow of fluid from the plasma into the tissues and increased lymphatic drainage (see below). It is only when the vascular stagnation is extreme that it is likely to impair tissue nutrition seriously and contribute to the necrosis which is commonly observed in severe inflammatory reactions. Such necrosis is more likely to result directly from the injury which has induced the inflammatory response, e.g. bacterial toxic action, thermal injury, etc.

Exudation of protein-rich fluid

Microscopic examination of inflamed tissues reveals an accumulation of extracellular fluid, i.e. interstitial oedema (Fig. 3.4). This can only have come from the blood plasma, and since it has been shown that the amount of fluid draining away from inflamed tissues by the lymphatics is also greatly increased, there is obviously a considerable rise in the net amount of fluid leaving the blood vessels. As illustrated in Fig. 3.5, the inflammatory exudate is also much richer in plasma proteins than is normal extracellular fluid (transudate) in the same tissue, indicating increased permeability of the vessels to macromolecules. These two features of exudation—increased loss of intravascular fluid and of plasma proteins—are best considered separately, for the factors involved in the passage of water and small solutes across the walls of microvessels, in both normal and inflamed tissues, differ from those concerned in the escape of molecules as large as the plasma proteins.

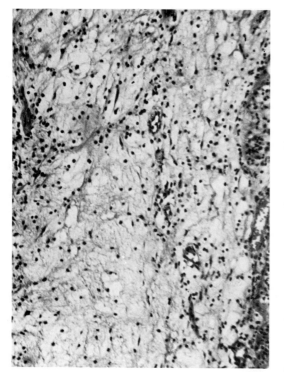

Fig. 3.4 Meso-appendix in acute appendicitis, showing inflammatory oedema with early leukocytic emigration. × 100.

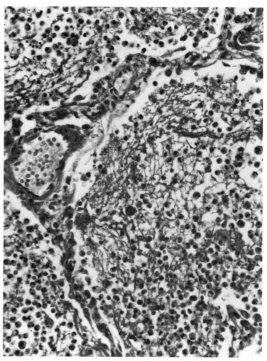

Fig. 3.5 Acute inflammation of the lung in pneumonia. The exudate, which fills the alveoli, is rich in plasma proteins, and this is illustrated by the fine network of fibrin (stained black) which has resulted from the clotting of exuded fibrinogen. (Weigert's fibrin stain.) × 150.

Escape of water and micromolecular solutes

In all tissues the capillaries and post-capillary venules are readily permeable to water and micromolecular solutes. For molecules above a molecular weight of 10 000 daltons, the permeability decreases sharply with molecular size, and molecules greater than 40 000 escape from the plasma in relatively small numbers. This applies particularly to the vessels in skeletal muscles, central nervous system, dermis and other connective tissues. In the liver, intestinal mucosa, exocrine and endocrine glands and the glomeruli, macromolecules escape more readily but still much less so than do micromolecules.

Our understanding of the mass movement of water and small solutes between plasma and extravascular fluid is based upon (*a*) the observations of Starling and of Landis on microfiltration, and (*b*) morphological considerations.

(a) Microfiltration theory

Starling (1896) proposed that the vascular endothelium behaves like a passive microfilter, across which the movement of fluid and electrolytes is determined by physical forces. On this theory the main force driving fluid out of vessels is the height of the hydrostatic pressure within the vessels above that in the extravascular space, and this is opposed by the height of the osmotic pressure of the plasma above that of the extravascular fluid. Thus at the arteriolar ends of capillaries the effective hydrostatic pressure would normally exceed the osmotic pressure and fluid should be forced out. At the venular ends of capillaries the osmotic pressure would exceed the hydrostatic pressure and fluid should be drawn into the capillary (Fig. 3.6). This theory received direct support from the work of an American medical student, Landis (1927), who devised techniques of meas-

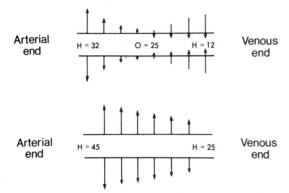

Fig. 3.6 Exchange of fluid across the walls of capillaries and venules. H and O represent the heights of the hydrostatic and osmotic pressure respectively (mmHg) of the plasma above the corresponding pressures of the extravascular space. The arrows indicate the net movement of fluid into and out of the vessels along their length. *Upper figure,* normal tissue: fluid movement across vessel walls approximates to equilibrium. *Lower figure,* acute inflammation: much more fluid leaves the vessels than returns to them.

The values of H and O are approximations. In inflammation, H may be less than indicated because of rise of pressure in the extravascular space, and O will also be reduced by escape of plasma proteins into the inflammatory exudate.

uring the hydrostatic pressure in individual small vessels, and of calculating the rate of diffusion of fluid into and out of the vessels. Landis showed that when inflammation was induced in the frog mesentery there was a rise in the hydrostatic pressure within the microcirculation which upset the balance between hydrostatic and osmotic forces, with a resultant net loss of fluid from the vessels. The escape of plasma proteins from inflamed vessels will tend to reduce the osmotic pressure difference between plasma and extravascular fluid and this may be sufficient to accentuate the loss of fluid (Fig. 3.6). These findings have now been confirmed in normal and inflamed mammalian tissues and, while Starling's views have required to be modified in detail to take account of the fluid exchange function of the post-capillary venules, his major suggestion —that *the walls of small vessels behave like a passive filter through which the exchange of fluid is determined by opposing haemodynamic and osmotic forces*—has been widely accepted.

(b) Morphological evidence

Acceptance of Starling's microfiltration theory and subsequent studies have suggested the existence, in the walls of microvessels, of a physiological system of small 'pores' of sufficient size to allow the escape of water and electrolytes, but impermeable to proteins and other macromolecules (Pappenheimer *et al.,* 1951).

There is strong evidence that the basement membrane of small vessels does not form a barrier to water or small molecular solutes and the effective filter thus appears to be in the endothelial layer. Electron microscopy of vascular endothelium suggests two possible routes of fluid transport across the endothelium. Firstly, endothelial cells contain small cytoplasmic vesicles (*micropinocytotic vesicles*), some of which open onto the inner or outer surface of the cell (Fig. 3.7). Simionescu *et al.* (1975) have shown that these vesicles may link up to form channels across the cytoplasmic barrier, through which peptides of below 2000 daltons are capable of passing. Constrictions in these channels may represent the small pores of the endothelial microfilter.

Secondly, fluid may escape *between endothelial cells.* Electron microscopy shows endothelial cell 'junctions' to be potential spaces containing amorphous material (Fig. 3.8). These spaces show constrictions which may act as the endothelial small pores.

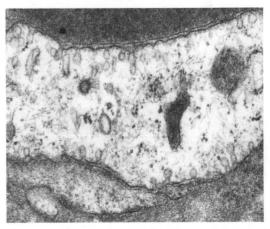

Fig. 3.7 Electron micrograph of part of a normal capillary endothelial cell in which micropinocytotic vesicles are seen in relation to both the inner and outer surfaces and also lying free in the cytoplasm. The capillary lumen is at the top of the field. × 50 000.

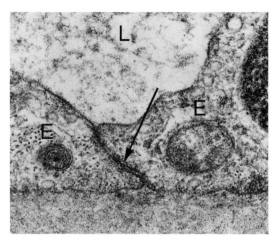

Fig. 3.8. Electron micrograph showing the narrow space (arrow), filled with amorphous material, between adjacent vascular endothelial cells (E). L is the lumen of the vessel. × 68 000.

There appears no doubt that fluid and micromolecular solutes can cross the endothelium by both the above routes but their relative importance is still uncertain.

Leakage of proteins from microvessels

While relatively permeable to water and small solutes, the walls of normal capillaries and venules exert a sieving effect on larger molecules, providing an increasingly effective barrier to macromolecules proportionate to their size. In connective tissues and voluntary muscle there is relatively little loss of albumin and even less of the larger plasma proteins.* Nevertheless some protein does escape from the microvessels of all tissues, and physiologists have postulated the existence of a second microfilter system of smaller numbers of larger 'pores' to account for this (Pappenheimer *et al.*, 1951). In an exercised limb, increased pressure and flow of blood through the small vessels of the muscles results in greatly increased flow of the lymph, and yet the total protein content of the lymph, which represents most of the protein escaping from the microvessels, is not in-creased. Active hyperaemia does not, therefore, account for the increased protein leakage from the microvessels in acute inflammation, which can be explained only by assuming an increase in the number of Pappenheimer's postulated large 'pores'.

The observation of leakage from individual vessels and the detection of Pappenheimer's large pores through which proteins leak out was accomplished by inducing acute inflammation and injecting intravascularly a suspension of carbon particles. The particles escape through the large pores and so label the leaking vessels, while the sites of leakage can be detected by electron microscopy. Using this technique, it was shown by Majno *et al.* (1961) that, when increased permeability was induced by histamine or other potential endogenous mediators (see below), the carbon particles escaped through large gaps which developed between adjacent endothelial cells (Fig. 3.9.). This has now been fully confirmed in acute inflammation induced in various tissues by various injurious agents. The gaps appear to be temporary, for injected colloidal material has also been observed deep to normal (i.e. 'tight') endothelial cell junctions in acutely inflamed tissue. Very occasionally, this has been observed in normal (non-inflamed) tissues, suggesting that transient gaps account also for the normal leakage of small amounts of protein.

Although plasma proteins of various molecular sizes appear in the acute inflammatory exudate, a sieving effect persists, the smaller proteins escaping more readily than the larger ones. Since the observed inter-endothelial cell gaps are much larger than the largest protein molecule, it is apparent that vascular basement membrane also acts as a relatively coarse filter to proteins which have leaked through the endothelium.

It is possible that some protein is normally transferred across the vascular endothelium in the micropinocytotic vesicles (see Fig. 3.7), but these have not been shown to increase in inflammation and are unlikely to be an important factor.

---

*In small vessels in many other tissues, e.g. glomeruli, glandular tissues, gut mucosa, the endothelial cells show zones of extreme thinning (fenestrae) while the vascular sinusoids of liver, bone marrow, etc., have relatively large endothelial defects. These features probably account for the relatively greater permeability of vessels in these tissues. Studies on acute inflammation have usually been made on the skin and voluntary muscle and are valid only for the 'continuous' (non-fenestrated) vessels of these tissues.

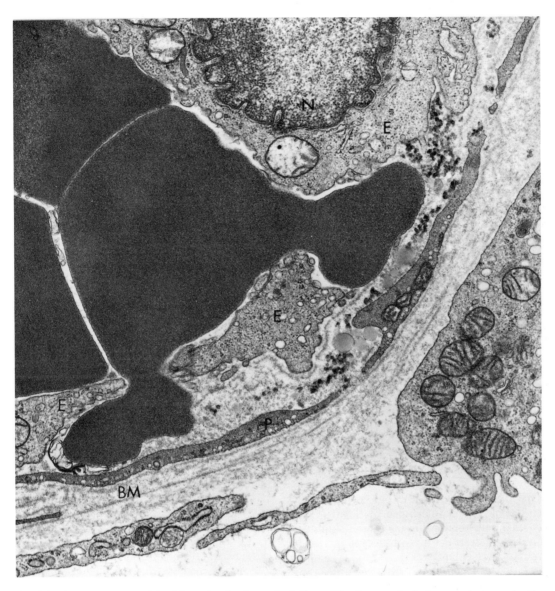

Fig. 3.9 Two gaps caused by histamine in the endothelium (E) of a venule (rat cremaster muscle, three minutes after a local injection of histamine). Red blood cells are very plastic and can easily 'flow' into endothelial gaps; this one is going to have a problem, because it is slipping out of two different gaps! Note the tight folds in the endothelial nucleus (N) (suggestive of cellular contraction). Because the basement membrane (BM) acts as a filter (beyond the endothelial gaps), many blood-borne particles accumulate in the venular wall: the dark granules are carbon black (India ink which had been injected intravenously); the larger, smooth, round bodies are chylomicrons. (P: pericyte.) × 29 700. (Dr. Isabelle Joris.)

In summary, *exchange of fluid and small solutes across the endothelium of capillaries and venules occurs by passive filtration either through the intercellular material or along channels formed by microvesicles which can bridge the endothelial cytoplasm. The increased leakage of fluid and electrolytes in acute inflammation is explained by the increased hydrostatic pressure of the blood in the small vessels in active hyperaemia: it depends on increased filtration pressure and not on increased permeability. Exudation of plasma proteins from the small vessels in acutely inflamed tissue requires an increase in permeability of the endothelium and this is provided by the reversible opening up of relatively large gaps between endothelial cells: such gaps probably explain also the physiological leakage of small amounts of proteins from normal vessels.*

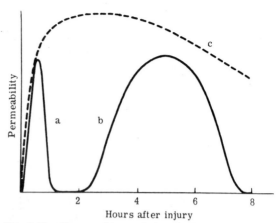

Fig. 3.10 Phases of increased vascular permeability following injury to the skin by application of heat. Following mild injury, there is immediate but transient increase in permeability (a): with moderate injury, this is followed by delayed prolonged increase in permeability (b), while severe injury causes immediate persistent increase (c). (Modified after the late Professor D. L. Wilhelm: *see* Zweifach, 1973–4.)

Phases of increased vascular permeability

In experimental studies of increased vascular permeability, acute inflammation has usually been induced by readily controlled injury, e.g. mild heat or injection of irritating chemicals. Increased permeability may be observed by use of colloidal carbon as mentioned above, but is more readily measured by administering an intravascular injection of either a dye such as Evans blue which binds to plasma proteins, or of plasma albumin labelled with a radioactive isotope. Blue discolouration of the tissue or accumulation of the isotope then indicates escape of protein from the blood vessels. By such techniques, it was shown by Sevitt (1958) that moderate thermal injury of the skin of a guinea-pig results in two phases of increased vascular permeability (Fig. 3.10). The first phase is *immediate and transient*, subsiding within about thirty minutes. The second phase is *delayed and prolonged,* starting after one to two hours, reaching a peak in about four hours and subsiding slowly. Milder thermal injury results only in the immediate transient phase, while severe injury induces *immediate persistent* increase in permeability continuing for twenty-four hours or more. These patterns, with some variations, have been demonstrated using thermal, chemical and bacterial toxic injury (Burke and Miles, 1958) to induce inflammation in various tissues and animal species.

Mechanisms of increased vascular permeability

The phases of increased vascular permeability described above have been further analysed by electron miscroscopy using colloidal carbon as a 'vascular marker' (p. 50) to indicate the sites of escape of proteins. During **the immediate transient phase**, *leakage occurs through the endothelium of venules only* (Fig. 3.11). Since all potential endogenous mediators so far investigated (e.g. by use of carbon marking) have been found to increase the permeability of venules, but not of capillaries, this finding suggests that the immediate transient phase is endogenously mediated. Moreover, when the zone of injury is sharply defined, as is the case when a hot metal tube is applied to the skin, *the increased venular permeability of this phase is seen to extend to the surrounding uninjured tissue,* (Fig. 3.12),which suggests diffusion of endogenous mediators. A third feature is that the endothelial cells of the leaking venules present changes like those described by Majno (see Ryan and Majno, 1977a) after injection of histamine: the cells appear plumper and their nuclei become more rounded and show crinkling of the nuclear membrane (Fig. 3.9). These features suggest that the endothelial cells contract, becoming shorter and fatter, and pull apart from one another, thus accounting for the observed gaps between cells. It is noteworthy that histamine and most of the other

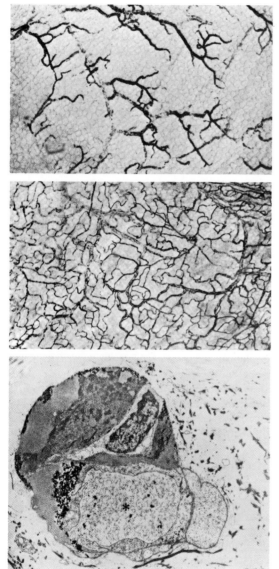

seemed heretical, but endothelial cells (and also polymorphs, monocytes and platelets) are now known to contain contractile proteins resembling actin and myosin and cytoplasmic microfibrils resembling those of smooth muscle cells. Accordingly, it seems likely that *endogenous mediators cause increased venular permeability by stimulating endothelial cells to contract.*

By contrast, in **the delayed persistent phase** of increased permeability induced by application of heat, *there is leakage of macromolecules from both venules and capillaries (Fig. 3.11) confined strictly to the zone of tissue injury (Fig. 3.12).* This observation was made by Hurley (1972) who concluded that this phase was not due to endogenous mediators but to *the delayed effect of direct injury on the endothelium,* a view supported by electron-microscopic evidence of endothelial injury (Fig. 3.11c). This conclusion is of considerable importance, for it follows that attempts to inhibit excessive prolonged leakage of plasma proteins, e.g. in extensive burns, should aim at diminishing the effects of endothelial injury rather than at the suppression of endogenous mediators. Hurley made the interesting observation that promethazine, which reduces the delayed injurious effect of carbon tetrachloride on the liver cells, also diminished the delayed prolonged phase of increased permeability following thermal injury. The **immediate prolonged increase in permeability** following more severe injury presents features

Fig. 3.11 Carbon labelling of vessels to demonstrate increased vascular permeability following thermal injury. *Upper*, the immediate transient phase, showing labelling of venules only. *Middle*, the delayed persistent phase, showing labelling of venules and capillaries. *Lower*, a dermal capillary showing endothelial injury: the lumen is marked by an asterisk. Note leakage of carbon. (By permission of Dr Guido Majno and the Upjohn Company.)

potential mediators of increased permeability are known to cause contraction of smooth muscle, e.g. in isolated intestine or uterus. A few years ago, the suggestion that endothelial cells can contract like smooth muscle cells would have

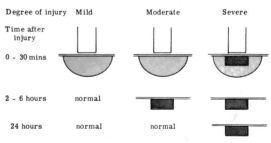

Fig. 3.12 The phases of increased vascular permeability following various degrees of heat injury to the skin by a hot tube. Two effects are observed. Firstly, an immediate transient increase in venular permeability (lightly shaded), due to release of histamine, etc.: this probably occurs with all degrees of injury short of necrosis and extends beyond the zone of injury. Secondly, more persistent injury (heavily shaded) results from direct heat injury to the endothelium of capillaries and venules: this is delayed in moderate injury and immediate in severe injury, and is confined to the zone of injury.

similar to those of the delayed prolonged phase, and is due to a greater degree of direct endothelial injury. Thrombosis may occur in the badly damaged vessels, but otherwise exudation continues until the damaged endothelial cells recover or are replaced. In injury severe enough to cause tissue necrosis, exudation does not, of course, occur in the dead tissue, but immediate persistent exudation occurs in the severely injured adjacent tissue.

Observations similar to those described above have been reported in experimental inflammation induced in various animal species by diverse injurious agents, e.g. x-irradiation, ultraviolet light, certain bacterial toxins and crushing injury. There are, however, exceptions: for example, the delayed persistent increase in permeability which occurs when carrageenan is applied to the cremaster muscle of the rat is confined to venules and appears to be endogenously mediated. Also, different tissues behave differently: for example, various types of injury to the skin of the rat result in increased permeability apparently due to direct injury, but the same agents applied to the rat diaphragm induce prolonged increase in permeability apparently due to endogenous mediators.

In summary: *exudation of protein-rich fluid in acute inflammation has been shown experimentally to occur in two phases—one immediate and transient, and the other delayed and prolonged. The immediate phase is due to release of histamine and other endogenous mediators which appear to cause contraction of venular endothelial cells, with consequent development of temporary gaps between them, through which protein-rich fluid escapes. Endogenous mediators may also play a role in the delayed phase, but in some instances there is strong evidence that the direct effect of the causal injury upon the capillary and venular endothelium is responsible for the intercellular gaps observed in both types of vessel in this phase.*

Endogenous mediators of increased vascular permeability

Although the work of Hurley and others has demonstrated that increased vascular permeability can and does result from the direct effects of injury on the vascular endothelium, it is apparent from the above account that endogenous mediators also contribute. A large and increasing number of endogenous compounds which can increase vascular permeability have indeed been demonstrated in effective concentrations in inflamed tissues and in inflammatory exudates. To prove that a particular compound is responsible for increased permeability it would be necessary also to demonstrate that specific suppression of its production or activity results in a reduction in increased permeability. This is difficult to achieve, for potential endogenous mediators are numerous and complex, and any procedure or antagonist which suppresses one is liable to interfere with others. Moreover, mediators differ in their effects on different animal species. For example, 5-hydroxytryptamine is much more effective in increasing venular permeability in rats and mice than in other mammalian species. However, the immediate transient phase is now widely regarded as being mediated largely by histamine for it is partly inhibited by low doses of relatively specific histamine antagonists, e.g. mepyramine maleate, and by prior histamine depletion, e.g. by Polymixin B. Apart from this, none of the potential mediators has yet been shown conclusively to be of practical importance in increasing vascular permeability. Accordingly, the following notes on their production and properties are intentionally brief.

Mediators derived from the plasma

These include various products of activation and interaction of four major 'cascade' systems—the **clotting**, **fibrinolytic**, **kinin** and **complement systems**. Each system has a number of components which include pro-enzymes, conversion of which to the active enzymes can trigger off the activation of subsequent components in the system, giving a chain or cascade reaction. Each system is complicated by the presence in the plasma of inhibitors and accelerators, and by positive and negative feedback mechanisms. Moreover some of the activation products of the individual systems can interact with the other systems. Fig. 3.13 is a gross over-simplification of these complexities. The clotting and fibrinolytic systems are described in more detail on pp. 234–5 in relation to thrombus formation and lysis, and the complement system on p. 142 in relation to its activation by antigen-antibody complexes.

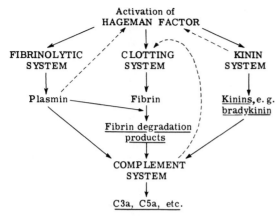

Fig. 3.13 A simplified version of the complex interactions between the fibrinolytic, clotting, kinin and
complement systems. The first three of these systems
are triggered off by activated Hageman factor and
products of their activation activate more Hageman
factor. The complement system can be activated by
products of the fibrinolytic and kinin systems. Products underlined cause active hyperaemia, increase
the permeability of venular endothelium, and some
are also chemotactic for leukocytes. Controlling and
inhibitory factors are not shown in the diagram.

As shown in Fig. 3.13, **Hageman factor** in the
plasma (traditionally factor XII of the clotting
system) plays a key role, for once activated it
can initiate activation of the clotting, fibrinolytic and kinin systems, each of which can, in
turn, activate more Hageman factor. *In vitro*,
Hageman factor is activated by contact with
negatively-charged surfaces, e.g. glass or
kaolin. *In vivo*, it is activated by contact with
various extracellular tissue elements, including
basement membrane, by bacterial endotoxin (p.
178) and by various proteolytic enzymes of the
kinin, clotting and fibrinolytic systems. It is
thus apparent that, once inflammation has developed, Hageman factor leaking through
endothelial gaps can become activated by contact with basement membrane and activation of
three of the major systems can ensue. Products
of the activity and interactions of these three
systems induce inter-endothelial cell gaps,
apparently by causing endothelial cell contraction: they include fibrinopeptides, fibrin
degradation products and kinins. In addition
(Fig. 3.13), activation products of the fibrinolytic and kinin systems can activate the complement system which also generates permeability-
increasing factors and which, in turn, can activate the clotting system. As mentioned earlier,

these permeability-increasing factors are also
capable of promoting active hyperaemia (p. 46).

In established inflammatory lesions, large
numbers of enzymes are released by tissue cells
and leukocytes. These include proteases, some
of which are capable of activating components
of the four major plasma systems shown in Fig.
3.13, and also of breaking down tissue and
plasma proteins into peptides, some of which
can themselves act as permeability-increasing
factors.

The kinin system was revealed largely by the work
of Miles and Wilhelm (1955). They detected a permeability-increasing factor (termed PF/dil) which
was generated spontaneously from diluted plasma in
a glass container. The system has been elucidated
mainly by the work of Cochrane and Wuepper and
their colleagues (Cochrane *et al.*, 1974). The main
components of the system are shown in Fig. 3.14.
Prekallikrein activator is a product of activated
Hageman factor. The other components of the
system are all present in the plasma, but enzymes
with kallikrein activity are present also in most
tissues and in urine and glandular secretions. Bradykinin is a nonapeptide derived from breakdown of
kininogen, a plasma glycoprotein, by the proteolytic
action of kallikrein. On injection, bradykinin causes
pain, active hyperaemia and increased venular permeability. Several closely related peptides have similar properties: they are rapidly destroyed by kini-
nases in the plasma and tissues, which also contain
kallikrein antagonists. The latter are commercially
available for therapeutic use.

The complement system is described more fully in
relation to hypersensitivity on p. 142-4. It consists
of a series of components termed C1, C2, etc., in the
plasma. Activation of the system generates agents
which increase venular permeability. These are
termed anaphylatoxins and include C3*a* and C5*a*
which are cleavage products of C3 and C5

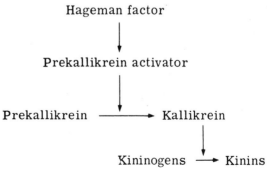

Fig. 3.14 The major components participating in
the cascade reaction of the kinin system.

respectively. They act mainly by liberating histamine from mast cells, but C5a is also strongly chemotactic for leukocytes (p. 60). Plasma contains a potent in-activator of these products (which may also inactiv-ate kinins).

In the complex environment of the inflammatory reaction there are a number of ways in which C3a and C5a may be generated: the main ones are as follows.

(a) In *bacterial infections*, the host's plasma may contain antibodies to antigenic components of the invading bacteria (perhaps developed during a previous infection): the union of such antibodies with the corresponding antigens can activate the complement system.

The endotoxins of Gram-negative bacteria can activate the complement system at the C3 stage. Also, some bacteria secrete proteases which are capable of cleaving C3 and C5.

(b) *Tissue injury* itself can also activate comple-ment, for the reaction of auto-antibodies (often present at low levels in the plasma) with the various corresponding tissue antigenic components released by tissue injury provides antigen-antibody complexes capable of acti-vating complement.

When injured, heart muscle, and probably other tissues, also release enzymes capable of cleaving C3 and C5.

(c) *Neutrophil polymorphs and macrophages* which have migrated into the tissues and are phago-cytosing tissue fragments or bacteria, etc., secrete lysosomal enzymes, some of which are capable of cleaving C3 and C5.

(d) As indicated above, some products of activa-tion of the other plasma cascade systems (clot-ting, fibrinolytic and kinin systems) are cap-able of activating the complement system.

Although the above observations do not establish that complement plays a part in non-immunological inflammatory reactions, this possibility is suggested also by the demonstration that animals depleted of plasma complement by various methods show im-paired inflammatory exudation following physical or chemical tissue injury. Since such animals react normally to injected histamine, kinins, etc., comple-ment appears to be of importance either as a source of mediators or by stimulating the production of mediators from other sources (Willoughby, Coote and Turk, 1969; Lewis and Turk, 1975).

Mediators released by cells

These are also numerous, but only a few have been characterised chemically. They include the following.

Histamine is stored in inactive form in the gran-ules of *mast cells*, which are present adjacent to blood vessels in most tissues, and also in basophil leuko-cytes and platelets. Active histamine is released from these cells by many substances and stimuli, including those which induce acute inflammation, e.g. heat, irradiation, irritating chemicals, toxins, venoms, by anaphylatoxins (p. 55), and by a lysosomal protein secreted by polymorphs in inflammatory exudates. Release of histamine from platelets is also stimulated by factors which cause platelet aggregation (p. 232). Its release in some types of immunological reaction is described in Chapter 6.

On local injection, histamine causes itching and pain, active hyperaemia and increased venular per-meability for approximately fifteen minutes, after which the vessels are said to become refractory for several hours to a further injection of histamine. Compounds which deplete the mast-cell store of his-tamine, and others which inhibit the venular re-sponse to histamine by competitive binding to endothelial-cell receptors, do not have important anti-inflammatory effects in low dosage, although they partly inhibit the immediate transient phase of increased vascular permeability.

5-hydroxytryptamine (serotonin) is present in most tissues. Rich sources include the cells of the chrom-affin system of the gastro-intestinal tract, the spleen and nervous tissue, mast cells and platelets. On injec-tion, 5-hydroxytryptamine, like histamine, causes a brief increase in venular permeability: it may par-ticipate in inflammatory reactions in rats and mice, which are particularly sensitive to it, but in other species, including man, it is unlikely to make an im-portant contribution to inflammation.

Prostaglandins are a group of long-chain hydroxy-fatty acids which are produced in most tissues by the action of an oxidase (PG-synthetase) on poly-unsaturated fatty acids such as arachidonic acid. They are rapidly catabolised and are not stored within the body. While they differ greatly in their properties, prostaglandins E1 and E2 have been isol-ated from inflammatory exudates in man and an-imals and shown to be capable of causing active hyperaemia, increased vascular permeability and possibly chemotaxis of polymorphs. They are also potent pyrogens when injected into the third ventricle and although small doses intradermally do not cause pain, they lower the pain threshold of nerve endings to histamine, 5-hydroxytryptamine and kinins. Control of their synthesis and release is obscure, but they have been detected in inflammatory exudates and are sec-reted by phagocytically active polymorphs. Firm evid-ence that prostaglandins play an important part in inflammation is scanty, but it is of interest that aspirin and related drugs, which have anti-inflammatory, anti-pyretic and analgesic properties, have been shown to be capable, in low concentrations, of inhibiting the production of prostaglandins, both *in vivo* and *in vitro*, by antagonising prostaglandin synthetase activity.

Neutrophil polymorphs and monocytes. As stated earlier, these cells migrate from the venules into the tissues in acute inflammation, and become more actively motile and phagocytic. During this activity, and also when these migrated cells are injured by bacterial toxins, etc., they release various lysosomal enzymes and other proteins, many of which participate in the activation of the plasma cascade systems (p. 55) or break down various plasma proteins into fragments which increase venular permeability. In addition, polymorphs secrete a factor which stimulates the release of histamine, etc. from mast cells and other factors which act directly on venules, increasing their permeability.

Conclusions. *The early (immediate transient) phase of increased venular permeability observed in mild inflammation is due partly to histamine release. There are many potential mediators of the later phase of increased venular permeability, but none has been implicated with certainty. It seems reasonable to conclude that the important process of exudation has been safeguarded by the development, during evolutionary selection, of multiple mediators of increased venular permeability, no single one of which is indispensible.*

Preoccupation with endogenous mediators should not be allowed to obscure the evidence provided by Hurley and others that, in some experimentally-induced inflammatory reactions, prolonged increase in permeability affects capillaries and venules and is due to direct endothelial injury (p. 53).

Emigration of leukocytes

The escape of cells from the blood vessels is a prominent feature of inflammation. Escape of erythrocytes is purely passive: they are forced out of capillaries and venules, through gaps between endothelial cells, by the hydrostatic pressure of the blood. Their escape in very large numbers is an indication of severe endothelial injury. By contrast, escape of **neutrophil polymorphs** and **monocytes** is an active process of great importance, and of particular significance in the defence against bacteria. It is independent of the endothelial gaps responsible for increased vascular permeability and involves two stages: firstly, the leukocyte becomes arrested on the surface of the vascular endothelium, and secondly it passes through the vessel wall.

In acute inflammatory lesions, neutrophil polymorphs migrate earlier and in much greater numbers than monocytes.

Margination of polymorphs

Arrest of neutrophil polymorphs on the vascular endothelium is often conspicuous in acute inflammation and is known as **pavementing** or **margination** of leukocytes. It is seen solely in venules and occurs with the slowing of the blood flow in the dilated vessels. In the earlier stage of rapid flow, blood in the arterioles and venules shows **axial streaming**, the cells being mainly in the central or axial columns of blood, separated from the vessel wall by a clear layer of plasma containing only occasional cells. This streaming is dependent on the rapid flow of blood and later, as the rate of flow decreases, axial streaming disappears. In particular, the leukocytes in the venules pass into the peripheral stream, where they can make contact with the endothelium. Neutrophil leukocytes making such contact tend to become arrested momentarily and then become detached and move on, or roll slowly along the endothelial surface. Eventually more and more of them become arrested for longer periods on the endothelium and they may form an almost continuous layer or may even become heaped up on one another (Fig. 3.15). The nature of adhesion between the leukocytic and endothelial cell surfaces is unknown: changes in the cell surfaces have not been detected by electron microscopy.

In recent studies, vascular endothelial injury in small vessels has been caused by a fine laser beam (5–15 μm diameter) during perfusion with saline coloured with a dye, and adhesion of leukocytes to the injured endothelium has been observed following restoration of blood flow. Since blood cells and plasma were excluded from the vessel during injury, pavementing can clearly result from endothelial injury alone, and does not require injury to the leukocytes.

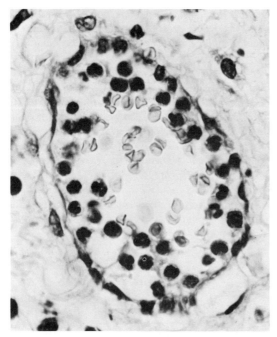

Fig. 3.15 Section of venule in acute inflammation, showing pavementing of polymorphonuclear leukocytes. × 1000.

Emigration of polymorphs

The 'pavemented' polymorph pushes out cytoplasmic pseudopodia and when one of these encounters the junction between two endothelial cells, it extends between them, disrupting the junction (Fig. 3.16), and the rest of the cell squeezes through: the intercellular junction reforms rapidly without significant leakage of plasma. The emigrating polymorph also passes through the basement membrane, which is repaired almost immediately. The mechanisms of disruption and repair of the endothelial cell junction and basement membrane are not known. Polymorphs take only a few minutes to pass these barriers; they then wander through the tissues and play a role in digestion and phagocytosis of fibrin, degenerate tissue and cell fragments and, most important in infections, in the destruction and removal of micro-organisms. The phagocytic function of leukocytes is considered on pp. 63 and 180.

Intensity of polymorph emigration in acute inflammation depends upon the nature and severity of the tissue injury. It is usually only moderate in physical injury unless infection supervenes. Inflammatory chemicals, including bacterial products, vary greatly in the degree of leukocytic emigration they induce. In the mild inflammatory reaction which occurs around tissue dying from acute ischaemia, i.e. an infarct (p. 246), the degree of polymorph emigration also varies greatly. In myocardial infarction, for example, there may be virtually no polymorph infiltration of the dead muscle, or large numbers may be present, particularly near the margin.

The outstanding examples of intense emigration of polymorphs are provided by bacterial infections: bacteria which, like *Strep. pyogenes*, *Staph. aureus* and *Strep. pneumoniae* are particularly active in this respect, are accordingly termed **pyogenic** (pus inducing) bacteria. Other bacteria, such as, *Salmonella typhi* (the cause of typhoid fever) and *Clostridium welchii* (a cause of gas gangrene), induce far less polymorph emigration, even though they cause severe inflammation. These special features are considered in more detail below and in Chapter 8, but it is worth noting here that differences between inflammatory reactions are not simply in degrees of severity: the nature of the injurious agent determines to some extent the relative degrees of the various features (exudation, emigration of leukocytes, etc.) of the reaction.

Chemotaxis

The migration of polymorphs through the walls of venules and their subsequent movement in the tissues has been widely assumed to be mediated by chemotaxis, a process in which cells move towards higher concentrations of certain substances termed **chemotactic agents** or **chemotaxins**. Such directed movement is not readily demonstrated *in vivo*, largely because it is difficult to establish and maintain gradients of concentration of test substances in living tissues. Nevertheless, time-lapse cinephotomicrography of inflamed tissues within rabbit ear chambers* has revealed that the movements

---

*The rabbit ear chamber consists of two thin, flat transparent plastic discs with a narrow space between and open around the edge. For use, it is sutured in a round hole punched in the pinna, and a layer of vascular connective tissue grows in to occupy the space. Inflammation can be induced in the connective tissue by various means and the changes examined microscopically *in vivo* (Fig. 4.5, p. 80).

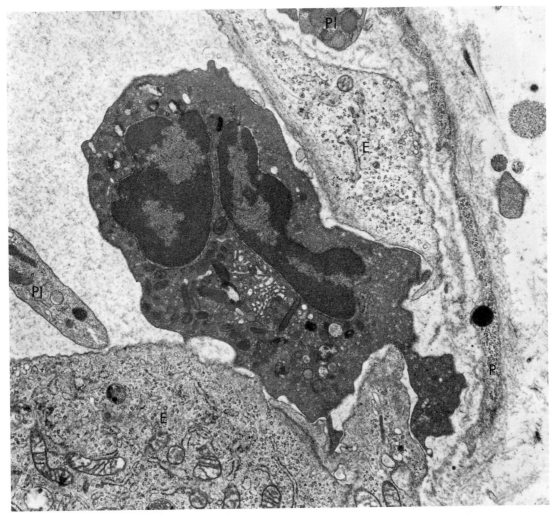

Fig. 3.16 A neutrophil polymorph caught in the act of emigrating out of a venule (rat omentum; experimental inflammation caused by sterile necrotic kidney tissue). Note the many fibrils in the endothelial cell at top; above it, part of a platelet (P1)—which must have slipped out earlier (not necessarily through the gap now being used by the neutrophil). (E: Endothelium; P: Pericyte; Pl: Platelet.) × 24 470. (Dr. Guido Majno.)

of polymorphs in pursuit of bacteria appear as purposeful as a dog following a scent.

Two methods have been used extensively to detect chemotactic agents. In the method of Boyden (1962) a suspension of leukocytes is separated by a millipore membrane from the test solution. If the latter contains chemotactic agents, the leukocytes migrate through the pores of the membrane (Fig. 3.17) and measurement of their rate of advance can provide a reliable assay of chemotactic activity. Precau-

tions must be taken, however, to exclude the effects of **chemokinetic agents,** which enhance random motility of leukocytes without influencing their directional motility. In the other method (Harris 1953), the suspension of leukocytes is incubated in a slide-coverslip preparation in the presence of a source of the agent being tested for chemotaxis; the movement of individual leukocytes is observed microscopically, usually by time-lapse cinephotomicrography.

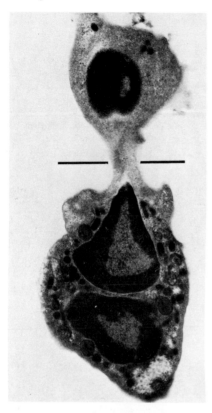

Fig. 3.17 Electron-micrograph of a neutrophil polymorph migrating through a millipore membrane in response to a chemotaxin. Most of the organelles have passed into the cytoplasm which, together with two lobes of the nucleus, has moved downwards through a pore, the site of which is indicated by the heavy line. × 14 300. (By courtesy of Dr. P. C. Wilkinson and Churchill-Livingstone.)

Chemotactic agents for neutrophil polymorphs

By use of the above methods, it has been shown that there are many substances which are chemotactic for neutrophil polymorphs *in vitro*. They include products of (*a*) the complement, clotting, fibrinolytic and kinin systems, (*b*) injured tissues, (*c*) micro-organisms, (*d*) polymorphs during phagocytic activity, and (*e*) partial digestion of proteins in the inflammatory exudate.

(a) The plasma cascade systems. Activation of the clotting, kinin and fibrinolytic systems, already discussed in relation to the mediation of increased vascular permeability (p. 54) results in chemotactic products. These include *fibrinopeptides, fibrin degradation products* and *kallikrein*.

Activation of the complement system also produces chemotaxins, the strongest of which is C5*a* (a cleavage product of C5): a complex of activated C5, 6 and 7 may also be chemotactic. Complement seems to be of particular importance in chemotaxis and accordingly its activation in inflammatory lesions, already considered on p. 55, is further commented on below.

(b) Tissue injury. Injured tissue cells release compounds which are directly chemotactic for polymorphs, including *prostaglandin E1* (which is also a potential mediator of increased vascular permeability), and enzymes which activate the complement system. The importance of complement as a source of chemotactic agents when tissue injury occurs is suggested by experiments in which necrosis of part of the myocardium was induced in rats by ligation of a coronary artery: emigration of polymorphs from the blood vessels at the margin of the infarct was found to be largely suppressed by prior depletion of the plasma C3 (Hill and Ward, 1971).

(c) Micro-organisms. Some bacteria secrete lipid or protein compounds which are directly chemotactic for polymorphs, for example, *Staph. aureus* and *Esch. coli.*

As described on p. 56, the reaction of microbial antigens with host antibodies can result in activation of complement, while bacterial endotoxins can directly activate complement at the C3 stage. Some bacteria also secrete proteolytic enzymes capable of cleaving C3 or C5.

Although viruses are not known to produce chemotactic agents, cells containing replicating virus have been shown to do so.

(d) Neutrophil polymorphs which have migrated into inflamed tissue secrete an agent which is chemotactic for other neutrophil polymorphs. Once they have become actively phagocytic, polymorphs secrete lysosomal enzymes, some of which are capable of cleaving C3 or C5. During phagocytic activity, polymorphs also secrete a substance which immobilises other polymorphs in the vicinity. These cells thus appear to have the means to ensure their continued replacement in an inflammatory lesion so long as tissue debris, bacteria, etc. are available for phagocytosis.

(e) Partly denatured proteins. The inflammatory exudate contains various proteolytic enzymes derived from injured tissue cells, from migrated polymorphs and from activation of the plasma cascade systems. Proteins in the exudate or released by cell injury are thus exposed to mild proteolysis, the effect of which in some instances (e.g. plasma albumin, immunoglobulin G and haemoglobin) is to render them chemotactic.

The above account, by no means comprehensive, may serve to indicate the complexity of chemotactic agents. These have been detected by *in-vitro* experiments, and the role of chemotaxis *in vivo* is not established. It is, however, very likely that it is important in the accumulation of leukocytes in inflammatory lesions, for *a correlation has been shown between the chemotactic properties of various compounds and their in-vivo capacity to induce migration of polymorphs.*

Conclusions. *In their number and complexity, chemotactic agents in acute inflammatory lesions resemble potential mediators of increased vascular permeability. Some agents have both properties, e.g. prostaglandin E1, complement products and fibrinopeptides. However, increased vascular permeability and emigration of polymorphs occur independently, often from different vessels and at different times during the inflammatory response. This is not surprising in view of the important role of direct endothelial injury in increased permeability.* (p. 53.)

The mechanism of chemotaxis

Chemotactic agents for polymorphs are many and diverse, and so it is unlikely that recognition of each depends on the existence of specific receptor sites on the cell surface. Wilkinson (1974) has suggested that hydrophobic chemical groups are important in conferring chemotactic properties, and this would explain why mild denaturation or proteolytic digestion of some proteins renders them chemotactic, for such treatment exposes hydrophobic groups. This proposal is supported also by the demonstration that coupling of non-polar (hydrophobic) groups to proteins renders them chemotactic, while polar groups are without this effect.

Polymorphs which have responded to a chemotactic agent become refractory to this and other chemotactic agents, although they can still phagocytose and kill bacteria. In explanation, it has been proposed that chemotactic agents operate by activating the enzyme serine esterase, which is present in inactive form on the cell surface. Once activated, the enzyme decays rapidly and is apparently not regenerated by the polymorph. In support of this possibility, agents which inhibit serine esterase suppress chemotactic responses. In preliminary experiments, Wilkinson *et al.* (1977) have made use of chemotactic agents labelled with a fluorescent dye. They have shown that such agents bind diffusely to the surface of responding cells, but after an hour or so the agent aggregates at one part of the cell surface and is then ingested by the cell. These changes are accompanied by loss of chemotactic responsiveness and immobilisation of the cell: they are consistent with removal from the cell surface of serine esterase or some other agent necessary for chemotaxis.

Movement of leukocytes is probably effected by the contraction of myofibrils formed by polymerisation of actin and myosin and attached to the inner side of the plasma membrane. Wilkinson (1974) has proposed that direction of movement is controlled by the cell's microtubule system and this is supported by the demonstration that colchicine, which inhibits the polymerisation of tubulin to form microtubules, renders the cell incapable of chemotactic responses without interfering with their random motility.

In most acute inflammatory lesions, **eosinophil polymorphs** emigrate from the vessels in relatively small numbers. They are reported to respond chemotactically to some bacterial products and to cleavage products of C5. Their behaviour in inflammation caused by allergy is described on p. 148.

Very few **basophil leukocytes** are observed in most acute inflammatory reactions.

Emigration of monocytes

Neutrophil polymorphs emigrate earlier and more rapidly than monocytes, so that in short-lived acute inflammation the peak of polymorph emigration has passed before monocytes emigrate in significant numbers. In more prolonged inflammation due to pyogenic bacterial infection, emigration of polymorphs continues until most of the bacteria have been destroyed, and only then do monocytes emigrate in large numbers. It is thus apparent that different factors control emigration of polymorphs and monocytes. Chemotactic responses of monocytes have not yet been investigated extensively, but it is apparent that both monocytes and macrophages are attracted by some of the agents which are chemotactic for polymorphs, for example some bacterial products, cleavage products of C5 and kallikrein.

In inflammation due to infection with some bacteria, e.g. *Myco. tuberculosis* and *S. typhi*, emigration of polymorphs is transient or absent, and most of the emigrating cells are monocytes and lymphocytes. The role of cell-mediated immunity in such responses is discussed in Chapter 7, but monocyte emigration also predominates in the experimentally-induced reaction to relatively inert foreign material, such as carrageenan and synthetic polymers, which are unlikely to invoke an immunological reaction. It is thus apparent that there are chemotactic agents which predominantly attract monocytes. One such is a lysosomal protein secreted by polymorphs during phagocytic activity, while a product of *Corynebacterium parvum* appears to be specifically chemotactic for monocytes: an intradermal injection of this bacterium induces emigration mainly of monocytes.

Lymphocytes and chemotaxis. There is recent evidence that lymphoid cells can respond chemotactically to some agents, while they are capable also of influencing migration and motility of polymorphs, monocytes and other lymphocytes (Chapter 6).

The lymphatics in acute inflammation

The smallest lymphatics are blind-ending tubes with a very thin endothelium and a fine, incomplete, i.e. discontinuous, basement membrane. Normally they are partly collapsed, but fine fibrils attach the outer surface of the endothelium to the collagen in the surrounding tissue, and swelling of the tissue by inflammatory exudate tenses these fibrils and *distends* the lymphatics. The endothelial cells overlap one another and their junctions are very easily separated: they appear to act as valves, allowing fluid to pass in but not out.

These features allow greatly increased lymph drainage from inflamed tissue. Exuded proteins are removed by the lymphatics, and red cells and leukocytes also pass into the lymphatics of inflamed tissue.

The filter function of the lymph nodes in inflammation is described in Chapter 18.

Effects of acute inflammation

Acute inflammation is classed as a pathological process although there is no doubt that its effects are, in general, beneficial. It helps to eliminate invasive micro-organisms, to limit the injurious effects of irritating chemicals and bacterial toxins, and participates in the removal of necrotic cells and tissue debris.

Like most beneficial biological processes, acute inflammation is not without its disadvantages: in some instances it appears to confer no obvious benefit, and in others it seems positively harmful.

Beneficial effects

These are conferred partly by the flow of exudate through the inflamed tissues and partly by the phagocytic and microbicidal effects of emigrated leukocytes.

The inflammatory exudate

The fluid exudate is protective in the following ways.

1. Dilution of toxins. When inflammation is caused by toxic chemicals, including bacterial toxins, the exudate diminishes local tissue injury by diluting the toxins and carrying them away by the lymphatics.

2. Protective antibodies. The proteins in the exudate include antibodies which have developed as a result of infection or immunisation and which are present in the individual's plasma. In acute inflammation due to infection, the exudate may thus contain antibodies which react with, and promote destruction of, the micro-organisms, or which neutralise their toxins. Antibodies promote killing of micro-organisms by rendering them susceptible to lysis by complement and destruction by phagocytes. This is described more fully in Chapter 7.

3. Fibrin formation. Fibrinogen in the exudate is converted to solid fibrin by the action of tissue thromboplastin. A network of deposited fibrin is commonly seen in inflamed tissues, and may form a mechanical barrier to the movement and spread of bacteria. It may also aid in their phagocytosis by leukocytes.

4. Promotion of immunity. Micro-organisms and toxins in the inflammatory lesions are carried by the exudate, either free or in phagocytes, to the local lymph nodes where they may stimulate an immune response. This provides antibodies and cellular mechanisms of defence which appear within a few days and may be maintained for years.

5. Cell nutrition. The flow of inflammatory

exudate brings with it glucose, oxygen, etc., and thus helps to supply the greatly increased numbers of cells: it also carries away their metabolic products.

Phagocytosis

The neutrophil polymorphs in inflammatory lesions are actively phagocytic. The emigrated monocytes are not at first so active, but they rapidly change into the larger, more active macrophages. The process of phagocytosis is similar for both polymorphs and macrophages, and resembles closely the engulfment of food particles by amoebae. First, the surface of the phagocyte attaches to the particle, e.g. bacterium, to be ingested. The cytoplasm then flows around the particle and envelops it in a **phagocytic vacuole.** Finally the plasma membrane enclosing the vacuole breaks away from the cell surface, and the membrane-lined vacuole lies free in the cytoplasm. The subsequent fate of the particle depends on its nature and on the host's response. Adjacent lysosomes fuse with the membrane of the phagocytic vacuole, and pour their contents into it, the vacuole now being termed a **phagolysosome** or **phagosome.** The particle is thus exposed to the lysosomal acid hydrolases, and these include such a wide range of enzymes that most biological material, including red cells, fibrin, collagen and ground substance, dead cells and cell components, are digested. By engulfing and digesting the debris of the inflammatory reaction, the phagocytes act as scavengers (Fig. 3.18). During phagocytic activity, polymorphs and macrophages also release lysosomal enzymes into the surrounding fluid where they contribute to the digestion and so removal of inflammatory debris: the digestion products include peptides, nucleotides, etc. which, by increasing vascular permeability and attracting leukocytes by chemotaxis, may enhance the inflammatory reaction.

Polymorphs and macrophages play a vital protective role in microbial infections. In most bacterial infections, the bacteria are eliminated rapidly by phagocytosis and other protective mechanisms. However, there are exceptions, and some micro-organisms live and even multiply in phagocytes. The factors concerned in these host/parasite relationships are considered in Chapter 7.

Neutrophil polymorphs are highly specialised cells; they are actively motile, rich in lysosomal enzymes, and respond to relatively early chemotactic stimuli in the inflammatory reaction. They have a rich store of glycogen, and enzyme systems which provide the energy required for motility and phagocytosis by glycolysis. The last property allows polymorphs to function in the low oxygen tension present in highly cellular inflammatory exudates.

Because of these properties, the polymorph is admirably suited to its role in early defence against acute bacterial infections: it arrives early on the scene and is aggressive in engulfing and killing bacteria. It is, however, an end-stage cell and is unable to re-synthesise the surface plasma membrane and granules (lysosomes) used up in these activities. In consequence it soon loses its granules, becomes ineffective and dies. The supply of polymorphs is, however, practically unlimited.

Monocytes are less actively motile and phagocytic than polymorphs. They provide a reserve of cells which, on emigration in an inflammatory lesion, change into macrophages: this involves increases in lysosomal enzymes, metabolic activity, motility, and phagocytic and microbicidal capacity. Like polymorphs, they have enzyme systems which supply the energy for this increased activity by anaerobic glycolysis, but they differ in having little stored glycogen and must therefore make use of glycogen released by polymorphs or glucose in the exudate as a source of energy. Macrophages can ingest and destroy inflammatory debris (dead cells, fibrin, tissue fragments, etc.—Fig. 3.18) and can envelop and sequester indigestible material, e.g. foreign bodies and certain micro-organisms, for long periods: they can synthesise plasma membrane, lysosomal enzymes and lysosomes and are capable of division and of long survival after phagocytic activity. These properties suit them particularly to sustained function in prolonged inflammatory reactions.

Harmful effects

Swelling of acutely inflamed tissues may have serious mechanical effects. For example, in acute laryngitis the lumen of the larynx may be so reduced as to interfere with breathing.

Acute inflammation of tissues which are

confined within a restricted space, and so cannot expand, results in a rise of tissue pressure which may impair function directly or may interfere with blood flow and so cause ischaemic injury. Examples include inflammation of the brain (encephalitis) and meningitis, both of which cause increased intracranial pressure sometimes leading to coma and death. Similarly acute bacterial infection of the bone marrow (osteomyelitis) raises the pressure in the medullary cavity and extensive ischaemic necrosis may occur. A third, painful example is acute inflammation of the testis, usually caused by mumps virus; the tough tunica albuginea prevents much expansion, and ischaemia results,

sometimes with permanent residual injury. Fortunately, both testes are seldom severely affected.

Some examples of inflammation are inappropriate and harmful. For example, most people encounter grass pollen in the air without ill effect, but others become sensitised to pollens and react by the acute conjunctivitis and rhinitis of hay fever. There is also a rare condition, angio-neurotic oedema, in which acute inflammatory lesions develop spontaneously in various tissues, including the gastro-intestinal tract. It is due to deficiency of a plasma factor which controls activation of complement, and the inflammatory lesions are apparently mediated by complement activation products.

Further stages of acute inflammation

The three common results of the acute inflammatory reaction are:

(*a*) Resolution, i.e. subsidence of the inflammatory changes and return of the tissue to normal.
(*b*) Progression to suppuration.
(*c*) Progression to a chronic phase with fibrosis.

Resolution

Termination of the injury which has caused acute inflammation is followed by reversal of the inflammatory changes, and provided that there has not been wholesale destruction, the tissue usually returns to normal. Cell and tissue debris are digested by enzymes in the exudate or by phagocytes (Fig. 3.18); pavementing and emigration of leukocytes cease; the vessel walls regain their normal permeability, and blood flow returns to normal. Most of the emigrated polymorphs probably die, while macrophages (emigrated monocytes) may pass to the draining lymph nodes. Inflammatory exudate drains away in the lymphatics, and normality is restored.

A striking example of resolution is presented by lobar pneumonia, an acute infection of the lung usually due to *Streptococcus pneumoniae*, in which typically the alveoli throughout a whole lobe become filled with a protein-rich exudate containing a fine network of fibrin and large numbers of neutrophil polymorphs (Fig.

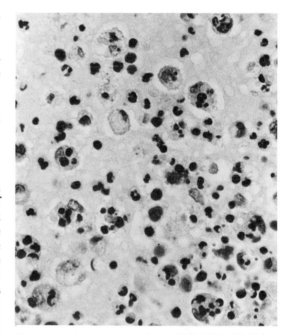

Fig. 3.18   A late stage of pyogenic bacterial infection, showing phagocytosis of polymorphs, red cells and debris by macrophages. × 510.

16.24, p. 468). Following destruction of the bacteria, usually after several days, polymorphs and macrophages complete the digestion of fibrin, dead cells and debris, the fluid exudate is removed partly by reabsorption and partly by coughing, and in most cases the lobe returns to normal.

Suppuration

Pyogenic bacteria (p. 58) cause acute inflammation in which emigration of polymorphs is intense, and in which local toxic injury is often severe enough to cause tissue necrosis at the centre of the lesion. The dead tissue is digested by the polymorph enzymes, leaving a space in the tissue filled with inflammatory exudate rich in polymorphs (Fig. 3.19) and containing also

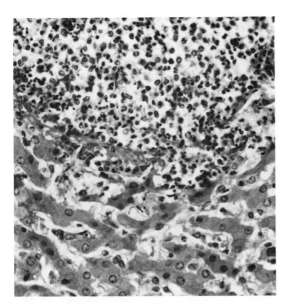

Fig. 3.19 Margin of an abscess cavity in the liver. In the upper part of the field the liver tissue has been destroyed and digested, leaving a space filled with purulent exudate. × 250.

bacteria, fragments of necrotic tissue, cell debris and fibrin. Such a cavity is termed an **abscess**, and the contained fluid, which may be creamy from its cell content and sticky from its high nucleic acid content (from dead polymorphs) is called **pus** or **purulent exudate**. Return to normal is no longer possible since tissue has been destroyed, and the abscess becomes enclosed in a wall of granulation tissue (the pyogenic membrane) which eventually matures to scar tissue. Pus can also form in a natural body cavity, such as the pleura or peritoneum, without tissue destruction, as a result of pyogenic bacterial infection.

A more detailed account of suppuration and its effects is given in Chapter 8.

Fibrosis in acute inflammation

Although acute inflammatory lesions frequently subside without leaving any significant residual changes, this is by no means always so. Formation of granulation tissue with consequent fibrosis or scarring is a common result. It complicates acute inflammation when there is necrosis of tissue or excessive deposition of fibrin and when acute inflammation persists and becomes chronic.

Tissue necrosis. Inflammation has been defined as the reaction to injury of *living* tissue, but many injuries, e.g. burns or bacterial infections, bring about necrosis of tissue. Obviously, inflammatory changes cannot occur in necrotic tissue, but inevitably the adjacent, surviving tissue is injured less severely and inflammation occurs in it. Accordingly, necrotic tissue is commonly present in the centre of acute inflammatory lesions. The occurrence of such wholesale necrosis of tissue, as distinct from necrosis of single cells, precludes the possibility of return to normal. If the dead tissue is superficial, as in a burn, it

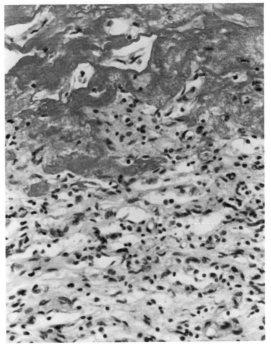

Fig. 3.20 A dense layer of fibrin on the pleural surface, showing organisation, i.e. replacement by vascular granulation tissue, extending from the underlying pleura. × 250.

usually becomes detached, leaving a gap in the surviving tissues. If deeper, it may be gradually replaced by granulation tissue (a process termed **organisation**), or it may be digested, as in suppurating infection, leaving an abscess cavity. In all three instances, granulation tissue grows from the adjacent living tissue, and matures to fibrous scar tissue.

It is worth noting that when tissue is excised, leaving a gap, or dies from ischaemia (lack of blood supply), its place is usually taken by fibrous tissue in the process of healing. The fibrosis which follows necrosis of tissue in acute inflammatory lesions is thus an example of healing.

Organisation of fibrin. The inflammatory exudate contains plasma proteins, including fibrinogen, and frequently this is converted to insoluble fibrin which is deposited in the inflamed tissue. Fine strands of fibrin (Fig. 3.5, p. 48) are readily digested by proteolytic enzymes in the exudate or removed by phagocytosis (p. 63). Larger deposits of fibrin, however, are not readily removed in this way, but, like dead tissue, are more gradually replaced by granulation tissue (Fig. 3.20) by the process of organisation, with consequent scarring. This is commonly seen in acute inflammation of a serous membrane, such as the pleura or pericardium (Fig. 3.21), when a thick layer of fibrin is deposited on the surface, and its subsequent organisation results in fibrous thickening.

Chronic inflammation. Progression of acute to chronic inflammation is described below.

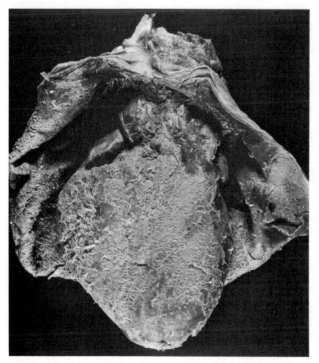
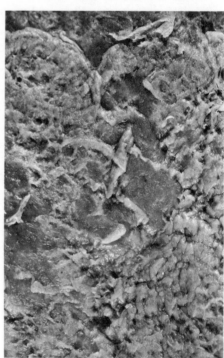

Fig. 3.21   Acute pericarditis, showing a thick, irregular deposit of fibrin on the pericardial surfaces. *Left,* × 0·7; *right,* × 3.

Chronic Inflammation

In contrast to tissue injury of short duration, which induces a brief or acute inflammatory reaction, prolonged tissue injury causes persistent, or chronic inflammation. There is, however, no generally accepted time limit beyond which an inflammatory lesion is regarded as chronic. To some extent, it depends on the nature of the disease process concerned: for example a whitlow lasting for several weeks might well be regarded as chronic, as compared with the usual short course, while tuberculous lesions showing extensive spread within weeks are regarded as acute in contrast to those which smoulder on for months or years.

An important feature of chronic inflammation is the production of vascular granulation tissue, which matures into fibrous tissue. Such **proliferative changes** are in contrast to the exudative changes of the acute inflammatory reaction, but when acute inflammation fails to resolve and becomes chronic, the two processes are commonly associated. Even in an early stage of acute inflammation, some proliferation of fibroblasts occurs and, in general, the more chronic the inflammatory reaction, the more pronounced are the proliferative changes, and the greater the degree of ultimate fibrous scarring.

Causes and types of chronic inflammation

Inflammation is a response to tissue injury and soon subsides when the causal injury ceases. Acute inflammation is elicited by relatively intense injury which is usually brief, but in some instances it may persist, although in less intense form, and there is progression from acute to chronic inflammation. There are also many agents, both microbial and inanimate, which cause tissue injury which is prolonged, but of low grade from the start.

Chronic inflammation may thus have an acute onset, or may develop more insidiously.

Chronic inflammation with an acute onset

The outstanding example of this is *bacterial infection*. Most acute bacterial infections are rapidly eliminated, and the tissue returns to normal or, if there has been tissue destruction or excessive fibrin deposition, replacement fibrosis and scarring ensue. But in some instances the infection is only partly subdued in the acute stage, the bacteria survive in relatively small numbers and so the inflammation progresses to a chronic stage. This is exemplified by bacillary dysentery (infection of the colon), in which

there is an acute exudative reaction in the mucosa of the colon. This may resolve or may progress to chronic inflammation in which the exudative changes are accompanied by patchy tissue destruction with ulceration of the mucosa, formation of granulation tissue and scarring. Another important example is provided by pyogenic infection of a bone which, unless treated early and effectively, is likely to cause extensive necrosis of the bone. Bacteria persist within the dead tissue, where they are protected from the host's defence mechanisms, and the infection may continue for years.

It is particularly in this form of chronic inflammation that the bacteria survive in foci and continue to promote an exudative reaction with emigration of polymorphs. From time to time the infection may flare up, with abscess formation. Such infected foci become enclosed in granulation tissue which may form large masses, and which, as it ages, becomes converted into dense fibrous tissue. The granulation tissue is infiltrated with polymorphs, as in the acute stage, but also with macrophages, and with lymphocytes and plasma cells which reflect the host's specific immune response to the infection.

Chronic inflammation of insidious onset

Agents which cause low-grade but persistent tissue injury, and thus promote this form of 'primary' chronic inflammation, fall into the following main classes.

(a) **Particulate material**. This is phagocytosed by macrophages. If it is bland, e.g. suture material (Fig. 3.25), or carbon dust deposited in the lungs from polluted air, there is little or no fibrous reaction and the change can scarcely be regarded as inflammatory. More irritating particles, such as silica, may also be inhaled or may enter the tissues in dirty wounds or in the form of talc formerly used to lubricate surgical gloves.* This also stimulates phagocytosis by macrophages, but the silica dissolves very slowly within the phagolysosomes, yielding silicic acid which injures the macrophages in such a way that they secrete lysosomal enzymes and eventually die. The supply of macrophages is, however, maintained by emigration of monocytes and, on

---

*Starch powder, currently in general use to lubricate surgical gloves, has also been reported to cause peritoneal inflammation in some cases following abdominal operation.

release from dead cells, the particles are ingested by fresh ones. These events are accompanied by formation of abundant dense fibrous tissue. The stimulus to fibrogenesis is not understood, but Allison has suggested that it is induced as a consequence of leakage of lysosomal enzymes (see Allison, 1978). He has demonstrated that various materials which induce such leakage when phagocytosed by macrophages in cell culture induce fibrosis *in vivo*.

The inflammatory response to fibrous silicates (asbestos) is similar to that of silica. Some other substances, e.g. particles of beryllium compounds, also promote chronic inflammatory lesions in which it seems likely that a state of hypersensitivity is involved (see below.)

(b) **Microbial infections.** Various bacteria and fungi cause chronic infections of insidious onset. Some of these organisms are remarkably non-toxic but can live and multiply within macrophages without destroying them. Unless the host develops a state of hypersensitivity to the organisms, the infected tissues become heavily infiltrated with macrophages containing huge numbers of the organisms. There is little or no fibrosis but such lesions are classed as chronic inflammation, partly because they are infections and partly because the host develops an antibody response which is reflected by the presence of lymphocytes and plasma cells, formerly regarded as 'chronic inflammatory cells', in and around the lesions. Examples include lepromatous leprosy (Fig. 8.20, p. 215) and leishmaniasis (p. 564).

Other bacteria, exemplified by the tubercle bacillus, are equally non-toxic but the features of the lesions are modified by the development of a state of **delayed hypersensitivity** by the host. This not only promotes killing of the bacteria by macrophages, but results also in tissue injury with necrosis, granulation tissue formation and scarring. The hypersensitivity reaction is a result of the host's immune response and is characterised by infiltration of the lesions with lymphocytes and increased numbers of macrophages which adopt a characteristic appearance and arrangement (Fig. 8.13, p. 209). Similar changes are seen in the tuberculoid form of leprosy and in the reaction to the eggs of schistosomal worms (Fig. 20.46, p. 698).

In many chronic infections, e.g. syphilis, there is tissue destruction, formation of granulation tissue and aggregation of macrophages, lymphocytes and plasma cells, but it is not yet known how much the destructive changes are due to toxic injury by the causal organism and how much they are the result of the host's hypersensitivity.

(c) **Hypersensitivity reactions.** The important part played by hypersensitivity reactions in some chronic infections is noted above. Hypersensitivity to normal tissue constituents also occurs and is responsible for chronic auto-immune thyroiditis, gastritis, etc. Such lesions produce important effects by destruction of the parenchyma of the affected organs.

A form of chronic inflammation of the skin, termed *contact dermatitis*, is also a manifestation of a hypersensitivity reaction: it occurs when various substances are absorbed into the skin, where they react with, and modify, host proteins: in consequence, the host develops immunity and a state of delayed hypersensitivity to the affected skin, and this results in an inflammatory rash which may be chronic if exposure to the chemical responsible for it is prolonged. A good example is the nickel used in thimbles and in the fasteners of women's underwear: slight solution of the nickel occurs on sweating and nickel compounds are absorbed and react with epidermal proteins.

(d) **Unknown agents.** In some chronic inflammatory diseases the causal agents remain unknown. Important examples are *sarcoidosis* (p. 216) which produces lesions somewhat similar to tuberculosis, and *ulcerative colitis* (p. 622) which may necessitate removal of the colon.

The appearances of chronic inflammatory lesions

From the examples given above, it will be apparent that chronic inflammation presents considerable histological variety. The features include foci of acute exudative inflammation, sometimes with active suppuration, infiltration with polymorphs, macrophages, lymphocytes and plasma cells, necrosis, and formation of granulation tissue and dense fibrous tissue. (Figs. 3.22—3.25, 3.28) Variations result from the relative prominence of each of these features, and on the site and distribution of the causal agent. Moreover, macrophages can present various appearances, not only dependent

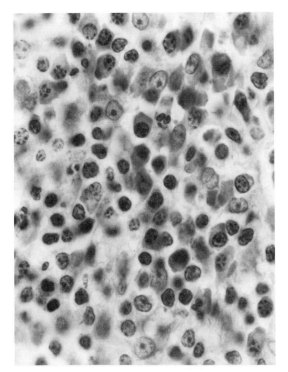

Fig 3.22 Chronic inflammation: showing the confusing variety of cells. In this instance, they include plasma cells, lymphocytes and occasional polymorphs, while the larger nuclei probably belong to macrophages and fibroblasts. × 820.

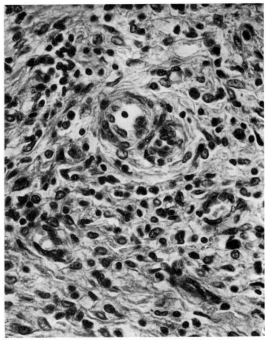

Fig. 3.24 Chronic inflammation. This field shows vascular fibrous tissue infiltrated mainly with lymphocytes. × 560.

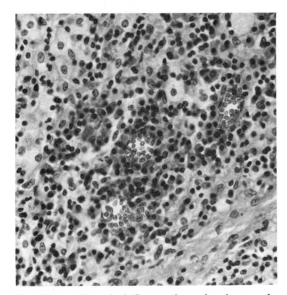

Fig. 3.23 Chronic inflammation: showing newly formed vascular fibrous tissue which is heavily infiltrated with macrophages (top left) lymphocytes and plasma cells. × 300.

on the numbers which accumulate, but also on their arrangement and adoption of striking morphological features (p. 73).

The macroscopic appearances are equally variable: abundant granulation or fibrous tissue can lead to tumour-like swellings or more diffuse enlargement; in other instances, loss of parenchyma and scarring are predominant, the tissue becoming firm and shrunken. If due to pyogenic infection, there may be sinus formation with leakage of pus from underlying abscesses, and even without suppuration, necrosis may occur and extend to the skin or a mucous membrane, with consequent ulceration.

In some examples, the gross and/or microscopic features are sufficiently characteristic to suggest a specific diagnosis, but there are dangerous pitfalls: for example, several agents can give rise to changes readily mistaken for tuberculosis. Accordingly, *a firm diagnosis usually depends on the recognition of a specific causal agent, or on other procedures such as serological tests for a particular infection.* Sometimes specific bacteria or fungi can be detected in the lesions by their morphology and staining properties, while anisotropic foreign material can be detected and sometimes identified by microscopic examination in polarised light (Fig. 3.25).

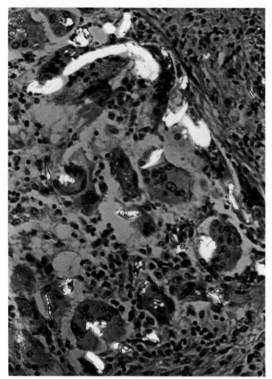

Fig. 3.25 Foreign-body giant cells in a chronic inflammatory reaction to suture material, viewed through partly crossed polarising films to show up the birefringent foreign material. × 250.

Granuloma and granulomatous inflammation

These terms are widely used, but with three different meanings,

Traditionally they are used to describe a chronic inflammatory lesion in the form of a mass and thus grossly resembling a tumour: hence the suffix-*oma* which is usually reserved for true tumours. Such inflammatory masses are usually due to infection (**infective granulomas**): they are usually composed largely of granulation and fibrous tissue, but may contain foci of suppuration, or may consist mainly of aggregated macrophages as in lepromatous leprosy.

Recently there has been an increasing tendency to limit the use of 'granuloma' to lesions composed largely of macrophages, or even to restrict it further to mean the collection of altered macrophages (epithelioid and giant cells) found in the tubercles of tuberculosis (Fig. 8.13, p. 209) and similar, non-tuberculous lesions. Since tubercles are often barely visible to the naked eye and do not contain granulation tissue, this is an important change of meaning which does, however, seem likely to be generally accepted. Meanwhile, it is advisable to indicate this usage by such terms as **macrophage granuloma**, **epithelioid cell** or **tuberculoid granuloma**.

Finally, a number of heterogeneous entities are called granulomas, e.g. *malignant granuloma of nose* or *midline granuloma*, (a lesion with histological features of chronic inflammation which resembles a tumour in its infiltration and destruction of tissue), *Wegener's granuloma* (due to a polyarteritis) and *eosinophil granuloma of bone* (a mass consisting mainly of eosinophil leukocytes). These terms are distinctive enough to avoid confusion.

Effects of chronic inflammation

When due to an infection, chronic inflammation is a protective process. Granulation tissue forms a barrier to bacteria and their toxins and provides numerous small vessels from which exudation and emigration of leukocytes can continue. In many instances, as explained above, chronic inflammation is due partly to a delayed hypersensitivity reaction to microorganisms. This is a defensive process which nevertheless causes tissue injury, and it is often difficult to know whether tissue injury is due to the invading bacteria or to the host's reaction to them. When chronic inflammation results from hypersensitivity to otherwise harmless chemicals, e.g. in contact dermatitis, it seems to subserve no useful function, and the same applies to the chronic inflammation of autoimmune thyroiditis, etc.

In some instances of chronic inflammation with features of hypersensitivity reactions, the causal agent is unknown, and although the inflammation causes tissue injury it may conceivably help to suppress a causal microorganism as yet unidentified. Sarcoidosis (p. 216), Crohn's disease (p. 620) and rheumatoid arthritis (p. 917) fall into this category.

The fibrous tissue which is formed in chronic inflammation may induce serious effects by constricting orifices and tubes—for example, the mitral valve in chronic rheumatic fever (p. 417) or the small intestine in Crohn's disease (p. 620). Chronic inflammation of internal organs is usually accompanied by loss of parenchymal cells, and this, together with irregular fibrosis, results in shrinkage, irregular scarring and distortion. Commonly the surface becomes uneven, with a fine or coarse granularity: this is particularly well seen in cirrhosis of the liver (Fig. 20.31, p. 685), where the irregularity is accentuated by proliferation and enlargement of surviving liver cells.

In some instances, the fibrous tissue produced in chronic inflammation may have a useful function: for example, walling off chronic infections, or strengthening the aorta weakened by loss of muscle and elastic tissue in various forms of arteritis.

Other causes of fibrosis

While fibrosis is an important feature of chronic inflammation, it may result from other causes. As stated above, fibrosis is the usual method of repair when tissue has been lost, and occurs in the removal of deposits of fibrin by organisation. Unless dissolved by fibrinolytic enzymes, thrombus in blood vessels is also replaced by fibrous tissue. These processes are dealt with in the next chapter.

When the blood supply to a part is gradually diminished by arterial disease, atrophy of the specialised cells may be accompanied by overgrowth of the supporting tissue. Similarly, death of tissue resulting from sudden occlusion of an artery, e.g. by thrombosis, is followed by replacement of the dead tissue by fibrous tissue. Patches of fibrosis of this nature are commonly seen in the myocardium. These effects of deficient blood supply (ischaemia) are described in Chapter 9.

Types of Cell in Inflammatory Lesions

Polymorphonuclear leukocytes

Neutrophil polymorphs. The origin and morphology of these cells are described on p. 184 *et seq*. Their migratory activity has already been considered and their roles in the defence against micro-organisms and in Arthus type hypersensitivity reactions are dealt with in later chapters.

Eosinophil polymorphs. The accumulation of these cells in inflammatory lesions is closely associated with hypersensitivity reactions, in which they may play a modulating role (p. 148). They are observed particularly in the lesions of bronchial asthma, in the tissues around metazoan parasites, in certain skin diseases, and in various lesions of the gastro-intestinal tract. Intense local accumulation of eosinophils is commonly associated with eosinophil leukocytosis in the blood and there is recent evidence to suggest that this is mediated by an immune response. The thymic-dependent lymphocytes which respond to antigenic stimulation, e.g. by a parasitic worm, in some way stimulate the proliferation of eosinophil precursors in the bone marrow.

Lymphoid cells

Lymphocytes accumulate in chronic inflammatory lesions and their presence in large numbers is suggestive of either a delayed hypersensitivity reaction or possibly of antibody-dependent lymphocyte cytotoxicity. These phenomena are described in Chapters 5 and 6.

The presence of **plasma cells** in inflamed tissues, as elsewhere, is indicative of antibody production: they do not usually appear until about a week after onset of inflammation and are present in greatest numbers in persistent lesions caused by bacteria. Their origin and function are described in Chapter 5.

Macrophages: the mononuclear phagocyte system

The terms **macrophage** and **mononuclear phagocyte** were applied by Metchnikoff, in 1905, to large phagocytic cells, which he distinguished from the smaller phagocytic neutrophil polymorph. In 1924, Aschoff described investigations on tissue cells based on vital staining, i.e. the ingestion of droplets of fluid (pinocytosis) containing non-toxic dyes bound to protein, and concentration of the dye in the cell cytoplasm. While many cells did this, Aschoff noted particularly intense staining of cells in the lining of vascular and lymphoid sinusoids, reticular cells of the spleen and lymph nodes, and scattered cells lying in connective tissues. He grouped these cells together under the term *reticulo-endothelial system*. From this grouping, the macrophages have emerged as cells which, although widely dispersed through the body, share a common origin and have certain well-defined functions. Accordingly the term 'mononuclear phagocyte system' is being used increasingly for macrophages and their precursor cells. The term 'reticulo-endothelial system' is no longer appropriate: reticular cells and endothelial cells lining blood vessels are quite distinct in their origin and functions.

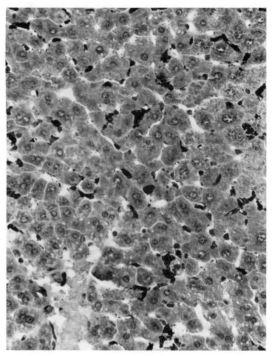

Fig. 3.26 Section of mouse liver following an intravascular injection of colloidal carbon. The hepatic macrophages (Kupffer cells) are black because of the large amount of carbon which they have phagocytosed. × 300.

Cells of the system

Macrophages may be recognised by the avidity with which they engulf particulate material of various kinds (Fig. 3.26) the firmness with which they adhere to a glass surface, both *in vivo* and *in vitro*, and their morphological differences from the other 'professional' phagocyte, the neutrophil polymorph.

Cells of the mononuclear phagocyte system are scattered widely throughout the body. In some sites they are normally inactive and inconspicuous but are capable, on stimulation, of enlargement, increased metabolism, and the active phagocytic role of the macrophage. Cells of the system include the following (van Furth *et al.*, 1975):

(1) The Kupffer cells, which form part of the lining of the hepatic sinusoids; similar cells in the vascular sinusoids of the bone marrow, spleen, adrenal cortex and adenohypophysis, and in the lymphatic sinuses of lymph nodes.

(2) Cells in the spaces of the network formed by the reticular cells in the medulla of lymph nodes and red pulp of the spleen.

(3) Cells on the surface of the serous cavities. These are particularly numerous in the omentum, where they are aggregated to form the 'milk spots'.

(4) Alveolar macrophages lying free on the surface of, and also within, the alveolar walls.

(5) Histiocytes in connective tissues, osteoclasts in bone, and microglial cells of central nervous tissue.

(6) The monocytes of the blood and their precursors (monoblasts and promonocytes) in the bone marrow.

Kinetics of mononuclear phagocytes

In experimental animal studies, it has been shown that the monocytes are produced in the bone marrow, circulate in the blood for a few days, and are the precursors of the cells listed in 1–5 above, which may persist for months or possibly years. The fate of the mononuclear phagocytes is not known. There is some evidence that they may re-enter the blood and pass to the lungs, to be excreted via the bronchi.

The kinetics of macrophages in inflammatory lesions have been studied extensively by Spector and others (see Spector and Mariano, 1975). In various types of granulomatous inflammation, and in various tissues, it has been shown that most of the macrophages are provided by migration of monocytes. Their life-span in chronic inflammatory lesions has been found to vary depending on the causal agent. With relatively strong cytotoxic agents, macrophage turnover is rapid, a continuous supply from the blood being necessary to maintain the macrophage population of the lesion. With more bland agents, turnover is much slower (i.e. weeks), and mitosis of macrophages in the lesion may be almost sufficient to maintain the population. Curiously, mitosis of macrophages from inflammatory lesions is accompanied by a high incidence of chromosomal abnormalities which, by precluding further divisions, must limit their local proliferation.

Morphology of macrophages

Macrophages are motile cells and can assume polarity and various shapes. They have an oval, indented or irregular nucleus, abundant cytoplasm rich in lysosomes, and surface microvilli (Fig. 3.27). Phagocytic vacuoles, if present, are helpful in their recognition. Macrophages vary greatly in size (Fig. 3.28): they are usually larger than monocytes, but in the resting state they may closely resemble lymphocytes (e.g. in the peritoneum) and distinction can be made by histochemical demonstration of macrophage cytoplasmic enzymes.

Monocytes may be regarded as immature macrophage precursors which, on stimulation, transform to macrophages. The change involves increase in motility, size and phagocytic activity: cytoplasmic RNA and lysosomes increase, and the nucleus becomes larger and less

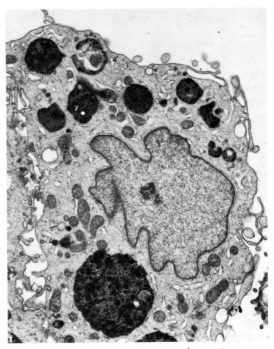

Fig. 3.27 An electron micrograph of part of a macrophage, showing microvilli (*top*) and a portion of the nucleus (*right centre*). The cytoplasmic dense bodies (black) are phagosomes formed by the fusion of lysosomes with phagocytic vacuoles and the 'empty' spaces are dilated endoplasmic reticulum. × 9000.

condensed. Similar changes have recently been demonstrated by Wynne *et al.* (1975) when inflammatory exudate is added to cultures of macrophages (Fig. 3.29).

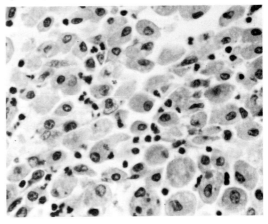

Fig. 3.28 Macrophages of various sizes in the wall of a chronically inflamed gallbladder. Note the ovoid or indented nucleus and abundant cytoplasm. × 405.

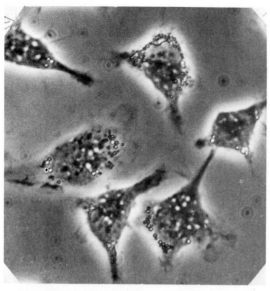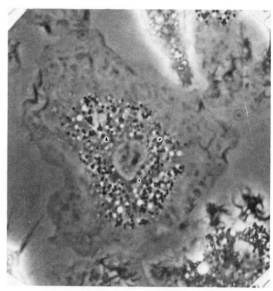

Fig. 3.29 Mouse peritoneal macrophages in culture, viewed by phase-contrast microscopy. Inflammatory exudate has been added to the culture shown on right. Note the increase in size, content of (phase-dense) lysosomes and (phase-lucent) vesicles and extensive cytoplasmic 'ruffling' of the stimulated cell. ×960. (Professor W. G. Spector and Mrs. Katherine M. Wynne.)

In chronic inflammatory lesions, macrophages may assume the special features of **epithelioid cells** or of **giant cells.** Change to epithelioid cells (so-called because they have some resemblance to epithelial cells) involves an increase in the amount of cytoplasm and in rough endoplasmic reticulum: epithelioid cells are not actively phagocytic, and they may have a secretory function.

The factors responsible for change of macrophages to epithelioid cells are not fully understood: it is seen in immunological reactions of delayed hypersensitivity type, and may therefore be mediated by lymphoid cells: the same factors may be concerned in formation of Langhans' giant cells (see below) for these are usually associated with epithelioid cells.

Giant cells. It is common to see macrophages with two or more nuclei, but they can fuse together to form very large giant cells with sometimes over 100 nuclei. Such cells are usually classified into **foreign-body giant cells,** which have irregularly scattered nuclei, and **Langhans' giant cells,** in which the nuclei are arranged peripherally (Fig. 3.30). Spector has studied giant-cell formation by monocytes in tissue culture. At first they resemble foreign-body giant cells, but may later develop the features of Langhans' cells.

The **osteoclasts**, which digest bone matrix in the process of bone resorption, appear to be formed by coalescence of monocytes, and thus represent specialised cells within the macrophage system. The influence of the local environment on macrophages is also illustrated by the alveolar macrophages, which require oxygen for full phagocytic activity, whereas macrophages elsewhere can produce the necessary energy solely by glycolysis under anaerobic conditions.

Macrophage functions

The major function of the macrophage is phagocytosis and destruction of micro-organisms and other harmful or unwanted material. The general features of their scavenging role in inflammation are considered on p. 63 and their protective role in infection on pp. 180–81. Macrophages also have the important physiological role of removing dead or effete cells. For example they are responsible for taking up degenerate erythrocytes: they break down the cell and its haemoglobin, and release the iron, etc. for reutilisation.

Macrophages are capable of ingesting large amounts of insoluble material (Fig. 3.26), and of retaining it for months or even years. This

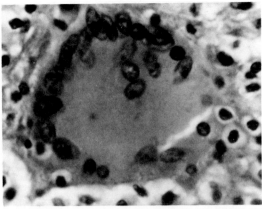

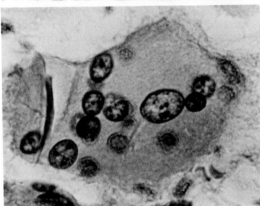

Fig. 3.30 Multinucleated giant cells formed by fusion of macrophages. The upper cell is a Langhans' giant cell in a tuberculous lesion: note the peripheral arrangement of the nuclei and abundant cytoplasm. The lower cell is a foreign-body giant cell: the nuclei vary in size and are irregularly distributed, and the cell has engulfed a fragment of suture material. × 750.

happens when, for various reasons, abnormal amounts of lipids (p. 28) or iron accumulate in various tissues, or when dust particles are inhaled in atmospheric pollution. These conditions of abnormal storage are described in later chapters, in relation to the organs and tissues they most affect.

Other functions of the mononuclear phagocytes include the secretion of factors which stimulate fibrosis (p. 68), production of some of the components of complement (p. 142), participation in immune responses (p. 134) and the production of endogenous pyrogen in pyrexia (p. 189), and of colony stimulating factor which promotes proliferation and maturation of polymorph and monocyte precursors (p. 187).

Other cells in inflammation

Serosal cells. In acute inflammation of a serous surface, cells on or near the surface enlarge and often pass into the exudate at an early stage. They include macrophages and endothelial lining cells. In more chronic inflammation, the latter cells may grow in clumps in the fluid exudate in the cavity, and may show nuclear abnormalities and mucin secretion. In aspirated fluid, they are sometimes very difficult to distinguish from cancer cells.

Fibroblasts are seen in most acute inflammatory lesions, but their presence in large numbers is associated with chronic inflammation and repair. They are considered in the next chapter.

References and Further Reading

Allison, A. C. (1978). Macrophage activation and nonspecific immunity. In *International Review of Experimental Pathology*, Vol. 18, pp. 304–346. Edited by G. W. Richter and M. A. Epstein. Academic Press, New York, San Francisco and London.

Boyden, S. (1962). The chemotactic effect of mixtures of antibody and antigen on polymorphonuclear leukocytes. *Journal of Experimental Medicine* **115**, 453–66.

Burke, J. R. and Miles, A. A. (1958). The sequence, of vascular events in early infective inflammation. *Journal of Pathology and Bacteriology* **76**, 1–19.

Cochrane, C. G. *et al.* (1974). Soluble mediators of injury of the microvasculature: Hageman factor and the kinin forming, intrinsic clotting and fibrinolytic systems. *Microcirculation Research* **8**, 112–21.

†Cohnheim, J. (1889). *Lectures in General Pathology*, Vol. 1., pp. 242 to at least 270. (English

†Mainly of historical interest.

translation). New Sydenham Society, London. (The classic account of the acute inflammatory reaction observed *in vivo*.)

*van Furth *et al.* (1975). Mononuclear phagocytes in human pathology—proposal for an approach to improved classification. pp. 1–15. In *Mononuclear Phagocytes in Immunity, Infection and Pathology*. pp. 1062. Ed. by R. van Furth. Blackwell Scientific Publications, Oxford. (A comprehensive multi-author text.)

Harris, H. (1953). Chemotaxis of granulocytes. *Journal of Pathology and Bacteriology* **66**, 135–46.

Hill, J. H. and Ward, P. A. (1971). The phlogistic role of C3 leukotactic fragments in myocardial infarction in rats. *Journal of Experimental Medicine* **133**, 885–900.

*Hurley, J. V. (1972). *Acute Inflammation*. pp. 137. Churchill Livingstone, Edinburgh. (A clear and interesting account suitable for the general reader.)

†Landis, E. M. (1927). Micro-injection studies of capillary permeability. 1. Factors in the production of capillary stasis. *American Journal of Physiology* **81**, 124–42.

*Lepow, I. H. and Ward, P. A. (Eds.) (1972) *Inflammation Mechanisms and Control*. pp. 388. Academic Press, New York and London. (Review articles on selected topics by some leading workers.)

Lewis, E. and Turk, J. L. (1975). Comparison of the effect of various antisera and cobra venom factor on inflammatory reactions in guinea-pig skin. *Journal of Pathology* **115**, 97–109.

†Lewis, T. (1927). *The blood vessels in the human skin and their responses*. pp. 322. Shaw and Sons, London.

Majno, G., Palade, G. E. and Schoefl, G. (1961). Studies in Inflammation. II. The site of action of histamine and serotonin along the vascular tree: a topographic study. *Journal of Biophysical and Biochemical Cytology* **11**, 607–26.

†Metchnikoff, E. (1905). *Immunity in Infective Diseases*. (English translation.) Cambridge University Press, London.

Miles, A. A. and Wilhelm, D. L. (1955). Enzyme-like globulins from serum reproducing the vascular phenomena of inflammation. I. An activable permeability factor and its inhibitor in guinea-pig serum. *British Journal of Experimental Pathology* **36**, 71–81.

Pappenheimer, J. R., Renkin, E. M. and Borrero, L. M. (1951). Filtration, diffusion and molecular sieving through peripheral capillary membranes. A contribution to the pore theory of capillary permeability. *American Journal of Physiology* **167**, 13–46.

*Ryan, G. B. and Majno, G. (1977a). Acute inflammation. *American Journal of Pathology* **86**, 185–276. (A detailed review with an extensive bibliography.)

*Ryan, G. B. and Majno, G. (1977b). *Inflammation*, pp. 80. Upjohn Company, Kalamazoo. (A beautifully illustrated, clear account, of convenient length for the general reader.)

Sevitt, S. (1958). Early and delayed oedema and increase in capillary permeability after burns of the skin. *Journal of Pathology and Bacteriology* **75**, 27–37.

Simionescu, N., Simionescu, M. and Palade, G. E. (1975). Permeability of muscle capillaries to small heme-peptides: evidence for the existence of patent transendothelial channels. *Journal of Cell Biology* **64**, 586–607.

Spector, W. G. and Mariano, M. (1975). Macrophage behaviour in experimental granulomas. pp. 927–42. In *Mononuclear Phagocytes in Immunity, Infection and Pathology*. pp. 1062. Ed. by R. van Furth. Blackwell Scientific Publications, Oxford. (A comprehensive multi-author text.)

†Starling, E. H. (1896). On the absorption of fluids from the connective tissue spaces. *Journal of Physiology* **19**, 312–26.

*Wilkinson, P. C. (1974). *Chemotaxis and Inflammation*. pp. 214. Churchill Livingstone, Edinburgh. (An authoritative account of chemotaxis including original observations by the author.)

Wilkinson, P. C., Russell, R. J. and Allan, R. B. (1977). Leucocytes and chemotaxis. *Agents and Actions*, suppl. 3, 61–70.

*Willoughby, D. A., Coote, E. and Turk, J. L. (1969). Complement in acute inflammation. *Journal of Pathology and Bacteriology* **97**, 295–305.

*Willoughby, D. A., Giroud, J. P. and Velo, G. P. (Eds.) (1977). *Perspectives in Inflammation, Future Trends and Developments*. pp. 638. M.P.T. Press Ltd., Lancaster, England. (Report of an international conference with accounts by many leading workers.)

Wynne, K. M., Spector, W. G. and Willoughby, D. A. (1975). Induction of DNA synthesis in rat macrophages *in vitro* by inflammatory exudate. *Nature* (Lond). **253**, 636–7.

*Zweifach, B. W. (Ed.) (1973–4). *The Inflammatory Process*, 3 vols. Academic Press, New York and London. (Accounts on most aspects of inflammation by leading workers.)

* General texts, reviews, and reports of symposia.
† Mainly of historical interest.

4

Healing (Repair) and Hypertrophy

Healing

Reaction of tissues to injury varies greatly in different species of animals and in different tissues. **Regeneration**, i.e. the replacement of a single type of parenchymatous cell by production of more cells of the same kind may be seen in man but different tissues vary in their regenerative capacity. A helpful guide to the expected reaction to damage of any tissue is given by the division of somatic cells into three types.

(a) Labile cells are those which under normal conditions continue to multiply throughout life and include epidermis, alimentary, respiratory and urinary tract epithelium, uterine endometrium and the haemopoietic bone marrow and lymphoid cells.

(b) Stable cells normally cease multiplication when growth ceases but retain mitotic ability during adult life so that some regeneration of damaged tissues may occur. This group includes liver, pancreas, renal tubular epithelium, thyroid and adrenal cortex.

(c) Permanent cells lose their mitotic ability in infancy and the classic example of this group is the neuron.

In many instances healing of an organ or tissue occurs by regeneration, the cells lost being replaced by proliferative activity of those remaining. However, when the injury involves a cell type inherently incapable of this or when other factors, e.g. interruption of blood supply, prevents restoration, healing occurs by the **formation of a fibrous scar** the development of which is best illustrated by the healing of a wound of skin and subcutaneous tissue.

Healing of skin wounds

Healing by first intention (primary union)

Primary union occurs when uninfected surgical incisions and other clean wounds without loss of tissue are closed promptly, e.g. by sutures. (Fig. 4.1A) It is characterised by the formation of only minimal amounts of granulation tissue. It is a rapid process and contrasts with healing by **secondary intention** which occurs in an open wound, the edges of which are not brought together by sutures (Fig. 4.1B). Wound infection also prevents healing by first intention. The sequence of events in healing by first inten-

tion is as follows: blood clots between the wound edges and on the surface where it dries to form a protective scab. While removal of clot and dead tissue is occurring, firstly by the action of polymorphs and later of macrophages, there is a rapid spread of epithelium beneath the scab to bridge the wound surface within the first two days. Within 3 to 5 days capillaries and fibroblasts grow in beneath the epithelium, and collagen formed by the fibroblasts begins to bind the wound edges together by the end of the first week, reaching a maximum in two or three weeks. Thereafter wound strength slowly increases over many months.

The wound clot and its removal

When an incision is made in the skin and subcutaneous tissue, blood escaping from cut vessels clots on the wound surface and fills the gap between the wound edges which, in sutured wounds, is narrow. The fibrin in the blood clot acts temporarily as a glue which holds the cut surfaces together, while the dehydrated blood clot on the surface forms a scab which effectively seals the wound. Excess of blood clot deeper in the wound delays healing, for it greatly increases the risk of infection and if not evacuated, will only slowly be converted to fibrous tissue (see organisation, p. 98). During the first 24 hours, there is a mild inflammatory reaction at the wound edges with exudation of fluid and migration of polymorphs and later of monocytes and lymphocytes. Blood clot is digested by enzymes from disintegrated polymorphs and this is aided from about the third day by macrophages, derived mainly from blood monocytes, which ingest and digest any remaining fibrin, red cells and cellular debris, converting macromolecules into useful amino acids and sugar. The macrophages, which are the dominant cell by 72 hours after wounding, probably also play an important part, perhaps along with platelets, in attracting fibroblast precursors into the wound and in stimulating their proliferation. They may also promote the formation of new blood vessels (see below). These changes represent the acute inflammatory (exudative) phase of response to injury and are usually mild unless infection supervenes.

Epithelial regeneration

The first tissue to bridge the incisional gap is the squamous epithelium of the epidermis. Within 24 hours and extending from 3–4 mm around the wound edge there is enlargement and flattening of the basal cells with loss of prominence of rete ridges. Two processes then contribute to the closure of the gap. Close to the cut edge, cells from the deeper part of the epithelium begin to slide over each other; they *migrate* out over the wound surface and become flattened to form a continuous advancing sheet. *Proliferation* also occurs, mainly among basal cells in the epidermis and pilosebaceous follicles adjacent to the wound. Mitosis is rarely seen in the migrating cells but occurs later in the new epithelium. While the

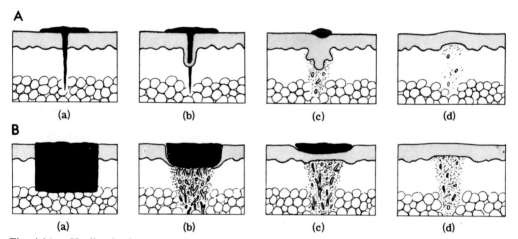

A

(a)   (b)   (c)   (d)

B

(a)   (b)   (c)   (d)

Fig. 4.1A.   Healing by first intention (sutured surgical incision). Immediately after injury (**a**) the wound fills with blood clot and a scab forms on the surface. Epithelium which has grown from each side of the wound joins together within about two days (**b**) and later forms a spur of epithelium. A little granulation tissue grows into the wound (**c**). The collagen formed by the fibroblasts in the granulation tissue unites the wound edges. The epithelial spur resorbs and the epithelium does not re-form rete ridges. The narrow fibrous scar gradually becomes less vascular (**d**).
Fig. 4.1 B.   Healing by second intention (open excised wound). After injury the wound fills with clot (**a**). Epithelium begins to extend under the clot and abundant granulation tissue grows into the base of the wound (**b**). Contraction of the wound occurs and the epithelium finally completely covers the base of the wound (**c**). The vascularity of this more bulky fibrous scar gradually diminishes (**d**).

advancing edge of the sheet of new epidermis consists of a single layer of flat cells, the older part at the periphery of the wound becomes stratified so that there is a gradient of thickness. The cells will only migrate over viable tissue. They burrow beneath the superficial part of the blood clot and wound debris, down the cut edges of the dermis; by their proteolytic enzymes, they cleave a path between dead and living collagen fibres (figs. 4.1A and 4.2). Within 48 hours the wound may be bridged by epithelium which rapidly becomes stratified but does not form rete ridges (Figs. 4.3, 4.8). Any epithelium which has grown down into the dermis is later resorbed (Fig. 4.1A).

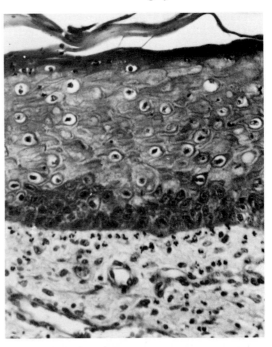

Fig. 4.3 Newly formed epithelium on healed ulcer. The epithelium is several cells thick, but there is little differentiation, and there is no formation of rete ridges. A similar appearance is seen in a healed surgical incision. × 400.

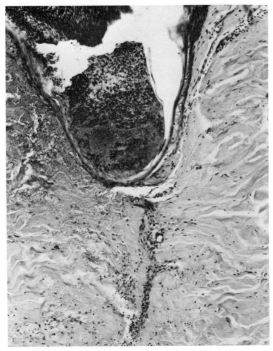

Fig. 4.2 Aseptic abdominal wound showing the stage of healing at five days. The incision is represented merely by a vertical cellular line. The round body on the surface is a small scab beneath which the epithelium has extended down to cover the dermis. × 105.

Suture tracks. Each suture track is a wound, with haemorrhage, death of cells and injury to skin appendages, and in consequence there is a slight inflammatory reaction and fibroblast proliferation (Fig. 4.4). Because the suture prevents closure of the surface epithelium the track is prone to infection and 'stitch abscesses' are commoner than sepsis of surgical incisions.

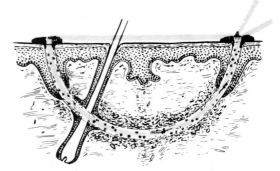

Fig. 4.4 Diagram of suture track a few days after wounding and before removal of sutures. In the centre of the picture the healed epithelium still forms a small projection into the dermis and beneath it the more cellular vertical line of the healing wound is seen.

The surface epithelium and that from a damaged hair follicle have grown along the suture track which is open to the skin surface and is lined by a layer of fibrin containing polymorphs. There is more vascular and fibroblastic proliferation around the suture track than around the original wound.

Epithelium also tends to grow down suture tracks from both ends (Fig. 4.4). Often much of the epithelium is avulsed when stitches are removed but some may remain and occasionally gives rise either to a small implantation cyst or to a subacute inflammatory reaction to keratin, which may simulate infection.

Repair of the dermis and subcutaneous tissue

These tissues heal by proliferation of new blood vessels and fibroblasts to form '**granulation tissue**', probably under the influence of stimulating factors released by macrophages. From about the third day, **vascular proliferation** is seen as capillary sprouts, which grow from blood vessels at the wound margins (Fig. 4.5), and advance up to 2 mm per day into the wound: the capillary sprouts are produced partly by rearrangement and migration of pre-existing endothelial cells and partly by their proliferation just behind the advancing tip. The sprouts are often solid at first, but they unite with one another or join a capillary already carrying blood and develop a lumen. These newly formed capillaries are very delicate (Fig. 4.12), have an incomplete basement membrane and behave as if acutely inflamed: they leak protein-rich fluid with escape of some red cells, and polymorphs emigrate from them. It has been observed in rabbits that if blood flow is not soon established through a new vessel then the lumen disappears, the vessel reverting to a solid cord which then breaks and the ends retract by sliding back of endothelial cells to the nearest vessel carrying blood. Within a few days of the establishment of circulation, some of the new vessels differentiate into arterioles and venules by the acquisition of muscle cells either by migration from pre-existing larger blood channels or by differentiation from mesenchymal cells.

Lymphatic channels are re-established in the same manner as blood vessels.

Fibrous tissue production. After the removal of blood, fibrin and dead cells from the wound, and simultaneously with the development of new blood vessels, long, spindle-shaped fibroblasts (Fig. 4.6a and b) stream from the perivas-

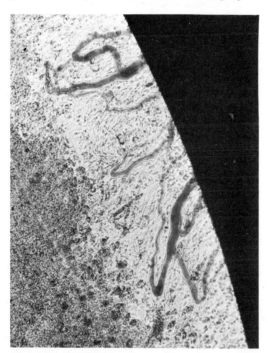

Fig. 4.5 Capillary loops growing into a blood clot in a transparent chamber embedded in a rabbit's ear, photographed *in vivo*. Similar but less marked vascular proliferation is seen in the healing of a simple surgical incision. The rounded dark objects are macrophages which are digesting the blood clot in advance of growing vessels. (The late Prof. Lord Florey.)

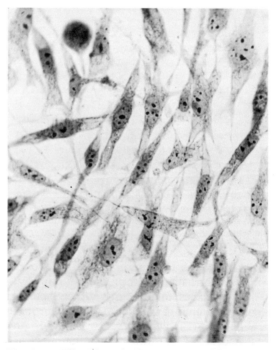

Fig. 4.6a Fibroblasts in tissue culture. (The late Dr. Janet S. F. Niven.)

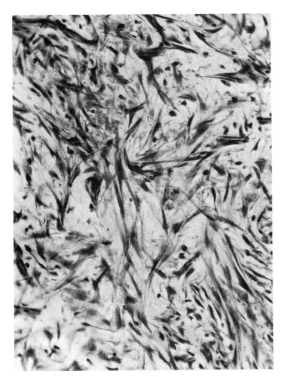

Fig. 4.6b Fibroblasts in a healing wound, showing the characteristic shape and early formation of collagen fibrils. × 350.

cular connective tissue and begin to proliferate and to move into the wound. Within a few days fibroblasts thus come to lie in the wound: they produce both type I and type III collagen (see below), synthesis being greatest at about 7 days. The collagen fibres come to lie across the incision line and help to unite the cut edges from about the end of the first week after injury. Proteoglycan ground substance, also secreted by the fibroblast, may play an important role in determining fibre size and direction and also later in enhancing crosslinks between collagen molecules (see below). By the third week the total amount of collagen in the wound has almost reached a maximum. In contrast, at this stage the tensile strength of the wound is still low, but it increases over many months by further intermolecular bonding between collagen fibrils and by remodelling of the anatomical configuration of the collagen in response to mechanical stress. Such remodelling involves collagen turnover, i.e. synthesis and lysis which occurs also in normal (unwounded) tissues (see below).

While healing of a wound by fibrous tissue is clearly beneficial, in some tissues it may also have harmful results, for example narrowing of the oesophagus, stenosis of the mitral valve, or stricture of the urethra. Attempts to modify the fibrotic process by inhibiting collagen formation, promoting its destruction or altering its metabolism by drugs so far have not been very effective.

Collagen synthesis. Collagen is synthesised and secreted by fibroblasts in soluble form, and deposited extracellularly. As with secretory proteins in general, the polypeptide chains of collagen (**pro-α-chains**) are formed on the ribosomes with N and C terminal extension peptides. A distinctive feature of collagen synthesis is the conversion of proline and lysine residues on the growing polypeptide chains to hydroxyproline and hydroxylysine residues. This enzymic hydroxylation requires Fe^{++}, O_2, ascorbic acid and α-ketoglutarate. Glycosylation of some of the hydroxylysine residues then occurs. In the cisternae of the endoplasmic reticulum pro-α-chains are converted to **pro-collagen** by the formation of disulphide bonds and they begin to assume a tri-helical structure. The pro-collagen molecules, of which there are several types, are stabilised by hydroxyproline and are secreted via the Golgi apparatus. Outside the cell the N and C extension peptides, which do not assume the helical form, are removed in some types of collagen by pro-collagen peptidase. This drastically alters the properties of the molecule which precipitates as **tropocollagen**. The tropocollagen molecules, which are rigid rods of 290 × 1·4 nm, align side by side, probably in fives, staggered at a quarter of their length to produce a fibril with a 64 nm periodicity on electron microscopy (Fig. 4.7). The acquisition of tensile strength of the fibrils is

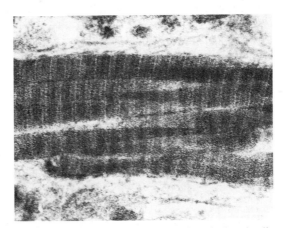

Fig. 4.7 Collagen fibres are seen here in longitudinal section. The characteristic, regular cross banding is evident. × 65 000.

Table 4.1   Types of collagen

Type	Molecular form	Tissue
I	Two identical chains $\alpha1(I)_2$ and one $\alpha2$	Dermis, tendon, bone, dentin, cornea (stains red with Van Gieson, green with Masson and blue with Mallory stains for collagen).
II	Three identical chains unique to itself $\alpha1(II)_3$.	Cartilage.
III	Three identical chains unique to itself $\alpha1(III)_3$	Embryonic dermis (and about 10–15% of adult) – early scar tissue, granulomas, cardiovascular tissue, synovial membrane (stains with silver nitrate as reticulin).
IV	Three identical chains unique to itself $\alpha1(IV)_3$ but perhaps a heterogeneous group	Basement membrane (almost amorphous and does not show the typical banded structure on electron-microscopy).

dependent on the formation of co-valent links, mainly of aldemine and keto type. Increase in strength results from further alterations in the extent and nature of intermolecular crosslinkage.

Types of collagen. There are at least four different types of collagen derived from different structural genes (see Table 4.1). All have the triple helical configuration and types I, II and III have an identical appearance, banded at 64 nm, on electron microscopy. (Fig. 4.7).

The time needed for their synthesis and secretion varies as does their susceptibility to the various collagenases bringing about collagen lysis. While many tissues contain more than one type of collagen (e.g. adult dermis contains type I and about 10–15% of type III), mixed fibres are not found. Initially in a healing scar there are more type III (**reticulin**) fibres than in adjacent skin but later these are replaced by type I fibres.

Collagen lysis. Collagenases are formed, at the site where they are required, e.g. in healing wounds, by macrophages, polymorphs and regenerating epidermal epithelium. The collagenase is secreted directly onto the fibre by a closely apposed cell and this splits the fibre so that fragments may be ingested by macrophages. Splitting is more likely to occur in fibres with few or unstable cross links. Within the phagosomes, the fragments are broken down to amino acids or small peptides. In the healing wound, lysis occurs in the early stage of cleaning up the damaged collagen at the wound face and for a depth of about 7 mm into the surrounding tissue. There is also breakdown and replacement of much of the collagen first formed: wound remodelling continues for six months to a year. If the balance between synthesis and lysis is upset by starvation, sepsis, or deficiency of specific protein or of oxygen, then the wound collagen may be extensively digested.

Events following primary wound healing

Once the wound has healed the young scar is commonly raised above the surface due to the underlying proliferative processes and is red as a result of increased vascularity. The blood vessels gradually decrease in number, probably in the manner already described, and the amount of collagen may also diminish. *Elastic fibres* are formed much later than collagen (Fig. 4.8). *Sensory nerves* may grow into the scar in about three weeks but specialised nerve endings such as Pacinian corpuscles do not re-form. The end result of healing by first intention should be a pale linear scar, level with the adjacent skin surface, but sometimes a **hypertrophic scar** or **keloid** forms (p. 342).

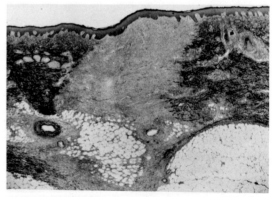

Fig. 4.8   Healed surgical wound of skin of 14 days' duration. The elastic fibres are stained black, and the healed wound is seen in the centre: it is composed of connective tissue in which elastic fibres have not yet formed. × 5.

Healing by second intention (secondary union)

Healing of an open gaping wound with loss of tissue or of an infected closed wound occurs by the formation of granulation tissue which grows from the base of the wound to fill the defect. The vascular and fibroblastic proliferation which together make up the granulation tissue are much more abundant and healing takes much longer than when it occurs by first intention (Fig. 4.1 B). Skin grafts are increasingly used to speed the healing of open wounds.

Clean open wounds. As in the closed wound there is haemorrhage and exudation of fibrin from the cut surfaces. This is soon followed by a much greater emigration of polymorphs and subsequently of macrophages, from vessels in the wound: by enzymic action and phagocytosis these cells soften and remove the fibrin and other debris. As in the incised wound, epithelial cells at the margins enlarge and begin to migrate down the walls of the wound in the first day or two after injury. Migration and proliferation together produce a sheet of cells which advances in a series of tongue-like projections beneath any remaining blood clot or exudate on the wound surface. As the single layer of cells moves inwards towards the wound centre, there is stratification of the cells near to the wound margin (Fig. 4.9). Since the denuded

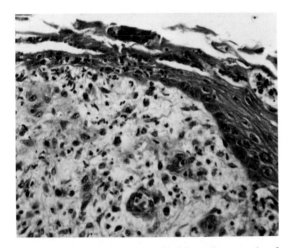

Fig. 4.9 Granulating wound with early growth of epithelium over the surface. The epithelium is growing from the right-hand side and tapers off as a thin layer. × 400.

area is large, the advancing epithelial sheet does not completely cover the wound until the granulation tissue from the base (see below) has started to fill the wound space. Care should always be taken, in removing adherent dressings from an open wound, because the delicate epithelium is easily ripped off. As soon as the wound surface is covered, epithelial cell migration ceases and proliferation, stratification and keratinisation are rapidly completed, though rete ridges are not re-formed.

When the full thickness of the skin is destroyed by a burn re-epithelialisation is slow for the cells, with the help of their collagenases, have to burrow beneath the thick layer of dead coagulated collagen. In contrast, in a burn which destroys only part of the skin thickness, in a superficial wound or the donor site of a 'split thickness' skin graft, re-epithelialisation is relatively rapid as proliferation of epithelium occurs not only from the wound edge but also from the cut mouth of each pilosebaceous follicle. In man, slower and less perfect epithelial regeneration occurs from sweat gland ducts. If skin appendages are destroyed they are not re-formed.

Although epithelium shows the first evidence of reparative activity, within a few days the pre-existing vessels in the wound bed produce vascular sprouts which grow upwards, forming loops and coils near the wound surface (Fig. 4.10), giving it a red, granular appearance—hence the term *'granulation tissue'* (Fig. 4.11.) From these new, more permeable vessels (Fig. 4.12), small haemorrhages occur and polymorphs migrate, reinforcing those already present in the exudate on the wound surface and helping to keep down bacterial growth. At the same time as the new capillaries form, fibroblasts, some of which are in mitosis, are seen in the base and walls of the wound, often running parallel to the new capillary walls (i.e. towards the wound surface). This fibrovascular granulation tissue continues to proliferate and to fill the wound space only until epithelium grows over its surface, when the exudative inflammatory changes and the migration of polymorphs also subside. Later the fibroblasts may become orientated parallel to the wound surface (Fig. 4.13) and about the end of the first week collagen is produced and rapidly increases in amount. If epithelialisation is delayed, e.g. by further trauma or infection, granulations may

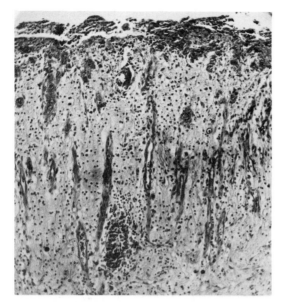

Fig. 4.10   Granulating wound showing the vertical lines of newly formed blood vessels. × 150.

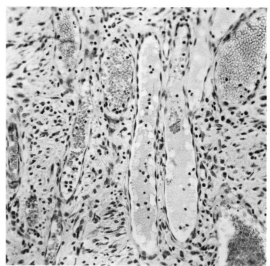

Fig. 4.12   Newly formed thin-walled blood vessels in a granulating wound, the surface of which is to the top. × 150.

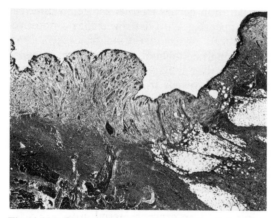

Fig. 4.11   Granulating wound of 12 days' duration. The advancing epithelial margin is seen as the dark surface layer on the right. Granulation tissue projects from the floor of the wound, and can be seen to contain many small blood vessels. × 10.

pout from the wound surface. Following healing, there is gradual retraction and disappearance of some of the new vascular channels and further crosslinking and remodelling of collagen (see above) which, over a period of months, becomes progressively less cellular.

Healing of an open, excised wound is aided by **contraction of the surface area** in sites where the skin is mobile and loosely attached to underlying tissue. All edges of the wound do not move together to the same extent, the degree of contraction being related to skin tension. This movement of the edges towards the centre of the wound is brought about by contraction of the fibroblasts which are now accordingly termed **myofibroblasts**. These cells develop temporarily a well-organised system of contractile cytoplasmic microfilaments resembling that of smooth muscle cells and responding to many pharmacological agents which contract smooth muscle. The bundles of parallel contractile microfilaments run longitudinally within the cells and are attached to the cell surface at sites where it is firmly adherent to other cells or to underlying tissue. Contraction of microfilament bundles in a meshwork of myofibroblasts in an open wound may thus pull together the wound edges, in which position they are stabilised by the deposition of collagen fibres. When desirable, as sometimes in flexor surfaces over joints, wound contraction may be inhibited by early skin grafting.

Infected wounds. The repair of infected wounds is accomplished by the same processes already described for clean, open wounds; that is, by the production of granulation tissue, but with a more pronounced acute inflammatory reaction, and also by formation of larger and more numerous blood vessels.

Open wounds, apart from those produced under aseptic surgical conditions, are almost

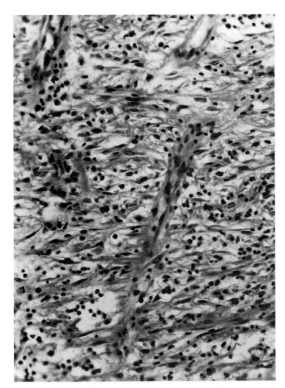

Fig. 4.13 Deeper part of granulating wound. *Below*, the collagen fibrils are being formed parallel to the surface; *above*, the vessels are seen running in a vertical direction. × 240.

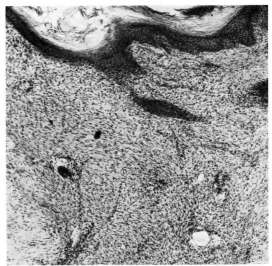

Fig. 4.14 Healing abdominal wound in which infection has delayed the process of healing. Note that the line of cellular tissue is much broader than in Fig. 4.2. × 75.

always contaminated by bacteria, and for this reason a careful surgical toilet should include removal of dead tissue, which promotes invasive bacterial growth; this *débridement* is an important part of treatment. Granulation tissue provides a good defence against bacteria because, being rich in small blood vessels, it can mount an effective inflammatory response. These local defensive factors may be aided by antibacterial therapy, which may permit early suture or skin grafting. If infection continues, however, more leukocytes pour into the surface exudate, which then becomes purulent. The result of acute infection on the healing processes is to inhibit both epithelial regeneration and proliferation of fibroblasts, so that healing is delayed. This delay and the greater tissue destruction result eventually in increased fibrous tissue and a larger and denser scar (Fig. 4.14).

Skin grafting. When a skin graft is placed on the recipient site it adheres to this new bed by fibrin and is nourished by diffusion of plasma from the raw surface. Within about three days

capillary buds growing from the recipient area begin to unite with those on the undersurface of the graft, while ingrowing fibroblasts produce collagen which anchors the graft more securely. Good vascularity of the bed without haematoma formation, control of pathogenic infection and close, undisturbed contact with the graft, promote a rapid 'take'.

Grafts from the same individual (autografts) persist indefinitely. Grafts from another individual (homografts) are accepted initially but are destroyed within a month or so by an immune reaction by the recipient; they are nevertheless useful to provide temporary cover of extensive raw surfaces, for example large burns, and help to prevent excessive contraction of the area.

Control mechanisms in healing

While the morphological changes of wound healing are well known, the factors controlling the various observed processes are controversial or unknown.

Control of cell movement. The covering of a wound surface by epithelium cannot be explained simply by movement due to '*growth pressure*'. While a burst of mitoses may displace adjacent cells by a concerted nudge, it is known that healing may occur without cell division and, in the skin, epithelial cell migration over the wound surfaces appears to precede proliferation. There is evidence from tissue culture that virtually all cells have the ability to move along a surface to which they can adhere. If two cultures of fibroblasts are made on a plane surface the cells grow out as a monolayer from each explant until they collide, when movement virtually ceases because the cells will almost never pile up on one another. This is known as **contact inhibition**. The same phenomenon may govern the covering of the surface of a wound by epithelial cells from around the margin. The concept of contact inhibition in regard to epidermal cells and fibroblasts helps to explain not only initiation of movement but also the direction of cells into the wounded area, especially since there is no evidence that chemotaxis applies to any cell other than leukocytes (and spermatozoa). Contact inhibition appears to be tissue specific in some degree, for if skin and oesophageal epithelium meet, although both are squamous, cell movement and proliferation continue and cells heap up at the junction.

Explantation of a fragment of adult tissue into a culture medium does not result in rapid migration, although the cells at the free edge of the fragment now lack contact with similar cells. If the tissue is first wounded a short time before excision however, migration is greatly increased and it seems that some factor in addition to loss of contact inhibition may be involved. There is some evidence to suggest that there is a change in the cell surface, causing a diminution of its adhesive properties, thus permitting mobilisation.

The stimulus to migration and proliferation. It has been suggested that the stimulus to wound healing and enhanced mitotic activity is mediated by growth promoters—**trephones** or 'wound hormones'—liberated by damaged cells. Tissue culture studies suggest that there may be a stimulating substance but this has never been shown to initiate cell migration or multiplication *in vivo* and at the moment the existence of a wound hormone derived from damaged cells and promoting healing in animals remains no more than a possibility.

It has been postulated that cells of epidermis and other tissues normally secrete a diffusible tissue-specific depressor of cell mitosis and that wounding may inhibit the production or effect of this depressor substance or **chalone**, thus allowing an increase in mitotic activity. This possibility is supported by the experimental finding that removal of skin from one side of a mouse's ear provokes a burst of mitotic activity in the intact epidermis of the other side, maximal opposite the middle of the defect rather than opposite the wound edges. There is also evidence for the production of a fibroblast chalone in tissue cultures. Acceptance of the validity of this important concept of cell-specific chalones has not been universal because no one has yet purified and biochemically characterised these compounds, although their existence was reported many years ago.

The concept of the chalone has interesting implications apart from those related to wound healing. Their postulated inhibitory action on mitoses in skin cultures is apparently potentiated by adrenalin, and the known cyclical fluctuation in adrenal function may thus account for the diurnal mitotic rhythm seen in many organs. The adrenalin-chalone complex appears to act after DNA synthesis is complete, just before prophase in the mitotic cycle. There is some evidence also to suggest that tumour cells (which proliferate abnormally) may fail to synthesise or release adequate concentrations of tissue-specific chalones.

Factors which impair healing

Healing may be influenced by local factors. Infection delays healing (p. 85) as does a poor local blood supply; wounds of the relatively avascular shin tend to unite more slowly than those of the highly vascular scalp or face. Defects in collagen formation may result from generalised deficiency of vitamin C or of sulphur-containing amino acids and also from an excess of glucocorticosteroids.

Deficiency of vitamin C (ascorbic acid) and sulphur-containing amino acids. Man, monkey and guinea-pig are unable to synthesise vitamin C, and in the guinea-pig impaired synthesis of wound collagen occurs after even a few days on a diet lacking the vitamin. In man, however, a much longer dietary deficiency is necessary before collagen formation is depressed, although this may occur before scurvy is clinically apparent (p. 889). Patients with multiple injuries or extensive burns readily become deficient in vitamin C unless intake is increased. Deficiency of the vitamin disturbs the synthesis of collagen at the stage of intracellular hydroxylation of amino acids so that most of the underhydroxylated collagen remains within the cell and the small amount that escapes is more readily degraded than normal collagen. As a result, although wound contraction is not impaired, the wound is weak and tends to break down after re-epithelialisation and apparent healing: this was a well-known complication of naval surgery on scorbutic sailors. In addition to the reduced amount and abnormality of the collagen formed in the wound, the new capillaries may be unduly fragile because of failure of formation of basement membrane (type IV collagen). Deficient galactosamine may alter the properties of the ground substance. Similar alteration in collagen production with loss of wound strength may be seen in starving animals deficient in the sulphur-containing amino acids such as methionine, which are essential for collagen synthesis. Even when starvation continues, some of the methionine required for wound healing may be obtained from endogenous tissue proteins but wound strength is increased by providing a diet adequate in protein. In well nourished individuals, protein and vitamin supplements will not speed healing or improve wound strength.

Excess of adrenal glucocorticoid hormones. Large doses of glucocorticoids, especially if given within the first few days after wounding, may suppress repair in experimental animals. In man the usual therapeutic doses seem to have little effect on healing of sutured incisions but may delay closure of open wounds with their higher energy requirements. Polymorphs and macrophages tend to be scanty, fibroblast proliferation and migration and the formation

of new blood vessels are all diminished, while epithelialisation and contraction are also deficient. In the steroid-treated patient there is a higher risk of wound infection and this is more likely to be undetected clinically. While the administration of vitamin A systemically or topically may counteract some steroid effects it does not restore wound contraction.

Zinc deficiency. Zinc is necessary for the synthesis of collagen. Oral supplements of zinc may promote wound healing in patients with zinc deficiency, but it is difficult to identify these patients since serum zinc levels may not reflect accurately the overall bodily status of zinc metabolism.

Healing of fractures

Healing in bones bears many resemblances to healing in soft tissues. Primary union of a fracture is however exceptional (p. 92), healing by the proliferation of callus (similar to wound healing by secondary intention) being the rule. There is initial haemorrhage and mild acute inflammation, followed by a proliferative or productive stage in which osteogenic cells play a vital part. Continuity between the bone fragments is first established by a mass of new bony trabeculae and sometimes cartilaginous tissue (**provisional callus**). This undergoes slow remodelling, with resorption and replacement so that, under favourable conditions, firm bony union is achieved. Sometimes restoration is so good that the fracture site is later hardly identifiable.

Early stages

A good deal of force is normally required to break a bone, the fragments are usually displaced, and in addition to a relatively small amount of haemorrhage between the bone ends much blood may seep into the tissues from ruptured vessels of the torn periosteum and adjacent soft tissues. In addition to haemorrhage, local inflammatory changes take place with hyperaemia and exudation of protein-rich fluid from which fibrin may be deposited. Polymorphs are scanty unless there is infection, and this is common only in **compound fractures**, i.e. when a bone fragment has torn the overlying skin or mucous membrane. Macrophages also

invade and phagocytose clot and tissue debris. Red blood cells are often removed rapidly from the fracture site, leaving a homogeneous mass of fibrin between the bone ends. A large amount of clot and debris between the bone fragments delays healing.

Bone necrosis occurs chiefly as a result of tearing of blood vessels in the medullary cavity, cortex and periosteum: the first recognisable histological evidence is observed within a day or two, the haemopoietic marrow cells showing loss of nuclear staining (Fig. 4.15). Fat released from dead marrow may be taken up by macrophages, and fat 'cysts' form, surrounded by foreign-body giant cells. Damage to the marrow may have serious results when globules of fat enter torn local venules and produce **fat emboli** in the pulmonary bed, brain and kidneys (p. 244). Because of its vascular arrangements the cortical bone usually suffers more extensive necrosis than the spongy medullary bone. The amount of bone necrosis depends especially on the local peculiarities of the blood supply; the talus, carpal scaphoid, and the femoral head following intracapsular fracture, are particularly liable to undergo extensive ischaemic necrosis. When there is splintering of bone (**comminuted fracture**) some of the fragments may lose their blood supply; they become necrotic and, if small, are eventually resorbed by osteoclasts. Bone death is recognisable histologically by loss of osteocytes from the bone lacunae (Fig. 4.15) but some cells may remain visible long after their death.

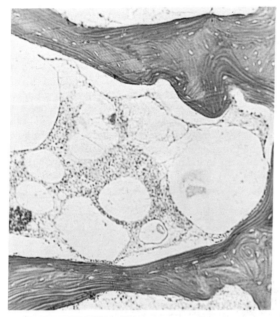

Fig. 4.15 The bone is necrotic and osteocytes have disappeared, leaving empty lacunae. Cell ghosts can be seen in the necrotic haemopoietic marrow. × 100.

Provisional callus formation

(a) **Periosteal reaction.** The cells of the inner layer of the periosteum proliferate in a fairly wide zone overlying the cortex of each fractured bone end. (Fig. 4.16). A cuff of bone trabeculae is formed around each bone end at right angles to the cortex and anchored to it ((b) in Fig. 4.17).

Further woven bone trabeculae (p. 875), less well orientated, form an irregular meshwork whose pattern at this stage is uninfluenced by stress. This formation of new bone is dependent on the blood supply, which derives partly from surviving periosteal vessels but largely from muscle and other surrounding soft tissues. Mixed with this cuff of new bone there are often nodules of hyaline cartilage which usually do not appear until bone formation is well under way (Fig. 4.17). The amount of cartilage which is formed in provisional callus varies greatly from one species to another. Small mammals such as mice, rats and rabbits tend to form chiefly cartilaginous callus while in man the amount, though variable, is less. Cartilage formation is thought to be promoted by a poor blood supply and by shearing

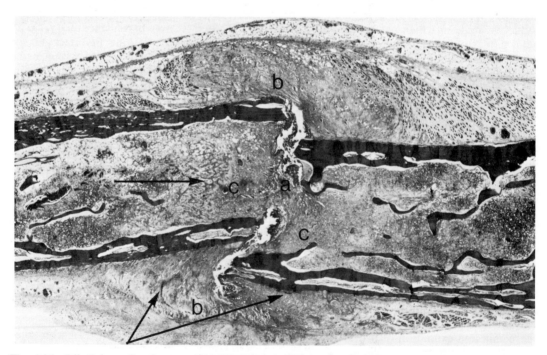

Fig. 4.16 Rib 7 days after fracture. The fracture gap (a) contains fibrin and extends into the adjacent soft tissue. A spindle of highly cellular tissue (b) has formed in the muscle around the fracture site but only a little new subperiosteal bone (arrows) and cartilage have formed as yet. Bone and marrow at the fracture site are dead (c) but there is some early revascularisation of the marrow and a little bony callus is beginning to form in the medullary cavity (arrow). × 10.

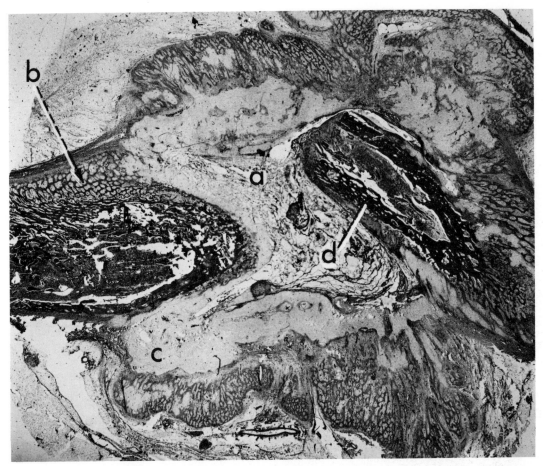

Fig. 4.17 Healing of displaced birth-fracture in the femur of a premature infant. The bone ends are cut obliquely. Bridging periosteal callus has formed but around the bone ends there is still a gap (a) which contains a meshwork of fibrin. The subperiosteal cuff of new bone is well seen at (b). The bridging callus consists partly of woven bone and partly of pale hyaline cartilage (c). The Haversian canals of the living cortex (d) are slightly enlarged by osteoclasis. × 5.

strains and stresses so that it is particularly abundant in poorly immobilised fractures: bone gradually replaces the cartilage by endochondral ossification.

The two enlarging cuffs of callus advance towards each other and finally unite to bridge the fracture line leaving a gap between the bone ends (Fig. 4.17). This 'bandage' of **external callus** helps to immobilise the fragments in an unstable or poorly fixed fracture.

The amount of bridging periosteal callus varies greatly in different sites and under different circumstances. In intracapsular fractures (i.e. within a joint capsule), such as subcapital fracture of the femoral neck, the periosteum is lacking and union is almost wholly dependent on **internal callus** formed by osteo-blasts lying in the medullary cavity (see below). By contrast, fractures of the shaft of large tubular bones, such as the femur and humerus, tend to form much external callus, internal callus in the relatively small medullary cavity not being striking. The formation of bulky external callus probably depends on plenty of surrounding undamaged muscle as a source of blood supply, for one of the causes of the difficulty in healing of fractures of the tibia is that they are partially covered by relatively avascular subcutaneous tissue and tend to form little callus. Poorly aligned fractures and those with much movement at the fracture site (e.g. the ribs and clavicle) are liable to produce abundant external callus, whereas fractures which are well immobilised by external or internal surgical fixation may unite with relatively little callus formation.

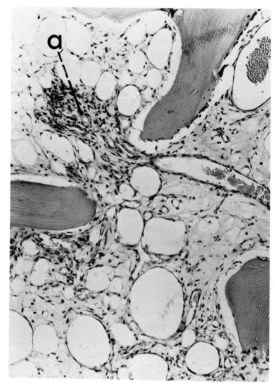

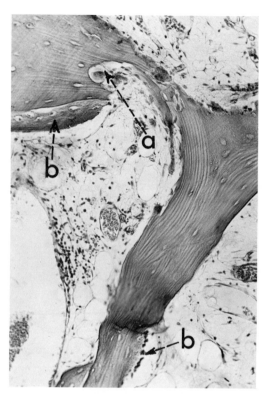

Fig. 4.18 Dead fatty marrow in the medullary cavity is being revascularised. A knot of proliferating capillaries is seen at (a). × 100.

Fig. 4.19 A dead medullary bone trabecula is being removed by osteoclasts at (a) and new bone is being laid down on the surface of dead bone at (b). × 120.

(b) Medullary reaction. The first evidence of healing is the advance of capillaries from the viable into the necrotic marrow (Fig. 4.18) closely followed by macrophages, fibroblasts and osteoblasts. The macrophages phagocytose and remove dead material, while osteoclasts begin to resorb dead spongy bone (Fig. 4.19) and the endosteal surface of the necrotic cortex. The osteoblasts produce new woven bone in the marrow spaces: the new bone is deposited partly on the surface of dead trabeculae which, when surrounded by new bone, may remain unresorbed for months or even years (Fig. 4.20).

In contrast with external callus, cartilage is rare in the medullary cavity, perhaps because it is a relatively vascular site and is protected from mechanical stress. It may form, however, when callus formation reaches the fracture gap (see below).

(c) Cortical reaction. The most striking reaction in the living cortex adjacent to the fracture is an increase in osteoclastic resorption with widening of the Haversian canals, presumably partly due to disuse atrophy (Fig. 4.21 and p. 39). This may be followed later by some osteoblastic activity. Similar changes are seen in the dead cortex of the bone ends once there has been revascularisation of the Haversian canals from adjacent vessels in viable bone or from periosteal and medullary vessels. The resorption of necrotic bone may widen the fracture gap.

The fracture gap

The periosteal (external) callus unites the fragments externally but not directly across the bone ends. As already stated, immediately after fracture, blood clot, exuded fibrin and bony debris fill the gap and this is attacked by macrophages and by osteoclasts. The fibrin clot, which usually persists between the bone ends (Figs. 4.16 and 4.17), is finally invaded by blood vessels and cellular tissue containing varying amounts of osteogenic cells and fibroblasts, so that bony union may occur in either of two ways.

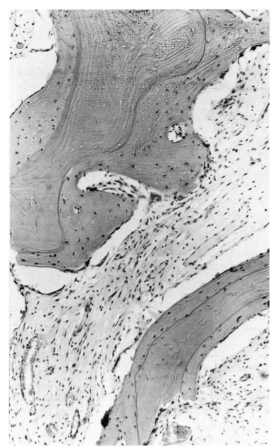

Fig. 4.20 Months after fracture dead bone trabeculae are still recognisable, covered by new living bone. × 70.

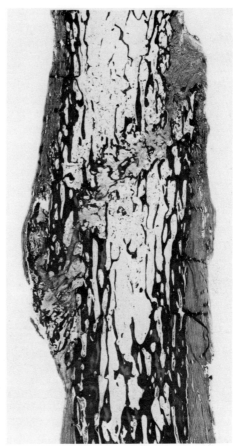

Fig. 4.21 This 12-week-old fracture of the distal fibula in an old man has formed a good deal of external callus medially (on the left). The fracture gap itself is filled with fibrous tissue in which a few trabeculae of metaplastic bone are forming. As a result of immobilisation and disuse the fibula is porotic with enlargement of Haversian canals. × 3.

(a) Direct ossification is brought about by osteogenic cells speading from medullary and periosteal callus. Cartilage may also be formed and is converted into bone. This process is relatively rapid and effective.

(b) Fibrous union may occur initially. Fibrous tissue grows in from medulla or periosteum or both, becomes densely collagenised, and only then much more slowly becomes ossified (Fig. 4.21). This slower type of union occurs especially when there is instability, separation by excessive traction or marked resorption of the bone ends, massive necrosis, a poor blood supply, extensive periosteal damage, comminution or infection. Sometimes conversion to bone following fibrous union is very slow (**delayed union**) and occasionally it fails to occur (**non-union**). In non-union the fibrous tissue may become very dense, hyaline and finally fibro-cartilaginous. The appearance of an area of eosinophilic fibrinoid necrosis is followed by a linear split which may enlarge and eventually develop a lining similar to synovium, thus forming a false joint (**pseudarthrosis**) (Fig. 4.22). The bone ends buried in the dense fibrous tissue tend to become very sclerotic.

Later stages: final remodelling

Once bony union has occurred and function has been regained, the bone begins to be remodelled in response to mechanical stresses. If the fracture has united at an angle new bone is incorporated on the concave side while

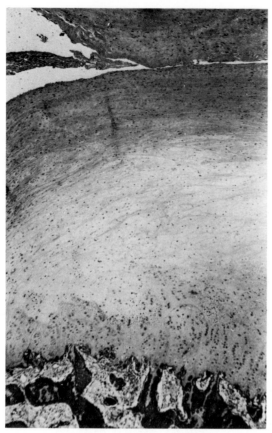

Fig. 4.22 Pseudarthrosis following fracture of the clavicle. The bone ends have become covered by cartilage. At the top of the picture a split in the cartilage has occurred giving a false joint. There is endochondral ossification of the proliferated cartilage in the lower part of the picture. × 40.

resorption occurs on the convex, so that the bone becomes straighter. In any event excessive callus is resorbed, slowly formed lamellar bone begins to replace the hastily laid down woven bone, and any remaining necrotic bone is removed and replaced (Fig. 4.23). The cortex is re-formed across the fracture gap and gradually medullary callus is removed and the marrow cavity is restored. The whole process may take about a year and is more rapid and complete in children.

General factors and bone healing.

Some of the local factors affecting bone healing have already been mentioned but, as in wound healing, general factors are also important. Lack of vitamin C results in depression of both fibroblastic and osteogenic activity so that collagen and bone production are both deficient. Glucocorticosteroids administered to animals with fractures also delay healing but it seems that they have little effect when given to patients in the usual therapeutic doses. In vitamin D deficiency abundant callus may form, but it fails to calcify, remaining soft until the deficiency is made good.

Primary union of fractures

Although primary union of soft tissues is the rule in clean sutured surgical incisions, primary union in bone is a curiosity. It entails bony union with the formation of only minimal amounts of callus and was first described in compression arthrodesis (i.e. excision of the joint) of the knee, the cancellous surfaces of femur and tibia being held together by compression clamps. Bony union occurs in about 4 weeks and biopsy shows only a thin line of new bone at the contact points of opposing trabeculae. While moderate compression forces may assist union of a fracture, rigid fixation and close apposition of surfaces are probably the major factors. Cortical fractures in dogs, produced by a very fine saw with minimal necrosis, and fixed by a compression plate, have united without periosteal callus. The necrotic ends of the cortical bone were not resorbed but blood vessels entered the Haversian canals and subsequently the bone ends in contact were joined by new osteones (Haversian systems) which involved both bone fragments. At the opposite cortex from the compression device a small amount of new bone, formed from the endosteal cells of the Haversian canals, filled the narrow gap between the fragments and was later replaced by osteones. The healing process is similar to normal bone remodelling. Although a patient with a rigidly fixed fracture can be mobilised early, the more extensive bone necrosis results in slow healing since it depends on the formation of medullary callus and the direct replacement of cortical osteones.

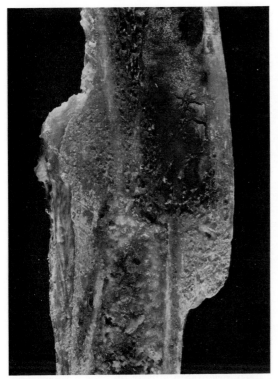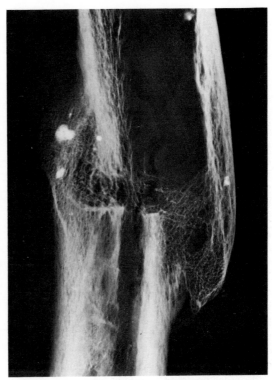

Fig. 4.23 This fracture through the midshaft of the femur united with anterior shift of the proximal fragment. Eighteen months after fracture there is firm bony union. The slab radiograph shows how the provisional callus has become remodelled along lines of stress with buttressing of the posterior and slightly concave part of the fracture line and some retubulation in the medullary canal at the fracture site.

Repair of some other tissues

Repair of articular cartilage

There is evidence that articular cartilage remains metabolically active throughout life, with continuous turnover of the proteoglycans and collagens of the matrix. Following injury, chondrocytes may proliferate to form cell clusters and there is an increase in proteoglycan turnover. However the capacity to form new collagen is limited and it is exceptional for these intrinsic reactions to produce any significant filling in of cartilage defects.

Extrinsic repair may occur by the growth of fibrous tissue over the articular surface from the joint margin. When there is loss of the full depth of the cartilage, fibrous tissue growing from the underlying marrow, through cracks in the exposed subchondral bone plate, may cover the bone end. This collagenous tissue may then acquire a more chondroid matrix, to become fibrocartilage, and is sometimes able to function reasonably well. However, the amount of new tissue formed by extrinsic repair is usually insufficient and of poor quality, especially when the defect is large, so that joint function is only partly restored and tends to deteriorate.

Repair of tendon

A good functional result following healing of a severed tendon requires a strong fibrous union between the ends without loss of a full range of gliding motion. In patients with sutured tendons, repair occurs by ingrowth of fibroblasts and blood vessels from surrounding connective tissue into the fibrin meshwork between the sutured ends. The cells, at first randomly arranged, later become orientated along the line of the tendon and produce collagen fibres. The amount of collagen synthesised is increased for some weeks after injury and, as in a healing wound, there is subsequent remodelling of the fibrous scar. The extrinsic source of vessels and cells during the healing process makes the formation of adhesions inevitable, but a good range of movement is retained when the adhesions are long and consist of loosely arranged areolar tissue. Restricted movement is associated with short adhesions containing large bundles of collagen fibres. Rough operative handling is thought to promote the formation of such adhesions, but little is known of other factors concerned.

Recent experimental evidence suggests that fibrocytes of tendon are not necessarily inert, but have the intrinsic potential for carrying out repair and remodelling without the formation of adhesions. It may be that it is the surgical suture of the severed ends which, by disturbing the local blood supply, impairs this response and makes healing dependent on extrinsic sources. Unfortunately suture is essential to hold the severed ends together and allow union to occur.

Repair of muscle

(a) Skeletal muscle. When muscle fibres are damaged, the sarcoplasm of dead fibres disintegrates, and this is followed by phagocytosis of the fragments by macrophages. Regeneration of muscle occurs in two ways. Firstly, by the formation of multinucleated sprouts (Fig. 4.24) from the surviving ends of injured fibres. It has been estimated that these sprouts advance into the damaged area at a rate of less than 1 mm/day. Secondly, by the growth of mononucleated myoblasts. The origin of these cells is controversial. Regeneration may be complete when the endomysial tube remains intact as in **Zenker's hyaline degeneration**. This condition may accompany severe toxic infections, especially typhoid fever, and tends to involve most severely the muscles of the abdominal wall, diaphragm and intercostals. When the connective and supporting tissue in muscle is also torn or destroyed, as in more severe injuries, regeneration is less well orientated and a

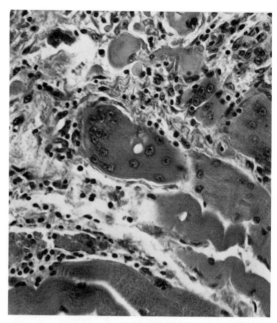

Fig. 4.24 Wounded skeletal muscle, showing sarcoplasmal sprouts with multiple nuclei. × 200.

scar composed of fibrovascular tissue and irregularly orientated muscle fibres is formed. This is seen, for example, in Volkmann's ischaemic contracture (p. 930)

(b) Visceral muscle (smooth muscle). The healing of visceral muscle, e.g. in surgical incisions in the bowel or uterus, occurs by fibrous repair. Although smooth muscle may be seen in recently differentiated arterioles (p. 80) and in atheromatous plaques (p. 367), its origin is uncertain and it may arise by migration of smooth muscle cells or by differentiation from other mesenchymal cells. Proliferation with mitotic activity is said to occur in the early months of the physiological uterine enlargement of pregnancy.

(c) Cardiac muscle. Destruction of cardiac muscle by infarction is repaired by fibrous tissue (Fig. 15.11, p. 405). Effective regeneration occurs in young patients with Coxsackie virus infections or diphtheria, where there is damage to individual fibres with preservation of the endomysium, a situation similar to that of Zenker's degeneration in skeletal muscle.

Repair of nervous tissue and nerves

Central nervous tissue. Once mature nerve cells of the brain, cord or ganglia are destroyed, they are not replaced by the proliferation of other nerve cells. There is also no useful regeneration of the axons in the central nervous system: indeed when an axon is severed at any point, the entire axon and the nerve cell body degenerate. Of the neuroglial cells, proliferation in response to tissue damage is restricted to astrocytes, this being referred to as gliosis (p. 728).

Regeneration of peripheral nerves. In contrast to the nerve cells and fibres in the central nervous system, peripheral nerves have considerable regenerative capacity.

When a nerve is transected, the axis cylinders distal to the cut undergo Wallerian degeneration, i.e. the axon and its myelin sheath break down and the debris is absorbed by macrophages. At the same time the Schwann cells proliferate within the neurilemmal sheath to form pathways along which the axons may regrow. Above the level of transection, myelin degeneration extends upwards only to the first or second node of Ranvier and the nerve cell body characteristically shows reversible changes (central chromatolysis p. 726). Axonal sprouts soon emerge from the proximal ends of the interrupted axis cylinders and, if the cut ends of the nerve are in close apposition, they grow into the distal part of the nerve and along the spaces formerly occupied by axis cylinders and now filled with proliferated Schwann cells. The axons grow at a rate of about 3 mm per day. These new axons, which at first are very thin, develop a new myelin sheath and then increase in diameter. They do, however, remain smaller than normal nerves unless they establish satisfactory end-organ connections and functional relationships. This takes some time, and restoration of function is accordingly slow and often imperfect.

A feature of regenerated nerves is that the internodal segments are shorter than in normal nerves.

The degree of functional recovery in a damaged peripheral nerve depends principally on the severity of the injury. If nerve fibres only are disrupted and the other components of the nerve trunk remain intact, as in a crush injury and sometimes in a stretching injury, regenerating axons can grow along their original endoneurial tubes, continuity of which is preserved and these fibres can re-establish their original end-organ relationships. If there is considerable disorganisation of the internal structure of individual nerve bundles within the nerve trunk, the continuity of endoneurial tubes is less likely to be preserved: fibrosis then occurs within the damaged segment and interferes with the growth of axons from the proximal segment of the damaged nerve. Some axons never traverse the fibrous barrier, while those that do almost never grow along their original endoneurial tubes. Thus many axons fail to reach their original end-organ and abnormal and incomplete innervation results. When there is subtotal or complete loss of continuity of the nerve trunk, the proliferation of axonal sprouts, fibroblasts and Schwann cells from the proximal end of the nerve results in the formation of a so-called **traumatic** or **stump neuroma** (Fig. 4.25).

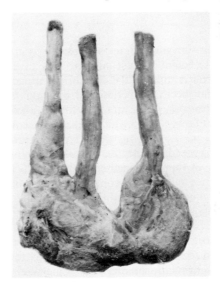

Fig. 4.25 Traumatic neuroma at severed proximal ends of nerves of an amputated arm.

In severely damaged nerves, surgical repair after excision of the involved segment or the traumatic neuroma is often the only hope of achieving any functional recovery, but some residual disability almost invariably persists.

Repair of mucosal surfaces

Cells which line mucosal surfaces, are being lost and replaced continuously throughout life and, like all surface epithelia, have a good potential for regeneration (Fig. 4.26). In general, the raw surface is first covered and only later is there differentiation into more specialised cells.

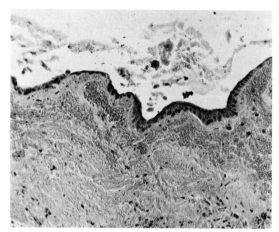

Fig. 4.26 Repair of lining of gallbladder after acute inflammatory desquamation. The epithelial cells extend as a thin flattened layer to reline the viscus. × 150.

(a) Gastro-intestinal tract mucosa. Physiological replacement of lost surface cells takes place by proliferation of the cells of the mucosal glandular necks. Experimental excision of an area of mucosa, in the stomach for instance, is rapidly followed by re-epithelialisation: epithelial cells of the mucous neck type migrate over the exposed connective tissue, forming first a layer of thin, flattened epithelium, which later becomes cubical or columnar. The epithelium of glands adjacent to the wound undergoes mitosis, as do surface cells, and this proliferation keeps up the supply of migrating cells until the surface is covered. Gland crypts reform by mucous cells growing down into the underlying granulation tissue and, some weeks later, specialised cells, e.g. parietal cells, differentiate from the mucous cells in the crypts. Failure of re-epithelialisation of chronic peptic ulcers (p. 613) is not fully understood. Wounds of the mucous membranes following surgical anastomosis heal readily, and the line between the two different types of mucosa remains sharp.

Rectal lesions heal slowly with formation of much granulation tissue, but the small and, to a lesser extent, the large bowel mucosae have a good capacity for regeneration (Fig. 19.51d, p. 624). Repeated ulceration and repair of the colon, as for instance in ulcerative colitis and bilharzial infestation, may lead to overgrowth of the reparative mucosa, producing polypoid projections (Fig. 19.69, p. 638).

(b) Respiratory tract mucosa. The basal cells of the tracheal and bronchial lining epithelium proliferate throughout life and replace loss of the surface ciliated epithelium. Many microbial infections result in loss of only part of the thickness of the pseudostratified columnar epithelium, and this is readily replaced by cell proliferation. Destruction of the whole thickness of the mucosa is followed by the usual pattern of migration and proliferation of cells which at first appear transitional and later become low columnar: eventually the superficial cells develop cilia. Destruction of subepithelial tissue or repeated damage, e.g. in chronic bronchitis, may result in less perfect regeneration, the ciliated cells being replaced by columnar non-ciliated mucus-secreting cells, and under very unfavourable circumstances, as in heavy cigarette smoking, metaplasia (p. 441) of the regenerating epithelium to squamous type may be seen.

(c) Urinary tract mucosa. The urinary tract mucosa, like the epidermis, responds to injury by movement and proliferation of cells. The transitional cell epithelium of the bladder has particularly good powers of rapid regeneration, all layers of the mucosa participating.

Repair of kidney

The glomerulus is a highly specialised unit and little effective regeneration follows damage. Lost renal substance is replaced by fibrous tissue. If the basement membrane of the tubules remains intact, damage to tubular epithelium may be followed by proliferation (Fig. 4.27) and slow migration of surviving cells to restore continuity. It is doubtful, however, whether, when the damaged cells are highly specialised, as in the proximal convoluted tubule, the regenerated cells have the same degree of functional efficiency.

Repair of the liver

The hepatic parenchymal cells form a fairly stable population, and few mitotic figures are seen in the normal liver. Replacement of normal 'wear-and-tear' cell loss is by division of neighbouring cells. Some replacement is effected by division of the nucleus and enlargement of the cell, which explains the occurrence of binucleate and multinucleate liver cells, particularly in elderly individuals.

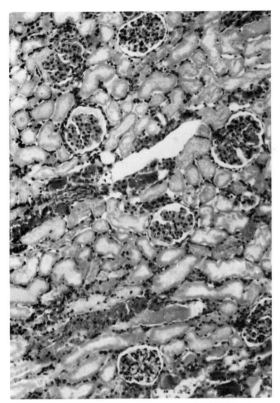

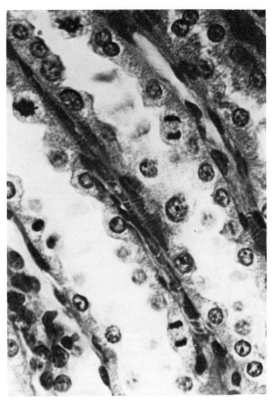

Fig. 4.27a Acute tubular necrosis in the rat. Note the anatomical normality of the glomeruli and the absence of nuclei in the dead tubular epithelial cells. × 150.

Fig. 4.27b Regeneration of renal tubular epithelium following acute tubular necrosis in the rat. Four mitotic figures are present. The adjacent regenerated cells are still of subnormal size. × 450.

Wounds of the liver are repaired by formation of connective tissue, with minimal replacement of parenchymal cells around the margin of the wound.

The outcome of liver cell necrosis depends on the distribution of the cells affected and also upon the presence or absence of an intact vascular system. Occlusion of hepatic arterial branches may be followed by infarction of liver tissue: as in most other tissues, coagulative necrosis occurs and the dead tissue is digested by macrophages and replaced by organisation (see below), eventually leaving a fibrous scar. Necrosis of individual liver cells scattered throughout the lobules, as in the typical attack of virus hepatitis, is followed by autolysis and disappearance of the dead cells, which are replaced by proliferation of surviving cells with restoration to normal. Even when there is destruction of all the parenchymal cells in the centres or mid-zones of the lobules the periportal cells proliferate and extend into the surviving vascular framework so

that normality is once again achieved. If, however, there is loss of most or all of the hepatocytes through the whole substance of the lobules, proliferation of the surviving hepatocytes leads only to irregular nodules of regeneration, the lobular pattern being lost. The vascular framework in the areas depleted of parenchymal cells becomes collapsed and scarred (Fig. 4.28).

The very high regenerative capacity of liver cells has been demonstrated by subjecting animals to excision of various amounts of liver tissue. After excision of two-thirds of the rat's liver, hypertrophy and hyperplasia in the remaining third result in restoration of a normal liver mass in 15–20 days. The capacity of the liver to regenerate in this way is maintained even when partial hepatectomy is performed monthly for up to one year.

The factors which regulate the extent of liver regeneration are not understood. When partial hepatectomy is performed upon one member of a pair of parabiotic rats, hepatocyte prolifera-

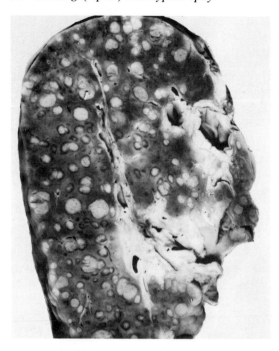

tion occurs in both animals. This and similar experiments suggest that a humoral mediating factor is responsible for hepatic regeneration. More recent studies in dogs suggest that a humoral growth-stimulating factor is responsible for hepatic regeneration and is released by regenerating liver. If the portal vein is divided and anastomosed to the inferior vena cava before partial hepatectomy, regeneration of parenchyma is impaired, and it thus seems that portal venous flow through the liver affects the degree of restoration. There is evidence that insulin plays a major role in maintaining normal functioning of liver cells and in promoting hepato-cellular proliferation. This makes good sense of the drainage of pancreatic venous blood to the liver and not to the systemic venous system.

Fig. 4.28 Following extensive liver necrosis there has been proliferation of surviving liver cells. These form the pale rounded nodules lying in a background of scar tissue from which dead liver cells have now disappeared.

Organisation

This means the replacement, by fibrous tissue, of solid, non-living material such as fibrin, clotted blood, intravascular thrombus and dead tissue. The process involves the gradual digestion of the material by macrophages. Since these phagocytic cells can only operate within a short distance of capillaries, removal of more than a small amount of dead material requires the ingrowth of capillaries and fibroblasts. This formation of granulation tissue is similar to that in healing, and the term organisation is used only when inanimate material is replaced by it.

An example already familiar is the removal of **fibrin deposited in acute inflammation** (p. 66). Thin strands of fibrin are rapidly phagocytosed and digested, but larger deposits, for example the thick layer which forms on the pleural surface in some cases of pleurisy, are removed more slowly by organisation. After the acute inflammation has subsided monocytes continue to emigrate from the vessels in the pleura underlying the adherent fibrin and

assume the features of macrophages: they begin to digest the fibrin by a combination of phagocytosis and release of lysosomal enzymes. Capillary sprouts develop from the superficial pleural vessels and grow into the spaces created by the macrophages (Fig. 4.29): they anastomose to form a network of capillaries, some of which enlarge and develop into arterioles and venules. The capillaries are accompanied by proliferating fibroblasts which produce collagen and ground substance. A thin layer of granulation tissue thus takes the place of the deepest part of the fibrin and gradually the process extends until all the fibrin has been replaced. Meanwhile, the granulation tissue slowly changes to less vascular, firm fibrous tissue. If the layer of fibrin has glued together the visceral and parietal pleura, organisation proceeds from both surfaces and meets in the middle: in consequence, the lung becomes firmly bound to the chest wall by fibrous tissue.

A second example of organisation is seen when haemorrhage occurs into the tissues and

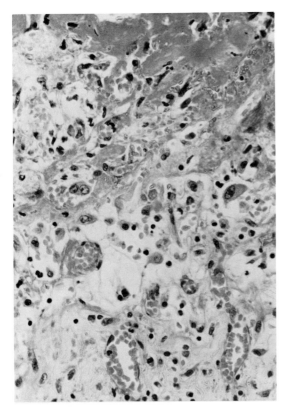

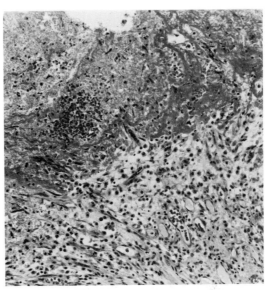

Fig. 4.30 Organisation of a haematoma after 7 days. Capillary sprouts are beginning to grow into the clot and there are also large numbers of macrophages at its margin. × 80.

Fig. 4.29 Dilated capillaries and fibroblasts are beginning to grow into the dense fibrin on the surface of the lung. × 400.

the escaped blood clots to form a solid mass, i.e. a **haematoma**. This is removed by organisation from the surrounding tissues (Fig. 4.30) and progresses to the centre of the clot, even-

tually leaving a fibrous scar. A patch of **necrotic tissue** (most commonly seen in the heart, brain, kidneys, etc. as the result of arterial blockage by thrombus, i.e. an infarct) is similarly removed by organisation with consequent scar formation.

When an artery or vein is blocked by **thrombus**, this is removed partly by organisation, but other processes are involved and the fate of thrombi is described on pp. 241–3.

Hypertrophy

Stimulation of the parenchymal cells of an organ, usually by increased functional demand or by hormones, results in an increase in the total mass of the parenchymal cells. This may be brought about by enlargement of the cells— **hypertrophy** or by an increase in their number—**hyperplasia**. The relative importance of the two processes varies in different organs. In some, e.g. the skeletal muscles, enlargement is purely by hypertrophy, but in most organs hypertrophy and hyperplasia both contribute.

(a) The response to increased functional demand

This is illustrated by the hypertrophied **muscles** of manual labourers and athletes; the individual fibres increase in thickness but not in number. Similarly, when extra work is demanded of the **heart** as a result of valvular disease or high blood pressure (Fig. 4.31), there may be much thickening of the muscular walls of those chambers which bear the brunt of the extra work. Narrowing of the mitral valve, for example, produces chiefly left atrial and right

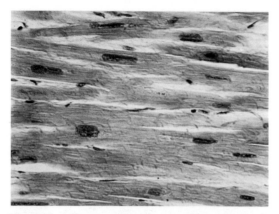

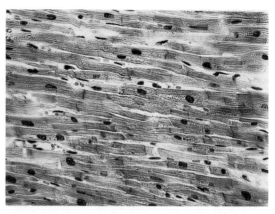

Fig. 4.31a Hypertrophied muscle fibres of heart in a case of arteriosclerosis with high blood pressure. × 250.

Fig. 4.31b Slightly atrophied heart muscle; to compare with Fig. 4.31a. × 250.

ventricular hypertrophy, whereas systemic hypertension gives rise predominantly to left ventricular hypertrophy (Fig. 15.1, p. 399). The heart may increase to twice the normal weight, the degree of hypertrophy being limited by the diffusion of oxygen and nutrients between the capillaries and the thickened fibres. **Smooth muscle** may also undergo hypertrophy, for example in the wall of the stomach in a patient with pyloric stenosis, in large bowel proximal to an obstructing tumour (Fig. 19.81, p. 653), or in the bladder when the outflow is narrowed by an enlarged prostate (Fig. 25.3, p. 992). The muscle in arterial walls also hypertrophies in response to long continued high blood pressure (Fig. 14.13, p. 371). The most striking hypertrophy is seen in the pregnant uterus, where a combination of increased functional demand and hormonal stimuli results in enlargement of fibres to more than a hundred times their original volume. In early pregnancy, there may be both hypertrophy and hyperplasia of muscle fibres. After parturition, the muscle fibres return to a normal size and this is seen also in hypertrophied heart muscle when the increased work stimulus is removed.

In some instances, the response to an increased demand is by a pure hyperplasia; for instance, blood loss is not followed by enlargement of red cells and leukocytes but by an increase in their production in the haemopoietic marrow (Fig. 17.9b, p. 517).

Compensatory hypertrophy may occur in the survivor of a pair of organs when one is removed. Following nephrectomy, the remaining kidney enlarges and, particularly in young patients, may double its weight. This is brought about by increase in the size of the nephron as a result of both hypertrophy and hyperplasia of the component cells of the glomeruli and tubules. Removal of one adrenal leads to hypertrophy of the cells of the opposite cortex, the medulla remaining unchanged. Following removal of a lung, the remaining lung enlarges but this is caused mainly by over-distension, which produces a lasting enlargement of the alveoli; only when it occurs in early life is there any formation of new alveoli. Compensatory hypertrophy is a widespread natural phenomenon, as illustrated in Fig. 4.32.

The testes are exceptional in that, in both man and animals, removal of one in adult life is not followed by enlargement of the other, the number of spermatozoa produced being reduced.

(b) Hypertrophy due to hormonal changes

A balanced activity of certain of the endocrine glands is essential for the normal growth and metabolism of the tissues and many of the examples of hypertrophy and hyperplasia already mentioned require the continued physiological action of the growth hormone of the anterior pituitary as well as an adequate blood supply. Excessive secretion of growth hormone (usually due to a tumour of the oxyphil cells of the anterior pituitary) results in adults in acromegaly (p. 1010) with bone enlargement and generalised organ and tissue hypertrophy. This is

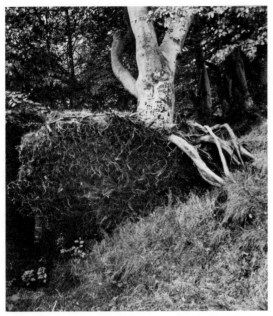

Fig. 4.32 This beech tree was largely uprooted by a gale six years before, and has since leant against its neighbour. It continues to survive because a few roots (on the right) have retained contact with the soil and have become greatly hypertrophied.

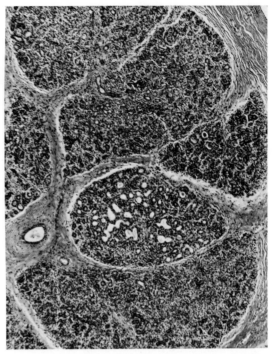

Fig. 4.33 Breast lobule in pregnancy showing marked hypertrophy and hyperplasia. × 50.

even more strikingly seen when the excess of hormone occurs in adolescence, before the skeleton matures; the result is gigantism (p. 1011). An example of physiological hormonal hypertrophy is the enlargement of the breasts in pregnancy, when the formation of mammary gland acini is stimulated chiefly by hormones from the corpus luteum or placenta (Fig. 4.33).

Further Reading

Guber, S. and Rudolph, R. (1978). The myofibroblast. *Surgery, Gynecology and Obstetrics* **146**, 641.

Hunt, T. K. and Van Winkle, W. Jr. (1976). *Fundamentals of Wound Management in Surgery. Wound Healing: Normal Repair.* Distributed by Smith Kline and French Laboratories.

Jackson, D. S. (1978). Collagens. In *Diseases of Connective Tissue*, pp. 44–8. Ed. by D. L. Gardner. Publ. by *Journal of Clinical Pathology*.

Matthews, P. and Richards, H. (1974). The repair potential of digital flexor tendons. An experimental study. *Journal of Bone and Joint Surgery* **56B**, 618.

McKibbin, B. (1978). The biology of fracture healing in long bones. *Journal of Bone and Joint Surgery* **60B**, 150.

Sevitt, S. (1970). Bone repair and fracture healing. *British Journal of Hospital Medicine* **3**, 693.

5

Immunophysiology: The Immune Response

Introduction

The invasion of the body by living organisms, including viruses, bacteria, and protozoan and metazoan parasites, presents a major threat to the stability of the internal milieu upon which Claude Bernard placed such importance. To counter this threat certain general defence mechanisms have evolved—a relatively impermeable epidermis, methods of ridding the body of noxious material, such as vomiting, diarrhoea and coughing, the dilution of irritants by increased flow of interstitial fluid in inflammatory oedema, and the destruction of particulate matter by phagocytic cells. In addition, there exists in vertebrates a special defence mechanism of immense potential which is mobilised when the body is invaded by foreign organisms and which is expressly and specifically adapted to overcome the effects of any particular invader. The special mechanism is called **acquired specific immunity** and its study—the science of **immunology**—is of great importance in the understanding and prevention of disease.

The phenomenon of acquired specific immunity has been recognised for centuries in that individuals who had survived an attack of certain clearly recognisable infectious diseases such as smallpox were known to be much less susceptible to the disease during a later epidemic. Such individuals could be said to show **immunity** (i.e. protection) against the disease, **acquired** inasmuch as it did not apparently exist before the first infection, and **specific** inasmuch as an attack of smallpox protected the individual against a further attack of smallpox but had no bearing on his susceptibility to later attacks of measles, diphtheria, etc.

This knowledge has been applied with great success to the prevention of infectious disease by prophylactic immunisation, a procedure in which a relatively harmless variant, or modified toxin, of a pathogenic organism is purposely introduced into the body; this results in the development of specific immunity such as would be encountered following recovery from the natural disease. The principle is well illustrated by Edward Jenner's use of fluid from the lesions of cowpox (vaccinia) to vaccinate against smallpox; it was known to Jenner that milkmaids who had had natural cowpox infection had developed not only markedly altered reactivity to re-infection with cowpox but also resistance to a first infection by smallpox, a closely related but much more serious disease. In this case the two viruses are so similar that immunity to one is effective also against the other.

When an individual has become immune following natural infection or prophylactic exposure to a pathogenic organism or its toxin he is said to be **actively immunised** against that organism. Specific resistance to infection can in many instances be conferred upon a non-immune individual by an alternative method, namely the injection of *serum* or *lymphoid cells* from an actively immune individual. The state of **passive immunity** so conferred is not due to transfer of the infecting organism or its toxin but to the transfer of the products of immunisation developed by the actively immunised donor of the serum or lymphoid cells. The *passive transfer* of immunity thus provides a way of analysing the factors which contribute to the immune state, and by transfer experiments it has been shown that in some instances specific immunity results from the presence in the serum of special globulins known as **antibodies**, while in other cases the immune state seems to be mediated directly by **specifically primed (sensitised) lymphocytes** without the participation of serum antibody. Serum containing one or more antibodies produced by active immunisation is termed **antiserum** or **immune serum**.

There is obviously considerable survival advantage in having the ability to acquire specific

102

immunity to pathogenic organisms or their toxins. Unfortunately the specifically altered reactivity produced by an immune response can lead to reactions which result in tissue injury. This can happen following exposure even to relatively harmless substances, such as grass pollen, which on subsequent contact causes a harmful and seemingly unnecessary inflammatory reaction in certain individuals. Such **acquired specific hypersensitivity** has in many cases been shown to be due to reactions of an immunological nature although with its connotation of protection the word 'immune' appears unsuitable. Because of this difficulty and the gradual way in which knowledge of the complex processes involved has unfolded, an elaborate but imprecise jargon relating to immunology has developed and many authors have used the same terms with different meanings. Von Pirquet, for example, coined the word **allergy** as a unifying term to indicate *altered* specific reactivity of all kinds, including both protective immune responses and also hypersensitivity. Despite this the words allergy and hypersensitivity are frequently used interchangeably.

In this book we follow the current common practice of using the words 'immune' and 'immunity' in two distinct ways: in one they are general terms to embrace all forms of specifically altered reactivity (i.e. allergy in von Pirquet's sense) and in the other they refer to specific protection against disease; we believe that the meaning implied will be evident from the context.

Antigens

An antigen is a substance which is **immunogenic**, i.e. capable of evoking an immune response: this may take two main forms.

(1) Antibody production, i.e. the appearance of globulin molecules which have the property of combining specifically with and remaining attached to antigen of the same kind as that which has led to their formation.

(2) Cell-mediated immunity, i.e. the production of specifically primed lymphocytes whose presence can be demonstrated *in vivo* by the development of a local inflammatory reaction appearing about 24 hours after intradermal injection of the antigen—a **delayed hypersensitivity reaction**.

Most antigenic stimuli evoke both cell-mediated immunity and antibody production. These responses take place in the lymphoid tissues, and their products, specifically primed lymphocytes and antibody, both capable of reacting with the antigen, are released into the bloodstream.

Under certain conditions, an antigenic stimulus may induce a state of **specific immunological tolerance**, i.e. non-responsiveness to subsequent challenge with the same antigen.

The term '*immunological reaction*' should not be confused with '*immune response*' as described above. An **immunological reaction** is the effect observed when the products of the immune response—antibody or primed lymphocytes—encounter and combine with the appropriate antigen *in vitro* or *in vivo*.

Factors affecting the immune response

The form taken by the immune response depends upon several factors including the nature of the antigen, the genetic constitution of the individual exposed to the antigen, the route by which the antigen enters the body and the dose administered. These factors are discussed below.

The nature of antigens. It is difficult to define precisely the properties which make a substance capable of evoking an immune response, but in general terms antigens are large molecules, usually of molecular weight exceeding 3000, fairly rigid in structure, and either protein or carbohydrate, with or without associated substances such as lipids. Antigen–antibody reactions appear to be the result largely of stereochemical interactions of molecules of complementary configurations, analogous to the interaction of lock and key. For this reason floppy molecules such as gelatin are poor antigens. Evidence will be presented later that immune responses follow the binding of antigen molecules to specific receptors on the surface of lymphocytes. It seems likely that, to trigger off an immune response, antigen must form a link between these surface receptors: this explains why most antigens are large molecules.

Although some small molecules, such as para-aminobenzoic acid, are not by themselves antigenic, they may become so if they are attached to larger molecules. Injection of *p*-aminobenzoic acid attached by diazotisation to serum albumin may result in formation of some antibody molecules which combine specifically with the *p*-aminobenzoic acid moiety and not with the albumin carrier protein. In these circumstances, *p*-aminobenzoic acid is said to be a **hapten**, i.e. a substance which is antigenic inasmuch as it can take part in an immunological reaction (in this case antigen–antibody combination) but which is not itself immunogenic, i.e. cannot by itself evoke an immune response (in this example, the formation of specific antibody) unless it is conjugated with macromolecular material. The existence of such simple haptens suggests that the antigenic specificity of large molecules may be determined by the three-dimensional configuration of small parts of these molecules (**antigenic determinant sites** or **epitopes**). Study of synthetic polypeptide and polysaccharide antigens has confirmed that specific antigenic determinant sites do consist of a few amino acids or monosaccharides, and it has been shown that most naturally-occurring macromolecules such as plasma albumin contain several antigenic determinant sites of differing specificity. Larger, complex antigenic particles, such as bacteria, contain a correspondingly greater number and variety of epitopes. Both antibody production and cell-mediated immunity evoked by antigenic material are correspondingly complex, each particular kind of epitope being potentially capable of inducing both types of response.

Genetic constitution of the individual. The repertoire of specific immune responses which an individual can mount depends on the selection of genes inherited from two distinct sets— the V genes which code for the various antigen binding sites found on different antibody molecules (pp. 126–8) and the Ir (immune reactivity) genes which are not linked with (i.e. on the same chromosome as) the genes coding for antibodies, but lie in the 'I' region of the major histocompatibility complex (p. 167). The genetic nature of the responsiveness is clearly shown by crossing inbred strains of mice which exhibit marked differences in their responses to immunisation with substances containing only one type of epitope, such as simple synthetic oligo-peptides. Inheritance of specific responsiveness to most natural antigens is difficult to demonstrate because of the multiplicity and variety of antigenic sites on natural macromolecules but the magnitude of response to these substances is controlled non-specifically by a number of genes, some affecting such characters as rate of antigen degradation by macrophages (pp. 134–6).

Genetic factors also play a large part in determining the antigenicity of tissues, and this field has become particularly important in the practice of blood transfusion and of tissue transplantation. The molecular composition of tissues, including potential antigenic sites, is, of course, genetically determined. In general, when tissues are injected or transplanted from one individual to another, the more genetically dissimilar or foreign the two individuals are to each other, the easier it is to induce antibody formation and cell-mediated immunity. For example, human red cells injected into rabbits evoke a wide variety of antibodies reacting with a corresponding variety of antigenic determinants on the human red cell; when, as in this case, the antigen is derived from a species other than that of the immunised animal (and this would include bacteria, etc.), it is called a **hetero-antigen** and the antibodies are **hetero-antibodies**. Injection or transplantation of one human with the red cells or tissue cells of another may result in the formation of antibodies to antigenic groups not shared by both individuals; e.g. human red cells containing the Rhesus antigen D (Rhesus positive cells) into a person whose cells do not contain this antigen (Rhesus negative) may result in the development of antibodies specific for D antigen; antigens which differ within a species are called **iso-antigens** and the corresponding antibodies **iso-antibodies**. In general, iso-antigens are much less numerous and less likely to evoke an immune response than hetero-antigens. Finally it should be noted that injection of an individual with his own cells (**auto-antigen**) results in **auto-antibody** formation or cell-mediated immunity only in exceptional cases; the subject of **auto-immunity** is considered further on p. 161. Unfortunately the prefixes used to indicate the relationship between individuals providing antigen and forming antibody are, by usage,

Table 5.1 Terminology of antigens, antibodies and tissue grafts

Relationship between donor and recipient	Genetic terminology	Antibody, antigen	Transplantation terminology
Same animal	—	Auto-antibody Auto-antigen	Autograft
Identical twins and inbred strain	Syngeneic (Isogeneic)	—	Isograft
Same outbred species or different inbred strains	Allogeneic	Iso-antibody Iso-antigen	Allograft (Homograft)
Different species	Heterogeneic Xenogeneic	Hetero-antibody Hetero-antigen	Xenograft (Heterograft)

different from those used in the more recent field of tissue transplantation, in which graft rejection is effected mainly by delayed hypersensitivity reactions. Table 5.1 summarises this confusing and irrational situation.

As stated above, the cells and tissues of an individual are antigenic when injected or grafted into an animal of another species or even into a different individual of the same species, yet with certain exceptions the individual does not react to the antigens of his own cells by the development of auto-antibody or delayed auto-hypersensitivity. Non-reactivity to auto-antigen is a general physiological principle described by Ehrlich as 'horror autotoxicus'. It may reflect absence of lymphoid cells with the genetic coding necessary for the synthetic processes associated with formation of antibody or cell-mediated immunity against most 'self' components, analogous to the inherited non-reactivity of certain strains of animals to synthetic polypeptide antigens. Burnet has,

however, suggested an attractive alternative explanation, that the various potential antigens in an individual's tissues do act on the cells responsible for immune reactions but that, instead of causing antibody formation or cell-mediated immunity, they lead during fetal life to specific immunological tolerance. The subject is, however, a complex one; it is considered more fully on p. 132.

Route of administration of antigen. In most cases antigens elicit an immunological response only when they are introduced parenterally (i.e. not through the alimentary canal) so that their macromolecular state and the configuration of their antigenic determinants are not destroyed by digestion in the gut. Traces of certain proteins, such as those in heterologous milk, may, in fact, be absorbed from the gut and bring about specific sensitisation, especially in infants. In general, however, antigens introduced via the portal circulation are less immunogenic than when adminstered by other routes.

Antibodies

Antibody molecules have the special property of combining specifically with antigen or hapten. In so doing they may cover up harmful areas on molecules of toxin, in which case they are said to be **antitoxins**, or their combination with cells such as bacteria may lead (with the help of complement—p. 144) to death and lysis of the bacteria (**bacteriolytic effect**) or phagocytosis by polymorphs and macrophages (**opsonic effect**). Chemically, antibodies belong to the **immunoglobulin (Ig)** proteins of the plasma (for-

merly called γ-globulins because of their predominant electrophoretic mobility); and there are five classes: IgG, IgM, IgA, IgD and IgE. All immunoglobulins are composed of one or more similar units, each unit consisting of two pairs of identical polypeptide chains (Fig. 5.1); one pair, termed the **heavy chains**, are about twice the size (molecular weight) of the other pair, which are termed the **light chains**. Digestion of an Ig molecule by papain breaks it into three fragments, of which two are identical and

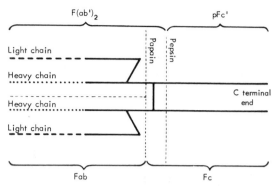

Fig. 5.1 Structure of monomeric immunoglobulin molecule. In any one molecule the two light chains have an identical amino-acid sequence and so also have the heavy chains. Each immunoglobulin class has a distinctive Fc piece (C terminal end of heavy chains). The amino-acid sequence of the interrupted portions of the light chains and dotted portions of heavy chains (the N-terminal ends) vary greatly among immunoglobulin molecules even of the same class and constitute the specific antigen-binding (Fab) sites, of which there are two on each molecule. The constitution of these variable regions of an Ig molecule is also known as the idiotype. (The light lines indicate separation of the molecules into an Fc and two Fab fragments by papain digestion, and into one F(ab′)₂ and two pFc′ fragments by pepsin.)

are termed **Fab** (antigen-binding fragments) because each contains a combining site for antigen. The third fragment consists of the C-terminal ends of the heavy chains, and is termed **Fc** fragment; it is readily obtained in crystalline (hence Fc) form. As shown in Fig. 5.1, digestion of IgG by pepsin frees two pFc′ fragments but leaves the two Fab fragments united by part of the Fc fragment as a single fragment—F(ab′)₂. Heavy chains differ structurally for each class of Ig, and the letters γ, μ, α, δ, ε, are used to indicate the heavy chains of IgG, IgM, IgA, etc. respectively. By contrast, there are only two types of light chain, κ and λ, in all Ig classes, and each Ig molecule has *either* κ *or* λ light chains. Differences in the behaviour of antibodies of the same specificity, but of different Ig classes, and of the four sub-classes of IgG (IgG 1–4), are determined by the properties of the Fc part of their heavy chains.

The combination of antibody with antigen is believed to be achieved by hydrogen bonding, electrostatic, hydrophobic and van der Waal's forces; all of these are effective over a very short range and hold separate molecules together only when they fit snugly. The specificity

of antigen–antibody union therefore depends on the antibody combining-site having a complementary shape to the antigenic determinant which permits the necessary close fit. The shape of the combining site is determined by the amino-acid sequence of the N-terminal ends of the heavy and, to a lesser extent, of the light chains. In view of what is now known of protein synthesis this is of great interest and of fundamental importance in elucidating how antigenic stimulation gives rise to specific antibody formation. In contrast to most other proteins, each one of which in a given individual is of uniform amino-acid sequence, the immunoglobulins in a serum show marked heterogeneity of their N-terminal regions (the **variable regions**), the number of variations amounting to millions. This variety is responsible for the great range of antibodies which can develop in response to stimulation by an enormous number of different antigens.

Some idea of the specificity of antibody–antigen union can be gained from study of antibody against chemically defined haptens. Landsteiner, for example, showed that antibody raised against para-aminobenzene sulphonic acid does not combine with the ortho-form but gives a weak reaction with meta-aminobenzene sulphonic acid (Fig. 5.2). The

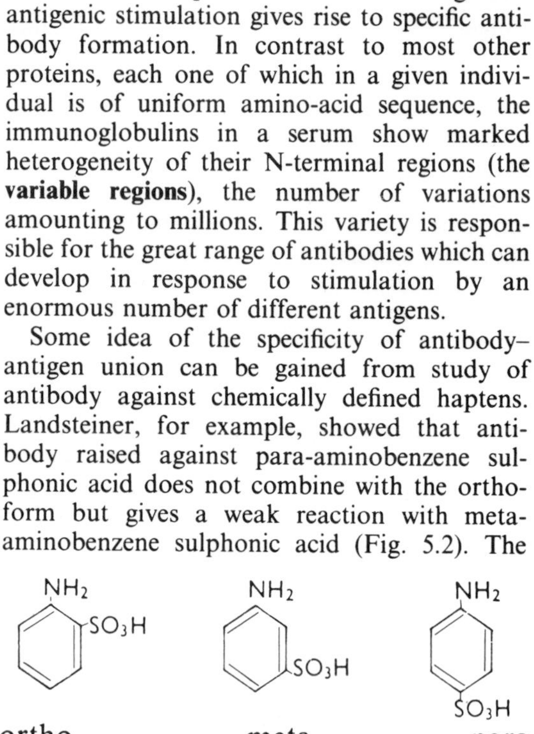

NH₂ ... SO₃H   NH₂ ... SO₃H   NH₂ ... SO₃H

ortho   meta   para

Fig. 5.2 Isomeric forms of aminobenzene sulphonic acid.

latter is called a cross reaction and it implies immunological reactivity with an antigen different from that which has led to the production of antibody. It results from the production of some antibody molecules which fit the cross reacting antigen sufficiently well to permit intermolecular attraction by short-range forces (see above). The closeness of fit between the antigen-binding sites of antibody with an antigen of given configuration can thus vary and this affects the firmness of combination; we therefore speak of high or low **affinity** of antibody for a given epitope. Cross reactions are generally of low affinity.

When an antiserum contains a variety of

antibodies reacting with multiple and often heterogeneous epitopes on a macromolecular antigen, the strength of the binding together of antigenic molecules by antibodies is referred to as the **avidity** of the antiserum; this is influenced not only by the affinities of each of the various antibodies reacting with individual epitopes, but also by the number of antigen–antibody linkages formed: although individual antibody–epitope linkages dissociate, those which fit snugly dissociate less readily than poorly-fitting linkages, and large numbers of firm linkages will result in the maintenance of avid binding.

Quite apart from their specific reactivity with antigens, antibodies of different classes possess properties which depend on the Fc part of the heavy (μ, γ, α, etc.) chains. These class distinctions are described on pp. 108–9.

The production of antibody

Injection of an antigen to which an individual has not previously been exposed results in a **primary antibody response**, i.e. the transient appearance in the blood of a small amount of specific antibody, mainly of IgM class, about seven days after the injection. Re-injection of the same antigen at a later date leads to a **secondary** or **anamnestic** (remembering) **response** in which large amounts of specific antibody, most of which is usually of IgG class, appear in the blood rapidly (in four days or so) and continue to be produced, although in gradually diminishing amounts, for weeks, months or even years. The greatly enhanced antibody production of the secondary response is the reason for the repeated injections of microbial antigens (vaccines) widely used in prophylactic immunisation.

Most of the antibody found in serum is produced by plasma cells in lymph nodes, spleen and bone marrow but some may also be formed by plasma cells in the lymphoid tissue of the gut and in the inflammatory lesion which forms around injected antigenic material. **Plasma cells** (Fig. 5.3) are ovoid cells, somewhat larger than small lymphocytes, and with a small round nucleus in which granules of chromatin are regularly spaced around the periphery, giving a 'cart-wheel' or 'clock-face' appearance. Their cytoplasm is basophilic and also pyroninophilic, indicating a high content

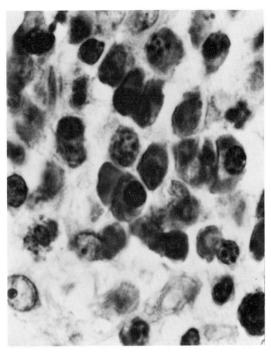

Fig. 5.3 Plasma cells in a lymph node draining a focus of infection. Note the eccentrically-placed, round nucleus with clumping of chromatin, and the deeply-stained (basophilic) cytoplasm showing, in some instances, a crescentic area of pallor alongside the nucleus. × 1000.

of ribonucleic acid, and electron microscopy (Fig. 5.4) reveals a large amount of complex rough endoplasmic reticulum of the type found in cells which synthesise and secrete protein. It has been shown by immunofluorescence that each plasma cell at any given time produces light chains together with heavy chains of only one immunoglobulin class (e.g. IgG or IgM). Furthermore, *following stimulation with two distinct antigens (e.g. diphtheria and tetanus toxins) individual plasma cells will produce antibody to one or the other but not to both of these antigens.*

An additional polypeptide, **the J chain**, is synthesised by plasma cells producing IgM and IgA. It links together the basic 4-chain units of IgM and IgA to form polymers (see below).

Properties of the immunoglobulin classes

The various immunoglobulin classes have different functions (beyond that of specific com-

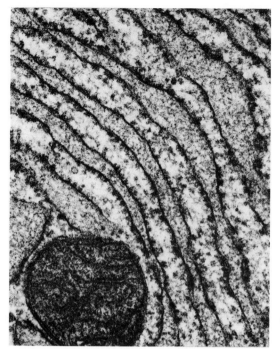

Fig. 5.4 Electron micrograph of part of the cytoplasm of a plasma cell, showing the abundant rough endoplasmic reticulum. Part of a mitochondrion is also included. × 108 000.

bination with antigen, which is common to all) and this is determined by the structure of the part of the heavy chains included in the Fc fragment.

When immunoglobulin of a particular class is injected into animals of another species it acts as an *antigen*, and antibodies specific for the light and for the heavy chains appear in the serum of the injected animal. Combination of the latter antibody with immunoglobulin *in vitro* provides a simple method of demonstrating the class to which a particular immunoglobulin belongs, for example by immunoelectrophoresis (p. 111).

Table 5.2 compares some of the features of the five known immunoglobulin classes. **IgG** is present in the plasma and extravascular spaces in the largest amount. IgG antitoxins are of importance because they combine with and neutralise toxins, thus protecting the individual from their harmful effects. There are receptors for the Fc part of IgG antibodies on polymorphs and macrophages which facilitate adherence and phagocytosis of the corresponding antigens. The reaction of IgG antibody with the

corresponding antigen can usually be demonstrated *in vitro* (see below): it can cross the human placenta and in this way passive immunity is transferred from mother to child. The four sub-classes of IgG (1–4) differ somewhat in their properties, e.g. capacity to acti-

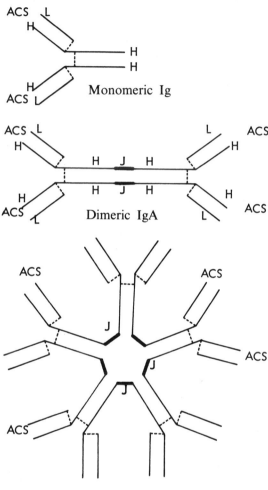

Fig. 5.5 The structure of immunoglobulins. The monomeric Ig molecule consists of two heavy and two light chains (*upper and Fig. 5.1*). IgA (*middle*) is secreted as a dimer, consisting of two monomeric units joined by J chains (heavy lines). Secretory IgA also contains a secretory piece (not shown). *Lower*, the pentameric IgM molecule, consisting of five monomers joined by J chains. Note that each unit has two antigen-combining sites (ACS), so that IgA dimer has four and IgM ten. (The heavy chains of Ig are angulated at the so-called hinge region, so that the unit molecule is Y-shaped: this is not shown in Fig. 5.1.)

vate complement (see below). These differences are referred to later in relation to topics in which they are of importance. **IgM**, a macroglobulin consisting of pentamers of the basic four-chain units or monomers (each of which has two antigen-combining sites) linked by J chains (Fig 5.5), is the first Ig class of antibody to be produced following the initial introduction of an antigen. Because of its 10 combining sites, it is usually of high avidity: it is especially effective in activating complement (see below), and its reactions are readily demonstrated *in vitro*. Except in inflammatory lesions, it is largely confined to the plasma, where it has an important function in destroying micro-organisms. The presence of IgM antibody, e.g. to rubella virus, indicates recent or continuing exposure to that antigen. **IgA** is secreted locally by plasma cells in the intestinal mucosa, the lacrimal glands, respiratory passages and salivary glands. It is secreted by the plasma cells in the form of a dimer, the two molecules being linked by a J chain. Such locally produced IgA is taken up by the glandular and lining epithelial cells of these tissues and coupled with a carbohydrate 'transport piece' which renders it more resistant to digestive enzymes. In this form it is secreted in the tears, saliva, alimentary and salivary mucus, etc. and forms a lining, sometimes referred to as 'antiseptic paint', over the alimentary and respiratory mucous membranes and conjunctiva. IgA activates complement by the alternative pathway and may enhance the bacteriolytic activity of lysozyme (p. 175). It is also present in the plasma in the form of monomers and dimers. **IgE** has the special property of attaching to tissue, particularly to mast cells and basophils, by means of its Fc fragment, leaving the specific combining sites (on the Fab fragments) available for union with antigen. If such union takes place, pharmacologically active substances such as histamine are released, with the production of an anaphylactic hypersensitivity reaction within a few minutes (p. 146). The biological properties of **IgD** are unknown, but it acts as a lymphocyte surface antigen-receptor (pp. 125, 128).

Table 5.2 Size and plasma (or serum) concentrations of immunoglobulins

Class	Molecular weight (daltons)	Degree of polymerisation	Concentration (normal serum) g/litre
IgG	150 000	Monomer	8–16
IgM	900 000	Pentamer	0·5–2
IgA	Mainly 150 000	Mono- and dimer	1·4–4
IgD	185 000	Monomer	0–0·4
IgE	200 000	Monomer	$2–45 \times 10^{-7}$

Demonstration of antigen–antibody reactions

This section and the following one on demonstration of cell-mediated immunity are largely of a technical nature and are intentionally brief. To some extent, they interrupt the account of the immune response which continues on p. 114. They do, however, illustrate the practical aspects of what might otherwise seem to be largely an academic subject. Accordingly, the reader is advised not to skip them.

The demonstration of antigen–antibody reactions is applicable equally to the detection and assay of antigen by means of a known antibody and of antibody by means of a known antigen.

Antigen–antibody reactions in vivo may be demonstrated in three ways.

(1) A potentially harmful antigenic substance may be rendered harmless by union with antibody and not have the expected effect. For example, in the Schick test, intradermal injection of a small amount of diphtheria toxin into the skin of a non-immune individual results in an area of inflammation. The diphtheria antitoxin present in an immunised individual neutralises the toxin and so suppresses the inflammation. Similarly, antibodies to pathogenic micro-organisms may be demonstrated by their capacity to protect experimental animals against a lethal dose of the micro-organism.

(2) A normally harmless stimulus may result in tissue injury, i.e. a hypersensitivity reaction. For example, inhalation of grass pollen may induce an attack of hay fever or asthma, mediated by its reaction with antibody specific

for grass pollen. In this instance, the antibody is usually of IgE class, but hypersensitivity reactions may result from the union *in vivo* of other classes of antibody with antigen: they are of considerable importance in disease processes and are described in Chapter 6.

(3) In the special instance of antibodies which react with antigenic constituents of the host cells, death of the target cell may result, e.g. destruction of lymphocytes by anti-lymphocyte serum. There are also rare examples of antibodies which alter the physiological activity of target cells, e.g. increased secretion of thyroxin as a result of the reaction of auto-antibody specific for the TSH-receptor of thyroid epithelium. By binding to the receptor, the antibody has the same effect as TSH.

Antigen–antibody reactions in vitro may be demonstrated in various ways, depending on the nature of the antigen and the type and amount of antibody present.

(1) Visible aggregation of antigen. Since each antibody molecule has at least two combining sites it can bind with two or more antigen molecules. If the antigen molecules contain several antigenic determinants, and if they are in solution, antibody can form cross-linkages between antigen molecules, uniting them in the form of a lattice (Fig. 5.6): if antigen and antibody molecules are present in optimal combining proportions the aggregates will be large (Fig. 5.6a) and visible as an insoluble precipitate (**precipitin reaction**). Lattice formation and therefore precipitation can be inhibited when an excessive amount of antigen saturates the combining sites on all the antibody molecules, and smaller complexes may then be formed (Fig. 5.6b). Conversely, when gross excess of antibody is present (Fig. 5.6c), each antigen combining site may fix a separate antibody molecule, and, once again, the complexes may be too small to form a visible precipitate (**prozone effect**). Optimum antigen–antibody proportions for lattice formation can readily be achieved by allowing antibody and antigen to diffuse towards each other through agar (Ouchterlony technique, Fig. 5.7). The interpretation of agar diffusion tests involving antiserum raised against a complex mixture of antigens (as when human serum is injected into rabbits) is facilitated by partial separation of the constituent antigens by electrophoresis prior to the precipitin reaction; this method, called

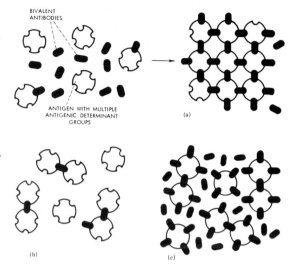

Fig. 5.6   The reaction of antigen and antibody (a) in optimal proportions to form large aggregates: (b) in antigen excess: (c) in antibody excess. In (b) and (c) small complexes are formed. In the case of soluble antigens, large aggregates form as in (a), and produce a precipitate, whereas with particulate antigens, e.g. bacteria, formation of aggregates is termed agglutination.

immunoelectrophoresis, is illustrated in Fig. 5.8.

When the antigen molecules are associated with a large particle, e.g. the antigenic determinants of the surface of a red cell or bacter-

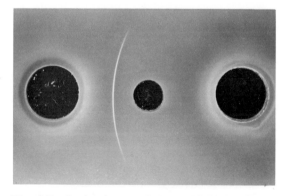

Fig. 5.7   Ouchterlony technique. The central well contains a solution of antigen. The well on the left contains the corresponding antiserum, and that on the right a negative control serum. A white line of precipitate, composed of antigen–antibody complex, has formed between the antigen and antibody wells. In this instance the antigen is thyroglobulin and the test detects auto-antibody to thyroglobulin in the serum of a patient with chronic thyroiditis.

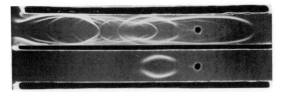

Fig. 5.8 An illustration of the use of immunoelectrophoresis to detect antigens. A mixture of antigens (in this case human serum in the upper well) is subjected to electrophoresis in agar. Antiserum (rabbit antiserum to whole human serum) is then placed in the trough and diffusion allowed to proceed. Each antigen reacts with the corresponding antibody to form an arc of precipitation, the position of which depends on the electrophoretic mobility of the antigen. Use of a single purified antigen (in this case the C3 component of human complement in the lower well) helps to determine whether that antigen is present in the mixture. The upper and middle troughs contain antiserum to whole human serum and the lower trough antiserum to human C3.

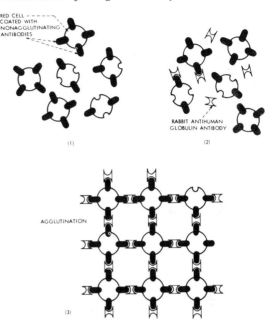

Fig. 5.9 Antigenic particles sensitised with a non-agglutinating antibody are agglutinated by antibody to immunoglobulin (antiglobulin reagent).

ium, or are adsorbed artificially onto red cells or latex particles, antibody causes aggregation of the particles (**agglutination reaction**). The visible aggregation of large particles such as bacteria can be effected by minute amounts of antibody.

(2) **Methods using anti-immunoglobulin.** In certain circumstances antibody combines with antigen without causing aggregation. This may occur if the spatial arrangement of the antigen (e.g. the Rhesus antigen on the surface of red cells) prevents the divalent IgG antibody molecule from combining simultaneously with antigenic determinant groups on two different red cells. In these circumstances, exposure of the Rhesus positive red cells to anti-Rhesus antibody merely results in their being coated with IgG. However, the coated cells can be agglutinated by antibody against IgG (**antiglobulin** or **Coombs' reaction**) (Fig. 5.9).

A similar principle is used in the **indirect immunofluorescence (indirect fluorescent antibody) technique** to detect insoluble antigen (e.g. bacterial capsular polysaccharide) in a histological section or smear. When this is exposed to antiserum the antibody combines with antigen without visible effect. The slide is washed to remove the antiserum, leaving only the specific antibody which is, of course, an immunoglobulin, attached to the antigen present in the section. Antibody to immunoglobulin, conjugated with a fluorescent dye such as

fluorescein isothiocyanate, is then applied to the section or smear and the site of antigen–antibody combination is visualised by the presence of the fluorescent antiglobulin when the section is examined microscopically with ultraviolet light (Figs. 5.10, 5.11). In the **direct immunofluorescence technique** the tissue or cells are washed to remove free immunoglobulins and treated directly with fluorescein-conjugated antiglobulin reagent. This demonstrates the binding of antibody (or the deposition of antigen-antibody complexes) *in vivo*. More recently, analogous techniques have been introduced in which antibody is labelled with the enzyme *peroxidase* instead of with a fluorescent dye; peroxidase can be localised as a dark deposit by ordinary light microscopy after appropriate histochemical treatment.

(3) **Methods using radioactive antigen.** In the Farr technique, which is valuable in measuring antibody to soluble antigen, excess antigen labelled with radioisotope is added to antiserum; the immunoglobulin (including antigen–antibody complexes) is then precipitated by 50 per cent saturation with ammonium sulphate. Provided that the free antigen (uncombined with antibody) is not salted out by this

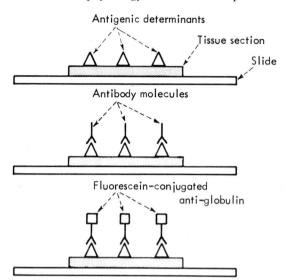

Fig. 5.10 The indirect immunofluorescence technique performed on a tissue section. *Top*, tissue section on slide. *Middle*, section treated with antibody (⋏) to a tissue constituent and washed: antibody molecules adhere to the tissue antigen. *Bottom*, section treated with fluorescein-conjugated antibody (☐) to immunoglobulin: sites of antigen–antibody reaction fluoresce in ultraviolet light.

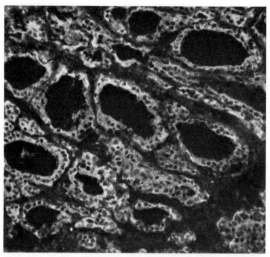

Fig. 5.11 A positive indirect immunofluorescence test for antibody to thyroid epithelium. A frozen section of thyroid tissue has been treated with the serum undergoing test (from a patient with chronic thyroiditis), followed by treatment with fluorescein-conjugated anti-human-IgG. Note fluorescence of the thyroid epithelial cytoplasm. (U.V. microscopy.)

procedure, the amount of radioactivity precipitated is proportional to the amount of antibody in the serum.

In the **antiglobulin coprecipitation technique** the amount of antibody to a given radioactive antigen can similarly be measured by precipitation with class-specific anti-Ig antibody instead of by a salting out procedure.

Numerous very sensitive radioimmunoassays have been devised for the measurement of antigen or antibody. For example, the concentration of insulin in the plasma may be measured by mixing the plasma with anti-insulin and radioactive insulin in standard amounts, and determining how much radioactive insulin is excluded, by the plasma insulin, from combining with antibody.

(4) Methods involving damage to cells. Antibody combined with antigen on the surface of intact cells such as bacteria or erythrocytes can damage the cell membrane and cause lysis (partial dissolution) of the cells which is readily demonstrable. The lysis is mediated by a complex group of at least twenty factors present in fresh normal serum and known collectively as **complement** (p. 142). These factors are activated by the Fc portions of IgM and IgG anti-

bodies which have combined with antigen, and once activated they give rise to a chain of enzyme reactions culminating in digestion of the cell membrane where the antibody is attached. In the course of the reaction complement is used up, or 'fixed'.

(5) Complement fixation. Complement is fixed in many antigen–antibody reactions in addition to those involving cell-surface antigens. Invisible antigen–antibody reactions can often be demonstrated indirectly by allowing them to occur in the presence of a measured amount of complement and subsequently adding an indicator system, namely red cells coated with a 'haemolytic' antibody i.e. one which causes red cell lysis only in the presence of complement. Fixation of complement by the invisible antigen–antibody reaction prevents haemolysis in the indicator system (Fig. 5.12). A more detailed account of complement is given on p. 142.

(6) Blocking antibody. In certain circumstances (usually poorly defined), antibody can combine invisibly with antigen which thereby becomes unavailable for participation in a subsequent visible immunological reaction such as agglutination or cytotoxic damage. The presence of blocking antibody in a serum can thus be demonstrated by a two-stage test.

Mix antigen and antibody	Add complement (C)	Add sensitised RBC
Positive test $Ag^x + Ab^x \longrightarrow Ag^x\!-\!Ab^x$ (union)	$+ C \longrightarrow Ag^x\!\!\underset{\underset{\text{(complement used up)}}{C}}{\rule{0pt}{1em}\top}\!\!Ab^x$	No lysis
Negative test $Ag^x + Ab^y \longrightarrow Ag^x + Ab^y$ (no union)	$+ C \longrightarrow Ag^x + Ab^y + C$ (complement not used)	Lysis

Fig. 5.12 The complement fixation reaction depends on the 'fixation' of complement by an antigen–antibody complex (upper line). The fixation of complement is demonstrated by non-lysis of subsequently added red cells coated with a haemolytic antibody. If there is no antigen–antibody reaction (lower line), complement is not used up and lyses the sensitised red cells.

Demonstration of cell-mediated immunity

As noted on p. 103, immune responses to most antigens induce not only the production of antibody but also cell-mediated immunity (CMI), i.e. the production of specifically primed lymphocytes which are capable of reacting with the inducing antigen. When such lymphocytes encounter the antigen, they release biologically-active compounds termed *lymphokines* (p. 157), one of which causes an acute inflammatory reaction, while another immobilises macrophages. The reacting lymphocytes also enlarge and undergo mitosis and stimulate mitosis in other lymphocytes. Tests for CMI are based on such changes. It is demonstrated most readily *in vivo* by intradermal injection of the antigen, which leads to an indurated erythematous lesion in the dermis maximal in 24–72 hours—the **delayed hypersensitivity reaction**. During the development of the lesion there is early but transient emigration of polymorphs, followed by an increasing accumulation of lymphocytes and some macrophages around venules, hair follicles and sweat glands: this is accompanied by inflammatory hyperaemia and oedema (Fig. 6.8, p. 158). CMI may also be demonstrated in animals by injecting the antigen into the cornea which becomes opaque 24–48 hours later as a result of migration of mononuclear cells into it. These sites are convenient for eliciting delayed hypersensitivity reactions, but all tissues are reactive, for the sensitised small lymphocytes circulate through the blood and lymphoid tissues and can migrate into any tissue.

A classical example of CMI is that which develops to tuberculoprotein in most individuals who are (or have been) infected with *Mycobacterium tuberculosis* or following inoculation with BCG (an attenuated strain of *Mycobacterium bovis*). The Mantoux test (p. 157), in which more or less purified tuberculoprotein is injected intradermally, is a classical delayed hypersensitivity reaction.

Skin tests with appropriate antigens may be used similarly to test for CMI to various other micro-organisms, including viruses and fungi. They are also useful to elicit CMI to certain simple chemicals which, when applied to the skin, act as haptens and by combining with skin proteins become immunogenic: examples include *p*-phenylene diamine (in some hair dyes) and nickel salts (derived from nickel clasps on underwear, etc.): once CMI has developed, further application of the chemical to the skin results in an inflammatory lesion known as *contact dermatitis*, which is simply a delayed hypersensitivity reaction.

CMI may also be demonstrated *in vitro* by observing the effect of the appropriate antigen on living cells from an immune individual. For example, if leukocytes are placed in a capillary tube immersed horizontally in tissue culture medium, the cells migrate from the open end of the tube: such migration is inhibited by adding the antigen to the tissue culture medium. Secondly, when lymphocytes from the blood of an immunised individual are maintained in culture in the presence of the antigen, a proportion of them transform into larger cells (lymphoblasts) with basophilic cytoplasm, synthesise DNA and undergo mitosis. Addition of radio-active thymidine to the culture medium and subsequent determination of its incorporation into DNA is a method of assessing the transformation. Such *in vitro* methods are being used increasingly to demonstrate CMI to various micro-organisms and other antigens.

A further method of determining the capacity of experimental animals to develop CMI consists in the application of a tissue allograft or xenograft; CMI normally develops to such foreign tissue and plays an important role in its destruction by the host: failure to reject a foreign skin graft is thus evidence of deficient CMI.

In experimental work it is sometimes useful to induce in animals CMI to soluble proteins and other antigens which, when injected alone, usually induce antibody production but only feeble CMI: the latter may be enhanced greatly by mixing the antigen with killed *Myco. tuberculosis*, other mycobacteria, or a peptidoglycolipid extracted from the walls of such organisms and injecting it in the form of an emulsion containing droplets of light mineral oil (Freund's type of 'adjuvant').

It should be noted that the demonstration of CMI *in vivo* is by elicitating a delayed hypersensitivity reaction which is a destructive lesion and may, if severe, progress to necrosis. Delayed hypersensitivity reactions occur naturally, e.g. in various infections and in contact dermatitis, and are responsible for most of the tissue injury in tuberculosis. CMI does, however, afford protection against various micro-organisms, notably viruses, fungi and many of the bacteria which cause chronic infections. This is well illustrated by children with congenital agammaglobulinaemia who cannot produce antibodies and yet overcome most viral infections normally unless they are also deficient in CMI.

The Cellular Basis of the Immune Response

So far, this account has concentrated mainly on describing the usual products of antigenic stimulation, i.e. antibodies and specifically-primed lymphocytes, capable of reacting with the antigen. We must now consider in detail the cellular events involved in these responses.

The cytology of immunological phenomena is complex but is worth studying in some detail, not only because of the vital importance of specific immunity, but also because it illustrates the complexity of the systems by which eukaryotic cells communicate with one another and co-ordinate their activities. Most of the advances have been based on the manipulation of cells and tissues of experimental animals, but the features of immune responses and of naturally occurring immunodeficiency states in man, the effects of therapeutic immunosuppression, and investigation of human lymphocytes *in vitro* all indicate that the same basic rules apply.

The main features of the cellular basis of antibody production and cell-mediated immunity may be summarised as follows.

1. Cell-mediated immunity and antibody production are both attributable to lymphocytes capable of recognising and responding specifically to the stimulus provided by an antigen, i.e. **specifically-responsive lymphocytes**.

2. At some stage in their development, lymphocytes become **'committed'**, i.e. capable of responding only to a particular antigenic determinant group, or to closely similar determinant groups. Lymphocyte populations thus consist of individual cells which differ in the antigens to which they can respond. In consequence, no one antigen can stimulate a response in more than a small proportion of them.

3. The specifically responsive lymphocytes which bring about cell-mediated immunity are **thymus-dependent** or **T lymphocytes**. They develop from stem cells in the thymus under the influence of a thymic hormone and many of them leave the thymus and reach the various other lymphoid tissues.

4. On encountering an antigen to which it is specifically responsive, the T lymphocyte proliferates in the lymphoid tissues to produce a clone of lymphocytes, all of which are capable of reacting with that antigen—**specifically-primed T lymphocytes**. These are responsible for delayed hypersensitivity reactions.

5. The specifically-responsive lymphocytes which bring about antibody production are **thymus-independent** and are termed **B lymphocytes**. In mammals, they develop from stem cells in the haemopoietic tissue from which many of them migrate and pass to the various other lymphoid tissues.

6. On encountering an antigen to which it is specifically responsive, the B lymphocyte, like the T lymphocyte, proliferates in the lymphoid tissues to form a clone of cells capable of reacting with that antigen. Some cells of the clone differentiate into plasma cells and secrete antibody which also is capable of reacting with the antigen. The plasma cells are thus derived from B lymphocytes.

7. Some of the lymphocytes produced by antigen-induced proliferation of T and B lymphocytes persist as **memory cells**. In other words, antigenic stimulation increases the number of T and B lymphocytes capable of reacting with that antigen, and some of these lymphocytes are long-lived and are responsible for a secondary response on subsequent stimulation by the antigen.

8. Although T lymphocytes do not give rise to antibody-producing plasma cells, they co-operate with B cells in antibody responses, and such co-operation enhances the production of antibody to most antigens, and is essential for some antibody responses. T lymphocytes can also have a suppressive effect on immune responses.

9. In some circumstances, antigenic stimulation results in neither antibody production nor cell-mediated immunity, but renders the individual specifically unresponsive to subsequent challenge by that antigen. This unresponsive state is termed **acquired immunological tolerance**. It provides an explanation of why we do not usually respond strongly to antigens in our own cells and tissues, and it plays an important role in successful transplantation of foreign cells and tissues.

These basic features of immune responses are considered more fully below.

The specifically responsive lymphocyte

For the development of specific immunity, it is necessary that cells should recognise specific determinant sites (epitopes) on antigenic molecules, and should respond to them in ways that lead to the production of antibodies and primed lymphocytes, both of which are capable of reacting specifically with the antigen. Much of the credit for demonstrating that these cells—the keystones of the immune response—are lymphocytes, is due to Gowans and others (see Gowans, 1966). They used techniques in which lymphocytes were removed from rats by thoracic duct drainage. By drainage for several days, the cell-free fluid being returned to the rat, depletion of a population of small lymphocytes was achieved and the depleted rats were found to be defective in their responses to antigenic stimulation. For example, when challenged by injection of sheep erythrocytes or tetanus toxoid they made poor antibody responses, and when grafted with skin from an allogeneic rat they did not reject the graft, indicating failure of the normal cell-mediated response to the graft antigens. These immunological deficiencies were corrected by injection of small lymphocytes from the thoracic duct of a normal rat, and when the donor had been previously immunised, e.g. by a skin allograft or an injection of sheep erythrocytes, the recipient showed the rapid and intense response to antigenic challenge which is characteristic of the secondary response. These observations suggested that small lymphocytes in thoracic duct lymph are essential for primary immune responses, and showed more conclusively that they include specifically responsive cells resulting from a previous immune response, i.e. immunological memory cells (thus explaining the rapidity of the secondary response). Gowans' findings have since been confirmed by many other workers and have been shown to apply to several mammalian and avian species. Animals depleted of lymphocytes by various other methods (p. 121) have also been shown to be immunologically deficient and the deficiency is corrected by injection of lymphocytes from normal animals. Moreover, in such experiments it has been shown by cell labelling techniques that the donated lymphocytes proliferate and give rise to the plasma cells which produce antibody and the lymphocytes responsible for cell-mediated immunity.

By such experiments, it has been firmly established that, *in both primary and secondary immune responses, the cells capable of recognising the antigen and of responding specifically to it by production of antibody or cell-mediated immunity, are lymphocytes.*

The origin of lymphocytes: the primary lymphoid organs

Evidence is presented below that the thymus is the original source of a major population of lymphocytes termed **thymus-dependent** or **T lymphocytes**, and that there is a second population of lymphocytes which, in birds, arises in a pouch-like outgrowth of the hind-gut, the *bursa of Fabricius*. In mammals, this second population, termed **B lymphocytes**, originates mainly, and probably solely, in the haemopoietic tissue. Production of lymphocytes in the thymus and haemopoietic tissue occurs spontaneously, being quite independent of antigenic stimulation, and they are commonly called the **primary lymphoid organs**.

The origin of T lymphocytes: the thymus

Development. The thymus develops from bilateral epithelial ingrowths of the endoderm of the 3rd and 4th branchial arches accompanied by mesenchyme which is probably of ectodermal origin. In most mammals, these ingrowths fuse to form a single organ. Meanwhile some of the haemopoietic stem cells, developing in the yolk sac and migrating into the blood, settle in the thymus where they proliferate rapidly and differentiate into lymphocytes. The thymus now appears as a lobulated organ (Fig. 5.13) in which the outer or cortical layer is crowded with proliferating lymphocytes lying in a network of epithelial cells. In the inner or medullary layer, lymphopoiesis is less active and there are aggregates of epithelial cells (Hassall's corpuscles).

Colonisation of the thymus by stem cells from the blood has been demonstrated by tissue-culture studies of embryonic thymic tissue and by thymus grafting experiments. For example, Le Douarin (1977) and others showed that when the epithelial thymus

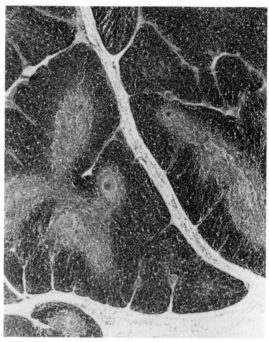

Fig. 5.13 Thymus in childhood, showing lobulation and division into cortex (darker areas) and medulla. × 30.

of an early Japanese quail embryo was implanted for two days in a chick embryo,* and then transferred back to a quail embryo, the lymphocytes first developing in it were of chick origin, derived from stem cells in the blood which settled in the graft during its sojourn in the chick embryo. Subsequently stem cells from the second (quail) host settled in the graft, and quail lymphocytes developed in it.

By other cell transfer experiments it has been shown that stem cells capable of colonising the thymus originate in haemopoietic tissue, appearing first in the yolk sac, then in the fetal liver and subsequently in the bone marrow.

Similar experiments with mice, using chromosomal morphological markers to distinguish between

*These two species were chosen because their lymphocytes can be distinguished morphologically.

donor and host lymphocytes, have led to the same conclusions.

Function. Until quite recently the thymus was an organ of mystery. Unlike the other lymphoid tissues (lymph nodes, spleen, tonsils, etc.) it is not a site of significant immune responses following exposure to antigen, and the proliferation of lymphocytes in the thymic cortex, which is maximal around the time of birth but continues throughout life, is quite independent of antigenic challenge. This suggested that the thymus supplies lymphocytes, but many lymphocytes produced in the cortex die *in situ*, their nuclear debris being conspicuous in macrophages, and export of thymic lymphocytes remained for long no more than a likely possibility. Nor did early studies of thymectomy elucidate thymic function, for no important immunological effects were observed.

The important clue to thymic function came from the observation by Good and his coworkers (1964) and others that congenital immunological deficiency states in man were sometimes associated with thymic abnormalities. Miller (1964) then demonstrated that mice thymectomised *at birth* failed to thrive and commonly died of a wasting disease since shown to be due mainly to infections. The thymectomised mice were shown to be defective in cell-mediated immune responses and in their antibody responses to some antigens. They were also deficient in lymphocytes in the blood, thoracic duct lymph, and parts of the lymph nodes, spleen, tonsils, etc. These deficiencies were soon shown to be prevented, or completely and permanently corrected, by a syngeneic thymus graft, while lymph node or spleen cells from normal mice were partially restorative. Similar deficiencies occur spontaneously in an inbred strain (*nu nu*) of mice with thymic aplasia.

It thus appears that, in mice, the presence of the thymus is necessary for the development of a major population of lymphocytes which are responsible for cell-mediated immune responses and which also influence antibody production. By preparation and use of suitable antisera, mouse thymocytes have been shown to exhibit various surface antigens, some of which (e.g. θ or Thy-1 antigens) are shared by many of the lymphocytes in the blood, lymph and other lymphoid tissues. It is these lymphocytes with 'thymic markers' which fail to develop following neonatal thymectomy or in *nu nu* mice;

accordingly they are termed the **thymus-dependent** or **T lymphocytes**, and mice lacking them are sometimes termed *'B' mice*.

The same immunological and T-cell deficiencies as occur in mice have been shown to follow neonatal thymectomy in several other species, and can be prevented or corrected by thymus grafts. In man, the T lymphocyte population develops long before birth, but congenital failure of thymic development (p. 170) is associated with the same features as neonatal thymectomy in mice.

It has also been demonstrated in a number of species that, in conditions much closer to the physiological state than in the experiments described above, the thymus supplies lymphocytes to the other lymphoid tissues. This was done by injecting ^{3}H-thymidine into the thymus, so that it became incorporated in the nuclei of dividing thymocytes: labelled lymphocytes were subsequently detected by auto-radiography in the other lymphoid tissues.

Thymic function in the adult. As the thymus slowly involutes following puberty, its lymphopoietic activity diminishes but does not cease entirely, even in old age. The diminishing importance of the thymus is illustrated by performing thymectomy in mice after the neonatal period: the longer it is delayed, the less its effect. This is clearly because the thymus provides much of the T-lymphocyte population shortly after birth. Even in adult mice, however, thymectomy has some effect, for a year or more later the mice show deficient cell-mediated immunity as illustrated by reduced capacity to reject a skin allograft. Similarly in man, thymectomy in young adults (performed therapeutically in patients with myasthenia gravis) has no immediate immunological effect, but defective cell-mediated immunity and a diminution in T lymphocytes in the blood has been reported in patients examined 15 or more years later.

In spite of its involuted state in the adult, the thymus remains capable of replacing the whole T-lymphocyte pool. This is demonstrated by subjecting mice to a dose of x-irradiation which destroys virtually all the body's lymphocytes and haemopoietic stem cells, and administering bone marrow cells to restore the haemopoietic tissue. Regeneration of the T lymphocytes (from haemopoietic stem cells) is dependent on the presence of the thymus and is prevented by concomitant thymectomy.

The thymus thus produces and exports T

lymphocytes (Fig. 5.14). This occurs maximally during fetal life or shortly after birth (depending on species). Thymectomy before production of the T-lymphocyte population results in a virtual absence of T cells and consequent severe immunological deficiencies. The thymus continues to supply T lymphocytes after birth but this function becomes progressively less important with age, the T-lymphocyte population, which includes much of the individual's immunological experience stored in memory cells, becoming increasingly self-sufficient.

Thymic lymphopoietic hormone. There is evidence that the thymus produces a hormone, '**thymosin**', which stimulates differentiation and proliferation of T lymphocytes. This was first suspected when implantation of thymic tissue enclosed in cell-proof diffusion chambers was found to restore partially the T-lymphocyte population of neonatally thymectomised mice. Subsequently, extracts of thymic tissue have been shown to have a similar effect, and similar activity has been detected in normal human and mouse plasma, but is absent following thymectomy. According to Bach, *et al.* (1975), the plasma activity in man decreases with age, an

observation which accords well with the normal process of thymic involution. It thus seems likely that production of T lymphocytes in the thymus is stimulated by the local effect of thymic hormone.

Although administration of thymus extract has some influence on differentiation of T lymphocytes in the thymectomised animal, there is no strong evidence that production of mature T lymphocytes from stem cells can occur without the thymus.

From electron-microscopic and other observations, the thymic epithelium seems the most likely source of thymosin.

The origin of B lymphocytes

In birds, the *bursa of Fabricius*, like the thymus, develops as an epithelial organ and is invaded in embryonic life by haemopoietic stem cells which proliferate and differentiate into lymphocytes: these, in turn, enter the blood and help to populate the lymph nodes, spleen, etc. They constitute a second major population of lymphocytes, termed **B lymphocytes** (B for bursa-dependent), and bursectomy of the embryo

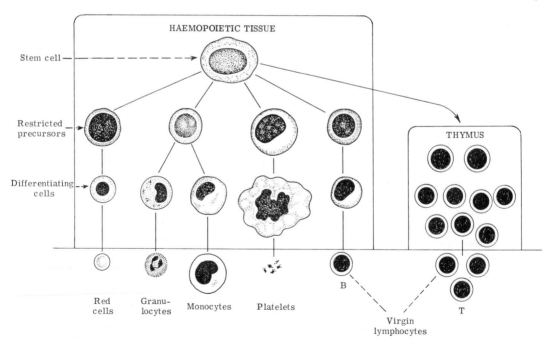

Fig. 5.14   In addition to differentiating into restricted precursors of red cells, granulocytes, monocytes and platelets, the haemopoietic stem cell differentiates into pre-B cells which undergo B-lymphopoiesis (in mammals within the haemopoietic tissue) and provide virgin B lymphocytes. Some stem cells pass into the blood and settle in the thymus, giving rise to virgin T lymphocytes.

results in failure to develop B lymphocytes. Such birds develop T cells normally, and can make cell-mediated immune responses, but they lack plasma cells and cannot make antibodies; accordingly, the plasma is devoid of immunoglobulins ('agammaglobulinaemia').

The haemopoietic marrow of mammals contains large numbers of lymphocytes which are rapidly labelled by ^{3}H-thymidine (p. 117), i.e. they are an actively dividing population, and the labelled immature cells mature into B lymphocytes, some of which can subsequently be detected in the lymph nodes, spleen, etc. *Haemopoietic tissue is thus a site of production of B lymphocytes from stem cells* (Fig. 5.14), *but it is not known whether it is the only site.*

Lymphocytes in the secondary lymphoid tissues, blood and lymphatics

In contrast to the primary lymphoid organs, in which generation of lymphocytes is independent of antigenic stimulation, *lymphocyte proliferation in the* **secondary lymphoid tissues** (*lymph nodes, spleen, tonsils, Peyer's patches, etc.*) *is a response to antigenic stimulation.*

The secondary lymphoid tissues receive from the primary lymphoid tissues T and B lymphocytes which have not yet responded to antigenic stimulation (**'virgin' lymphocytes**). When antigen is introduced into the body, those virgin lymphocytes capable of responding to it undergo a clonal proliferation, giving rise to the effector and memory cells of the primary immune response. The **effector cells** are those cells responsible for the defensive mechanisms of specific immunity; they include the plasma cells which secrete antibody and the cytotoxic T lymphocytes which react directly with antigen and mediate the delayed hypersensitivity reaction. **Memory cells** of T and B origin are small lymphocytes specifically primed to react with the antigen which has induced their production. On second or subsequent introduction of a particular antigen into the body, the immune response is augmented by participation of T and B memory lymphocytes in the secondary lymphoid tissues: these cells give rise to large numbers of effector cells and also memory cells, and are responsible for the rapidity and intensity of secondary immune responses.

The secondary lymphoid tissues (lymph nodes, spleen, tonsils, Peyer's patches, etc.) contain a complex mixture of T and B cells, and the situation is further complicated by the continuous redistribution of lymphocytes via the blood and lymphatics. Considerable progress has, however, been made in defining and identifying the major lymphocyte subpopulations in the secondary lymphoid tissues and the blood, and in elucidating their lifespan, function and migratory behaviour. The main features are described briefly in the following sections, but first it is necessary to note some of the methods of recognising T and B lymphocytes.

Identification of T and B lymphocytes

Although morphologically similar, T and B lymphocytes differ in a number of ways. It is, however, important to appreciate that the features of both types of cell change during their life cycle. The situation is further complicated by the existence of subsets of lymphocytes with features not characteristic of either T or B cells, the nature of which is uncertain. Some of the features used for identification are summarised below.

Surface antigens. Depending on their degree of maturity, the lymphocytes of various species, including man, may be identified by hetero-antisera specific for T and B cells. Such antisera may be used to identify individual cells by immunofluorescence or, together with complement, to destroy either T or B cells *in vivo* or *in vitro*.

Intracellular esterase activity is readily demonstrable in T, but not in B, lymphocytes.

Response to mitogens. A number of substances induce mitosis preferentially in T or B cells. For example, phytohaemagglutinin and concanavalin A induce mitosis mainly in T cells while bacterial lipopolysaccharides induce B-cell mitosis. Using these and other reagents, *in vitro* mitotic activity may be assessed by incorporation of ^{3}H-thymidine, but these tests are used mainly as indirect indications of T or B cell functional activity and are unsuited to identifying individual lymphocytes.

Surface immunoglobulin. As they mature in the haemopoietic marrow, B lymphocytes develop surface immunoglobulin; this is detectable in both virgin and memory B cells, and also up to a late stage of differentiation of B cells into plasma cells. Surface Ig may be detected by use of anti-Ig antisera (Fig. 5.15).

Receptors for Fc. B cells and K cells (see below) have surface receptors for the Fc part of IgG which has been aggregated by heat or complexed to an antigen. Fc receptors may be demonstrated by the binding of antibody-sensitised red cells to form rosettes (Fig. 5.16) or fluorescein-labelled antigen–antibody complexes. Some T cells also develop receptors for the Fc of IgG, and these are also a feature of monocytes, macrophages and polymorphonuclear leukocytes. Monocytes and polymorphs and some B cells also bind complement component C3b. On incubation *in vitro*, some T cells develop receptors for the Fc part of IgM.

Receptors for red cells. Human thymocytes and T lymphocytes are capable of binding sheep red cells *in vitro* to form rosettes (Fig. 5.16). This is a chance finding, the significance of which is obscure.

In our experience, approximately 70 per cent of human blood lymphocytes form rosettes with sheep red cells; about 28 per cent form Fc rosettes with antibody-sensitised red cells, and of these rather less than half are B cells (positive for surface Ig) and the remainder ('null' cells) include the K-cell population (p. 152).

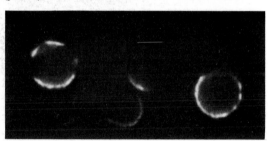

Fig. 5.15 The demonstration of surface Ig in human B lymphocytes by immunofluorescence, using labelled anti-Ig. Surface Ig is seen in four cells: it is forming aggregates on the cell surface, and in the upper central cell exhibits 'capping' (p. 125).

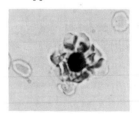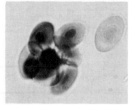

Fig. 5.16 Use of rosette formation to detect lymphocyte surface markers. **a**, a T lymphocyte binding sheep red cells. **b**, a lymphocyte binding (chicken) red cells sensitised with IgG antibody, indicating that the lymphocyte has surface receptors for the Fc of IgG.

Electron microscopy reveals differences between T and B cells, but some cells have features intermediate between the two.

The long-lived recirculating lymphocytes

In their experiments on rats, Gowans and others (p. 115) showed that when thoracic duct drainage was continued for several days, the number of small lymphocytes in thoracic duct lymph fell rapidly and the lymph nodes and spleen became partially depleted of small lymphocytes. They also showed that lymphocyte depletion was prevented by re-injecting the lymphocytes *intravenously*, and that when the cells were radio-labelled before return to the animal, most of the labelled cells reappeared *in the thoracic duct lymph* within the next few days. It was thus demonstrated that large numbers of small lymphocytes recirculate continuously between the blood, secondary lymphoid tissues and major lymphatics. This has since been shown to apply also to the mouse, sheep, bovines and man. Curiously, recirculation of lymphocytes is much less apparent in the pig.

Normally, about 80 per cent of the thoracic duct small lymphocytes are T cells and the rest are B cells. In thoracic duct drainage, the number of T cells removed falls rapidly, while the fall in numbers of B cells is much slower. Correspondingly, the lymph nodes, spleen and blood are depleted of T cells rapidly and of B cells slowly. In the mouse, this difference in depletion rate has been shown to be due partly to the greater rapidity of T-lymphocyte recirculation, and partly to the longer lifespan of T cells. By contrast, B lymphocytes recirculate more slowly and have a shorter lifespan.

The pathway and lifespan of recirculating T lymphocytes

The recirculating pathway of T lymphocytes has been elucidated by Parrott and de Sousa (1971) and other workers, usually by injecting intravenously lymphocytes radio-labelled with ³H-thymidine or ³H-uridine (which is incorporated into RNA) and following their distribution in the body by autoradiography of tissue sections or smears. Such experiments have shown that T lymphocytes in the blood gain entrance to the lymph nodes by migrating

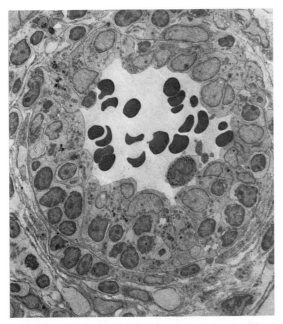

Fig. 5.17 Electron micrograph of a post-capillary venule in a Peyer's patch from a rat, showing a lymphocyte on the luminal surface, several lying between endothelial cells, and others in the surrounding sheath. × 1200. (Dr. Gutta I. Schoefl.)

through the walls of post-capillary venules in the **paracortex** (also termed **deep cortex**) of the nodes. These venules have unusually tall endothelial cells, and the migrating lymphocytes pass between them (Fig. 5.17) to enter the paracortex, which contains mainly T lymphocytes and has been termed the **T-dependent zone** of lymph nodes. In neonatally thymectomised or athymic (*nu nu*) mice, these zones lack lymphocytes (Fig. 5.18) and similar depletion is produced by thoracic duct drainage or by destroying T lymphocytes by a heterologous anti-lymphocyte serum. Similar depletion of the T-dependent zones is observed in children with congenital thymic aplasia (p. 170). From the paracortex, the lymphocytes migrate to the medullary sinuses, and thus to the efferent lymphatic. They then pass via the lymphatics to the blood, thus completing the cycle (Fig. 5.19). T lymphocytes pursue a similar course through T-dependent zones of the tonsils, Peyer's patches and Malpighian bodies (white pulp) of the spleen. In the mouse, they pass through the Malpighian bodies of the spleen in about 6 hours and through the lymph nodes in about 18 hours.

T lymphocytes also leave the blood, although

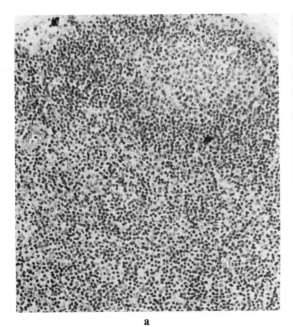

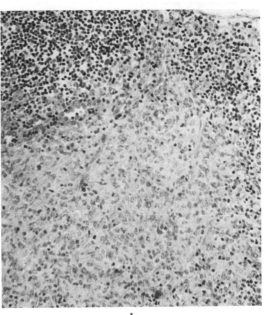

a   b

Fig. 5.18 Mouse lymph nodes, showing the influence of the thymus on the histological appearances. **a**, normal lymph node, showing a cortical follicle (top right), and the deep cortex which occupies the lower two thirds of the field. **b**, lymph node from an athymic mouse: the superficial cortex shows little abnormality, but the deep cortex is almost devoid of lymphoid cells and consists largely of 'reticulum cells'. × 150. (Professor D. M. V. Parrott and Dr. M. A. B. de Sousa.)

in smaller numbers, in the various non-lymphoid tissues of the body and return to the draining lymph nodes via the afferent lymphatics.

As explained on p. 119, the recirculating small T lymphocytes include memory cells derived from a previous antigenic stimulus. Recent work suggests that virgin lymphocytes supplied by the thymus do not join the pool directly.

In the mouse, the number of virgin T lymphocytes leaving the thymus is much greater than the number entering the recirculating T-lymphocyte pool. When the nuclei of thymic cortical lymphocytes are radio-labelled by injecting ^{3}H-thymidine directly into the thymus, labelled cells can be detected subsequently in the Malpighian bodies of the spleen, but only a few appear in the lymph nodes or thoracic duct lymph. Such cells do not, however, accumulate progressively in the spleen, and most of them apparently die within a few days of leaving the thymus. It has been suggested that, to avoid this fate, the virgin T lymphocyte must encounter an antigen to which it can respond; it then undergoes proliferation and provides effector cells and memory cells. This is supported by the fact that gnotobiotic animals (reared from birth in a germ-free state) fail to develop the recirculating T-lymphocyte pool, although lymphopoiesis in the thymus proceeds normally and some short-lived T lymphocytes (presumably virgin cells) can be detected in the spleen. They may circulate between the blood and lymph nodes, spleen, etc. during their short lifespan, but this has not been established with certainty.

It thus appears likely that the recirculating T-lymphocyte pool consists mainly of memory cells. This being so, they would be expected to be long-lived: this has been confirmed by administering injections of ^{3}H-thymidine over periods of several weeks and observing the rate of labelling of T lymphocytes in the recirculating pool (usually by autoradiography of cells in the thoracic duct or blood), and the duration of their persistence after stopping the injections. In mice it has been estimated that their lifespan is approximately 6 months: in rats it appears to exceed 1 year. The lifespan of human T lymphocytes is not known, but it is thought to be many years. This is based on the finding of lymphocytes with chromosomal abnormalities incompatible with successful mitosis in the blood of patients treated by radiotherapy many years before (Fig. 2.30, p. 37). Analysis of small lymphocytes in the blood,

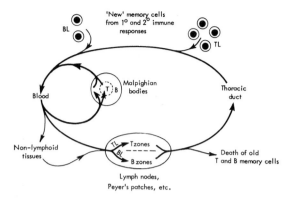

Fig. 5.19 The recirculation pathway of long-lived T lymphocytes (TL) and B lymphocytes (BL).

lymph nodes and thoracic duct has shown that 70–80 per cent of them are cells of the recirculating T-lymphocyte pool, and the degree of depletion effected by prolonged thoracic duct drainage agrees with this estimate.

A small percentage of T cells in the blood and thoracic duct are not small lymphocytes but larger 'blast' cells. These have arisen in the proliferative responses to various antigenic stimuli: experimental studies suggest that many of them settle and die in the secondary lymphoid tissues, notably those lining the gut, while a few differentiate into small lymphocytes and join the recirculating pool.

The pathway and lifespan of recirculating B lymphocytes

Most, if not all, of the small B lymphocytes in the blood, thoracic duct and secondary lymphoid tissues are recirculating cells. This has been established by experiments similar to those described above for T cells. They appear to leave the blood by the same route as T lymphocytes, i.e. via the post-capillary venules in lymph nodes, tonsils, Peyer's patches, etc., but they then come to occupy **B-dependent zones** of these secondary lymphoid tissues: in the lymph nodes they pass into and through the superficial cortex (cortical nodules—Fig. 5.30, p. 136) and medulla, and leave by the efferent lymphatic to return to the blood (Fig. 5.19). In the spleen they pass into the peripheral zone of the Malpighian bodies and presumably leave by the venous sinuses of the red pulp. These B-cell zones are depleted by thoracic duct drainage, but this takes longer than T-cell depletion because the small B lymphocytes recirculate less actively, and their lifespan (in mice approximately 6 weeks) is distinctly shorter than that of recirculating T lymphocytes.

There are occasional large B 'blast' cells in the thoracic duct and blood: these cells have arisen in the proliferative response to various antigenic stimuli: many of them differentiate into plasma cells, some in the lamina propria of the gut where they produce IgA antibodies, others in the lymph nodes, etc. where they mostly produce antibodies of other classes.

As with the T cells, it is unlikely that virgin B lymphocytes leaving the primary lymphoid organ (in mammals the haemopoietic marrow) enter directly into the recirculating lymphocyte pool. The number of B lymphocytes leaving the marrow appears to exceed greatly the number of lymphocytes entering the recirculating pool. Like virgin T cells, many apparently die quickly, probably in the spleen, and it may be that the recirculating B lymphocytes are mainly memory cells resulting from proliferation of those virgin cells which meet an antigen to which they can respond by proliferation.

Accordingly, the recirculating T and B lymphocytes, which make up the great majority of small lymphocytes in the secondary lymphoid organs, blood and lymphatics, are likely to consist mainly of relatively long-lived memory cells.

Once antigen has been encountered, the primary immune response will have resulted in addition of specifically responsive T and B memory cells to the recirculating lymphocyte pool. On subsequent encounter with the same antigen, it is these memory cells which are responsible for the rapid and enhanced secondary antibody response and strong cell-mediated immunity (Fig. 5.20).

In both primary and secondary antibody responses, the proliferating B cells differentiate into effector cells (antibody-producing end-stage plasma cells) and B memory cells which

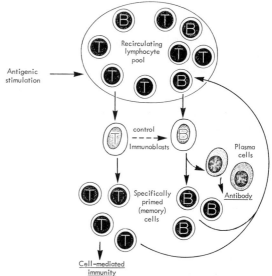

Fig. 5.20 The secondary immune response. The appropriately primed T and B memory cells in the recirculating lymphocyte pool proliferate in the secondary lymphoid tissues, providing memory cells (which re-join the recirculating pool) and effector cells. The effector B cell is the plasma cell. The effector T cells include proliferating 'blast' cells and probably also the T memory cells (see p. 119). The primary response is similar, but depends on relatively few virgin T and B lymphocytes responsive to the antigen, and so is slower and smaller than the secondary response.

join the re-circulating pool. In T-cell responses, the distinction between effector and memory cells is not so clear cut: the effector T cell is capable of producing lymphokines on reacting with the appropriate antigen, and of killing target cells (e.g. of allografts) which incorporate the antigen in their surface membrane. Both the proliferating blast cells of the cell-mediated immune response and the T memory cells which result from the response are capable of these effector functions.

The specific response of individual lymphocytes to antigenic stimulation

During their maturation in the sheltered environment of the primary lymphoid organs, individual lymphocytes differentiate in such a way that each one becomes capable of responding to only a narrow range of antigenic determinants or epitopes. The result is a continu-

ous supply of virgin lymphocytes of such considerable diversity that no matter what or how many natural or artificially-prepared foreign antigens are introduced into the body, there are likely to be some lymphocytes capable of mounting a specific immune response against each sort of determinant on each antigenic molecule. The restricted responsiveness and diversity of lymphocytes also ensures that only a very small proportion of the available lymphocytes can respond to any one antigen, so that immune responses to many different antigens can proceed simultaneously. The development of this restricted responsiveness of individual lymphocytes comes about by changes in the cell's DNA: it occurs in both B and T lymphocytes and is heritable and irreversible, so that when a mature virgin lymphocyte meets an antigen to which it can respond, it does so by proliferation and all the cells of the resulting clone have the same restricted specificity of response (Fig. 5.21). Encounter with an antigen thus leads to an increase in the number of lymphocytes which can respond to it. Some of the cells so produced are long-lived memory lymphocytes, which, on subsequently encountering the same or a closely similar antigen, also undergo proliferation. The result is that large numbers of responsive lymphocytes are available for those antigens which are encountered frequently.

The evidence for this restricted potential of lymphocytes, and its mechanism, must now be considered. B lymphocytes have yielded up some of the secrets of their behaviour more readily than T lymphocytes, and although they are influenced by T cells, it is convenient to consider B-cell responses before T-cell responses.

The response of B lymphocytes to antigenic stimulation

Antigenic stimulation induces proliferation of B lymphocytes in the secondary lymphoid tissues. In lymph nodes, for example, this is seen in the germinal centres of the superficial cortex where responding B lymphocytes enlarge to become **B 'blast' cells** (B immunoblasts) with increase in both nuclear DNA and cytoplasm: the latter becomes rich in RNA and so is basophilic in its staining properties (Fig. 5.22). By successive divisions, large numbers of cells are produced, some of which differentiate into **plasmablasts**, with abundant rough endoplasmic reticulum (p. 107) and finally give rise to mature **plasma cells** which synthesise and secrete antibody (Figs. 5.3, 5.4, p. 108): others differentiate into **B-memory cells** and join the recirculating pool of long-lived small lymphocytes (Fig. 5.20).

Both virgin and memory B lymphocytes respond as described above to antigenic stimulation (Fig. 5.22). The primary response does not produce very much antibody, presumably because it depends entirely on virgin lymphocytes, relatively few of which are capable of responding to any particular antigen. The primary response does, however, provide memory cells, and these account for the much greater amount of antibody produced in the secondary response.

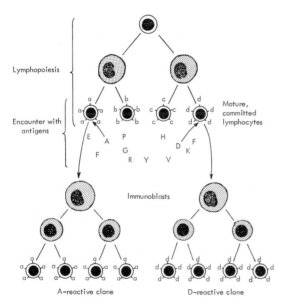

Fig. 5.21 The clonal selection theory of immune response. During lymphopoiesis, each developing T or B cell becomes committed to respond to a narrow range of antigenic determinants: this is reflected by the specificity of the antigen receptors (a, b, c, etc.) on its surface. For example, lymphocytes with hypothetical 'a' receptors can bind an antigen 'A', but not 'D' or 'E', etc. Binding of an antigen stimulates a lymphocyte to proliferate, producing a clone of lymphocytes with identical commitment.

How B lymphocytes recognise antigens

To respond to an antigen, a lymphocyte must have surface receptors capable of recognising antigen to which the cell can respond, and union of antigen with surface receptors must stimulate the response. In fact, when lymphocytes from a normal individual are incubated with an antigen which has been labelled,

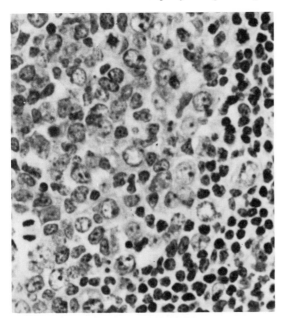

Fig. 5.22 Segment of a germinal centre showing proliferating B 'blast' cells with large pale nuclei and abundant cytoplasm. The centre is surrounded by tightly packed small lymphocytes. × 850.

for example with ^{131}I or fluorescein, the labelled antigens can be demonstrated to bind to the surface of very small proportions of both T and B lymphocytes. If the donor has previously encountered that antigen, the number of antigenbinding lymphocytes is increased, but is still only a very small proportion of the total.

The B lymphocyte has on its surface molecules of immunoglobulin (SIg), which float in the lipid of the cell membrane with the Fab end of the molecules projecting from it, and there is now no doubt that these act as the specific antigen receptors on B cells. Some of the evidence for this is summarised below.

Firstly, treatment of B lymphocytes with an anti-immunoglobulin (anti-Ig) inhibits antigen binding.

Secondly, evidence has been provided by the 'capping' phenomenon. When B lymphocytes are treated with a labelled antigen, the SIg molecules of those cells which bind the antigen become aggregated into clumps and finally in a single mass or 'cap' at one part of the surface: the effect is the same as that induced by treating B cells with anti-immunoglobulin (Fig. 5.15, p. 120). When capping is induced by antigen, the cap can be shown to contain *all* the antigen bound to the cell surface and *all* the SIg molecules, thus demonstrating that all the SIg molecules react with the antigen.

The significance of antigen binding by the surface Ig of B cells

Those B cells which can bind a particular antigen are responsible for the antibody response to that antigen. This has been demonstrated by passing lymphocytes through a column of inert material coated with antigen. The cells which bind the antigen are retained and are thus separated from non-binding lymphocytes. The separated cells may be tested for antibody response either *in vitro* or by administering them to an animal whose own lymphocytes have been destroyed (e.g. by x-irradiation) and then challenging the animal with the same and other antigens. Such experiments have shown that the antigen-binding cells can mount an antibody response to the same antigen. The non-antigen-binding population does not respond to the same antigen, but responds normally to other antigens. These findings suggest that the SIg molecules of B lymphocytes represent a sample of the specific antibody which that cell and its descendants can synthesise and secrete. This is further supported by the observations outlined below on individual clones of proliferating cells.

The sequences of amino acids in the variable regions of the light and heavy chains of the immunoglobulin (Ig) molecule, including the antigen-combining sites (Fig. 5.1, p. 106) constitute what is known as the **idiotype** of the molecule and are responsible for its specificity as an antibody. The idiotype of the molecule might be expected also to exhibit specific *antigenic* properties, but this is difficult to establish because normal Ig, e.g. in serum, is a mixture of enormous numbers of antibodies, each with its own idiotype. However, some B-cell lymphoid tumours, for example myeloma, differentiate into plasma cells and secrete molecules of Ig which are identical for any one such tumour. This can only be explained by concluding that the Ig is **monoclonal**, i.e. that the tumour arises from clonal proliferation of a B cell already committed to production of Ig of a particular idiotype. *It follows that the commitment of a B cell to production of Ig of a particular idiotype, i.e. of a particular antibody, is transmitted to its descendants.*

In some of these Ig-secreting tumours, the tumour cells resemble normal B lymphocytes in having surface Ig (SIg), and this has provided an opportunity to compare the secretory and surface Ig of a B-cell clone. When the mono-clonal Ig (obtainable from the patient's serum) is injected into a rabbit, the antiserum contains antibodies to the variable regions, and these **anti-idiotype antibodies** react with, and cause complete capping of, the SIg of the tumour cells (p. 120). This is strong evidence that B-cell SIg has the same idiotype as the antibody sec-reted by that cell and its descendants. There is now evidence that this applies also to normal (i.e. non-neoplastic) B cells, for by injecting mice of a selected inbred strain with a poly-saccharide of limited antigenicity, relatively few lymphocytes are stimulated to clonal prolifera-tion and antibody production, and it has been possible to demonstrate that an anti-idiotype antibody reacts with both the free antibody and the SIg of the cell clone responsible for it. Accordingly, it may be concluded that *the sur-face Ig of normal B lymphocytes represents a sample of the specific antibody which that cell or its descendants can produce in response to an antigenic stimulus.*

How B lymphocytes develop specific responsive-ness and diversity

From the preceding sections it is apparent that, at some stage in its development, each B lym-phocyte becomes committed to producing anti-body of a particular specificity. Since the speci-ficity of antibody depends on the sequence of amino acids in the variable regions of the poly-peptide chains, it is a reflection of the sequen-ces of the bases in the DNA of the genes coding for immunoglobulin synthesis. Commitment of the lymphocyte thus implies that it becomes restricted to coding for only one particular sequence for the variable regions of the heavy chain and one sequence for the variable regions of the light chain. Since all the B cells of a pro-liferating clone are committed to produce the same antibody, commitment must be heritable and irreversible through many cell generations. But individual lymphocytes become specifically committed to produce *different* antibodies, thus providing the great diversity of the antibody response.

We must therefore conclude that either (a) the genome of the individual contains large numbers of alternative genes for the variable parts of the Ig chains (V genes), and that commitment involves the restriction to coding for one light and one heavy chain V gene, or (b) the genome of the individual contains relatively few V genes, and different se-quences of bases develop by somatic mutation during early lymphopoiesis (Jerne, 1971). It has not been established with certainty which of these two theor-ies of diversity is the correct one, but present evi-dence favours the former (which is assumed in this account), i.e. that the genome of the individual con-tains sufficient V genes to account for the whole re-pertoire of antibodies which the individual is capable of producing (**the germ line theory**), and each B lym-phocyte becomes committed to specific antibody production by restriction of coding to one V gene for each Ig chain.

It is known that each Ig chain is synthesised as a single unit, by translation of messenger RNA carrying the code for the constant and variable regions of the whole chain. It is now believed that the gene selection responsible for lymphocytic commitment and diversity is brought about by the mechanism illustrated for heavy chain synthesis in Fig. 5.23. The heavy chain V genes (VH genes) form a continuous series and by formation and exclusion of a loop of random length, a particular VH gene seg-ment is brought into apposition with the gene segment coding for the constant part of the heavy chain (Cμ, Cγ, etc.). Once this has occur-red, the adjacent V and C genes act as a single cistron, and the sequence of amino acids in the variable regions of the heavy chain of Ig pro-duced by that cell and its descendants is irrevo-cably decided.

Recently this mechanism of rearrangement of gene segments has been shown to operate in the formation of Ig light chains, in which three DNA segments come together to form the whole chain (Fig. 5.24). The antibody specifi-city is decided by random combination of a VL and a 'J' gene segment,*with which the C seg-ment also combines to complete the cistron.† In the mouse κ chains there are approximately 1000 VL gene segments and 10 'J' segments, giving a repertoire of 10^4 amino-acid se-

---

*The sequences of DNA which encode the antigen-combining component of light chains have recently been shown to be divided into VL gene segments and J segments. The J segments are quite unrelated to the J chains which bind together monomeric IgA and IgM to form polymers.

†Separation of segments of a single gene on the DNA strand of the chromosome has been shown also in relation to production of ovalbumin and other proteins and may apply to eukaryotic proteins in general.

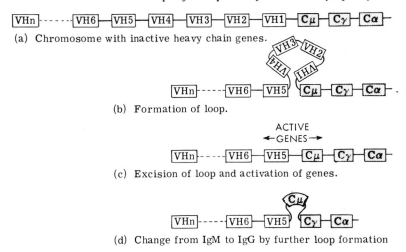

(a) Chromosome with inactive heavy chain genes.

(b) Formation of loop.

ACTIVE
←GENES→

(c) Excision of loop and activation of genes.

(d) Change from IgM to IgG by further loop formation

Fig. 5.23 Model of chromosome with genes for the variable region (VH1, VH2 ... VHn) and constant region (Cμ, Cγ, Cα) of heavy chains, showing selection of a single VH gene by formation and removal of a DNA loop. In this example, the cell becomes committed to synthesis of heavy chains with a variable region containing the amino-acid sequence determined by VH5. At first IgM is synthesised, but removal of a loop containing Cμ leads to subsequent synthesis of IgG with the same specificity (determined by VH5).

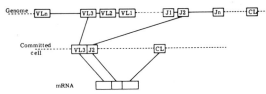

Fig. 5.24 Gene segments involved in coding for immunoglobulin light chain. The variable region is determined by selection of one of approximately 1000 VL gene segments; these are separated from 10 or so J gene segments which also determine part of the variable regions. The J segments are separated from the (C) segment which codes for the constant region. Committment of the cell depends on random apposition (by looping) of one VL and one J segment. The superfluous bases between the J and C segments are transcribed but the corresponding part of the messenger RNA (mRNA) is excised, leaving a continuous mRNA strand coding for the whole light chain. (Modified from Williamson, 1979).

quences. The specificity of antibody depends on the variable regions of light and heavy chains, and if we assume a similar variability (10^4) for the mouse heavy chain, this gives a total repertoire of 10^8 different antibodies, which agrees fairly closely with most estimates based on analyses of the antibodies which develop in response to one particular antigenic determinant. (See Williamson, 1979).

The theory of random selection of gene segments coding for the variable parts of Ig which form the specific antigen receptors explains not only the specificity of immune responses but also the multiplicity of antibodies which, as mentioned above, are produced, even in response to a simple antigen with only one type of determinant. The antigen stimulates all those B lymphocytes whose specific surface receptors can bind it sufficiently firmly and each of these cells gives rise to a clone of plasma cells producing its own distinctive antibody molecules. The result is a mixture of diverse antibodies, some of which can bind the antigen more firmly than others, but the total effect of which is exquisite specificity. If the antigen is administered repeatedly in small doses it is taken up mainly by those lymphocytes which can bind it most firmly and as these proliferate the result predicted would be a progressive increase in the avidity (p. 107) of the antibody, which is indeed what happens.

It is now widely accepted that commitment of B lymphocytes occurs spontaneously, probably during lymphopoiesis in the sheltered environment of the haemopoietic tissue, and is not dependent on encounter with an antigen. This view appears to have been held as early as 1908 by Ehrlich, but was for long ignored in favour of the *instructive theory* which postulated that antigenic material was taken up by antibody-producing cells and instructed the cell to make antibody by acting as a template on which the antibody was moulded. Ehrlich's view was revived by Jerne (1955) and by Burnet (1959) as the **clonal** or **cell selection theory** (Fig. 5.21, p. 124). Once it was established that antibody specificity was determined by the sequence of amino acids in the Ig chains, the instructive theory became untenable, and the evidence in favour of the clonal selection theory, some of which has been outlined in the preceding account, is now overwhelming.

The classes of antibody produced by B cells

The class of Ig synthesised by a B cell will depend on which C-gene segment is linked to the selected VH gene, and change of production from one class to another, e.g. IgM to IgG, probably involves similar looping and exclusion of C-gene segments as shown in Fig. 5.23. It is noteworthy that the class of Ig synthesised (embodied in the Fc portion of the heavy chains) may change during the development of a clone of antibody-producing cells, but the light chain type and idiotype do not change.

During maturation in the haemopoietic marrow, B cells pass through a stage in which they synthesise and secrete small amounts of monomeric IgM. This is followed by the appearance of monomeric IgM on the surface membrane. In the primary immune response, the proliferating B lymphocytes have mainly surface IgM, and differentiate into plasma cells which secrete IgM antibody. Later in the response some of the proliferating B cells develop into plasma cells which secrete IgG and other classes of antibody. Memory B lymphocytes (long-lived small B lymphocytes of the recirculating pool—p. 122) have mainly IgD on their surface membrane, but give rise predominantly to plasma cells which secrete IgG or IgA antibodies, as observed in the secondary response.

The response of T cells to antigenic stimulation

Antigenic stimulation induces proliferation of responsive T lymphocytes: the proliferating cells (like responding B cells) become enlarged and acquire abundant basophilic (RNA-rich) cytoplasm (Fig. 5.25): they are termed **T 'blast' cells** or **T immunoblasts**. They pass through a succession of divisions during which they

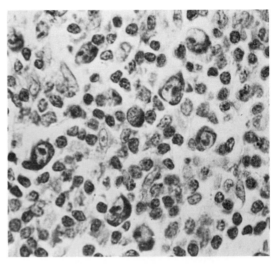

Fig. 5.25 Large lymphoid cells with enlarged nucleus and pyroninophilic cytoplasm (*immunoblasts*) in a human lymph node removed 6 days after a skin allograft. Methyl green pyronin stain. × 480. (Professor D. M. V. Parrott and Dr. M. A. B. de Sousa.)

differentiate into small T lymphocytes capable of binding the antigen which has induced their production. T-cell proliferation takes place in the T-dependent zones of the secondary lymphoid tissues (p. 121).

Like B lymphocytes, T lymphocytes become committed to respond to a narrow range of antigenic stimuli, and this occurs without antigenic stimulation, probably during lymphocytic maturation in the thymus. Another similarity is that the T lymphocyte recognises antigens by means of surface receptors, but the nature of these is uncertain. The T cell has not been shown to synthesise Ig at any stage of its development, and conventional Ig cannot be detected on its surface.* Yet T cells show specific antigen-binding properties, and the development of cell-mediated immunity depends on such antigen binding. It still remains possible, however, that the T-cell antigen receptor consists of amino-acid sequences which are the products of VH and VL genes, i.e. the variable regions of Ig molecules, for these are not detectable by conventional anti-Ig. Support for this view has been provided by the following experiments.

By administering to inbred mice or rats an antigen which in these animals stimulates only a few T and B

---

*When blood is withdrawn and allowed to cool, plasma IgG adheres to the surface of T lymphocytes, but dissociates readily at 37 °C.

lymphocytes to clonal proliferation, it has been possible to isolate antibody of a particular idiotype (p. 125) and to prepare an anti-idiotype antibody. In such experiments it has been shown that the anti-idiotype antibody reacts with the receptors of both T- and B-cell clones, which suggests strongly that they are identical, and since the B-cell receptors are known to be the variable ends of Ig molecules, it seems likely that the T-cell receptors are also of this nature. Alternatively, T-cell receptors could be determined by a set of genes analogous to, but distinct from, the V genes which code for B cells: possible contenders are the *Ir* (immune response) *genes* (p. 167) which somehow influence T-cell-dependent responses.

The remainder of the T-cell receptor molecule, corresponding to the constant regions of Ig, has not been shown to be any of the known classes of Ig (μ, γ, etc.), and its nature is unknown. The C genes of B cells thus appear to be represented in T cells by another gene, or series of genes, of unknown nature. Accepting this assumption, the commitment of T lymphocytes can be explained by the same looping and exclusion mechanisms illustrated in Fig. 5.23.

In summary, *T lymphocytes owe their specific responsiveness to antigen to the presence on their surface of antigen-specific receptors. Unlike the specific (SIg) receptors of B cells, the T-cell receptors are not whole Ig molecules, but in some instances their antigen-binding sites have been shown to be similar (and possibly identical) to the idiotypes of SIg. The part of the T-cell receptor corresponding to the Fc of SIg is, however, of unknown nature.*

Control of the immune response

So far, this account might suggest that antibody and cell-mediated immune responses arise when B or T lymphocytes respectively encounter an antigen to which they can respond. In fact, immune responses are far more complicated than this, and although antigenic stimulation is obviously of central importance in triggering them off, the nature of the antigen, its molecular size and density and variety of determinant sites are only some of the factors concerned. Account must be taken of many other factors which can enhance, suppress or modify immune responses. Some of these are outlined briefly below.

T-dependent and T-independent antibody responses. Animals deficient in T cells (e.g. 'B' mice, p. 117) are unable to mount antibody responses to many antigens, including foreign proteins. B cells require the co-operation of T cells to produce antibodies to such antigens, which accordingly are called **thymus-dependent antigens**. Some antigens, however, do stimulate 'B' mice to antibody production: these so-called **thymus-independent antigens** are usually of very high molecular weight, with large numbers of one or more particular antigenic determinants, e.g. bacterial lipopolysaccharide, pneumococcal capsular polysaccharide or artificially prepared polymers. It appears that, by binding to, and so linking up, large numbers of the surface Ig receptors on a B cell, such antigens can provide the necessary stimulus for clonal proliferation and antibody production (Fig. 5.26). By contrast, smaller molecules, or globular proteins which display a variety of antigenic determinants without a high concentration of any one determinant, would be expected to bind less strongly to B cells and to occupy fewer surface receptor sites: this may be why they cannot stimulate an antibody response without the help of T cells.

The helper function of T cells in antibody responses has been elucidated by complexing a hapten (e.g. dinitrophenyl) to a foreign carrier protein. Using this system, Mitchison (1971) and others have shown that an antibody response to the hapten is dependent on the development of cell-mediated immunity to the carrier protein. It seems likely that the binding of molecules of the protein to primed T lymphocytes renders the hapten-protein complex

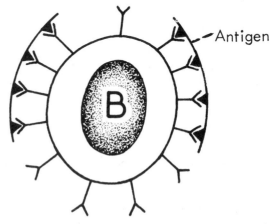

Fig. 5.26 T-independent antibody response induced by an antigen with large numbers of a particular type of antigenic determinant (epitope) which effectively links the surface Ig antigen receptors of an appropriate B cell and stimulates it to respond.

immunogenic to B cells, perhaps by presenting the hapten to B cells in such a way that it effectively links together the B cell receptors (Fig. 5.27b). Alternatively, it could be that the T cell binding the protein carrier transmits an additional stimulatory signal to the B cell binding the hapten. Some evidence for this 'second signal' hypothesis is provided by the demonstration that T cells binding and responding to a quite separate antigen (or to mitogens—p.

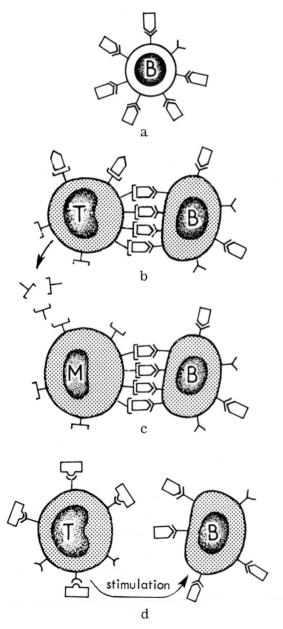

119) can be of some help to the B cell in its response (Fig. 5.27d). It is also possible that the T cell responding to the protein carrier transfers receptor sites to macrophages, and thus confers on them specific helper capacity (Fig. 5.27c).

Whatever the mechanism of T-cell co-operation in antibody production, it has been shown to be a property of memory T cells and, as indicated above, can be antigen-specific or non-specific. Specific T-cell co-operation is essential for optimal primary and secondary antibody responses to most protein antigens, and even those immune responses which can occur without T-cell help are usually limited mainly to production of antibodies of IgM class. The co-operation of T cells appears to be necessary for the production of large amounts of IgG antibody, as in the secondary response. Indeed, there is evidence that the formation of B-memory lymphocytes is less dependent on T-cell help than is the production of antibody-producing plasma cells. The degree of helper T-cell activity in the response of inbred strains of mice to highly artificial T-dependent antigens has been shown to involve the so-called Ir (immune response) genes which lie within the major histocompatibility gene complex (p. 167). While it is possible that Ir genes code for specific antigen receptors on the surface of T cells, there is increasing evidence that many genes of the major histocompatibility complex are concerned with the co-operation of T cells with B cells and with macrophages (Munro and Waldmann, 1978).

Suppressor T cells. In addition to T cells which co-operate in the antibody response, it is

Fig. 5.27 Possible mechanisms of co-operation of T cells in antibody production by B cells. In **a**, a B lymphocyte has bound an antigen by a particular type of determinant, but is not stimulated by it because it has not cross-linked the specific antigen receptors. If a T cell also binds the same antigen by a different determinant, as in **b**, it may effectively cross-link the B-lymphocyte receptors and thus stimulate it (indicated here by 'blast' transformation of the B cell). Alternately the T-cell antigen receptors may be transferred to macrophages **c** which then become capable of co-operating in B-cell stimulation. Lastly, a T cell which has bound an independent antigen, as in **d** can also provide a stimulus to the B lymphocyte. In all these forms of co-operation, the stimulating T cell has itself been stimulated to 'blast' transformation, and indeed the last form of co-operation can be provided by a T cell which has been stimulated non-specifically, e.g. by phytohaemagglutinin.

now known that subsets of T cells have a suppressive effect on B cells. This explains why the antibody response to thymus-independent antigens is often greater in T-deficient animals. In lepromatous leprosy and some other chronic infections, very high titres of antibodies to the causal agent are commonly observed and may well be due to the lack of suppressor T-cell control, for failure of cell-mediated immunity (and therefore of T-cell function) to the microorganism is a feature in such cases.

The helper and suppressor activities of T cells are complex, and it seems likely that the T cells responsible are distinct sub-sets rather than stages in the differentiation of one series of T cells. The complexity is increased by recent evidence that helper T cells (and probably suppressor T cells) exert some control over T cell, as well as B cell, immune responses.

Antibodies. The immune response to an antigen can be partially or even completely inhibited by injection of the corresponding antibody either before or shortly after administration of the antigen. Part of the inhibitory effect is due to rapid phagocytosis and destruction of much of the antigen following its union with the injected antibody. There is, however, evidence that antibody can exert an additional inhibitory effect, which is not due to destruction of antigen, and may involve receptors on suppressor T cells for the Fc of IgG. The inhibitory effects of antibodies are of practical importance in prophylactic immunisation of infants, for maternal IgG antibodies cross the human placenta and may interfere with the response to vaccines during the first few months of infancy. The inhibitory effects of antibody are now used extensively to prevent immunisation of the rhesus-negative mother by a rhesus-positive fetus (p. 151).

Anti-idiotype antibodies. As explained earlier (p. 104), most antigens are of exceedingly complex structure, and each stimulates large numbers of different T and B cells to clonal proliferation. In consequence, the antibody produced is really a mixture of large numbers of different antibodies, each the product of a clone of B lymphocytes. Even antigens with a single type of determinant usually stimulate clonal proliferation of many different lymphocytes, and a mixture of antibodies results (p. 127). In spite of this heterogeneity of the antibody response, there is evidence that the variable parts of the antibody molecules resulting from any particular clonal proliferation may act as *antigens* in the host and stimulate the development of anti-idiotype antibodies (p. 126). These can bind to the antigen receptors of the corresponding B- and T-cell clones (p. 129) or of the corresponding antibody molecules, and in so doing can exert a regulatory effect on the cells of the clones. Depending on various factors, they may either enhance or suppress further clonal proliferation and differentiation, and thus exert some control over the immune response. Such control does not stop at this level, for there is now evidence that the anti-idiotype antibodies also act as antigens and may stimulate the development of further anti-idiotype antibodies (anti-anti-idiotypes), and so on.

It is thus becoming increasingly apparent that immune responses, like many other biological processes, are not regulated by a simple feedback mechanism, but by a complexity of factors, the outcome being determined by the total effect of all the stimulatory and inhibitory factors involved.

In conclusion, *the production by B cells of antibodies to many antigens is dependent on the co-operation of T cells. Such help is provided optimally by T cells which have responded to the same antigen. There is evidence that T cells may also suppress the immune response of both B and T cells, and that they play a major role in controlling the intensity of immune responses. Antibody itself is also capable of suppressing the immune response to the corresponding antigen, and anti-idiotype antibodies can both enhance and inhibit clonal proliferation of both T and B cells with receptors of the corresponding idiotype.*

Transfer factor

Since 1948, Lawrence has reported investigations which suggest that cell-free extracts of human leukocytes can transfer cell-mediated immunity to non-immunised recipients, and that the responsible agent, transfer factor, has a molecular weight of about 3000 (see Lawrence, 1969). Attempts to demonstrate transfer factor in experimental animals have, in general, been disappointing, but it must be appreciated that, in general, man and other primates show much stronger cell-mediated immune responses and DHS reactions than do lower animals.

Recently, a number of reports have appeared on the therapeutic use of transfer factor in the treatment of patients with resistant infections due to immunodeficiencies, and with various diseases of obscure causation (e.g. sarcoidosis, connective tissue diseases and tumours). The degree of success achieved has varied greatly, and it is difficult to draw conclusions. The existence of human transfer factor which enhances immune responses is no longer in doubt, although its mode of action is obscure and its antigen-specificity has not been widely accepted.

Acquired immunological tolerance

In some circumstances, exposure to antigen does not result in an immune response, but in the development of unresponsiveness (tolerance) of the individual to that particular antigen, although responses to other antigens remain normal. In addition to true or 'classical' tolerance, suppressor T cells and antibody are both capable of inhibiting specific immune responses (see above), and thus may bring about a state resembling true tolerance.

Classical immunological tolerance. When living cells or tissues are exchanged between genetically dissimilar individuals, the host develops an immune response which results in destruction of the transplanted cells. Yet in 1945 Owen, an American veterinary surgeon, detected red cells of two distinct groups in some bovines, and noted that such animals were always derived from a twin pregnancy. Apparently there is sometimes placental vascular anastomosis between dizygotic twin cattle, with consequent admixture of their blood during early fetal life. Circulating haemopoietic stem cells from each fetus settle in the other and remain functional so that each twin subsequently produces red cells, etc. from its own and from its twin's stem cells.

This observation—that allogeneic cells introduced into the embryo were not rejected by the host—led Burnet and Fenner (1949) to postulate that antigenic challenge during fetal life could result in specific unresponsiveness rather than an immune response. Burnet failed to substantiate this because of an unlucky choice of antigen/host combination. It was, however, subsequently confirmed by Medawar and his co-workers, who showed that injection of living cells from a mouse of one inbred strain (say Y) into a *neonatal* mouse of another inbred strain (X) induced immune unresponsiveness to cells of the donor strain. Thus when the treated

mouse matured, it failed to reject a skin graft from a Y mouse, although capable of rejecting normally skin from a mouse of an unrelated strain (Z) (Fig. 5.28). The likely explanation of this form of **'classical' tolerance** is that, on encountering an antigen to which it can respond, the immature lymphoid cell is either destroyed

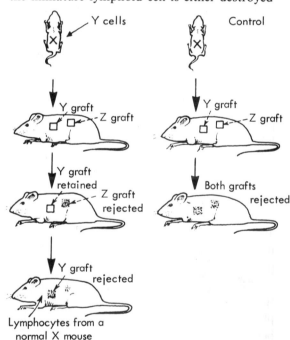

Fig. 5.28 Immunological tolerance to allogeneic cells. A neonatal 'X' strain mouse (top left) injected with strain 'Y' cells becomes tolerant to 'Y' 'transplant' antigens, as shown by retention of a subsequent 'Y' skin graft. It rejects an unrelated ('Z' strain) graft normally. Injection of lymphocytes from a normal 'X' mouse results in rejection of the 'Y' graft. (In practice, injection of lymphocytes or haemopoietic cells is commonly used to induce tolerance in such experiments: this raises the complication of the graft versus host reaction (p. 167) which, for the sake of simplicity, has been ignored in this illustration.)

or rendered irreversibly unresponsive. This is supported by the additional finding that when the tolerant X mouse bearing a Y skin graft is injected with lymphocytes from a normal adult X mouse, the Y graft is rejected, i.e. tolerance is abolished.

Tolerance may be induced also to foreign proteins by injecting them into the fetal or neonatal animal, but to maintain such tolerance it is necessary to administer repeated injections of the antigen. Thus classical tolerance is maintained only so long as the antigen persists in the host. As an explanation, it is suggested that, when lymphocytes become committed to recognise a particular antigen, they pass through an immature stage during which encounter with the antigen promotes their death or non-responsiveness: if antigen is continuously present it will 'catch' potentially responsive lymphocytes at this stage and tolerance will persist. Mature lymphocytes are more likely to mount an immune response on encountering the antigen. It follows that widely spaced pulses of antigen should favour an immune response, as indeed they do.

Although tolerance is most readily induced in immature animals, adults may also be rendered tolerant and Mitchison (1967) showed that this could be achieved by administering repeated injections of either very low or very high doses of antigen to adult mice. Intermediate doses induced an immune response. The explanation is that tolerance is readily induced in T lymphocytes by very small or very large doses of antigen, while B-lymphocyte tolerance is induced only by very large doses of antigen (Fig. 5.29). It follows that high dosage suppresses both the T-cell response (cell-mediated immunity) and the B-cell response (antibody production). If the antigen is T-dependent (p. 129), as in Mitchison's experiment, then low dosage, by inducing T-cell tolerance, will inhibit also the antibody response. For T-independent antigens, however, low dosage will induce suppression of cell-mediated immunity but there will still be antibody production: this is sometimes termed **split tolerance** or **immune deviation**.

In fact, the situation is more complex than stated above, for any particular antigenic determinant will be bound by many lymphocytes with different specific receptors (p. 127). Some of these cells will have receptors which make a 'good fit' with the antigen

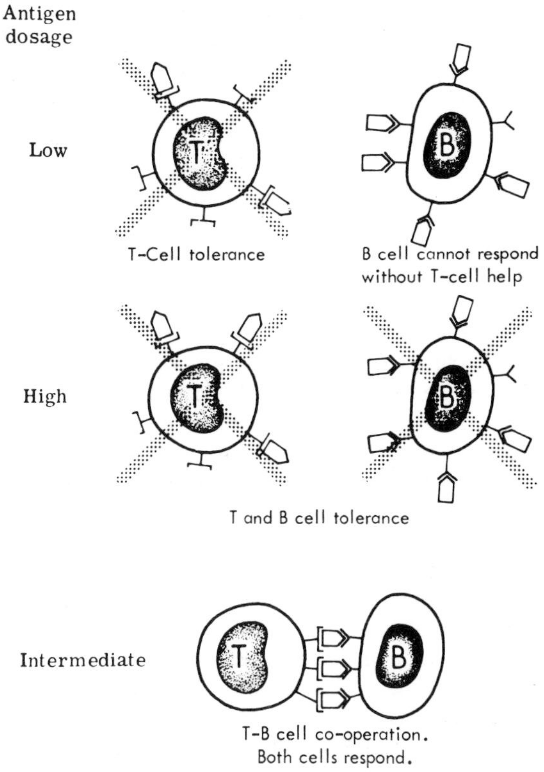

Antigen dosage

Low

T–Cell tolerance

B cell cannot respond without T-cell help

High

T and B cell tolerance

Intermediate

T–B cell co-operation. Both cells respond.

Fig. 5.29 The induction of immunological tolerance to a 'thymic-dependent' antigen by administration of very small or very large amounts of the antigen.

and bind it firmly; others will bind it less well because it fits their receptors poorly. These factors will influence not only the amount of antibody produced, but also its avidity. A high concentration of antigen which induces non-responsiveness of strongly-binding cells may stimulate an immune response in those binding the antigen less firmly, with consequent production of a relatively small amount of antibody of poor avidity. The same considerations apply to T lymphocytes, and accordingly tolerance is not an all-or-nothing phenomenon. Any antigenic stimulus is likely, in fact, to induce tolerance in some potentially responsive lymphocytes and an immune response in others.

Well-established tolerance to an antigen can sometimes be broken down by administering the antigen incorporated in Freund's adjuvant (p. 114) or by administering a closely related cross-reacting antigen. The mode of action of Freund's adjuvant is uncertain, but abolition of tolerance by a closely related antigen is probably explained by Mitchison's work with hapten bound to a protein carrier. As already noted (p. 129), he showed that antibody production to the hapten is dependent on a T-cell response to antigenic determinants of the carrier protein. If T-cell tolerance to the carrier is induced by low dosage of the hapten-carrier complex, then, as explained above, the antibody response will also be suppressed. If now the same hapten coupled to another protein is injected into the animal, T cells will respond to the new carrier protein and in doing so will provide the co-operation needed by B cells to respond to the hapten. Native proteins each possess various antigenic determinants and by regarding any particular type of determinant as equivalent to the hapten in Mitchison's experiments, we can explain the breakdown of B-cell tolerance by administration of a closely related cross-reacting antigen.

Conditions resembling classical tolerance. So far in this account, tolerance has been explained on the basis of a direct and permanent suppression of T cells, and sometimes of B cells also, by a particular antigenic stimulus. However, it was shown by Gershon and Kondo (1971) that the thoracic duct lymphocytes of a mouse rendered tolerant to a particular antigen could confer tolerance on a normal animal of the same strain. This is now regarded as due to the development of suppressor T cells capable of inhibiting T- and B-cell responses to a particular antigen. A form of unresponsiveness to an antigen can also be induced by administration of the corresponding antibody shortly before or after antigenic stimulation (p. 131).

The significance of immunological tolerance. The capacity of the immunity system to develop immune responses to countless antigens carries with it the danger of responding similarly to one's own normal body constituents, i.e. by auto-immunisation. The ease with which classical tolerance can be induced to specific antigens during fetal and neonatal life is believed to be the major safeguard against auto-immunisation, but it is not always effective and some diseases are attributable to auto-immunity (p. 161). Also B cells with surface Ig

capable of binding self-constituents, e.g. thyroglobulin or DNA, have been detected in the blood of some normal individuals, indicating a capacity for auto-antibody formation; this is apparently held in check in most individuals either by lack of T-helper cells, or by a dominating influence of suppressor T cells, and there is evidence that deficiency of the latter is a feature of auto-immune diseases.

As described above, tolerance may also develop towards the antigens of *foreign* cells or proteins introduced into the animal during fetal or neonatal life, and this can apply also to micro-organisms, with consequent persistence of infection, e.g. lymphocytic choriomeningitis of mice (p. 183).

The fact that tolerance to foreign antigens can be induced throughout life offers a promising approach to the therapeutic transplantation of foreign tissues, for the induction of specific tolerance to antigens of the donor tissue would obviously be preferable to the use of drugs which bring about a general depression of the host's immunity system to all antigens, including those of pathogenic micro-organisms. In fact, administration of such drugs (e.g. azathioprine, glucocorticoids, etc.) together with an antigen facilitates the induction of tolerance in the adult, and this is probably of importance in clinical renal transplantation, in which the dosage of immunosuppressive drugs can be gradually reduced without rejection of the kidney. Some form of tolerance develops to the alloantigens of the transplant: this may either be 'classical' tolerance, as described above, or it may be due to production of specific suppressor T cells or of 'blocking' or 'enhancing' antibody, which suppresses further immune responses, including cell-mediated immunity, to the transplant antigens (p. 167).

Macrophages and the immune response

When antigenic foreign macromolecular or finely particulate material penetrates into the body, much of it is engulfed by macrophages. Most of the ingested antigen is digested within phagolysosomes and destroyed, but some antigenic material becomes bound to the plasma membrane and a small proportion persists within the macrophage where it is protected in some unknown way from digestion and is slowly secreted. Both forms of antigenic material—surface and secretory—persist for at least 2 weeks in immunogenic form (see below).

Macrophages can bind and engulf antigen without the assistance of antibody, but if IgG antibody is present (from previous immunisation) and combines with the antigen to form immune complexes, binding is greatly enhanced because macrophages, like polymorphs and some lymphocytes, have surface receptors for the Fc of the IgG in the complexes. Macrophages do not have receptors for IgM, but when IgM antibody reacts with antigen, complement is activated and the binding of the antigen–antibody complexes is then enhanced by surface receptors for the C3b component of complement (p. 181). Some sub-classes of IgG antibody are cytophilic for macrophages, i.e. they bind to the macrophage surface in the absence of antigen, and will enhance the binding of antigen subsequently encountered. These mechanisms of antigen binding are summarised in Fig. 7.2, p. 180.

The immunogenicity of macrophage-associated antigen. When living macrophages are incubated with an antigen *in vitro* and washed to remove free antigen, they induce an immune response when injected into a syngeneic animal. If the antigen is weak, i.e. induces a poor immune response when injected alone, prior processing by macrophages considerably enhances its immunogenicity. Similar experiments suggest that macrophage-associated antigen enhances both primary and secondary antibody and cell-mediated immune responses: it is particularly effective in stimulating the production of B-memory cells and so primes the individual for a secondary response. Both the number of B lymphocytes responding to a weak antigen and the number of cells resulting from the clonal proliferation of each stimulated B cell are increased by macrophage participation. Macrophage activity does not, however, overcome the need for helper T cells in T-dependent antibody responses, nor does it induce immune responses in animals which have acquired immunological tolerance to the antigen.

There is recent evidence that macrophages secrete various non-antigenic products which influence lymphocyte responses to antigen, and also that macrophages can bind a product (? antigen receptors) of responding T lymphocytes (Fig. 5.27c, p. 130).
Trapping of lymphocytes by macrophage-associated antigen. When macrophages are treated *in vitro* with antigens and then washed free of unbound antigen

and added to a suspension of lymphocytes, a small proportion of the lymphocytes bind to individual macrophages to form clusters. The number of clusters is much greater when the lymphocytes are taken from an animal previously immunised with the same antigen, and it may thus be concluded that specifically-responsive lymphocytes, including memory cells, bind to the surface-bound antigen on the macrophage, from which they receive antigenic stimulation. The clusters contain T and B lymphocytes and it may be that, by attracting both types of cell, the macrophage promotes T–B cell co-operation in the immune response.

The distribution of antigen within the body depends on the route of entry and on the amount and nature of the antigen. When a small amount of antigen is introduced into the skin, it is taken up mainly by macrophages in the draining lymph nodes. Antigen entering the bloodstream is taken up by macrophages in the spleen and liver and also in various lymph nodes. These patterns of distribution are, however, influenced by whether the antigen is in solution or in particulate form, and by the presence or absence of antibodies resulting from a previous exposure to the antigen.

The virgin lymphocytes responsible for a primary immune response are believed to lie mainly in the spleen and lymph nodes (p. 122) where they presumably encounter the macrophage-bound antigen, although the possibility that these short-lived cells recirculate has not been ruled out. The secondary response is due to the presence, in the recirculating lymphocyte pool, of T and B memory cells responsive to the antigen (p. 123), and within a day or so of introduction of the antigen these specifically responsive memory cells aggregate at the sites of the macrophage-associated antigen, i.e. in the spleen and/or lymph nodes, and so disappear from the recirculating pool. Electron-microscopic studies have shown aggregates of lymphocytes around antigen-containing macrophages, similar to the *in vitro* clusters described above. In some instances, antigen persists locally in a non-lymphoid tissue, where its presence stimulates a macrophage reaction followed by aggregation of lymphocytes and a local immune response (p. 139).

Dendritic germinal-centre cells are not true macrophages, for they are of mesodermal origin. Their property of binding antigen–antibody complexes is described on p. 138.

Conclusions. *By destroying excess antigen and presenting the remainder in strongly immunogenic form, macrophages may inhibit the development of immunological tolerance and enhance the immune response. By their prolonged retention of antigen within the secondary lymphoid* *tissues, macrophages afford good opportunity for responsive T and B cells of the recirculating lymphocyte pool to encounter and respond to the antigenic stimulus. They thus help to ensure that* *the immunological experience of the individual, represented by T and B memory cells, is brought to bear on any foreign antigen entering the body.*

Histological Features of the Immune Response

The cellular events of immune responses take place mainly in the secondary lymphoid organs, i.e. the lymph nodes, Malpighian bodies of the spleen, tonsils and gut-associated lymphoid tissues. Study of the morphological changes of immune responses is not easy, for the large numbers of micro-organisms in the alimentary and upper respiratory tracts, and on the other exposed mucous membranes, provide continual antigenic stimuli which ensure that the immunity system is never completely inactive. The maintenance of animals in a germ-free environment from birth onwards is helpful, but technically exacting, and does not ensure complete freedom from antigenic stimulation: thus 'germ-free' mice are likely to be infected with mouse leukaemia virus, and do, in fact, show evidence of immune responses in their lymphoid tissues. There is also great regional variation in lymph node responses: when the antigenic stimulus is localised, e.g. in vaccination, the draining lymph nodes usually show the greatest response, but there may be marked differences, even between adjacent nodes.

Study of the lymphoid tissues in animals rendered deficient of T cells (e.g. by neonatal thymectomy, anti-lymphocyte serum or thoracic duct drainage), in fowls rendered B-cell deficient by bursectomy, and in patients with major congenital immunodeficiencies, has helped to distinguish between the histological features of the T-cell-mediated immune response and those of the B cell antibody response.

Lymph nodes

Normal structure. The lymph node consists of cortex, medulla and lymph sinuses (Fig. 5.30). The cortex occupies the superficial part of the node except at the hilar region: the medulla lies centrally, but extends to the hilum. The framework of the node consists of a net-

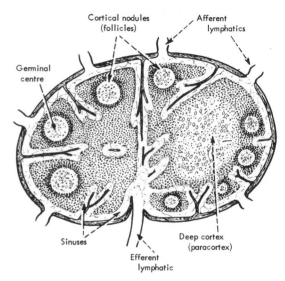

Fig. 5.30   Diagram of a lymph node, portraying the superficial cortex with nodules and germinal centres, and on the right an ill-defined area of deep cortex.

work of fine reticulin fibrils which are covered by the cytoplasm of elongated, flat reticulum cells with branching cytoplasmic processes. Many different names have been suggested for these cells, but their origin, nature and function are unknown. The sinuses are simply channels in the reticular framework, and they also are lined and traversed by reticulum cells. Macrophages are present in varying concentrations in all parts of the lymph nodes, including the lumen and walls of the sinuses.

Most of the free cells in the node are lymphocytes, and small lymphocytes usually predominate. In the cortex, the lymphocytes are closely arranged, and *the superficial part of the cortex* consists of foci, termed *primary nodules*, in which lymphocytes are more closely packed. In a stimulated node, as described below, a focus of lymphopoiesis, termed a *germinal centre*, may develop within the primary nodules. The *deeper cortex*, sometimes termed the *paracortex*, consists of ill-defined uniform areas of cortical tissue lying between the superficial cortex and medulla (Fig. 5.31): in the stimulated node, there may be intense proliferation of lymphoid cells here, and this may result in one or more large cellular zones which compress the medulla of the node.

Lymph arriving at the node by the afferent lymphatics enters the peripheral sinus which surrounds the lymphoid tissue of the node and communicates at the hilum with the efferent lymphatic. From the peripheral sinus, cortical sinuses pass radially inwards to the medulla, running between the superficial cortical nodules and penetrating the deep cortex. In the medulla the lymph sinuses are numerous and the lymphoid tissue lies between them as the *medullary cords*: the medullary sinuses unite to form the efferent lymphatic.

The lymph nodes have two major functions. One of these is the interception and removal of abnormal or foreign material in the lymph stream passing through them, and is described on pp. 568–9, 573: the other is the production

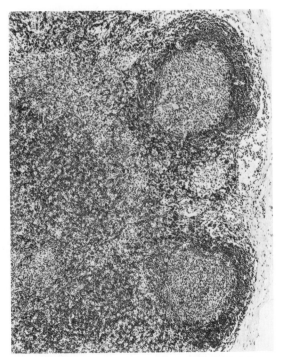

Fig. 5.31 Part of the cortex of a lymph node, showing two large cortical nodules (follicles) with germinal centres. The ill-defined area to the left of these consists of deep cortex. × 40.

of immune responses, the histological features of which are described below.

Immune responses in lymph nodes

(a) Cell-mediated immune responses. In lymph nodes draining the site of an antigenic stimulus of a kind which induces this type of response, e.g. an allogeneic skin graft or application to the skin of the hapten dinitrochlorobenzene, the most conspicuous early change is the appearance of large basophilic (and pyroninophilic) **T 'blast' cells** or **immunoblasts** in the deep cortex of the node. These cells appear 2 days or so after antigenic stimulation; they multiply rapidly and are maximal at about 5 days. Small lymphocytes also increase in number in the deep cortex, which becomes enlarged and conspicuous, causing appreciable increase in size of the node. If the antigenic stimulation is not prolonged, the immunoblasts disappear after a further few days, the main feature then being an increased number of small lymphocytes in the deep cortex.

As explained on p. 121, the deep cortex is in the pathway of the recirculating T lymphocytes, which are responsible for cell-mediated immune responses, and the appearance of immunoblasts and subsequently small lymphocytes in the deep cortex represents the clonal proliferation of specifically responsive T cells following antigenic stimulation. The responsive cells may have encountered antigen in the tissues and passed to the lymph nodes, or antigenic material, either free or carried by macrophages, may have reached the draining nodes and there stimulated appropriately responsive cells among the recirculating lymphocytes passing through the deep cortex. The use of tritiated-thymidine labelling has shown that the T immunoblasts in the deep cortex proliferate to produce small T lymphocytes, and that these appear in the recirculating lymphocyte pool at about the time of development of cell-mediated immunity: recirculation will allow such 'primed' cells to encounter, and react with, the corresponding antigen almost anywhere in the body, a factor of obvious importance in combating infections.

(b) Antibody production involves the proliferation of B lymphocytes to provide B memory cells and the plasma cells which synthesise and secrete antibody. As with T cells, the recirculation of B lymphocytes provides opportunity for their encounter with antigens in most of the tissues of the body. The main site of cell proliferation observed during antibody responses is in the superficial cortical nodules, which develop large spherical or ovoid **germinal centres** (Fig. 5.22), consisting of actively dividing, large basophilic B immunoblasts. **Plasma cells** appear in increasing numbers deep to the germinal centres and in the medullary cords, which are the main site of antibody production. During the early stages of the primary response neither antigen nor immunoglobulins are readily demonstrable in the cells of the germinal centres but, as antibody appears, antigen–antibody complexes become bound to the surface of the large **dendritic cells** of the germinal centres, and may persist there for many weeks. The nature of the dendritic cells, and the role of their surface complexes in antibody production, are not known; it is tempting to assume that the complexes provide a persistent antigenic stimulus to B cells, with consequent development of plasma cells which pass to the medulla and produce antibody, but this lacks proof. Small numbers of macrophages are also present in the germinal centres and contain ingested pyknotic nuclear material, the significance of which is unknown.

Although the function of the germinal centres is still uncertain, the intensity of mitotic activity within them during antibody responses suggests that they are the major site of clonal proliferation of specifically responsive B cells.

During antibody responses, which are often most pronounced in the lymph nodes draining the site containing antigen, the proliferating B cells differentiate into both plasma cells and memory B cells. Some of the B immunoblasts leave the nodes via the efferent lymphatic, and are distributed by the blood to other lymph nodes, etc., to the haemopoietic marrow, the lamina propria of the gut, and to the inflammatory reaction which may develop if antigen persists at the site of its introduction in the tissues (see below). Presumably these migrant cells also give rise to both plasma cells and B memory cells.

Although the histological features of cell-mediated immune responses and antibody production are described above separately, it must be emphasised that many antigenic stimuli induce both responses, and indeed the control of antibody responses by helper and suppressor T cells (p. 129) requires the combined form of response, although the site of T–B cell interaction in the lymphoid tissues is not known.

Immune responses in other lymphoid tissues

Spleen. The structure of the spleen is described briefly on p. 561. Immune responses take place in the Malpighian bodies in which the area immediately adjacent to the central arteriole is occupied by T lymphocytes of the recirculating pool, and corresponds to the deep cortex of lymph nodes. The more peripheral lymphoid tissue is occupied by recirculating B lymphocytes: it corresponds to the superficial cortex of lymph nodes and is the site of formation of germinal centres during antibody production. Antibody-producing plasma cells appear at the periphery of the Malpighian bodies and pass into the adjacent red pulp.

Immune responses in the spleen occur particularly when antigenic material gains entrance to the blood stream, and present morphological appearances similar to those which have been described for the lymph nodes.

Gut-associated lymphoid tissues. The solitary lymphoid follicles and Peyer's patches of the gut and the lymphoid tissue of the appendix all have T- and B-cell areas, and are in the pathway of long-lived T and B lymphocytes (probably mostly or all memory cells—p. 123). The gut lymphoid tissue has no afferent lymphatics but lies immediately beneath the surface epithelium which in these sites is cuboidal and includes specialised 'M' cells which have a complex folded surface. Antigen in the gut lumen, including whole bacteria, can penetrate the overlying epithelium and stimulate an immune response in both T and B cells, with the usual histological changes, including germinal centre formation. The B cells of these lymphoid tissues do not specialise in the production of IgA antibodies, this being the function of plasma cells lying in the lamina propria of the gut mucosa and derived from other lymphoid tissues by way of the major lymphatics and blood (p. 123).

The thymus. As already indicated, the thymus is a site of T-cell lymphopoiesis. It is not an important site of immune responses, but occasional germinal centres and plasma cells are demonstrable in the medulla of the thymus in a significant percentage of people dying suddenly or after a short illness: this suggests that B lymphocytes, presumably entering the thymus from the blood, are capable of mounting an antibody response. Thymic germinal centres are rarely seen in patients dying after a chronic illness, perhaps because there has been increased secretion of adrenal glucocorticoids, which results in thymic and lymphoid atrophy. Thymic germinal centres are, however, numerous in many cases of myasthenia gravis (p. 936), and occur also in the connective tissue diseases.

Immune responses in non-lymphoid tissues

In intensive and prolonged antibody responses, plasma cells may be widespread in various tissues, including the haemopoietic marrow, which can be an important site of antibody production. When antigen gains entrance to non-lymphoid tissues, some of it is carried, either free or by macrophages, to the local lymph nodes where an immune response occurs. If, however, the antigen persists in its original site, as in chronic infections, skin allografts and locally-injected antigen of low solubility, then specifically primed T and B cells derived from the immune response in the lymph nodes may enter the tissue and respond specifically to the antigen: thus after 2 weeks or so there may be numerous plasma cells and also proliferating T lymphoblasts. Macrophages also accumulate and may play a role in the local immune response by processing the antigen (p. 134). If the antigen persists locally for some weeks, lymphoid tissue with germinal centres and T-cell areas may develop, i.e. ectopic secondary lymphoid tissue. This is seen also in the thyroid, etc. in the organ-specific autoimmune diseases (p. 162), and in the synovial membrane of joints in rheumatoid arthritis (Fig. 23.52, p. 918).

References

Bach, J.-F., Dardenne, M., Pleau, J.-M. and Bach, A. A. (1975). Isolation, biochemical characteristics and biological activity of a circulating thymic hormone in the mouse and in the human. *Annals of the New York Academy of Science* **249**, 186–210.

Burnet, F. M. (1959). *The Clonal Selection Theory of Acquired Immunity*. Cambridge University Press, Cambridge.

Burnet, F. M. and Fenner, F. (1949). p. 76 in *The Production of Antibodies*, 2nd edn. pp. 142. Macmillan and Co. Ltd., London.

Gershon, R. K. and Kondo, K. (1971). Infectious immunological tolerance. *Immunology* **21**, 903–14.

Good, R. A., Martinez, C. and Gabrielsen, Ann E. (1964). Clinical considerations of the thymus in immunobiology. In *The Thymus in Immunobiology*, pp. 3–47. Ed. by R. A. Good and Ann E. Gabrielsen. Harper and Row, New York.

Gowans, J. L. (1966). Life-span, recirculation and transformation of lymphocytes. *International Review of Experimental Pathology* **5**, 1–78.

Jerne, N. K. (1955). The natural-selection theory of antibody production. *Proceedings of the National Academy of Science (N.Y.)* **41**, 849–57.

Jerne, N. K. (1971). The somatic generation of immune recognition. *European Journal of Immunology* **1**, 1–9.

Lawrence, H. S. (1969). Transfer factor. *Advances in Immunology* **11**, 196–266.

Le Douarin, N. M. (1977). Ontogeny of primary lymphoid organs. In *B and T Cells in Immune Recognition*, pp. 1–19. Ed. by F. Loor and G. E. Roelants. John Wiley and Sons Ltd., Chichester.

Miller, J. F. A. P. (1964). Effect of thymic ablation and replacement. In *The Thymus in Immunobiology*, pp. 436–60. Ed. by R. A. Good and Ann E. Gabrielsen. Harper and Row, New York.

Mitchison, N. A. (1967). Immunological paralysis as a dosage phenomenon. In *Regulation of the Antibody Response*, pp. 54–63. Ed. by B. Cinader, pp. 400. C. C. Thomas, Springfield.

Mitchison, N. A. (1971). The carrier effect in the secondary response to hapten-protein conjugates. *European Journal of Immunology* **1**, 10–27.

Munro, A. and Waldmann, H. (1978). The major histocompatibility system and the immune response. *British Medical Bulletin*, **34**, 253–78.

Owen, R. D. (1945). Immunogenetic consequences of vascular anastomoses between bovine twins. *Science* **102**, 400–1.

Parrott, D. M. V. and de Sousa, M. A. B. (1971). Thymus-dependent and thymus-independent populations: origin, migratory patterns and lifespan. *Clinical and Experimental Immunology* **8**, 663–84.

Williamson, A. R. (1979) Control of antibody formation: certain uncertainties. *Journal of Clinical Pathology*. Supplement (Royal College of Pathologists) **13**, 76–84.

Further Reading

Advances in Immunology. Vols. 1–28. (1961–1980). Academic Press, New York. (A continuing series of comprehensive articles on major immunological topics by leading authorities.)

Bowry, T. R. (1977). *Immunology Simplified*, pp. 223. African Medical and Research Foundation. (A clear and brief account of basic and clinical immunology.)

Herbert, W. J. and Wilkinson, P. C. (Eds.) (1977). *A Dictionary of Immunology*, 2nd edn., pp. 194. Blackwell Scientific, Oxford. (A most helpful compilation of brief descriptions of terms used in immunology.)

Loor, F. and Roelants, G. E. (Eds.) (1977). *B and T Cells in Immune Recognition*, pp. 504. John Wiley and Sons, Chichester. (A collection of articles, by leading workers, on the development and functions of lymphocytes.)

Roitt, I. M. (1977). *Essential Immunology*, 3rd edn., pp. 334. Blackwell Scientific, Oxford. (A clearly written and beautifully illustrated account of basic and clinical immunology.)

Turk, John (Ed.) *Current Topics in Immunology Series*. Edward Arnold, London. (A series of monographs on basic and clinical aspects of important immunological topics.)

See also bibliography for Chapter 6.

6

Immunopathology

This chapter is devoted entirely to disease processes which have an immunological basis. It falls naturally into two parts. First, the **hypersensitivity reactions** which are of an immunological nature. It should be noted that this use of the term hypersensitivity is somewhat restricted. It does not include those conditions in which the subject is abnormally sensitive to a drug as a result of genetically determined deficiency of an enzyme system necessary for metabolising the drug or because of failure to excrete the drug or its metabolites, e.g. in diseases of the liver or kidneys: this type of undue responsiveness is termed *idiosyncrasy* and is not dealt with here.

The second main section of the chapter describes the **immunological deficiencies**, i.e. congenital or acquired conditions in which the subject is incapable of the normal range of immunological responses and as a result is unduly susceptible to infection.

Hypersensitivity Reactions

In most instances, hypersensitivity may be defined as a state in which the introduction of an antigen into the body elicits an unduly severe immunological reaction. It follows previous exposure to the antigen and is a consequence of the development of an immune response, i.e. production of antibodies or sensitised lymphocytes reactive with the antigen. *It is this reaction between the antigen and products of the immune response which produces the lesions of the hypersensitivity disease processes.*

Hypersensitivity reactions may be localised to the site of entry of the antigen, or generalised: the local reactions are mainly of an inflammatory nature, but may also include spasm of smooth muscle. The generalised effects include fever, shock, gastrointestinal and pulmonary disturbances, and sometimes fatal circulatory collapse. One of the earliest examples of hypersensitivity was provided by Richet and Partier (1902) who observed that intravenous injection of small amounts of extracts of sea anemone into dogs was harmless, but a second injection some weeks later was quickly followed by a violent and sometimes fatal reaction with dyspnoea, vomiting, defaecation, micturition and collapse. Since this early report, which illustrates the acute and severe nature of some hypersensitivity reactions, a great deal has been learned, and hypersensitivity reactions may now be classified into four major types (see below).

The definition of hypersensitivity given above refers solely to **foreign antigens** entering the body from outside. However, the term includes also the conditions commonly known as the **autoimmune diseases**, in which antibodies or sensitised lymphocytes appear which are capable of reacting with a normal cell or tissue constituent *in vivo*, with consequent pathological changes. Hypersensitivity reactions may result also from passive immunisation, for example when antibody is produced in the mother by active immunisation by fetal red cells, and crosses the placenta in a subsequent pregnancy to gain entrance to the fetal circulation. Another special example of hypersensitivity of increasing importance is **the rejection process in allogeneic or heterogeneic tissue transplants**. The increasing diversity and use of drugs has also provided an important group of **drug hypersensitivities** and the same applies to the expanding number of chemicals used domestically and in industry.

The four major types of hypersensitivity reactions are described briefly below and then each is dealt with in more detail. They have been elucidated very largely by animal experiments. Hypersensitivity reactions in man, whether they occur naturally or as a result of transplantation, or from administration of a drug, tend to be complex and often involve more than one of the four types.

Atopic, anaphylactic or type 1 reactions occur in individuals who are predisposed to develop increased amounts of IgE class antibodies in response to antigenic stimuli. IgE antibody binds to mast cells, and subsequent union of the corresponding antigen triggers off release of histamine, etc., from the sensitised mast cells, giving rise to a local inflammatory reaction and smooth muscle spasm, or to a more generalised reaction. Examples include hay fever and asthma.

Cytotoxic antibody or type 2 reactions occur when antibody develops which is capable of reacting with surface antigens of cells. As a result, the cells are injured by subsequent complement activation, phagocytosis, etc. Examples include destruction of red cells and platelets by auto-antibodies to their surface components.

Immune-complex, Arthus-type or type 3 reactions are caused by the reaction of antibody, usually of IgG class, with the corresponding soluble antigen. This can occur locally (Arthus reaction) or in the blood. In either case, immune complexes are deposited in the walls of blood vessels, where they activate complement and induce vascular injury.

Delayed hypersensitivity or type 4 reactions occur when the primed T lymphocytes, which develop during the cell-mediated immune response, encounter the corresponding antigen. The specifically reactive T lymphocytes transform to blast cells and secrete a number of factors (lymphokines) which mediate an acute inflammatory reaction, aggregation of more lymphocytes and monocytes, and sometimes necrosis. The tuberculin skin test is a good example.

It should be noted that type 1 and 2 reactions occur in subjects predisposed to unusual immune responses, while types 3 and 4 are the result of immune responses of which all normal individuals are capable.

Before considering types of hypersensitivity in detail, this is a convenient place to give accounts of two systems, the profound importance of which is becoming increasingly apparent. The first is the **complement system**, which was for long regarded as being concerned solely in relation to antigen–antibody reactions, but is now known to participate in many other processes, e.g. in inflammation, blood clotting and fibrinolysis. The second is the **cyclic nucleotide system**, in which the levels of cyclic AMP and GMP within the cell play an important role in most of the functions of animal cells: its role in controlling the release of mast cell products, which is outlined briefly below, is involved in some forms of hypersensitivity, but is only one illustration of its much wider importance.

The complement system

This consists of at least 18 proteins which make up about 10 per cent of the total protein of the plasma. Many of the components are synthesised by monocytes and macrophages and increased macrophage activity, as in inflammation, is accompanied by enhanced production of some complement components.

Eleven of the complement components are termed C1–C9 (C1 is a complex of three factors, C1q, C1r and C1s), and when complement is activated by an antigen–antibody reaction these components react in sequential or cascade fashion in the order 1 to 9 except for C4 which is now known to react sequentially between C1 and C2. Such activation is termed the **classical pathway**. A second method of activation, termed the **alternative pathway**, is also initiated by antigen–antibody complexes and by certain bacteria without the necessity for an antigen–antibody reaction: it involves at least four additional factors—factors B, D, P (properdin) and C3b—and triggers off the sequential reaction at the C3 stage, so that C1, 4 and 2 are not involved. Various proteolytic enzymes present in inflammatory exudates and participating in the clotting and kinin systems can also activate the complement reaction at the C1 or C3 stages (p. 55). Compliment activation is modulated by spontaneous decay of some of the activated components and by a number of inhibitory factors, the best known of which are CĪ-INH which inhibits CĪ† and C3b-INA and β1H, both of which inhibit C3b activity.

The classical pathway (Fig. 6.1) is initiated when IgG or IgM antibody reacts with antigen. As shown in Fig. 6.1, three of the stages of the pathway involve enzyme reactions, and since one molecule of enzyme can cleave many molecules of substrate, the sequential reaction is amplified as it progresses. Such amplification is, however, opposed by the rapid spontaneous decay of some of the activated components and by various inhibitory factors.

The alternative pathway. It is probable that there is continuous triggering of the classical pathway, perhaps by low concentrations of antigen–antibody complexes resulting from absorption of small amounts of environmental antigens or by low-grade plasmin activity. Such

complement activation is largely held in check by C1-INH, but presumably provides some C3b, which is an essential factor in the alternative pathway (Fig. 6.1). Normally, the alternative pathway is held in check by C3b-INA and β1H, both of which are necessary to prevent uncontrolled cleavage of C3 by this pathway, and agents which trigger off the alternative pathway do so by interfering with the inhibitory function of C3b-INA and/or β1H. The lipopolysaccharide cell wall material (including endotoxin) of various bacteria is the most important activator of the alternative pathway; it probably acts by binding C3b and rendering it resistant to the action of these inhibitors. The alternative pathway is also activated by IgA antibody–antigen complexes, and since C3b is the limiting factor in the alternative pathway, its production in the classical pathway also promotes alternative pathway activity.

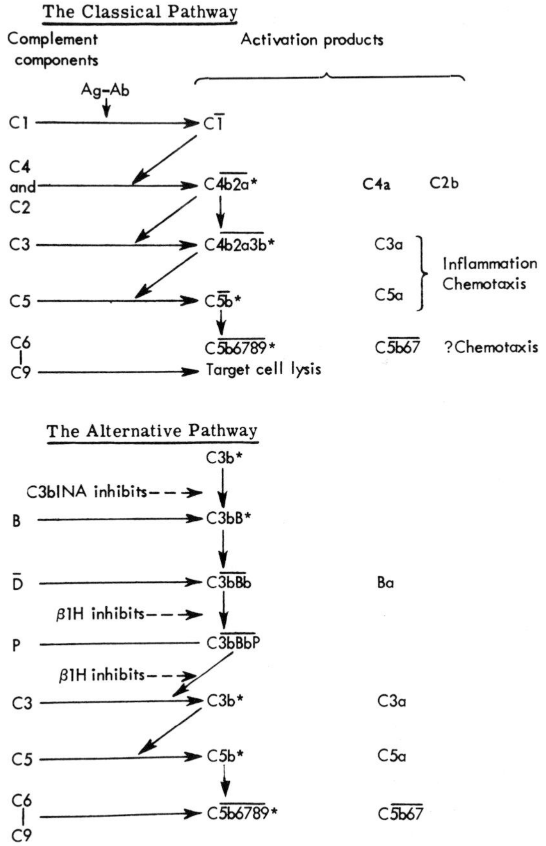

Fig. 6.1 Activation of complement. **The classical pathway** is initiated when C1, which is a pro-enzyme, is activated by binding to the Fc of IgG or IgM antibody complexed with antigen (Ag–Ab). The active enzyme CĪ (activated components of the system are indicated by overlining) cleaves both C4 and C2 into small fragments (C4a and C2b) and large fragments (C4b and C2a). The large fragments unite to form a second enzyme C4b2a which cleaves C3 into C3a and C3b. The large fragment, C3b, binds to C4b2a to form a third enzyme, C4b2a3b, which cleaves C5 into C5a and C5b. C6 and C7 then bind to C5b, forming a stable complex, C5b67. C8 binds to this complex which in turn binds C9 to form the C5b-9 lytic complex.

The alternative pathway requires C3b for its initiation: this is provided by continuous spontaneous low-grade activity of the classical pathway, or by splitting of C3 by plasmin, the kinin or clotting systems, or by various proteolytic enzymes released by polymorphs, injured tissue cells, etc. C3b is inactivated by C3bINA and β1H, but is protected by the binding of B (and probably also by endotoxin). D splits B in this complex, releasing Ba, leaving C3bBb which binds P (properdin) to form a complex which splits C3, producing more C3b: this amplifies the alternative pathway activation and also contributes to an enzyme complex which splits C5 to provide C5b. The reaction then proceeds as in the later stages of the classical pathway.

* Those activated components and complexes which bind to cell surfaces are marked with an asterisk.

† Activated components of the complement system are indicated by overlining, e.g. CĪ.

Biologically active products of complement. When complement is activated by either pathway, some of the activation products are released into the surrounding fluid. Of these, C3a and C5a influence the behaviour of various cells. They stimulate mast cells and basophils to release histamine and other vasoactive amines and thus induce vascular exudative changes as in acute inflammation. In these effects, C5a is far more potent than C3a. C5a is also chemotactic for neutrophil polymorphs and monocytes and so promotes emigration and accumulation of these cells. C3a and C5a are commonly, though inappropriately, termed *anaphylatoxins* (p. 55). When complement is activated by particulate material, e.g. microorganisms or host cells sensitised with antibody, or certain bacteria alone, some of the activation products, indicated in Fig. 6.1 by an asterisk, bind to the surface of the target cell and promote its destruction by two methods. Firstly, polymorphs and macrophages have surface receptors for C3b, adherence of which to the target cell (*immune adherence*) thus promotes the binding of polymorphs and macrophages and favours phagocytosis and destruction of the target cell. Secondly, completion of the complement cascade results in the insertion of the C5b-9 complex into the target cell plasma membrane which is consequently injured, sometimes causing cell death. The mode of injury is not fully understood, but in electron micrographs apparent holes develop in the cell membrane (Fig. 2.10, p. 18), the cell absorbs water and electrolytes, swells up and ruptures.

When complement is activated by either pathway, C5b is released and may adhere to adjacent cells not involved in the initial activation. The C5b-9 complex may then build up on these 'innocent' cells, causing their death. This is known as **bystander cell lysis** or **reactive lysis.**

The pathological importance of complement. As explained earlier (pp. 44–61), complement is a source of *mediators of the acute inflammatory reaction* and appears to be of importance in the inflammation induced by various non-immunologic stimuli. The role of complement in types 2 and 3 hypersensitivity reactions is discussed later in this chapter.

Probably the most important role of complement is in killing micro-organisms and rendering them susceptible to ingestion and killing by phagocytes (pp. 180–2).

Complement deficiency. Genetically-determined deficiency of one or other of the complement components is rare. Deficiency of an early component (C1, C4 or C2) does not usually give rise to disease, presumably because activation can still occur by the alternative pathway. Deficiency of a later component usually results in an increased susceptibility to bacterial infection.

The best known genetic abnormality of complement is deficiency of C$\bar{1}$-INH which results in uncontrolled activation of complement and the inflammatory lesions of hereditary angiooedema (p. 254).

Detection of complement components. The measurement of total haemolytic complement activity present in serum is performed traditionally by determining the concentration of serum required to cause lysis of 50% of a suspension of red cells sensitised with antibody (p. 112). Techniques are, however, available to measure individual complement components, and also their activation products: such tests are now in routine use to detect evidence of activation of complement *in vivo* in various diseases, and to distinguish between activation by the classical and alternative pathways.

The cyclic nucleotides

The integrity of multicellular organisms is obviously dependent on co-ordinated function of their individual cells. This involves systems of communication between cells by the nervous system, and the responsiveness of cells to the levels of hormones and various other solutes in the extracellular fluid. A major advance in the understanding of how cells respond to such signals has been provided by the discovery that many cell functions are controlled by the concentration of cyclic nucleotides in the cytosol (see Larner, 1977). The effects of these compounds are illustrated here by the role they play in release of stored products by mast cells, a phenomenon of importance in type 1 hypersensitivity.

The release of histamine and other vasoactive agents stored in mast cell granules has already been discussed in relation to the increased vascular permeability of acute inflammation. It is triggered off by various physical and chemical agents. In type 1 hypersensitivity, degranulation of mast cells (and basophil leukocytes) occurs when molecules of antigen combine with molecules of IgE class antibody bound to the mast cell surface (see below). β-adrenergic receptor blockade also has the same effect, while β-adrenergic stimulation, e.g. by isoprenaline, salbutamol and adrenaline, inhibits mast cell degranulation (Fig. 6.2). Stimulation or blockade of α receptors and cholinergic receptors also influence mast cell degranulation. It is thus apparent that many agents have an effect on this important function of mast cells. It now appears that they operate through a common pathway—by raising or lowering the levels of cyclic nucleotides in the cytosol of the mast cell.

Agents which stimulate β receptors activate an enzyme, adenyl cyclase, which lies at the inner surface of the cell membrane, and this results in increased production of cyclic adenosine monophosphate (cAMP) which suppresses release of stored products of the mast cell, while β-adrenergic blockade inhibits adenyl cyclase with consequent fall in cAMP level and the stored products are released. Stimulation or blockade of the α-adrenergic receptors have the opposite effects. Agents which react with the cholinergic receptors influence the activity of guanyl cyclase which in turn affects the level in the cytosol of a second nucleotide, cyclic guanosine monophosphate (cGMP). In general, cAMP and cGMP have opposite effects on cell function, and it appears to be the ratio of the two which is of importance. Thus a fall in cAMP and/or a rise in cGMP favour degranulation. The cyclic nucleotides are inactivated by intracellular phosphodiesterases, and many agents, including some of those mentioned above, also influence the levels of the cyclic nucleotides by affecting the activity of these enzymes.

Not only do cAMP and cGMP have opposite effects on the cell, but some agents which lower the level of one increase the other. This may be mediated by an effect on the permeability of the cell membrane for Ca^{++} or on the distribution of Ca^{++} within the cell, for a rise of Ca^{++} in the cytosol inhibits adenyl cyclase activity and activates cAMP-phosphodiesterase, thus decreasing cAMP: it has the opposite effect on cGMP.

Although the mast cell has been used to illustrate the importance of the cyclic nucleotides, they are of equal importance in all cells, exerting an influence on cell division, motility, secretion, etc. A fall in cAMP and rise in cGMP is

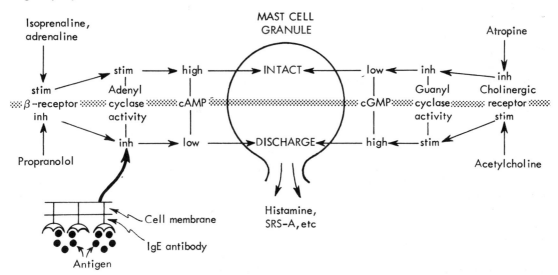

Fig. 6.2 Discharge of mast-cell and basophil-leukocyte granules, showing the relationship between the levels of the cyclic nucleotides (cAMP and cGMP) in the cytosol and release of products stored in the cell granules. Stimulation (stim) and inhibition (inh) of β-adrenergic and cholinergic cell surface receptors influence the activity of adenyl and guanyl cyclases and thus the levels of cAMP and cGMP in the cytosol. The attachment of antigen to cell-bound IgE antibody inhibits adenyl cyclase and causes discharge of the granules. Although α-adrenergic receptors (not shown) also influence the levels of cyclic nucleotides, the mechanism has not been elucidated. Note that the pathways above the hatched lines stabilise mast cell granules and those below stimulate their discharge.

associated with mitosis. In many glandular cells, the same change is associated also with secretory activity, although in some instances, e.g. the cells of the adenohypophysis and the thyroid epithelium, secretion is induced by a rise in cAMP and a fall in cGMP.

Atopy (anaphylactic, 'immediate' or type 1) hypersensitivity

Approximately 10% of the population suffers from this type of hypersensitivity, although in most of these the symptoms are mild and occasional. The commonest manifestations of atopy are **hay fever** and **extrinsic asthma**, which tend to run in families and are sometimes preceded by **atopic eczema** in infancy and childhood. The sufferer from hay fever develops acute inflammation of the nasal and conjunctival mucous membrane with sneezing and nasal and lacrimal hypersecretion within minutes of exposure to an atmosphere containing the causal agent (usually grass or other pollens). Similarly, an acute attack of asthma, with difficult wheezing respiration due to narrowing of the airways by bronchospasm and mucous secretion, develops rapidly when the asthmatic inhales the agent to which he is hypersensitive, e.g. house dust or animal dander. Atopic individuals, particularly in childhood, may also suffer from '**food allergies**' in which absorption of antigenic constituents of certain foods, e.g. milk or eggs, promotes an acute reaction in the gut with colicky pain, vomiting and diarrhoea.

Urticaria, consisting of acute inflammatory lesions of the skin with wealing due to dermal oedema, is common in atopic subjects and also occurs alone as an acute or chronic condition.

In addition to local disturbances, atopic patients sometimes develop **acute systemic anaphylaxis** (anaphylactic shock) with dyspnoea, urticaria, convulsions, prostration and sometimes death. Generalised reactions occur when the responsible agent is absorbed in amounts which produce a significant level in the blood. Fortunately, severe anaphylactic shock is rare, but it sometimes occurs in hypersensitivity to drugs, notably penicillin, and to the venoms of stinging insects.

Skin tests and provocation tests. Diagnosis of atopy depends firstly on an accurate clinical history, which usually suggests that acute attacks result from exposure to a particular environmental antigen. To confirm the state of hypersensitivity, dilute solutions of the suspected antigens (which are commercially available) may be placed on the skin and pricked in with a needle. A positive result is indicated by a local weal and flare reaction, developing within a few minutes (Fig. 6.3) and lasting for an hour or so. Hence the term 'immediate type' hypersensitivity. Although of diagnostic help, skin tests are not infallible. The atopic individual tends to give positive reactions not only to the environmental antigen(s) responsible for attacks of atopy, but also to various others. Also, in a proportion of cases the skin test is negative although the history is very suggestive of atopy to that antigen. A more reliable indication of the causal role of a particular antigen is provided by provocation tests, for example bronchial challenge by controlled inhalation of the suspected antigen by the asthmatic, and nasal application for the hay-fever patient: an acute attack implicates the test antigen. In all such tests, careful precautions must be taken to avoid provoking a severe reaction.

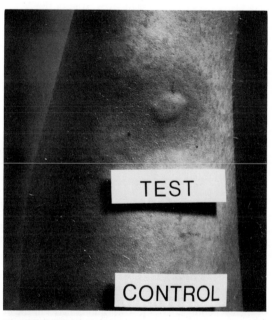

Fig. 6.3 Skin test showing immediate (type I) hypersensitivity reaction. The patient was an asthmatic and the test was performed by intradermal injection of an extract of house dust. Note the oedema and wide zone of reddening. Photograph taken 10 minutes after injection. (Dr. Ian McKay.)

The mechanism of atopic hypersensitivity

Passive transfer of immediate type hypersensitivity was demonstrated beautifully 60 years ago by the classical investigation of the two German doctors, Prausnitz and Küstner. Küstner himself regularly developed hypersensitivity reactions immediately after eating fish, and intradermal injection of an extract of cooked fish induced an immediate-type reaction. Injection of a small amount of Küstner's serum intradermally into Prausnitz induced a local state of hypersensitivity, for when cooked fish muscle extract was injected intradermally 24 hours later at the same site an immediate-type reaction occurred, whereas other skin sites were negative.

Passive transfer has been confirmed repeatedly with serum from atopic subjects: it has been shown to be antigen-specific, and the interval between the two injections can be prolonged to 3–4 weeks, demonstrating that the serum factor (reagin—see below) binds to some tissue element in the skin.

Temporary atopic hypersensitivity has also been observed in recipients of blood from atopic donors: the recipient exhibits positive skin tests and may develop clinical atopy if exposed to the relevant antigen(s). Evidence that reagin sticks to various tissues and not just to skin has been provided by the demonstration that fresh bronchial tissue removed from an atopic subject undergoes contraction of the smooth muscle when exposed to the appropriate antigen, and it has been shown that normal tissues of various types can be sensitised passively by the serum of atopic individuals.

Reaginic antibody: IgE. Being antigen-specific, the serum factor responsible for passive transfer of atopy has long been regarded as an antibody, and known as **reagin** or **reaginic antibody**. It has proved difficult to characterise, for it is present in serum in only trace amounts, and is relatively instable; also it is **homocytotropic**, *i.e.* binds to the tissues of man or related primates, but not to tissues of other genera: this restricts its detection by passive transfer to experiments on man and some monkeys. However, it was eventually shown by Ishizaka *et al.* (1966) to be due to an immunoglobulin of a distinct 'new' class, since termed IgE. Patients with IgE-producing mye-lomas (plasma-cell tumours) have provided a rich source of IgE. Using this material, it was shown that when a solution of IgE or of its Fc component was injected into the skin it was found to block the tissue sites of attachment of reaginic antibody, and so inhibited the Prausnitz–Küstner reaction at the same site. This is strong confirmation that reaginic antibodies are of IgE class, and shows that fixation to tissues is a property of their Fc component. Antibody specific for myeloma IgE is now used to assay the level of IgE in serum and also as the basis of the *in-vitro* assay of specific IgE antibodies, e.g. by the 'radio-allergosorbent test' (RAST). Raised levels of IgE, and of IgE class antibodies to the relevant antigens, have been detected in the serum and nasal secretions, etc., but such *in-vitro* tests have so far contributed little to clinical practice.

Role of mast cells and basophil leukocytes. Mast cells are widely distributed in most tissues, and are particularly numerous adjacent to small blood vessels. Basophil leukocytes resemble mast cells in appearance and function; like other leukocytes, they can respond to chemotaxins and migrate from the blood into the tissues. Both mast cells and basophils have large basophilic cytoplasmic granules which can be discharged by various stimuli, e.g. the various causal agents of acute inflammation, and which release histamine and other vaso-active compounds.

Many mammalian species are capable of developing immediate-type hypersensitivity reactions similar to atopic reactions in man, and animal studies have demonstrated that reaginic antibody binds firmly by its Fc component to surface receptors of mast cells and basophils. This leaves the Fab ends of the antibody free to react with the corresponding antigen, and when this occurs, cross-linking of surface-bound antibody molecules by the antigen results in degranulation via the cyclic-nucleotide pathways (p. 145), and the discharged granules in turn release their stored histamine and other vaso-active agents which bring about vascular hyperaemia and exudation (Fig. 6.4). Prior depletion of mast cell and basophil mediators by such compounds as 48/80 inhibits the immediate hypersensitivity reaction in animals, as does the administration of histamine antagonists.

Although atopy in man differs in certain

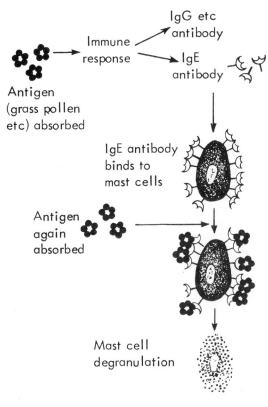

Antigen
(grass pollen
etc) absorbed

Immune response → IgG etc antibody
→ IgE antibody

IgE antibody binds to mast cells

Antigen again absorbed

Mast cell degranulation

Histamine etc.

Fig. 6.4 The mechanism of atopic reactions. IgE antibody to pollens, etc., binds by its Fc component to mast cells (and basophil leukocytes), and subsequently absorbed antigen triggers off the sensitised mast cells (probably by linking together antibody molecules on their surface) to release histamine, etc.

respects from experimental immediate-type hypersensitivity in animals, and has not been so thoroughly studied at cellular level, there is nevertheless strong evidence for the mechanism summarised in Fig. 6.4. Human basophil leukocytes have been shown to bind IgE antibodies and to be degranulated by subsequent addition of antigens. Mast cells in monkey lung have been shown to bind human IgE, subsequent cross-linking of which causes the cells to release histamines, etc. (Ishizaka, Ishizaka and Tomioka, 1972). I am unaware of similar work on human mast cells, but it has been shown that human lung tissue removed surgically from an atopic subject (who had developed bronchial carcinoma) yielded histamine and SRS-A (the slow reacting substance of anaphylaxis) when perfused with fluid containing a solution of the appropriate antigen. The main source of these two vaso-active agents in man are the mast cells and basophils. **SRS-A** is a lipid which increases vascular permeability and induces more prolonged spasm of bronchial smooth muscle than does histamine. Other factors released by mast-cells and basophils include two tetrapeptides known collectively as **ECF-A** (the eosinophil chemotactic factor of anaphylaxis) and possibly prostaglandins.

The role of eosinophil leukocytes. Acute atopic reactions are characterised by vascular hyperaemia, exudation, and emigration of eosinophil polymorphs into the affected mucous membrane. The role of eosinophils has long remained a mystery, but evidence is accumulating that they modulate the intensity of atopic reactions. Experimentally-induced immediate-type hypersensitivity reactions in rats are enhanced by injection of an anti-eosinophil serum which depletes the blood of eosinophils, and these cells not only secrete histaminase and arylsulphatase, which inactivate histamine and SRS-A respectively, but there is also evidence that they may inhibit both mast-cell degranulation and restoration of degranulated mast cells. The eosinophil also plays a defensive role against parasitic worms (see below).

Other immunological factors. Although IgE antibody is the important mediating agent of atopy, it may not be the only such factor. There is recent evidence that IgG4 antibody (p. 108) can mediate a complement-dependent form of immediate type hypersensitivity, although it has not yet been proved that this second mechanism plays a significant role in human atopy. The antibody response is not restricted to IgE: other classes of antibody are also produced and in some atopic subjects the immediate reaction is followed by an Arthus (type 3) hypersensitivity reaction due to the formation of antigen–antibody complexes and possibly also by a delayed-hypersensitivity (type 4) reaction, due to primed T lymphocytes, in some cases. These later reactions, which may cause difficulty in detecting the responsible antigen(s), have been demonstrated most readily by provocation tests.

Atopic hypersensitivity can often be reduced, but seldom abolished, by subcutaneous injection of the responsible antigen in a slowly soluble (e.g. alum precipitated) form. The mechanism of such **hyposensitisation** is not known, but it has been shown to lead to a fall in IgE antibody and a rise in IgG antibody in the serum over the next few months. It is thought that the IgG antibody has a 'blocking' effect by reacting with naturally-absorbed antigen, thus preventing its combination with IgE antibody bound to mast cells. Hyposensitisation is not always successful, and the outcome is not predictable. There is, moreover, a possibility that, by stimulating the production of IgG antibody, the procedure may predispose the individual to immune complex disease (p. 152). The possible role of IgA antibodies in atopy is discussed below.

Predisposition to atopy

The occurrence of atopy in several generations of some families suggests a genetic predisposition. In general, atopic subjects have higher total serum IgE levels, and produce more IgE antibody in response to antigenic stimulation, than control subjects. Accordingly it seems likely that the genetic factor determines the intensity of IgE responses. Some support for this is provided by the finding of an association, in some families predisposed to atopy, between the IgE response to ragweed antigen (commonly a cause of hay fever) and the possession of particular HLA antigens.

Although atopy is attributable to the reaction between antigens and IgE antibodies, there must be other important factors, for in some cases the skin tests do not correlate with provocation tests nor with the occurrence of clinical atopy. One possibility is that the affected mucous membranes, e.g the nasal mucosa in hay fever subjects and the bronchial mucosa in asthmatics, are unduly permeable to small antigenic molecules (most of those which induce atopy have a molecular weight of 40 000 or less), but the evidence for this is not convincing. Related to this is the possible importance of the IgA antibody response and the secretion of IgA by mucous membranes. It has been shown that injection of IgA antibody into rats inhibits the absorption of inhaled or injected antigens. Most atopic subjects have normal serum IgA levels, but it has been reported that intranasal application of antigen results in the appearance of less IgA antibody and more IgE antibody in the nasal secretion in hay-fever subjects than in controls (Butcher, Salvaggio

and Leslie, 1975). It is also of great interest that assay of the serum IgA levels of the infants of atopic parents has shown that those with a low level of IgA at three months of age are more liable subsequently to develop atopic eczema (Taylor *et al.*, 1973) and probably also asthma (Soothill, personal communication). The same group of workers has also reported that avoidance of the environmental antigens which commonly cause atopy (including dairy products) during the first six months of life reduces the incidence of atopic eczema in infants with an atopic predisposition (Matthew *et al.*, 1977).

It has also been reported that T-cell depletion in rats enhances IgE antibody responses. In atopic subjects, there is no good evidence of a T-cell deficiency, although children with the rare Wiskott-Aldrich syndrome (p. 171), who have a congenital T-cell deficiency, are prone to develop atopy.

There is also evidence that parasympathetic bronchoconstrictor nerve endings between the bronchial epithelial cells are unduly irritable in asthmatics. These nerve endings are triggered by various stimuli, possibly including antigen–antibody complexes, and it has been postulated that an asthmatic attack may be initiated by formation of such complexes with consequent stimulation of cholinergic mast cell receptors and degranulation (Fig. 6.2). From these various observations, it is apparent that a number of abnormalities in the pathway between the exposure of the mucosa to antigens and the reaction of submucosal blood vessels, mucous glands and smooth muscle of the bronchi could be involved in atopy, but none have been demonstrated with certainty to be of importance.

It is noteworthy that in African communities with a high rate of infestation with parasitic worms, IgE levels are also high, although atopy is uncommon. Infestation with worms or injection of worm extracts has been shown in animals to increase the IgE antibody response to various antigens. IgE antibody is important in the defence against worms, and it has been suggested that, by binding to mast cells, antiparasitic IgE antibody, if present in relatively high concentration, excludes the binding of other IgE antibodies and thus protects against atopy. This would account for the higher incidence of atopy in populations with a low level of parasitic infestation, and it may be that elimination of most of our parasites has exposed us to the harmful effects of IgE antibody responses to various otherwise harmless environmental antigens.

Cytotoxic antibody (type 2) reactions

The only distinctive feature of this type of hypersensitivity reaction is that it is mediated by antibodies which cause injury to cells by combining specifically with antigenic determinants on their surface. With few exceptions, the targets of cytotoxic antibodies are the cells of the blood. Such injury has been investigated mainly in man, in whom it may occur in the following circumstances.

1. Auto-antibodies may develop which are reactive with normal antigenic constituents on the surface of cells. This unexplained breakdown of self-tolerance may occur in isolation or as a feature of systemic lupus erythematosus (p. 164) and is sometimes associated with a number of infections and with lymphocyte neoplasia.

2. Drug-induced cytotoxic antibodies. Some drugs or their metabolites bind to the surface of one or other type of cell: if such a drug is haptenic, it induces an antibody response, and the reaction of antibody with the cell-bound hapten may bring about destruction of the cell.

3. Iso-antibodies can cause injury to cells of the blood following blood transfusion or transplantation of haemopoietic or lymphoid tissue. Maternal iso-antibodies of IgG class may also pass through the placenta and injure the cells of the fetus.

Cytotoxic antibodies to cells of the blood

Cytotoxic auto-antibodies. The classical example is *auto-immune haemolytic anaemia* in which red cell injury is brought about by auto-antibody reactive with various antigenic determinants inherent in the surface of red cells. The antibody may be of IgG or IgM class, and can be detected on the red cell surface by the antiglobulin test (p. 111). When present in low concentration on the cell surface, IgG may have little or no effect. In higher concentration, it promotes the binding of the red cell to macrophages which have receptors for the Fc of IgG; such binding may result in injury to the red cell membrane or to phagocytosis and destruction of the red cell by macrophages, mostly in the red pulp of the spleen and the hepatic sinusoids. IgG antibody can also activate complement and cause intravascular lysis of the cells: this requires pairs of IgG antibody molecules bound to closely adjacent antigenic sites on the red cell surface. IgM antibodies, even in low concentration, often cause red cell destruction by intravascular lysis: single IgM molecules binding to two or more antigenic determinant sites on the red cell surface are capable of activating complement. Complement activation also promotes binding of the red cells to macrophages (by the C3b receptors of the latter), while IgM antibody can also cause agglutination of red cells, particularly where the circulation is slow, as in the red pulp of the spleen; both these effects result in intrasplenic destruction of red cells.

Idiopathic thrombocytopenic purpura is caused by auto-antibody which reacts with the surface components of normal platelets, with similarly destructive effects. The frequency with which splenectomy is followed by a rapid rise in the platelet count indicates the importance of the splenic macrophages in the increased platelet destruction.

Auto-antibodies to leukocytes may be a cause of leukopenia (reduced numbers of leukocytes) but this is difficult to prove, partly because such auto-antibodies must usually be sought by testing the patient's serum with leukocytes from another individual, and iso-antibodies to leukocytes are a common snag. Secondly, leukocytes tend to bind IgG non-specifically and give a false-positive antiglobulin test.

Drug-induced cytotoxic antibodies. Some drugs or their metabolites are capable of binding to the surface of red cells, leukocytes or platelets and acting as haptens. Antibody develops and binds to the hapten on the cell surface, and cell injury and destruction may then result, as in the case of auto-antibodies (see above). A good example of this is provided by penicillin, the benzyl-penicilloyl degradation product of which binds firmly to red cells. Most people who have received penicillin have some antibody (usually IgM) to the penicilloyl group, but after prolonged heavy dosage, high titres of IgG antibody develop in some patients and this brings about the destruction (mostly by splenic phagocytosis) of sensitised red cells. Some drugs, for example rifampicin, result in platelet destruction by an immunological reaction; this may be due to its binding to the platelet surface and acting as a hapten, as described above, but it seems more likely that it forms complexes with antibody in the plasma and that it is the binding of such complexes to Fc receptors of the platelets which causes their destruction (p. 160).

A very few drugs can induce the development of *auto-antibodies*: for example, patients receiving α-methyldopa for a few months often develop auto-antibodies to surface antigens on their red cells, detectable by the direct antiglobulin test: there is no evidence that the antibodies react with drug-derived antigens, for they are true auto-antibodies and react with the patient's and other individuals' red cells. In most instances, there is insufficient antibody to cause significant red cell destruction, but approximately 1 per cent of patients develop a haemolytic anaemia which gradually disappears on withdrawing the drug; the mechanism of auto-immunisation is obscure.

Cytotoxic iso-antibodies. In blood transfusion, administration of red cells possessing the A or B surface iso-antigens to an individual whose plasma contains the natural anti-A or anti-B iso-antibodies usually results in rapid destruction of the donated red cells. These natural antibodies are of IgM class and so complement fixation and lysis of the incompatible red cells results. There are literally dozens of other red cell iso-antigens, but normally the corresponding antibodies appear in the plasma only after blood transfusion or pregnancy (see below). After the ABO groups, the Rhesus (Rh) system of iso-antigens is of most importance in man. Transfusion of red cells possessing Rh antigens which are not present in the recipient's red cells often results in development of the corresponding Rh antibody, following which the transfused cells are destroyed abnormally rapidly in the spleen. During labour (or abortion) some fetal red cells enter the mother's circulation, and, if Rh-incompatible (which depends on the father's Rh group) they sometimes stimulate development of Rh antibodies.

The Rh antibodies are particularly important in pregnancy, because they are usually mainly of IgG class, and so can cross the placenta. If the pregnant woman has developed Rh antibodies, as a result of a previous pregnancy or blood transfusion, they enter the fetal circulation and, if the fetal red cells possess the corresponding Rh antigens, abnormal destruction results in fetal death or anaemia (Fig. 6.5). Once an individual has developed Rh antibodies, from either pregnancy or transfusion, subsequently transfused Rh-positive red cells are liable to be destroyed rapidly. The development of Rh antibodies can very often be prevented by injecting Rh antibody into the Rh-negative woman within 48 hours after termination of an Rh-incompatible pregnancy.

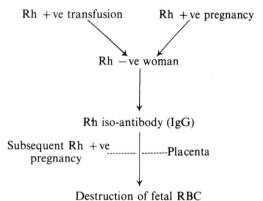

Fig. 6.5 Haemolytic disease of the newborn. Fetal red cell destruction is brought about by maternal isoantibody which has developed as a result of previous Rh +ve pregnancy or transfusion of Rh +ve blood.

In common with tissue cells, the leukocytes and platelets have antigens belonging to the HLA and other 'transplant antigen' systems (p. 166). This is seldom of importance in blood transfusion unless the aim is to supply these cell types to a deficient recipient. Blood transfusion and pregnancy do, however, stimulate the development of HLA and other antibodies, and subsequently transferred platelets or leukocytes may be destroyed rapidly. Such iso-immunisation is of importance if subsequent transplantation, e.g. of a kidney, is performed (p. 846), and maternal iso-antibodies to platelets may also cause thrombocytopenia in the fetus.

Auto-antibodies to tissue constituents

Auto-antibodies which react with components of tissue cells *in vitro* are demonstrable in the serum of patients with various diseases (p. 161), but the available evidence suggests that they are not usually a major cause of cell injury. In some instances, this is because they react with intracellular, as opposed to surface constituents, of the target cells. A good example is antibody to deoxyribonucleoprotein, which is present in the plasma of patients with systemic lupus erythematosus: it can react with, and lead to destruction of, the nuclei of dead cells, but does not reach the nuclei of living cells.

There are, however, two examples of auto-antibodies which react with cell surface receptors and have a profound effect on the target tissue cells. One is a thyroid auto-antibody, which reacts with the TSH receptor of thyroid epithelium and, like TSH itself, stimulates the cell to increased function and proliferation: this is the cause of *Graves' disease*, the common type of hyperthyroidism. The other is an antibody to the acetylcholine receptor in skeletal muscle cells: it blocks the receptor and thus causes the muscle weakness of *myasthenia gravis* (p. 936). A third example of a harmful auto-antibody is found in a small proportion of sterile men: it reacts with spermatozoa and may be present in sufficient concentration in seminal fluid to impair their motility.

Although 'cytotoxic' implies injury to cells, type 2 hypersensitivity is sometimes extended to include antibody-induced injury to extracellular tissue elements. The best known example of this is the rare type of glomerulonephritis in which auto-antibody develops to glomerular capillary basement membrane. Union of this antibody with the inner surface of the basement membrane is followed by activation of complement, as in the Arthus reaction, and a destructive inflammatory lesion results in the glomeruli (p. 832).

Antibody-dependent lymphocyte cytotoxicity

When a suspension of living cells is treated with an IgG class antibody which reacts with their surface membrane, and normal lymphocytes (e.g. from the peripheral blood of a normal individual) are added, some of the lymphocytes bind to the surface of the sensitised cells and bring about their destruction: this probably involves penetration of the target cell membrane by the lymphocyte (Reid *et al.*, 1979). The cytotoxic lymphocytes, sometimes called K cells (p. 120), do not have surface Ig, and so are not B lymphocytes: they may be a subset of T cells or a third type of lymphocyte.

The importance of this type of cell injury in man is not known, but there is evidence suggesting that it contributes to the destruction of tumour cells in experimental animals.

Immune complex, Arthus-type (type 3) reactions

These result from formation of immune complexes by union of antigen with free IgG or IgM antibody with consequent activation ('fixation') of complement. This leads, in turn, to acute inflammation with accumulation of polymorphs and aggregation of platelets. The polymorphs phagocytose the immune complexes and release lysosomal enzymes which cause tissue injury and aggravate the inflammatory response directly and by activating the kinin, clotting and plasmin systems (Fig. 3.13, p. 55). Depending on the distribution of antigen, the reaction may be localised to a particular tissue, and is then termed an Arthus reaction, or immune complexes may form in the blood, producing a generalised reaction commonly known as 'serum sickness' or circulating immune-complex disease.

The local or Arthus reaction

This was described in 1903 by Arthus, who injected rabbits repeatedly with horse serum. When the animals had developed a high level of circulating antibodies to horse serum proteins, he noticed that a subcutaneous injection of horse serum induced a local acute inflammatory reaction, developing over a few hours and sometimes progressing to necrosis. It has since been shown that the reaction may be induced by local injection of a soluble antigen into various tissues in animals with a high level of the corresponding precipitating antibody in their blood. It can be induced also in animals immunised passively by intravenous injection of precipitating antibody (passive Arthus reaction). Localisation of the reaction depends on precipitation of all the antigen in the tissues around the injection site, and thus on a high titre of precipitating antibody in the plasma.

Histological features. Microscopy of the Arthus reaction shows the typical changes of acute inflammation with congestion of small vessels, inflammatory exudation, and marked pavementing and emigration of neutrophil polymorphs. There may be aggregation of platelets in the small vessels and, depending on the severity, haemorrhages and thrombosis, and necrosis extending from the walls of small vessels to surrounding tissues.

Mechanism. Immunofluorescence techniques have demonstrated precipitates of antigen–antibody complexes in the lesion, particularly in the walls of venules. Fixed components of complement may also be detected in the precipitates. The Arthus reaction is largely suppressed in animals by depletion either of neutrophil polymorphs, e.g. by nitrogen mustard, or of complement, e.g. by cobra-venom factor; the intensity of the reaction is reduced by administration of corticosteroids. From such evidence it has been deduced that the reaction is brought about as follows (see also Fig. 6.6). Immune complex formation and deposition in the walls of venules leads to activation of complement, the products of which include **anaphylatoxins*** (C3a and C5a) which bring about acute inflammation by releasing histamine, etc., from mast cells. C5a, and possibly other complement products, are chemotactic for polymorphs, which consequently migrate into the vessel walls and surrounding tissues in large numbers and phagocytose the immune complexes. In so doing, they release lysosomal enzymes and cationic proteins which cause further tissue damage, digest proteins with production of kinins and other vaso-active peptides, and thus aggravate the inflammatory reaction. Platelet aggregation occurs in the damaged vessels and initiates thrombosis with consequent ischaemic necrosis.

The Arthus reaction in man was commonly seen in the days when crude preparations of horse antitoxic globulin or whole antitoxic serum was administered in the prevention and treatment of diphtheria, tetanus, etc. This resulted in the development of precipitating antibodies to horse proteins and a subsequent subcutaneous or intramuscular injection of horse globulin or serum elicited an Arthus reaction. More recently, it has been shown that the Arthus reaction is the basis of **extrinsic allergic alveolitis**, a good example of which is 'farmer's lung'. The farm worker inhales large numbers of the spores of bacteria growing in mouldy

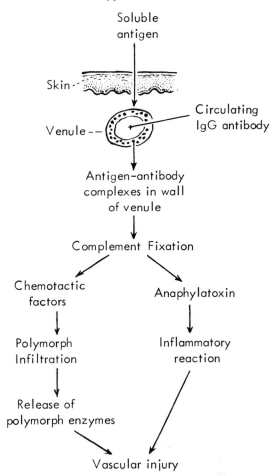

Fig. 6.6 Mechanism of the Arthus reaction. Local injection of soluble antigen into an animal with a high plasma level of the corresponding antibody of IgG class results in union of antigen and antibody in the walls of venules. Complement reacts with the antigen–antibody complexes, and reaction products of complement induce inflammation and polymorph infiltration. The release of polymorph enzymes brings about vascular and tissue injury.

hay; bacterial antigen is absorbed via the alveolar walls and stimulates antibody production. Subsequent inhalation of the spores induces an acute Arthus reaction in the alveolar walls. It has become apparent that individuals with precipitating antibody in their serum vary greatly in their susceptibility to farmer's lung: there is some evidence suggesting that IgE antibody is also necessary, and that the Arthus reaction is

---

* The term *anaphylatoxin* is unfortunate, because products of complement fixation do not participate in classical anaphylaxis in man, which is due to IgE antibodies.

triggered off by an initial atopic reaction which allows escape of antibodies of IgG class into the vessel walls. As in the rabbit, Arthus reactions in man are inhibited by administration of glucocorticoids.

Circulating immune-complex disease: serum sickness

In man, antigen–antibody complexes are formed in the plasma, both as a result of administration of foreign proteins and haptenic drugs, and also in a number of natural diseases, particularly infections. Serious effects result from their deposition in the walls of blood vessels, especially in the glomeruli, but also in the skin and the walls of arteries. Local lesions develop at these sites and, depending on the duration of deposition, may be acute and self-limiting, recurrent or chronic.

Experimental basis. The basis of this form of hypersensitivity has been elucidated by Dixon, Cochrane and others (see Cochrane, 1973), mainly in rabbits. After a single injection of a large amount of antigen, e.g. bovine serum albumin, no harmful effects occur until, after several days, antibody is produced. As it appears, it combines with antigen still present in the plasma, forming immune complexes. Initially antigen is present in relative excess and its union with antibody produces small soluble complexes (Fig. 5.6, p. 110) which are not readily phagocytosed and so persist in the circulation. As antibody increases, intermediate-sized soluble, and then large, insoluble complexes are formed, and after a few days free antibody can be detected. The larger aggregates of immune complex are rapidly taken up and destroyed by phagocytic leukocytes and by macrophages in the liver, spleen, etc. Accordingly, in a rabbit producing a lot of precipitating antibody, complexes disappear from the plasma in a few days (Fig. 6.7). During this period, however, in which soluble complexes formed in antigen excess are present in the circulation, their presence triggers off a series of reactions leading to release of histamine and other vasoactive agents, with consequent increase in vascular permeability. This in turn allows the soluble complexes, along with plasma proteins, to leak out between the endothelial cells of various blood vessels. At the sites of leakage, complexes are trapped and

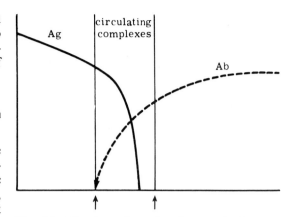

Fig. 6.7 The formation of antigen–antibody complexes in the circulation. Injection of antigen is followed after some days by the appearance of antibody in the plasma: during the next few days, the concentration of antigen falls sharply and antigen antibody complexes are present in the plasma.

accumulate between the endothelium and basement membrane, where their presence results in vascular injury.

The mechanism of increase in vascular permeability, as in inflammation, is complicated, and varies in different species. In the rabbit, in which most of the reservoir of histamine in the blood is in the platelets, histamine release appears to be due mainly to union of antigen with IgE antibody bound to basophil leukocytes (i.e. a type 1 hypersensitivity reaction): this induces release of a factor which causes the platelets to aggregate and discharge their histamine. Other mechanisms of release of histamine from platelets involve activation of complement by the complexes and participation of neutrophil polymorphs.

In the experiment described above, in which rabbits are given a single injection of an antigen, immune complexes in the blood are deposited beneath the vascular endothelium, particularly in the glomerular capillaries, the small vessels in the joints and skin, in the endocardium, and focally in various arteries. The deposited complexes continue to fix complement, and, except in the glomeruli, this triggers off an Arthus-type reaction, with acute inflammation, infiltration of polymorphs, and sometimes thrombosis and necrosis. The reaction is particularly intense in the arterial lesions, which may extend to involve the whole thickness of the wall. Activation of complement and polymorphs results in phagocytosis of the deposited complexes within 48 hours, so that, although intense, the reaction is brief. Like the local Arthus reaction, it can be suppressed by prior depletion of polymorphs or complement. In the glomeruli, complexes deposited within or on the epithelial side of the capillary basement membrane fix complement, and yet inflammation is relatively mild and polymorphs are scanty: an obvious explanation is the one-way flow of filtrate from the capillary lumen to the urinary space, which presumably washes away the anaphylatoxins and chemotaxins produced by complement activation. Complexes persist in the glomeruli for many days, and cause glomerular injury by some unexplained mechanism, with resultant proteinuria.

Chronic immune-complex disease can be produced in rabbits by giving daily intravenous injections of soluble antigen in amounts sufficient to provide a period of relative antigen excess over antibody in the plasma after each injection. In contrast to acute serum sickness, the complexes are deposited solely in the glomerular capillaries, where they give rise to lesions resembling various forms of progressive glomerulonephritis in man. Deposition of immune complexes is also influenced by the nature of the antigen and quality of the antibody. Unless there is gross antigen excess, precipitating antibody forms large insoluble complexes which, as stated above, are rapidly phagocytosed and cause little or no injury, so that antigen excess is necessary for formation of smaller, pathogenic complexes. Antibodies which can only react with very few determinant sites on the antigen molecule and have poor avidity (p. 107) also form soluble complexes, even when present in relative excess. Accordingly, some antigen–antibody complexes can produce lesions even when there is a relative excess of antibody in the blood.

Circulating immune-complex disease in man results from injection of heterologous immunoglobulin (now an uncommon cause) and administration of potentially haptenic drugs. It also occurs naturally in systemic lupus erythematosus, in which auto-immune complexes are formed, and in various infections. The formation of immune complexes in the blood may produce both a *general reaction*, and lesions in the glomeruli and elsewhere resulting from *complex deposition in the walls of blood vessels*.

The acute generalised reaction. In its extreme form, for example when a large amount of foreign protein is injected into an individual with a high titre of the corresponding antibody in the plasma, the rapid formation of high concentrations of immune complexes in the plasma may induce a rapid collapse: this is attributable to intense activation of complement, release of polymorph lysosomal enzymes, etc., and activation of the kinin, clotting and plasmin systems. The clinical features are similar to those of anaphylactic shock (p. 146). When a foreign protein is injected for the first time, classical serum sickness develops 7–10 days later, when production of antibody results in the formation of immune complexes in the plasma. It is a short febrile illness characterised by intense itching of the skin and urticaria, swelling of peripheral joints, and enlargement of lymph nodes. Histamine antagonists bring partial relief. Examination of the serum reveals abnormally low levels of complement components and the presence of products of complement activation. Immune complexes are also demonstrable, although the available techniques are not entirely satisfactory. The polymorph count is at first low, but later raised. After recovery, free antibody appears in the serum. These features indicate that immune complexes form in the blood, activate complement, and trigger off the release of vaso-active agents, including histamine. Phagocytosis of circulating complexes probably results in degeneration and disappearance of most of the polymorphs, and also in the release of endogeneous pyrogen and thus the development of fever (p. 189).

The mechanism of release of histamine, etc. involves the anaphylatoxins of complement, release of polymorph lysosomes, activation of Hageman factor and production of kinins. It may also be that, as in the rabbit, basophil polymorphs or mast cells sensitised with IgE antibody are involved. This possibility is supported by the frequency of bronchospasm suggestive of atopy, and by the occasional severe circulatory collapse as in generalised anaphylaxis.

The typical attack of serum sickness which followed injection of crude antisera is now uncommon, but similar reactions can follow administration of drugs which can confer antigenicity to plasma proteins, and the severe form of dengue fever is due largely to circulating virus antigen–antibody complexes. In spirochaetal infections, including syphilis, and in lepromatous leprosy and some other chronic bacterial infections, the first dose of treatment by an effective drug may kill very large numbers of micro-organisms and so release microbial antigen, which, depending on the level of circulating antibody and the amount of antigen released, either forms complexes in the blood or induces local Arthus reactions in the lesions. The features of the reaction (*the Jarisch–Herxheimer reaction*) suggest that both phenomena may occur.

Immune-complex deposition is an important cause of glomerulonephritis in man. The typical acute glomerulonephritis following a streptococcal throat infection resembles that of acute serum sickness in the rabbit. It develops when antibody to streptococcal antigen enters the blood and immune complexes are formed and deposited in the glomerular capillaries. Other infections and drug hypersensitivities can have the same effect, and more chronic glomerular injury occurs from prolonged or intermittent immune-complex formation in quartan malaria, lepromatous leprosy and some other chronic infections. In systemic lupus erythematosus, auto-antibodies develop which react with various cellular constituents, e.g. DNA, and complexes formed in the blood are deposited in small vessels in the skin, glomeruli and elsewhere. In most types of human immune-complex glomerulonephritis, however, the nature of the antigen is unknown: the various patterns of disease depend partly on the size of the circulating complexes and the duration and rate of their deposition, and there is also evidence that antigen may be deposited in the glomerular capillary walls, followed by the binding of circulating antibody to form complexes.

Arterial lesions due to complex deposition are less common in man, and their nature is usually difficult to prove because, as in the rabbit, the immune complexes are phagocytosed rapidly by polymorphs. Nevertheless, the focal lesions of polyarteritis nodosa and some other forms of arteritis appear to be of this nature, and surface antigen of the hepatitis B virus has been implicated in some cases.

In many patients with immune complex disease, IgM antibodies develop which are capable of reacting with IgG. These 'rheumatoid factors' react most avidly with the IgG in immune complexes, and may cause circulatory disturbances by increasing the viscosity of the blood, or aggravate the injury caused by deposited immune complexes. The IgM–IgG complexes often precipitate in cooled serum, and are then termed cryoglobulins.

The lesions produced by immune complex deposition in the kidneys and elsewhere are described in more detail in the appropriate chapters.

Delayed hypersensitivity (DHS or type 4) reactions

Antibody production and cell-mediated immunity are both parts of the normal immune response to most antigens. The union of antibodies with antigens can result in the hypersensitivity reactions described above. Delayed hypersensitivity (DHS) does not involve antibody, but is mediated by the specifically-primed T lymphocytes produced in the cell-mediated immune response. By means of their specific surface receptors, these cells can bind to the antigen which has stimulated their production, and this results in tissue injury characterised by a slowly developing inflammatory reaction—hence *delayed* hypersensitivity.

The reaction of primed T lymphocytes with microbial antigens is an essential defence mechanism against many pathogenic bacteria, viruses and fungi, etc.: the DHS reaction promotes their destruction, and the accompanying tissue injury is the price which must be paid for this protection. Cell-mediated immunity to tumour-cell antigens is known to develop in some cancer patients, and is being intensively investigated in the hope that it may be utilised for the effective destruction of tumours by DHS reactions.

Cell-mediated immunity develops also against harmless foreign antigens, body constituents modified by foreign haptens, against transplanted allogeneic cells or tissues, and sometimes even against the individual's own apparently normal tissue cells. In these circumstances, unwanted DHS reactions occur, resulting respectively in contact dermatitis, rejection of transplants, and auto-immune disease.

Morphological features

The DHS reaction can occur in any part of the body where primed T lymphocytes encounter the corresponding antigen. Its induction in the skin is used as a test for cell-mediated immunity to various antigens, the classical example being **the tuberculin reaction** in which a small amount of tuberculoprotein ('purified protein derivative' or PPD) is applied to the skin or injected intradermally as in the Mantoux test. This has no effect in non-immune individuals, but in subjects who have developed cell-mediated immunity to tuberculoprotein as a result of tuberculosis or immunisation with BCG (attenuated *Mycobacterium bovis*) the typical delayed inflammatory reaction appears in 12–24 hours and persists for 48 hours or more. The skin becomes reddened and a firm central nodule appears. In a highly sensitised individual, necrosis and ulceration may follow.

Microscopically, the major features are microvascular congestion, accumulation of lymphocytes in and around the small vessels, and swelling of the collagen, apparently due to inflammatory oedema. At the height of the reaction there is intense infiltration with lymphocytes and occasional macrophages, both in and around the capillaries and venules, particularly round the sweat glands and hair follicles (Fig. 6.8). These are the features of the DHS reaction to a soluble protein in man. In animals, accumulation of polymorphs and macrophages, in addition to lymphocytes, is much more prominent. The morphological features of DHS reactions in infections are complicated by the injuries inflicted directly by the micro-organisms or their toxins and by other types of hypersensitivity reactions. A glance at the microscopic appearances of various inflammatory lesions in which DHS is a prominent feature will show considerable differences (e.g. tuberculosis, p. 209; tuberculoid leprosy, p. 215; typhoid fever, p. 10, and contact dermatitis, p. 161). In general, infiltration with macrophages, lymphocytes and lymphoblasts is prominent. The macrophages may also change to epithelioid cells, fuse to form giant cells and undergo necrosis.

The mechanism of DHS reactions

DHS reactions occur when specifically-primed T lymphocytes (memory T lymphocytes) encounter antigen with which they can react. To encounter antigen in the tissues, specifically responsive T lymphocytes must leave the blood in the vicinity of the antigen, and the factors involved in such emigration are largely unknown.

Circulating T lymphocytes are known to wander through many tissues (p. 121), and there is also evidence that specifically-primed lymphocytes respond chemotactically to the corresponding antigen (Wilkinson *et al.*, 1977), but it is not known whether they are T and/or B cells, nor whether they respond chemotactically *in vivo*. In animal experiments involving passive transfer of radio-labelled lymphocytes, it has been shown that the lymphocytes which aggregate at the site of a delayed hypersensitivity reaction are recently-divided cells and pre-mitotic immunoblasts. In these experiments it was also shown that only a small proportion of the cells accumulating at the test site were specifically primed to the antigen. It still remains undecided whether specifically-primed T lymphocytes are attracted preferentially to the antigen site, and by release of lymphokines (see below) attract other lymphocytes, or whether any recently-divided or stimulated lymphocytes are attracted to the site of injection of any antigen or other, non-specific tissue injury.

Having encountered and bound antigen by means of its surface receptor, the specifically primed T lymphocyte is stimulated to enlarge and synthesise DNA, transforming into an immunoblast: it also secretes a number of soluble compounds known as *lymphokines*, which are described below. When the antigen is a surface component of a living cell, the T lymphocyte may bind to and kill the target cell: such direct cytotoxicity is of importance in the rejection of allografts (p. 166) and killing of virus-infected cells (p. 195) and tumour cells (p. 315), and probably plays a major pathogenic role in the organ-specific auto-immune diseases (p. 162).

There has been much discussion on the relationship between various functional types of T cells—memory cells, helper and suppressor cells, cytotoxic cells and lymphokine secretors. Until their inter-relationship becomes clearer, it is reasonable to adopt the view, as a working hypothesis, that T memory cells can develop any of these functions.

Lymphokines. As noted above, memory T lymphocytes react with the corresponding antigen and secrete soluble compounds termed lymphokines. The reaction may conveniently be elicited by adding antigen to a suspension of lymphocytes and the supernate examined for lymphokines by a combination of *in-vitro* and *in-vivo* tests. By such means, the following pro-

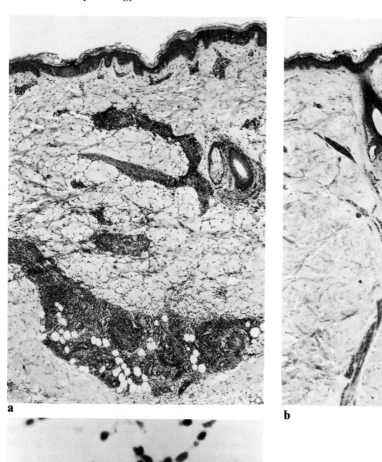

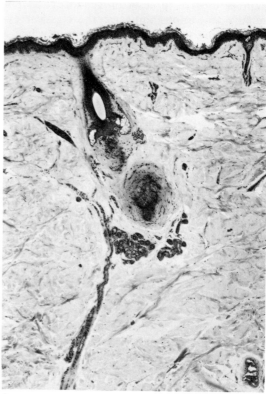

Fig. 6.8 Positive **a** and negative **b** Mantoux tests. Note the heavy cellular infiltrate around the sweat glands and pilo-sebaceous units in **a**. This distribution is determined by the vascularity of the skin appendages. × 43. At higher magnification **c**, the infiltrating cells are seen to be mostly lymphocytes, which are aggregated around the small blood vessels. × 470. (The late Dr. Janet Niven.)

perties of lymphokines have been demonstrated.

1. Induction of acute inflammation. Intradermal injection demonstrates a factor which induces congestion of small blood vessels and inflammatory oedema. This could account for these features in the DHS reaction.

2. Effects on mononuclear phagocytes. These are complex, but there is evidence for the following.

(*a*) *A chemotactic factor.* This induces chemotaxis of monocytes or macrophages *in vitro* and emigration of monocytes *in vivo*: it may account for accumulation of macrophages in DHS reactions.

(*b*) *A macrophage immobilising factor*, demonstrable by its inhibitory effect on the migration of macrophages, e.g. from the open end of a horizontal capillary tube. When the tube is immersed in tissue culture fluid, addition of this factor to the fluid inhibits migration. It may also play a role in the accumulation of macrophages in DHS reactions.

(*c*) *A macrophage activating factor*, which increases the metabolic activity of macrophages and enhances their mobility and capacity to phagocytose and kill micro-organisms. This microbicidal effect has been demonstrated *in vitro* and *in vivo*.

(*d*) *A specific macrophage-arming factor* (*SMAF*) has been demonstrated in experimentally-induced cell-mediated immunity to tumour cells. The DHS reaction between primed T cells and tumour cells releases a factor which confers on macrophages enhanced killing properties specific for the tumour cells. This factor differs from (*c*) above in that it is antigen-specific.

3. Other factors. Another factor released when primed T cells react with antigen is cytotoxic for tissue cells, and may contribute to the necrosis commonly seen in DHS reactions. This is distinct from the antigen-specific killing of target cells by T lymphocytes mentioned above, which requires close contact.

Other lymphokines are chemotactic for lymphocytes and induce mitosis of lymphocytes: these properties may explain why so many of the lymphocytes in DHS reactions are not specifically primed to react with the antigen which has induced the reaction (see above).

Elucidation of these important factors is still at an early stage. Their importance as mediators of the changes seen in DHS reactions is suggested by their detection not only in reactions in test tubes, but also in extracts of DHS reaction sites.

Man and other primates show, in general, much stronger cell-mediated immune responses and DHS reactions than do lower animals. It is therefore unwise to assume that the findings for guinea-pigs, etc., are applicable to man. Lawrence's transfer factor (p. 131) may be important in cellular immunity and DHS reactions in man, in whom it is far more readily demonstrable, and has a much more lasting effect, than any counterpart in guinea-pigs, etc.

Until recently, it was widely assumed that the presence of lymphocytes in a hypersensitivity reaction was a good indication of a DHS component, but B lymphocytes can and do migrate into sites of antigen (hence the presence of plasma cells in many infections): also it is now known that so-called K cells (p. 152), which have the appearances of small lymphocytes, may bind by surface Fc receptors to target cells sensitised with IgG class antibody and bring about their destruction. The *in vivo* significance of this co-operative cytotoxic effect of antibody and K lymphocytes is not yet known. The presence of macrophages in hypersensitivity reactions is not necessarily indicative of DHS, for they are attracted also by antigen-antibody complexes and by non-antigenic foreign and endogenous material (pp. 61–2, 67).

Systemic effects of DHS reactions

Although this account has concentrated on local DHS reactions, systemic reactions also occur. For example, injection of relatively large amounts of tuberculoprotein into an individual who has developed cell-mediated immunity to it results not only in a severe localised DHS reaction at the injection site, but also fever, malaise and a fall in the level of circulating lymphocytes. If the individual has active tuberculosis, the DHS reaction of the lesion is also aggravated, with extension of necrosis. These effects are known collectively as the *Koch phenomenon* after Robert Koch* who first described them. They are probably attributable to

---

* The German bacteriologist who, in 1882, discovered the tubercle bacillus and showed it to be the cause of tuberculosis.

the release of lymphokines following the reaction between tuberculoprotein and specifically primed T cells in the blood, lymphoid tissues and tuberculous lesions. The fever of the Koch phenomenon and of active tuberculosis is probably a secondary effect, due to release of endogenous pyrogen (p. 189) by macrophages activated by lymphokines. The Koch phenomenon is not observed in individuals who have not developed cell-mediated immunity to tuberculoprotein.

Hypersensitivity to drugs and chemicals

Most drugs and chemicals which cause hypersensitivity reactions do so because they or their metabolic products combine with host proteins and act as haptens. At first sight, this seems to contradict the observation that haptens can only stimulate an immune response when combined with *foreign* carrier proteins to which the recipient develops cell-mediated immunity (p. 129). The explanation is that the many drugs and chemicals which cause hypersensitivity reactions not only act as haptens, but alter the configuration of the protein molecules with which they combine, thus rendering them 'foreign'.

The type of hypersensitivity reaction which results will then depend on the nature of the immune response, the particular cell or tissue constituent with which the hapten has complexed, the route of administration and dose, etc. In individuals with a tendency to atopy, reaginic antibodies may develop, and further administration of the hapten can then induce *a type 1 reaction*, e.g. asthma or hay fever if the hapten is inhaled as a vapour or airborne suspension, an immediate inflammatory reaction if it is applied locally, or a generalised anaphylactic reaction if a large amount of hapten is absorbed by any route. Anaphylactic reactions to penicillin and related compounds are not uncommon, and have resulted in a number of deaths: in most instances the hypersensitivity is directed towards the penicilloyl degradation product of penicillin. The development of IgG class antibody to a haptenic drug or chemical can give rise to *local reactions of Arthus type* (*type 3*) when the hapten is localised to one particular area within the tissues, or can lead to formation of complexes of hapten and antibody within the plasma, with the risk of circulating immune-complex disease (p. 155).

A number of drugs which act as haptens stimulate the production of antibodies which, although not cytotoxic, can bring about destruction of red cells, leukocytes or platelets. For reasons unknown, complexes of these drugs with antibody bind to cells of the blood, and although such binding is often loose, activation of complement by the drug-antibody complex results in C5b and subsequent complement components building up on the cell surface to produce the haemolytic C5b-9 complex (p. 144), with consequent 'bystander' or 'reactive' cytolysis: the binding of immune complexes and complement components also promotes phagocytosis of the cells in the spleen. Drugs which form complexes with these effects include sulphonamides, phenacetin, chlorpromazine and rifampicin, but the list is long and differs for red cells, leukocytes and platelets.

Thirdly, binding of a haptenic drug or drug metabolite to red cells, leukocytes or platelets may render the cells susceptible to injury by antibody to the drug (*cytotoxic (type 2) antibody reaction*—p. 150). It is not known whether tissue cells are injured in this way.

Lastly, cell-mediated immunity may develop towards the hapten–protein complex, and, as described above, subsequent absorption of the haptenic compound gives rise to *a delayed hypersensitivity (type 4) reaction*. This is seen in *contact dermatitis* in which relatively simple chemicals behave as haptens: they are absorbed into the body, often through the skin, and combine with tissue proteins. Cell-mediated immunity develops against the modified proteins, and subsequent skin contact with the same chemical induces a delayed hypersensitivity reaction (Fig. 6.9), causing inflammatory lesions with cellular infiltration, predominantly lymphocytic, and oedema which affects both the dermis and epidermis and progresses to formation of vesicles. The substances capable of inducing this condition are very numerous, and include particularly chemicals which combine firmly with proteins, e.g. dyes, chrome salts, formalin and various derivatives of benzene. Reactions which appear to be of this type occur commonly in women in relation to nickel fasteners on underclothes, some of the nickel being dissolved by acid sweat and absorbed

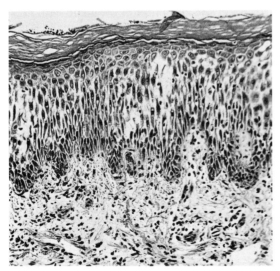

Fig. 6.9 Contact dermatitis. Note oedema of epidermis and perivascular infiltration of lymphocytes in the dermis. The patient had developed hypersensitivity to chromium salts used as a hardener in cement. × 110.

presumably as nickel salts which can combine with skin proteins. Contact with some plants, e.g. poison ivy and primulas is another common cause, and cases also occur from the use of hair dyes, such as paraphenylene diamine, which, of course, bind firmly to keratin. Contact dermatitis results also from application of various medicaments to the skin. It is noteworthy that any individual can be sensitised to various chemicals, and contact dermatitis can thus be induced, but nevertheless some people appear to develop it more readily than others. This is seen in the use of various adhesive surgical dressings which usually produce no reaction but in some instances lead to contact dermatitis, and a similar effect may result from wearing rubber face masks.

It is important to appreciate that the above account is an oversimplification. In many instances, hypersensitivity to drugs or chemicals is extremely complex and the clinical features often conflict with the results of the various available tests for hypersensitivity. With the ever-increasing number of chemicals used therapeutically and in industry, it is not surprising that hypersensitivity reactions, particularly those manifested in the skin and mucous membranes, are becoming increasingly common. Apart from the possession of highly reactive

groups by which they can bind to proteins, it is not yet known what properties of a substance are related to the likelihood of its stimulating the development of hypersensitivity. Individuals predisposed to atopy and patients with systemic lupus erythematosus are prone to develop drug hypersensitivities, but, apart from this, predisposition to drug reaction is quite unpredictable.

Auto-immunity and auto-immune diseases

Some confusion exists over the definitions of auto-antibodies and auto-immune diseases. **Auto-antibodies** *may be defined as antibodies which react with the individual's own normal body constituents* (which may accordingly be termed **auto-antigens**). This definition excludes antibodies which react only with body constituents which have been altered, for example by a haptenic drug, and so have become 'foreign' to the individual (see above). The definition does not, however, assume that normal body constituents have necessarily stimulated the production of the auto-antibodies. For example *Streptococcus pyogenes* possesses antigens similar to constituents of human myocardium and a streptococcal pharyngitis can induce antibodies which react with normal myocardium (p. 415): these qualify as auto-antibodies. Within this definition, *auto-antibodies to several cell products or constituents are quite commonly present in the serum of individuals both with and without clinical evidence of disease*: they include, for example, antibodies to thyroglobulin, to thyroid epithelial cells, to gastric parietal cells and to the deoxyribonucleoprotein of cell nuclei. These antibodies all react *in vitro* with the individual's own body constituents and with those obtained from others, so that they are acceptable as true auto-antibodies.

Although auto-immunisation occurs without clinical disease, it is strongly associated with a number of diseases. For example, most apparently normal individuals with thyroid auto-antibodies have been shown to have sub-clinical chronic thyroiditis, and patients with more severe, clinically apparent chronic thyroiditis usually have high titres of thyroid antibodies. Similarly, high titres of antibodies to deoxyribonucleoprotein occur especially in patients with the connective tissue diseases, and particularly in systemic lupus erythematosus.

Cell-mediated auto-immunity has also been demonstrated by in vitro tests in some diseases. For example thyroid auto-antigens inhibit the migration of leukocytes (p. 113) of patients with chronic thyroiditis.

It is thus apparent that, in some diseases, there is evidence of auto-immunisation against particular body constituents. These are the so-called **auto-immune diseases**. In most, there is still a lingering doubt that the lesions are due to immunological reactions against the target auto-antigens; in some instances this probability is supported by production of similar lesions by auto-immunisation of animals, or by investigations on naturally-occurring auto-immune diseases in inbred strains of animals.

There are also a number of examples in which auto-antibodies develop as a result of tissue injury and appear to be without pathogenic effect, an example being auto-antibodies to myocardial cells which frequently develop following ischaemic necrosis of the myocardium; presumably antigen is released by the dead muscle cells and stimulates an immune response.

Auto-immune diseases may be classified into: (1) a group of organ-specific diseases affecting glandular tissues; (2) systemic lupus erythematosus and possibly the other connective tissue diseases; and (3) a number of miscellaneous diseases which do not fit readily into either of the above classes.

The organ-specific auto-immune diseases

These are characterised by chronic inflammatory destruction of a particular glandular tissue accompanied by the presence in the plasma of auto-antibodies which react specifically with normal cellular components of the target tissue. The tissues affected include the thyroid, gastric mucosa, adrenal cortex, parathyroid glands and cells of the pancreatic islets of Langerhans. The main features are exemplified by **chronic auto-immune thyroiditis**, in which infiltration of the thyroid gland by lymphocytes, plasma cells and macrophages is accompanied by glandular epithelial destruction and fibrosis. These changes may be focal and are then sub-clinical and usually non-progressive, or they may be diffuse, giving rise to either thyroid enlargement, sometimes with hypofunction (*Hashimoto's thyroiditis*), or de-

struction and shrinkage of the gland with gross hypofunction (*primary myxoedema*). Auto-antibodies to normal thyroid constituents are detectable in the serum in virtually all cases of Hashimoto's thyroiditis, and in most cases of primary myxoedema and sub-clinical thyroiditis. They include antibodies reactive with: (1) thyroglobulin, often in sufficient concentration to give a precipitin reaction (Fig. 5.7, p. 110); (2) a second constituent of thyroid colloid; and (3) cell membrane constituents ('microsomes') of thyroid epithelium—the so-called thyroid microsomal antibody (Fig. 5.11, p. 112). Chronic thyroiditis occurs much more often in women than in men, and the incidence increases with age. Over 10 per cent of middle-aged or elderly women have one or more thyroid antibodies and some degree of chronic thyroiditis. There is a general correlation between the presence and titres of the serum antibodies and the extensiveness and activity of the thyroiditis, but the correlation is by no means exact for any one antibody or any combination of antibodies.

As mentioned earlier, a fourth thyroid antibody, which reacts with the TSH receptors of thyroid epithelial cells, is responsible for the hyperthyroidism of Graves' disease which is usually accompanied by focal auto-immune thyroiditis.

Chronic auto-immune gastritis, affecting the acid-secreting mucosa of the gastric fundus, has many points of resemblance to chronic thyroiditis. It affects women more often than men, and the incidence increases with age. In most cases, the serum contains 'microsomal' antibody to gastric parietal cells and, in a minority of cases, antibodies to the intrinsic factor essential to absorption of vitamin B_{12}. The affected mucosa is infiltrated with lymphocytes, plasma cells and macrophages, and all grades of destruction of chief and parietal cells are observed. In most cases, the gastritis is mild and sub-clinical, and progresses very slowly, but in some cases it progresses more rapidly to diffuse atrophy of the mucosa (like the thyroid in primary myxoedema) and parietal cell deficiency then results in achlorhydria and lack of intrinsic factor, the latter leading in some cases to B_{12} deficiency and pernicious anaemia.

Auto-immune adrenalitis is a much less common condition; it is, however, the major cause of adrenal cortical atrophy and functional deficiency (Addison's disease). The serum commonly contains 'microsomal' auto-antibody to a cell-membrane constituent of adrenocortical epithelium. **Primary hypoparathyroidism** is rare: specific auto-antibodies are demonstrable in the serum in some cases, and the parathyroid glands are shrunken and extremely difficult to find at necropsy.

In addition to their morphological and serological similarities, each of these diseases tends to have a high familial incidence, and moreover the diseases tend to occur in association, both within affected families and in individuals. For example, patients with Hashimoto's thyroiditis have a high incidence of gastric antibody and a particular tendency to develop pernicious anaemia, while thyroid and gastric antibodies, sometimes associated with the corresponding clinical diseases, are unduly common in patients with auto-immune Addison's disease or primary hypoparathyroidism: even these two latter rare diseases have been found to be particularly associated with one another.

Insulin-dependent (type I) diabetes differs from the other organ-specific auto-immune diseases in affecting children and young adults, and there is recent evidence suggesting that it may be initiated by a viral infection. Auto-antibodies to cells of the islets of Langerhans are detectable in the serum in nearly all early cases. The islets at first show lymphocytic infiltration and later become atrophic.

Pathogenesis and aetiology. It has not been proved that these diseases are the result of auto-hypersensitivity reactions, an alternative explanation being that the glandular destruction is due to some other (unknown) agent, and that auto-antibodies develop as a secondary phenomenon. In favour of an auto-immune pathogenesis, auto-antibodies do not, in general, result from destruction of tissue. For example, thyroid injury by large doses of radio-iodine or viral thyroiditis does not stimulate the production of thyroid antibodies, although if antibodies are already present their titres may increase: nor does recurrent alcoholic gastritis result in gastric antibodies. Secondly, organ-specific lesions resembling those of the human diseases, but usually reversible, can be induced experimentally in animals by injections of homogenates of the organ (e.g. thyroid or adrenal) incorporated in Freund's adjuvant. The adjuvant enhances immune responses, particularly those dependent on T lymphocytes (p. 129) and passive transfer of lymphocytes and antibody suggest that cell-mediated immunity is a more important cause of tissue injury than auto-antibodies in these experimental conditions. There are, however, exceptions, one being the chronic thyroiditis which develops spontaneously in an inbred obese strain of chickens: it is accompanied by thyroid auto-antibodies and is more severe in chickens rendered deficient in T cells by thymectomy after hatching, but is prevented by depriving the birds of B cells by early bursectomy (p. 118). The same results apply to artificially-induced auto-immune thyroiditis in ordinary chickens.

In the human diseases, the respective roles of auto-antibodies and cell-mediated immunity in the organ-specific auto-immune diseases are not known. It is noteworthy that in the two examples of diseases in which the function of tissue cells are known to be affected by auto-antibodies (thyrotoxicosis and myasthenia gravis—p. 152), the antigen is a receptor projecting from the surface of the target cell. Thyroid microsomal antibody has been shown, in the presence of complement, to be cytotoxic for thyroid epithelial cells in culture, but only if the cells are first treated with trypsin, and it may be that such treatment is necessary to expose the cell membrane auto-antigen. There is no evidence of thyroid injury in the infants of mothers with Hashimoto's thyroiditis although in some cases high concentrations of thyroid antibodies of IgG class are transferred to the fetal circulation.

It is difficult, in man, to investigate the pathogenic role of cell-mediated auto-immunity, for while macrophage migration inhibition tests (p. 159) suggest that this develops, the evidence is not conclusive, and in any case does not indicate that it causes tissue destruction. The lesions are typically infiltrated with lymphocytes, which suggests a delayed hypersensitivity reaction, but could also represent an antibody-dependent (type 2) cytotoxic reaction (p. 152). Also, there are usually some, and often many, plasma cells in the lesions, and locally produced antibody might have a cytotoxic effect. In spite of the rather flimsy nature of the evidence, there is a fairly general belief that the lesions of these diseases are mediated largely by delayed hypersensitivity reactions.

The familial incidence of the organ-specific auto-immune diseases suggests a genetic predisposing factor, and this is supported by the greater concordance in monozygotic than in dizygotic twins (i.e. if one twin has the disease, the other is more likely to develop it if they are monozygotic). The studies on twins indicate that there must also be environmental predisposing factors, and these have been the subject of speculation, but with little advance. One thyroid auto-antigen, thyroglobulin, is normally present in low concentration in the plasma, and appears to induce 'low-dosage' tolerance of T cells (p. 133): potentially responsive B cells have been demonstrated in normal individuals, but probably they require T-cell co-operation to produce antibody. If this applies to the other auto-antigens in these diseases, then breakdown of T-cell tolerance must be necessary for cell-mediated auto-immunity and auto-antibody production. It has been suggested that T-cell tolerance might be broken by modification of cell constituents by drugs, by microbial products, or by disorders of metabolism, but so far there is no evidence for any of these possibilities in the organ-specific auto-immune diseases. Another possibility is the defective functioning of suppressor T cells (pp. 130, 134).

The connective tissue diseases

Systemic lupus erythematosus. This is one of the so-called connective tissue diseases. It is characterised by acute and chronic inflammatory lesions in many organs and tissues, and by the occurrence in the plasma of various auto-antibodies, most of which react with normal constituents common to most types of cell in the body. The sites of lesions include the skin, muscles, joints, glomeruli, heart and blood vessels, but the distribution varies greatly and may be even wider. Auto-antibody to deoxyribonucleoprotein is nearly always demonstrable in the serum by immuno-fluorescence tests (Fig. 6.10), and antibodies to DNA, RNA and various cytoplasmic cellular constituents are commonly present. There may also be cytotoxic auto-antibodies to red cells, platelets and leukocytes and antibodies to clotting factors in the plasma.

The auto-antibodies to nuclear and cytoplasmic constituents are not cytotoxic, and many of them occur in other diseases and, usually in low titre, in some normal subjects. The corresponding auto-antigens may, however, be released by breakdown of cells, and immune-complex (type 3) reactions can then

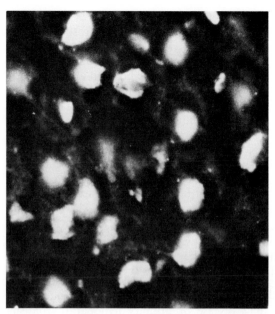

Fig. 6.10 Antibody to deoxyribonucleoprotein demonstrated by the immunofluorescence technique. Note the diffuse nuclear fluorescence. × 775. (Professor J. Swanson Beck.)

result. In fact, most of the pathological features of SLE can be explained on the basis of deposition of circulating immune complexes in the walls of small blood vessels. Disease activity correlates fairly closely with the concentration of anti-DNA in the plasma (measured by DNA binding capacity of the serum) and low levels of serum complement. The glomerular lesions (p. 813) are due to deposition of immune complexes in the glomerular capillary basement membrane and subsequent complement fixation, and this process is responsible also for at least some of the lesions in the skin and elsewhere. Auto-antibodies to native (double-stranded) DNA are virtually specific for SLE and their complexes with DNA contribute significantly to the renal lesions. Antibodies to denatured (single-stranded) DNA occur also in other diseases and do not correlate so closely with disease activity.

The familial occurrence of SLE, and of the various auto-antibodies associated with SLE, raises the possibility of genetic factors, and the spontaneous development of a very similar disease in the F1 hybrid of the NZB and NZW inbred strains of mice developed in New Zealand by Bielchowsky, provides a genetically-determined model.

There is also circumstantial evidence that a virus infection may be involved in SLE. Virus-like particles have been observed in the renal lesions, and are regularly discernible in the tissues of NZ mice. When maintained in tissue culture, lymphoid cells from these mice release C type RNA virus particles which *in vivo* stimulate the development of antibodies reactive with host DNA and RNA. It is possible that this virus, which is responsible for lymphoid neoplasia in mice, modifies the lymphoid cells in some way which predisposes them to auto-immune responses. There is also evidence that the SLE-like disease of NZ hybrid mice is related to thymic deficiency: 'thymic hormone' levels (p. 118) fall at a relatively early age in these mice (and are low in patients with SLE), and the disease in mice is accelerated by neonatal thymectomy and inhibited by injection of thymocytes from young mice. These observations, and the demonstration that animals rendered immunologically tolerant to an antigen develop suppressor T cells which are capable, on transfer to a normal animal, of inhibiting the immune response to that antigen (p. 134), raise the possibility that auto-immune responses are normally inhibited by suppressor T cells, and that auto-immune diseases arise particularly in individuals with T-cell deficiences. In SLE, which occurs most commonly in women of reproductive age, serum antibody levels to some viruses are unusually high, and cell-mediated immune responses are impaired, suggesting that suppressor T-cell function may be deficient. It is therefore of considerable interest that antibody cytotoxic for a subset of T lymphocytes has been demonstrated in the serum of patients with SLE and occurs also in their close household contacts, including spouses (suggesting a causal viral infection?). The possibility that this auto-antibody destroys suppressor T cells could explain the large numbers of auto-antibody responses observed in this disease. Antibody claimed to be cytotoxic for suppressor T cells has also been detected in NZ mice.

Rheumatoid arthritis (RA). Because of its high incidence and disabling effects, this is the most important of the connective tissue diseases. The main feature is a destructive polyarthritis, in which the synovial membrane is infiltrated with lymphocytes, macrophages and plasma cells. Immune complexes and activated complement components are present in the synovial fluid and are deposited in the synovial membrane. In most cases, the serum contains **rheumatoid factors**: these are immunoglobulins (usually IgM) which behave as antibodies to auto-antigenic components of IgG. Rheumatoid factors react only weakly with native IgG, but strongly with IgG which has been heat-

denatured, and with IgG antibody coupled with the corresponding antigen. Experimental evidence suggests that rheumatoid factors develop when IgG antibody forms immune complexes: binding with antigen alters the IgG molecule and renders it auto-antigenic.

The aetiology and pathogenesis of RA are discussed on p. 939. It appears that inflammatory changes are brought about as a result of activation of complement by antigen-antibody complexes. Initially such complexes might be provided by antibody reacting with a postulated infective agent. Subsequently, complexes are formed by IgG rheumatoid factor which reacts with its own Fc component (Fig. 23.70, p. 939). RA may thus be an Arthus (type 3) reaction, but there are other possibilities, including a delayed hypersensitivity (type 4) reaction between specifically primed T lymphocytes and synovial lining cells.

Polyarthritis is not uncommon in SLE, but is seldom so severe or destructive as rheumatoid arthritis. This and other associations do not indicate an auto-immune pathogenesis for rheumatoid arthritis, but merely suggest that common genetic and possibly environmental factors predispose to both conditions.

The other connective tissue diseases are dealt with in the relevant systematic chapters. Apart from the variable occurrence of anti-nuclear and other auto-antibodies, there is little evidence to suggest an auto-immune pathogenesis.

Other auto-immune diseases

Auto-immune destruction of red cells, leukocytes and platelets by cytotoxic antibodies (p. 150) may occur in isolation, or in association with systemic lupus erythematosus. The pathogenic effects of auto-antibodies in *Graves' disease* and *myasthenia gravis* have already been mentioned (p. 163).

Other diseases in which auto-immunity may be significant include *ulcerative colitis*, in which the intestinal epithelium may be the target cell of an auto-immune response and some types of chronic liver disease, notably *primary biliary cirrhosis* and virus-negative *chronic active hepatitis*, in which there is evidence of auto-immunity to components of bile-duct epithelium and hepatocytes respectively. Various other diseases could be mentioned, but as the list lengthens, the evidence becomes progressively weaker.

Rejection of transplanted tissues

The treatment of burns by skin grafting is a well-established procedure. The epidermis of *autologous grafts* extends to cover the denuded area and survives indefinitely, while *allogeneic grafts* become established, but invariably undergo necrosis within two or three weeks. Evidence that this rejection process is mediated by an immunological reaction on the part of the host was first provided by Gibson and Medawar in 1943. In a series of important experiments, Medawar and his colleagues went on to lay the foundations of transplant immunology. They showed that skin grafts between syngeneic* mice were accepted permanently, while allogeneic grafts stimulated an immune response in the host and were consequently destroyed ('rejected') 1–3 weeks after grafting. They also showed that mice injected at birth with allogeneic cells would subsequently accept permanently a skin graft from the same donor strain and that this state of unresponsiveness—the first experimental demonstration of acquired immunological tolerance (p. 132)—could be abolished, with consequent rejection of the skin graft, by injection of host-strain lymphocytes from a normal mouse or from one that had previously rejected a graft from the allogeneic strain. Lymphocytes from the latter mouse induced more rapid and intense graft rejection, showing that, as a result of previously rejecting an allograft, it had developed persistent immunity, manifested by the reactivity of its lymphoid cells. This early work suggested the importance of cell-mediated immunity in allograft rejection. It is true that antibodies also developed in the recipients of allografts, but their injection into tolerant animals bearing an appropriate allograft did not result in rejection.

Medawar's major observations and conclusions have been confirmed in experiments involving transplantation of various tissues in many vertebrate species. The mechanism of rejection is complex, but in most situations cell-mediated immunity plays a major role and the graft is destroyed mainly by a delayed hypersensitivity (type 4) reaction. Specifically-primed T lymphocytes bind to 'transplant' antigens on the surface of the graft cells (see below)

and bring about their destruction. The mechanism of such cytotoxic activity is not known. The specifically-reactive T lymphocytes also release lymphokines (p. 157), which activate macrophages, and possibly also a specific macrophage-arming factor (SMAF) which enables macrophages to bind specifically to the transplant antigens of the graft cells and destroy them. In organs such as the kidney, which are transplanted by connecting the major blood vessels of the graft to host vessels, injury may result also from a cytotoxic antibody (type 2) reaction (p. 150).

Transplant antigens: the HLA system. The cells of probably all vertebrates possess numerous surface iso-antigens, termed transplant antigens. In several species, including man, a major system of strong antigens, characteristic for each species and determined by multiple alleles at a complex locus, has been demonstrated. In man, this is the HLA system of antigens, so called because the antigens were first detected in human leukocytes. Each individual inherits HLA antigens from each parent as shown in Fig. 6.11.

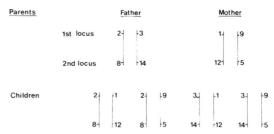

Fig. 6.11 The major histocompatibility complex in man contains a number of allelic genes, at loci close together on the same chromosome (No. 6). The diagram shows the mode of inheritance of genes of the first two loci, which code respectively for one antigen of the HLA-A series (antigens 1, 2, 3, 9, 10, 11, 28 and 29) and one antigen of the HLA-B series (antigens 5, 7, 8, 12, 13, 14, 18 and 27). The individual thus inherits a pair of antigens (one from each parent) in each series. Because of their close linkage, the genes, and so the antigens, are inherited in 'sets', so that siblings with the same antigens in one series (e.g. the same HLA-A antigens) are likely to have the same antigens in the other series. This is shown above for HLA-A and HLA-B antigens, but it applies also to the HLA-C and -D antigens, and explains why there is a 25 per cent chance that two siblings will inherit identical sets of antigens. Transplantation between such siblings is usually highly successful.

* For terminology, see p. 105.

In rats and mice, the major transplant antigens are the main factors in determining the intensity of the iso-immune response, and thus of rejection, following transplantation. In human renal transplantation, matching has so far been limited by the availability of suitable antisera and has been restricted largely to HLA-A and -B antigens which (together with HLA-C antigens) are detectable by means of antisera (see below). Another group of HLA antigens (the D or LD antigens) determined by alleles at a fourth locus were not detected by antisera (although these are now becoming available) but by the mixed lymphocyte reaction, in which a mixture of lymphocytes from two individuals is incubated and a positive reaction is indicated by DNA synthesis and 'blast' cell transformation. Such transformation represents a reaction of T lymphocytes induced by HLA-D antigens on the B lymphocytes (of the other individual). By treating the lymphocytes of one individual with mitomycin before mixing, they are rendered unresponsive and any reaction then represents the response of the T cells of the other individual (the 'one-way' mixed lymphocyte reaction). As explained in Fig. 6.11, the close proximity of all the HLA loci on the chromosome 6 ensures that siblings who have inherited the same HLA-A and -B antigens will also almost always have the same C and D antigens, and will thus be closely histocompatible. By contrast, it is very difficult to find complete HLA identity among unrelated individuals.

Because it codes for strong histocompatibility antigens, the HLA region on chromosome 6 has been termed the *major histocompatibility complex* (MHC). Similar complexes are found in mice and other higher vertebrates. In addition to the HLA (or in the mouse the H2) loci, the MHC contains Ir genes which determine the strength of the thymus-dependent antibody responses to particular antigens: they influence co-operation between T and B cells and also degradation of antigen by macrophages.

Graft versus host reaction. If normal lymphoid cells are injected into an allogeneic host, they will be destroyed unless the host is immunologically deficient or tolerant and cannot mount a rejection reaction. In these circumstances, the grafted cells may survive and mount an immune response against the host, with a consequent **graft-versus-host (G.v.H.)** reaction. This occurs when allogeneic lymphocytes from an adult mouse are injected into neonates or into mice rendered immunodeficient, e.g. by thymectomy and x-irradiation, and when an F1 hybrid mouse is injected with lymphocytes of either parental strain. The G.v.H. reaction is complex and includes splenomegaly, lymph node enlargement, haemolytic anaemia and predisposition to infections. When induced in the neonate, these changes, together with impairment of growth, have been termed *runt disease*. In man, G.v.H. disease may result from infusion of lymphoid or haemopoietic cells into patients with T-cell deficiency, e.g. following intensive cytotoxic therapy for leukaemia: it presents as anorexia, diarrhoea, dermatitis and liver failure.

Human renal transplantation

Many thousands of kidneys have been transplanted in the past few years to patients with irreversible renal failure. The major obstacle is immunological rejection of the graft and, except for transplants between identical twins, it is essential to protect the graft by administration of immunosuppressive drugs such as glucocorticoids, azathioprine or actinomycin C. Initially, high dosage is necessary to prevent acute rejection, but the dosage can gradually be reduced, in some cases to very low levels, without rejection occurring. This indicates that the host becomes increasingly less responsive to the graft antigens. One possible explanation is that the continued release of antigens by the graft, together with immunosuppression, results in specific immunological tolerance. Another is that the host develops 'enhancing' antibodies (p. 134) which protect the graft by suppressing the cell-mediated immune response or by combining with graft antigens and so concealing them from specifically responsive T lymphocytes. Administration of iso-antibodies reactive with antigens of the grafted tissue has been shown to prolong graft survival in animals, and there is preliminary evidence that administration of HLA antibodies may have a similar enhancing effect in human renal transplantation, although such antibodies (presumably in larger amounts) can also cause immediate rejection (p. 846).

While on large doses of immunosuppressive

drugs, transplant patients are very liable to develop infections, both with virulent pathogens and with opportunistic micro-organisms such as *Cytomegalovirus*, *Pneumocystis carinii* and various fungi.

In spite of these problems, approximately 50 per cent of the transplants have done well and are functioning some years later.

The pathological features of rejection of renal transplants are described on p. 846.

Tissue typing. At present, tissue typing is usually performed by a cytotoxicity test, using typing antisera and complement, upon cells of the individual to be typed: if the cells possess the corresponding iso-antigen, they will be killed (Fig. 2.2, p. 10). All tissue cells, leukocytes and platelets (but not red cells) possess HLA antigens, and it is convenient to use blood lymphocytes for typing. HLA antisera are obtained from recipients of blood transfusions or previous transplants, or from parous women, some of whom have developed antibodies to HLA antigens of the fetus. By testing with a panel of lymphocytes of known HLA phenotypes, and suitable absorption to remove unwanted antigens, specific HLA antisera can be provided.

There is no doubt that renal allografts have a better chance of surviving when the donor and recipient are closely matched for HLA antigens. The effect is greatest in grafting between siblings of identical HLA-A and -B antigens because, as explained on p. 167, they are also very likely to have identical C and D antigens, and over 90 per cent of kidneys are functioning well one year later. Even with close matching between unrelated donors and recipients, the figure is only about 60 per cent because identity at all four HLA loci is unlikely. Testing for histocompatibility of HLA-D antigens by the mixed lymphocyte reaction takes 4 days or so, and is usually impracticable. In addition to the HLA antigen, there are loci on other chromosomes determining weaker transplant antigens, and even grafts between HLA-identical siblings will be rejected unless the recipient receives immunosuppressive therapy.

For reasons explained on p. 846, it is essential to ensure ABO compatibility in human renal transplantation, and to test the recipient's serum for cytotoxic antibody to donor cells.

Transplantation of other tissues

Infusion of **haemopoietic cells**, which include pluripotent stem cells (p. 118), is a logical treatment for infants with congenital deficiency of haemopoietic stem cells, for patients with certain forms of aplastic anaemia, and for children treated for acute leukaemia by cytotoxic drugs in doses which destroy their haemopoietic and lymphoid cells. The depressed immune responsiveness of such patients reduces the risk of rejection of the donated cells, but immunocompetent T lymphocytes in the donation are very liable to respond to transplant antigens of the host, causing a fatal *graft-versus-host reaction* (see above). It is thus essential to use as donor an HLA-identical sibling.

Successful **corneal allografting** has long been practised without immunosuppression of the recipient. This is because the cornea is avascular and therefore a 'protected site' in which the graft does not induce an immune response in the recipient. If, as sometimes happens, blood vessels extend into the grafted cornea, then rejection occurs.

In allografts of **blood vessels** and **tendon**, the cells either die from ischaemia or are destroyed by a rejection reaction, but the collagen and elastic fibres persist, and are repopulated with host cells and vessels: thus the use of stored vessel or tendon is equally, if not more effective. Similarly, the cells of **bone grafts** die, but the matrix may provide the desired mechanical effect (p. 875). The use of **cartilage grafts** in plastic surgery is of considerable interest: both the cells and the matrix of allografts may survive for long periods without inducing a rejection reaction. This is due to the avascular nature of cartilage, and to the matrix which allows diffusion of nutrients and metabolites between graft chondrocytes and host, but acts as an 'immunological barrier' between them.

Another exception to the general phenomenon of allograft rejection is provided by nature's allograft, **pregnancy**. The trophoblast, of fetal origin, is bathed in maternal blood, and yet it is tolerated for nine months, in spite of the presence of incompatible (paternal) transplant antigens in the fetal cells. There is slight depression of maternal immune responsiveness during pregnancy, but the mother does not develop specific immunological tolerance to the fetus. The most likely explanation of failure to reject the fetus appears to be that the cells of the syncytiotrophoblast are coated with a layer of mucopolysaccharide, which provides an 'immunological barrier'. As already mentioned, pregnancy commonly results in the development of maternal antibodies to the transplant antigens of the fetus, but this is without apparent effect.

Immunological Deficiency States

There are a large number of conditions in which the normal defence mechanisms against invasive micro-organisms are impaired. For most purposes it is useful to classify such deficiencies into two major groups. Firstly, deficiencies of non-specific resistance, as in diabetes mellitus, impaired function of neutrophil polymorphs (p. 513), etc. This miscellaneous group is dealt with under the appropriate diseases: it includes also lesions which impair resistance locally, for example obstruction of hollow viscera, as in the urinary tract or air passages, and ischaemia of the lower limb leading to gangrene.

In the second major group, which is discussed here, impaired resistance is due to defects in specific immunological responsiveness. These are best classified into primary and secondary types, and also in relation to the type of immunological defect present.

In the group of *primary conditions*, the immunological deficiency becomes manifest usually, but not always, in early childhood, and in most of the conditions there is good evidence that the defect is genetically determined. Other abnormalities, e.g. thrombocytopenia in the Wiskott–Aldrich syndrome, or hypoparathyroidism in the DiGeorge syndrome, may accompany the immunological defect, giving rise to characteristic disease complexes, but the immunological deficiency is not secondary to the other parts of the syndrome. By contrast, the *secondary immunological deficiences* occur at any age, are not genetically-determined, and the immunological defects are the result of injury to the lymphoid tissues, either by various disease processes, particularly lymphoid neoplasia, or by immunosuppressive agents.

The type of immunological defect present determines the clinical picture and form of therapy required. The division of lymphoid cells into two major classes—thymic-dependent (T) and thymic-independent (B)—has been dealt with in Chapter 5. Its validity in man is demonstrated by the occurrence of immunodeficiency states affecting mainly T-cell function, with depression of cell-mediated immune responses, or mainly B-cell function, with depression of antibody production: combined deficiencies, affecting both T- and B-cell function, are also observed. Such well-defined immunodeficiencies occur as primary, congenital defects, but they are rare. Less serious and less clearly-defined deficiencies also occur, both as congenital and acquired conditions.

Primary immunological deficiencies

(1) Deficiency of B-cell function. This group is exemplified by **infantile sex-linked agammaglobulinaemia**, which was the first to be described and is sometimes known as the **Bruton type of agammaglobulinaemia** after its discoverer. The major abnormality is a virtually complete inability to produce the three major classes of immunoglobulins—IgG, IgM and IgA. In consequence, there is little or no antibody production in response to infections or immunisation procedures, and the normal blood group iso-antibodies are usually not detectable. The condition is observed nearly always in boys, being transmitted by a gene defect in the X chromosome (sex-linked recessive). Symptoms usually arise in the second year of life, protection before that being provided by maternal antibodies of IgG class transmitted to the fetus. The defect results in unusually frequent and serious bacterial infections, particularly those due to the pyogenic bacteria, and including respiratory and pulmonary infections, meningitis and septicaemia. 'Opportunistic' infections (p. 174), e.g. pneumonia due to the protozoon, *Pneumocystis carinii*, also occur, and candidiasis is common. The infections respond to appropriate antibiotics, and diagnosis depends upon the demonstration of the near-absence of serum IgG (below 0·5 g/litre), IgM and IgA (below 3×10^{-2} g/litre). Deficiency of IgG cannot be demonstrated until the maternal IgG has fallen to a low level—usually by about 8 months old, although very low levels of the other two immunoglobulins are observed before this time, since they do not cross the placenta.

The lymph nodes and tonsils are small, and biopsy reveals an absence of germinal centres and plasma cells, while rectal biopsy reveals absence of plasma cells in the mucosa. The blood lymphocytes are not greatly diminished, but B lymphocytes are virtually absent. The thymus is normal, and cell-mediated immune responses are not impaired. Accordingly, the responses to BCG and vaccinial immunisation are normal and afford protection, and virus infections in general occur with the same frequency and clinical features as in normal children. Chronic polyarthritis, closely resembling rheumatoid arthritis, is of common occurrence.

The effectiveness of regular injections of human IgG in preventing infections has increased the importance of early diagnosis. It is important to distinguish the Bruton type of agammaglobulinaemia, which requires life-long therapy, from **transient hypogammaglobulinaemia**. This latter condition presents similar clinical features and morphological changes in the lymphoid tissues, but is merely a delay, and not a permanent failure, of the capacity to produce immunoglobulins. It is familial, relatively common, and more frequent and severe in infants born prematurely: it affects both sexes, and the defect disappears within the first three years of life. In most cases, severe immunoglobulin deficiency is limited to IgG, and normal levels of IgM and IgA in the serum may help to distinguish it from the Bruton type.

There are a number of less well-defined conditions which appear to fall within this group. In all of them, there is defective production of one or more classes of immunoglobulins, impairment of antibody production, and relatively normal cell-mediated immune responses. The evidence favouring a genetic predisposition, and a particular mode of genetic transmission, varies in the different types. In some forms, the immunological deficiency does not become manifest until adult life, and yet the disease tends to occur in families, and often exhibits a familial association with other immunological disturbances, e.g. hypergammaglobulinaemia and systemic lupus erythematosus. Some patients with such late-onset immunoglobulin deficiency also develop auto-immune diseases such as pernicious anaemia and connective tissue diseases, but without demonstrable auto-antibodies.

(2) Deficiency of T-cell function. An example of this group is provided by the rare **DiGeorge syndrome**, in which there is almost complete failure of development of the thymus and parathyroids from the third and fourth branchial arches.

In those infants who survive the neonatal period, immunoglobulin production appears normal, although antibody responses, at least to some antigens, are impaired, probably because of lack of helper T cells. The lymph nodes contain plasma cells and germinal centres, but the paracortical (thymus-dependent) areas are deficient in small lymphocytes, and the number of circulating lymphocytes, although variable, is low in some cases. The condition may affect infants of both sexes, and there is no evidence for a genetic predisposition. Affected infants can deal perfectly well with pyogenic bacteria, but suffer from 'opportunistic' infections, e.g. by *Pneumocystis carinii* (p. 474) and fungi and also from severe virus infections. Impairment of cell-mediated immunity is demonstrable by failure to develop contact hypersensitivity to agents such as dinitrochlorobenzene (p. 137) and immunisation with live vaccines is liable to give rise to fatal generalised infections. The condition is fatal: in some instances life has been prolonged by transplantation of thymic tissue, but the problem here is to prevent rejection of the grafted thymus by the host T lymphocytes which generate under its influence.

(3) Combined immunological deficiency. In **alymphocytic agammaglobulinaemia**, sometimes termed the **Swiss type of agammaglobulinaemia**, both the thymus-dependent and -independent immunity systems fail to develop. The thymus is hypoplastic and deficient in Hassall's corpuscles and small lymphocytes, the lymph nodes are extremely small and lacking in germinal centres, lymphocytes and plasma cells, and circulating lymphocytes are scanty. There is a near-absence of the three main classes of immunoglobulins from the serum, and both antibody production and cell-mediated immunity are grossly defective. The condition is transmitted as an autosomal recessive character, and affected infants show retarded growth, recurrent bacterial and virus infections, and response to antibiotics and chemotherapy is poor. Immunisation with living viruses is likely to prove fatal, and the condition usually results in death during the first or second year. The basic defect appears to lie in the haemopoietic stem cells (p. 118), which fail to undergo lymphopoiesis.

Combined immunological deficiency occurs also in **reticular dysgenesis**, in which there is a deficiency of haemopoietic stem cells, resulting in failure of lymphopoiesis and haemopoiesis: death usually occurs before or shortly after birth.

In both these conditions, the deficiencies are restored by infusion of haemopoietic cells, which include stem cells, but unless the donor is an HLA-identical sibling there is a grave risk of fatal graft-versus-host reaction (p. 167).

(4) Other primary immunological deficiencies are mostly of obscure nature. In **ataxia telangiectasia** there are widespread vascular defects resulting in dilatation of small vessels (telangiectases), and an insidiously-developing immunodeficiency with depression of cell-mediated immunity and low levels of IgE and IgA in the blood. The IgG level is also low in some cases. Recurrent infections of the paranasal sinuses and lungs are the most common consequences of the immunological defect. In some instances the thymus has been found to be poorly developed and lacking in Hassall's corpuscles. The condition appears to be determined genetically by an autosomal recessive gene.

Another condition in which immunodeficiency develops insidiously is the **Wiskott–Aldrich syndrome** in which the platelets are abnormal or reduced in number. There is progressive depletion of lymphocytes in the blood and in the T-dependent areas of the lymphoid tissues. The blood levels of IgM and IgA gradually fall and cell-mediated immunity declines. The condition is determined by a sex-linked genetic defect and affects boys: atopic eczema, attacks of diarrhoea and recurrent infections are common features. Recent reports suggest that administration of Lawrence's transfer factor has a restorative effect on the immunodeficiencies in this condition, in which the thymus appears normal or is slightly diminished in size.

Secondary immunological deficiencies

These are conditions in which the immunity system develops and functions normally but becomes defective from the direct or indirect effect of various disease processes or immunosuppressive agents. Causal conditions include malnutrition, certain infections, various forms of cancer and renal failure.

Susceptibility to infections is a well-known feature of malnutrition, but it is only recently that **protein deficiency**, both experimental and in man, has been demonstrated to impair cell-mediated immune responsiveness. *Because of its prevalence in many parts of the world, this is probably the most important cause of immunodeficiency.*

Depression of cell-mediated immunity may be a feature of various **acute virus infections**, but has been demonstrated most clearly in measles and infectious mononucleosis, in both of which a temporary depression of cell-mediated immunity has been shown by skin tests (e.g. to tuberculoprotein) becoming negative, and by impaired responsiveness of lymphocytes to stimulation *in vitro* by antigens or phytomitogens (see below).

Impaired cell-mediated immunity occurs also in some **bacterial and protozoal infections** in which there is extensive colonisation of the macrophage system, e.g. lepromatous leprosy and leishmaniasis. T-cell function is depressed also in **sarcoidosis**, a condition of unknown cause characterised by tubercle-like granulomas of the lymphoid and various other tissues.

Patients with **advanced cancer** commonly have depression of both T and B cell function: without doubt, this is a result of cancer, although there is evidence that the incidence of cancer (of both the lymphoid and epithelial tissues) is increased in patients who survive with primary immunodeficiencies and in patients on long-term immunosuppressive therapy, e.g. following renal transplantation.

Immunodeficiencies are particularly common in patients with **lymphoid neoplasia (lymphoma)**. In chronic lymphocytic leukaemia, there is very often deficient T and B cell function; this may be due to crowding of the lymphoid tissues, marrow and blood with neoplastic (usually B) lymphocytes. It is, however, of interest that immunosuppression is an early effect of infection with the retraviruses, which induce lymphomas in animals, and it is likely that human chronic lymphocytic leukaemia (and some other lymphomas) are also virus-induced. Depression of antibody levels is a feature of multiple myeloma, a plasma-cell tumour usually confined to the bone marrow; the high levels of Ig secreted by the myeloma cells increase the rate of Ig catabolism and may also depress antibody responses.

In a third lymphoid neoplasm, Hodgkin's disease, the lymphoid tissues are often extensively infiltrated, and T-cell deficiency is then the usual result: tuberculosis or virus infection (e.g. varicella zoster) may prove fatal.

The immunodeficiency of **renal failure** affects T-cell, and probably also B-cell, function. This is important in renal transplantation because it helps initially to prevent rejection of the transplanted kidney.

Assessment of immunological function

In cases of suspected immunodeficiency, information can be obtained from examination of the blood to determine: (*a*) the levels of the various classes of Ig; (*b*) the presence and titres of ABO blood group antibodies; and (*c*) the proportions and numbers of T and B lymphocytes.

The responsiveness of lymphocytes to stimulation by antigens, e.g. tuberculoprotein, and to phytomitogens, gives some indication of function. Blast-cell transformation occurs when normal blood lymphocytes are cultured in the presence of phytohaemagglutinin (PHA) or concanavalin A (con-A), both of which stimulate T cells, pokeweed mitogen (PWM) which stimulates both T and B cells, and bacterial endotoxin, which stimulates B cells.

Other tests include assay of antibodies against commonly encountered antigens, and cell-mediated immunity may be investigated by skin tests or *in vitro* techniques (p. 113). Finally, antigens may be administered and the responses measured, but live vaccines should not be used for this purpose in subjects who may not be able to eliminate even attenuated micro-organisms.

With increasing use of immunosuppressive and cytotoxic drugs—cortisone, azathioprene, cyclophosphamide, etc., and also radiotherapy, infections due to immunodeficiencies are becoming common, and often limiting factors in renal transplantation and the treatment of various forms of cancer and other fatal diseases. Some of these agents destroy not only lymphocytes, but also polymorphs and macrophages, and thus depress resistance to infection in more than one way.

References

Butcher, B. T., Salvaggio, J. E. and Leslie, G. A. (1975). Secretory and humoral immunogenic response of atopic and non-atopic individuals to intra-nasally administered antigen. *Clinical Allergy* 1, 33.

Cochrane, C. G. and Koffler, D. (1973). Immune complex disease in experimental animals and man. *Advances in Immunology*, Vol. 16, pp. 186–264. Academic Press, New York and London.

Gibson, T. and Medawar, P. B. (1943).The fate of skin homographs in man. *Journal of Anatomy*, **77**, 299–310.

Ishizaka, K., Ishizaka, T. and Hombrook, M. M. (1966). Physico-chemical properties of reaginic antibody. V. Correlation of reagin activity with γE-globulin antibody. *Journal of Immunology* **97**, 840–53.

Ishizaka, T., Ishizaka, K. and Tomioka, H. (1972). Release of histamine and slow reacting substance of anaphylaxis (SRS-A) by IgE—anti-IgE reactions on monkey mast cells. *Journal of Immunology* **108**, 513–20.

Larner, J. L. (1977). *Cyclic Nucleotide Metabolism*, pp. 52. In *Current Contents Series*, Upjohn Co., Kalamazoo, Michigan.

Matthew, D. J., Norman, A. P., Taylor, B., Turner, M. W. and Soothill, J. F. (1977). Prevention of eczema. *Lancet* i, 111–13.

Reid, F. M., Sandilands, G. P., Gray, K. G. and Anderson, J. R. (1979). Lymphocyte emperipolesis revisited. *Immunology* **36**, 367–72.

Taylor, B., Norman, A. P., Orgel, H. A., Turner, M. W., Stokes, C. R. and Soothill, J. F. (1973). Transient IgA deficiency and infantile atopy. *Lancet* i, 111–13.

Wilkinson, P. C., Parrott, D. M. V., Russell, R. J. and Sless, F. (1977). Antigen-induced locomotor responses in lymphocytes. *Journal of Experimental Medicine* **145**, 1158–68.

Further Reading

Gell, P. G. H., Coombs, R. R. A. and Lachmann, P. J. (Eds.) (1975). *Clinical Aspects of Immunology*, 3rd edn., pp. 1754. Blackwell Scientific, Oxford. (Extensive reviews by leading workers.)

Holborow, E. J. and Reeves, W. G. (Eds.) (1978). *Immunology in Medicine*, pp. 1185. Academic Press, London; Grune and Stratton, New York. (A comprehensive but readable account of disease processes with an immunological basis.)

Irvine, James (Ed.) (1979). *Medical Immunology*, pp. 506. Teviot Scientific Publications, Edinburgh. (An up-to-date readable account by leading workers.)

Miescher, P. A. and Müller-Eberhard, H. J. (Eds.) (1976). *Textbook of Immunopathology*, 2nd edn., pp. 1118. Grune and Stratton, New York, San Francisco and London. (Extensive reviews by leading workers.)

Rose, N. R., Milgrom, F. and van Oss, C. J. (Eds.) (1978). *Principles of Immunology*, 2nd edn., pp. 544. Macmillan Publishing Co. Inc., New York. (An up-to-date account by leading workers.)

The HLA System (1978). *British Medical Bulletin* **34**, pp. 213–316. (A series of review articles on biological and clinical aspects of the system.)

See also Bibliography for Chapter 5 (pp. 139–40).

7

Host—Parasite Relationships

Throughout evolutionary development, many species have adapted to a parasitic existence, living in or on the surface of a host of another species, from which they derive warmth, nourishment and mobility. The relationship is not necessarily harmful to the host, and may be advantageous. For example, various relatively harmless bacteria colonise the skin of man and help to exclude more harmful bacteria, while reabsorption of bile pigment from the gut and the production of vitamin K depend largely on the metabolic activities of the intestinal bacterial flora. These normal inhabitants of the skin and mucous membranes are called **commensals**. Other parasites, termed **pathogens**, are less well adapted and by injuring the host endanger their own survival: they include many species of micro-organisms (microbes) including viruses, bacteria, fungi and protozoa and also metazoa of various sizes. The terms **pathogenicity** and **virulence** are commonly used synonymously to indicate the capacity of a particular micro-organism to cause disease.

Although it is important to distinguish between commensals and pathogens, the distinction is not absolute, for many commensals are only harmless so long as they are kept at bay by the host's defence mechanisms. In immunodeficiency states, for example, various normally harmless microbes may behave as 'opportunistic' pathogens. Similarly, a breach of local defence mechanisms, even in a normal individual, may allow commensals to cause severe infections, an example being *Escherichia coli*, which normally inhabits the gut: this bacterium may be introduced into the urinary tract by catheterisation of the bladder, and may then cause severe acute pyogenic inflammation, even extending into the kidneys. Local abnormalities in the host may also predispose to injury by commensals: for instance, heart valves which have been scarred and distorted by rheumatic

fever are readily colonised by *Streptococcus viridans*, a bacterium which lives in the mouth and finds its way into the blood following tooth extraction, or even when the teeth are brushed vigorously. In normal individuals it is quickly eliminated, but it can settle and multiply in the distorted valve cusps, causing bacterial endocarditis. Because the distinction between pathogens and commensals is not sharp, it is helpful to use the term **infection** to indicate the presence of a particular type of micro-organism in a part of the body where it is normally absent, and where, if allowed to multiply, it is likely to be harmful, i.e. to cause **infective disease**.

As implied above, most infective diseases depend on penetration of the host's tissues by micro-organisms, and the factors concerned in such invasion provide the first major topic of this chapter. Following invasion, the microbes may be eliminated without causing obvious disease (inapparent infection) or clinical disease of any grade of severity may follow: the factors determining these events form a second major topic. Lastly, two important reactions to infection, neutrophil leukocytosis and fever, will be considered.

The subject of infective disease is extremely complex, involving as it does a consideration of the relationships between man and numerous species and strains of micro-organisms. The following account is limited to a brief outline of the subject.

Factors determining invasion

The skin and mucous membranes are exposed to many different types of micro-organisms present in expired droplets in the air, in dust particles, and in food and water. The skin and various mucous membranes on which these organisms settle have properties which render

174

them suitable for the survival and sometimes multiplication of certain organisms, but inhospitable to others. In some instances, the requirements of a particular microbe for growth *in vitro* help to explain its colonisation of particular parts of the surface of the body, but many of the factors determining such colonisation are still unknown, and indeed the predilection of certain bacteria for a particular host species is in most instances quite unexplained. Nevertheless, certain factors are known to be of great importance in limiting or preventing invasion by many types of microbes, and these must be considered briefly.

Barriers to invasion

(a) **Mechanical barriers.** The superficial keratinised layer of the epidermis is an excellent mechanical barrier to microbial invasion, and provided it is kept clean and dry, direct invasion is extremely unlikely. Penetration may however occur when dirt is allowed to accumulate on the skin and particularly in moist warm areas subject to friction, such as the axillae and sub-mammary folds. In many skin diseases which result in exudation with loss or sogginess of the keratin layer, bacterial and fungal infections are common complications. The conjunctival, oral, respiratory-tract and gastro-intestinal mucosae, covered as they are by a film of mucous or serous secretion, also present a formidable barrier to many microorganisms, although some can penetrate the epithelium readily, e.g. influenza virus, rhinoviruses.

Wounds and ulcers of the skin and mucous membranes open up pathways for bacterial invasion and are obviously important causes of infection. Burns are particularly liable to become heavily infected because the dead superficial tissue provides a good medium for coliform bacilli, staphylococci, pyocyanea and many other bacteria. In the mouth, tooth extraction and tonsillectomy inevitably lead to bacterial invasion, and tonsillectomy has been shown to predispose to invasion by the virus of poliomyelitis in the post-operative period. Vitamin A and C deficiencies also impair the resistance of the mucous membranes and skin to bacterial invasion.

Some parasitic organisms have evolved a life cycle in which they multiply in insect vectors and are introduced to man and other hosts by the insect bite, thus penetrating the major barrier of the skin. Examples include the protozoa which cause malaria, the metazoan filarial worms, and the virus of yellow fever, all of which are transmitted by mosquitoes. *Yersinia pestis*, the cause of bubonic plague (the Black Death), is transmitted by the flea of the black rat, and the rickettsiae which cause typhus are spread by ticks, mites and lice. Rabies virus enters the tissues by the bite of a rabid animal.

(b) **Glandular secretions.** The secretions of glands opening on to the skin surface play an important role by maintaining the integrity of the skin, and also by providing an environment in which many types of bacteria cannot survive for long. The acidity of the sweat and the long-chain unsaturated fatty acids produced by the action of commensal bacteria on sebaceous secretion both exert a selective bactericidal effect, and consequently the bacterial flora of the skin surface tends to be rather constant: it has been shown that some types of pathogenic bacteria, when placed on the skin, are virtually all destroyed within an hour or two. The secretions of mucous membranes possess similar qualities. **Lysozyme**, an enzyme which digests the mucopeptide of bacterial cell walls, is present in high concentration in the lacrimal gland secretion and probably exerts an important protective effect in the conjunctival sac: it is secreted also by the salivary and nasal glands but in much smaller amounts. **Antibodies of IgA class**, modified by addition of a 'transport piece' so that they are resistant to digestive enzymes, are present in saliva, tears, intestinal contents, respiratory tract mucus, milk and urine (p. 109). Provided that IgA antibody has developed against a particular organism as a result of previous infection, it will be represented in these secretions. This is of importance in preventing invasion by certain viruses, for the virus may encounter the antibody in the surface mucus and be neutralised by it: its significance in relation to bacterial invasion is less certain, although there is evidence that IgA antibody may render bacteria highly susceptible to the lytic action of lysozyme, and it also activates complement by the alternative pathway.

The acidity of the gastric juice is effective in killing most types of microbes ingested in food or water; but hypochlorhydria due to chronic gastritis is common, and minor illnesses and even emotional stresses can reduce temporarily the acidity of the juice. In general, those microbes which cause intestinal infections, such as the salmonellae and dysentery bacilli, are relatively acid-resistant. *Entamoeba histolytica*, the cause of amoebic dysentery, produces cysts which resist the gastric juice and pass through the stomach before hatching out and invading the wall of the colon.

The normal acidity of the urine contributes to the defences of the urinary tract against infection. Also there is a mucosal factor which eliminates bacteria in contact with the urinary tract epithelium but its nature and mechanism are not understood.

(c) Secretion currents. The continuous flow of tears over the the surface of the conjunctiva has an important effect in the removal of contaminating bacteria, which are carried rapidly into the nasopharynx. In the nose and mouth also, the secretions covering the mucosa flow towards the pharynx and hence to the stomach, carrying with them residual food particles, bacteria, etc. The importance of the saliva is illustrated by the oral infections and severe dental caries which accompany loss of salivary secretion in Sjøgren's syndrome (p. 594). The lacrimal secretion is also diminished, and conjunctival infections result. The importance of removal of contaminating bacteria by the saliva may explain the common occurrence of infection in the crypts of the tonsils and also in the periodontal sulci, for once bacteria gain entrance to these spaces, they are out of the main stream of salivary flow.

In the respiratory tract there is a continuous flow of mucus upwards over the surface of the bronchial and tracheal mucosa: inhaled particles are caught up and removed in this stream, and the air is almost sterile by the time it reaches the respiratory bronchioles. This defence mechanism is dependent on a normal production of mucous secretion and on the integrity of the ciliated respiratory epithelium. Most of the micro-organisms capable of invading the respiratory mucosa in spite of mucociliary flow are enabled to do so by having surface components which allow them to bind to respiratory epithelium: such organisms include influenza virus, *Mycoplasma pneumoniae*, rhinoviruses (common cold) and *Bordetella pertussis* (whooping cough). Other microorganisms are less likely to cause respiratory in-

fections unless the mucosa is first damaged. Such damage may be caused by the virus of influenza which parasitises the respiratory epithelium, interfering with its protective function: as a result, secondary bacterial infection invariably develops, and by extending into the alveoli may give rise to pneumonia. The integrity of the respiratory mucosa is also seriously impaired in chronic bronchitis, most commonly due to cigarette smoking but also to atmospheric pollution: this leads to metaplasia, the ciliated epithelium being replaced by goblet cells in the smaller bronchi. There is increase in the amount of secretion, which also becomes more viscous, and this tends to stagnate and become infected.

Intestinal pathogens, such as the salmonellae of 'food poisoning' and the shigellae of bacillary dysentery, induce an acute inflammatory reaction in the intestinal mucosa: diarrhoea results from the increased peristalsis and exudation, and repeated evacuation of the gut helps to get rid of the offending bacteria.

The flow of urine is of importance in preventing growth and spread of any bacteria gaining entrance to the urinary tract by the urethra, and any abnormality resulting in stagnation of urine or incomplete emptying of the bladder, particularly if chronic, e.g. obstruction by an enlarged prostate, predisposes to infection.

(d) Bacterial commensals. In spite of the defence mechanisms described above, the skin, mouth, nasal cavity, conjunctival sac and intestines are all colonised by bacteria of various types. The local environment provided by each of these various surfaces favours the survival of particular types of bacteria and thus each regional surface develops its own flora. In their usual site of colonisation, most of these commensals are non-pathogenic, and they tend to prevent the establishment of other types of microbes, including pathogens, by competing for nutrients and by release of metabolic products which are toxic to other organisms.

In normal circumstances the bacterial florae of the various surfaces are remarkably stable, but if they are disturbed, colonisation by pathogens may result: hence the common occurrence of fungal infections of the pharynx in patients on antibiotic therapy, and the production of lesions by the toxin of *Clostridium difficile* in pseudomembranous colitis which may arise when the normal flora is depressed by broad-spectrum antibiotics. 'Seeding' of the gut with non-pathogenic bacteria has achieved some success in preventing the overgrowth of pathogens in neonates and in patients treated by antibiotics.

(e) Phagocytes. There is evidence that phagocytic cells migrate on to the surface of various mucous membranes: for example neutrophil polymorphs pass through the thin epithelium lining the depths of the tonsillar crypts, and macrophages pass into the alveoli of the lungs. In both these sites the migrant cells have been shown to phagocytose particles on the surface of the mucosa and this may play a role in preventing invasion.

Invasive capacity of micro-organisms

Micro-organisms vary greatly in their capacity to invade the host's defensive barriers. Most bacteria cause injury only after invading the host's tissues, but some are virtually incapable of invasion and yet can produce disease. For example, *Clostridium tetani*, the cause of tetanus, flourishes only in dead tissue, foreign material and exudate in wounds, but its toxin is absorbed and has serious effects on the nervous system. *Vibrio cholerae* does not invade the mucous membrane of the small intestine, but secretes a toxin which, by disturbing the control of fluid transport across the epithelium, causes severe dehydration. Other organisms, and particularly some viruses, are very highly invasive and infect virtually all individuals who have not previously encountered or been immunised against them, e.g. the viruses of morbilli (measles) and rubella (german measles). Examples of highly invasive bacteria include *Yersinia pestis* (the cause of plague), *Salmonella typhi* (typhoid fever) and the brucellae (undulant fever), all of which regularly invade the bloodstream. However, a great many bacteria lie intermediate between these extremes in their invasive capacity. This includes the more important pyogenic bacteria which are commonly present in the nose or throat, or on the skin. Their presence is often harmless, but disturbances of defence mechanisms may allow them to invade and cause lesions.

In general, bacteria of high invasive capacity are also highly pathogenic, but there is little correlation between the invasive capacity and pathogenicity of viruses. For example, poliovirus invades readily but only a small proportion of infected individuals develop clinical disease, and non-pathogenic strains are administered orally to produce infection and immunity. Also the protozoon *Toxoplasma gondii* is highly invasive and yet, apart from the lesions it causes in fetal life, it is of low pathogenicity.

Pathogenic effects of micro-organisms

Bacteria which have invaded the host tissues may be destroyed without causing clinically apparent disease, may promote a local inflammatory lesion, or may spread to other parts of the body and produce widespread lesions. The two major ways in which bacteria are known to cause pathological changes are firstly by the production of toxins, and secondly by promoting hypersensitivity reactions on the part of the host.

Viruses cause injury by invading the host's cells and utilising the cellular synthetic processes for their own replication. The colonised cells may be destroyed directly by the replicating virus, or as a result of an immunological host reaction (probably mainly delayed hypersensitivity).

Bacterial toxins

These are of two main types, exotoxins and endotoxins.

Exotoxins are secreted by living bacteria: they are simple proteins, are often extremely potent, and vary considerably in their biological effects upon the host. They are antigenically specific and their biological activity is usually neutralised by union with antibody. Many pathogenic bacteria produce a number of different exotoxins when cultured *in vitro*. Thus *Streptococcus pyogenes* and *Staphylococcus aureus*, two of the most important pyogenic bacteria, produce haemolysins and hyaluronidases. *Strep. pyogenes* also produces a leukocidin which kills leukocytes, and *Staph. aureus* a coagulase which clots fibrinogen. Some exotoxins are injurious to virtually all types of host cell and their effects thus depend on their concentration and distribution. *Corynebacterium diphtheriae*, the cause of diphtheria, secretes such a toxin and at the site of infection, usually the pharynx, it causes local tissue necrosis. Less florid but still severe cell injury is far more widespread and is reflected morphologically in fatty change and necrosis of the parenchymal cells of the various organs: in severe cases, death may result from its effect upon the myocardium (Fig. 7.1). The mechanism of injury by this particular toxin is known (p. 8): other toxins with a similarly widespread effect are produced by many of the pathogenic Gram + ve bacteria but in most instances the mechanism of toxic action is not known. Some have enzymic activity, e.g. phosphatases, proteases, lipases. Some bacteria produce toxins which act specifically on one type of tissue, e.g. the neurotoxins of *Cl. botulinum* interfere with the production of acetylcholine at cholinergic synapses in the peripheral nervous system, and cause a flaccid paralysis, while the neurotoxin of *Cl. tetani* has a contrasting effect on the synapses in the central nervous system, resulting in widespread tetanic muscular contractions in response to slight local stimuli.

Attempts to equate the pathogenic effects of

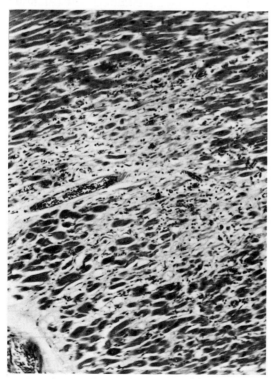

Fig. 7.1 Heart muscle in fatal diphtheria, showing destruction and disappearance of muscle fibres and a light inflammatory cellular infiltrate. × 115.

a particular micro-organism with its toxins have encountered difficulties: not only are many toxins produced by a single strain of bacteria but different samples of a toxin, even in highly purified form, may have different biological properties. Also toxins vary greatly in their effects on hosts of different species, and experimental observations are not necessarily applicable to man. Finally, production or nonproduction of toxin by bacteria growing *in vitro* does not necessarily indicate a similar behaviour *in vivo*. It is a feature of exotoxins that their biological effects are neutralised by the corresponding antitoxin, and in some instances, e.g. diphtheria and tetanus, prior administration of the antitoxin or active immunisation by injection of *toxoid* (inactivated toxin which maintains its immunogenicity) will protect animals against the effects of injection of the toxin and man against the disease. Thus in some instances, particular toxins have been incriminated beyond all reasonable doubt as the pathogenic agents responsible for the disease; in others, it seems most likely that toxins are responsible, but there remains the possibility that the bacteria may have other, at present unknown, pathogenic properties in addition to toxin production.

Endotoxins are structural elements of bacteria and are released only when the bacterium dies. They are constituents of the cell wall of Gram-negative bacteria, and are complexes of phospholipid (lipid A), polysaccharide and protein. The endotoxins produced by different Gram-negative bacteria are antigenically different but they all have the same biological effects and the active component resides in lipid A. Endotoxin is responsible for fever, activation of complement by the alternative pathway (p. 143), intravascular conversion of fibrinogen to fibrin, vascular lesions and cellular necrosis in various organs. In small dosage it causes a neutrophil leukocytosis, in large amounts a leukopenia followed by a leukocytosis. In severe Gram-negative bacterial infections, a state of shock develops with some or all of the above features—'septic' or 'endotoxic' shock (p. 264). Because they produce fever, endotoxins are sometimes termed *pyrogens*. They are heatstable and unless special precautions are taken are liable to contaminate apparatus used for haemodialysis, etc., and fluids prepared for parenteral administration.

Hypersensitivity reactions to micro-organisms

Virtually all microbial infections stimulate immune responses by the host, and the reaction of the antibodies or primed T lymphocytes with microbial antigens can result in hypersensitivity of various types. Atopic (type 1) reactions, such as urticaria, are a common feature of infestation by parasitic worms, even in individuals not otherwise predisposed to atopy, and microbial infections sometimes cause atopic reactions in individuals predisposed to this type of hypersensitivity. Cytotoxic antibody (type 2) reactions may, in theory, result from the cross-reaction of microbial-induced antibodies with host cells, a possible example being rheumatic fever, in which antibodies to *Strep. pyogenes* react with heart muscle cells. Immune complex (type 3) reactions are important complications of some infections. Local Arthus reactions occur when microbial antigens in infected tissues react with antibodies in the plasma. Immune complexes are deposited in the walls of small blood vessels. Circulating immune-complex disease occurs when microbial antigens enter the blood, immune complexes then being formed in the plasma, resulting in an acute febrile reaction and/or deposition of the complexes in small blood vessels, notably in the glomeruli where they are responsible for glomerulonephritis (p. 156). The acute generalised reaction is seen in the severe form of dengue fever which occurs in people who have had a previous, usually mild infection with the virus. On re-infection (possibly with another strain of the virus) large amounts of viral antigen encounter antibody in the plasma, triggering off the complement, clotting, plasmin and kinin systems (p. 55) and causing a profound state of shock. Other examples of infections giving rise to immune-complex reactions, and the way in which lesions are produced, are described on pp. 154–6.

Cell-mediated immunity is an important defence mechanism in various infections. The lymphokines released when primed T cells react with microbial antigens (p. 158) are responsible for both destruction of micro-organisms by macrophages and the tissue injury of delayed (type 4) hypersensitivity. Consequently, the two phenomena are commonly associated. The classical example is tuberculosis, in which cell-mediated immunity develops to tuberculoprotein, and is largely responsible for the lesions of this disease. *Myco. tuberculosis* has not been shown to produce toxins and can colonise macrophages in culture without causing apparent injury: addition of primed T lymphocytes reactive with tuberculoprotein results in destruction of macrophages and their ingested micro-organisms. The morphological features of tuberculosis, described in the next chapter, can all be explained on the basis of delayed hypersensitivity. Leprosy is another disease in which delayed hypersensitivity plays a major role. In some cases, cell-mediated immunity is weak or absent and *Myco. leprae* multiply progressively, mostly within macrophages. Like tubercle bacilli, they cause little or no cell injury, and the lesions consist of enlarging nodules composed of macrophages containing large numbers of *Myco. leprae*. In other cases, strong cell-mediated immunity develops, and the bacteria are kept partly in check. Very few are demonstrable in the lesions, but delayed hypersensitivity results in tissue necrosis and fibrosis (p. 215). This is a good example of the dual effect of cell-mediated immunity—it limits the numbers of micro-organisms, but also causes injury of host tissues.

Delayed hypersensitivity reactions are commonly prominent in fungal, viral and chronic bacterial infections. They are probably involved also in some of the skin lesions of chickenpox, measles, etc. but firm evidence on the pathogenesis of the skin rashes in these conditions is remarkably scanty.

Defence mechanisms in infections

When micro-organisms have invaded the tissues, there are three major defensive reactions which tend to limit their multiplication and spread, and bring about their destruction: these are the inflammatory reaction, phagocytic activity and specific immune reactions.

The inflammatory reaction

The acute inflammatory reaction. The defensive role of this reaction has been considered in Chapter 3. Without doubt, it is of considerable importance, and *those infections which are accompanied by acute inflammation at the site of invasion are more likely to remain localised than those in which invasion is accomplished without* *local injury or reaction*. The pyogenic bacteria are a common cause of the former type of infection, while silent invasion is illustrated by *Treponema pallidum*, the cause of syphilis, which spreads widely through the body before the appearance of a local lesion at the site of entry. Other bacteria which may enter the body silently and spread widely include *Neisseria meningitidis*, a cause of acute meningitis, and brucellae, the cause of undulant fever. Many of the parasites transmitted by biting insects, such as the plasmodia which cause malaria, produce generalised infection without a significant local reaction, and many viruses invade the body and produce viraemia without first producing local inflammation.

Chronic inflammatory change also plays a defensive role by exposing the micro-organisms to phagocytes, antibodies and effector T lymphocytes, and by surrounding them with a layer of granulation tissue which has been shown to be an effective barrier to bacteria. In the more prolonged infections, such as tuberculosis, surviving micro-organisms may be effectively confined within a zone of dense fibrosis resulting from chronic inflammatory change.

Phagocytosis and killing of micro-organisms

A general account of phagocytosis has been given on p. 63, and we are concerned here with factors which determine the capacity of neutrophil polymorphs and macrophages to phagocytose and subsequently kill micro-organisms. Bacteria differ greatly in their resistance to these processes, and such resistance is often an important factor in their pathogenicity.

The inflammatory and immune responses are important host factors favouring phagocytosis and killing of micro-organisms. They help to provide an environment favourable to phagocytosis, render the micro-organism more susceptible to phagocytosis, and increase the phagocytic and killing activities of phagocytes. These factors are illustrated for macrophages in Fig. 7.2. Emigration of polymorphs and monocytes is part of the inflammatory reaction, and the inflammatory exudate opens up tissue spaces in which the emigrated phagocytes can move. Immunoglobulins and components of complement enter infected tissues in the inflammatory exudate; if specific antibodies are present, they may aid phagocytosis by rendering the micro-organisms more susceptible to phagocytic ingestion (opsonisation), or by neutralising toxins harmful to phagocytes. The reaction of antibodies usually activates complement, which may kill micro-organisms directly, or favour their destruction by enhancing the inflammatory reaction and chemotaxis of phagocytes (pp. 55, 60).

Both polymorphs and macrophages have

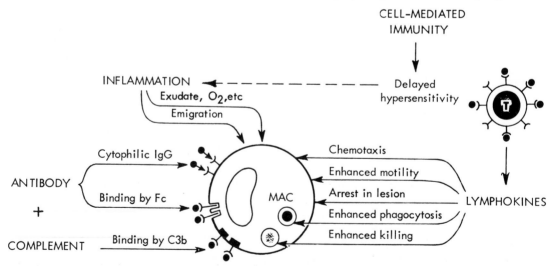

Fig. 7.2 The ways in which the inflammatory reaction, delayed hypersensitivity and antibodies promote the emigration and aggregation of macrophages at the site of infection and enhance their binding, phagocytic and killing capacities for micro-organisms (represented by black spheres). Y represents specific receptors for microbial antigens on T or B lymphocytes and also antibodies binding by various receptors to the surface of macrophages.

surface receptors for the Fc component of IgG antibodies, and this facilitates surface binding and subsequent phagocytosis of microbes sensitised with IgG antibodies (Fig. 7.2): they also have surface receptors for the C3b component of reacted complement but, surprisingly, while complement fixation by antibody-sensitised bacteria enhances binding to the phagocyte, it apparently does not enhance phagocytosis. IgM antibodies are opsonic, particularly for micro-organisms with a non-protein capsule, but their opsonic effect is not due to specific binding to phagocytes, which do not have surface receptors for Fc of IgM.

Cell-mediated immunity is particularly effective in destroying microbes which invade host cells. The lymphokines released when primed T cells react with antigen include factors which promote inflammation, accumulation of macrophages and lymphocytes, and enhance, both specifically and non-specifically, the phagocytosis and killing of ingested micro-organisms by macrophages (see below).

The mechanisms of killing of micro-organisms by phagocytes are complex. Unlike phagocytosis, which occurs readily under anaerobic conditions, killing is accompanied by increased oxygen uptake. In **polymorphs**, oxygen is converted by NADPH into superoxide ($^-O_2$) by removal of an electron; some of this is converted into hydrogen peroxide (H_2O_2) and singlet oxygen ($'O_2$), which has an unstable distribution of electrons around the two nuclei, is also produced. All these forms of highly reactive oxygen are produced within the phagosome, the membrane of which protects the host cell from their effects. They react with the wall of the phagocytosed micro-organism and are highly lethal to many bacteria, viruses and fungi. Hydrogen peroxide also co-operates with myeloperoxidase which, together with halogen ions, forms a system which attacks the microbial cell wall.

In addition to the above mechanisms, the low pH within phagosomes is unfavourable to many micro-organisms, and other lysosomal products exert a harmful effect, notably cationic lysosomal proteins which injure microbial cell walls, lactoferrin (an iron-binding protein), and lysozyme which has a synergistic lytic effect with complement.

Macrophages lack myeloperoxidase, cationic microbicidal proteins and lactoferrin. They are nevertheless capable of producing microbicidal forms of oxygen and they are activated by bacterial products and by the lymphokines produced by T lymphocytes in delayed hypersensitivity reactions (p. 158); their motility, phagocytic activity, lysosomal enzymes and killing capacity are all increased as a result.

Microbial resistance to phagocytes. In general, those bacteria which develop a non-protein capsule, e.g. the anthrax bacillus or smooth strains of *Strep. pneumoniae* and *Haemophilus influenzae*, are not readily phagocytosed. Some bacterial products are chemotactic, but *Strep. pyogenes* and some other bacteria secrete toxins which injure phagocytic (and other) cells and so inhibit phagocytosis. Other bacterial products, e.g. the endotoxins of Gram-negative bacteria, enhance the phagocytic activity of polymorphs and macrophages in low concentrations, but inhibit it in higher concentrations. *Staphylococcus aureus* secretes a factor ('Protein A') which partially inhibits phagocytosis of bacteria sensitised by antibody, possibly by blocking their binding to the Fc receptors of phagocytes (see above).

A number of micro-organisms undergo phagocytosis but are able to resist the microbicidal activity of phagocytes and even multiply within them. A good example is provided by the gonococcus (the cause of gonorrhoea) which colonises neutrophil polymorphs (Fig. 7.3). Some

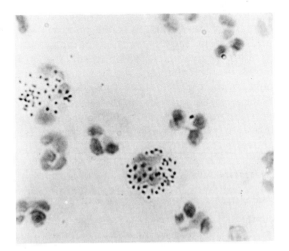

Fig. 7.3 Smear of urethral exudate in acute gonorrhoea. Two polymorphs contain large numbers of gonococci, and show degenerative changes. Other polymorphs contain few or no bacteria and appear relatively healthy. (Gram stain.) × 1200.

viruses undergo phagocytosis by macrophages, but can bind to the phagosomal wall and pass into the cytosol of the host cell. A number of organisms succeed in preventing the fusion of lysosomes with the phagocytic vacuole, and so protect themselves from lysosomal microbicidal products: this is observed with tubercle bacilli ingested by macrophages in culture and with the protozoon *Toxoplasma gondii* and the fungus *Aspergillus flavus*, all of which cause chronic infections in man. In other instances, the organism can flourish within phagosomes, e.g. the brucellae which cause undulant fever. Other organisms have a suppressive effect on cell-mediated immunity and persist within macrophages which are handicapped by lack of the enhancing effects of T-cell lymphokines on their microbicidal activity. This includes the leprosy bacillus and some protozoa.

The immune response

The several ways in which antibodies and cell-mediated immunity help to destroy micro-organisms have been described in this and preceding chapters, and may be summarised as follows. **Antibodies** of IgA class are important in preventing the invasion of mucous membranes by viruses and probably by some bacteria (p. 175). IgM and IgG antibodies can neutralise bacterial toxins, agglutinate and immobilise micro-organisms (p. 108), and prevent cell invasion by viruses: by activating complement, they may cause lysis of microbial cell walls without the intervention of phagocytes (p. 144). Activation of complement also promotes the inflammatory reaction and attracts polymorphs by chemotaxis (pp. 55, 60). Antibodies, particularly those of IgG class, also opsonise micro-organisms, thus favouring their ingestion and destruction by phagocytes (see above).

When the primed T lymphocytes produced by **cell-mediated immune responses** react with microbial antigens, they release lymphokines which induce the inflammatory and other changes of the delayed hypersensitivity reaction (p. 158). In addition to exerting chemotactic and immobilising effects on macrophages, lymphokines include a macrophage-activating factor which increases their killing capacity for ingested micro-organisms, and a second factor—the specific macrophage-arming factor—which enables macrophages to kill allogeneic target cells and may also mediate destruction of micro-organisms.

One of the main purposes of this summary is to emphasise the complex relationships and synergism between the inflammatory response, phagocytosis, and immunological reactions, which together provide a closely interwoven system of defence against micro-organisms.

Interferon (p. 194) is probably mainly responsible for arresting virus infections, yet children with congenital T-cell deficiencies tend to develop progressive virus infections. This could be attributable to loss of the interferon which is produced by T cells responding to antigen, although many other types of cell are capable of producing interferon.

Microbial resistance to the host's immune response. Micro-organisms which colonise host cells are protected from **antibody** in the plasma and tissue fluids, and can persist in spite of a strong antibody response. This is illustrated by the brucellae of undulant fever, the protozoon *Leishmania donovani* which causes leishmaniasis, and some fungi, all of which can survive in macrophages. This mode of protection is particularly successful for organisms which do not kill the host macrophage nor prevent its division. As obligatory intracellular parasites, viruses are protected from antibodies once they have established an infection, although many of them are prevented by antibody from invading the host and spreading by the bloodstream. Those viruses which are integrated into the host cell genome (p. 302) may not provide an antigenic stimulus unless they replicate, and indeed have been shown in various species of animals to be transmitted from generation to generation via the host's germ cells.

To survive, intracellular micro-organisms must also protect themselves against the host's **cell-mediated immune response** and many of them do this by exerting a suppressive effect on cell-mediated immunity in general. This is observed in a number of viral infections, including measles, mumps, infection with the Epstein–Barr virus (the cause of glandular fever), and the animal leukaemia viruses which colonise lymphoid cells. It is also a feature of lepromatous leprosy (p. 216), leishmaniasis (p. 564) and malaria (p. 305).

In some infective diseases, sufficient microbial antigen is produced to overwhelm the immune response. This is seen in severe acute cases of meningococcal septicaemia and meningitis, in which free bacterial polysaccharide antigen can be detected in the serum and CSF (a test used in diagnosis), and also in acute pneumococcal pneumonia or septicaemia. Another example is provided by the B hepatitis virus (p. 670) which replicates in the liver and produces large amounts of viral envelope: in carriers, free viral surface antigen can be demonstrated in the serum. The cell-mediated immune response can also be overwhelmed in extensive infections, for example in widespread tuberculosis or acute tuberculous bronchopneumonia; in these conditions the skin test with tuberculoprotein, which is based on a delayed hypersensitivity reaction (p. 157), becomes negative.

Another ingenious method of circumventing the host's immune response is by **antigenic variation**. The best-known examples are relapsing fever, caused by *Borrelia recurrentis* and trypanosomiasis caused by flagellate protozoa. Both of these organisms stimulate an antibody response to which they are susceptible, but they possess a number of genes coding for antigenically-distinct surface coat material. Although the great majority are destroyed by the host's antibody response, occasional organisms operate another gene for surface coat production and arise as resistant variants with consequent relapse, and so the diseases are characterised by successive recurrences. The influenza virus is notorious for producing mutant strains which are responsible for fresh outbreaks in the population.

Another elegant method of protection is illustrated by the group of parasitic trematodes termed *Schistosomes*. These parasites enter the body as a larval form or schistosomule, which stimulates an immune response in the host, but the larvae rapidly become coated with host blood-group substances and so provide themselves with an immunological cloak which they maintain during development and adult life. The immune response is partly effective in destroying schistosomules subsequently entering the body, before they become coated, and further infection is thus usually avoided. Unfortunately many of the eggs produced by the adults are arrested in the host tissues and elicit a delayed hypersensitivity reaction resulting in a chronic inflammatory lesion, notably in the liver (p. 698).

Mention should also be made of the possibility of a micro-organism inducing in the host **specific immunological tolerance** to its own antigens. This occurs when mice are infected via the ovum with lymphocytic choriomeningitis virus. The virus induces tolerance and persists into adult life, notably in the ependyma and cells lining the meninges· little or no harmful effects result until tolerance partly breaks down and the development of antibodies is followed by deposition of antigen-antibody complexes in the glomeruli and elsewhere. If a mouse is first infected some time after birth, it develops choriomeningitis due to the development of cell-mediated immunity and a consequent delayed hypersensivity reaction with viral antigens. A parallel in man has not been demonstrated. Tolerance might arise also from **molecular mimicry**, in which a micro-organism possesses surface antigens closely similar to host antigens. Some of the coliform bacilli in the gut have been shown to share a common antigen with colonic epithelium, and antibodies induced by various bacteria react with particular transplant (HLA) antigens of man. Such antigenic similarities have not been shown to influence infections, but individuals possessing particular HLA antigens have been found to be unduly prone to certain infections. For example, Reiter's syndrome (p. 988) due to a chlamydia, occurs especially in people with HLA-B27, and tolerance or genetically-determined inability to respond to a particular microbial antigen remain as possibilities.

Antibacterial drug therapy

In many types of bacterial infection, antibiotic drugs are capable of killing the bacteria or suppressing their multiplication, and thus tip the balance in favour of the host and terminate the infection. Antibiotic therapy is not, however, without risk. Apart from their toxic side-effects and the induction of hypersensitivity reactions, antibiotics can, as already mentioned, encourage the multiplication of resistant strains of bacteria. Such resistance may be determined by orthodox genetic bacterial inheritance, but one form of resistance can be transmitted from resistant to susceptible bacteria by transfer of *plasmids* (extra-chromosomal genetic factors) from antibiotic-resistant bacteria. Antibiotic therapy has, in some circumstances, resulted in a great increase in the incidence of antibiotic-resistant infections, particularly among hospital patients, and this emphasises the importance of avoiding their indiscriminate use.

Diminished resistance to infection

There is a wide range of individual 'natural' resistance to microbial infections among apparently normal individuals. This is largely unexplained, but it is apparent that variations in susceptibility to some infections are related to the individual's 'transplant' iso-antigens (see above). In passing, it is worth noting that similar associations with HLA antigens have recently been claimed for many diverse diseases of obscure nature, e.g. disseminated sclerosis, the connective tissue diseases and lymphoid neoplasia. These observations may throw light on genetic factors in disease, and help to explain the nature of 'constitutional' predisposition and resistance.

Impaired resistance to infection can occur in many ways. Examples of defects in local barriers to invasion have been given earlier in this chapter. Normal phagocytic function, immune responsiveness and complement function are all essential factors contributing to the range of protective mechanisms. A serious fall in the number of polymorphs in the blood, as in agranulocytosis, predisposes to bacterial invasion and severe, spreading infections, e.g. of the pharynx and intestine, by both commensals and more highly pathogenic bacteria. Genetically-determined defects of polymorph function also predispose to bacterial infection. These polymorph abnormalities are considered in Chapter 17. There are also many diseases which impair specific immune responses; they include the rare congenital immunological deficiency states and also acquired diseases which involve the lymphoid tissues and affect their immunological functions (pp. 169–72).

In other diseases, predisposition to infection is well known but unexplained. A good example is diabetes mellitus, in which boils and urinary tract infections are common and there is a predisposition to tuberculosis: it may be that phagocytic activity, which requires the energy provided by glycolysis, is impaired by the defective carbohydrate metabolism of diabetes.

Two important reactions to infection are leukocytosis and fever, accounts of which follow.

Polymorphonuclear Leukocytosis

The number of neutrophil polymorphs in the blood, normally $2.5–7.5 \times 10^9$/litre in older children and adults, increases in various pathological conditions. The increase is a controlled reaction and when the cause subsides the leukocyte count returns to the normal level for that individual. This account deals with the causes and mechanisms of such a neutrophil leukocytosis and with the changes in the haemopoietic marrow responsible for increased leukocyte production. The proliferation of leukocytes in myeloid leukaemia is neoplastic rather than reactive and is described in Chapter 16.

Causes

Neutrophil leukocytosis occurs in association with acute inflammatory reactions, tissue necrosis, thrombosis, haemorrhage, acute lysis of red cells, and sometimes cancer. A mild polymorph leukocytosis occurs in pregnancy and also results from strenuous exercise, severe mental stress, and from injection of glucocorticoids, corticotrophin or adrenaline. By far the commonest cause in clinical medicine is inflammation due to bacterial infection, and in general the degree of leukocytosis correlates with the size of the inflammatory lesion and the intensity of polymorph emigration in the infected tissues. Pyogenic infections, due for example to virulent staphylococci, streptococci, pneumococci or coliform bacilli, are accompanied by a brisk leukocytosis, the height of which depends partly on the duration and partly on the extent of the infection. A boil or acute appendicitis may induce a moderate rise, e.g. to 10×10^9 polymorphs per litre, while a large abscess, acute bacterial pneumonia or general peritonitis are commonly accompanied by a count of $20 \times 10^9/l$ or more. In some severe infections with pyogenic bacteria, e.g. streptococcal septicaemia or pneumococcal pneumonia, there may be absence of leukocytosis, or even leukopenia, and this usually indicates overwhelming toxaemia and is a bad prognostic sign. In some severe infections, e.g. gas gangrene due to *Cl. welchii*, polymorph emigration is less intense, and the increase in polymorphs in the blood is less marked, while the acute inflammatory lesions of the intestine caused by the typhoid and paratyphoid bacilli are virtually devoid of polymorphs (Fig. 7.4) and there is actually a fall in the number of polymorphs in the blood. Many virus infections, particularly in the early stages, are also accompanied by a neutrophil leukopenia.

Necrosis of tissue, for example myocardial infarction, causes a slight or moderate neutrophil leukocytosis, and extensive thrombosis, e.g. in the leg veins, or severe haemorrhage, both have a similar effect.

Leukocytosis may develop within a few hours of the onset of a bacterial infection and is of diagnostic value. This early rise is due partly to release of many polymorphs which normally lie marginated in the venules of the lungs and elsewhere, and partly to release of polymorphs lying in the sinusoids of the haemopoietic marrow. Soon, however, there is an increased rate of formation of polymorphs in the marrow and the leukocytosis is thus maintained. It appears from recent observations that the life of the neutrophil polymorph in the

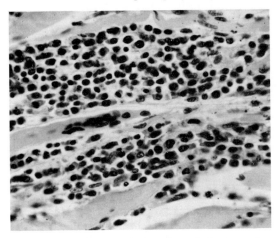

Fig. 7.4 Inflammatory infiltration of the muscular layer of the small intestine in typhoid fever, showing mononuclear cells and absence of polymorphs. × 150.

blood is probably not more than 12 hours, and since there are approximately 5 litres of blood containing about 4×10^9 polymorphs per litre, the normal daily production must be at least 4×10^{10}. In a suppurating infection, ten times this number may be lost daily for weeks or months in the pus discharging from an abscess, while at the same time the blood level may be maintained at 20×10^9/litre or more. It is thus apparent that the output of polymorphs is capable of enormous and sustained increase, and the process responsible for this is hyperplasia of the bone marrow, considered below.

Production of polymorphs (Granulopoiesis)

In the normal adult, production of the granulocyte or myeloid series of leukocytes is restricted to the haemopoietic marrow, where it occurs along with the production of red cells, platelets and monocytes. All these cells, and also lymphocytes (p. 118), originate from *haemopoietic stem cells*, which give rise to more stem cells and also to cells of more restricted potential: some are progenitors of red cells, others of megakaryocytes, while recent observations have demonstrated progenitor cells capable of giving rise to both polymorphs and monocytes (see below).

Because of their basic role in haemopoiesis, haemopoietic stem cells are dealt with in the chapter on blood (p. 504).

Stages of granulopoiesis. The earliest recognisable granulocyte precursor is termed a myeloblast: small numbers of these are present in normal haemopoietic marrow and they divide to give rise to a population of cells which undergo successive multiplications and form the largest cell population in the marrow. This proliferation is accompanied by a continuous process of differentiation up to the granulocyte stage: representative stages are illustrated in Fig. 7.5. Throughout the process the ratio of cytoplasm to nucleus increases and after initial enlargement up to the early myelocyte stage, diminution in size is a feature of differentiation. In the primitive stages the nucleus is large, ovoid or indented, and the chromatin is finely distributed. Gradually the nucleus shrinks, becoming more deeply staining, and eventually it becomes elongated giving the 'band form', followed by division into lobes, the number of which increases during the late stages of matur-

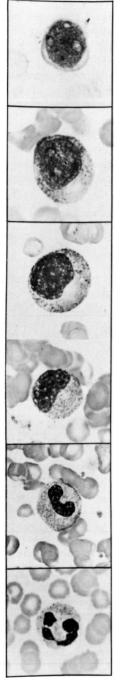

Myeloblast: non-granular (oxidase-negative), basophilic cytoplasm (rich in RNA); nucleus roughly spherical, with dispersed chromatin (euchromatin), and containing 2 or more nucleoli. 10–18 μm diameter.

Promyelocyte: a few primary (oxidase positive) cytoplasmic granules; basophilic cytoplasm; nucleus spherical, still with dispersed chromatin and nucleoli. 12–18 μm diameter.

Myelocytes: cytoplasm less basophilic; primary granules disappear and secondary granules develop—they are strongly oxidase-positive and specific (neutrophil, eosinophil or basophil). Nucleus spherical or ovoid with some condensation of chromatin (heterochromatin). Active mitosis occurs at this stage. 12–18 μm diameter.

Metamyelocyte: cytoplasm only faintly basophilic (poor in RNA), with many specific granules and no primitive granules. Nucleus becoming elongated, smaller and more condensed. 12–15 μm diameter.

Polymorphonuclear leukocyte: cytoplasm as in metamyelocytes; nucleus smaller, and chromatin more condensed, at first horse-shoe shaped, later lobulated. 10–15 μm diameter.

Fig. 7.5 Cells in haemopoietic marrow representing stages of granulopoiesis: from the myelocyte stage, only neutrophil cells are illustrated. Leishman stain × 1000. (Dr. R. Brooke Hogg.)

ation of the polymorph in the marrow and in the blood. In preparations stained by a Romanowsky dye (e.g. Leishman's, Wright's, Jenner's or Giemsa stains), the cytoplasmic changes are as described in Fig. 7.5: from the myelocyte stage, there is not sufficient RNA to impart strong basophilia, and the cytoplasm is pale blue. Lysosomal granules appear in the cytoplasm in the promyelocyte stage: at first they are large and stained reddish-blue, but in the myelocyte stage these early granules are gradually replaced by granules specific for neutrophil, eosinophil or basophil polymorphs. In the neutrophil myelocytes the granules are small and are stained reddish or purple: in the eosinophil they are larger and bright orange, while in the basophil they are large and dark blue. These characteristic granules persist in the three types of mature granulocytes or polymorphs. In an early neutrophil leukocytosis there is an increased proportion of young cells and even myelocytes may appear in the blood.

Leukocytosis is brought about by hyperplasia, (i.e. an increase in the number of cells), in the haemopoietic marrow, and the proportion of myeloid cells, and particularly of myelocytes, is increased. This is termed a *granulopoietic reaction* and is analogous to the erythroblastic reaction in response to an increased requirement of red cells, e.g. after haemorrhage. The fat cells normally present in haemopoietic (red) marrow diminish in number as the cellularity increases (Fig. 7.6) and also foci of haemopoietic tissue arising from stem cells appear in the yellow fatty marrow of the long bones. These foci extend rapidly and in a severe prolonged suppurating infection much of the yellow marrow in the shafts of the femur and other long bones may be replaced by red marrow, the change starting in the upper ends of the bones and extending downwards. All the cellular constituents of normal marrow are present in this newly formed haemopoietic tissue, but myelocytes and later forms predominate (Figs. 7.7, 7.8).

Factors controlling granulopoiesis. It has long been known that many substances promote a neutrophil leukocytosis when injected into animals: they include peptones, digestion products of nucleic acids, and metabolic products and extracts of bacteria. Such observations have not helped much in the elucidation of the mechanisms of leukocytosis, but investigations

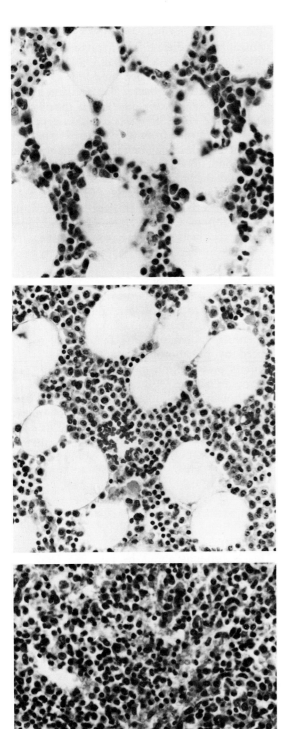

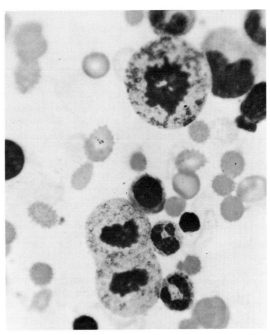

Fig. 7.7 Smear preparation of sternal marrow during a granulopoietic reaction. Note granular myelocytes in mitosis and various stages of transition to polymorphonuclear leukocytes. × 600.

involving the culture of marrow cells *in vitro* have proved more successful. When cultured in a suitable semi-solid medium, the growth of myeloid cells requires the presence of a factor **(colony stimulating activity or CSA)** which stimulates the proliferation of individual cells to form discrete colonies. At first, the proliferating cells are mainly or entirely granulocyte precursors, but as the numbers increase some of the cells differentiate into polymorphs and others into monocytes. Since such colonies are derived from single cells, this is good evidence of a common precursor of polymorphs and monocytes. CSA can be extracted from most tissues (including haemopoietic marrow) and is present in the serum and urine. It is now known to be produced by monocytes, macro-

Fig. 7.6 Sections of haemopoietic marrow illustrating hyperplasia associated with neutrophil leukocytosis. *Top*, normal marrow. *Middle*, marrow showing increased cellularity in a patient with leukocytosis of short duration. *Bottom*, marked hyperplasia of marrow in a patient with prolonged leukocytosis: the fat cells have been replaced by haemopoietic cells. × 315.

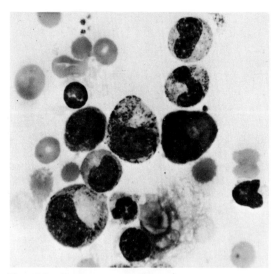

Fig. 7.8 Smear preparation of marrow showing finely granular myelocytes and transitions to polymorphonuclear leukocytes. × 1000.

phages, vascular endothelium and stimulated lymphocytes. Assay of CSA by its effect on marrow culture is difficult and complex. This is probably because it is produced by monocytes in the culture, and in heavily seeded cultures sufficient CSA is produced to promote colony formation. It now seems likely that local production of CSA in haemopoietic marrow is important in the physiological production of neutrophil polymorphs and monocytes. Mature neutrophils produce a factor (possibly lactoferrin) which inhibits leukopoiesis and thus provides a negative feedback mechanism. Shortly after an injection of bacterial endotoxin, a **polymorph releasing factor** appears in the plasma, and has the effect of releasing mature neutrophil polymorphs from the marrow sinusoids into the blood. It may be that, by thus reducing the production of the neutrophil inhibitory factor in the marrow, this allows hyperplasia with production and release of more granulocytes. Bacterial endotoxin also increases the production of CSA by monocytes in culture and *in vivo*, and so it may reduce the negative feedback in the marrow and also directly stimulate leukopoiesis.

Other factors of possible importance include a lipoprotein present in normal plasma which, when added to marrow cell cultures, is said to increase the production of monocytes at the expense of polymorphs. A factor is also produced by polymorphs in culture fluid which inhibits proliferation of early polymorph precursors in culture.

Although these observations promise considerable advances in our understanding of polymorph production, their relevance to natural neutrophil leukocytosis in man is still not known.

Pyrexia (Fever)

In this account, *pyrexia* and *fever* are used synonymously to mean a rise in the internal temperature of the body ('core temperature') to levels above the normal range. Traditionally, *fever* is also used in the nomenclature of various diseases (usually infections) in which pyrexia is a prominent feature, e.g. typhoid fever, yellow fever and cerebrospinal fever. Doubtless both these usages will continue.

Body temperature is controlled partly by reflexes initiated by the thermo-sensory nerve endings in the skin, and partly by a central control mechanism in the hypothalamus.

The peripheral reflex control mechanism can be demonstrated simply by observing a fall in the temperature of the skin of the left hand when the right hand is immersed in cold water. This is brought about by impulses from the cold receptors in the chilled skin (of the right hand) which stimulate sympathetic vasoconstrictor fibres supplying the skin and subcutaneous tissues in general. The result is a reduction in heat loss and maintenance (or even rise) of the core temperature. This experiment works when the blood flow through the right arm is arrested by a pressure cuff, and so is not dependent on the temperature of the blood reaching the hypothalamus. In experimental animals, the reflex can be elicited even when the spinal cord has been transected at a higher level, and so is not attributable to sensory impulses reaching the brain.

The central thermo-regulatory mechanism may, for practical purposes, be likened to a thermostat. The thermo-sensory centre, shown in animals to be in the anterior hypothalamus, responds to variations in the temperature of the blood flowing through it, and may be demonstrated experimentally by direct heating of the anterior hypothalamus, which results in a fall in the core temperature. Signals from the thermo-sensory centre influence the activity of other hypothalamic centres which regulate the physiological processes responsible for heat production and heat loss, thus controlling the core temperature. It is not known how the thermo-sensory centre responds to variations in local temperature. Experimental studies suggest that release of catecholamines and 5-hydroxy-tryptamine by nerve endings in the anterior hypothalamus are important in the control of temperature in extreme environmental conditions, and that there are marked species differences in the influence of these monoamines on body temperature. Under moderate environmental conditions, however, their depletion or inhibition does not seriously influence temperature control.

Fever accompanying infections and various other pathological conditions is attributable to a humoral effect on the hypothalamic thermo-sensory centre (analogous to the thermostat being set high). It is important to distinguish this from conditions in which the centre is functioning normally but, for various reasons, heat loss cannot keep pace with heat gain, and so the body temperature rises, e.g. during vigorous exercise in a hot, moist atmosphere.

Disturbances of the thermo-sensory centre

It has long been realised that injection of dead bacteria or bacterial products induces fever. A number of such products, termed **exogenous pyrogens**, have been detected in filtrates of cultures of various bacteria and fungi, but the *endotoxins* of Gram-negative bacteria have been most extensively investigated. On injection into rabbits, these phospholipid-polysaccharide-protein complexes or lipid A (p. 178) induce fever in about 1 hour, and this is followed by a refractory period in which further injections of endotoxin are ineffectual. Following injection of endotoxin or other exogenous pyrogen into rabbits, a second pyrogenic factor appears in the plasma; this causes fever in about 20 minutes following injection

into a second rabbit, and differs from endotoxin in being pyrogenic in rabbits rendered refractory to endotoxin. This second pyrogen, now called **endogenous** (or **leukocyte**) **pyrogen (EP)**, has also been detected in the plasma of animals in the early stages of febrile bacterial and viral infections. It is produced when suspensions of human or rabbit polymorphs or monocytes are stimulated by endotoxin or by readily phagocytosed material such as dead bacteria or antigen–antibody complexes, and when macrophages are activated by lymphocytes in delayed hypersensitivity reactions (p. 159). Synthesis of RNA and protein is necessary for EP production, which in polymorphs starts about 2 hours after stimulation: monocytes take longer but secrete much more EP than polymorphs, and the EPs produced by the two cell types differ in their molecular weights. Polymorphs and macrophages obtained from inflammatory exudates produce EP *spontaneously* when incubated in culture medium, indicating that they have been stimulated *in vivo*.

These various observations suggest that many of the agents capable of inducing fever act by stimulating production of EP. In addition to its production by human leukocytes *in vitro*, EP has been demonstrated in inflammatory exudates in man. Its detection in human plasma during infective fevers has proved difficult, but this is not surprising because fever can be induced in man by injection of amounts of EP too small to provide a detectable level in the recipient's plasma. EP has, however, been demonstrated in human plasma at the onset of a bout of malarial fever. Further investigations on EP would be greatly helped by a more sensitive method for its detection than that depending on production of fever in experimental animals.

The fever which accompanies tissue destruction, e.g. myocardial infarction, or necrotic tumours, is probably also mediated by EP released by phagocytes in the inflammatory reaction to the necrotic tissue, although it may be that tissue cells can also release pyrogens.

Effector mechanisms of fever (Fig. 7.9)

Although fever cannot be regarded as a physiological reaction, it is nevertheless brought about by stimulation of the physiological mech-

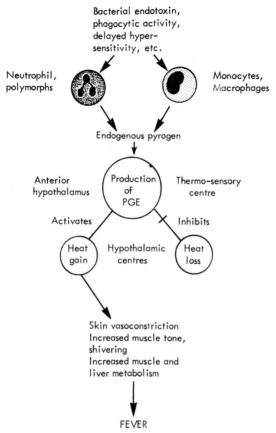

Bacterial endotoxin,
phagocytic activity,
delayed hyper-
sensitivity, etc.

Neutrophil,
polymorphs

Monocytes,
Macrophages

Endogenous pyrogen

Anterior
hypothalamus

Production
of
PGE

Thermo-sensory
centre

Activates

Inhibits

Heat
gain

Hypothalamic
centres

Heat
loss

Skin vasoconstriction
Increased muscle tone,
shivering
Increased muscle and
liver metabolism

FEVER

Fig. 7.9 The probable mechanism of fever in bacterial infections, etc.

anisms for heat production and inhibition of those responsible for heat loss. For example, the shivering which accompanies a sharp rise of temperature is the normal response to a cold environment, and is associated with increased catabolic activity and heat production in the skeletal muscles. The coldness and pallor of the skin at the onset of fever are due to cutaneous vasoconstriction and, together with 'gooseflesh' (contraction of the pilo-erector muscles) and inhibition of sweating, are part of the normal heat-saving reaction to cold. Heat production is also increased in fever, as it is in a cold climate, by increased metabolic activity, particularly in the skeletal muscles (see above) and liver. This is mediated in part by stimulation of the sympathetic system and increased catecholamine secretion, and eventually thyroid activity may increase. A high caloric diet is

necessary to provide the fuel needed to maintain the body at temperatures above normal, failing which catabolism of endogenous fat and protein increases, resulting in a negative nitrogen balance and, especially in children, keto-acidosis. These catabolic activities account for the wasting commonly seen in patients with prolonged fever,* and the metabolic status in fever is, in fact, closely similar to that following injury (p. 265): in both, a warm environment and a high caloric intake, including increased protein, are beneficial.

Not only is the 'thermostat set high' in fever, but it is unstable, so that the temperature commonly fluctuates, and is readily affected by environmental conditions. As described above, a rise of temperature is achieved by increasing heat production and reducing heat loss by physiological mechanisms. Conversely, a fall of temperature, either during or at the end of a fever, is accomplished by reduction in catabolism and by cutaneous vasodilatation and sweating. The skin is flushed, warm and moist, and the patient feels hot. During fever, the degree of increased metabolic activity, etc. will depend largely on the environmental conditions and, in a chilling environment, on the degree of insulation of the body by clothing.

Heat production and loss are regulated by centres in the posterior hypothalamus, including one which influences activity of the sympathetic system, and a second which appears to control muscle tone and induction of shivering. When injected into the anterior hypothalamus, EP induces fever within minutes. It now appears likely that EP does not act on the thermo-sensory centre directly, but by stimulating the production of prostagladins of the E series (PGE) in various parts of the brain, including the anterior hypothalamus. This view is supported by the following observations. (1) High levels of PGE are present in the cerebrospinal fluid during fever induced by endotoxin. (2) Injection of minute amounts of PGE_1 or E_2 induce fever in various species when injected directly into the anterior hypothalamus or third ventricle. (3) Aspirin-like drugs, which inhibit the synthesis of prostaglandins (p. 56) prevent the induction of fever by endotoxin (or by EP) but have no effect on fever induced by PGE. In the cat, PGE_2 is mainly involved, but other

---

* The old adage 'starve a fever; feed a cold' had little metabolic justification.

prostaglandins may be concerned in other species.

The role of prostaglandins explains the fever associated with induction of labour in pregnant women by an infusion of PGE_2; it would account also for the antipyretic effect of aspirin and similar drugs.

Cortisone is also antipyretic, but its inhibitory effect on production of EP by leukocytes stimulated by endotoxin, etc., probably accounts for this.

Effects of fever

The ill-effects of fever include general malaise, anorexia and increased catabolism. When the temperature rises to 41·6°C (107°F), there is a danger of direct thermal injury to various tissues, and particularly to cerebral neurones. In general, there is no evidence that fever has a beneficial effect, and its reduction by antipyretic drugs or by cooling the body does not seem to influence the course of infections. Apart from the spirochaete of syphilis and gonococcus (the cause of gonorrhoea), micro-organisms in culture do not appear to be adversely affected by moderate rises in temperature. The effects of fever on viruses are complex and require further investigation.

The spontaneous movement of neutrophil polymorphs *in vitro* and their response to a chemotactic stimulus are most rapid at 40°C (104°F), and fever may thus enhance the defensive role of these cells in infections.

Other causes of fever

Lesions of the hypothalamus may cause fever by interfering with the functioning of either the thermo-sensory centre or the hypothalamic areas which regulate heat loss and heat production. In experimental animals, injury of the anterior hypothalamus often causes pyrexia, while injury of the posterior hypothalamus may induce hypothermia. In man, haemorrhage in the pons is often accompanied by fever, and lesions between the hypothalamus and upper cervical cord interfere with tracts controlling heat loss and production, rendering the individual less able to respond to environmental temperature changes, etc.

Fever may occur in the absence of any disturbance of the thermo-sensory mechanism in conditions where the physiological mechanisms of heat loss cannot keep pace with heat production. This occurs in *thyrotoxicosis*, in which excess secretion of thyroid hormone stimulates general metabolism and physical activity and thus increases heat production. In normal subjects, vigorous exercise or a hot moist environment may both cause fever, and the combination is particularly likely to do so. Obviously, heat loss is influenced by the temperature and humidity of the atmosphere, air currents and insulation by clothing. These factors affect loss of heat by conduction, convection, radiation and evaporation, and also by the cooling effect of inspired air. Sweating is a major mechanism of heat loss, but is only effective if the sweat evaporates on the skin surface, thus extracting the latent heat of vaporisation. Excessive sweating may, however, cause dehydration and, if water is restored, salt deficiency. Also, marked cutaneous vasodilatation may impair the circulation. These various factors are associated in combinations which give rise to several clinical syndromes, the chief of which are as follows.

1. Heat exhaustion results from physical activity in a hot climate, particularly if the atmosphere is moist. Vasodilatation in the skin and skeletal muscles creates a relative oligaemia, i.e. the filling of the enlarged vascular bed reduces the return of blood to the right side of the heart, and so cardiac output falls. Literally, there is not enough blood to go round. The heart rate increases and the blood pressure falls, giving a fast weak pulse, dyspnoea and other signs of circulatory insufficiency. The skin is hot and damp, and the subject feels tired and becomes confused. Rest and restoration of fluid usually bring rapid improvement.

2. Dehydration exhaustion. When dehydration due to excessive sweating, reduced fluid intake, etc., accompanies heat exhaustion, all the features of circulatory failure are exaggerated by actual, in addition to relative, reduction in the blood volume. Dehydration in a hot dry climate is also increased by loss of fluid through the epidermis, which is not entirely impervious. The core temperature may be very high and collapse and sudden death may occur.

3. Heat stroke. In the two conditions mentioned above, heat-losing mechanisms operate, but are inadequate. In heat stroke, exercise in a hot environment, with consequent fever, leads in some way to a breakdown of the control mechanisms, so that the heat-losing mechanisms remain inactive, and the temperature continues to rise and may reach 43°C (109°F). At this temperature, brain injury is accompanied by coma and convulsions, and death or permanent brain injury results.

4. Heat cramps. Painful cramps in the muscles are the result of salt deficiency. This is liable to occur when there is excessive loss of water and salt by sweating and only the water is replaced.

5. Malignant hyperpyrexia. This is an unusual complication of general anaesthesia, usually with suxamethonium but also with other agents. During the anaesthesia, muscle tone increases and the temperature rises rapidly, often to above 42°C (107·5°F). Cyanosis, shock and keto-acidosis develop and death may occur from cardiac arrest unless the condition is recognised and treated. The underlying metabolic predisposition is not understood, but in some instances has been shown to run in families in which a raised level of plasma creatine phosphokinase has been reported.

Hypothermia

This may be defined as a fall in the core temperature of the body to below 35°C (95°F). It has no particular relevance to host–parasite relationships and is considered here simply because the processes involved in temperature control, described above in relation to fever, are equally important in hypothermia.

Hypothermia occurs when heat production fails to keep pace with heat loss. In robust adults, this occurs only in conditions of extreme heat loss, such as immersion in the sea or exposure on mountains. However, factors which interfere with heat production predispose to hypothermia in less rigorous environmental conditions. Because of their relatively large surface area and thin layer of insulating fat, infants, particularly if premature, are especially liable to it. Old people, especially women, living in cold surroundings on an inadequate diet, are particularly prone to develop hypothermia in winter. Predisposing diseases include hypothyroidism, generalised skin diseases, psychiatric disturbances and conditions which impair consciousness, metabolic or physical activity, e.g. alcoholism, narcotic drugs, paralysis, severe trauma and general states of disability.

Pathology. In general, metabolic processes decline rapidly below 33°C (91°F) and the cardiac output, blood pressure and respiratory rate fall. Fluid leaks from the microvessels with consequent haemoconcentration and increased blood viscosity. Blood flow to the tissues is further impaired by peripheral vasoconstriction; hypoxia and CO_2 retention increase and a combination of respiratory and metabolic acidosis develops. Below 25°C (77°F), the thermoregulatory mechanism ceases to function, and death results from cardiac arrest.

The changes found at necropsy include venous thrombosis, multiple small infarcts in various organs, pulmonary haemorrhages and bronchopneumonia. Acute pancreatitis is a common complication in patients who survive.

Induction of hypothermia to reduce the metabolic requirements of the brain and other organs was formerly practised in surgical procedures involving interruption of the circulation, but it carries a risk of ventricular fibrillation and is now used only occasionally in association with a pump to maintain the circulation.

Further Reading

Mims, C. A. (1976). *The Pathogenesis of Infectious Disease*, pp. 246. Academic Press, London and New York; Grune and Stratton, New York.

See also bibliography for Chapter 8 (pp. 224–5).

8

Types of Infection

Within living memory, infective disease was the major cause of death throughout the world, and the elimination or reduction in the incidence of most of the important infections largely accounts for the greatly increased lifespan in technologically advanced communities. Many factors have contributed to this decline of serious infections: they include improved standards of community and personal hygiene, better nutrition and housing, prophylactic immunisation and antimicrobial therapeutic agents.

In spite of these great triumphs, infective disease is still of considerable importance: it remains the major cause of death in many tropical and subtropical countries where, in addition to bacterial and viral infections, protozoal and metazoal parasites account for a great deal of illness. Even in countries where infections have been greatly reduced, many problems remain. The common cold is as common as ever, and upper respiratory virus infections are the major cause of absenteeism from school, office and factory. The rise in the volume and speed of world travel has increased greatly the risk of epidemics of influenza, cholera, etc. Even antibiotics have not proved an unmixed blessing, for their use has resulted in the spread of resistant pathogenic bacteria, particularly in hospitals. There are, moreover, a number of important diseases which may eventually prove to be due to infections, for example rheumatoid arthritis, multiple sclerosis, ulcerative colitis and sarcoidosis. Virus infections may also prove to be important causal factors of the lymphoid neoplasms, including Burkitt's lymphoma and lymphatic leukaemia, and of other forms of cancer.

This chapter gives a brief account of the various types of infection and describes some of the more important examples. As with other forms of disease, the effects of infection depend not only on the nature of the lesion, but also on its site in the body, and for this reason the special features of infection of the lungs, kidneys, brain, etc., are described in the appropriate systematic chapters.

Virus Infections

Of all the pathogenic organisms which affect man, viruses show the most extreme degree of parasitism. In the extracellular state viruses are metabolically inert and depend absolutely on the metabolism of the host cell for their replication. Basically, all viruses consist of a protein shell or **capsid** surrounding and protecting the nucleic acid—which may be either DNA or RNA. The **virion** or complete infectious particle of some viruses has an additional outer layer, or **envelope**, partially derived from the plasma membrane of the host cell. When a virus enters a susceptible host cell, the nucleic acid is released from the capsid and becomes functionally active: it is either transcribed into messenger RNA, or acts itself as messenger RNA, which re-directs the synthetic pathways of the host cell to manufacture components for new virus particles. This involves the replication of nucleic acid molecules and the production of proteins which include both the nonstructural proteins (e.g. enzymes) necessary for viral replicative processes and also the structural proteins which become incorporated in the capsid of new virus particles.

Apart from those viruses which enter the

host by the bite of an insect (e.g. yellow fever), or in the case of rabies virus by the bite of an animal, all parasitic viruses must enter the body by invading the surface epithelial cells of some part of the body. In many instances the site of initial infection is in the respiratory or alimentary tracts.

In man, most virus infections are mild and are followed by complete recovery. Many infections are entirely symptomless and immunity to reinfection is acquired without serious disturbance at the time of primary infection. Although latent infection with virus may continue for months or occasionally even for years, viruses do not form a non-invasive flora in the way that some bacteria do. A few virus infections, such as smallpox, regularly cause serious disease and even viruses such as *herpes simplex* or the enteroviruses, which generally cause mild or symptomless infection, may occasionally give rise to severe disease in an unusually susceptible host (Fig. 21.40, p. 756). Viral infections, especially of the respiratory tract, are extremely common in the community and are, in general, more frequent in childhood than in adult life.

Viruses are structurally simple parasites and do not produce disease by the elaboration of toxins as bacteria do. Lesions in viral infections are due to direct invasion of body tissues with subsequent cell damage due to the effect of viral replication in the host cells. In most clinically-apparent virus infections, replication of the virus is accompanied by death of the infected cell (Fig. 8.1). Some viruses induce fusion between infected and adjacent non-infected cells, with the formation of multinucleated giant cells, for example the Warthin–Finkeldey cell of measles (Fig. 18.8, p. 572). Such giant cells usually die, at least in tissue culture preparations, but their formation may be important in allowing virus to spread without entering the surrounding medium. There is increasing evidence that the immune response of the host may sometimes play an important role in causing lesions—for example in the development of bronchiolitis due to respiratory syncytial virus, which may be at least partly due to a hypersensitivity reaction in the lungs of the host. In arbovirus encephalitis, it has been postulated on the basis of some results of animal experiments that the lesions may be due to virus–antibody complexes inducing a type 3 hypersensitivity reaction rather than to the

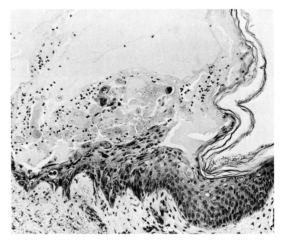

Fig. 8.1 Part of a vesicular skin lesion in varicella, illustrating virus-induced cell injury. The virus has replicated in the epidermal cells, resulting in cell death. The resulting epidermal defect has then become distended with inflammatory exudate, forming the vesicle. Note the swelling and hyperchromatic nuclei of the colonised epidermal cells, lying free in the vesicle and in the underlying epidermis. × 96. (The late Professor J. A. Milne.)

direct effect of the virus on the cells of the brain.

Unlike some bacterial infections, *virus diseases are not usually accompanied by a polymorphonuclear leukocytosis, but a lymphocytosis is common.* Most are associated with fever, and rash and lymphadenopathy are quite commonly seen. In the acute phase of virus infection a protein, **interferon**, can be detected in the blood and tissues. Interferon is released from cells in response to virus infection and when taken up by other cells makes them refractory to virus infection. Although the production of interferon is induced by virus, the protein itself is a species-specific cellular protein. It is not virus-specific in its antiviral effect but inhibits virtually all viruses. *Interferon production is an important host defence mechanism against virus infection and is probably the major factor in bringing about recovery from acute virus infections.* Although specific neutralising antibody is responsible for immunity to re-infection, it begins to appear in the bloodstream only when the acute infection is subsiding. It is notable that infants with immunological deficiencies resulting in impairment of T-lymphocyte function (p. 170 *et seq.*) are prone to develop chronic progressive vaccinia (vaccinia gangrenosa) following vaccination, and chronic infection with measles virus has also been reported. This provides evidence that cell-mediated immunity plays an important role in limiting viral lesions in normal individuals.

Distribution of lesions in virus infections

In some instances, the main lesion is at the site of the initial infection. For example, the virus responsible for influenza gives rise to a localised infection which spreads rapidly throughout the epithelial lining of the larger air passages of the respiratory tract. This results in epithelial necrosis of varying extent, and the cell injury and loss results in acute inflammatory oedema, which is the major clinical feature of influenza. The severity of the illness depends on the extent of epithelial necrosis, but secondary bacterial infection of the damaged mucosa is also of importance, especially in major epidemics. Influenza virus may enter the bloodstream, but appears unable to replicate successfully in the cells of other tissues. Other examples of virus infections which remain localised, and produce lesions mostly at the site of initial infection, are molluscum contagiosum (p. 1054) and the common cold.

In many other instances, the initial infection is clinically silent, but the virus invades various other tissues and organs and produces characteristic lesions in them. Thus in varicella the initial infection is probably in the respiratory tract. From there the virus spreads widely, invading the blood (viraemia) and many other tissues and organs. The characteristic vesicular lesions in the skin are due to invasion of the epidermal cells, and are one manifestation of the systemic infection. Suppuration of the skin lesions (pustulation) is due to secondary bacterial infection. The childhood fevers, e.g. measles, mumps, rubella (and also smallpox) are other examples of generalised virus diseases which follow initial infection *via* the respiratory tract.

Because of the mode of virus spread in varicella, the incubation period between initial infection and appearance of symptoms is about 14 days, and it may be even longer in some other exanthemas, e.g. measles and mumps. *Poliovirus* also spreads in a complex fashion within the body: following ingestion of the virus, there is an initial infection of the Peyer's patches in the small intestine. The virus then spreads to the regional lymph nodes, and in some instances produces viraemia. In a few individuals (e.g. about 1 per cent of those infected with poliovirus type 1) the organism invades the anterior horn cells of the spinal cord (Figs. 21.44 and 21.45, p. 759), causing paralytic poliomyelitis. The intestinal infection is clinically silent, but it nevertheless results in the development of antibody in the blood and in the appearance of IgA antibody in the gastrointestinal tract (p. 175): immunity is thus provided against subsequent infection with the same type of poliovirus.

Persistent virus infections are known to occur in man. Herpes simplex virus, for example, remains latent within the trigeminal ganglion but becomes activated from time to time, e.g. during pneumonia or other febrile illness, to produce vesicles around the mouth. Varicella virus also commonly remains latent, and may subsequently become active and replicate within the cells of the dorsal root ganglia to produce an attack of zoster (Fig. 21.43, p. 757).

There is considerable interest at present in **slow virus infections**, which may be defined as virus diseases having a long incubation period, in some instances years, and a prolonged and progressive course. Such diseases have been demonstrated to occur in certain animals, e.g. Aleutian disease of the mink, and it seems very likely that kuru (p. 761) and Creutzfeldt–Jakob disease are examples in man. The agent of scrapie, a widespread chronic disease of sheep, is most unusual in its remarkable resistance to heat and viricidal chemicals.

Active immunity can readily be produced by the administration of attenuated viruses, e.g. Sabin poliovirus vaccine, measles and yellow fever vaccines, and also—although somewhat less effectively—by inactivated viruses, e.g. influenza and rabies vaccines. Naturally-acquired immunity after virus infection is generally lifelong and is due to the development in the blood of antibodies which neutralise the infectivity of viruses. However, in a few virus diseases, reinfections or repeated infections are common. This may be due to the existence of numerous serologically distinct strains of virus, e.g. the common cold, or to the virus undergoing antigenic variation, e.g. influenza. In the case of certain viruses, and especially herpes simplex and varicella-zoster viruses, reactivation of virus in the tissues despite the presence of circulating antibody is not uncommon. The recurrences of infection are probably due to the ability of these viruses to remain latent within cells and to spread on re-activation directly through cell walls to infect neighbouring cells. The presence of antibodies in people who have experienced a virus infection can be demonstrated by various *in-vitro* tests such as complement fixation, haemagglutination-inhibition and neutralisation tests.

The possible role of virus infections in neoplasia is considered in Chapter 11.

Acute Bacterial Infections

The several processes which constitute the acute inflammatory reaction have been described in Chapter 3. They are basically the same in all acute inflammatory reactions, including those due to bacterial infections, but they differ in detail depending on the properties of the causal agent and the special features of the tissue involved. In some lesions, for example, inflammatory oedema may be unusually severe, while in others emigration of polymorphs or fibrin deposition may be predominant. In consequence of these variations, some acute inflammatory lesions, usually due to infections, present sufficiently characteristic appearances to warrant the use of the following descriptive terms.

Catarrhal inflammation. Acute inflammation of a mucous membrane is accompanied by glandular secretion, usually of thin watery fluid. Injury to the surface epithelium, together with inflammatory exudation from the superficial underlying vessels, results in detachment of the epithelial cells, either singly or in sheets (Fig. 8.2), and the detached cells are carried away in the mixture of secretion and exudate. When the infection subsides, the epithelium is quickly restored by proliferation of surviving cells, although prolonged or recurrent catarrhal infections may result in formation of granulation tissue and eventually fibrosis, and alteration of the epithelium to a less specialised or sometimes to squamous type.

The best known example of acute catarrhal inflammation—the common cold or coryza—is initiated by virus infection of the nasal mucosa, but various pathogenic bacteria multiply on the inflamed mucosa and aggravate the inflammatory reaction. The mixture of secretion and exudate then becomes increasingly viscid and turbid due to emigration of increasing numbers of polymorphs until it may consist of

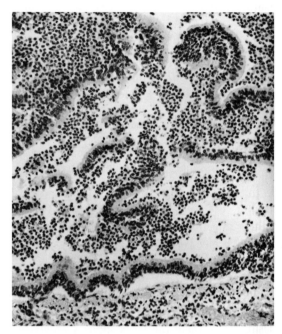

Fig. 8.2 Wall of bronchus in acute inflammation, showing desquamation of epithelium and polymorphonuclear leukocytic infiltration. × 250.

a mixture of mucus and pus: the inflammation, initially catarrhal, thus becomes *muco-purulent*. Catarrhal bronchitis (Fig. 8.2) is seen in mild influenza and, as in the common cold, the initial virus infection is often complicated by bacterial infections, with similar effects. Bacterial infection also induces catarrhal inflammation, for example of the colon in bacillary dysentery of moderate severity, and chemically-induced inflammation, such as that induced by inhalation of formalin or other irritating gases or vapours, may also be catarrhal.

Pseudo-membranous inflammation. This is usually due to bacteria which have a low invasive capacity but grow on the surface of a mucous membrane and produce exotoxins which cause superficial necrosis and acute inflammation of the underlying tissue. As the exudate passes to the surface, the fibrinogen in it clots within the necrotic surface layer. The fibrin and dead tissue together form the *false (pseudo-) membrane*, which contains also the causal bacteria, polymorphs and erythrocytes. Eventually the digestive activity of polymorph enzymes at the junction of living and dead tissue results in loosening and detachment of the pseudo-membrane; when the micro-organisms are destroyed, healing occurs, sometimes with some scarring. Examples of this type of inflammation are provided by diphtheria, usually affecting the pharynx or larynx (Fig. 8.3), and in the colon the more severe examples of bacillary dysentery.

Serous inflammation. This consists of acute inflammation in which there is copious fluid exudation but emigration of leukocytes and escape of red cells are minimal. The tissues become grossly oedematous and when the

lining membrane of a body cavity, e.g. the pleura, is involved, the 'serous' exudate accumulates in the cavity. Serous inflammation is seen in the early stages of many acute bacterial infections, and particularly in infection by *Clostridium oedematiens*, one of the causal organisms of gas gangrene.

The terms **fibrinous** and **haemorrhagic** are also applied to inflammation, to indicate respectively marked fibrin deposition and escape of red cells.

Two important variants of acute bacterial infections with special features—**pyogenic infections** and **gas gangrene**—are described below.

Pyogenic infections: suppuration

In many acute bacterial infections, emigration of polymorphs is intense, and these cells accumulate in huge numbers in the inflamed tissues. If, as commonly happens, tissue necrosis also occurs, then the dead tissue is digested and a cavity is formed which contains polymorph-rich (**purulent**) exudate, or **pus** (Figs. 8.4, 8.5). Such a cavity is called an **abscess** and the process of abscess formation is termed **suppuration**. The adjective **pyogenic** is applied to bacteria which cause suppuration. Pyogenic bacterial infection of a natural body cavity, such as a joint, the peritoneum or subarachnoid space, results in accumulation of pus in the cavity without the necessity for tissue necrosis and digestion.

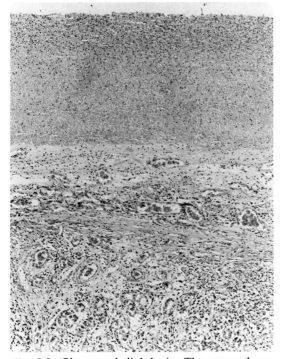

Fig. 8.3 Pharyngeal diphtheria. The mucosal surface (top) is coated with a false membrane composed of dead epithelium and fibrinous exudate. The underlying connective tissue shows acute inflammatory congestion. × 85.

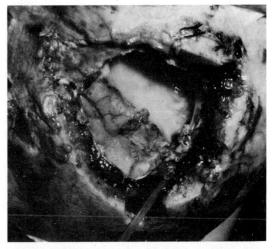

Fig. 8.4 Abscess of brain. Part of the skull has been removed surgically and a cavity containing pus is seen in the brain. (Photographed at necropsy.)

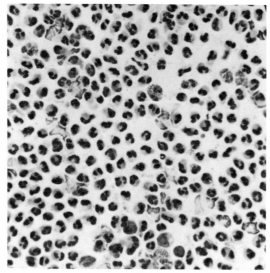

Fig. 8.5   Smear of pus. Most of the cells are neutrophil polymorphs: some are undergoing autolysis. × 400.

Suppuration

Initially, a pyogenic bacterial infection shows the usual features of acute inflammation: as it progresses, local bacterial spread results in enlargement of the lesion, and unless the bacteria are destroyed rapidly, the tissue in the centre of the lesion undergoes necrosis. This is probably due mainly to the high concentrations of powerful toxins produced by pyogenic bacteria, but the pressure of inflammatory oedema, slowing of the blood flow, and sometimes thrombosis due to endothelial injury may also be important. The central necrotic tissue becomes infiltrated with polymorphs from the surrounding inflamed tissue, and during the process of phagocytosis and subsequent degeneration, these cells release lysosomal enzymes which digest the dead cells and tissue framework. Gradually a space, or abscess cavity, is formed containing fluid exudate rich in polymorphs, fragments of necrotic tissue, sometimes fibrin clots (from fibrinogen in the exudate), red cells and, of course, bacteria.

Necrosis of tissue and abscess formation favour multiplication of the causal bacteria. In acutely inflamed tissue, the continuous flow of exudate from small blood vessels into the tissue spaces and its removal by lymphatics is important in host defence (p. 62). In an abscess, however, the exudate is relatively stagnant: some fluid can exude into the space from the surrounding inflamed tissue, but lymphatic drainage is inadequate. The intense migration of polymorphs into the abscess cavity also increases its contents, and in consequence the hydrostatic pressure in the cavity rises. The stagnant exudate in the abscess is a suitable growth medium for most pyogenic bacteria, and so they multiply and produce toxins which, by devitalisation of the surrounding living tissue, result in extension of the necrosis and enlargement of the abscess. Because of its raised pressure, the pus in an abscess tends to extend along tissue planes of least mechanical resistance; if present, for example, in the kidney, it may extend radially within and around the tubules, and may also burst through the capsule and spread extensively in the loose perinephric fatty tissue. An abscess forming near the skin, a mucous membrane or a serosal cavity, tends to extend towards the surface and rupture, discharging its pus.

If the growth of bacteria is checked, either by the natural defence mechanisms alone or with the help of antimicrobial drugs, the abscess stops enlarging, and becomes enclosed in a layer of granulation tissue (the *pyogenic membrane*) which grows from the surrounding inflamed tissue. Commonly, bacteria persist in the pus for a long time and the granulation tissue extends inwards while its outer part gradually matures to fibrous tissue. A long-standing abscess thus becomes enclosed in dense scar tissue which progressively thickens and, as long as the bacteria persist, is lined on its inner side by a layer of granulation tissue showing the changes of acute inflammation (Fig. 8.6). In the innermost granulation tissue, emigration of polymorphs may be conspicuous, while further out there may be plasma cells, lymphocytes and macrophages.

Extension of an abscess is accompanied by increase in toxaemia, fever and neutrophil leukocytosis, and rupture into a serosal cavity may result in extensive infection, e.g. generalised peritonitis or pleurisy. This is sometimes prevented, however, for as the abscess extends towards the cavity, fibrin in the inflammatory exudate glues adjacent viscera to the inflamed serosa, and by the time the abscess reaches the surface, that part of the cavity may be walled off. When an abscess ruptures through the skin or into the alimentary tract, the pus discharges

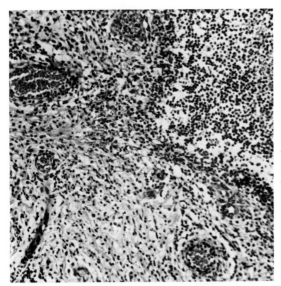

Fig. 8.6 Wall of an abscess. The abscess cavity is seen at the top right. The wall consists of vascular granulation tissue showing an inflammatory reaction. × 120.

and the release of pressure allows free flow of exudate from the surrounding tissue into the abscess cavity: this favours elimination of the bacteria, not only by their removal in the discharging exudate, but also by the protective mechanisms afforded by a free flow of exudate (p. 62). Accordingly, surgical incision and drainage of an abscess is an important therapeutic measure: by promoting bacterial elimination and destruction, it allows the abscess cavity to heal with minimal scarring. The pressure in an abscess is well illustrated by the spurting out of pus when it is incised, but needs no emphasis for anyone who has experienced the throbbing pain of an apical tooth abscess.

Abscesses which are not drained, and which do not discharge naturally, may persist for months or even years and become surrounded by dense scar tissue. The bacteria may eventually be destroyed, and if the cavity is still small it may be gradually filled by granulation and eventually scar tissue. The pus in larger abscess cavities may be slowly transformed to clear fluid as the cell debris, etc. is removed by macrophages, leaving a cyst-like cavity which cannot collapse because of the surrounding rigid fibrous tissue. Occasionally the pus becomes inspissated to a solid, lipid-rich crumbly material, and deposition of calcium salts converts this into a stony hard mass which

may finally be replaced by bone. Even when an abscess is drained or discharges naturally, bacteria may persist in the cavity and drainage track, particularly if sufficient fibrosis has occurred to prevent its collapse.

Perhaps the commonest example of an abscess is a **boil (furuncle)**. It occurs most often in the dense dermal connective tissue at the back of the neck. The causal organism, *Staphylococcus aureus*, invades *via* the hair follicles or sebaceous ducts and sets up an acute inflammatory swelling. It spreads locally in the dermis, and necrosis of a patch of skin at the centre of the lesion results from toxic action and the vascular factors outlined above: polymorphs migrate from the surrounding inflamed tissue and digest the periphery of the necrotic 'core', which thus becomes separated from the lining tissue by a layer of pus. When separation is complete, the core is discharged, leaving an ulcer (Fig. 8.7). This is usually followed by elimination of the staphylococci, and the ulcer heals, leaving a pitted scar. In some instances, particularly in individuals with impaired resistance to infection, e.g. untreated diabetics, the infection may spread extensively in the dermal and underlying soft tissue of the neck, giving rise to a **carbuncle** consisting of a complex loculated abscess, or several separate abscesses, with multiple discharging sinuses (Fig. 8.8).

Suppuration in a serous cavity presents the same general features as an abscess developing in a solid tissue, and the principles of treatment are the same.

Composition of pus. As indicated above, pus consists of an accumulation of inflammatory exudate containing very large numbers of neutrophil polymorphs which give it an opaque appearance. Many of the polymorphs in recently formed pus are living, but the life of polymorphs which have emigrated is probably 12 hours or less, and in old pus most of the cells are dead and in various stages of degeneration and digestion. Release of DNA from these cells accounts for the sticky, slimy nature of pus. Some red cells are usually present, particularly in newly formed pus, and also fragments of tissue debris: fibrin may be present as free fragments, or may form a layer lining the wall of the cavity. In old pus, the number of macrophages increases and cholesterol crystals and globules of fat, derived

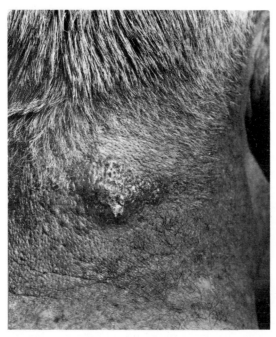 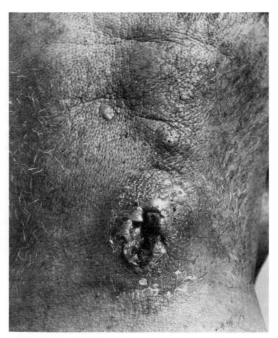

Fig. 8.7 Furuncle ('boil'). *Left*, the centre of the lesion is necrotic and about to be discharged. *Right*, the necrotic core has been discharged, leaving a ragged ulcer. × 1. (The late Professor J. A. Milne.)

from degenerated cells and perhaps from blood lipids, gradually accumulate.

Bacterial infection of the blood

It is customary to classify the presence of bacteria in the blood into **bacteraemia**, **septicaemia** and **pyaemia**. The distinction between the three is not sharp, but they are none the less useful terms. In bacteraemia, bacteria are present in the blood in relatively small numbers but do not multiply significantly. Septicaemia and pyaemia are much more serious conditions in which bacteria, usually of high pathogenicity, multiply in the blood.

Only very rarely are bacteria present in the blood in sufficient numbers to be detected by direct microscopy, culture of the blood being necessary for their detection.

Bacteraemia. Small numbers of bacteria of low virulence are present from time to time in the blood of normal subjects, or in individuals with minor, often subclinical lesions. *Streptococcus viridans* may be cultured from the blood after vigorous brushing of the teeth, particularly if there is dental sepsis, and it is likely that occasional intestinal bacteria enter the portal circulation. Because of its high content

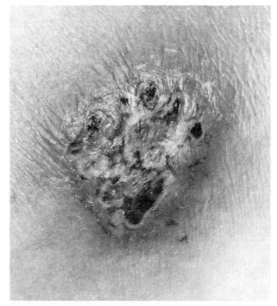

Fig. 8.8 Carbuncle: the foci of suppuration have extended to the overlying skin and discharged pus at several places. × 1. (The late Professor J. A. Milne.)

of antibodies and complement, and the large numbers of circulating phagocytes and sinus-lining macrophages in the liver, spleen, etc., the blood is a hostile environment to most micro-organisms, and although bacteria may multiply in local infections, those entering the blood are usually destroyed rapidly. Even in more serious and extensive localised infections, such as pneumococcal pneumonia or *Escherichia coli* infections of the urinary tract, bacteria can sometimes be detected by blood culture, but usually they fail to multiply significantly in the blood and disappear from it when, or even before, the local infection subsides. This applies also to the bacteria which enter the blood-stream as a regular feature of certain diseases, for example typhoid fever and brucellosis (undulant fever).

Bacteraemia is of some importance, for whenever they enter the blood, bacteria may settle in various parts of the body and cause lesions, for example suppurative meningitis or arthritis in pneumococcal pneumonia, and periostitis due to *Salmonella typhi* in typhoid fever.

Septicaemia means the presence and multiplication of bacteria in the blood, and is applied especially to the rapid multiplication of highly pathogenic bacteria, e.g. the pyogenic cocci or the plague bacillus, *Yersinia pestis*. The term thus implies a serious infection with profound toxaemia, in which the bacteria have overwhelmed the host defences.

In some instances it is difficult to distinguish between bacteraemia and septicaemia. For example, *Escherichia coli* causes infection of the peritoneal cavity, urinary and genital tracts: blood infection may occur, particularly as a complication of generalised peritonitis, but it is often not clear whether the bacteria are multiplying in the blood or are continuously entering it, e.g. from the infected peritoneum.

Multiple small haemorrhages may occur in septicaemia (Fig. 21.27, p. 747), due either to capillary endothelial damage from the severe toxaemia or to multiple minute metastatic foci of bacterial growth. The number of neutrophil polymorphs in the blood may be raised, although in overwhelmingly severe septicaemia they may be diminished and show toxic granulation (p. 512). The spleen is often enlarged and congested, and may contain large numbers of polymorphs. If the septicaemia is not rapidly fatal, foci of suppuration may develop in various parts of the body as a result of local invasion by blood-bourne bacteria.

Pyaemia. In localised pyogenic infections, toxic injury to the endothelium of veins in-

volved in the lesion may result in thrombosis: bacteria multiply in the thrombus, which then becomes heavily infiltrated by polymorphs and broken down by their digestive enzymes. Small fragments of the softened septic thrombus may then break away and be carried off in the blood (**pyaemia**—literally, pus in the blood). Where they become impacted in small vessels, they cause local injury both by obstructing the vessels and by the release of toxins from their contained bacteria: a combination of necrosis, haemorrhage and suppuration results, with formation of multiple **pyaemic abscesses** in the various tissues, their distribution depending on the site of the original septic thrombosis. Pyaemic abscesses are typically surrounded by a zone of haemorrhage (Fig. 8.9). Microscopy of an early lesion may show a central zone of necrosis often containing huge numbers of bacteria (Fig. 8.10); this is surrounded by a zone of suppuration and an outermost zone of acutely inflamed, often haemorrhagic tissue. As the lesions progress, the necrotic tissue is digested, and apart from their multiplicity and widespread distribution, they become indistinguishable from non-haematogenous abscesses. In septic thrombosis of major veins, larger fragments may be released into the circulation, and

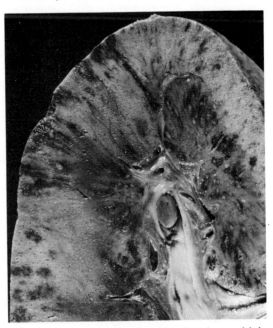

Fig. 8.9 The kidney in pyaemia, showing multiple small abscesses which are seen as pale areas surrounded by dark haemorrhagic zones.

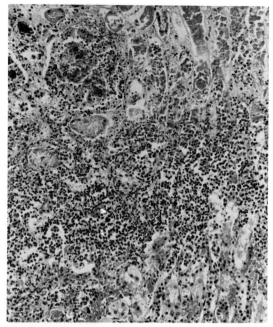

Fig. 8.10 Pyaemic abscess of kidney in a case of staphylococcal pyaemia. Infarcted tissue (*above*) is separated from congested living tissue (*below*) by a zone of suppuration. The dark patches in a glomerulus are masses of staphylococci, and have probably increased after death. × 65.

by impacting in arteries give rise to correspondingly larger foci of necrosis and suppuration (**septic infarcts**).

Septic thrombosis of systemic veins results especially, but not exclusively, in pyaemic abscesses in the lungs, while septic thrombosis in pulmonary veins results in pyaemic abscesses mainly in the systemic arterial distribution. In acute bacterial endocarditis, in which septic thrombus forms on the infected valve cusps, the distribution of pyaemic lesions depends on the particular heart valves involved. Septic thrombus of a portal venous tributary, e.g. in acute appendicitis, gives rise to **portal pyaemia**, with abscesses mainly in the liver.

Inevitably, bacteria are released from septic thrombus in pyaemia, and frank septicaemia commonly supervenes.

Septicaemia and pyaemia were formerly most often due to the pyogenic cocci. The incidence has, however, been greatly reduced by antibiotic therapy, and bacterial infections which are less readily eliminated by antibiotics have increased in relative importance, *Escherichia coli* now being the commonest cause of blood infections in general hospital practice. In states of lowered resistance to bacterial infection, e.g. agranulocytosis, immunodeficiencies and therapeutic immunosuppression, blood infection is a particular hazard. Because of impaired defence mechanisms, bacteria normally of relatively low resistance may cause septicaemia and pyaemia in these conditions.

The common pyogenic bacteria

Pyogenic infections in man are most commonly caused by *Staphylococcus aureus* and *Streptococcus pyogenes*. *Staphylococcus aureus* is the usual cause of boils, carbuncles and septic lesions of the fingers: the infection usually remains localised, although suppurating lymphadenitis may occur in the local nodes, and unless treatment is effective, septicaemia and pyaemia may occur. Some types of *Staph. aureus* are resistant to penicillin and sometimes to other antibiotics. Symptomless nasopharyngeal carriers of resistant types are commonly responsible for outbreaks of infection of surgical wounds, burns, etc., in hospital: phage typing has proved of great value in tracing the source of such outbreaks. Staphylococci are also a cause of pneumonia complicating influenza and other virus infections of the respiratory tract, and may produce a fulminating enteritis in patients receiving broad-spectrum antibiotics. The staphylococcal lesion shows the usual features of acute inflammation, and unless checked by antibiotic therapy it frequently progresses to suppuration and discharges a thick creamy pus.

Streptococcus pyogenes commonly produces acute pharyngitis and tonsillitis, 'septic fingers', otitis media and mastoiditis, also extensive inflammation of the subcutaneous connective tissues (*cellulitis*), and *erysipelas*, a spreading infection of the dermis producing a raised, red, painful lesion of the skin, usually of the face, with a well-defined margin. Before the introduction of antiseptics, *Strep pyogenes* was a very common and important cause of fatal peritonitis or septicaemia arising from infection of the genital tract following childbirth. It can also cause fatal septicaemia resulting from a minor injury, e.g. a finger prick sustained by the surgeon or pathologist dealing with a streptococcal infection.

The differences between infections due to

staphylococci and streptococci are partly explicable by their toxins (p. 177). Staphylococcal infections show a greater tendency to remain localised, possibly due in part to the production of staphylocoagulase which clots fibrinogen, producing a deposit of fibrin which may help to limit spread of the organisms and promote their phagocytosis. Streptococcal lesions tend to spread, possibly due partly to the production of hyaluronidase, which digests hyaluronic acid and thus liquefies the ground substance of connective tissues. *Streptococcus pyogenes* also produces fibrinolysins, and leukocidins which kill polymorphs.

Other pyogenic bacteria include *Strep. pneumoniae* (the common cause of lobar pneumonia) which may be complicated by metastatic blood-borne lesions, e.g. suppurative meningitis or arthritis; *Neisseria meningitidis* (meningococcus) which invades the nasopharynx, often silently, and produces a septicaemia or bacteraemia with the subsequent development of meningitis; *Neisseria gonorrhoeae* (gonococcus), transmitted by coitus and producing an acute urethritis, etc.

The intestinal commensals are important causes of pyogenic infections in the abdomen, e.g. appendicitis, diverticulitis and peritonitis, and in the lungs; they also infect surgical and other wounds, bedsores, burns and ulcers of the skin. They include *Escherichia coli*, *Bacteroides*, anaerobic streptococci, *Proteus*, *Pseudomonas pyocyanea* and *Klebsiella*, and may cause infections singly and in various combinations. These organisms are of particular importance in debilitated and immunosuppressed patients. All of them, but especially *Esch. coli* and *Bacterioides*, give rise to septicaemia and pyaemia, with severe septic shock (p. 264).

Gangrene

Definition. The term gangrene means digestion of dead tissue by saprophytic bacteria, i.e. bacteria which are incapable of invading and multiplying in living tissues. Many types of bacteria, often present in various combinations, may participate, and breakdown of tissue proteins, carbohydrates and fat may result in simple end-products: volatile products and gases may be formed, giving the foul odour of putrefaction, and the same changes are observed in putrefaction of meat, etc. Gas production may give rise to emphysematous crackling on palpation. The changes in colour—dark-brown or greenish-brown, and sometimes almost black—are due to changes in haemoglobin, and are most conspicuous when the dead tissue contains a lot of blood.

Gangrene may be either *primary* or *secondary*. The difference lies in the cause of the tissue necrosis. In primary gangrene it is brought about by the toxins of bacteria (which may then invade and digest the dead tissue). In secondary gangrene, necrosis is due to some other cause—usually loss of blood supply from vascular obstruction or tissue laceration—and saprophytic bacteria then digest the dead tissue.

Primary gangrene

This includes *gas gangrene* which results from infection with specific *clostridia*, and gangrene brought about by various other bacteria.

Gas gangrene is caused by a group of anaerobic sporulating bacteria, the *Clostridia*, of which the three most important are *Cl. welchii*, *Cl. oedematiens* and *Cl. septicum*. These organisms are intestinal commensals in man and animals; their spores are widespread, and are liable to contaminate wounds. Being anaerobic and saprophytic, they cannot multiply in living, oxygenated tissue, but they flourish in blood-soaked foreign material and dead tissue in dirty puncture or lacerated wounds such as are caused by road accidents and by shrapnel. Given such a favourable environment, the *Clostridia* produce exotoxins which diffuse into and kill the adjacent tissues and these in turn are invaded, so that the process spreads rapidly, particularly along the length of skeletal muscles (Fig. 8.11). Gas gangrene is most often due to *Cl. welchii*. Before the muscle and other tissues are killed, they become intensely oedematous, are extremely painful, and appear swollen and pink. Microscopically, emigration of leukocytes is minimal. Among a number of toxins, *Cl. welchii* produces a lecithinase (α toxin) which by its action on phospholipids lyses cell and mitochondrial membranes, also hyaluronidase and collagenase which digest ground substance and collagen respectively and may promote the rapid spread of infection. *Cl. welchii* ferments sugars, producing H_2 and CO_2 which collect as bubbles in the dead tissues,

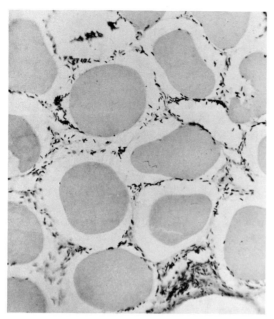

Fig. 8.11 Skeletal muscle in gas gangrene. The muscle fibres are necrotic and their nuclei have disappeared. Large numbers of *Cl. welchii* are present in the dead tissue, mainly in the endomysium. × 400.

rendering them crepitant on palpation. The subcutaneous tissue and skin are also involved, and the affected part, often a limb, may burst open as a result of the swelling of oedema fluid and pressure of gas. The dead tissues are commonly invaded by a mixture of other organisms present in the original wound, and these may play a major role in putrefaction. Gas gangrene may complicate intestinal lesions, e.g. appendicitis or strangulation of the gut (p. 643), clostridia being present in the intestine; it occurs also as a puerperal infection of the uterus from contamination via the perineum.

In addition to the rapidly spreading local lesion, gas gangrene is accompanied by acute haemolysis and a severe toxaemia which affects all the internal organs, and death results from peripheral vascular collapse. Spread by the blood stream may occur as a late, usually terminal event. In consequence all the tissues at necropsy may contain large numbers of clostridia, with extensive digestive changes.*

The clostridia of gas gangrene may also cause infection of subcutaneous tissue (cellulitis) without affecting the underlying muscle, or may grow in dirty wounds, producing a foul discharge but without either severe toxaemia or invasion of the surrounding tissues.

Production of toxin by *Cl. welchii* growing in contaminated food is also one cause of toxic gastroenteritis which is self-limiting and does not involve clostridial invasion of the gut wall.

If lacerated wounds are treated by early excision of the devitalised tissue, and toxic action is controlled by the use of antitoxic sera, clostridial infections are unlikely to establish themselves. Antibiotics have also contributed greatly to the prevention of gas gangrene by inhibiting the growth of clostridia.

Other examples of primary gangrene. In gas gangrene we have an example of primary gangrene caused by members of a group of clostridia whose toxins kill the tissue and, sometimes in association with other anaerobes, digest it. Primary gangrene can be caused by many other bacteria and mixtures of bacteria. For example, inhalation of dirty water in partial drowning, or of foul discharge from an ulcerated and infected cancer of the larynx, or from an oesophageal cancer which has ulcerated into the trachea, can each cause a gangrenous infection of the lungs in which various bacteria and fungi participate.

Gangrenous infection is particularly liable to develop in debilitated individuals and in those whose resistance to infection is lowered by various diseases; for example gangrenous pharyngitis or colitis may develop in patients with agranulocytosis, who lack the defences provided by neutrophil polymorphs. Diabetics also, unless their carbohydrate metabolism is adequately controlled, are particularly susceptible to infections, and gangrene may supervene. The following two unusual forms of primary gangrene also deserve mention.

'Meleney's post-operative synergistic gangrene.' This is a slowly spreading infection of the skin and subcutaneous tissue of the chest or abdominal wall; it starts at the site of an operation wound and usually the operation has been performed to deal with a focus of sepsis in the chest or abdomen. The spreading edge of the lesion is acutely inflamed and

---

* When necropsy is performed after a body has remained for a day or more in a warm environment, putrefactive changes, including bubbles of gas, may be seen in various tissues and especially in the liver and other abdominal viscera. This is due to agonal and post-mortem spread and growth of *Cl. welchii* etc. present in the gut. It is seen especially in obese or oedematous subjects dying from any cause and must not be confused with gas gangrene.

appears red and swollen: as it spreads, the central zone becomes darker and finally gangrenous, followed by sloughing to leave an ulcerated area with a granulating base. The lesion may spread relentlessly to involve much of the trunk. It is usually caused by a synergistic combination of *Staphylococcus aureus* and a streptococcus, but other combinations may have a similar effect.

Noma (*cancrum oris*) is a gangrenous condition occasionally seen in poorly nourished children and tends to complicate debilitating infections; it begins on the gum margin and spreads to the cheek, where an inflammatory patch of dusky red appearance forms and then becomes darker in colour and ultimately gangrenous. The condition is caused by bacteria of the genus *Bacteroides* (anaerobic bacilli present in huge numbers in the intestine and also part of the normal flora of the mouth) together with *Borrelia vincenti*, another mouth commensal. Deficient intake of the vitamin B complex, especially of nicotinic acid, is a predisposing factor.

Secondary gangrene

This is usually the result of ischaemic necrosis (from loss of blood supply) followed by invasion and digestion of the dead tissue by putrefactive micro-organisms. It is seen most often in the foot and leg, and in the intestine. As explained below, it occurs in two forms—'wet' and 'dry' gangrene.

Gangrene of the leg. Infarction of toes, a foot, or the lower leg is not uncommon as the result of arterial occlusion (Fig. 2.6, p. 12), the collateral circulation being insufficient to keep the part alive. This is caused by arterial thrombosis complicating advanced atheroma (p. 238), which is very common in old people and tends to be particularly severe in diabetics (hence the terms '*senile*' and '*diabetic*' *gangrene*). It may occur also in early or middle adult life in patients with thrombo-angiitis obliterans, a disease which affects multiple arterial branches, especially in the lower limbs. Another occasional cause is the symmetrical spasmodic contraction of arteries in Raynaud's disease.

If there is much subcutaneous fat, and particularly when the limb is oedematous, as in congestive heart failure, **wet gangrene** commonly supervenes in the infarcted tissues, with blebs of fluid in the skin, sometimes gas production, and rapid putrefaction: there is no sharp line of demarcation between dead and living tissue, and indeed gangrene may spread proximally beyond the tissues originally affected When infarction occurs in a non-oedematous leg, particularly when there is little subcutaneous fat and when gradual arterial occlusion has preceded the actual infarction, so-called **dry gangrene** is liable to ensue: the skin becomes cold and waxen, the haemoglobin diffuses out of the veins and produces reddish-purple staining of the dead tissues, which then become brownish-red and ultimately almost black, and the dead tissue gradually dries out and shrinks (*mummification*).

Use of the term dry gangrene is controversial. Commonly, mummification occurs with little or no putrefaction. Saprophytic organisms are, however, usually present in small numbers, particularly adjacent to the junction with living tissue, where the dead tissue remains moist. If amputation is not performed, putrefaction becomes established at this site, and a process of slow putrefactive ulceration penetrates the soft tissues, ultimately down to the bone.

Secondary gangrene of the intestine occurs when the blood supply to part of the intestine is arrested by thrombosis of the mesenteric arteries or when a loop of intestine becomes impacted in a hernial sac. In the latter case, secretion of fluid and gas production by bacteria in the lumen result in a rise of pressure in the entrapped loop, with consequent interference with blood flow. In both cases, the impaired blood flow results in necrosis of the wall of the intestine, which is invaded by putrefactive bacteria from the lumen, becomes gangrenous, and ruptures unless removed without delay. While the intestine is dying, the wall becomes swollen and at first red and then black from fluid and red cells escaping from the small vessels. The features are thus those of wet gangrene. Ischaemic necrosis of other organs, e.g. the pancreas, may also progress to wet gangrene if it becomes infected with putrefying bacteria from the gut.

Anthrax

Anthrax is a fatal epizootic disease of animals, particularly cattle and sheep, caused by a large Gram-positive sporulating bacillus, the spores of which can survive for 50 years or more in soil.* In herbivores the disease is contracted by

---

* The island of Gruinard, off the West Coast of Scotland, is still contaminated with anthrax spores deposited experimentally during the 1939–45 war.

ingestion of spores and causes a severe acute enteritis with a terminal septicaemia: the excreta and secretions are highly infective. More chronic, localised lesions can also occur in animals. In man, *B. anthracis* is of low infectivity, but acute lesions occur in the skin from direct contact with infected material, or more rarely internally from inhalation or ingestion of spores.

The factors determining the virulence of the bacillus include a capsular polypeptide rich in D-glutamic acid, which renders the organism resistant to phagocytosis, and a complex exotoxin which promotes increased vascular permeability, causing gross inflammatory oedema. Death can result from hypovolaemic shock due to local and generalised exudative loss of plasma fluid.

Cutaneous anthrax (malignant pustule) of man occurs from direct contact with animal material, e.g. carcasses, hides or bristles in shaving brushes. Although many imported hides are contaminated with spores, anthrax is rare among those handling them. The organism probably enters through a minor abrasion, and a painful papule forms and becomes blistered:

it is surrounded by a zone of intense congestion and oedema. Central haemorrhage and necrosis follow, resulting in a black crust (Fig. 8.12). Leukocytic emigration is usually scanty. Spread may occur to the regional lymph nodes, which become enlarged, oedematous and haemorrhagic. Although uncommon, the condition is an important example of a serious, sometimes fatal infection which can be effectively treated if diagnosed early.

Respiratory anthrax occurs from inhaling spores, usually from hides or wool. A localised lesion develops in the lower trachea or larger bronchi: it consists of a patch of haemorrhagic, ulcerated mucosa with intense oedema, involvement of hilar and mediastinal lymph nodes, extension to the lungs and haemorrhagic pleural and pericardial effusions: the prognosis is poor.

Intestinal anthrax is rare in man. It consists of one or more haemorrhagic foci in the wall of the upper small intestine, with central necrosis, gross oedematous swelling and involvement of the mesenteric lymph nodes.

Septicaemia and a haemorrhagic meningitis may occur in man, but are rare.

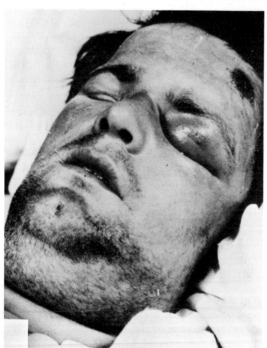 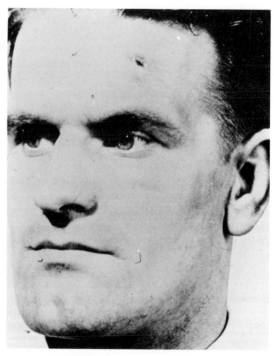

Fig. 8.12 Anthrax. *Left*, before treatment. The malignant pustule is seen on the forehead. Note the gross and extensive inflammatory oedema. *Right*, following treatment. (By kind permission of Dr. W. M. Jamieson and the Editor of *Medicine*.)

Chronic Bacterial Infections (Infective Granulomas)*

Under this heading may be included the many infections which give rise to chronic inflammation without a conspicuous exudative reaction, but usually with production of granulation tissue which eventually progresses to fibrosis. The general features of chronic inflammation have been described on pp. 67–71 and a more detailed account of the production of granulation tissue is given on pp. 80–7. The following account describes briefly some of the more important chronic infections. Because of its wide prevalence and tuberculous-like features, sarcoidosis is also included here, although there is no evidence that it is an infection.

Tuberculosis

Formerly one of the great killing diseases of temperate climates, tuberculosis is now much less common in Western Europe and North America. It is, however, prevalent in communities with a poor standard of living, and still ranks among the world's most important diseases. The disease illustrates well various basic features of bacterial infection, and in particular the importance of the reaction of the host in determining the nature of the lesions, and the spread of infection within the body. The causal mycobacteria, or tubercle bacilli, are aerobic Gram-positive bacilli with a waxy cell wall which renders them difficult to stain. Once the stain has penetrated the cell wall, however, it is also difficult to remove, and the mycobacteria are sometimes referred to as acid- and alcohol-fast bacteria, since they resist decolourisation by mineral acids and alcohol, as in the Zeihl–Neelsen stain. Tubercle bacilli grow slowly in culture; they are highly pathogenic for the guinea-pig, inoculation of which has been much used for their detection when present in small numbers in sputum, etc. In man, they usually cause chronic disease but can also produce a much more acute and even rapidly fatal infection. In addition to the tubercle bacilli, of which there are two major types causing human disease (see below), the

mycobacteria include the lepra bacillus which causes leprosy, and there are also various ill-defined organisms, sometimes termed *anonymous* or *atypical mycobacteria*, which cause lesions in the skin, lymph nodes, lungs and elsewhere.

Epidemiology

The two types of tubercle bacillus mainly responsible for disease in man are the human type. *Mycobacterium tuberculosis*, and the bovine type *Mycobacterium bovis.* The *human type* is the more important: infection with it is usually contracted by inhalation, and the initial or primary lesion is nearly always in the lungs. Patients with chronic pulmonary tuberculosis provide the reservoir of infection and spread the disease by exhaling infected droplets and by coughing up infected sputum. The organism is resistant to drying and can survive for long periods in dust, inhalation of which is the usual method of contracting the disease. Infection of the tonsils or of the intestine can also occur from swallowing the human type of tubercle bacillus in contaminated dust, or the bovine type of bacillus in contaminated milk from cows with tuberculous mastitis.

Several factors are responsible for the declining incidence of tuberculosis in Western Europe and North America. Firstly, the rising standard of nutrition and housing: there is no doubt that under-nourishment predisposes to tuberculosis and impairs the resistance of the individual who has contracted the disease. Overcrowding and inadequate personal and domestic hygiene are also of importance in spreading the disease in the home and in public transport and meeting places, etc. The environment of a subject coughing up the organism is likely to be heavily contaminated, and spread within families is especially common, giving rise to both pulmonary and alimentary infections.

Since the 1939–45 war, the use of specific chemotherapeutic bactericidal agents has also helped to reduce the incidence of the disease

---

* As stated on p. 70, there is an increasing tendency to restrict *granuloma* to inflammatory lesions consisting of aggregates of macrophages. I have preferred to use *macrophage granuloma* to describe such a lesion, and to retain the traditional usage of *granuloma* to mean any chronic inflammatory lesion.

by diminishing greatly the infectivity of patients with chronic pulmonary tuberculosis. Mass miniature radiography has revealed unsuspected cases of tuberculosis in the community, and protection against infection has been provided by means of BCG vaccination.

In countries where the disease is rife, infants and young children are particularly at risk, and in this country the mortality rate in children contracting the infection before the age of 3 years was formerly very high. Those who overcome the infection develop partial resistance to the organism, but may become re-infected and develop chronic pulmonary tuberculosis in adult life. The bacteria may survive for many years in dormant lesions, without clinical manifestations, and these may become active as a result of malnutrition, as in war or famine, as a complication of other debilitating diseases such as diabetes mellitus, or from administration of corticosteroids or other immunosuppressive agents. In Western Europe, a high proportion of 'new' cases are middle-aged or old and have had dormant lesions for many years from the time when the disease was much commoner. It is, however, relatively common among Asian immigrants, younger age groups being affected. *Mycobacterium bovis* causes mastitis in cattle, and is transmitted to man by consuming infected milk and milk products. Infection results usually by way of the gut or tonsils. In many countries, bovine infection in man has been eradicated by pasteurisation of milk, which kills the organism, and by tuberculin testing of cattle and elimination of infected cows. The avian tubercle bacillus (*Myco. avium*) is a rare cause of disease in man.

Hypersensitivity and immunity

The immune response to the tubercle bacillus provides the classical example of cell-mediated immunity, i.e. the production of specifically primed T lymphocytes which are capable of reacting directly with antigenic protein of the mycobacterium. The mechanism of this type of response, and the state of delayed hypersensitivity which results from it, have been described in Chapters 5 and 6 respectively. It is not understood why cell-mediated immunity is the dominant type of immune response to the

tubercle bacillus, but it may be of significance that mycobacteria, living or dead, have a powerful enhancing effect on the cell-mediated immune response to antigens in general, and this forms the basis of their use in Freund's adjuvant (p. 114). Whatever the explanation of its adjuvant effect, infection with tubercle bacilli results, within two weeks or so, in the development of a high degree of cell-mediated immunity to a protein fraction (tuberculoprotein) of the organism* and the subsequent course of the infection and the features of the lesions are profoundly influenced by the hypersensitivity state. The specifically primed T cells react with tuberculoprotein, and release the various lymphokines described on p. 158. The results are both beneficial and harmful. *The tubercle bacillus has not been shown to produce any direct toxic effect, and can survive and multiply within macrophages in tissue culture without harm to the cultured cells. Indeed, it is likely that the tissue injury resulting from tuberculous infection is due mainly or entirely to the delayed hypersensitivity reaction against the bacteria.* Nevertheless, without an immune response, multiplication of the organism would presumably continue unchecked. The delayed hypersensitivity reaction is therefore to be regarded as protective in reducing or eliminating the infection, but at the same time injurious to the tissues. Interpretation of the features of the lesions of tuberculosis in terms of delayed hypersensitivity is attempted in the account of structural changes (below).

Although antibodies to mycobacterial antigens develop in tuberculosis, they do not appear to influence the course of the infection, and have not provided a useful diagnostic test.

Tuberculin skin testing. This is carried out by intradermal injection of very small amounts of tuberculoprotein, as in the *Mantoux test*. In individuals who are, or have previously been, infected, a delayed hypersensitivity reaction develops, the features of which are described on p. 157. In some patients with very severe tuberculosis, the test is negative, presumably because the large amount of tuberculoprotein being released from the lesions has overwhelmed the state of hypersensitivity. Tuberculin skin tests give positive reactions in infections with both

* This state of hypersensitivity was demonstrated by Robert Koch (1891), using a crude preparation termed 'old tuberculin'. A more refined preparation is termed 'purified protein derivative' (PPD).

human and bovine types of tubercle bacillus, and with other types of mycobacteria. For this reason they may be positive in individuals infected with *Mycobacterium leprae*. Positive tests are also observed in healthy inhabitants of tropical and sub-tropical countries, apparently as a result of previous sub-clinical infection with other mycobacteria.

Immunisation against tuberculosis. Protective immunisation requires the induction of cell-mediated immunity to tuberculoprotein, and this is most effectively achieved by injecting living mycobacteria. Attenuated strains of the bovine type, e.g. *bacille Calmette-Guérin* (BCG), or other non-human strains such as *Myco. muris* (the vole bacillus), are used for this purpose. Cell-mediated immunity develops, with consequent delayed hypersensitivity reactions at the site of injection and sometimes also in the draining lymph nodes which may become infected. The attenuated bacilli are destroyed and the lesions heal, but the cell-mediated immunity persists.

Structural changes

When a guinea-pig is inoculated with *Myco. tuberculosis* there is little reaction during the first day or so apart from local infiltration with neutrophil polymorphs, which soon disappear. During the next few days, macrophages migrate into the area and ingest the bacteria without bringing about their destruction. After ten days or so, lymphocytes begin to appear in the lesion, and macrophages derived mainly from monocytes of the blood aggregate in increasing numbers to form a minute nodule consisting of a macrophage granuloma. These very early stages of infection cannot, of course, be observed in man, but the subsequent changes are closely similar in man and the guinea-pig. The macrophages enlarge and change to **epithelioid cells** (p. 74). Small lymphocytes accumulate around the margin of the nodule, which is then termed a **tubercle** and becomes visible to the naked eye about 3 weeks after the onset. In the central part of the lesion, multinucleated **Langhans' giant cells** (p. 74) are formed by fusion of epithelioid cells (Fig. 8.13). As the tubercle enlarges, the epithelioid and giant cells in the central part undergo necrosis (Fig. 8.14): the cells lose their outline and nuclear staining and become fused into a homogeneous or

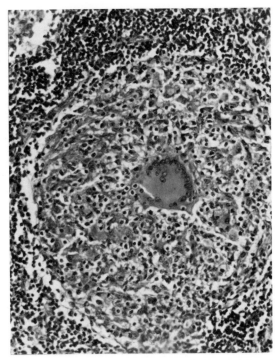

Fig. 8.13 An early tubercle, consisting mainly of epithelioid cells, some of which have fused to form a Langhans' giant cell. Lymphocytes are scattered among the epithelioid cells and are numerous around the periphery. × 174.

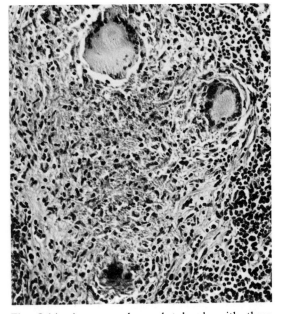

Fig. 8.14 A more advanced tubercle with three giant cells and early necrosis among the most centrally-placed epithelioid cells. × 150.

slightly granular material, which may also contain fibrin from vascular exudation. The tubercle thus comes to consist of a necrotic centre, surrounded by epithelioid and sometimes giant cells (Fig. 8.15), with a peripheral aggregation of small lymphocytes. The necrotic material is creamy-white, and resembles cream cheese in appearance and consistence—hence the terms **caseation** and **caseous material**.

The initial accumulation of macrophages and phagocytosis of tubercle bacilli occur before there is any immune response and are seen also in the reaction to particles of various non-antigenic foreign materials. Lymphocytic infiltration, however, follows the development of cell-mediated immunity and some of the cells are specifically primed T-cells which, by releasing various lymphokines (p. 159) contribute to the arrival of more macrophages by chemotaxis, and to their arrest around the tubercle bacilli by migration-inhibition factor: macrophage-activating factor may transform the macrophages to epithelioid cells, and may mediate the destruction of phagocytosed bacilli. The T-cell cytotoxic factor presumably accounts for the necrosis of macrophages at the centre of the lesion, although the tubercle follicle is avascular and ischaemia may also be important. It

has been shown in animal experiments that many of the lymphocytes in the tuberculous lesion are not specifically primed cells resulting from the cell-mediated immune response (p. 157): they may be attracted to the site of infection by a chemotactic lymphokine, but their significance in the lesion is obscure.

The further course of the infection depends on several factors, including the infecting dose and virulence of the organism and also the degree of resistance of the host. What determines virulence in strains of tubercle bacilli is not understood, but the so-called virulent strains are those which are capable of relatively rapid multiplication *in vivo*. If bacterial multiplication is checked, tubercles are replaced by fibrous tissue. If the bacteria continue to multiply in the lesions, they may escape and gain a foothold in the surrounding tissues, with further tubercle formation. A cluster of tubercles may thus arise, and as these enlarge, they become confluent, and the central areas of caseous necrosis eventually unite to give a large caseous patch with tubercles around the periphery. Such lesions may reach several centimetres in diameter. When they arise in the lungs, they seldom reach this size without involving the wall of a bronchus, and the caseous material is then discharged, leaving a tuberculous cavity (Fig. 8.16). In other tissues, and particularly in the kidneys and in lesions of bone

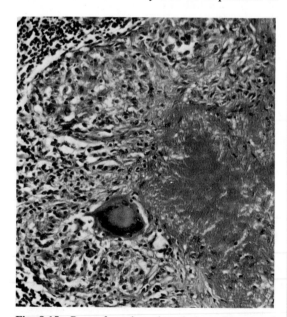

Fig. 8.15 Part of a tuberculous lesion with central caseation (*right*) and surrounding epithelioid cells with giant-cell formation. Note the structureless appearance of the caseous material. × 150.

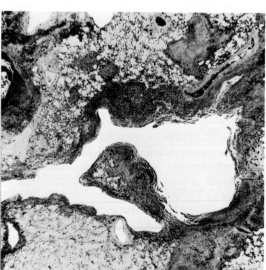

Fig. 8.16 Formation of a tuberculous cavity. The lesion has ulcerated into a bronchus and the caseous material is discharging. × 4.

extending into the surrounding soft tissues, caseous material may be invaded by neutrophil polymorphs, with resultant liquefaction ('tuberculous pus'). Such a lesion used to be called a **cold abscess**, because it is not accompanied by the acute inflammatory features of a pyogenic abscess. The softened caseous material may track through the tissues and may eventually reach a surface and discharge.

Some tuberculous lesions present more acute features than those described above. For example, rapid dissemination may occur by the air passages throughout the lung, resulting in multiple scattered lesions. Microscopy then shows extensive filling of the alveoli with large rounded macrophages (Fig. 8.17); these cells rapidly undergo fatty change and necrosis, and the lesions enlarge and coalesce with little or no attempt at healing. If it infects the subarachnoid space, usually by way of the bloodstream, the tubercle bacillus multiplies rapidly in the cerebrospinal fluid and the meningitis is of acute exudative inflammatory type with deposition of fibrin and accumulation initially of neutrophil polymorphs and later of macrophages and lymphocytes. Tubercles are usually poorly formed, and involvement of the walls of arteries and veins lying in the subarachnoid space may cause severe narrowing of their lumina by endarteritis (Fig. 21.33, p. 751) or occlusion by thrombosis. The lesions which result from infection of the pleural and peritoneal cavities are also commonly exudative, with a serous or serofibrinous exudate, and when the pericardium is involved the exudate may be rich in fibrin and is often haemorrhagic, presumably as a result of the mechanical effect of the heart beat.

Primary and reinfection tuberculosis

Infection of an individual who has not been previously infected or immunised gives rise to the **primary lesion** at the portal of entry in the lung, tonsil or small intestine. This usually remains small, and commonly heals without becoming detectable. Early spread of bacteria to the regional lymph nodes is, however, the rule, and their rapid multiplication may occur in the affected nodes, i.e. at the root of the lung (Fig. 16.29, p. 476), in the neck or in the mesentery, depending on the site of the primary lesion. The combination of the primary lesion and

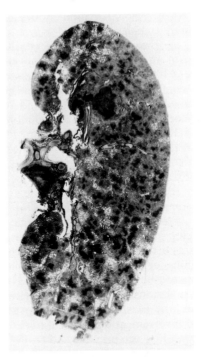

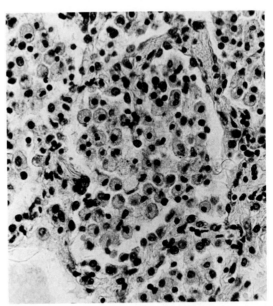

Fig. 8.17 Acute tuberculous bronchopneumonia. *Above*, Primary pulmonary tuberculosis in a child. The infection has spread by the bronchi and has caused widespread lesions which are becoming confluent and have undergone central caseation (dark areas). *Below*, the lesions consist initially of accumulations of macrophages and lymphocytes in the alveoli. The macrophages undergo fatty change and appear 'foamy': necrosis then supervenes. × 370.

enlarged, caseous regional lymph nodes is called the **primary complex.**

Reinfection or **chronic tuberculosis** results from infection of an individual who has overcome a primary infection or been immunised by BCG. The reinfection lesion is usually in the apex of one or other lung and may extend to give a large local lesion with one or more cavities (Fig. 8.18). There is usually little or no involvement of the local lymph nodes. Reinfection lesions occur also in the tonsils, small intestine, pharynx and skin, again without much involvement of the regional nodes, but these are relatively uncommon sites. Individuals with reinfection tuberculosis of the lungs may, however, develop lesions in the larynx, mouth and intestines as a result of endogenous infection by coughing up and swallowing sputum containing tubercle bacilli (Fig. 19.59, p. 633). These metastatic lesions resemble those of reinfection tuberculosis in spreading locally with minimal or no involvement of the local nodes.

The differences between primary and reinfection tuberculosis appear to depend mainly on the spread of the bacilli to the local lymph nodes and their multiplication there in the early

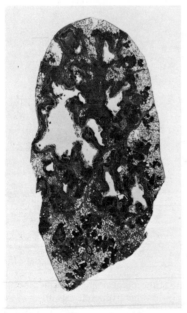

Fig. 8.18 Apical part of the lung showing chronic (reinfection) tuberculosis. The infection has extended to form coalescing lesions with central caseation and peripheral fibrosis. The caseous material in the larger lesions has discharged *via* the bronchi, leaving several cavities with fibrous walls. × 0·7.

stages of the primary infection, before the development of a high level of cell mediated immunity.

Although the term 'reinfection tuberculosis' is commonly used for chronic tuberculosis occurring usually in adults, it may well be that, in some cases, tubercle bacilli have persisted in a healed primary lesion and eventually multiply and produce the 'reinfection'.

The spread of infection within the body is discussed below, but more detailed accounts of the resulting lesions are given in the chapters on regional pathology, e.g. pulmonary tuberculosis, pp. 475 *et seq.*

Amyloid disease (p. 269) is an important complication of chronic tuberculosis.

Spread of infection

Tuberculous infection is very prone to spread by lymphatics and to produce lesions in lymph nodes. This occurs especially in the early stages of the primary infection, with resulting involvement of the draining lymph nodes, and infection may spread from these to adjacent nodes or groups of nodes, e.g. in the mediastinum. In chronic (i.e. reinfection) tuberculosis, lymphatic spread is usually localised to the tissue immediately around the lesions, the draining lymph nodes seldom being severely involved. This limitation of lymphatic spread is probably attributable to the modified behaviour of macrophages which results from delayed hypersensitivity. There is experimental evidence that lymphatic spread results from ingestion and transport of *Myco. tuberculosis* by macrophages, and the T-cell factors which convert macrophages into 'killer' cells and interfere with their migration from the lesion are likely to impede such spread.

Spread also occurs by the bloodstream. This is seen notably in **acute miliary tuberculosis**, in which large numbers of bacteria enter the blood and give rise to multiple scattered tubercles in the various organs. The condition arises most commonly in primary tuberculosis and is due usually to involvement of a vein by the large caseating lymph node lesions of the primary complex—in most cases the pulmonary hilar nodes: the caseating process extends into the wall of an adjacent vein, usually one of the pulmonary veins, and caseous material containing large numbers of mycobacteria is then discharged into the circulation. The resulting lesions are particularly numerous in the liver, kidneys and spleen. They consist of tubercles of fairly uniform size, and without specific therapy death usually results from tuberculous meningitis after about a month, at which time the tubercles are of approx. 1–2 mm diameter (Fig. 16.31, p. 479): they are rather poorly developed, often without giant cells, but with central necrosis (Fig. 8.19) and are termed **miliary tubercles** (latin *milium*—millet seed). In some instances, the bacteria escape into a systemic vein, either directly or by involvement of the thoracic duct, and as a result the number of miliary lesions in the lungs far exceeds those in other organs. When a relatively small number of tubercle bacilli gain entrance to the bloodstream, few tubercles are produced in the various organs, and since the patient may survive much longer than is the case in untreated acute miliary tuberculosis, the lesions may become larger. One or more large metastatic lesions may also occur, for example in the bones, joints, kidneys, epididymes or fallopian tubes, and less commonly in the brain. Although in heavily infected communities blood-borne lesions arise most commonly as a complication of the primary tuberculous complex in young children, in countries where the disease has been largely eradicated they are uncommon and are now seen mostly in older patients with reinfection tuberculosis, particularly in advanced cases. Haematogenous lesions are also observed when tuberculosis is complicated by other debilitating diseases, or as a result of corticosteroid or other immuno-suppressive therapy.

Spread of tuberculous infection occurs also along hollow viscera and in body cavities. In the lungs, spread by the bronchi is of great importance. Mycobacteria coughed up in sputum may settle and give rise to lesions in the larynx and intestine. Spread may occur from the fallopian tubes to the endometrium, and from the kidney to the urinary tract, and dissemination may occur within the pleural, pericardial and peritoneal cavities and, in tuberculous meningitis, within the subarchnoid space and ventricles of the brain.

Healing of tuberculous lesions

The healing of tubercles or larger tuberculous lesions is dependent on the elimination or

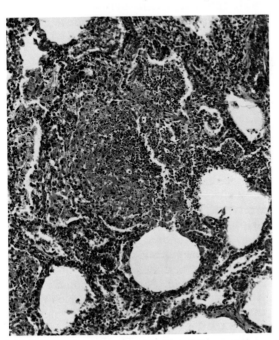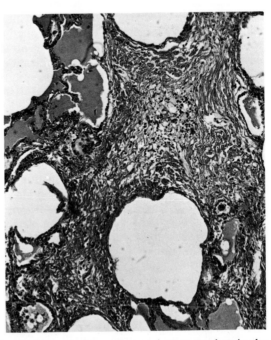

Fig. 8.19 On the left is shown a miliary tubercle of lung with central caseation and acute exudate in the surrounding alveoli from a patient with untreated miliary tuberculosis; on the right a fibrous scar containing a few lymphocytes, the remains of a miliary tubercle after specific chemotherapy. × 100.

reduction in numbers of mycobacteria. Healing is brought about by formation, around the lesions, of reticulin fibres, progressing to more dense fibrosis. If caseation is slight or absent, as in early tubercles, the whole lesion may be gradually replaced by fibrous tissue, leaving a scar (Fig. 8.19), but extensive patches of caseation usually persist and become encapsulated in fibrous tissue. Slow progressive deposition of calcium salts commonly occurs in the caseous material, which eventually may become stony hard and clearly visible in radiographs: in some instances the calcified material may be replaced by bone, which may even develop spaces containing haemopoietic marrow. The course of the disease depends on the balance between bacterial multiplication, with extension and caseation of the lesions, and the reactive processes involved in killing the bacteria, preventing their spread, and promoting a fibroblastic reaction.

The effects of drugs. The course and prognosis of tuberculosis have been radically changed by effective specific chemotherapy, which has also greatly modified the appearance of tuberculous lesions. When healing occurs 'naturally', i.e. without specific chemotherapy, large caseous lesions become walled off first by cellular tubercles and then by new-formed fibrous tissue, which penetrates the outer zone of tubercles and finally encapsulates the central caseous mass. Dense fibrosis and calcification complete the process: there is little resolution. Effective drug therapy is accompanied successively by resolution of the surrounding exudative lesions, increased vascularity, reversion of the epithelioid cells to foamy macrophages, formation of granulation tissue, absorption of necrotic and caseous material, and finally by healing with the production of minimal amounts of fibrous tissue. Combined therapy thus strikingly modifies the outcome; early lesions may clear up almost completely without residual effects and chronic caseous and fibrotic pulmonary lesions with excavation are transformed to smooth-walled cavities, which may become lined by epithelium.

Because of the spontaneous occurrence of mutant tubercle bacilli resistant to one or more drugs, it is now accepted practice to administer a combination of three drugs, usually isonicotinic acid hydrazide (isoniazid), rifampicin and ethambutol. Because the tubercle bacillus multiplies relatively slowly, it may take some months for the selective advantage conferred by drug therapy on a resistant mutant to be reflected in clinical deterioration, and repeated bacteriological examinations, e.g. of sputum, are therefore important during treatment.

Leprosy

It is estimated that there are some 10 million people with leprosy throughout the world and approximately 100 000 new cases are registered annually. The disease now occurs mainly in those tropical and sub-tropical countries with poor living standards, although it was formerly quite common in Europe and North America. The causal organism, *Mycobacterium leprae*, was the first bacterial pathogen to be seen and described in a human disease. It is an acid-fast bacillus, demonstrable by a modified Ziehl–Neelsen staining technique: it has not yet been grown in culture and does not cause natural disease in species other than man, although it causes a local lesion when injected into the mouse foot-pad and spreading infection in animals in which cell-mediated immunity has been depressed by neonatal thymectomy or anti-lymphocyte serum. *Infectivity is low, and although the bacillus is often present in large numbers in the nasal and oral secretions of patients, only a small percentage of long-term close contacts develop the disease.*

The leprosy bacillus appears to be highly temperature-dependent, for it produces lesions mainly in colder parts of the body, namely the skin, especially of the nose, lobes of the ears and extremities, the anterior part of the eye, the nasopharynx, mouth and upper respiratory tract, superficial lymph nodes and testes. It also has a predilection for nerves; it always involves the small nerve twigs in the skin and often larger superficial nerves.

Host resistance is dependent mainly on the cell-mediated response to *Myco. leprae*. In **lepromatous leprosy** this is depressed, and the lesions progress relentlessly and contain huge numbers of bacilli. A strong response is associated with **tuberculoid leprosy**, in which the lesions contain relatively few bacilli, and may become stationary or subside.

Lepromatous leprosy. The lesions consist of aggregates of macrophages (Fig. 8.20), containing huge numbers of lepra bacilli lying parallel

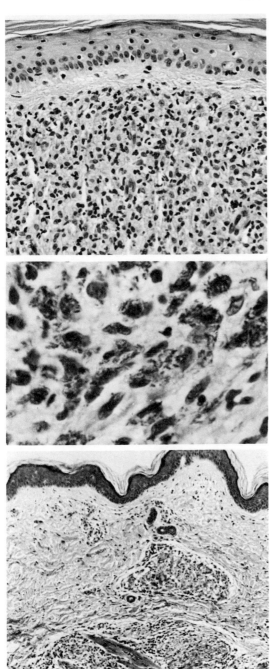

in bundles or aggregated to form large acid-fast masses (globi). In the absence of cell-mediated immunity, the bacilli are not destroyed, and multiply within the macrophages which have ingested them. Like tubercle bacilli, they appear to be non-toxigenic and macrophages containing large numbers of organisms show little evidence of injury apart from fatty change. Lymphocytes are scanty or absent, and tissue injury is probably due mainly to pressure. However, the skin lesions become very extensive and may ulcerate and become secondarily infected with various bacteria. Similar changes are seen in the oral, nasal and upper respiratory lesions. In spite of extensive involvement of superficial nerves, anaesthesia, trophic changes and paralysis are often late features of the disease. The internal organs are rarely seriously involved, although small clusters of macrophages containing lepra bacilli may occur in the liver, spleen, etc.

Tuberculoid leprosy. The lesions resemble those of tuberculosis, consisting of tubercle-like follicles (Fig. 8.20) and more extensive infiltrates of epithelioid and Langhans' giant-cells (both of which are modified macrophages) and lymphocytes. Necrosis occurs but is inconspicuous and leprosy bacilli are often difficult to find. Nerve injury due to scarring occurs early, and patches of hypopigmentation and sensory loss are often presenting features. The internal organs are seldom involved.

Forms of leprosy intermediate between lepromatous and tuberculoid are commonly encountered. In some instances, lesions of both types may be present (**borderline** or **dimorphous leprosy**), and such cases may progress in either direction. Drug therapy helps to convert lepromatous to tuberculoid leprosy, and to cure the latter.

Immunological reactions in leprosy. Intradermal injection of lepromin, an antigenic extract of *Myco. leprae*, elicits a delayed hypersensitivity reaction, resembling the tuberculin reaction, in individuals with tuberculoid leprosy: the reaction occurs also in individuals with cell-mediated immunity to the tubercle bacillus and

Fig. 8.20 Leprosy. *Above*, part of a skin nodule in lepromatous leprosy. The lesion is a macrophage granuloma: lymphocytes are scanty and necrosis has not occurred. × 60.
Middle, part of the same lesion, stained by Triff's method for acid-fast bacilli: the macrophages contain numerous *Myco. leprae*. × 650.

Below, skin lesions in tuberculoid leprosy, composed of epithelioid cells, giant cells and lymphocytes. Such lesions contain few bacilli. × 64. (The late Professor J. A. Milne.)

other mycobacteria. A later granulomatous lesion (the Mitsuda reaction) may develop within 4 weeks: this also is not diagnostic of leprosy. The test is usually negative in lepromatous leprosy, and becomes positive if the patient converts, spontaneously or as a result of drug therapy, to tuberculoid leprosy. These observations are supported by parallel results of *in-vitro* tests for cell-mediated immunity, and together with the morphological features of the disease indicate that *tuberculoid lesions are modified by a delayed hypersensitivity reaction to the lepra bacilli, whereas lepromatous lesions represent the growth of the bacilli in the absence of delayed hypersensitivity*.

Failure of cell-mediated immunity in lepromatous leprosy is not fully explained. The lymph nodes show lymphocyte depletion of the T-dependent zones, i.e. paracortex, and diminution of T lymphocytes in the blood has been reported. A plasma factor which depresses T lymphocyte function has also been described.

There is usually a high titre of antibody to *Myco. leprae* in the serum of patients with lepromatous leprosy, but this seems to afford little protection: drug therapy results in destruction of large numbers of bacilli, and release of antigen may then give rise to an acute Arthus reaction in the lesions (**erythema nodosum leprosum**) or generalised immune complex disease with glomerulonephritis (pp. 155–6). Another complication is amyloid disease.

Sarcoidosis

This disease, which is of unknown causation, is characterised by multiple granulomatous lesions, and may affect lymph nodes, lungs, skin, spleen, eyes, salivary glands, liver and bones, particularly of the hands and feet. It is of world-wide distribution, but with great geographical variation in incidence. It occurs over a wide age range, but most commonly in young adults, and is much more common in negroes than whites in the U.S.A., and in immigrants than natives in Great Britain. The highest reported incidence is in Sweden.

The disease most commonly gives rise to enlarged mediastinal and pulmonary hilar lymph nodes, often without symptoms, but sometimes accompanied by fever. Other groups of lymph nodes are often affected and minute lesions in the lungs may present an x-ray picture resembling that of miliary tuberculosis. Sarcoid lesions also occur in the skin and occasionally erythema induratum (p. 1065) develops and may be the presenting clinical feature. Microscopically, the sarcoid lesions consist of tubercle-like follicles composed of epithelioid cells with occasional giant cells and scanty peripheral lymphocytes (Fig. 8.21 and Fig. 18.10, p. 574). The giant cells may contain curious calcium-rich star-shaped or conchoid inclusions (*asteroid* or *Schaumann bodies*). Unlike tuberculosis, the lesions do not undergo caseation although there may be a little central necrosis.

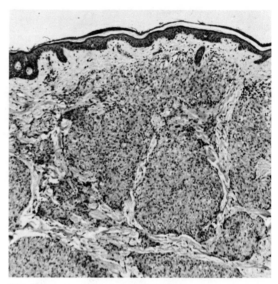

Fig. 8.21 Sarcoidosis of skin. The lesions consist of aggregates of epithelioid cells with relatively few lymphocytes. In contrast to tuberculosis, there is little or no necrosis. × 80.

The course of the disease is unpredictable: it may be acute or chronic, and temporary or permanent remission may occur spontaneously. It can cause blindness by involving the uveal tract, and is occasionally fatal, usually as a result of fibrosis of the pulmonary lesions with consequent right ventricular heart failure, or as a result of intercurrent infections. Hypercalcaemia may develop with consequent renal damage.

Diagnosis. Non-caseating epithelioid-cell granulomas, with or without giant-cell inclusions, are not diagnostic of sarcoidosis: they occur in various conditions including tuberculosis, various fungal infections, syphilis, brucellosis and berylliosis. The diagnosis of sarcoidosis thus depends also on the clinical features, the distribution of the lesions, and on excluding the above possibilities. Sarcoid-like follicles are occasionally found incidentally in surgical and necropsy material and are of unknown significance.

Intradermal injection of a sterile suspension prepared from sarcoid lesions (**Kveim test**) leads to the development of a lesion becoming maximal in about six weeks and having the histological features of sarcoidosis. The test is positive in most cases of sarcoidosis, but conflicting results have been reported in some other conditions, notably Crohn's disease (p. 620). During the course of sarcoidosis, tuberculin tests are negative in most cases even when these are known to have been previously positive and cell-mediated immunity in general is impaired. A fall in circulating T lymphocytes and a depressed response of T cells to PHA and other mitogens (p. 172) have also been reported. The capacity to produce antibodies, however, is normal or even increased.

Aetiology. The significance of these immunological features is obscure. The sarcoid lesion, consisting of epithelioid cells and lymphocytes, is itself suggestive of a delayed hypersensitivity reaction, although no exogenous antigen has been shown to be involved.

Subsequent development of tuberculosis has been observed in some patients, but sarcoidosis seems unlikely to be a modified form of tuberculosis, because depression of delayed hypersensitivity (as in sarcoidosis) would be expected to be associated with a florid form of tuberculosis. Also, the condition is not aggravated, and is sometimes improved, by administration of steroids. Various other aetiological factors have been suggested, but with little good supporting evidence.

Syphilis

Historical note

It is generally believed that syphilis was introduced into Europe on the return of the Spanish sailors of Columbus from America and that by the end of 1494 it had spread throughout Spain and along the Mediterranean coast into Italy. Within a century it had become widespread throughout Europe, having been carried everywhere by the mercenary troops returning to their own countries after the Siege of Naples (1495). At this time syphilis was clearly recognised as a new disease and its manifestations became so well known that Shakespeare was able to give a remarkably accurate (although anachronistic) account of them in *Timon of Athens* (Act IV, Scene 3). Absence of syphilis from the Old World is supported by the complete lack of evidence of the disease in skeletal remains dating back from 1494, whereas bones found in ancient tombs in Central America bear clear indications of the disease. The name comes from a poem composed in 1530 by Girolamo Frascatoro, a Verona physician, in which Syphilis, a swineherd, offended Apollo, who inflicted him with the disease.

General features

Formerly common, syphilis is now relatively infrequent in Western Europe: recent reports show some increase, particularly among homosexuals, but the rise is much less than for gonorrhoea. Syphilis is an important **venereal disease**, i.e. it is usually contracted by coitus and the primary lesion then develops on the external genitals. Rarely, extragenital infection occurs on the lip, tongue or breast and also on the fingers from handling infective lesions. The causal agent is a small motile spiral microorganism or spirochaete, *Treponema pallidum*. It dies rapidly on drying and even if kept moist does not survive for long outside the body. Accordingly, infection is usually by direct contact, the presence of a minute abrasion or crack in the skin apparently facilitating invasion. The disease has a distinct *incubation period*, followed by a *primary lesion* and then a *febrile secondary stage* with skin eruptions, and this is sometimes followed by a *tertiary stage*, with localised lesions, and by a late stage of *neurosyphilis*. It is convenient to give a general survey of the course of the untreated disease at this point. The special features of the individual lesions will be considered in the appropriate systematic chapters.

'Stages' of syphilis

The primary sore. The primary sore or chancre (Fig. 8.22) appears usually on the external genitals, after an incubation period of 2–12 (usually 3–4) weeks, as a small, slowly growing, hard, pale brownish-red, usually painless nodule. The centre ulcerates and there may be some exudate which, in a skin lesion, is usually scanty and forms a crust. When the lesion is on

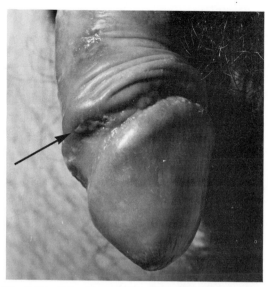

Fig. 8.22 Primary syphilitic chancre of penis. The lesion is seen as a swelling with (in this instance) central necrosis and ulceration: it is situated in the coronal sulcus and involves the reflection of the prepuce.

a mucous surface and the part is not kept clean, there may be more extensive ulceration, and various organisms, sometimes including other spirochaetes, are present in addition to *Tr. pallidum*. The ulcer persists for some weeks, during which the inguinal lymph nodes, usually on both sides, become somewhat enlarged and hard. *Treponema pallidum* is often detectable in the exudate of the ulcerated chancre, either by dark-ground microscopy or by fluorescence microscopy, using fluorescein-labelled antibody: if this fails, it may be demonstrable in fluid withdrawn by puncture of the enlarged lymph nodes. *Dissemination by the blood takes place before the appearance of the primary lesion*, and syphilis has been accidentally transmitted by transfusion of blood withdrawn before the primary lesion had appeared in the donor.

The primary chancre subsides spontaneously after a few weeks, leaving a slight scar. In a significant proportion of cases, it does not develop or passes unnoticed.

Secondary lesions appear at a variable interval, usually from 2–3 months after infection; they include multiple symmetrical lesions of the skin and squamous mucous membranes. The skin rash may be macular, papular or pustular, the palms of the hands and soles of the feet being commonly involved. Lesions of the hair follicles in the scalp lead to loss of the hair—*alopecia*. In the vulva, anus and perineum, flat raised papules sometimes develop—*condylomata lata*—and are intensely infective: they must not be confused with *condylomata acuminata*, the so-called venereal warts, which are of viral nature. The buccal and pharyngeal mucosa shows white, shining patches caused by thickening of the keratinised layer, and these break down, giving '*snail-track ulcers*'. General slight enlargement of lymph nodes is also common and is most easily detected in the superficial nodes. The secondary lesions are usually accompanied by fever, anaemia and general malaise. After some months all these features disappear spontaneously and the disease becomes latent.

Tertiary lesions appear irregularly, especially in the internal organs, skin and mucous membranes; they are few in number but usually much larger than the primary and secondary lesions, and lead to serious and permanent damage. They rarely appear within the first few years, and sometimes only after many years. Tertiary lesions are characterised by diffuse chronic inflammation, often with central necrosis, and extensive formation of granulation tissue. If necrosis is present, the lesion is termed a **gumma**. The central necrotic portion is dull yellowish, firm and rubbery; this is surrounded by a more translucent capsule of young connective tissue which has often a very irregular outline (Fig. 25.8, p. 996). Tertiary lesions may occur in any tissue, but especially in the liver, testes and bones. They cause extensive destruction, e.g. in the nasal bones with loss of the bridge of the nose and perforation of the palate, ulceration and destruction of the larynx, creeping ulcers in the skin, etc. Of special importance are the cardiovascular lesions. All tertiary lesions tend to heal eventually, and much distortion of the organs and interference with function may result from scarring.

Neurosyphilis. Lastly, in a small proportion of cases there occur two important nervous diseases, *tabes dorsalis* and *general paralysis*. They are due to the actual presence of the spirochaetes in the central nervous system.

Microscopic appearances

The main feature of the early **chancre** is heavy cellular infiltration of the dermis (Fig. 8.23)

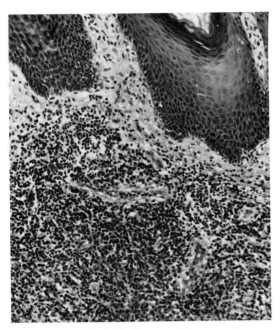

Fig. 8.23 Primary syphilitic chancre, showing the heavy cellular infiltration of the dermis. Most of the infiltrating cells (not readily identified at this magnification) are lymphocytes and plasma cells. × 120.

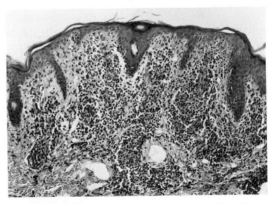

Fig. 8.24 Papular syphilitic rash, showing abundant cellular infiltration of the corium. Note also the hyperkeratosis. × 115.

with lymphocytes, plasma cells and occasional macrophages, which are mainly responsible for the hardness and swelling. At the periphery, the infiltrating cells lie mainly around the small vessels (periarteritis). Later, ulceration occurs with exudative inflammation and formation of granulation tissue. *The histological features are not diagnostic without the demonstration of Tr. pallidum, which requires special staining techniques.** After a time the cellular infiltration gradually diminishes and only a little thickening of the fibrous stroma remains. There is usually little or no residual scarring unless there has been much ulceration.

In the **secondary lesions** in the skin and mucous membranes the main changes are vascular engorgement and infiltration, mainly of plasma cells, but also lymphocytes and macrophages (Fig. 8.24). Cellular infiltration occurs also around and into the hair follicles, and the hairs may fall out. All these disseminated lesions of the skin and mucous membranes usually subside naturally, i.e. without specific therapy, and without scarring.

The **gumma** of the **tertiary stage** consists of

parenchymal necrosis, surrounded by a layer of connective tissue infiltrated with lymphocytes and plasma cells (Fig. 8.25). Eventual healing is accompanied by shrinkage, considerable scarring and distortion. Another common type of lesion is chronic interstitial inflammation or fibrosis, often spreading extensively, and sometimes containing foci of gummatous necrosis. In the necrotic tissue, the structural outlines may be preserved for a long time, the cells not having the same tendency to fuse into amorphous material as is seen in caseous tuberculosis. Giant cells may be present in the granulation

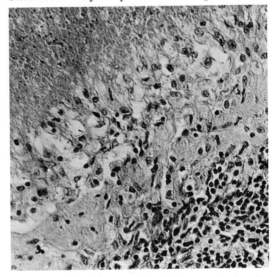

Fig. 8.25 Section of part of a gumma, showing the necrotic centre (*upper left*), bounded by connective tissue heavily infiltrated with lymphocytes. × 250.

* *Tr. pallidum* is argyrophilic (p. 648) and is thus stained by Levaditi's and similar methods based on deposition of silver.

tissue at the periphery, but they are usually smaller than in tuberculosis, and there are no well-formed follicles. Nevertheless the histological diagnosis between the two diseases may be difficult. The important **vascular lesions** of syphilis are described later; those in the larger arteries are due to the presence of spirochaetes in the adventitial sheath and media: they give rise to cellular infiltrations like those described above, and some medial necrosis may follow.

The number of spirochaetes in gummatous lesions is small, and the necrosis seems to be due either to ischaemia resulting from endarteritis of small vessels, or to a hypersensitivity reaction, possibly of delayed type.

A non-venereal form, termed *endemic syphilis* occurs in children in parts of Africa and India, and a similar condition, *bejel* affects young children in Arab countries.

Congenital syphilis

The first pregnancy after untreated infection is likely to terminate prematurely with a macerated fetus, in the tissues of which spirochaetes are abundant. The parenchymatous organs show diffuse proliferation of fibroblasts with minute foci of necrosis—miliary gummas—and there is severe damage to the liver, lungs, pancreas, etc. In subsequent pregnancies the effects are progressively less severe. The next child may be born alive with lesions of congenital syphilis, including a papular rash around mouth and nose, on the buttocks, palms of hands and soles of feet. Disease of the nasal bones and mucosa leads to 'snuffles' and interference with feeding. Syphilitic hepatitis with jaundice, splenomegaly, and lesions in the bones are also common. Later a characteristic deformity appears in the incisor teeth, which are peg-shaped with notched edges (Hutchinson's teeth) and there is also pitting of the first permanent molars. Still later, neurosyphilis may develop and also intestitial keratitis causing corneal opacity and blindness. Pregnancy has a curiously ameliorating effect on syphilitic lesions in the mother, who may appear healthy in spite of producing syphilitic offspring.

Immunology of syphilis

At least three distinct antibodies develop in syphilis, and their detection in the serum is of considerable diagnostic value. The older tests are based on the detection of antibody reactive with the diphosphatidylglycerol component of phospholipids of mitochondrial membranes. Alcoholic extract of beef heart muscle ('*cardiolipin*') is employed as antigen, but extracts of various normal animal and human tissues may also be used. Antibody is demonstrable by various precipitation (flocculation) techniques, e.g. the Kahn, Kline or VDRL (venereal disease research laboratory) tests, or by the Wassermann test which is based on complement fixation (p. 112). These are the so-called **standard tests for syphilis**: they are useful screening tests, antibody being detectable from an early stage, but are not specific for syphilis, **false positive reactions** occurring in various conditions, including many acute infections, malaria, infectious mononucleosis, mycoplasmal pneumonia, trypanosomiasis, leprosy and systemic lupus erythematosus. The tests are also positive occasionally in apparently normal individuals, particularly during pregnancy. It is not understood why antibody to diphosphatidylglycerol develops in syphilis: it fulfils the criteria of an autoantibody (p. 161), and the false positive reactions may result from auto-immunisation as a result of tissue destruction from causes other than syphilis, with release of cellular constituents.

A second antibody, which reacts with group antigen common to various species of treponemes, may be detected by a complement-fixation test, using as antigen non-pathogenic treponemes which grow readily in culture; this is also used as a screening test but is not specific for syphilis.

Confirmatory tests for syphilis depend on the demonstration of antibody specific for *Tr. pallidum* by (a) the treponemal immobilisation test in which the patient's serum is added to a suspension of living *Tr. pallidum* and antibody is indicated by immobilisation of the treponemes, or (b) the fluorescent antibody technique in which binding of antibody to *Tr. pallidum* is demonstrated by means of fluorescein-labelled anti-immunoglobulin (p. 111).

Antibody tests usually become positive a week or so after the appearance of the primary lesion: they are virtually always positive in the secondary stage, following which the percentage of positives falls. In neurosyphilis, antibody is more likely to be detected in the cerebrospinal fluid than in the serum.

Following cure, the antibody tests become negative, although the specific treponemal antibodies may persist for some years.

The protective role of specific immunity in syphilis is suggested by the overwhelming infection which sometimes occurs in the immunologically immature fetus. Some of the features of secondary syphilis, including the widespread skin lesions and occurrence of arthralgia and occasionally glomerulonephritis, are probably due to the union of large amounts of treponemal antigen with circulating antibody, to form immune complexes (pp. 155–6). In both congenital and secondary syphilis, lymphocyte depletion in the T-dependent areas of the spleen and lymph nodes, and depressed T-cell function, have been reported.

Other treponemal diseases

Two other diseases caused by treponemes occur in tropical countries. One is **yaws**, which resembles syphilis but is non-venereal and rarely causes cardiovascular or neurological disease. The causal agent, *Tr. pertenuae* cannot be distinguished from *Tr. pallidum* and infection with either confers immunity to both: the distinction from syphilis is based on clinical features. The second condition is **pinta**, another non-venereal chronic disease somewhat resembling syphilis: it is caused by *Tr. carateum* which does not confer immunity to syphilis.

Other pathogenic spirochaetes

These include the **Borreliae**, which are transmitted by lice and ticks, and cause **relapsing fever** (p. 696) and the **Leptospirae** which infest rodents, etc., and cause febrile illnesses, the best known being Weil's disease (p. 695).

Actinomycosis

This disease is produced by organisms which are normal commensals in the mouth and gut and only occasionally invade the tissues to produce infection. The actinomyces are branching bacteria which grow in the tissues to produce characteristic radiate colonies, sometimes visible macroscopically. In man, the micro-aerophilic *Actinomyces israelii* is the chief pathogen, but occasionally aerobic organisms—*Nocardia*—are involved, and also other species,

which grow more diffusely. In bovines, in which actinomycosis due to *Actino. bovis* is common, the lesions are localised and are large granulomatous masses which occur especially in and around the jaw. In man the disease usually affects children and young adults, more often males than females, and agricultural workers appear to be particularly at risk. The lesions are of a more suppurative type, and in about 70 per cent of cases are in the region of the mouth or jaws, the parasite gaining entrance commonly from a tooth socket following extraction or from a carious tooth. In 15 per cent the infection is in the appendix or caecal region, from which spread by the blood stream to the liver may occur; in about 10 per cent the initial lesion is in the lung and in 5 per cent it is subcutaneous. The lesion is usually a chronic suppurative one, with formation of multiple abscesses, each containing one or more colonies of the organism—the so-called honeycomb abscess. Fibrous septa between the abscesses are lined by granulation tissue which contains many foamy cells—macrophages laden with lipid—giving the lining of each abscess a yellowish colour. In the centre is pus containing actinomyces colonies (Fig. 8.26), which are sometimes visible by naked eye as small yellow or grey, gritty granules ('sulphur granules').

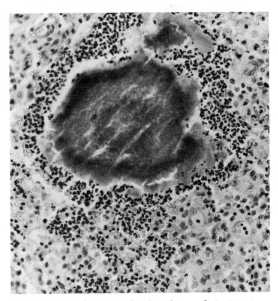

Fig. 8.26 Actinomycosis. A colony of *Actinomyces israelii* in a small abscess, the wall of which consists of granulation tissue heavily infiltrated with lipid-laden (foamy) macrophages. × 190.

Lesions of the face and neck, originating about the jaw, may produce much granulation tissue in which many small foci of suppuration persist and discharge through the skin, resulting in multiple sinuses. The infection spreads directly through the tissues but does not usually involve the regional lymph nodes; if untreated it tends to invade the bloodstream, giving rise to pyaemia with secondary abscesses in the liver, lungs and other organs.

Other Types of Infection

Rickettsial infections

The rickettsiae are micro-organisms of various shapes, smaller than bacteria but resembling them in their structural and metabolic features, including presence of a cell wall. They are obligatory intracellular parasites and infect many species including arthropods, birds and mammals. Several species of rickettsiae cause disease in man: in most instances they enter the body by the bites of infected ticks or mites, or from infected louse or flea faeces being scratched into the skin. The organisms enter and multiply in the endothelium of the capillaries and other small blood vessels; they are at first localised to the site of infection, but blood dissemination occurs during the incubation period and endothelial involvement then becomes widespread. Capillary obstruction from endothelial swelling or thrombosis occurs, with resultant necrosis in heavily involved tissues, and a mixed cell reaction develops, including polymorphs, macrophages, lymphocytes and plasma cells.

The rickettsial diseases include **endemic (murine) typhus**, caused by *R. mooseri* and transmitted by the rat flea; **epidemic typhus** (*R. prowazeki*) and **trench fever** (*R. quintana*) which are spread by the body louse: the **spotted fever** group (*R. rickettsi*, etc.) transmitted from various animals to man by the bites of infected ticks or mites, and finally **scrub typhus** (*R. tsutsugamuchi*), transmitted from rodents to man by a mite. Epidemic and endemic typhus are of world-wide distribution: the epidemic disease occurs in crowded louse-infested communities, and is common in times of war, earthquakes and other major disasters. Man is the only known reservoir of infection of *R. prowazeki*, which can persist for years as a latent infection and cause relapse ('*recrudescent typhus*' or *Brill–Zinsser disease*): such cases are responsible for fresh outbreaks.

Various forms of spotted fever are related to particular localities.

The rickettsial diseases vary in their severity and pathological detail: in all, the small blood vessels are involved, and lesions tend to result especially in the brain, heart and skin. Infected material is particularly dangerous to laboratory workers, and diagnosis is usually made by demonstrating a rising titre of antibody, either in the patient or in laboratory animals inoculated with the patient's blood, etc. Only *R. quintana* has been cultured successfully in cell-free media.

Q fever is a typhus-like illness caused by the *Coxiella burneti* which closely resembles the rickettsiae but differs from them in its antigenicity and in being much more resistant to drying, etc. and in being capable of both intracellular and extracellular growth. It is a parasite of domesticated animals of worldwide distribution and man is infected by inhalation of droplets while attending to animal births or by drinking infected milk, etc. Q fever usually presents as a 'non-bacterial' pneumonia, although lesions may occur in the brain and other organs. *Cox. burneti* may also colonise the valves of the heart, producing a form of infective endocarditis.

Diagnosis is usually based on a rising titre of antibody, but demonstration of *Cox. burneti* in the blood by guinea-pig inoculation is sometimes necessary.

Mycoplasmal infections

Mycoplasmas are very small filamentous or coccobacillary micro-organisms which lack a cell wall but can be grown in cell-free media and are classed as bacteria. They are distributed widely and are pathogenic to many animal and plant species. In man only one species, *Mycoplasma pneumoniae*, has been shown conclusively to be pathogenic, although other mycoplasmas have been isolated from the lesions of various other diseases. A major difficulty arises from their ubiquity and the consequent contamination of culture media; they can pass through bacteria-retaining filters and are also liable to contaminate cell cultures used in virology and for other purposes.

Mycoplasma pneumoniae is the cause of one form of 'non-bacterial' pneumonia, which is endemic in most parts of the world and also occurs as outbreaks, particularly in children. The organism disseminates in the body and may cause a meningo-encephalitis. The immune response includes the production of an antibody which cross-reacts at low temperatures with a human red cell antigen, and is responsible in some cases for acute haemolysis.

Chlamydial infections

The chlamydiae are a group of spherical micro-organisms intermediate in size between the larger viruses and bacteria. They are obligatory intracellular parasites, but otherwise resemble bacteria far more closely than viruses. The vegetative form multiplies by binary fission, and infection is spread by a smaller compact spore-like form (elementary body) which can survive, but not divide, extracellularly.

These organisms are enzootic in certain birds, including the psittacines (parrot family), and also cause infections in sheep, goats and cattle. In man, they are responsible for the sexually transmitted disease **lymphogranuloma inguinale**, for eye infections, the most important being **trachoma**, and for pulmonary infection (**ornithosis**) which results from inhalation of the organism. The initial reaction to chlamydial infection is granulomatous, with accumulation of macrophages and lymphoid cells, necrosis, formation of granulation tissue and scarring. In lymphogranuloma inguinale a small ulcerating primary lesion develops in the genitalia, but the draining lymph nodes become grossly involved and prolonged suppuration and extensive scarring result. Similar lesions occur extragenitally in cat-scratch disease, but the causal agent is uncertain.

Both antibodies and cell-mediated immunity develop in chlamydial infections, the latter probably being the more important in the elimination of the infection. These diseases are considered more fully in the appropriate systematic chapters.

Yeasts and fungi (*Eumycetes*)

Yeasts and fungi are primitive eukaryotic micro-organisms which are now usually classified as neither plant nor animal. They are mainly saprophytic and make an important contribution to the breakdown of dead animal and plant tissues. Only a few of the very many known species are pathogenic to man, and with some exceptions the lesions are superficial and not serious. Good examples of such infection are athlete's foot and thrush (candidiasis). However, in drug addicts, severely ill patients, and particularly in those with T-cell deficiency or on immunosuppressive therapy, some of the fungi can cause more extensive or even systemic infections.

Fungi grow typically as filamentous branching hyphae which form an interlacing mycelium; they produce spores, commonly on projecting (aerial) hyphae. Yeasts consist of simple spherical or ovoid cells which multiply by budding, but the distinction from fungi is not sharp, for the so-called dimorphic fungi can assume the form of either hyphae or yeasts, depending on the environmental conditions.

In general, superficial infections with yeasts or fungi promote a mild inflammatory reaction. The reactions to deeper and more extensive infections vary considerably depending on the nature of the parasite and the host responses: they include necrosis, abscess formation, granulation tissue, and aggregation of macrophages, lymphocytes and plasma cells. In some instances, an epithelioid and giant-cell reaction results in appearances similar to those of tuberculosis, and various hypersensitivity reactions may contribute to the pathological changes. Host defence appears to be mediated largely by cell-mediated immunity.

In superficial infections, diagnosis can often be made from the appearance of the lesion, supported by microscopy of skin or mucosal scrapings, but cultivation on suitable media is sometimes necessary.

Some examples of yeast and fungal infections are described briefly below.

Candidiasis. *Candida albicans* is normally present in the mouth and intestine, and on the surface of moist areas of the skin. Superficial invasion and proliferation results in white patches (**thrush**) consisting of yeast forms and elongated cells (pseudohyphae), with mild inflammation of the affected tissue. It occurs in the vagina, particularly in pregnancy, and in the mouth, particularly in infants and in patients on oral antibiotic therapy. More extensive local and systemic infections occur in debilitated, immunodeficient or immunosuppressed patients. *Muco-cutaneous candidiasis*, affecting principally the face, scalp and mouth, is a chronic and extremely disfiguring condition when it affects children with various grades of T-cell deficiency. In some cases, administration of transfer factor (p. 131) has been followed by remarkable and sometimes prolonged remission. Oesophageal thrush (Fig. 19.18, p. 599) is a common finding at necropsy in subjects who have died following a chronic debilitating disease.

Systemic candidiasis is rare; the lesions consist of multiple small abscesses, resembling those of pyaemia, and are usually most numerous in the kidneys.

Aspergillosis. The spores of various species of

aspergillus, which are filamentous fungi (Fig. 16.32, p. 481), are present in the atmosphere, and large numbers are inhaled, particularly by agricultural workers: clinical infection is, however, uncommon. It is largely confined to the bronchi and lungs and is usually due to *Aspergillus fumigatus*. In most cases there are predisposing factors, such as steroid therapy or the presence in the lungs of bronchiectatic or old tuberculous cavities in which large aspergillus colonies may develop. The fungus may be more aggressive, and produce suppurating and granulating lesions in the lungs: occasionally it invades blood vessels, causing septic thrombosis, and a pyaemic condition.

The immune response includes antibodies and cell-mediated immunity, and complex hypersensitivity reactions may result. In Northern Sudan, a tumour-like granuloma occurs in the paranasal sinuses and orbit.

Histoplasmosis. This is caused by the dimorphic fungus, *Histoplasma capsulatum*, and occurs in many parts of the world, including some parts of North America and Europe. In Africa, most cases are due to *H. duboisii*. Infection usually results from inhalation of spores, which are present in soil and in the faeces of dogs, cats, rodents, bats and birds. In man, pulmonary lesions are most common; they may be single or multiple and usually heal and become calcified. The hilar lymph nodes are often involved. Progressive lung disease sometimes develops and resembles chronic pulmonary tuberculosis in its effects. The organism multiplies in macrophages, in which it is seen as multiple small yeast-like bodies with a double contour: aggregates of macrophages undergo caseous necrosis. In disseminated infection the macrophages throughout the body are colonised and large lesions occur in the liver, spleen, adrenals, marrow, etc.

In areas of high incidence, skin tests with an extract of *H. capsulatum* elicit a delayed hypersensitivity reaction in most individuals, indicating that a high percentage of the population has developed immunity.

Cryptococcosis is caused by the yeast *Cryptococcus neoformans*, which grows in the droppings of pigeons and other birds. Infection in man occurs sporadically throughout the world. It probably results from inhalation of the organism, and produces a localised granulomatous pulmonary lesion: this may heal or extend, and spread may occur by the bloodstream, resulting in widespread granulomatous lesions mostly in the skin, lymph nodes and bones. A chronic meningitis also occurs, in which masses of yeast are seen macroscopically as gelatinous material.

Sporotrichosis is caused by a dimorphic fungus, *Sporothrix schenckii*, which is saprophytic on plants and is present in soil. Infection in man results from accidental inoculation of wounds or minor trauma. Chronic suppurating lesions develop locally and along the line of the draining lymphatics, but systemic infection is rare.

Protozoal and metazoal parasites

Most of the serious diseases caused by protozoan and metazoan parasites are now largely confined to tropical and sub-tropical countries, where they are responsible for an enormous amount of suffering. Because of the increase in world travel, however, these diseases are now encountered more often in visitors and immigrants to temperate areas, and an awareness of this is of major diagnostic importance.

The nature of the parasites, their life cycles and the features of the diseases they cause, are so varied that few useful generalisations can be made, and accordingly the more important individual diseases are described briefly in later chapters, under the systems in which they produce their major effects.

Further Reading

Christie, A. B. (1974). *Infectious Diseases: Epidemiology and Clinical Practice*, 2nd edn., pp. 1095. Churchill–Livingstone, Edinburgh, London and New York. (A highly readable text, dealing with all aspects of infectious disease.)

Collee, J. G. (1976). *Applied Medical Microbiology*, pp. 121. Blackwell Scientific, Oxford. (A short text for students.)

Davis, B. D., Dulbecco, R., Eisen, H. N., Guinsberg, H. S. and Wood, W. B. (1973). *Principles of Microbiology and Immunology*, 2nd edn., pp. 1562. Harper and Rowe, New York. (A comprehensive, well-written text.)

Duguid, J. P., Marmion, B. P. and Swain, R. H. A. (1978). *Medical Microbiology, Vol. 1*, 13th edn., pp. 666. Churchill–Livingstone, Edinburgh, London and New York. (A book for undergraduate and postgraduate students.)

Freeman, Bob A. (Ed.) (1979). *Burrows' Textbook of Microbiology*, 21st edn., pp. 1138. Saunders,

Philadelphia, London and Toronto. (A multi-author text with a major contribution by the editor. Readable and well-illustrated.)

Timbury, M. C. (1978). *Notes on Medical Virology*, 6th edn., pp. 138. Churchill–Livingstone, Edinburgh, London and New York. (A short text for students.)

Tyrrell, David A. J., Phillips, Ian, Goodwin, Stewart C. and Blowers, Robert (1979). *Microbial Disease: the use of the laboratory in diagnosis, therapy and control*, pp. 340. Edward Arnold, London. (A clearly-written book which relates clinical problems with laboratory practice.)

Wilson, G. S. and Miles, A. A. (Eds.) (1975). *Topley and Wilson's Principles and Practice of Bacteriology, Virology and Immunity*, 6th edn., Vols. 1 and 2, pp. 2848. Edward Arnold, London. (A comprehensive text for practising bacteriologists).

9

Disturbances of Blood Flow and Body Fluids

Disturbances of the flow of blood are intimately associated with lesions which affect the functioning of the heart and blood vessels: such lesions will be considered systematically in later chapters. Meanwhile it is useful to outline the main features of disturbances in total and local blood flow, the processes of thrombosis and clotting of the blood, and the disturbances in composition and volume of the body fluids. Accordingly, this chapter provides a general account of these phenomena.

Changes in Flow and Distribution of the Blood

Increase in total blood flow

This occurs when a sufficient number of arterioles relax to result in significant increase in the rate of passage of blood from the arterial to the venous compartment of the circulation. Physiological examples include the active hyperaemia in the skeletal muscles during physical activity and in the splanchnic circulation during digestion of a heavy meal. Pathological conditions causing an increase in total blood flow include the following.

(a) **Hypoxia,** which consists of significant fall in the amount of oxygen delivered to the tissues. This occurs in anaemia, i.e. a reduction in the amount of haemoglobin in the blood. In severe anaemia, cardiac output increases, but not enough to compensate for the reduced oxygen carrying capacity of the blood, and the tissues suffer from **anaemic hypoxia.**

Hypoxia occurs also when, as a result of various abnormalities of pulmonary function, the arterial blood is not fully oxygenated (**hypoxic hypoxia**). In lesions which interfere with pulmonary ventilation, the situation is complicated by increased P_{CO_2} of the blood, which, together with lowered P_{O_2}, is termed **asphyxia.** Congenital abnormalities of the heart or great vessels which result in mixing of venous and arterial blood can also cause hypoxic hypoxia.

Increased cardiac output is a feature of these various conditions, but it does not, of course, occur in heart failure, in which **ischaemic hypoxia** results from diminished perfusion of the tissues due to failing capacity of the heart to maintain the circulation.

(b) **Increased metabolic activity.** The general body metabolism is increased in hyperthyroidism (thyrotoxicosis), in fever, and convalescence from severe injury. The increased metabolism in these conditions is associated with an increased total blood flow.

(c) **Arterio-venous shunts.** A single large communication (fistula) between an artery and vein, such as sometimes results from trauma, allows the transfer of part of the cardiac output to the venous side of the circulation, and so reduces the amount of arterial blood available for tissue perfusion.

(d) **Extensive active hyperaemia.** In generalised inflammatory conditions of the skin, the active hyperaemia is sufficiently extensive to cause a significant increase in total blood flow. Similarly, a chronic increase in total blood flow occurs in Paget's disease affecting several large bones. In this condition, the marrow cavity of the affected bones is replaced by vascular granulation tissue, with local increase in blood flow. Also, there is persistent reflex active hyperaemia of the overlying skin and soft tissues, and the total blood flow is consequently increased (see Singer *et al.*, 1978).

(e) Liver failure. The cause of increased blood flow in liver failure is uncertain: it may be due to the vasodilator effects of accumulated metabolites, or of compounds absorbed from the gut, which are normally removed from the blood by the liver cells.

In these various conditions, increased cardiac output is associated with a lowering of arteriolar tone: the pulse is bounding (of high amplitude) and the skin is warm and pink. The mechanism of these changes is complex and not fully understood: the autonomic nervous system, vasomotor centres, adrenal cortex and medulla, local effects of tissue metabolites, baro- and chemo-receptors, are all involved. If long continued, as in untreated hyperthyroidism, the increased work of the heart is likely to lead to *'high-output' cardiac failure*, particularly in older people and especially if the heart is already handicapped by coronary artery disease or other abnormalities.

Locally increased blood flow

The outstanding example of a pathological increase in local blood flow is **acute inflammation,** in which arteriolar dilatation results in active hyperaemia (p. 45) and the characteristic warmth and erythema of the inflamed tissue. Active hyperaemia occurs also **following a period of temporary obstruction of the circulation**: this is important when the local circulation is arrested to facilitate a surgical operation, e.g. on a limb, for hyperaemia develops gradually, and small vessels which do not bleed immediately after the circulation is restored may subsequently do so.

Reduction in total blood flow

This is a feature of **heart failure**, in which the heart is incapable of maintaining the normal output. The condition may occur acutely, usually as a result of myocardial infarction, or chronic heart failure may result from inadequate function of the myocardium, usually due to coronary artery disease or to increased workload as in valvular lesions or pulmonary or systemic arterial hypertension. Chronic heart failure is often progressive; the heart is incapable initially of supplying the increased output required during physical activity, etc., but eventually it may fail to maintain an adequate circulation even at rest.

Reduced cardiac output is also the major feature of the acute condition of **shock,** in which grossly inadequate tissue perfusion can be fatal (pp. 260–5).

The cardiac output is also reduced in states of **general metabolic depression**, the commonest example being hypothyroidism, but in this instance it simply reflects the reduced requirements for tissue perfusion and is not of pathogenic importance.

The serious effects of heart failure are due very largely to **defective tissue perfusion,** which impairs the functions of all the organs. There are, however, two important structural effects: one is **general venous congestion**, from which the term **congestive heart failure** is derived: it is described below. The other is an increase in extravascular fluid, giving rise to **oedema**, which is described on pp. 253 *et seq*.

Local reduction in blood flow (local ischaemia)

This is of extreme importance since it accounts for a high proportion of cardiac and cerebral disease. Reduction of flow is usually due to **arterial narrowing**, or **complete obstruction by thrombosis or embolism**. These latter processes are described on pp. 235–45, and local ischaemia on pp. 245–51.

Local ischaemia can result also from *venous obstruction*, when it is accompanied by local venous congestion and commonly by oedema.

Venous congestion

When the heart fails to expel the normal amount of blood, arteriolar tone in general increases and a greater proportion of the blood accumulates in the venous compartment, which is readily distensible. This, together with an increase in blood volume (the mechanism of which is poorly understood) causes the veins to become engorged with blood. **Systemic venous congestion**, i.e. engorgement of the systemic veins, is most severe when the failure is predominantly of the right ventricle, as occurs in narrowing (stenosis) of the pulmonary valve orifice and in various diseases of the lungs which interfere with pulmonary blood flow.

Pulmonary venous congestion develops when there is failure of the left ventricle, as in many cases of coronary artery disease or systemic arterial hypertension: it occurs also when mitral valve stenosis restricts the flow of blood into the left ventricle, and may be present for many years without the development of heart failure. In both conditions, there is a rise in pulmonary arterial pressure due to hypertrophy and increased tone of the pulmonary arterioles, often leading to right ventricular failure and systemic venous congestion.

Venous congestion may also be localised to parts of the systemic circulation as a result of obstruction to the venous outflow. Such **localised venous congestion** is commonly seen as a result of thrombosis of the leg veins, often extending up to and involving the femoral vein. It occurs in the spleen and gastro-intestinal tract when portal venous flow is obstructed, as in cirrhosis of the liver. Various other veins may be obstructed, either by thrombosis or by pressure or constriction by a tumour or by scar tissue.

Systemic venous congestion

As explained above, this usually results from heart failure and, depending on the nature of the heart lesion, may be acute or chronic. In both instances, the outlook depends on the reversibility or otherwise of the cardiac failure: if this persists for long, the morphological changes of chronic venous congestion are striking, but it must be emphasised that *the congestive element is less important than the inadequate tissue perfusion of heart failure.*

The systemic veins can dilate to accommodate more blood without an immediate rise of venous pressure, but as the congestion increases, the pressure rises. This may be demonstrated directly by venous catheterisation, but commonly it is apparent from pulsation of the veins in the neck when the patient is sitting or standing. Normally, the neck veins in these postures are partly collapsed and do not pulsate visibly, the pressure in them being slightly below atmospheric. When venous pressure rises, however, the veins in the lower part of the neck are distended, and they pulsate at about the level where the blood is at atmospheric pressure.

Because of the reduced blood flow in heart failure, the degree of oxygen dissociation in the capillaries is greater than normal, and in vascular tissues there may be sufficient reduced haemoglobin to give the purple-blue colour of **cyanosis**: this is seen, for example, in the lips and buccal mucosa. When there is also systemic venous congestion, the distension of the venules and capillaries with sluggishly-flowing oxygen-deficient blood increases the degree of cyanosis. Venous congestion may be present without oedema, but oedema usually accompanies severe congestive heart failure: it is most marked in the lower parts of the body, and chronic hypoxia and the increased venous pressure are probably both contributory factors.

Structural changes of systemic venous congestion. Apart from gravity-dependent oedema (p. 255), the structural changes in systemic venous congestion are most obvious in the abdominal viscera. The **liver** may be moderately enlarged and is often tender and palpable. Microscopically, the centrilobular veins* are dis-

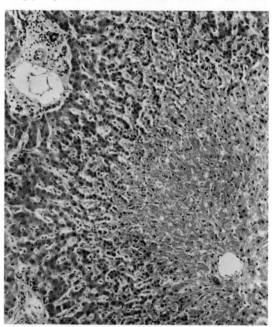

Fig. 9.1 Liver in chronic venous congestion, showing centrilobular atrophy and disappearance of liver cells accompanied by dilatation of sinusoids (rt. side of figure). × 105.

---

* The relationship between the traditional liver *lobule* and the *acinus*, the newer concept of the structural unit of the liver, is described on p. 661.

tended and the central part of each lobule consists of distended sinusoids, the hepatocytes having undergone atrophy and disappeared (Fig. 9.1). Macroscopically, this results in accentuation of the lobular pattern, the dark, congested centrilobular areas contrasting with the paler, sometimes fatty peripheral lobular cells (Fig. 9.2). Because of its similarity to the

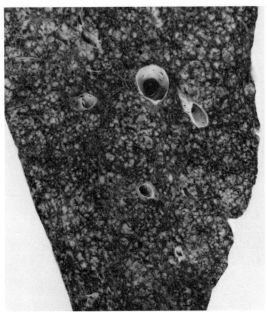

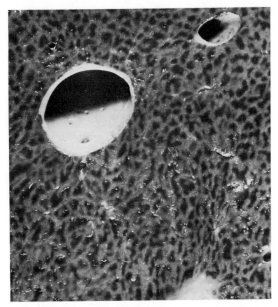

Fig. 9.2 The cut surface of the liver in chronic venous congestion. The congested centrilobular zones are dark, and contrast with the pale peripheral-lobular zones, giving the nutmeg-like appearance. × 1·8.

surface of a nutmeg cut longitudinally, this appearance has long been described by pathologists as 'nutmeg liver'. In some cases, and particularly when there have been recurrent periods of congestive heart failure, centrilobular fibrosis occurs and nodules of hyperplastic parenchyma result from compensatory proliferation of surviving hepatocytes. The liver then appears diffusely irregular (Fig. 9.3): although commonly termed *cardiac cirrhosis*, these changes differ from true cirrhosis and do not progress to liver failure.

The **spleen** may be enlarged up to 250 g. It feels firm and maintains its firmness and shape on slicing, little blood escaping from the cut surface. The red pulp is congested and appears almost black: the Malpighian bodies may be visible as contrasting pale spots. Microscopy

Fig. 9.3 Nodules of hyperplasia in the liver in chronic venous congestion, giving the irregular appearances of so-called cardiac cirrhosis. × 1.

shows congestion of the venous sinuses in the red pulp, with some thickening of the reticulin framework and atrophy of the medullary cords (Fig. 9.4). More marked congestion of the

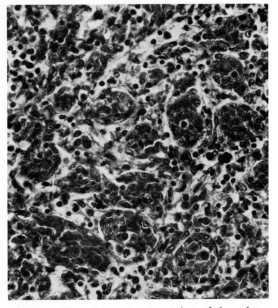

Fig. 9.4 Chronic venous congestion of the spleen. The vascular sinuses are distended with blood, and the intervening medullary cords are relatively inconspicuous. × 250.

spleen is seen in portal venous hypertension (p. 692).

The **kidneys** may be slightly enlarged and the medulla is particularly dark and congested; congestion is less obvious in the cortex, and appears as dark radial streaking (Fig. 9.5).

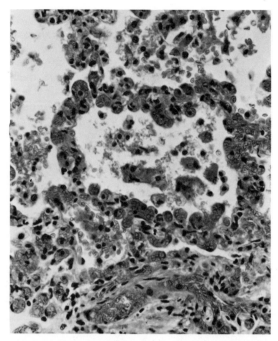

Fig. 9.6 Chronic pulmonary congestion, showing thickening of the alveolar walls, capillary congestion, and free (iron-containing) macrophages in the alveolar spaces. × 210.

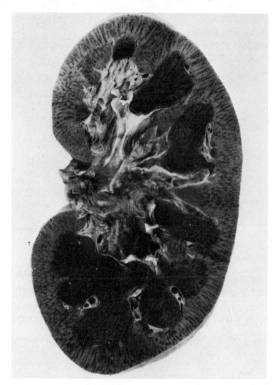

Fig. 9.5 Kidney in chronic venous congestion, showing the intense vascular engorgement, particularly of the medulla. × 0·7.

These changes in the abdominal viscera are without serious effects: there may be mild or sub-clinical jaundice, and some red cells and protein in the urine, but the underlying condition of cardiac insufficiency is far more important.

In venous congestion of the **lungs**, the pulmonary venules and alveolar capillaries are engorged with blood (Fig. 9.6) and their walls become thickened. Red cells escape into the alveoli, sometimes resulting in bloodstained sputum, but many of them are broken down by alveolar macrophages, which come to contain large amounts of haemosiderin. The macrophages accumulate in the alveoli around respiratory bronchioles (Fig. 10.10, p. 279) and as haemosiderin is gradually released, the reticulin

fibres in the alveolar walls become encrusted with it and fibrous thickening occurs. These changes result in increased firmness and give the lung a brown appearance (*brown induration*). The fine structural changes of pulmonary venous congestion are described on p. 457.

Many patients with chronic pulmonary congestion suffer from attacks of pulmonary oedema. They also develop pulmonary hypertension with its associated vascular changes (pp. 454–7). The iron-laden macrophages may be found in the sputum: they have been termed 'heart failure' cells, but are often present in pulmonary venous congestion, e.g. in mitral stenosis, for years before heart failure supervenes.

Local venous congestion

As mentioned above, this results from mechanical interference with the venous drainage of blood from an organ, limb, etc. The effects depend on the rapidity, degree and duration of obstruction and also on the local vascular arrangements.

Acute venous obstruction, e.g. by thrombosis or by a ligature does not usually cause complete arrest of blood flow because in most parts of the body there is sufficient venous anastamosis to carry the blood away from the drainage area affected. In a few places, e.g. in the intestine, venous anastomosis is inadequate: the tissue becomes swollen, engorged with blood, and haemorrhagic due to rupture of small vessels. Ischaemic necrosis (venous infarction, p. 248) then develops.

In most sites, acute venous obstruction has less serious effects, and acute congestion either subsides or becomes chronic. This is illustrated by thrombosis of the deep veins of the leg, which is the commonest example of local venous obstruction, and often extends up to the femoral vein and even beyond. The limb may become cold, cyanosed and oedematous, but there is nearly always sufficient anastomosis to prevent infarction. The effects tend to subside gradually, partly because the anastomotic channels increase in calibre, and partly because the size of the thrombus is reduced by contraction and by digestion by plasmin. The lumen of the occluded vessel is often largely restored, and blood flow increases. Eventually, organisation and recanalisation of residual thrombus may further restore blood flow, but in spite of these changes, deep vein thrombosis, if extensive, sometimes results in chronic venous obstruction and persistent oedema of the limb. Venous valves may be put out of action if they are caught up in an organising thrombus, and this may also be a source of persistent trouble.

Chronic venous obstruction may result from thrombosis, as mentioned above, or from compression or invasion of a vein by tumour, or constriction by fibrous tissue. When obstruction develops gradually, collateral veins enlarge (Fig. 9.7) and drainage is often well maintained.

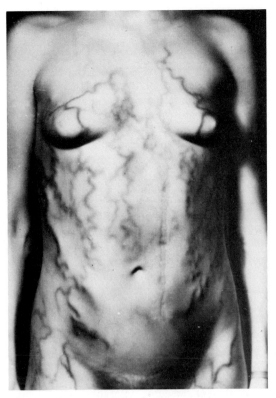

Fig. 9.7 Infra-red photograph showing enlargement of superficial veins to establish collateral circulation in a patient with obstruction of the inferior vena cava. (Dr. G. Watkinson.)

In chronic portal venous obstruction, which is an important effect of cirrhosis of the liver, the veins connecting the portal venous tributaries with systemic veins become enlarged and help to drain the portal system, but one such group of anastomotic veins, which run longitudinally in the submucosa of the lower oesophagus (Fig. 19.22, p. 604), is liable to rupture, causing serious or fatal haemorrhage.

Haemostasis and Thrombosis

It is essential that the blood should remain fluid within the cardiovascular system, and yet should be capable of *local haemostasis* by forming a solid adherent plug to prevent excessive bleeding from an injury to a vessel wall. The vital importance of these properties of blood is reflected in the complexity of the systems involved.

The repair of vascular injury

Injuries of vessel walls can be classified as major, when tissue is torn or cut and blood vessels are severed, and as minor 'wear-and-tear' defects which result from normal activities. **The minor defects** are presumably due to injury or loss of individual endothelial cells with consequent exposure of collagen, elastin, etc. Such lesions are repaired almost instantaneously by adherence of platelets, followed by growth of endothelium over the adherent platelets to restore the integrity of the vessel wall. The importance of platelets is illustrated by the spontaneous haemorrhages which occur from the microvessels in severe thrombocytopenia (a reduction in the number of platelets). The role of fibrin deposition is illustrated by the haemorrhages into joints (haemarthroses) in severe haemophilia, a hereditary condition in which the coagulation or clotting process (formation of solid fibrin) is defective. Evidently the small vessels in the joints are normally exposed to degrees of injury which, although minor, cannot be repaired by platelets alone.

More severe injury results in partial or complete severance of larger vessels. Loss of blood is diminished temporarily by **vasoconstriction**: platelets stick to the collagen fibres of the torn edge of the vessel wall and, together with deposition of fibrin strands, gradually build up to form a mass—the **haemostatic plug**, which may close the gap in the vessel and prevent further bleeding. Vascular endothelium extends to cover the haemostatic plug which is then gradually removed by the process of organisation and proliferation of smooth muscle cells, the sub-endothelial gap thus being permanently repaired.

The factors involved in haemostasis

As explained above, vascular defects are repaired initially by formation of a haemostatic plug. This is an example of *thrombosis* (intravascular formation of solid material or *thrombus* from the constituents of the blood). In order to understand such beneficial haemostasis, and also disorders which upset the normal balance between the fluidity of the blood and its capacity to undergo thrombosis, it is necessary to consider in more detail the major factors involved: these are the *platelets, vascular endothelium*, the *clotting* or *coagulation process* which leads to deposition of fibrin, and the *plasmin system* which digests fibrin.

Platelet function

In normal blood, platelets circulate as single disc-like fragments of cytoplasm lined by a plasma membrane. They do not adhere to normal endothelium but, as stated above, if endothelium is lost they adhere to the exposed collagen fibres. Adherent platelets undergo structural changes and discharge the contents of their storage granules (Fig. 9.8)—*the platelet release reaction*; these include adenosine diphosphate (ADP), 5-hydroxytryptamine, platelet factor 3, thromboxane A_2, stable prosta-

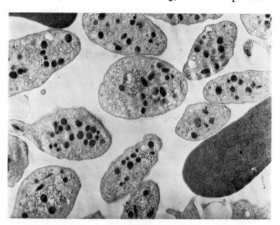

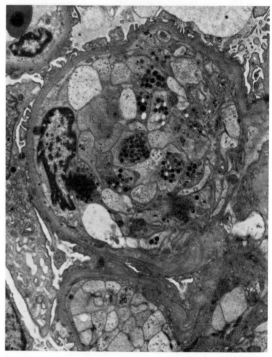

Fig. 9.8 Electron-micrographs of platelets. *Above*, free platelets in suspension, showing the dense storage granules. $\times 8000$. *Below*, two glomerular capillaries plugged by aggregated platelets, most of which have discharged their granules. $\times 3000$.

glandins, and a factor which stimulates proliferation of smooth muscle cells. These platelet products have at least three important effects. Firstly, thromboxane A_2, 5-HT and some stable prostaglandins, e.g. F_1, promote local vascular contraction. Secondly, ADP and thromboxane A_2 both cause free platelets to alter shape, throw out pseudopodia, and adhere to one another and to those already adherent to the vessel wall: the release reaction continues and the result is the rapid development of the platelet mass. Thirdly, platelet factor 3 (and also factors released from injured tissue) initiates the clotting mechanism: this results in deposition of strands of fibrin which reinforce the platelet plug. Fibrin and thrombin (another product of the clotting system) both tend to promote further deposition of platelets.

Platelet function may be studied in various ways, e.g. by assessment of the percentage of platelets in a given sample which adhere to a standard column of glass beads through which the blood is passed, or the aggregation of platelets in plasma following the addition of aggregating substances such as ADP. These techniques have shown that there are a number of syndromes in which, although platelet counts are normal, platelet function is abnormal. Conditions with deficient platelet function include uraemia, the primary thrombocytopathies and hereditary haemorrhagic telangiectasia (p. 557): increased platelet adhesiveness and aggregation have been found in diseases associated with thrombo-embolic phenomena such as ischaemic heart disease, peripheral vascular disease and venous thrombosis. In the puerperium and following surgical operations, platelet adhesiveness is increased, the effect being maximal around the tenth post-operative day. This contributes to the post-operative thrombotic tendency.

Prostacyclin and thromboxane A_2. In the past five years intense interest has developed in the influence of prostaglandins on platelet function and thrombosis. This has been stimulated by the discovery of prostacyclin (PGI_2) and thromboxane A_2, both of which are highly unstable prostaglandins with half lives of about 2 minutes and 30 seconds respectively. They are derived from arachidonic acid, a polyunsaturated long-chain fatty acid which is produced from linoleic acid and is a constituent of the phospholipid of cell membranes. All cells also possess in their membrane prostaglandin (PG) synthetase

(cyclo-oxygenase), which converts arachidonic acid into unstable cyclic endoperoxides. As shown in Fig. 9.9, the endoperoxides, in turn, can be converted into prostacyclin, thromboxane A_2, and stable prostaglandins (PGE_2, etc.). Vascular endothelium is rich in prostacyclin synthetase and so produces mainly prostacyclin, whereas platelets convert endoperoxides mainly into thromboxane A_2.

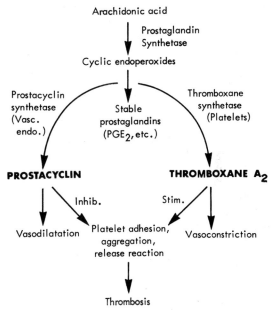

Fig. 9.9. The production of the unstable prostaglandins—prostacyclin and thromboxane A_2—by vascular endothelium and platelets respectively, and their effects on the adhesion, aggregation and release reaction of platelets.

The role of thromboxane A_2 in promoting haemostasis is described above. There seems no doubt that it plays an important role in platelet aggregation and thrombosis. Inhibition of its production by aspirin in low dosage or imidazole derivatives (both of which inhibit thromboxane synthetase) renders platelets less readily adhesive and prolongs the bleeding time from a minor puncture wound. Prostacyclin has antagonistic effects: it causes vasodilatation and inhibits aggregation of platelets, disperses pre-formed platelet aggregates, and so inhibits thrombosis. It now seems very likely that these effects on platelets are mediated via the cyclic nucleotide system (p. 144), prostacyclin stimulating adenyl cyclase and thus increasing cAMP, thromboxane A_2 having the opposite effect. Platelet aggregation and the release reaction are promoted by a low cAMP and inhibited by a high cAMP level.

It has been proposed by Moncada and Vane (1979) that prostacyclin exerts both a local and systemic control on platelet function. Its production by vascular endothelium may be of importance in preventing adhesion of platelets to normal endothelium. Mild physical or chemical injury to endothelium stimulates prostacyclin synthetase and so production of prostacyclin. Such injury may be sufficient to allow platelet adhesion to the damaged wall, thus effecting repair, but without the building up of a platelet aggregate, which is prevented by very low levels of prostacyclin.

The postulated systemic homoeostatic role of prostacyclin is attributed to its continuous release into the blood passing through the lungs. It is suggested that this maintains a level of cAMP in the free platelets which modulates their tendency to aggregate. There is, however, evidence that small loose aggregates of circulating platelets do sometimes occur, and this may be a cause of transient neurological symptoms in old people (p. 743).

These proposals are of potential importance in the use of drugs to influence thrombosis. For example aspirin, which is under trial in the prevention of coronary artery thrombosis, would be expected to inhibit thrombosis if given in low dosage, for this inhibits thromboxane synthetase; larger doses, which also inhibit prostaglandin synthetase, would be expected to interfere with production of both prostacyclin and thromboxane A_2 (Fig. 9.9), and thus have less or no inhibitory effect on platelet aggregation and thrombosis. There is some evidence in support of this (Masotti *et al.*, 1979).

The unstable prostaglandins are obviously of interest in relation to the thrombogenic theory of atheroma (p. 367).

The coagulation (clotting) mechanism

By clotting is meant the conversion of fibrinogen to solid fibrin. This is the result of a complex series of reactions involving sequential activation of a large number of clotting factors most of which have been purified, although the relative importance of the various parts of the system is not yet clear. Not only is the system complex, but most of the major factors have been numbered (I to XIII, Table 9.1) in the order of their discovery, and not in the order of their participation. The clotting process up to the activation of factor X can occur by two main routes, the *intrinsic* and *extrinsic pathways*. After this stage, there is a *common pathway* leading to the formation of fibrin. The complexity of the process is indicated by Fig. 9.10 which is a simplified scheme.

The intrinsic pathway results in clotting without the participation of factors released from

Table 9.1   International classification of the plasma coagulation factors (Roman numerals), together with their commonly-used names. The term 'factor VI', formerly applied to an intermediate product, is no longer used.

Factor I	Fibrinogen
Factor II	Prothrombin
Factor III	Tissue factor
Factor IV	Calcium
Factor V	Proaccelerin
Factor VII	Proconvertin
Factor VIII	Antihaemophilic globulin
Factor IX	Plasma thromboplastin component or Christmas factor
Factor X	Stuart–Prower factor
Factor XI	Plasma thromboplastin antecedent
Factor XII	Hageman factor
Factor XIII	Fibrin stabilising factor (plasma transglutaminase)

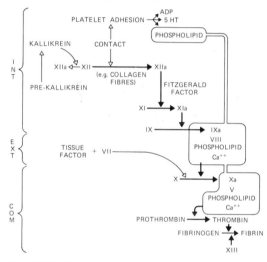

Fig. 9.10   The reactions involved in the clotting mechanisms. INT, intrinsic pathway; EXT, extrinsic pathway; COM, common pathway.

injured tissues. It occurs when blood is placed in a tube and is probably involved in minor vascular injury and when blood stagnates in a blood vessel. It is initiated by contact of factor XII (Hageman factor) with a foreign surface or with collagen. Activated factor XII (termed XIIa)* is an esterolytic enzyme which, together with another factor (Fitzgerald factor), converts factor XI to XIa; this, in turn, activates factor IX. Factor X is then activated by a reaction involving IXa, Ca^{++}, phospholipid and factor VIII (antihaemophilic factor).

The extrinsic pathway is activated by tissue injury. It is triggered by a lipoprotein complex

* The activated factors are indicated by the suffix 'a'.

(tissue factor 3 or thrombokinase), which activates factor VII: this in turn activates factor X.

The common pathway. Factor Xa, produced by either of the above routes, is a serine esterase which forms a complex with factor V and phospholipid in the presence of Ca^{++}: this complex converts factor II (prothrombin) to IIa (thrombin) which converts fibrinogen to fibrin monomer. Factor XIII then polymerises fibrin monomer to form insoluble fibrin.

The clotting process is influenced by a number of *amplifying and inhibiting reactions.* For example, in the intrinsic system activated Hageman factor (XIIa) converts prekallikrein (a component of the kinin system) to kallikrein, which activates more Hageman factor, while factor VII, which participates in the extrinsic pathway, is activated by a number of other factors—thrombin, XIIa, kallikrein, IXa and plasmin (see below). For the various activation steps there are specific inhibitors which modulate the clotting process and help to prevent inadvertent thrombosis.

The fibrinolytic (plasmin) system

This is shown diagrammatically in Fig. 9.11. Its activation results in the production of *plasmin*, a proteolytic enzyme which digests fibrin to soluble fibrin degradation products (FDP). Plasminogen is a β-globulin in the plasma. It is activated by a factor in vascular endothelium, by tissue factors, factor XIIa, and various bacterial products and chemicals. Plasmin digests not only fibrin, but also factors V, VIII and II (prothrombin): its activation and enzymic activity are controlled by a number of inhibitors in plasma, notably α_2-macroglobulin and α_1-antitrypsin.

Plasminogen binds selectively to polymerising fibrin and is then converted to active plasmin by activators which diffuse into the clot or thrombus where the effect of inhibitors is weak. Plasmin activity in the plasma is prevented by the presence of factors which both inhibit its formation and suppress its activity. It is, however, possible to prevent such inhibition by administration of urokinase or streptokinase. Increased plasmin activity of the plasma is found after exercise or emotional stress, and also following surgical operations and other trauma.

Plasminogen (inactive plasma globulin)

Activators——→

Plasmin (proteolytic enzyme)

Fibrin——→soluble products

Fig. 9.11 The fibrinolytic enzyme system.

The fibrinolytic enzyme system is probably in dynamic equilibrium with the blood clotting system, the two acting together to maintain an intact and patent vascular tree. According to this hypothesis the coagulation and fibrinolytic systems may both be continuously active, the former laying down fibrin where needed on the endothelium to seal any deficiencies which may occur, and the latter removing such deposits after they have served their haemostatic function.

As explained in earlier chapters (e.g. p. 54) there are complex inter-relationships between the clotting, kinin, plasmin and complement systems, none of which can now be regarded in isolation.

Pathological Thrombosis

Thrombosis is defined as the formation of a solid or semi-solid mass from the constituents of the blood within the vascular system during life. Coagulation, i.e. deposition of fibrin, is involved in the formation of all thrombi except perhaps the minute deposits of platelets which maintain vascular integrity (p. 232). As already noted, the composition of thrombus is determined very largely by the rate of flow of the blood from which it forms.

Appearances and composition of thrombi

As a general rule, thrombus forming in rapidly flowing blood, e.g. in an artery, consists mainly of aggregated platelets, with some fibrin; it enlarges slowly and is firm and pale, varying from greyish white to pale red, and is commonly called *pale thrombus*. The proportion of fibrin deposited in pale thrombus depends partly on the rate of blood flow, to which it has an inverse relationship. At the other extreme, thrombus forming in stagnant blood, e.g. adjacent to a complete occlusion of a blood vessel, is indistinguishable from blood which has been allowed to clot *in vitro*: the thrombus is soft, dark *red*, gelatinous and consists of strands of fibrin lying among the elements of whole blood (Fig. 9.12). It may retract from the vessel wall, revealing a smooth, shiny surface. Between these two extremes we have *mixed thrombi* which form in slowly flowing blood, usually in veins, and consist of alternating layers of platelet aggregates and red thrombus. The mixture may be intimate and only recognisable on microscopy: Fig. 9.13 shows such a thrombus in which spaces between masses of aggregated platelets are filled by a fibrin network containing leukocytes and some red cells. In other instances, veins may be filled with columns of red thrombus but with platelet aggregates at points of anastomosis. The formation of such thrombi is explained on p. 240. Except in recently formed thrombi, it is not easy to recognise ag-

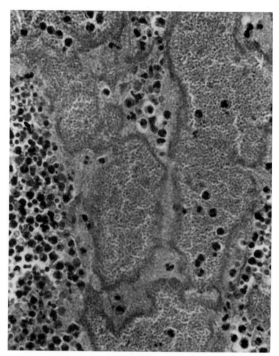

Fig. 9.13 Mixed thrombus, about 12 hours old, showing dense masses of granular material, composed mainly of platelets, fibrin strands and collections of leukocytes. × 336.

gregated platelets, for they soon lose their outlines, presenting microscopically a granular or structureless appearance. Immunofluorescence studies and electron microscopy (Fig. 9.8) have, however, helped in their recognition.

Sites and predisposing factors of thrombosis

The three major predisposing factors are:

(*a*) *local abnormalities in the walls of blood vessels or of the heart*

(*b*) *slowing and other disturbances of blood flow*

(*c*) *changes in the blood favouring platelet aggregation and fibrin formation.*

The roles of these three factors in the formation of thrombi in the heart, arteries and veins are considered below.

(a) Cardiac thrombosis

Thrombi may form on the walls of any of the chambers of the heart, and also on the valve cusps.

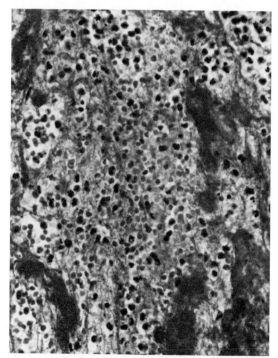

Fig. 9.12 Red thrombus, consisting of strands of fibrin lying among red cells, leucocytes and platelets. In this instance the proportion of entrapped red cells is much lower than in blood clot, indicating that there has been some flow of blood during thrombosis. × 305.

In the atria, thrombosis is commonest in the appendices, especially that of the right atrium, in cases of heart failure with atrial dilatation (Fig. 15.25, p. 417). Stagnation of blood is the important causal factor and this is accentuated by atrial fibrillation, which commonly occurs in such patients and is very liable to be complicated by atrial thrombosis: the thrombus is usually red and is moulded to the irregular wall of the atrium.

Rarely, small flattened globular thrombi form in either the atria or ventricles. They are pale, composed mainly of platelets and may show central softening. In mitral stenosis, a rounded thrombus may develop in the left atrium. It may exceed 3 cm in diameter and become detached to lie free: it is a rare cause of sudden obstruction of the circulation—the so-called 'ball valve thrombus'. The vegetations which form **on the heart valves** in certain diseases are essentially thrombi. In rheumatic fever the valve cusps are damaged along the line of apposition, and deposition of platelets and fibrin results in the formation of minute pinkish-grey bead-like vegetations (Fig. 9.14 and Fig. 15.22, p. 413): in infective endocarditis the cusps are damaged by microbial infection and much more fibrin is deposited, containing interspersed leukocytes; the vegetations are consequently larger, softer and more friable (Fig. 9.15). **In the ventricles**, mural thrombosis commonly occurs on the endocardium overlying an infarct (i.e. a patch of ischaemic necrosis of the heart wall—Fig. 9.16). Depending on the size of the infarct, the thrombus may be large or small. It forms a flat reddish—or, if older, a brown—patch attached to the endocardium. Probably the important factors in its formation are the disturbances in blood flow caused by lack of pulsation in the dead muscle and also diffusion of factor III (tissue thromboplastin) from the dead tissue.

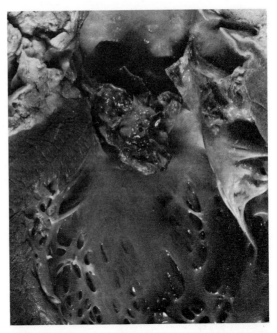

Fig. 9.15 Bacterial endocarditis. The root of the aorta has been cut open and the wall folded back to display the large irregular thrombotic vegetations which have formed on, and are obscuring, the aortic valve cusps.

At necropsy, **clots formed after death** are usually to be found in the chambers of the heart. They are soft and dark red with a glistening surface and are not firmly adherent to the endocardium. Occasionally the red cells settle before coagulation occurs and the upper (usually anterior) part of the clot is then yellow and gelatinous. Thrombi may form rapidly as the circulation is failing immediately before death. They are yellow or pinkish with a glistening surface and have a somewhat stringy appearance (Fig. 9.17). Such **agonal thrombi** originate at

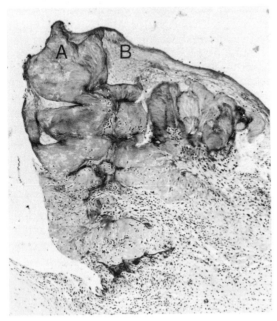

Fig. 9.14 Rheumatic vegetation on a cusp of the mitral valve. The vegetation consists mainly of dense hyaline material (A) composed of fused platelets, and fibrin coagulum (B). × 60.

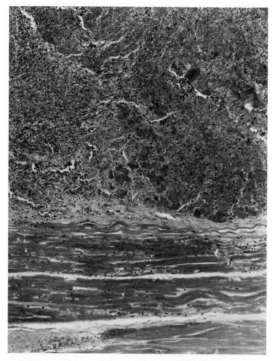

Fig. 9.16 Mural thrombus (*above*) which has formed on the ventricular endocardium over a myocardial infarct. Note the necrotic myocardium (*below*). × 120.

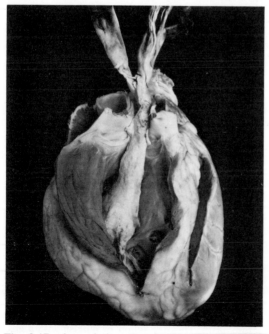

Fig. 9.17 Agonal thrombus in the right ventricle, extending along the pulmonary artery. × ½.

the apex of the ventricle to which they are attached and may extend through the valve orifice. They are composed mainly of fibrin, which separates out from the sluggishly moving blood before death, and may occur in either or both ventricles, although they are commoner in the right side of the heart.

(b) Arterial thrombosis

Probably because of the rapid flow of blood, arterial thrombosis is uncommon in the absence of a local lesion of the vessel wall. In affluent communities, **atheroma** is by far the commonest predisposing local lesion. It consists of multiple patches of fibrous thickening and lipid deposition in the intima of arteries of various sizes. *In the aorta*, atheroma is commonly severe and results in gross distortion and unevenness of the wall. When blood is flowing smoothly in a normal vessel, the particulate elements are separated from the vascular endothelium by a layer of almost pure plasma, but atheromatous plaques, by causing irregularities of the wall, result in turbulent flow, and platelets can then impinge on the wall. This alone probably predisposes to thrombosis, but because of the rapid flow of blood, thrombosis is often not superadded. Frequently, however, atheromatous patches ulcerate, and thrombosis supervenes. In the aorta the thrombi are usually *mural*, i.e. the ulcerated atheromatous patch becomes coated by thrombus which does not extend to occlude the lumen (Fig. 9.18). Thrombosis also complicates atheroma in *medium-sized and smaller arteries*, particularly those supplying the heart and brain. Because of their relatively small calibre, which is further reduced by the atheromatous plaques, thrombi readily occlude these vessels completely and ischaemic necrosis commonly occurs in the deprived tissues. This is described later in the section on infarction and also in the appropriate systematic chapters. When there is gross **localised dilatation (aneurysm)** of the wall of the heart, aorta or other arteries, stagnation and eddying of the blood usually result in some thrombosis. The thrombus may have a laminated appearance and may come to fill the aneurysmal sac (Fig. 9.19). **Inflammatory lesions** in the walls of arteries (pp. 377–83) also cause thrombosis: contributory factors may be irregularities of the wall, injury to or loss of the vascular endothelium, and release of tissue thromboplastin. In **severe arterial hypertension**,

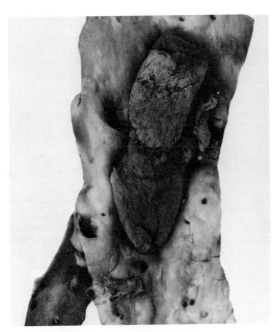

Fig. 9.18 Part of the abdominal aorta opened up to show a large thrombus which has formed over atheromatous patches. The dull, pale, shaggy thrombus consists mostly of fibrin and platelets.

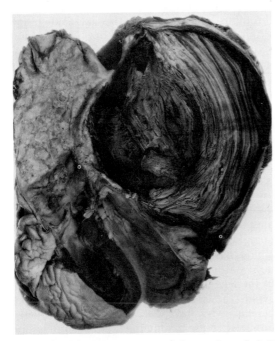

Fig. 9.19 A large aneurysm of the aortic arch (c.f. size of heart). The aneurysmal sac has become largely filled by laminated thrombus.

necrosis of the walls of small arteries and arterioles is commonly followed by thrombosis.

(c) Venous thrombosis

Apart from varicosity of the leg veins, diseases of the veins are uncommon, and although venous blood flow is slow, occlusion of veins in general occurs less frequently, and is usually less serious, than occlusion of arteries. The most important exception is *thrombosis of the veins of the lower limbs*, which is very common in bedridden patients, and is the usual cause of serious or fatal pulmonary embolism (see below): less often, thrombosis occurs in the *pelvic veins*, and this also may cause pulmonary embolism.

Thrombosis of leg veins usually starts in deep veins of the leg, most often within the calf muscles (Fig. 9.20), from where it may extend progressively to the posterior tibial and popliteal veins, the femoral (Fig. 9.21) and iliac veins and occasionally to the inferior vena cava. In some instances, it may start more proximally than the calf, or several thrombi may form in the calf and thigh veins.

Extension of the thrombus is sometimes very rapid, the whole length appearing as soft red thrombus: this probably occurs when flow of

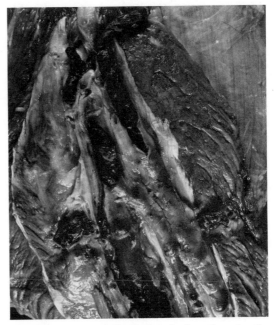

Fig. 9.20 Recently-formed red thrombus in the deep veins of the leg.

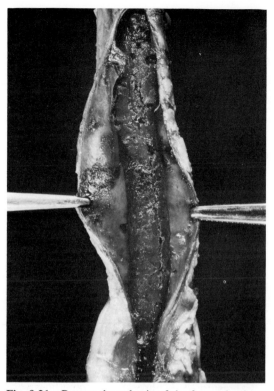

Fig. 9.21 Recent thrombosis of the femoral vein.

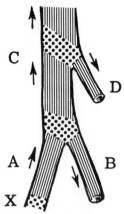

Fig. 9.22 Diagram showing the mode of extension of venous thrombosis. Thrombus occludes a small vein (A) at point X, and red thrombus (lined areas) rapidly extends in the stagnant column of blood up to the entrance of the next tributary (B), where platelet deposition forms a cap of pale thrombus (dotted areas): when this occludes the junction of A and B, red thrombus extends rapidly up to the entrance of the next tributary (C), and so on. Red thrombus also forms in each tributary as its entrance to the major channel is occluded. (Arrows show direction of spread of thrombosis.)

blood is very slow, and the thrombus resembles blood clot, being soft and red and readily detached from the vessel wall to reveal a red glistening surface or a paler, dull appearance due to deposition of platelets and fibrin. In other instances, probably where the blood flow is less sluggish, thrombosis extends more slowly, as depicted in Fig. 9.22. The initial thrombus formed in the calf veins occludes the lumen and for some distance proximal to the occlusion flow is virtually arrested. This column of blood is rapidly converted into red thrombus as far as the next proximal venous tributary. Blood from this tributary continues to flow into the affected vessel and for a time arrests the formation of red thrombus. However, platelets in the moving column of blood coming from the tributary are deposited on the proximal end of the red thrombus, which thus becomes capped with more slowly formed pale thrombus consisting mainly of platelets and strands of fibrin. This may eventually occlude the entrance of the tributary, again producing stagnation, and so red thrombus forms and extends proximally to the next tributary. So the process continues with

thrombus extending into larger, more proximal veins. Once a tributary has been occluded, red thrombus also forms in the stagnant blood within it and so the thrombus in the main venous trunks comes to have branches extending into the tributaries. Leg vein thrombosis tends to occur especially in patients lying immobile in the supine position, and impairment of blood flow by pressure on the calves appears to be an important predisposing factor. It is particularly common after an abdominal operation, severe injury, myocardial infarction, and in patients with congestive heart failure. There is an increased risk during pregnancy and following childbirth. Venous return from the lower part of the body is normally aided by muscular movements of the legs and by the pumping action which ensues from use of the abdominal muscles and diaphragm in respiration, and in all the above conditions immobility of the legs interferes with the normal flow. To avoid the pain of abdominal movements, patients who have had an abdominal operation tend to use mainly the thoracic muscles for respiration, and this is a further factor in impairing venous return from the legs. There is good evidence that thrombosis usually starts in the small leg veins *during* surgical operations. Extension into the large veins usually occurs over the next two weeks, when platelet numbers and adhesiveness and prothrombin levels are highest, and as in childbirth and myocardial infarction, pulmonary embolism is commonest around ten days after the event. The main factors predisposing to venous thrombosis in congestive heart failure are venous stagnation and immobility.

Leg vein thrombosis and embolism (see below) of large or small pulmonary arteries is an exceedingly common finding at necropsy on middle-aged and old patients (in our experience over 30 per cent). Recent reports on the prophylactic use of repeated small doses of heparin indicate that this reduces considerably both venous thrombosis and pulmonary embolism, but in surgical cases such therapy is more effective if started at the time of operation. It is partly to prevent venous thrombosis that patients are encouraged to leave their beds as soon as practicable after operation, childbirth, etc., and while bedridden to carry out muscular exercises and to practise abdominal respiration.

Thrombosis of the pelvic veins after operation, etc., is less common than leg-vein thrombosis. It is seen especially after childbirth when the uterine blood flow diminishes considerably, predisposing to thrombosis in the hypertrophied uterine veins. Puerperal sepsis is also a predisposing factor in some cases. Pelvic venous thrombosis may also originate in haemorrhoids or in the prostatic venous plexus and is a complication of operations on the pelvic organs, particularly if there is sepsis. Extension to large veins, including the internal and common iliacs, may complicate pelvic venous thrombosis and fatal pulmonary embolism may follow.

Other causes of venous thrombosis include *malnutrition, severe debilitating infections* and *wasting diseases* such as cancer. When associated with these conditions it is sometimes called **marantic thrombosis** and in severely debilitated infants and young children may affect the superior longitudinal sinus (Fig. 9.32, p. 249). Venous thrombosis is also prone to occur in **some disorders of the blood**, for example leukaemia and polycythaemia vera (excessive numbers of red cells, leukocytes and platelets). **Inflammation of veins (phlebitis)** also promotes

thrombosis: this may occur as a *migrating thrombophlebitis*, affecting various veins throughout the body: it is usually of obscure aetiology (p. 391), but is sometimes associated with cancer of the internal organs, particularly the pancreas. The thrombi are usually firmly adherent and embolism is unusual. In *septic venous thrombosis*, however, fragments of infected thrombus may break away and give rise to pyaemia (p. 201).

(d) Capillary thrombosis

Thrombosis in capillaries and venules commonly occurs in severe acute inflammatory lesions. It is due partly to endothelial damage and partly to haemoconcentration, the thrombi being composed mainly of packed red cells.

In the Arthus reaction, in which thrombosis of small vessels is often prominent, the endothelial injury is attributable mainly to release of enzymes by neutrophil polymorphs (p. 153).

Fibrin thrombi can be found in the capillaries in some patients dying of disseminated intravascular coagulation (p. 264), although in some cases they are absent, presumably as a result of fibrinolytic activity.

The fate of thrombi

Like other abnormal digestible material deposited in the body, thrombus is removed by enzymic action, and the success of such removal depends on the degree of restoration of the lumen of the thrombosed vessel.

The processes involved in removal of thrombus are (a) contraction of the thrombus, (b) digestion by plasmin and the proteolytic enzymes of neutrophil polymorphs trapped in the thrombus, and (c) organisation, involving digestion by macrophages and formation of fibrovascular tissue. The relative importance and effects of these processes depend on the type of thrombus and the site of its formation.

Occlusive venous thrombi are usually formed mainly of soft red thrombus which contracts well. Where it remains attached to the vessel wall, it becomes invaded by fibroblasts and macrophages, along with capillaries which are probably derived from the plexus of vessels external to the internal elastic lamina (vasa vasorum).

This ingrowth of granulation tissue does not often occur around the whole circumference of the vessel, usually being confined to sites where thrombosis has caused secondary damage to the intimal endothelium. Elsewhere around the wall, fluid-filled pockets may form where thrombus has retracted from the vessel wall or has been digested by the local action of plasmin. This is particularly prominent in the thrombus around the valve cusps of the vein. The cells of the intimal endothelium migrate and proliferate rapidly to cover the free surface of the thrombus, and also penetrate into it. This results in both fragmentation of the thrombus into tiny endothelial covered nodules and in the formation of small capillary channels, many of which are probably blind-ending, while a few link up with capillaries growing into the thrombus from the vein wall. The thrombus is also partially resorbed by the action of macrophages and sometimes the centre is softened by the enzymes from groups of dead polymorphs which have migrated from the thin-walled vessels. In this way, by the joining up of pockets, by fragmentation, resorption and softening of thrombus, a lumen may be restored leaving a thickened fibrovascular intimal plaque or a meshwork of fibrous strands marking the site of granulation tissue ingrowth with subsequent fibrosis. Occasionally, however, and perhaps when the thrombus is especially dense and slowly formed, it remains adherent to the whole circumference of the vein: pockets are not formed and significant recanalisation fails to occur. The thrombus is then replaced by granulation tissue which becomes increasingly collagenous, the vein eventually being reduced to a solid, shrunken cord without a lumen.

Occlusive arterial thrombi are usually formed more slowly and are more dense than venous thrombi; they contain a higher proportion of platelets and fibrin and are less readily digested. Also arterial endothelium is a relatively poor source of plasminogen activator and, possibly because of these factors, formation of pockets between the thrombus and arterial wall occurs much less than in veins. Consequently, the thrombus remains largely in contact with the artery wall and its removal takes place mainly by organisation. Macrophages migrate into the margin of the thrombus and gradually digest it. This is accompanied by invasion by fibroblasts from the intima and by new capil-

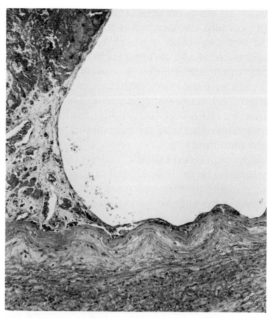

Fig. 9.23 Endothelium has grown over the surface of this partially organised thrombus adherent to an artery wall. × 40.

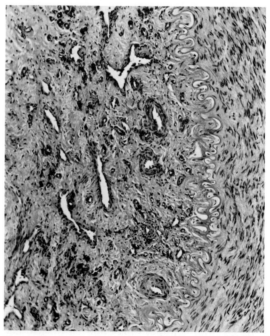

Fig. 9.24 Part of an artery showing the results of organisation of thrombus. The lumen was originally to the left of the internal elastic lamina, which runs vertically near the right margin. The lumen is now filled with vascular fibrous tissue in which some of the new capillaries have enlarged and acquired muscle to become arterioles. × 115.

laries which develop from the arterial endothelium, including that which grows over the ends of the thrombus (Fig. 9.23). The vasa vasorum probably play no part if the internal lamina is intact. The thrombus is thus gradually replaced by fibrovascular tissue and the length of vessel affected may eventually become a fibrous cord. The newly-formed capillaries anastomose and may develop into larger vessels extending through the length of the occlusion (Fig. 9.24), but such **recanalisation** does not often restore effective blood flow.

Mural thrombus. Thrombus may form on a part of the wall of a vessel (or of the chambers of the heart) without extending to fill the lumen. Such mural thrombi are rapidly covered with endothelium from the surrounding intima. Fibrinolysis, fragmentation, resorption and enzymatic breakdown probably all play a part in removing some of the thrombus, while granulation tissue grows in from the underlying wall and organises the remainder.

Embolism

By embolism is meant the transference of abnormal material by the bloodstream and its impaction in a vessel. The impacted material is called an **embolus**. In most cases it is a fragment of thrombus, although fragments of material from ulcerating atheromatous plaques of the aorta quite commonly form emboli in more distal arteries. A fragment of a tumour growing into a vein may also break off and form an embolus, and there may be embolism of the capillaries by fat globules, air bubbles or even groups of parenchymal cells. The site of embolism will, of course, depend on the source of the embolus. Thus embolism of the pulmonary arteries and their branches is secondary to thrombosis in the systemic veins or in the right side of the heart. Rarely, where there is a patent foramen ovale, an embolus may pass from the right side of the heart to the left atrium and thus be carried to the systemic circulation; (*crossed* or *paradoxical embolism*). With this rare exception, emboli occurring in the systemic circulation are derived from thrombi formed in the left side of the heart, from thrombotic vegetations on the aortic and mitral valves, and from thrombi or detached portions of atheromatous plaques in the aorta or large arteries. Emboli carried from tributaries of the portal vein lodge, of course, in the portal branches in the liver.

Effects of embolism

Systemic arterial emboli. The results are simply those of mechanical plugging and vary according to the site of the embolus, as described in pp. 245 *et seq.*

Pulmonary embolism is a very common and important event: it results from the detachment of a thrombus in a systemic vein, usually in the lower limb. Such thrombi form in conditions which have already been described (p. 240) and in any of them pulmonary embolism may result. It is most common around the tenth day after operation, and may cause sudden death. A large thrombus may become detached *en masse* and be carried to the right side of the heart, causing a sudden blockage of the pulmonary trunk or one of its divisions, death usually occurring at once or after a short period of pulmonary distress. Such fatal emboli are most often derived from the femoral and iliac venous trunk, characteristically forming a cylinder about 1 cm in diameter and as much as 30 cm long, which is found at necropsy coiled up like a snake in the pulmonary artery and right ventricle (Fig. 9.25). Depending on their size, less gross fragments of thrombus impact in the major or minor pulmonary arteries. When the patient has lived some time after the embolism, a varying amount of haemorrhagic infarction may be present in the parts supplied by the blocked vessels. Infarction, however, is never co-extensive with the area of distribution, and usually there is none.

Multiple small pulmonary emboli, impacting over a period of time, can rarely cause chronic pulmonary hypertension.

Septic emboli. With the widespread use of antibiotics, septic emboli, containing pyogenic bacteria, have become relatively uncommon.

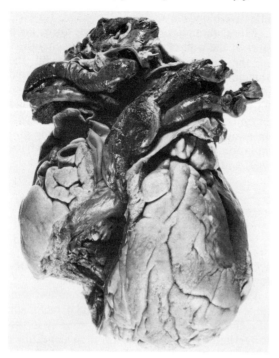

Fig. 9.25 Massive pulmonary embolism. Thrombus from the femoral vein has become detached and impacted in the pulmonary trunk and its right and left branches, causing sudden death.

Where they impact, such emboli may cause abscess formation, and the multiple abscesses of pyaemia develop in this way. An infective embolus occasionally weakens the arterial wall and gives rise to an aneurysm—*mycotic aneurysm*. In various septicaemic and pyaemic conditions, capillaries here and there may be plugged by organisms, most frequently pyogenic cocci, or by impaction of a small fragment of infected thrombus, the organisms then growing along the capillaries. The number of bacteria seen in necropsy material may have been greatly increased by growth after death.

Embolism from tumours. This is of two kinds. One or a few cells of the tumour may enter the bloodstream and impact in a capillary in some distant organ. In other instances there may be growth of a tumour into a large vein, and a larger fragment may become detached and impact in a vessel, e.g. a branch of the pulmonary artery or of the portal vein. Both of these processes can result in metastatic tumours.

Fat embolism. Entrance of fat into the circulation results from laceration of veins surrounded by adipose tissue. It probably occurs

after all fractures with laceration of adipose tissue, in caisson disease (p. 779) and as a complication of a fatty liver. In most instances the phenomenon is of no clinical importance but when the amount of fat entering the circulation is large, as in fractures of long bones, the **fat embolus syndrome** may develop within the following 3 days. The syndrome includes mental confusion, fever, dyspnoea, tachycardia, a petechial rash and sometimes cyanosis, haemoptysis, coma and death. It appears to be due largely to hypoxia resulting from pulmonary fat emboli complicated by oedema and haemorrhage. Fat may, however, pass through the lungs into the systemic circulation and cause emboli in the brain, giving rise to multiple small haemorrhages, in the kidneys (Fig. 9.26), and in the skin. There may also be thrombocytopenia. In patients who recover, there is usually no residual disability.

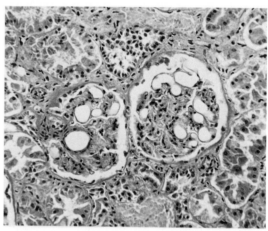

Fig. 9.26 Fat embolism of glomerular capillaries in a case of caisson disease. The globules of fat (dissolved out in processing the tissue) have impacted in glomerular capillaries and caused great distension. ×170. (Professor A. C. Lendrum.)

Air embolism. This occurs when air is aspirated into a severed vein, especially a large vein near the heart, but air may also enter the circulation in fatal amounts during blood transfusion if positive pressure is used without due care. The frequency and seriousness of the condition have probably been exaggerated. The air may produce effects in two ways. It may become mixed with the blood in the right ventricle, forming a froth which is not readily expelled and interferes with ventricular filling, or the bubbles of air may become arrested in the pulmonary arterioles and lead to the mechanical effects of embolism. When air enters the circulation it is absorbed rapidly, and to produce serious results the sudden entrance of over 100 ml is usually necessary; less than this has provoked alarming symptoms, but recovery has occurred after as much as 300 ml. Injury to the spinal cord and bones can result from formation of bubbles of nitrogen in caisson disease, which develops in divers, etc., from too rapid decompression from a high atmospheric pressure (p. 779).

At necropsy, bubbles of gas are sometimes found in the blood, due to the action of the *Clostridium welchii* after death; this should not be mistaken for air embolism.

Parenchymal-cell embolism. In certain conditions special types of cells form emboli in the pulmonary vessels, for example the megakaryocytes of the bone marrow in severe infections, the syncytial cells from the placenta, and hepatocytes after laceration of the liver. Such cellular emboli are without serious effect, the cells in all probability disintegrating. By contrast, the entry of **amniotic fluid** into the maternal circulation during prolonged or obstructed labour may cause serious effects in two ways. Firstly, it may produce extensive and sometimes fatal embolism of the pulmonary circulation by fetal squames, vernix and meconium. Secondly, it may bring about both widespread intravascular fibrin formation and activation of the plasminogen fibrinolytic system, with the result that there is severe hypofibrinogenaemia, and dangerous post-partum haemorrhage commonly results.

Local Ischaemia

Complete arterial occlusion

The term **ischaemic** is applied to tissue in which the blood flow has ceased (complete ischaemia) or is abnormally low (partial ischaemia). Ischaemia localised to an organ, a part of the body, or a patch of tissue, is usually due to obstruction to arterial blood flow.

By far the commonest and most important causes of complete arterial occlusion are thrombosis and embolism; other causes include proliferative changes in the intima of small arteries, and also arterial spasm as in Raynaud's disease or ergot poisoning.

When an artery is obstructed the result depends on the extent of **collateral circulation**, *i.e. alternative vascular routes by which blood can reach the deprived tissue.* The arterial anastomoses in the limbs are such that blockage of any one artery does not usually result in severe ischaemia provided that the other arteries are not seriously diseased. Similarly, there are effective collateral arteries in the integument and muscles of the trunk. In the internal organs, however, the anatomical arrangement of many of the vessels does not allow a sufficient anastomic supply, and severe ischaemia follows arterial occlusion. When an artery of a limb is suddenly obstructed in a healthy subject, there is an immediate drop in the blood pressure beyond the obstruction, and the circulation is brought almost to a standstill; the arteries then contract and the part contains less blood than normally. Soon, however, the anastomotic arteries dilate and blood thus bypasses the obstruction to enter the vessels of the affected part, through which a flow of blood is gradually established and increased until ultimately it may approach normal. Thus in a healthy subject the femoral artery may be ligated without permanent damage resulting. The limb becomes cold and numb, and some time elapses before the pulse returns at the ankle; and it is much longer before complete muscular power is restored. The collateral vessels remain dilated and maintain the circulation, and in response to the sustained rise in blood flow there occurs a thickening of their walls, with increase of the muscular and elastic tissue corresponding with the enlarged lumen; in other words, the collateral vessels become permanently enlarged or hypertrophied. An outstanding example is seen in the rare congenital localised stenosis (*coarctation*) of the aorta beyond the arch, in which the vessels linking the arteries of the head and neck with those of the trunk and legs become enormously enlarged during life and supply most of the blood to the lower part of the body.

The development of an efficient collateral circulation often depends on dilatation of healthy anastomotic arteries, and on a healthy heart. If, however, the collateral arteries are diseased, e.g. atheromatous, fibrosed or calcified, they are unlikely to dilate sufficiently to supply the necessary amount of blood to the ischaemic part, and a varying amount of necrosis will follow. Accordingly, in middle-aged or old people with atheroma, etc., blockage of the main artery of a limb, or even of a large branch, may be followed by death of the tissues supplied by the obstructed vessel, the condition of 'senile' gangrene resulting (p. 205). Multiple emboli in the arteries of the lower limbs (usually resulting from aortic atheroma) or spreading thrombosis, as in thromboangiitis obliterans (p. 378), may also lead to ischaemia and gangrene, even in young adults.

Infarction

Certain arteries of internal organs have imperfect anastomoses and their obstruction is always followed by serious results. Such arteries are called **end arteries**, and they may have no anastomosis, e.g. the splenic artery, or only capillary anastomosis, e.g. the branches of the renal artery, or arterial anastomosis insufficient to keep the part alive, e.g. the superior mesenteric artery. Obstruction of such vessels leads to ischaemia, usually sufficient to cause tissue necrosis. *The term* **infarct** *is applied to the altered area which has lost its blood supply, and use of the term implies that the tissue has undergone ischaemic necrosis.* During the process of infarction, the small blood vessels in the dying tissue may become engorged with blood from either retrograde flow or anastomosing small vessels. This engorgement, often accompanied by haemorrhages, results in the so-called *red* or *haemorrhagic* infarct. In other instances, little blood enters the dying tissues and a *pale* infarct develops. Pale infarcts occur in organs where there is little or no anastomosis, e.g. heart and kidneys; while in organs where there is some anastomosis, e.g. the intestine, and the lungs, red infarcts are found. Infarction means literally a stuffing-in, and was originally applied to the haemorrhagic type, which appeared stuffed with blood. When

pale infarcts were found to have a similar cause, the term was applied to them also.

Infarction is usually the result of acute occlusion of an artery by thrombosis or embolism. In the coronary arteries, atheroma with thrombosis is common, and is the usual cause of infarction of the myocardium; in the brain, thrombosis and embolism are both of importance but infarction can also result from hypotension; in the lungs, kidneys and spleen embolism is a commoner cause than thrombosis.

Features of infarcts in various sites. In the kidneys, spleen and lungs, the vascular arrangements are such that most infarcts are roughly wedge- or cone-shaped, the apex lying most deeply, in the vicinity of the occluded artery, and the infarct enlarging as it extends peripherally, the base being visible as a necrotic area on the surface of the organ (Figs. 9.27 and 9.30). The coronary arteries pass inwards from

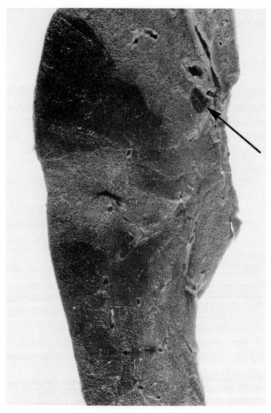

Fig. 9.27 Two haemorrhagic infarcts of lung, seen on section as dark wedge-shaped areas, widening towards the pleural surface (*left*). Note the pulmonary artery occluded by thrombus (*arrow*) beyond the apex of the upper infarct. × 1·3.

the epicardium, and accordingly myocardial infarcts involve especially the inner part of the wall, although commonly the whole thickness undergoes infarction.

In the **brain** a reduction in blood flow sufficiently severe to produce infarction is usually due to atheroma of the cerebral arteries or of major arteries in the neck that supply the brain, i.e. the internal carotid and vertebral arteries. The artery may be occluded by thrombus formed on an atheromatous patch or by an embolus, but stenosis alone, by severely impairing blood flow through the artery, may cause ischaemic damage in the brain. Indeed cerebral infarction may occur even when the arteries supplying the brain are normal. This sometimes results from a profound fall in cerebral blood flow due, for example, to an episode of severe hypotension. The sites of infarction of the brain depend on the cause of the ischaemia. When a major cerebral artery is blocked, infarction obviously occurs within the territory supplied by it, but blockage of the internal carotid or vertebral arteries, or a hypotensive episode, results in infarction in the so-called *boundary zones* (p. 743) at the margins of the territories supplied by the major cerebral arteries. Even when a major cerebral artery is completely occluded by thrombosis or embolism, there is considerable variation in the size of the infarct. This is due mainly to the efficiency of the potential collateral circulation through arteries on the surface of the brain and through the circle of Willis, both of which link the major cerebral arterial territories. A cerebral infarct may be pale or haemorrhagic. As the dead tissue soon breaks down and becomes soft, a cerebral infarct is often referred to as a *softening*. Thereafter, over a period of weeks or months, the necrotic tissue is gradually removed by phagocytes. The final result is a cystic shrunken area in the brain (see Figs. 21.25, 21.26, p. 744).

The central artery of the **retina** is an endartery, and its obstruction causes retinal infarction, with loss of sight in the eye.

In the **heart**, obstruction of a coronary artery or a major branch gives rise to infarction of the ventricular myocardium; it is usually somewhat irregular in form and pale, but may show congestion and haemorrhage at the margin (Fig. 15.9, p. 404).

Obstruction of even a large branch of a **pulmonary artery** does not always result in infarction. Experimentally-induced pulmonary emboli in otherwise healthy dogs do not usually cause infarction, some additional general impairment of pulmonary blood flow being required for infarction to result from the emboli, e.g. constriction of the pulmonary venous drainage. Similarly in man, a raised pulmonary venous pressure, due to mitral stenosis or heart failure, or to lung disease causing obliteration of pulmonary capillaries, predisposes to the development of infarction following pulmonary embolism. The subject is discussed more fully on pp. 458–60.

Pulmonary infarcts are typically wedge-shaped, with the base projecting slightly on the pleural surface (Fig. 9.27). They are firm and haemorrhagic (Fig. 9.28). In some instances, pulmonary arterial occlusion results in a wedge-shaped haemorrhagic patch without necrosis, and resolution may then occur, but when there is ischaemic necrosis, i.e. infarction, organisation and scarring follow in patients who survive for more than a few weeks.

Infarcts of the **spleen** are common and result usually from embolism. They are usually reddish at first and occasionally haemorrhagic, but soon become pale (Fig. 9.29) and yellow. In the **kidneys**, infarcts seen at necropsy are pale, with a deep red periphery due to congestion and

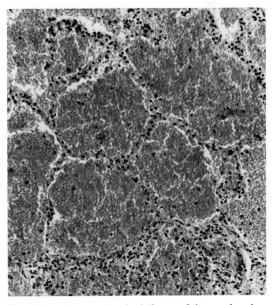

Fig. 9.28 Haemorrhagic infarct of lung, showing alveoli filled with red cells. × 115.

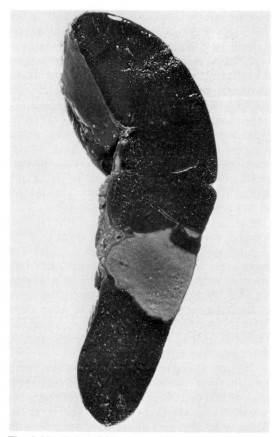

Fig. 9.29   Pale infarct of the spleen.

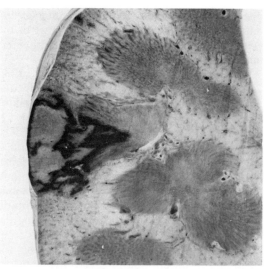

Fig. 9.30   Infarct of kidney, showing pale necrotic centre with haemorrhagic margin. × 1·2.

haemorrhage. The pale portion involves chiefly the cortex, the affected part in the medulla being usually red and haemorrhagic (Fig. 9.30), but small infarcts may be haemorrhagic throughout. When an arterial branch in a kidney is blocked experimentally, the area supplied becomes at first swollen and red throughout owing to general congestion. Thereafter, the dying kidney cells take up water (p. 12), and their swelling expresses blood from the central part of the infarct, which thus becomes pale. At the periphery and in the medulla the hyperaemia and stasis persist, the ischaemic capillaries rupture, and haemorrhage occurs into the tissues.

Blocking of the superior mesenteric artery produces a haemorrhagic infarct of the **intestine** (Fig. 19.72, p. 645), which rapidly progresses to gangrene. Death usually results unless the infarcted intestine is removed surgically without undue delay. Obstruction of the inferior mesenteric artery may be without serious effect, but sometimes causes ischaemic colitis.

Haemorrhagic infarction of the intestine, following obstruction of the superior mesenteric artery, has been studied experimentally in dogs. When this artery is ligated there is at first an arrest of the intestinal blood flow, accompanied by a contraction of the muscular coats of the intestine. This soon passes off and blood flows into the vessels of the ischaemic segment from the arterial anastomoses, but is inadequate to restore the circulation. The capillaries and small veins become engorged and finally stasis occurs and there is diffuse haemorrhage into the wall of the intestine and its lumen. Complete deprivation of blood from 5–10 cm of the bowel was found to lead to haemorrhagic infarction.

In the **liver**, obstruction of a branch of the portal vein is not followed by infarction, owing to the supply of blood from the hepatic artery. The obstruction does, however, reduce the blood flow sufficiently to cause atrophy and loss of hepatic parenchymal cells, and the sinusoids become dilated, so that the lesion appears dark red and shrunken (Fig. 9.31). Obstruction of the hepatic artery or of its branches may result in infarction of the liver (p. 664).

'Venous infarction'. Obstruction of a vein is an uncommon cause of arrest of blood flow through the tissue it drains, partly because in most tissues there is sufficient anastomosis to maintain venous drainage, and partly because

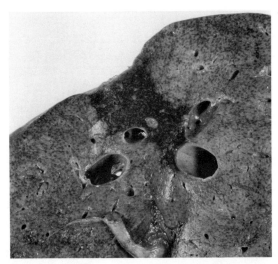

Fig. 9.31 A depressed red patch in the liver due to loss of parenchymal cells and sinusoidal congestion following thrombosis of a portal venous branch (not shown).

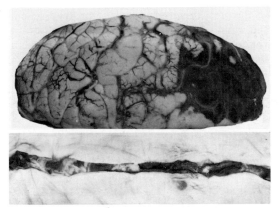

Fig. 9.32 Thrombosis of the superior longitudinal sinus (shown below), resulting in intense engorgement of the cerebral cortical veins and haemorrhage over the frontal lobe.

thrombosis of veins in internal organs is relatively rare, and emboli cannot, of course, impact in veins (except in portal venous systems, as in the liver). When venous infarction does occur the infarct is intensely engorged, oedematous and haemorrhagic. Marantic thrombosis of the superior longitudinal sinus sometimes occurs in severely debilitated children: the engorged cerebral cortical veins may rupture (Fig. 9.32), and there may be patches of haemorrhagic infarction of the cortex. Thrombosis of the mesenteric veins extending down to the smaller tributaries causes infarction of the intestine, which progresses to gangrene. Venous infarction is also seen occasionally in the liver as a result of extension of hepatic cancer into the hepatic veins. The best examples of venous infarction are, however, seen in the adrenals, which have several arteries but drain through a single large vein.

The susceptibility of tissues to ischaemia. The extent of infarction is usually less than that of the tissue supplied by the occluded artery, collateral circulation supplying the tissue at the periphery of the area. The size of the infarct resulting from occlusion of a particular artery may thus vary greatly, depending on whether the collateral arteries are healthy and capable of dilatation. The extent of necrosis is determined also by the capacity of the tissue to withstand ischaemia. As a general rule, *the*

parenchymal cells of the internal organs, which operate at a high metabolic rate, are relatively susceptible to ischaemia, whereas the supporting tissues—connective and fatty tissue and bone, are much less susceptible. The neurones of the central nervous system are perhaps the most susceptible cells of all, and cannot withstand deprivation of blood supply for more than a very few minutes. Glial cells are somewhat less demanding in their requirements, and accordingly at the margin of a brain infarct there is a zone in which partial ischaemia is followed by restoration of the circulation by collaterals; this results in death of the neurones, while the glial cells persist and undergo reactive proliferation. Hepatic parenchymal cells are also highly susceptible to ischaemia and, as described above, thrombosis of a portal venous branch is commonly followed by atrophy and loss of liver cells with survival and dilatation of the sinusoids. The renal tubular epithelium has also a low resistance to ischaemia, and while in the central part of a recent renal infarct all the cells are dead, at the periphery there is a zone in which the glomeruli and intertubular capillaries have survived while the tubular epithelium has died.

Changes following infarction. The autolytic changes which follow infarction have been described on pp. 11–13. Depending on the nature of the tissue, and whether or not it is oedematous or haemorrhagic, the infarct may remain firm (*coagulative necrosis*) or soften (*colliquative necrosis*).

From an early stage of infarction, products

of the breakdown of ischaemic or dead cells at the edge of the infarct diffuse into the surrounding tissue and promote a mild **acute inflammatory reaction**, with exudation of fluid from the vessels and migration of neutrophil polymorphs into the peripheral dead tissue. This, together with ischaemia of their walls, accounts for the dilatation of the small vessels and haemorrhage at the margin of the infarct. The acute reaction soon passes off, and the emigrated polymorphs die. The dead tissue stimulates a reaction similar to that around a foreign body: within a few days a zone of vascular **granulation tissue** forms around the infarct and the dead tissue is gradually organised. Macrophages migrate into and digest it from the periphery inwards; they are accompanied by new capillary buds and fibroblasts, so that the granulation tissue extends centrally, and as it matures into fibrous tissue the infarct is gradually converted to a **scar**. Extravasated red cells soon lose their outlines, and the pigment is slowly absorbed, although haemorrhagic infarcts, e.g. in the lungs, remain brown for a long time, and macrophages containing haemosiderin may long remain in and around the scar tissue. Loss of parenchymal cells and contraction of the fibrous tissue results in shrinkage; thus an old infarct of the myocardium presents the appearance of fibrosis and thinning of the ventricular wall (Fig. 15.11, p. 405). In solid organs, old scarred infarcts result in surface depressions, and when they are multiple, e.g. from repeated emboli in the branches of the renal arteries, the surfaces may be puckered and deformed by the scarring.

Septic infarcts. Multiple infarcts due to emboli containing pyogenic bacteria are an essential feature of pyaemia (p. 201) and thus a complication of acute bacterial endocarditis, acute osteomyelitis, carbuncle, etc. The bacteria may extend into, and multiply in, the dead tissue, and this results in an acute inflammatory reaction in the tissue around the margin of the infarct; thus the central dead tissue becomes surrounded by a ring of suppuration (Fig. 9.33).

The effects of infarction. The effects of infarction on function depend largely on the location and size of the infarct. In organs such as the kidneys, which have a large functional reserve, extensive or multiple infarctions of

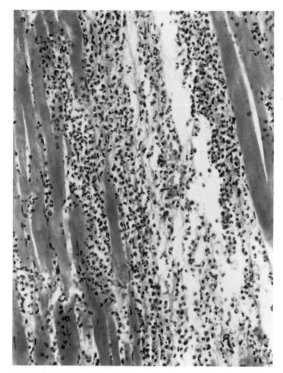

Fig. 9.33 Suppuration at the margin of a septic infarct of the heart. The necrotic myocardium (*right*) is becoming separated from the adjacent living tissue (*left*) by a purulent exudate. × 175.

both kidneys are necessary to bring about any serious disturbance of function, and serious impairment of liver function also requires very extensive infarction. By contrast, single infarcts of the myocardium are commonly sufficiently large to reduce seriously the functional reserve of the heart, and cause heart failure; infarcts involving the conducting system of the heart may cause heart block, and occlusion of a coronary arterial branch not uncommonly causes death from ventricular fibrillation before infarction has become apparent. Infarcts of the brain are a major cause of serious dysfunction, and even a small one involving the internal capsule is followed by hemiplegia. As already explained, infarction of lung tissue tends to occur especially in association with embarrassment of the pulmonary circulation, and for this reason recent pulmonary infarcts are quite commonly observed at necropsy of patients dying of heart failure.

The effects of infarcts are considered more fully later, in the systematic chapters.

Partial arterial obstruction

Chronic narrowing of the lumen of arteries is very common, and is usually caused by atheroma (p. 363). It brings about the serious effect of ischaemic atrophy of specialised cells with accompanying overgrowth of fibrous tissue, for example in the myocardium and the kidneys. Atheromatous narrowing of the arteries which supply the brain predisposes to focal loss of neurons or to actual infarction (p. 742): these events are particularly liable to occur during hypotensive episodes and no doubt contribute to intellectual deterioration in old age. Prevalence of atheroma in the elderly is an important cause of senile mental changes. Multiple or extensive atheromatous narrowing of the lumen is common in the arteries of the lower limbs, and the resulting chronic ischaemia brings about various trophic changes, and also limping, and cramp-like ischaemic pain, induced by walking (*intermittent claudication*). Narrowing of the smallest arteries and arterioles—*arteriolosclerosis*—occurs commonly in the abdominal viscera and central nervous system as an ageing effect, and results particularly from arterial hypertension: it is usually most severe in the afferent arterioles of the glomeruli, where it brings about glomerular sclerosis. These regional changes are, however, more appropriately considered in relation to the various systems and organs.

Disturbances of Water and Salt Balance

Water and salt deficiency

The water content of the average male body, estimated by the deuterium method, is about 62 per cent, and that of the female about 52 per cent, the sex difference being accounted for by the higher fat content in females. A man weighing 70 kg contains about 42 litres and this is distributed as 30 litres of *intracellular* water and 12 litres of *extracellular* water; the latter is subdivided into about 3 litres of *intravascular* fluid, the plasma, and about 9 litres of *interstitial* fluid which is distinguished from the intravascular and intracellular fluids by its very low protein content. The extracellular fluids contain practically all the sodium (except for that associated with collagen and that forming part of bone mineral), balanced chiefly by chloride and bicarbonate ions, whereas the intracellular fluid is almost devoid of sodium and chloride, its proteinate, sulphate and phosphate anions being balanced by potassium and magnesium. It is essential that the interstitial fluid should remain isotonic with the intravascular and intracellular fluids, and it contains a higher concentration of electrolytes which balances the colloid osmotic pressure of their proteins. Reductions in the water and salt content of the body are generally associated, but disproportionate depletion of either water or salt causes disturbances of the normal equilibrium which require different treatment. Deficiency of water tends to cause hypertonicity of the extracellular fluids so that water is withdrawn from the cells, which thus share in *primary dehydration*. Conversely, in relative salt depletion the extracellular fluids tend to become hypotonic, but this effect is minimised partly by increased renal excretion of water and partly by diffusion of water from the interstitial fluid into the cells with maintenance of isotonicity. Thus in salt deficiency the extracellular fluids are reduced in volume, but the administration of water or glucose solution without salt is actually harmful as it merely dilutes further the extracellular fluids and increases the diffusion of water into cells. *It is curious that whereas the need for water is normally indicated by thirst, in man there appears to be no urgent warning sensation when salt is lacking.*

Dehydration may be brought about in various ways and in minor degrees is very common. In hospital patients it is seen most often as a result of insufficient intake owing to physical weakness, coma and pyrexia. The urine is reduced in volume (500 ml) and is highly concentrated, the specific gravity rising to 1·040 or more. The plasma levels of Na^+, Cl^- and urea increase, probably as the result of diminished renal filtration, although the plasma volume is maintained relatively well by withdrawal of intracellular water and by active retention of Na^+

and excretion of K^+ under the influence of the renin–angiotensin–aldosterone system (p. 258) which is stimulated by the diminished blood volume—the so-called reaction of dehydration. More severe dehydration occurs under exceptional conditions, e.g. in people shipwrecked or lost in the desert, and then the deficiency of body water may ultimately reach over 12 per cent of body weight and amount to nearly 10 litres. Death is thought to be due to rise in the osmotic pressure of the cells. In children the ratio of body surface to weight is higher than in adults so that cutaneous losses of water are proportionately greater; also children cannot produce such a high concentration of urine as can adults. As a result, lack of fluid has a more severe effect in infants and young children than in adults.

Salt depletion is a commoner cause of serious effects than is water depletion, and also is more liable to remain unrecognised. Excessive loss of sodium chloride from the body occurs in various conditions and is commonly only one factor in complex fluid and electrolyte disturbances. Pure loss of salt results from excessive sweating when water is consumed freely, e.g. in the tropics or when working in a very hot atmosphere. It gives rise to a state of 'heat exhaustion' which necessitates the administration of large amounts of salt as well as of water, the consumption of water alone being liable to produce severe cramps. Clinically, vomiting and diarrhoea are the most important causes of combined water and salt depletion: the former is complicated by alkalosis due to loss of H^+, and the latter by acidosis from loss of the alkaline secretions of the small intestine. If water alone is restored the picture of pure salt depletion follows: lowering of the osmotic pressure of the extracellular fluid leads to renal excretion of water and to increased osmotic absorption of water by the tissue cells. In consequence, there is severe depletion of the extracellular fluid and circulatory collapse (*shock*) soon supervenes. The effects of this *secondary extracellular dehydration* are actually more serious than those of the disturbed acid–base balance which may develop from disproportionate loss of sodium or chloride ions, though the latter condition at one time received more attention. The symptoms of salt depletion when water is consumed freely include lassitude, weakness, giddiness, fainting attacks and cramps; also anorexia, nausea and vomiting occur and tend to set up a vicious circle. Marked loss of weight and mental confusion may occur also. The plasma concentration of sodium, normally about 137–148 mmol/litre, falls to 130–120 mmol/litre or less. The chloride and bicarbonate concentrations are also reduced *in toto* but their ratio varies with the presence of complicating acidosis or alkalosis. The blood is concentrated, with a rise in haemoglobin, haematocrit value and in plasma proteins. The urine contains little or no sodium or chloride except when the salt depletion is due to renal loss, as in Addison's disease or diabetic ketosis. The blood urea rises, often to over 17 mmol/litre (100 mg per 100 ml), owing mainly to reduced renal blood flow and diminution in the volume of glomerular filtrate—*pre-renal uraemia* (p. 847).

Combined deficiency of water and salt is more common clinically than of either separately. Vomiting and diarrhoea are probably its most frequent cause. If water is ingested and retained, salt deficiency will predominate, as described above, but without fluid intake water loss exceeds salt loss. In such combined deficiency, the extracellular fluid therefore tends to become hypertonic and consequently fluid is withdrawn from the cells; this leads to symptoms of salt depletion (see above) and unless corrected may cause acute circulatory failure. The rise in blood urea often leads to the erroneous diagnosis of uraemia due to renal failure, but the administration of water and salt in adequate amounts may completely relieve the symptoms.

Regulation of the water content of the blood and urine is normally carried out by the kidneys, which in turn are controlled largely by secretion of antidiuretic hormone by the neurohypophysis: this regulates resorption of water in the distal renal tubule. The neurohypophysis is so highly sensitive to the osmotic influence of sodium chloride that an alteration of 1 per cent in the osmotic pressure of the arterial blood can bring about a tenfold variation in the excretion of water, and the osmotic pressure of the extracellular fluids is thus very precisely controlled. Failure of this mechanism is seen in diabetes insipidus (p. 1015), in which there is intense polyuria approaching maximum water excretion. An analogous situation in respect of excessive salt excretion results from failure of the secretion of adequate amounts of aldosterone by the adrenal cortex, e.g. in Addison's disease, in which the cortex is largely destroyed. Uncontrolled sodium loss in the urine leads to fall of the plasma sodium to far below the level at which it normally ceases to be excreted. In consequence serious depletion of the body's store of sodium is brought about and this, if uncorrected, contributes greatly to the severe crises of Addison's disease and the tendency to acute circulatory collapse (p. 1044). Other hormones also play minor parts in the regulation of water and salt excretion, e.g. ovarian hormones can cause a distinct retention of water, as is seen in the late phase of the menstrual cycle and in pregnancy.

The pathology of generalised oedema has to be viewed against this background of water and salt balance. Maintenance of osmotic equilibrium is more important for life and is therefore regulated more exactly than the total volume of fluid in the body or within any of its compartments. Most importance was formerly attached to the chloride anion, but it is now recognised that the sodium cation is even more significant in regulating the amount of body fluid in the extracellular compartment of the tissues, and that sodium is intimately concerned in the pathogenesis of oedema.

Water and salt retention: oedema

Oedema is an abnormal increase in the amount of interstitial fluid. It may be localised, e.g. in an organ, limb, etc., or more generalised. In generalised oedema there is usually accumulation of fluid also in the serous cavities (hydrothorax, ascites, etc.). When oedema affects the skin and subcutaneous tissue swelling may be obvious, and momentary pressure will produce a depression ('pitting') which disappears in a few seconds as the oedema fluid returns to the tissue.

Control of interstitial fluid. The total exchange between the plasma and interstitial fluid is probably of the order of 7000 litres of fluid daily. In individual tissues exchange fluctuates with the physiological changes in blood flow. It is generally accepted that the interchange of fluid between the capillaries and venules and the tissue spaces can be explained on a physical basis, the distribution of fluid within and outside the vessels being regulated mainly by a

balance of the two processes of filtration and osmosis (pp. 48–9). The permeability of the capillary walls varies in different regions and also under different conditions of physiological activity in any one region, but the filtrate in all situations normally contains at least a small amount of protein, probably not exceeding 0·5 per cent in the more permeable areas such as the liver, and less than 0·1 per cent in the less permeable areas such as the limbs. In the normal exchange of interstitial fluid between vessels and tissue spaces most of the filtrate is returned to the circulation by the veins and only a small amount by the lymphatics, but most of the protein escaping from the vessels is carried away in the lymphatic fluid, the protein content of which therefore varies greatly in different parts of the body, depending on the permeability of the capillaries in the area drained: for example, the hepatic lymph is very rich in protein (3–5 per cent).

Water retention. It is important to appreciate that, regardless of its cause, generalised oedema represents retention of water and does not arise from a mere redistribution of the body fluids. In an adult, an increase of weight of about 5 kg invariably precedes the appearance of clinically recognisable generalised oedema, a fact utilised in the attention paid to the weight during pregnancy. Indeed generalised oedema can be regarded as a method of disposing of excess fluid which cannot be discharged by the usual channels, in order to regulate the blood volume. The body appears to tolerate badly an increase in the volume of the intravascular fluid; the excess is shunted into the interstitial spaces where its presence requires the simultaneous retention of a sufficient quantity of electrolytes, chiefly salt, to equalise the osmotic pressure of this fluid with that of the cells and of the plasma. The osmotic effect of the intracellular and plasma proteins is balanced by a higher concentration of electrolytes—chiefly salt—in the interstitial fluid. It is unlikely that increase of capillary permeability to macromolecules plays any major part in the common forms of generalised oedema, for the protein content of oedema fluid is not sufficiently high to suggest this possibility. Also, there is no gross fall in the blood volume, as might be expected if exudation of protein-rich plasma fluid was an important factor. In rare cases, cyclical oedema has been accompanied by hypovolaemia, and it has been suggested that the oedema of hypothermia may be related to an increase of factors such as bradykinin, which increase capillary permeability.

Local oedema

Active hyperaemia: inflammatory oedema. Active hyperaemia occurs in acute inflammation, in which the exudation of protein-rich fluid from the capillaries and venules gives rise to inflammatory oedema: as indicated in Chapter 3, major factors in the production of inflammatory oedema are increased hydrostatic pressure in the small vessels with dilatation and increased vascular permeability.

Active hyperaemia of lesser degree occurs also under physiological conditions, for example in the skeletal muscles during exercise, in the gastro-intestinal tract during digestion, and in the skin as an important mechanism of heat loss: the increase in interstitial fluid resulting from such physiological hyperaemia is, however, removed by the lymphatics and oedema does not result.

Oedema is a prominent feature of some types of **hypersensitivity reactions**, for example in hay fever, urticaria, the Arthus and delayed hypersensitivity reactions. These are all described in Chapter 6, and it is sufficient to state here that the oedema is of inflammatory nature, due to active hyperaemia and increased vascular permeability.

Urticaria consists of erythema, itching and wealing (which is sharply localised oedema) of the skin: it is very common, but occurs usually in mild form, with only occasional transient attacks. In some instances, however, attacks are frequent, severe, or more persistent. Although there is often a clear association with eating a particular food or taking a drug (especially aspirin), there is little firm evidence of an immunological hypersensitivity basis in most cases, and the underlying nature of the condition is usually unknown. Histamine antagonists are often beneficial, but in therapeutic dosage these agents have various other effects in addition to anti-histamine activity. Except when it occurs as part of an anaphylactic attack, urticaria is seldom dangerous.

Hereditary angio-oedema. This rare condition is characterised by attacks of acute localised oedema, most often affecting the skin of the face and trunk, but sometimes the larynx: acute abdominal pain, vomiting and diarrhoea can also occur as a result of oedema of a segment of gut, and some patients have undergone several abdominal operations. Death from laryngeal oedema is common in some affected families.

The condition is due to a genetically-determined (autosomal dominant) abnormality of an inhibitor of the activated first component of complement (C1-INH). In some cases there is insufficient inhibitor, in others it is qualitatively abnormal. The oedema is possibly due mainly to a kinin-like fraction of activated C2, and transfusion of fresh normal plasma (which contains the inhibitor) is of temporary value in both prevention and treatment of attacks.

Oedema may occur in severe cases of **zoster** (shingles) and is apparently a trophic effect due to inflammatory change in the posterior root ganglia. If the nerve lesion is unilateral, as it usually is, the oedema stops short in the midline of the body.

Local venous congestion and oedema. In a healthy animal, acute venous congestion produced by ligation of a large venous trunk does not usually lead to oedema, although there is an increased filtration of water and electrolytes owing to the heightened capillary pressure, and also an increase in the amount of protein leaving the vessels. Consequently there is increased flow of lymph containing a lowered concentration, but increased amount, of protein, and oedema does not usually develop. If, however, along with the ligation of the vein the vasomotor nerves supplying the part are cut, the intracapillary pressure is still further increased and localised oedema follows. Similarly, the application of an elastic band to a limb may merely produce venous congestion with increased lymph flow unless the band is tightened sufficiently to prevent the flow of lymph from the part, when oedema will result. These findings indicate that some other factor in addition to acute venous congestion is usually necessary for the production of oedema. In clinical cases, however, local venous congestion often lasts much longer than in the experimental animal, and this may possibly explain the common occurrence of oedema.

In acute venous obstruction there must be sufficient anastomotic drainage of venous blood to permit the circulation to continue; otherwise stasis, thrombosis and haemorrhagic infarction would follow as is seen in mesenteric venous thrombosis. After a time readjustment of the circulation occurs and arterial inflow diminishes. This leads to a reduction in tissue perfusion until, in time, the collateral circulation increases sufficiently to re-establish normal drainage. Until that stage is reached, the combination of venous congestion, tissue hypoxia and accumulation of metabolites may, by increasing capillary hydrostatic pressure and permeability, result in local oedema.

The oedema of chronic lymphatic obstruction, e.g. that produced by cancer, chronic inflammation, radiotherapy, filariasis, etc. (p. 393), is usually of the non-pitting type, i.e. the swollen tissues do not yield readily to pressure. A characteristic feature of chronic lymphatic oedema is the development of elephantiasis due to overgrowth of the connective tissue in the skin and subcutaneous tissue. Since the plasma protein normally present in the interstitial fluid is returned to the blood by the lymphatics, chronic lymphatic obstruction results in the accumulation of protein in the tissues while most of the water and electrolytes are taken up by the venules as usual. This accumulated protein may, in some unknown way, be responsible for stimulating the connective tissue cells to increased production of collagen.

Lymphatic oedema of the legs also occurs as a primary condition which is sometimes hereditary (Milroy's disease) and is believed to be due to a congenital abnormality of the lymphatics. The legs become permanently thickened.

General oedema

Cardiac oedema is apt to develop at a late stage in cases of **right ventricular failure** with long-standing systemic venous congestion. It appears first in the most dependent parts of the body and gradually extends upwards. Thus it is usually noticed first round the ankles, and pitting may be elicited by pressure over the lower end of the tibia. When the condition is advanced, the limbs become greatly swollen, the skin is tense and vesicles may form. Accumulation of fluid may occur also in the serous cavities.

As indicated above, increased transudation from congested, dilated capillaries is not sufficient to produce oedema experimentally be-

cause the excess fluid is removed by the lymphatics. When, however, heart failure becomes severe, the diminution in cardiac output adversely affects renal function which depends upon normal renal blood flow. The kidneys can compensate to some extent for reduced blood supply by increasing the proportion of fluid filtered off in the glomeruli; this is probably mediated by increased tone in the efferent arterioles. The volume of urine is reduced and it is highly concentrated, indicating that there is excessive tubular re-absorption of water. The mechanism of this excessive re-absorption is not fully understood, but the reduced renal blood flow may stimulate the juxta-glomerular cells to secrete excess of renin, and this in turn will enhance the secretion of aldosterone by the adrenal cortex, with consequent re-absorption of sodium by the renal tubules. The effect of sodium retention is to stimulate secretion of anti-diuretic hormone by the neurohypophysis, and so more water is re-absorbed in the renal collecting tubules. This mechanism has been demonstrated to play a role in some, but not all, cases of cardiac oedema (p. 258). The stimulus to this secondary aldosteronism is not fully understood, as it occurs among different types of heart failure, both in low output and in high output types. The great increase in body weight confirms the enormous amount of fluid retained in the oedematous tissues in some cardiac cases, and the importance of water and salt retention is shown by the effect of diuretics in diminishing the oedema. Reduction in the intake of sodium chloride in the diet has sometimes a markedly diuretic effect, water being eliminated with preservation of the isotonic state of the oedema fluid.

Other factors may play a part in the genesis of cardiac oedema, e.g. the accumulation in the tissues of waste products which by their osmotic action will tend to attract more water from the blood. There is also evidence that chronic hypoxia increases capillary permeability, although this view is not supported by the protein content of the oedema fluid, which is usually about 0·5 per cent or less. The fundamental cause of cardiac oedema appears, however, to lie in the faulty elimination of fluid consequent upon the deranged renal circulation. The distribution of the retained fluid in the tissues is determined by gravity because, with the reduction in cardiac power, the circulation is unable to absorb the tissue fluid and return it to the right heart against the hydrostatic pressure of the column of venous blood in the dependent parts. The distribution of oedema fluid is influenced also by the degree to which different tissues can be distended without a significant rise in tissue pressure.

In **failure of the left ventricle** of the heart, venous congestion occurs mainly in the lungs so long as the right ventricle continues to beat forcibly: pulmonary oedema may then develop without generalised oedema (p. 398).

Renal oedema. Generalised oedema occurs in various diseases which affect the glomeruli including some types of glomerulonephritis, and also in acute renal failure due to injury to the renal tubules. The pathological changes in these conditions are described in Chapter 22. However, an understanding of the factors likely to be involved in the production of the various types of renal oedema depends not so much on a knowledge of the detailed structural changes but rather on the associated functional disturbances. Accordingly, renal diseases which give rise to oedema may be classified into the following three groups.

(1) Conditions in which all the glomeruli are affected, with reduction in renal blood flow and in glomerular filtration. This group is exemplified by *acute diffuse glomerulonephritis* and *rapidly progressive glomerulonephritis*. There is usually a rise in blood pressure and blood urea level, and production of a diminished amount of concentrated urine containing moderate amounts of protein. The oedema in these conditions is not influenced by gravity to the same extent as is cardiac oedema and is often noticed first in the loose connective tissues, e.g. of the eyelids and face: in ambulant patients, however, gravity is seen to have some effect. The protein content of the oedema fluid is usually less than 0·5 per cent and the oedema therefore cannot be attributed to increased capillary permeability. Also the proteinuria is usually only moderate and the loss does not result in any significant reduction in the levels of the plasma proteins. The blood volume is normal or increased, and the oedema seems likely to be due to excessive re-absorption of salt and water in the renal tubules. The factors responsible for this excessive re-absorption are not, however, clearly defined. The renin–angiotensin–aldosterone system

may be implicated, but even this is uncertain.

(2) *The nephrotic syndrome.* In some renal diseases there is persistent and heavy loss of plasma proteins, particularly albumin, in the urine: when this exceeds about 10 g daily, the plasma albumin level falls considerably and this is accompanied by generalised oedema which often becomes very severe. This condition is known as the nephrotic syndrome. As in other types of renal oedema, the distribution of the tissue fluid is not so dependent on gravity as in cardiac oedema. In patients with nephrotic syndrome, the blood pressure is often not raised and there is commonly no rise in the blood urea, indicating that renal blood flow and glomerular filtration rates are approximately normal. The nephrotic syndrome may arise in a large number of conditions: in some it is regularly present, for example in *glomerulonephritis* of *minimal-change* and *membranous* types (q.v.). It is a common result of *amyloid disease* involving the glomeruli; it occasionally complicates other types of glomerulonephritis and the glomerular lesions of diabetes mellitus and various other diseases. *In all these conditions, its development is dependent on excessive loss of plasma albumin into the glomerular filtrate.*

Glomerular leakage of protein exhibits a molecular sieving effect, the amount of plasma albumin which escapes being disproportionately great because of its relatively small molecular size. Also because of its small size and its relatively high concentration in the plasma, albumin is the protein mainly responsible for the osmotic pressure of the plasma, and consequently, in states of severe hypoalbuminaemia, the amount of fluid leaving the capillaries and venules throughout the body greatly exceeds the amount drawn back into them by osmosis. Accordingly, the plasma volume tends to fall and this brings into play the renin–angiotensin–aldosterone mechanism, resulting in increased re-absorption of sodium and water from the renal tubules: this tends, in turn, to dilute the plasma protein still further and so transudation into the tissues remains excessive; a vicious circle is set up and continues to operate so long as gross albuminuria persists. As would be expected, the oedema fluid in the nephrotic syndrome has a very low protein content, and there is no evidence of general increased capillary permeability for macro-molecules.

The importance of protein loss and hypo-albuminaemia is confirmed by the appearance of similar gross oedema in protein-losing enteropathy (p. 639) in which the kidneys are normal and there is gross loss of plasma protein into the gut. The participation of the renin–angiotensin–aldosterone mechanism is demonstrated by the very high plasma levels of aldosterone found in the nephrotic syndrome.

(3) In *acute tubular injury*, the tubules lose their capacity for selective re-absorption and concentration of the glomerular filtrate. Consequently, most of the filtrate is re-absorbed and the small amount of urine produced approximates in its composition to a protein-free filtrate of plasma. There is retention of water and electrolytes and a progressive rise in blood urea. Apart from loss by sweating, vomiting, etc., most of the fluid taken by mouth is retained in the body and unless it is seriously restricted, gross oedema develops.

Acute tubular injury may result from shock or certain chemical poisons (p. 848). In some cases of acute renal failure following shock, the tubules show no convincing evidence of necrosis in a renal biopsy, and it now appears that hyperactivity of the renin–angiotensin–aldosterone system may be of importance (p. 850).

In the various forms of renal disease which are complicated by arterial hypertension, cardiac failure is liable to develop with consequent generalised or pulmonary oedema.

Nutritional oedema

Generalised oedema may clearly be caused by malnutrition. Protein insufficiency seems to be the main factor, and the extreme example is termed kwashiorkor (p. 667). Examination of the plasma shows a marked fall in glucose, lipids and proteins, the last being sometimes reduced to half the normal. It seems likely that a fall in osmotic pressure of the plasma is the most important factor in the production of the oedema, but no strict parallelism has been found, some cases failing to become oedematous in spite of severe depletion of serum albumin, while others show gross oedema with plasma protein levels within normal limits; also the oedema may disappear before there is any significant rise in the colloid osmotic pressure of the plasma. Nutritional oedema is commonly associated with xerophthalmia, a condition in which opacity with ulceration of the cornea occurs, as a result of deficiency in fat-soluble

vitamin A; possibly lack of the vitamin B complex is also concerned, and the 'wet' (oedematous) form of beri-beri is perhaps related. A similar form of oedema has been observed in infants when there has been excess of carbohydrates in the diet with marked deficiency in other foodstuffs. In all such examples of nutritional oedema, the problem is a complex one, and the relative importance of the various factors outlined above varies in individual cases.

Oedema may occur in patients with chronic wasting diseases, e.g. cancer, tuberculosis, etc., and is due mainly to cardiac failure, although fall in the plasma proteins is a contributory factor in some cases.

Pulmonary oedema

The osmotic pressure of the plasma (25 mm Hg) is substantially greater than the normal hydrostatic pressure in the pulmonary capillaries (8–10 mm Hg). Consequently, the development of oedema of the lungs usually requires a considerable rise in the hydrostatic pressure. As elsewhere, this occurs, together with increased vascular permeability, in acute inflammatory lesions, and inflammatory oedema is pronounced in severe influenza and lobar pneumonia, etc.

Pulmonary oedema can be produced readily in healthy dogs by interfering with the flow of pulmonary venous blood, for example by compressing the left atrium or ventricle, or constricting the aorta. Similarly, in man, it occurs in left ventricular failure, as in some cases of myocardial infarction and in systemic hypertension. In this latter condition, acute pulmonary oedema comes on especially when the patient is lying down, probably due to improved venous return from the legs, and perhaps also to increase in the blood volume by reabsorption of oedema fluid from the legs when recumbent. The attack is usually relieved by sitting up. Chronic pulmonary congestion, as, for example, in stenosis of the mitral valve, is not alone sufficient to produce pulmonary oedema in man. This is probably because reflex increase in tone of the hypertrophied pulmonary arterioles protects the pulmonary capillary bed from excessive rise in pressure. However, the situation is precarious, and pulmonary oedema is prone to result from physical exertion or other factors which increase the pulmonary blood flow. Chronic pulmonary oedema may occur as part of generalised renal oedema, particularly when there is, in addition, systemic hypertension, as in acute glomer-ulonephritis. Another important cause is over-loading of the circulation by rapid transfusion of blood to patients with severe anaemia. Finally, pulmonary oedema occurs in some cases of increased intracranial pressure, most commonly in head injury or intracranial haem-orrhage.

Apart from the above causes, oedema of the posterobasal parts of the lungs is a very common finding at necropsy, particularly in old people and where death is due to a toxic condition or has been preceded by coma. The oedema fluid is very prone to become infected by a mixture of bacteria, usually of low viru-lence, producing *hypostatic pneumonia* which, if untreated, is likely to be the immediate cause of death.

Depending on the causal factors, pulmonary oedema may be confined within the alveolar walls, i.e. interstitial oedema, or the fluid may pour into the alveolar spaces. The factors con-cerned are considered on pp. 451–4.

The renin–angiotensin–aldosterone system

Renin is an enzyme, stored and probably formed in the renal juxta-glomerular apparatus; it is present in high concentration in the cytoplasmic granules of cells of the wall of the terminal part of the afferent glomerular arterioles. The adjacent macula densa, a plaque of specialised epithelial lining cells in the wall of the distal convoluted tubule, is probably a sensory device, regulating the release of renin in response to changes in the composition of the fluid in the tub-ular lumen (Fig. 9.34).

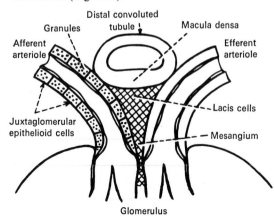

Fig. 9.34 Diagram of the juxta-glomerular apparatus.

Renin-substrate (angiotensinogen) is present in the α_2-globulin fraction of plasma and also in renal lymph.

The initial product of the action of renin on its substrate is an inactive decapeptide, angiotensin I, which is converted in the circulation to the active octapeptide, angiotensin II. This conversion takes place largely in the pulmonary circulation, but it occurs also in the kidneys and this is of considerable importance in considering the possible direct renal actions of angiotensin.

Renin is normally present in higher concentration in renal lymph than in renal venous plasma, but be-cause of the much higher rate of renal plasma flow, secretion into the renal vein is greater than that into lymph.

Effects of renin. Renin, by way of angiotensin, has three principal actions:

(*a*) Aldosterone-stimulating.
(*b*) Pressor, mediated mainly by peripheral vaso-constriction.
(*c*) A direct renal effect, modifying urinary output of water and electrolytes.

Other actions, which hitherto have been less fully studied, are the central stimulation of thirst, release of catecholamines and vasopressin.

The relative dominance of the three principal actions mentioned above is much modified by the prevailing sodium status. Sodium deprivation, for example, enhances the aldosterone-stimulating effect, while minimising the pressor action, so that a marked rise in circulating renin, angiotensin II, and aldosterone occurs with little or no increase in arter-ial blood pressure.

The renal effects of administered angiotensin vary widely according to the dosage, the prevailing sodium status, arterial pressure, and species. At most doses which can safely be given to normal man, an-giotensin reduces renal excretion of sodium and water, and this effect is enhanced by severe sodium depletion, as in untreated Addison's disease. By con-trast, in hypertension, irrespective of aetiology, and also in hepatic cirrhosis with ascites, angiotensin usually increases water and sodium loss.

Secondary hyperaldosteronism. The renin-angiotensin–aldosterone system is stimulated, and high circulating levels of all three components may be found, in sodium depletion, whether due to dietary sodium restriction, sodium-losing renal disease, diu-retics or purgatives: haemorrhage produces a similar response. Because in these situations the increase in aldosterone is thought to be a consequence of a rise in renin, these are regarded as examples of 'secon-dary' hyperaldosteronism.

Secondary hyperaldosteronism develops in some, but by no means all, cases of *untreated congestive heart failure*, in *hepatic cirrhosis with ascites*, and in *the nephrotic syndrome.* It may seem paradoxical that patients with these oedematous states, with their retention of sodium and water, should react as though sodium-deprived. The explanation lies probably in that the excess sodium is principally extravascular, and thus not capable of recognition by the kidney. The kidney therefore responds as in sodium deprivation; hence plasma renin and angiotensin, and in consequence, aldosterone, are elevated.

Renal artery stenosis is another instance in which the kidney probably receives a stimulus to increased renin release which is inappropriate to the overall requirements of the body. The old belief that renal artery constriction, by leading to increased circulating renin and angiotensin, is simply and directly responsible for hypertension *via* the pressor effect of angiotensin (p. 375) is a considerable oversimplification. It is clear, however, that in many cases of severe renal artery stenosis with hypertension, both renin and aldosterone are increased. A similar mechanism—possibly multiple intrarenal arterial lesions—may be the cause of the secondary hyperaldosteronism which often accompanies the malignant phase of hypertension, irrespective of aetiology. In advanced chronic renal disease with renal failure, occasionally such severe elevation of renin and aldosterone levels may occur that hypertension cannot be controlled until both diseased kidneys have been excised. This could well be an instance where sufficient angiotensin is circulating to have a direct pressor effect. However, angiotensin II also raises blood pressure by a slower-developing mechanism: infusion of angiotensin II at a rate too low to have a direct vasoconstrictor effect raises the blood pressure gradually and sometimes markedly. Some workers consider that this second effect is more important in renal artery stenosis than the direct vasoconstrictor effect of angiotensin II.

A particularly interesting form of secondary hyperaldosteronism is found in the rare condition of renin-secreting renal tumour, which occurs mainly in young patients.

In normal pregnancy, plasma levels of renin, renin-substrate, angiotensin II and aldosterone are all increased. This is an instance of physiological secondary hyperaldosteronism.

Other patterns of variation in circulating renin and aldosterone are readily predictable. Sodium loading, or the administration of sodium-retaining substances such as DOC, fluorocortisone, carbenoxolone or liquorice, depress circulating renin and aldosterone.

Primary hyperaldosteronism. An adrenocortical adenoma secreting an excess of aldosterone will lead to sodium retention, and thus to the combination of renin suppression with elevated aldosterone. This is known as *'primary'* hyperaldosteronism (p. 1041). The same combination will also be seen in any situation where excess aldosterone secretion is stimulated by mechanisms other than the renin–angiotensin system.

Hypoaldosteronism. In Addison's disease, the sodium deficiency stimulates marked secretion of renin, but aldosterone production remains deficient despite this stimulus, because the diseased adrenal cortex is unable to respond appropriately.

Primary renin deficiency, found mainly in elderly patients, is accompanied by selective aldosterone deficiency, cortisol secretion being normal.

Direct effects of renin and angiotensin on the kidney. The renal actions of angiotensin, although undoubted, are difficult to study in isolation from the pressor and aldosterone-stimulating effects. It has been suggested that phylogenetically, renin and angiotensin may have appeared initially as components of a purely intrarenal sodium-conserving system, and that the peripheral pressor and aldosterone-stimulating actions evolved as subsequent refinements and modifications, perhaps made necessary by a terrestrial, as opposed to an aquatic or semi-aquatic, habitat.

As mentioned earlier, a small proportion of angiotensin I can be converted to angiotensin II within the kidney. The major site of such conversion is, however, the lungs, and it has been suggested that this is an adaptation preventing the accumulation of dangerously high levels of angiotensin II within the kidney. When renal blood flow is impaired, the direct renal effect of angiotensin II may be initially beneficial, preserving glomerular filtration rate, possibly by a tonic action on efferent glomerular arterioles. However, with further elevation of angiotensin II, this beneficial effect is lost, and renal failure with tubular necrosis ensues.

Many years ago Goormaghtigh suggested that a renal effect of renin might be responsible for the reduced renal blood flow and oliguria of acute renal failure (see p. 850) and that acute renal failure might be the pathological extreme of the process outlined above. This is now supported by the demonstration that very large doses of angiotensin II can produce acute renal failure with tubular necrosis in experimental animals. A wide variety of stimuli causing increases in renin secretion predispose to acute renal failure with or without renal tubular necrosis. These include cardiac failure, sodium depletion, pregnancy, haemorrhage, Addison's disease and renal artery occlusion. Conversely, sodium loading and renal denervation reduce renin levels and are thought to protect against acute renal failure.

Shock

Definition and nature of shock. Shock is the name given to the complex series of changes which result from an acute fall in cardiac output.

These changes include regulatory mechanisms which are beneficial in that they tend to maintain the circulation, particularly to those organs with the most vital and urgent perfusion requirements—the heart and the central nervous system. Unless the circulating blood volume can be restored without undue delay, the diminished blood flow through most of the tissues results in widespread impairment of cell functions, and this, together with the compensatory circulatory changes, is responsible for the clinical features of shock.

A clear distinction should be made between shock and the *fainting* or *vaso-vagal* attack. The latter is immediate, can result from all grades of injury, from severe pain, or from psychogenic stimuli such as a fright or witnessing an accident or surgical operation. Fainting is characterised by pallor, sweating, weakness, a slow pulse, marked fall in blood pressure and loss of consciousness; vomiting and convulsions may also occur. These changes last only a few minutes and recovery is rapid. The fainting attack is mentioned here because it used to be known as 'primary shock'. In fact, it is quite distinct from shock, and should not be confused with it.

Causes and types of shock

The three major causes of shock are:

1. Reduction of blood volume, which induces **hypovolaemic shock**: examples include *severe haemorrhage*, *extensive vascular exudation* as in burns, and conditions such as severe vomiting and diarrhoea, which cause *dehydration*.

2. Acute cardiac failure (cardiogenic shock), due most often to myocardial infarction.

3. Severe infections, usually with bacteraemia or septicaemia, which induce **septic shock**.

Although all three major types have many features in common, they also differ in important ways. It is also important to emphasise that the longer shock persists, the more complicated it becomes, and in advanced shock all three factors—hypovolaemia, cardiac insufficiency and

bacterial infection—are often combined. It is convenient to give first an account of hypovolaemic shock, and then to describe the special features of the other types.

The nature and features of *anaphylactic shock* and of the shock-like state of *acute immune-complex disease* are described on pp. 146 and 155 respectively.

Hypovolaemic shock

This results most commonly from **acute severe haemorrhage**, due to trauma, to involvement of blood vessels in disease processes, or to a haemorrhagic disorder. Another important cause is **severe burning**, in which hypovolaemia results from inflammatory exudation of plasma fluid from the damaged small blood vessels in the vicinity of extensive burns. Thirdly, hypovolaemic shock can develop in **severe acute dehydration**, for example in association with a gastric or intestinal fistula, gastroenteritis or cholera.

Clinical features

The shocked patient is often restless and confused, has a pale, cold, sweaty skin, often with peripheral cyanosis, a rapid weak pulse, a low blood pressure, increased rate and depth of respiration, and may become drowsy and confused and finally comatose.

Haemorrhagic and traumatic shock

A normal healthy adult can lose 500 ml of blood, i.e. about 10 per cent of the blood volume, without any significant disability; the blood volume is almost restored within a few hours, although replacement of plasma proteins takes a day or two, and restoration of red cells takes much longer. Loss of 25 per cent of the blood (about 1250 ml) results in significant hypovolaemia over the next 36 hours, while a rapid loss of about half the blood volume so reduces the circulation that death is likely unless the blood volume is restored therapeutically.

Early changes. Acute hypovolaemia results in a reduced central (systemic) venous pressure and so a diminished flow of blood into the right atrium. The stroke volume is thus lowered and the cardiac output and arterial blood pressure fall. These haemodynamic changes trigger off peripheral and central baro-receptors with consequent sympathico-adrenal stimulation, and there is a huge increase in the levels of catecholamines in the plasma, sometimes by over 200 times. As a result of impaired renal perfusion, there is also intense secretion of renin and so a great increase of angiotensin II in the plasma (pp. 258–9).

The combined effects of these massive amounts of vasoactive agents result in an increase in the tone of the systemic veins, so that in spite of their reduced content of blood, central venous pressure and right atrial filling are partially restored, the heart rate increases, and cardiac output tends to rise towards normal. The high levels of catecholamines and angiotensin also cause constriction of the arterioles and venules in the skin, splanchnic area, and indeed most of the tissues of the body, so that peripheral resistance is increased, and even without treatment *the blood pressure may be partially or fully restored, although tissue perfusion is low.* The heart and central nervous system do not suffer to the same extent as the other tissues because they can autoregulate their own perfusion: their small blood vessels do not contract in response to noradrenaline, etc., but have an inherent property of relaxing when the blood pressure falls and contracting when it rises. In consequence of this autoregulatory mechanism, *cerebral and coronary blood flow are maintained close to normal levels at blood pressures down to 50 mm Hg.* At this pressure, arteriolar relaxation is maximal and perfusion rapidly falls off at lower pressures.

This, then, is the haemodynamic status in early shock. Compensating changes have tended to keep up the cardiac output and blood pressure, and the brain and heart are preferentially supplied with blood at the expense of diminished perfusion of the other tissues. If less than 25 per cent of the blood has been lost, and if there are no serious complicating factors (see below), the blood volume will rise naturally: vasoconstriction of the arterioles is greater than in the venules, so that the pressure in the capillaries is low and extravascular fluid passes into them (p. 49), and the high levels of angiotensin II stimulate adrenal secretion of aldosterone,

which promotes retention of salt and water. The circulation is nevertheless precarious, and further bleeding, major surgery to deal with the causal injury or bleeding vessel, severe pain, or the development of infection, will all tend to increase the circulatory deficit. *It is therefore important, in all save the mildest cases, to restore the blood volume by intravenous administration of fluid.* The nature of the fluid is not so important as the avoidance of delay: buffered saline or macromolecular solutions (plasma, dextran, etc.) are both effective initially, but macromolecular solutions have the advantage of maintaining the osmotic pressure of the plasma, thus tending to hold fluid in circulation, and are usually used for losses of around 25 per cent or more of the blood. It is also important to maintain the haematocrit at around 30 per cent in order to minimise tissue hypoxia, and matched blood (or in an urgent situation Group O Rh negative blood) are normally administered if haemorrhage has exceeded 25 per cent of the blood volume. Some estimate of the volume of fluids required can be made from the amount of blood lost, the clinical state, and the severity and nature of injury, but account must also be taken of internal haemorrhage, e.g. into the gastro-intestinal tract or around a fracture. The haemoglobin and haematocrit levels are not reliable guides to the degree of hypovolaemia during the first 36 hours. In the absence of cardiac insufficiency, a low blood pressure is an indication of hypovolaemia in early shock, but because of the compensatory mechanisms described above, it may be normal or nearly so in patients with serious hypovolaemia. A low central venous pressure is often, although not always, a useful indication of hypovolaemia, and if possible this should be monitored in all except mild cases of shock.

Although the peripheral vasoconstriction of shock serves a compensatory function, it is also harmful by reducing general tissue perfusion and it may, by increasing peripheral resistance, induce heart failure (see below). In some cases, the blood pressure may rise above normal, and the vasoconstriction may persist in spite of restoration of the blood volume. Drugs which promote vasodilatation (e.g. thymoxamine, sodium nitroprusside) are therefore sometimes beneficial, but only when steps have been taken to restore the blood volume: in the hypovolaemic patient they are liable to cause further circulatory collapse.

The changes of advanced shock. If shock persists, the widespread arteriolar constriction gradually passes off, but venular constriction is more persistent and capillary pressure rises with consequent loss of fluid into the extravascular space and further fall in blood volume. At this late stage of shock, the capillaries are congested with slowly-flowing blood, and *cyanosis* may be apparent. The general reduction in blood supply to the tissues is aggravated by a number of complex factors brought about by changes in the blood itself and by the injury to vascular endothelium and tissue cells resulting from perfusion failure. Some of the changes are as follows:

(*a*) *Viscosity of the blood* is increased by the haemoconcentration resulting from loss of capillary fluid. This leads to sludging of the red cells and rouleaux formation (p. 47) and these effects are increased by the rise in plasma fibrinogen which follows haemorrhage.

(*b*) *Release of thromboplastin* (Factor III) from hypoxic endothelium and tissue cells results in the production of thrombin (p. 234), which promotes aggregation of platelets and occasionally intravascular formation of fibrin. Aggregated platelets release adenosine diphosphate and thromboxane A_2 which cause further platelet aggregation.

(*c*) *Neutrophil polymorphs* adhere to the injured vascular endothelium of small vessels.

(*d*) *Hypoxic injury* results in release of lysosomal enzymes and secretory products into the blood. Proteolytic enzymes, e.g. trypsin from the pancreas, may activate the kinin system and thus further embarrass the circulation by causing vasodilatation and increased permeability. Production of the prostaglandins may also be increased: those of the E group have a kinin-like effect, while the F group may increase the resistance to pulmonary blood flow.

Metabolic disturbances. The hypoxia of shock interferes profoundly with cell metabolism. It prevents the entrance of pyruvic acid into the citric acid cycle and in consequence lactic acid accumulates and glucose passes out of the hypoxic cells, leading to insulin-resistant

hyperglycaemia and increased glycogenolysis. These metabolic disturbances together with high levels of catecholamines, result in a rise of fatty acids and amino acids in the plasma. Impaired carbohydrate metabolism results in a fall in production of adenosine triphosphate and so energy is not available for many cell functions, including the sodium pump: *potassium leaves the cells and sodium and water enter and cause swelling: these effects, sometimes termed the 'sick cell syndrome' (p. 19) may, by lowering the level of blood sodium, lead to inappropriate administration of salt.*

Metabolic acidosis, with rise in blood lactic acid, contributes to the hyperventilation of shock.

Organ function in shock. While all the organs are affected in shock, respiratory and cardiac failure are commonly of life-threatening importance. Quite apart from cardiogenic shock (see below), **acute heart failure**, first of the left and then of both ventricles, may develop in severe hypovolaemic or septic shock, and is particularly common in older patients with pre-existing coronary artery disease. The increased load on the heart resulting from peripheral vasoconstriction and its treatment with vasodilator drugs has been considered above. A factor which reduces myocardial contractility (*myocardial depressant factor*) has been detected in the plasma of shocked patients who subsequently died of cardiac failure: it is believed to be released from the pancreas. The impaired blood flow of severe shock, together with activation of the clotting mechanism, predispose to coronary thrombosis in patients with coronary artery disease. If operation is necessary, anaesthetic drugs may also impair cardiac function. Monitoring of the cardiac filling* and systemic arterial pressures, and particularly of changes in them during intravascular administration of fluid, helps to distinguish between hypovolaemia and cardiac insufficiency in shock. In some cases, drugs such as dopamine or digitalis, which increase myocardial contractility, are beneficial.

Disturbance of gas exchange in the **lungs** is another important complication of shock, and can be assessed by comparing the mixed venous and arterial oxygen tensions. Improvement

---

* The central venous pressure is used as a measure of the right heart filling pressure and the pulmonary artery 'wedge' pressure as an indication of the left heart filling pressure.

usually follows restoration of the blood volume, together with intermittent positive-pressure ventilation if necessary, but in some cases pulmonary function continues to deteriorate due to a combination of causes—pulmonary oedema, alveolar collapse, intra-vascular fibrin formation, embolism, infection, etc., known collectively as **shock lung** (p. 454), and death is then likely to result largely from the additional burden of respiratory failure.

Perfusion of the **kidneys** in shock is directly proportional to the blood pressure. Production of urine ceases at about 50 mm Hg and if the pressure remains low for some hours, focal hypoxic injury to the tubular epithelium may be associated with acute renal failure which persists for days or weeks after recovery from shock (p. 849). Renal damage is particularly common in shock associated with crush injury, childbirth, incompatible blood transfusion or severe infection.

Because of its autoregulatory mechanism, blood flow to the **brain** is relatively well-maintained unless the blood pressure falls below 50 mm Hg. Even a brief period of more severe hypotension can cause severe ischaemic brain damage (p. 247). Ischaemic centrilobular necrosis of liver cells may also occur, although liver failure is seldom prominent.

Other causes of hypovolaemic shock

Burns. In burning or scalding, necrosis of the more superficial tissues is accompanied by a lesser degree of injury to the underlying tissues, the reaction to which is acute inflammation. The small vessels dilate and their permeability increases, so that there is exudation of protein-rich fluid. When the area involved is extensive (10 per cent or more of the skin surface), the loss of fluid is severe enough to induce hypovol-aemia and shock. The changes are similar to those following haemorrhage but hypovolae-mia develops more slowly, haemoconcentration is more pronounced, with its attendant sludging and rouleaux formation, there is usually a marked leukocytosis, and the state of shock may recur or increase on the second or third days, possibly as a result of infection or absorption of breakdown products from the necrotic tissue. The principles of treatment of burn shock are the same as for haemorrhagic

shock, but the loss is of plasma rather than whole blood, so that plasma transfusions are used initially. Some destruction of red cells does however, occur in the burned area, and in very extensive burning severe anaemia may develop, necessitating blood transfusion. Another important complication of burning is bacterial infection, the dead tissue providing a good culture medium from which bacteria commonly invade the underlying tissue and bloodstream. Streptococci and staphylococci were formerly the most important invaders, but with antibiotic therapy Gram-ve bacilli, and especially *Pseudomonas aeruginosa*, now pre-dominate. The features of septic shock commonly supervene, and sepsis is now the major cause of death from burns.

Dehydration, if severe, causes hypovolaemic shock, although the blood volume is reduced relatively less than the extravascular fluid, and the effects of cellular dehydration are regarded as the usual cause of death (p. 252).

Cardiogenic shock

Acute lesions of the heart may severely reduce cardiac output and the subsequent haemo-dynamic and other changes are similar to those in hypovolaemic shock. The cardiac filling pressures are, however, raised, and although the clinical features—pallor, weak rapid pulse, sweating, etc.—are the same as in hypovolae-mia, intravenous administration of fluids, which is beneficial in selected cases, must proceed with caution.

The commonest cause is myocardial infarc-tion, and although only a small proportion of patients with this condition develop the full picture of shock, the mortality from this com-plication is very high even if facilities are avail-able for intensive therapy. Other conditions which can cause cardiogenic shock include rup-ture of a valve cusp, major arrhythmias, and cardiac tamponade due to haemopericardium (resulting from direct trauma or as a complica-tion of a ruptured myocardial infarct). Al-though not strictly cardiogenic shock, acute obstruction to blood flow by pulmonary emboli can result in a similar condition. As already indicated, cardiac insufficiency can develop as a complication of haemorrhagic and other types of shock.

Septic shock

Some patients with septicaemia or extensive localised infections, such as general peritonitis, pass into a state of shock which resembles that of hypovolaemia, but is often more prolonged, with a higher incidence of serious complications, and an overall mortality exceeding 50 per cent.

Septic shock is a common complication of infected burns, and of surgical operations, manipulations or instrumentation on the uro-genital, gastro-intestinal and biliary tracts. It occurs also in patients with immunodeficiency states, such as leukaemia and lymphomas, and as a complication of cytotoxic drugs or immunosuppressive therapy. Many such patients are dehydrated, and this is an important predisposing factor.

In a patient with known sepsis, high fever and symptoms and signs of shock, the diagnosis is not difficult, but in many patients, especially the elderly and following surgical procedures, septic shock develops insidiously, often without fever, and there may be an initial 'hyperdynamic' stage in which cardiac output is increased, the blood pressure reduced, peripheral resistance low, and the skin warm: these features may be due to bacteria-mediated release of kinins and other vaso-active agents. More often circulatory changes are similar from the onset to those of hypovolaemia, with pallor, sweating, cold extremities, increased peripheral resistance and reduced cardiac output, etc. Septic shock is particularly difficult to reverse and, as with other forms of shock, the longer it persists the more refractory it becomes. Tissue hypoxia results in widespread derangement of cell function, and features of multi-organ failure often develop. **Respiratory failure** due to 'shock lung' is often combined with **cardiac failure** and arrhythmias. **Acute renal failure** is also very common, although (as in hypovolaemic shock) many of its serious effects develop after recovery from shock.

Disseminated intravascular coagulation (p. 556) is more prone to develop in septic than in hypovolaemic shock. It interferes further with organ perfusion and may greatly aggravate pulmonary failure, or may, by consumption of clotting factors and activation of the plasmin system, progress to a bleeding state with widespread haemorrhage, e.g. from the gastro-intestinal mucosa.

Treatment of septic shock is based on elimination of the causal infection, restoration of the circulation, and correction of hypoxaemic metabolic acidosis and electrolyte imbalance. Antibiotic therapy cannot usually await the results of bacteriological culture of the blood etc. and tests for sensitivity, although it may need to be subsequently modified according to the bacteriological findings. The choice and rate of administration of intravascular fluids will depend on the results of monitoring procedures and haematological and biochemical tests. These include monitoring the cardiac filling and systemic arterial pressures, and frequent assay of the blood gases and pH, plasma electrolytes and osmolality, platelet counts and haematocrit. It may also be necessary to assay the status of the coagulation and plasmin systems. Intermittent positive-pressure ventilation, instituted at an early stage, has been shown to decrease the risk of the development of pulmonary failure, and drugs which increase cardiac output and tissue perfusion may be of value. The prognosis depends very much on the availability of experienced staff and facilities.

Aetiology. The microbial factors responsible for septic shock are by no means fully elucidated. With widespread use of antibiotics, the aerobic Gram-ve bacilli have replaced the pyogenic cocci as the major cause of septicaemia and bacteraemia. The organisms most commonly responsible include *Esch. coli*, *Proteus*, *Klebsiella* and in cases of burns *Pseudomonas aeruginosa*. About 50 per cent of patients with blood infection by these bacteria develop septic shock. Bacteroides (the anaerobic non-sporing bacilli which constitute over 99 per cent of the faecal flora) have been recognised quite recently as an important cause of blood infection, and about 30 per cent of cases are complicated by shock. All these Gram-ve bacteria release endotoxins when they die, and there is a widespread belief that endotoxin is a major cause of the manifestations of septic shock. Animals injected with endotoxin present many of the features of septic shock, including disseminated intravascular coagulation (the so-called *Schwartzman reaction*), and endotoxin has been detected in the blood of shocked patients with Gram-ve septicaemia by means of the limulus test (in which endotoxin is detected by its property of clotting a lysate of the blood amoebocytes of *Limulus polyphemus*, the horse-shoe crab). The limulus test is, however, time-consuming and, unless performed by an expert, can be misleading.

Endotoxin may induce the features of septic shock by a combination of its known effects, including activation of complement by the alternative pathway (p. 143), by promoting intravascular clotting, by its cytotoxic effects on neutrophil polymorphs, or possibly by promoting the production of kinins, prostaglandins, etc.

Severe shock sometimes develops in patients with fungal or acute virus infections, and in some instances immune-complex formation may be involved.

Other causes of shock

Some cases of shock do not fall into any of the three major types described above. For example, escape of gastric or duodenal juice into the peritoneal cavity, via a perforated peptic ulcer, causes severe shock, and so does acute haemorrhagic pancreatitis (which is non-bacterial), and the drinking of many poisons. In these conditions, it is likely that shock is chemically-induced, but there may also be severe pain which, without doubt, aggravates shock.

Severe shock results from transfusion of strongly incompatible blood to which the recipient has iso-antibodies; also in acute circulating immune complex disease (p. 155) and acute generalised anaphylaxis (p. 146).

Morphological changes in shock

The morphological changes in patients dying from shock are often inconspicuous. In spite of the fundamental disturbances of cell function, the parenchymal cells in general usually show only swelling and sometimes fatty change. In addition to the causal changes—injury, haemorrhage, coronary thrombosis, septicaemia, etc.—there may be various pulmonary changes, including oedema, congestion, hyaline membrane formation, collapse and bronchopneumonia (p. 454). The kidneys usually show the pallor and cortical swelling of acute tubular injury (p. 848) and there may be centrilobular hepatic necrosis. If the patient has survived sufficiently long for its recognition, there may be

acute ischaemic necrosis in the 'boundary' zones of the brain (pp. 745–6). Features of disseminated intravascular coagulation include widespread haemorrhages, and microscopy may reveal fibrin thrombi in the small vessels, especially in the lungs and kidneys (Fig. 9.35). The adrenals show the lipid depletion of the 'stress' reaction (p. 1039), but occasionally there is a combination of haemorrhage and necrosis, particularly in septic shock associated with meningococcal septicaemia.

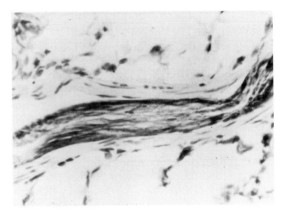

Fig. 9.35 Fibrin thrombus in a small pulmonary vessel in a case of disseminated intravascular coagulation. × 200.

Metabolism after injury

The metabolic disturbances associated with shock (p. 262) include incomplete carbohydrate catabolism, metabolic acidosis, disturbed protein and fat metabolism and a rise in the blood levels of glucose, amino acids and fatty acids. These changes were demonstrated experimentally by Cuthbertson, who termed them the *'ebb phase'*. Energy production is consequently depressed, and there is a general disorder of cellular metabolic processes. These changes are liable to develop in the first days following a severe injury, burn or surgical operation. Following the period of shock (or 2–3 days after such injury when shock has been prevented), the metabolism changes to a *'flow phase'* in which there is increased energy (and heat) production, due largely to breakdown of depot fat and protein, with consequent loss of weight and a negative nitrogen balance. During this period, which may persist for days to months depending on the severity of the injury, carbohydrate catabolism is complete and there is no metabolic acidosis unless carbohydrate intake is low. The mechanism of the increased

metabolic activity, which resembles that in fever, is uncertain, but weight loss can be minimised by a high calorie, high protein diet, and a warm environment.

Blood Groups and Blood Transfusion

Before administering a blood transfusion, it is essential to make sure that the donor's red cells are compatible to the patient, and in particular that the patient's plasma does not contain iso-antibodies reactive with surface antigens on the donor's red cells. The ABO blood group system is of outstanding importance, for iso-antibodies are normally present in the plasma (see Table 9.2) and their reaction with incompatible transfused red cells usually causes a severe haemolytic reaction with fever, shock, often acute renal failure and sometimes death. The rhesus (Rh) blood group system comes next in importance. Unlike the ABO system, Rh iso-antibodies are not usually present in the plasma, but they sometimes develop as a result of an Rh-incompatible blood transfusion or pregnancy.

For blood transfusion, the patient's ABO and Rh types should be determined and blood of the same type should be selected for transfusion. In addition, it is necessary to perform a *compatibility* or *cross-matching* test in which the donor's red cells are incubated in the recipient's serum at 37°C, and the cells are then examined for agglutination and also by the antiglobulin test (p. 111) to detect non-agglutinating (IgG) antibodies in the recipient's serum. The purpose of this procedure is to detect (1) technical or clerical errors in grouping and in collection and storage of the donor's blood,

and (2) the presence of unusual iso-antibodies in the recipient's plasma.

As a life-saving measure, it may be appropriate to transfuse Group O, Rh−ve blood to a patient of unknown group, but it is usually preferable to administer plasma while grouping procedures are being performed, and in any case a direct cross-matching procedure should always be performed.

Incompatibility can also arise when a donor's blood contains high titre antibodies reactive with the patient's red cells. Transfusion reactions from this cause are not usually severe because the donor's plasma (and thus the antibody) is diluted *in vivo* by the recipient's plasma. Screening tests for high titre ABO antibodies are not performed by most transfusion centres, and if donor and recipient are of the same ABO and Rh type the danger is largely excluded.

The ABO groups

Individuals can be classified into four groups by the presence or absence of A and B antigens on their red cells and of anti-A and anti-B antibodies in their plasma (or serum). Table 9.2 shows the features of the four groups.

Standardised anti-A and anti-B serum (from selected subjects of group B and A respectively)

Table 9.2   The four ABO blood groups

Blood group	Red cell antigens	Iso-antibodies in serum	Can accept blood of group	Can donate to patients of group	Incidence in Britain* (%)
AB	AB	nil	all groups	AB	3
A	A	anti-B	A, O	A, AB	42
B	B	anti-A	B, O	B, AB	8
O	O	anti-A + anti-B	O	all groups	47

*The frequencies of the four groups vary greatly in different ethnic groups.

are used to determine the group to which any individual belongs. If the red cells are agglutinated by both sera the blood belongs to group AB, if agglutinated by group B serum alone the blood belongs to group A, if by group A serum alone to group B, and if by neither serum, it belongs to group O. Since the serum of group AB does not agglutinate the red cells of any of the groups an individual of group AB can receive the red cells of any other group and is thus a 'universal recipient'. The cells of an individual of group O are not agglutinated by the serum of any group; the red cells can be transfused into an individual of any group and such persons are known as 'universal donors'.

The three blood group substances A, B and O are determined by allelic genes, one from each parent, so that there are six genotypes (AA, BB, AB, AO, BO and OO). O substance, however, is for practical purposes non-antigenic, and accordingly grouping is based on the presence or absence of A and B, giving the four phenotypes, which were first detected by Landsteiner. The iso-antibodies are mainly of IgM class, and develop after birth, apparently as a result of exposure to bacterial and other substances antigenically similar to A and B. Group A (or B) individuals are immunologically tolerant to A (or B) and so do not develop the corresponding antibodies.

The Rhesus (Rh) groups

The Rh blood group system was discovered by Landsteiner and Wiener (1940), who were interested in the antigens of human and animal red cells, and noted that guinea-pig or rabbit antisera to the red cells of *Macacus rhesus* monkeys agglutinated the red cells of 84 per cent of white Americans; accordingly, these 84 per cent were called Rh-positive, and the 16 per cent of non-reactors, Rh-negative. The human Rh system is, however, more complex, and further elucidation has come from the use of iso-antibodies which, unlike the ABO antibodies, are not routinely present in human serum, but develop in about 50 per cent of Rh−ve subjects transfused with Rh+ve blood, and in about 5 per cent of Rh−ve women as a result of an Rh+ve pregnancy (p. 151). Once Rh antibodies have developed, a subsequent Rh+ve blood transfusion is likely to cause an acute reaction with immune destruction of the trans-

fused red cells by a cytotoxic antibody (type II) reaction, while an Rh+ve fetus is liable to suffer from haemolytic disease of the newborn (p. 527).

Rhesus iso-antibodies may be of either IgM or IgG class: their demonstration requires incubation with appropriate red cells at 37 °C. Since IgG antibodies sensitise the red cells without agglutinating them, their detection is usually effected by use of the antiglobulin reaction (p. 111) and by methods which render red cells agglutinable by Rh antibodies, e.g. treating the red cells with papain or suspending them in a concentrated albumin solution.

Rh sub-groups. In simple terms, Rh blood group antigens are determined by three pairs of allelic genes, one of which codes for antigens C and c, one for D and d and the third for E and e. As the genes are closely linked, they are transmitted as haplotypic 'sets' which may be expressed as CDe, cde, etc., or by a set of symbols (R_1, r, etc.). The frequency of the eight possible haplotypes varies considerably in different peoples: their frequency in this country, together with the alternative symbols are shown in table 9.3

Table 9.3 The major Rh haplotypes and their frequency in Britain.

Haplotype	Abbreviation	Frequency*†
CDe	R_1	0·420
cde	r	0·389
cDE	R_2	0·141
cDe	R_0	0·026
cdE	r″	0·012
Cde	r′	0·010
CDE	R_z	very rare
CdE	r_y	very rare

* The frequency varies greatly in different ethnic groups.
† The frequency of any given *genotype* is obtained by multiplying together the frequencies of the two haplotypes as given here: thus CDe/cde occurs in 0·420 × 0·389 = approx. 16 per cent of the population of Britain, and cde/cde in 0·389² = 15 per cent. Reversing the calculation gives an estimate of gene frequency for known genotype frequencies.

Each individual inherits one of these sets from each parent, and his red cells may thus have from 3 to 6 different Rh antigens. In practice, iso-immunisation develops mainly when an individual of genotype cde/cde receives red cells which are D-positive. Accordingly, individuals whose red cells possess D are termed *Rh-positive* and those without D (i.e. with dd) are termed *Rh-negative*. In Caucasian stock, about 15 per cent of individuals are cde/cde (hence the frequency of cde as calculated in the table is $\sqrt{\frac{15}{100}} = 0.389$). Rh−ve individuals with other genotypes are comparatively rare.

There is also a significant risk of the development of anti-C when C+ cells are transfused to an Rh−ve individual, and it is common practice to use a mixture of anti-C and anti-D for Rh grouping. Iso-immunisation may also result when c+ or e+ blood is transfused to CC or EE individuals respectively, but d+ blood does not iso-immunise DD individuals.

The Rh system is, in fact, much more complex than has been suggested above: a fourth antigen, G, is closely associated with C and D, and further antigens, determined by variants of the common allelic genes or joint products of the genes, also occur.

Other blood group systems

In addition to the ABO and Rh groups many other blood group systems are known, but like the Rh group natural iso-antibodies are absent, and the sera that detect these groups are obtained mostly from persons immunised by transfusion or by pregnancy. These groups only rarely bring about iso-immunisation. Nevertheless the greatly increased use of blood transfusion necessitates their consideration and identification when a cross-matching test reveals an unexpected antibody.

References

Masotti, G., Poggesi, L., Galanti, G., Abbate, R. and Neri Serneri, G. G. (1979). Differential inhibition of prostacyclin production and platelet aggregation by aspirin. *Lancet* **ii**, 1213–6.

Moncada, S. and Vane, J. R. (1979). Arachidonic acid metabolites and the interactions between platelets and blood-vessel walls. *New England Journal of Medicine* **300**, 1142–7.

Sevitt, S. (1973). The mechanisms of canalisation of deep vein thrombosis. *Journal of Pathology* **110**, 153–65.

Sevitt, S. (1973). The vascularisation of deep vein thrombi and their fibrous residue: a post-mortem angiographic study. *Journal of Pathology* **111**, 1–11.

Singer, F. R., Schiller, A. L., Pyle, E. B. and Krane, S. M. (1978). Paget's disease of bone. In *Metabolic Bone Disease*, Vol. 2, pp. 548–9. Ed. by L. V. Avioli and S. M. Krane. Academic Press, New York, London and San Francisco.

Further Reading

Mollison, P. L. (1978). *Blood Transfusion in Clinical Medicine*, 6th edn. pp. 896. Blackwell Scientific, Oxford.

Race, R. R. and Sanger, Ruth (1975). *Blood Groups in Man*, 6th edn. pp. 682. Blackwell Scientific, Oxford.

Sevitt, S. (1974). *Reactions to Injury and Burns and their Clinical Importance*, pp. 256. Heinemann Medical, London.

Thomas, D. (Ed.) (1977). Haemostasis. *British Medical Bulletin* **33**, 118–288. (Reviews by leading workers.)

Thomas, D. (Ed.) (1978). Thrombosis. *British Medical Bulletin* **34**, 101–207. (Reviews by leading workers.)

10

Miscellaneous Tissue Degenerations and Deposits

The degenerative changes which result from cellular injury, and the intracellular accumulation of lipids and glycogen resulting from certain disorders of metabolism, have been dealt with in Chapter 1. In the present chapter we describe a group of changes which, although heterogeneous, consist of either the accumulation in the tissues of various substances—amyloid material, mucus, pigmented compounds, calcium deposits and urates—or tissue degenerations which usually affect the stroma of supporting tissues, and are recognised by their microscopic appearances but are ill-defined chemically.

Amyloidosis

Amyloid is a predominantly extracellular fibrillar material composed essentially of protein: it is deposited in various tissues in a number of diseases. Extensive deposits are visible by naked eye, causing enlargement of the involved organ and giving it a waxy appearance (Fig. 10.1). In

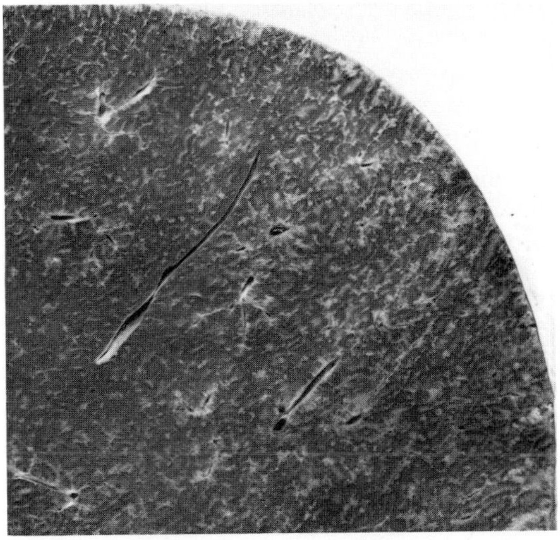

Fig. 10.1 Amyloidosis of liver. The amyloid material renders the organ firm, and gives it a dark, homogeneous appearance. × 1.

sections stained by haematoxylin and eosin amyloid is seen as a homogeneous, pink, refractile material. Electron microscopy shows it to consist of filaments of 7·5 nm diameter (Fig. 10.2), which can be dissociated into several protofibrils and are often twisted together in pairs.

Methods of demonstrating amyloid

The wide variety of methods currently used to demonstrate the presence of amyloid is an indication of their lack of specificity. Large deposits of amyloid are usually demonstrable by all the methods. If the amount of amyloid present is small, however, the results with each method vary from case to case and identification is correspondingly difficult; for this reason it is usual to use several methods, the best known of which are as follows.

(1) Lugol's iodine. Amyloid has a strong affinity for iodine (hence its name) and this forms the basis for a useful macroscopic test (Fig. 22.51, p. 842). When Lugol's iodine solution is poured over tissue, the amyloid is stained deep brown in contrast to the normal tissue which is only lightly stained. Congested tissues should first be rinsed free of excess blood as this obscures the test.

(2) Congo red. This stain may be used on gross specimens and sections for microscopy. Formerly the

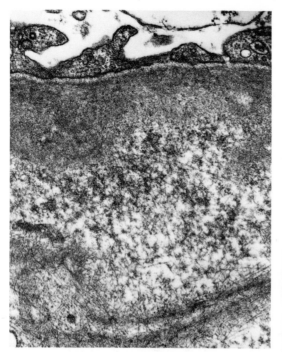

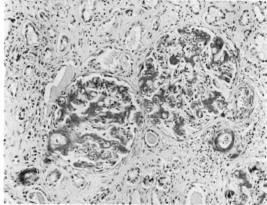

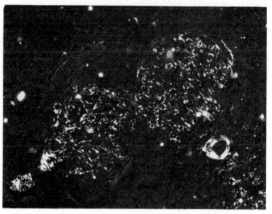

Fig. 10.2 Electron micrograph showing renal amyloidosis. The field shows glomerular capillary basement membrane on the outer side of which (above) the foot processes of the epithelium have fused to form a continuous layer. The inner part of the basement membrane is irregularly permeated by amyloid which also occupies the sub-endothelial space (lower half of the field) and is seen as fine filaments. × 39 000.

Fig. 10.3 The kidney in amyloidosis, stained by Congo red. The glomerular capillaries and the arterioles are affected. *Above*, viewed by ordinary light: the amyloid is seen as homogeneous material. *Below*, viewed by crossed polarising films, showing birefringence of the amyloid. × 105.

rate of disappearance from the serum of an intravenously injected solution of congo red was used as a clinical test for amyloidosis but owing to severe reactions and lack of accuracy it was abandoned. In polarised light amyloid stained by congo red shows a green birefringence, and this is the most reliable technique (apart from electron microscopy) for demonstrating amyloid (Fig. 10.3).

(3) Rosaniline dyes. These include gentian violet, methyl violet and crystal violet; they stain amyloid reddish while other tissue elements appear purple. This phenomenon of a dye reacting with a tissue constituent and undergoing a colour change is called *metachromasia*: it is believed that in this instance it is due to selective binding of impurities in the dyes by amyloid fibrils.

(4) Fluorescent dyes. Thioflavine-T binds to amyloid and its presence is demonstrated by fluorescence microscopy. The reaction is not, however, entirely specific for amyloid.

The deposition and effects of amyloid

Amyloid is deposited extracellularly, and first appears in the walls of small vessels, both arterial and venous, in relation to the basement membrane of capillaries and vascular sinusoids, and also of epithelial structures, e.g. the renal tubular basement membrane.

When present in small amounts, amyloid has little effect on the organs, with the exception of the kidneys in which quite early glomerular deposition may result in proteinuria (see below). Involved small vessels tend to be susceptible to trauma and to bleed readily, giving rise to petechial haemorrhages.

In greater amounts, amyloid causes enlargement of the organs and imparts to them a firm rubbery consistency and a slightly translucent, waxy appearance. The major features of involvement of the individual organs are as follows.

Amyloid produces effects by pressure on adjacent cells and by interfering with the normal transfer of water and solutes across the walls of affected small blood vessels.

The **liver** is firm and elastic and may be palpable during life. Amyloid appears to be deposited first in the space of Disse (between the sinusoidal endothelium and the hepatocytes) and as it increases forms a continuous network between the sinusoids and columns of liver cells. The change usually begins in the sinusoids of the intermediate zones of the lobules: it may become very extensive and produce marked atrophy of the liver cells (Fig. 10.4). Even at an advanced stage, liver function is not usually severely impaired.

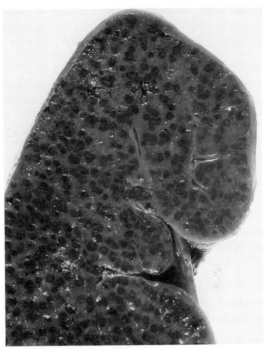

Fig. 10.5 Amyloid spleen of 'sago' type, i.e. affecting the Malpighian bodies.

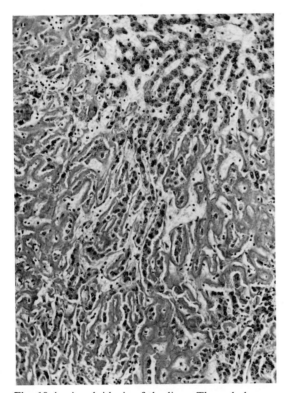

Fig. 10.4 Amyloidosis of the liver. The pale homogeneous amyloid substance extends around the walls of the sinusoids, enclosing the columns of liver cells, which are undergoing atrophy. The zone around the central vein (*top right*) is least affected. × 115.

The **spleen** shows two distinct patterns of involvement. In one the Malpighian bodies are changed to translucent globules by amyloid deposition in their reticulum (Fig. 10.5); hence the term 'sago spleen'. In this form splenomegaly is not marked. In the diffuse form, the change affects reticulum of the red pulp, walls of venous sinuses, and many of the small arteries; the spleen may be palpable and weigh up to 1 kg. The explanation of the two distributions is not known.

Amyloidosis of the **kidneys** is particularly important because of its effect on renal function. Deposition occurs upon the basement membranes of the tubules and in the walls of arterioles (Fig. 10.3) and venules, but the most important site is in relation to the glomerular capillary basement membrane (Figs. 10.2, 22.49 and 22.50, p. 842): amyloid is deposited initially on the endothelial side of the basement membrane, but extends through it to accumulate also on the epithelial side. The glomerular capillaries are rendered abnormally permeable to macromolecules, with consequent heavy proteinuria and nephrotic syndrome (p. 256).

Eventually many of the glomerular capillaries are obliterated, the kidneys become scarred and shrunken and chronic renal failure develops.

In the **stomach** and **intestines**, amyloid deposits may be widespread and this leads to atrophic changes in the mucosa. Diarrhoea may result from severe involvement of the gut, but even in its absence amyloid material is often demonstrable in rectal biopsy material, providing a useful diagnostic measure. Gingival biopsy is also useful, although less often diagnostic than rectal biopsy.

Other organs. Deposits of amyloid may also be found in the adrenals, heart, thyroid, skin and lymph nodes, and indeed in almost any tissue.

In the **heart**, it is deposited subendocardially and irregularly between myocardial fibres. Even when it has caused heart failure, there may be nothing to suggest its presence on naked-eye examination, but sometimes the ventricular myocardium is thickened and firm.

Classification of amyloidosis

Amyloidosis has been classified in several ways, none of which is entirely satisfactory. This is largely because, whichever method of classification is used, there is considerable overlap in the features which distinguish the different types, and while general rules can be applied, many exceptions are encountered. It seems at present more appropriate to distinguish between the two major types of amyloid material now known to exist, and also between generalised and localised amyloidosis. Lastly, the familial forms of amyloidosis are sufficiently distinctive to place in a separate group.

The two forms of amyloid material will be discussed later. Suffice it to say now that one form may be derived from a plasma protein but its real nature is uncertain and it is best termed AUO (*amyloid of unknown origin*); the other form is derived from the light chains of immunoglobulin and is conveniently termed AIO (*amyloid of immunoglobulin origin*).

Amyloidosis due to AUO. This is the classical form of **secondary amyloidosis** and develops in diseases characterised by chronic destructive inflammatory lesions and in certain forms of cancer. It is a common complication of tuberculosis, lepromatous leprosy, syphilis,

chronic bacterial osteitis, bronchiectasis and chronic suppurative pyelonephritis. These conditions have become amenable to treatment, and are less commonly seen as causes of amyloidosis in developed countries. Amyloid of unknown origin is also seen as a complication of rheumatoid and other forms of chronic arthritis, in which it can be detected at necropsy in about 20 per cent of cases, in Hodgkin's disease (a neoplastic condition, probably of macrophages), and occasionally in chronic ulcerative conditions of the skin (e.g. bedsores) or of the intestine (e.g. Crohn's disease), systemic lupus erythematosus and carcinomas.

The amyloid material is deposited most often and in greater amount in the liver, spleen, kidneys and adrenals, but has a wide distribution and some degree of involvement of the alimentary tract and lymph nodes is common. The major cause of death is renal failure.

Amyloid of unknown origin is usually typical in its staining reactions, being readily demonstrated by the methods outlined above.

Amyloidosis due to AIO. This occurs in approximately 15 per cent of patients with multiple myeloma (a neoplasm of the bone marrow of plasma cell type), in which the amyloid is almost certainly derived from light chains secreted by the neoplastic plasma cells; it may also complicate other neoplastic conditions of plasma cell type. It also occurs as a **primary condition**, almost always in old people: in some such cases, there is evidence of a latent form of plasma cell neoplasia, but in others no predisposing cause can be found. Typically, the distribution differs from that of AUO amyloidosis, the tissues severely affected being, in order of frequency, the heart, alimentary tract (including the tongue), skin, skeletal muscles, spleen, kidneys, liver and lungs. Death commonly results from myocardial failure, often with arrhythmias. Careful microscopic examination of necropsy material reveals minor degrees of this form of amyloidosis in a small percentage of old people dying from various causes.

Amyloid of immunoglobulin origin is often atypical in its staining reactions, and when present in small amounts it may be difficult to demonstrate convincingly.

Localised amyloidosis, restricted to one organ or tissue, is relatively common in the larynx where it gives rise to small tumour-like nodules. It may be restricted to the skin, bronchi, lungs, heart or urinary bladder, and is a rare cause of enlargement of the thyroid. It occurs also in the pancreatic islets in many diabetics, and as a feature of certain tumours, e.g. medullary thyroid cancer, islet cell pancreatic tumours and phaeochromocytomas of the adrenal medulla.

Genetically-determined amyloidosis. Several familial forms of amyloidosis have been described. The best known are familial mediterranean fever and primary familial amyloidosis.

Familial mediterranean fever is found principally in Mediterranean Jews and Armenians and is inherited as an autosomal recessive disease. In its most typical form, recurrent fever is associated with pain in chest, abdomen, joints and skin; amyloidosis supervenes, causing death by renal involvement, but affecting also the spleen, lungs and liver. Variants of the disease are recognised in which the amyloidosis becomes apparent before the other features.

Primary familial amyloidosis. This is least rare in parts of Portugal and is inherited as an autosomal dominant. The disease presents in the 3rd and 4th decades with increasing leg weakness and loss of reflexes. Subsequently sphincteric disturbances and malabsorption from intestinal involvement lead to death within 10 years.

Many other rare syndromes have been described in individual families, each with a particular distribution of amyloid deposition.

The nature and aetiology of amyloidosis

The essential constituent of amyloid is the protein which forms the fibrils seen on electron microscopy. Investigation of AIO, including amino-acid sequencing and immunological analysis, has shown it to have a molecular weight of 5000 to 18 000 and to consist of the N-terminal parts of immunoglobulin light chains. In any particular case, the amyloid is of *either* λ or, less commonly, of κ type (p. 106) and amino-acid sequencing indicates homogeneity of the polypeptide chains, which is strong evidence that *it is produced by a clone of plasma cells.* Amyloid from different patients shows differences in its amino-acid sequences. It is significant that nearly all patients with multiple myeloma complicated by amyloid have free light chains in their plasma and urine, and that partial proteolytic digestion of light chains *in vitro* produces a breakdown product which assumes the structure of amyloid filaments.

Analysis of AUO has shown it to be homo-geneous in each individual case, but there is disagreement on whether it too consists of a part of the immunoglobulin molecule. On balance, this appears to be unlikely, and antibodies to AUO have been reported to cross react with a trace protein present in the plasma, the concentration of which increases in old age. It may be that AUO is a breakdown product of this.

A characteristic feature of amyloid, revealed by x-ray diffraction analysis, is that the polypeptide molecules have a β-pleated configuration, which is unusual for mammalian polypeptides, and may explain its chemically inert nature, insolubility and poor antigenicity. It is of interest that, on enzymic digestion, a number of polypeptides, including insulin, glucagon and calcitonin yield fragments which can assume this configuration and adopt a fibrillar structure resembling amyloid. It may be that the polypeptide hormones are the source of the amyloid forming in pancreatic islets, islet-cell tumours and medullary cancer of the thyroid (which secretes calcitonin). In general, however, the sites of early deposition of amyloid suggest that it is derived from a constituent of the plasma which escapes from small vessels and is possibly converted to amyloid by the digestive enzymes of phagocytic cells.

Minor components of amyloid include a second protein ('P') which constitutes about 5 per cent of both major types of amyloid. It is readily soluble and is removed from amyloid during processing of tissue; *in vitro* it forms pentamers with a ring-like structure which become stacked (like red cells in rouleaux) to form rods with periodic cross-marking. It was suggested recently that P protein is a constituent of the first component of complement but this now seems doubtful. Amyloid also contains mucopolysaccharides, lipoproteins and fibrin in trace amounts, but it is likely that these have either been trapped by amyloid as it is deposited or are plasma constituents which have permeated it.

Amyloid is readily induced in animals by prolonged antigenic stimulation or oral administration of casein, and its deposition is enhanced by thymectomy and by immunosuppressive agents. Although human amyloid is associated with conditions which involve the immunity system, there is no common immunological disturbance: for example, in lepromatous leprosy cell-mediated immunity is depressed, whereas in tuberculosis it is normal or enhanced. This does not accord with the suggestion that amyloidosis results from T-cell depression and B-cell stimulation (Scheinberg and Cathcart, 1976).

There is some evidence that amyloid may be resorbed following effective treatment of the causal disease, but renal amyloid is persistent and steroid therapy has not, in general, proved beneficial.

Hyaline and Fibrinoid Changes

The term *hyalin** is applied to material of homogeneous, refractile, usually eosinophilic appearance seen on microscopy of stained tissue sections. It is purely descriptive, and many different formed tissue elements, as well as cell cytoplasm, may assume a hyaline appearance. In most instance the chemical basis of hyaline change is not known, although fibrin and amyloid both have a hyaline appearance. The collagen and background material of old dense fibrous tissue and the walls of aged blood vessels are often hyaline and because of its association with age this is often called *hyaline degeneration*. In the kidney and other organs, the walls of arterioles usually become thickened and hyaline in arterial hypertension (Fig. 22.6, p. 810), and glomeruli injured by chronic ischaemia became converted to hyaline balls (Fig. 22.7, p. 810). These changes occur also in diabetic nephropathy, and are believed to be due to accumulation of substances leaking out from the blood—*plasmatic vasculosis* (see below). There are many conditions in which abnormal amounts of plasma proteins leak into the glomerular filtrate; part of the protein is resorbed by the tubular epithelium where it is seen as eosinophil refractile droplets (Fig. 22.25, p. 824) commonly termed *hyaline droplets*. Protein may also coagulate in the tubular lumen and is then secreted in the urine as cylindrical '*hyaline casts*'. In virus hepatitis, damaged liver cells may appear hyaline (Fig. 20.14, p. 674) and '*Mallory's hyalin*' appears in the hepatocyte cytoplasm in alcoholic and certain other forms of liver cell injury. In Cushing's syndrome, hyaline material is seen in the basophil cells of the pituitary (*Crooke's hyaline change*—Fig. 26.4, p. 1011). Necrotic tissue, e.g. myocardium, and fused platelets in thrombi (Fig. 9.14, p. 237) may also appear hyaline.

These examples serve to show that hyaline material and its pathological associations are widely heterogeneous. It is nevertheless sometimes of diagnostic value, as will be seen from the many examples which crop up in the systematic chapters.

A second term, **fibrinoid change**, has long been used to describe impregnation of tissues with hyaline material which is brightly eosinophilic and has other staining properties similar to those of fibrin. The term became popular in the 1940s when fibrinoid change (incorrectly regarded as diagnostic of hypersensitivity reactions) was noted to be a common feature of the so-called collagen or connective-tissue diseases. More recently, immunofluorescence staining, and to a lesser extent electron microscopy, have provided more specific techniques for identifying fibrin in tissue sections, and have shown fibrin to be present in some, but not all, 'fibrinoid' lesions: in some instances the eosinophilic hyalin is due to ground-substance mucopolysaccharides; in others its nature remains unknown.

Deposition of fibrin in the tissues results from vascular exudation of fibrinogen, which is converted to fibrin by the action of tissue thromboplastin. If the injury causing the exudation is severe, there may also be death of tissue cells, and the changes are then traditionally known as *fibrinoid necrosis*. Examples of this are seen in many acute inflammatory lesions including the Arthus reaction (Fig. 14.28, p. 381), in some infarcts (in which plasma exudes from the ischaemic blood vessels) (Figs. 2.3, p. 10 and 2.5, p. 11), in the arteriolar lessions of malignant hypertension (Fig. 14.18, p. 374) and in the necrotic base of peptic ulcers. Fibrin is detectable in some fibrinoid lesions of the connective-tissue diseases, e.g. in some examples of the subcutaneous nodules of rheumatoid arthritis (Fig. 23.53a, p. 918).

* From the Greek '*hyalos*', meaning glass.

Deposited fibrin is usually removed by the action of plasmin or by phagocytic cells. It has, however, been demonstrated in slowly developing, permanent hyaline changes in the walls of arterioles and glomeruli in plasmatic vasculosis and this supports the view of Lendrum (1969) and others that such hyaline change results from an exudative process (see also p. 809).

Corpora amylacea. Under this term are included a number of rounded or oval hyaline structures, which may stain deeply with iodine, hence the name. They sometimes show concentric lamination and may undergo calcification. Such structures form in various situations and they cannot be regarded as all of the same nature. They are often a prominent feature within the acini of the prostate in the elderly; they occur also in the lungs, in old blood clots, and sometimes in tumours.

In the nervous system they are very common; e.g. in old age, in chronic degenerative lesions, and in the region of old infarcts and haemorrhages. They vary greatly in size, the smallest being spherical and homogeneous, and these usually stain deeply with haematoxylin. They appear to form simply by a deposition, in the intercellular spaces, of organic material containing acid mucopolysaccharides in globular form, but their exact composition is not known. They are of no importance except as a manifestation of the degenerative condition with which they are associated.

Mucins and Myxomatous Change

Mucins consist of complexes of proteins with carbohydrates and mucopolysaccharides. They are characterised by their slimy nature and histologically by their affinity for basic dyes and metachromasia with thiazine dyes such as toluidine blue. Most mucins are precipitated by acetic acid.

Mucins are secreted by various glandular epithelia and also by fibroblasts, osteoblasts and chondroblasts as important constituents of the ground substance of the various connective tissues. Both epithelial and connective tissue mucins are mixtures of *glycoproteins*, which are rich in hexose polymers and are stained pink in the PAS method, and *mucoproteins* in which the mucopolysaccharide is rich in hexosamines and which stain metachromatically with toluidine blue at low pH.

Disturbances of epithelial mucin secretion are not of much pathological importance except in *fibrocystic disease of the pancreas* (p. 721) in which an abnormality of mucus secretion occurs in the glands of the intestine, pancreas, bile ducts, bronchi and sweat glands. The thick mucin secreted obstructs the ducts, with subsequent gland atrophy and loss of function.

Obstruction of the ducts of small mucus-secreting glands, e.g. in the mouth, results in the development of mucin-filled cysts, and obstruction of the cystic duct may result in distension of the gallbladder with mucin—the so-called *mucocele* (Fig. 20.67, p. 711). Chronic irritation of a mucous membrane may result in increase in the number and activity of mucin-secreting cells, as in chronic bronchitis in which there is abundant mucous sputum. Some epithelial tumours secrete mucin, and its detection in relation to tumour cells is sometimes of help in determining the origin of the tumour.

The mucopolysaccharides of **connective tissue mucins** include hyaluronic acid, chondroitin, chondroitin sulphates and other sulphated compounds. They form the ground substances of fibrous tissue, cartilage and bone, and also joint fluid. In the soft tissues, the ground substance is largely in the form of a gel, but in acute inflammatory lesions the mucopolysaccharides are depolymerised, with conversion mainly to a fluid phase, which is more readily permeable to exudate and cells of the inflammatory reaction. Some bacteria also secrete hyaluronidase and other enzymes which may facilitate their spread in the tissues.

Some connective tissue tumours secrete abundant mucin, which appears as a basophilic stroma; they are called *myxomas* (Fig. 13.6, p. 343) and an increase in mucoid ground substance of connective tissue, so that it comes to resemble myxoid tissue of the fetus and umbilical cord, is termed **myxomatous** or **myxoid change**. It occurs in the aortic media in *Erdheim's medial degeneration* (Fig. 14.34, p. 386), and also, together with similar changes in other connective tissues, in *Marfan's syndrome*: in both conditions the inner part of the weakened aortic wall may rupture and blood may track along the media (dissecting aneurysm). Myxomatous change is also seen in the valve cusps of the heart and sometimes results in stretching and incompetence of the valves.

Production of ground substance is influenced by hormones; there is a generalised increase, for example, in *hypothyroidism* giving rise to the term **myxoedema**: the bloated appearance of the face is due to myxomatous change in the dermis, and the croaky voice is due to the same change in the larynx. Curiously, myxomatous change is seen in the pre-tibial region in some cases of thyrotoxicosis (hyperthyroidism).

There are also a number of defects of mucopolysaccharide metabolism—the **muco-polysaccharidoses**—which are inherited as Mendelian recessive characters. Excess mucopolysaccharides accumulate in various types of cell, and are excreted in the urine. The conditions are distinguished by the chemical nature and distribution of the material. The best known example is *Hurler's syndrome* or *gargoylism*, the major features of which include dwarfism, skeletal deformities, a characteristic facies, mental deficiency, corneal opacities and hepatomegaly.

Melanin Pigmentation

The melanins are iron-free sulphur-containing pigments varying in colour from pale yellow to deep brown. They are formed intracellularly from colourless precursors—melanogens—and are very stable substances, resistant to acids and many other reagents, but soluble in strong alkalis; they can be bleached by powerful oxidising agents such as potassium permanganate or hydrogen peroxide. They are related to the aromatic compounds, tyrosine, phenylalanine and tryptophane and may be formed from such substances by oxidation. On treating sections of skin with dihydroxyphenylalanine (dopa), 'dopa-positive' cells in the epidermis oxidise this substance by means of an enzyme like tyrosinase and become blackened in consequence. The only cells in the skin which are 'dopa-positive' *in vivo* are the *dendritic cells*, or *melanocytes*, which lie extended between the basal cells of the epidermis (Fig. 10.6); they are the only melanin-producing cells in the skin and fine granules of melanin in their dendrites are taken up by pinocytosis of the tips of the dendrites, into adjacent epidermal cells and also into certain phagocytic cells (*melanophores*) in the dermis which may thus become heavily laden with coarse pigment granules. Melanin granules possess the capacity to reduce certain silver salts, e.g. ammoniacal silver nitrate, with consequent deposition of metallic silver; melanin can thus be blackened in histological preparations, scanty or light-coloured granules being rendered conspicuous. This property is widely used histochemically. It is now known that the dendritic cells are of neuro-ectodermal origin, being derived from the cells of the embryonic neural crest, as are also the melanocytes of the squamous mucous membranes, the meninges, choroid and adrenals. This view harmonises well with the evidence about the origin of the naevus cells of pigmented moles from neuro-ectodermal cells and also accords with the

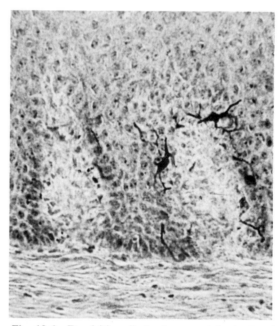

Fig. 10.6　Dendritic cells (melanocytes) in the basal part of the epidermis. (Dopa reaction.) × 220.

experimental work of Billingham and Medawar on the behaviour of melanocytes in skin autotransplants. This work seems to have rendered untenable the alternative view that melanocytes are modified basal epidermal cells. The Langerhans cells of the epidermis are now regarded as macrophages and may play a part in the control of keratinisation. Darkening of the skin on exposure to ultraviolet radiation is brought about first by migration of the melanin granules and subsequent darkening of their colour; later there is increased formation of pigment, apparently by the activity of the dendritic cells, which under further stimulation may increase in number.

In **Addison's disease**, which results from destruction of the adrenal cortex (p. 1044), there occurs a general increase in melanin pigmentation of the skin, especially in areas exposed to light and in areas normally pigmented. There may also be pigmentary deposition on the inner surface of the cheeks on a line corresponding to the junction of the teeth, and on the sides of the tongue, the position being apparently determined by irritation. In the skin the pigment is in the form of very fine brownish granules in the deeper layers of the rete Malpighii, and is present also as coarser granules, chiefly within macrophages in the underlying cutis, the appearance and distribution resembling those in the negro skin. The pigmentation in Addison's disease represents an increase of normal pigment, and occurs under the influence of the melanocyte-stimulating hormone of the pituitary (MSH) which is released in excess in the absence of adrenal inhibition (p. 1044).

Chloasma is a condition observed principally during pregnancy, and occasionally in association with ovarian disease, in which pigmented patches occur in the skin of the face, and the pigmented parts, e.g. the nipples, may become darker under the influence of oestrogenic and melanocyte-stimulating hormones. A similar condition has been described in women taking oral contraceptives.

Leukoderma (vitiligo) denotes patchy depigmentation of skin and this may be accompanied by increase of pigment in the intervening areas. In the affected areas the dendritic cells are of abnormal structure and have lost their capacity to oxidise dopa to form pigment.

Irregular pigmentation of the skin is common in chronic arsenical poisoning and in neurofibromatosis. In haemochromatosis also, the colour of the skin is due partly to deposition of haemosiderin in the cutis, notably around the sweat glands (p. 282), but also to increase in melanin. A striking degree of melanotic pigmentation of the oral and labial mucosa occurs in association with familial multiple polyposis of the small intestine, especially the jejunum (Peutz-Jeghers syndrome): the disorder is transmitted as a Mendelian dominant. The control of pigment metabolism in the skin is obscure, but it is known to be affected by exposure to light, chronic irritation and increased vascularity, activity of endocrine glands including the adrenals, pituitary and ovaries, and nervous influences.

Pigmented tumours. Melanin pigment is formed in large amount in the melanotic tumours which arise in the skin and in the pigmented coats of the eye, and most analyses have been carried out on the pigment from such tumours. The urine of patients suffering from extensive melanotic tumours occasionally contains a melanogen which darkens on exposure to the oxygen of the air.

Melanosis coli. This is a rather uncommon condition characterised by varying degrees of brownish to black pigmentation of the mucosa of the colon, beginning in the caecum and ascending colon, and sometimes extending to the anus. The pigment is contained mainly in macrophages in the lamina propria; it is absent from the epithelial cells. The condition is commonest when there has been intestinal stasis or chronic obstruction, and it is now recognised to be the result of absorption of aromatic products from the gut. This is commonly associated with the prolonged use of anthracene-derived purgatives, e.g. cascara, and the pigment consists of derivatives of anthraquinone combined with products of protein decomposition. The pigment resembles melanin in its reactions, but differs from it in being autofluorescent, weakly PAS-positive, and weakly sudanophilic. The cells containing pigment are dopa-negative.

Ochronosis. In this very rare condition, cartilages, capsules of joints and other soft tissues assume a dark brown or almost black colour, owing to pigment deposition. The pigment resembles melanin in some of its properties but does not reduce silver nitrate. In virtually all cases of ochronosis, alkaptonuria is present, a condition in which homogentisic acid (2,5-hydroxyphenylacetic acid) is excreted by the kidneys and causes the urine to blacken on standing owing to oxidation, especially alkaline urine. Homogentisic acid is formed from tyrosine and phenylalanine. Normally it is converted to malylacetoacetic acid by homogentisic acid oxidase in the liver and kidneys, but alkaptonurics lack this enzyme, and consequently homogentisic acid is not metabolised normally, but is oxidised into pigment and deposited in the tissues, producing ochronosis. The metabolic defect in alkaptonuria is inherited as an autosomal recessive character. In the early days of antiseptic surgery ochronosis occasionally followed the use of carbolic dressings for a long time, and the pigment is believed to be formed from the absorbed carbolic acid. This has been called *exogenous ochronosis*.

Pigments Derived from Haemoglobin

At the end of their life span, red cells are taken up by macrophages in the spleen, marrow, etc. Intracellular breakdown of haemoglobin (Hb) begins with opening of the porphyrin system of haem, the four pyrrole nuclei and globin now forming a long-chain molecule (choleglobin). The globin and iron are then split off and the residual *biliverdin* pigment, consisting of four pyrrole rings, is reduced to *bilirubin* and passes into the plasma where it is bound mainly to albumin. The bilirubin is taken up by the hepatocytes, dissociated from the protein, and is conjugated with glucuronic acid and excreted as bilirubin glucuronides in the bile. The iron which is split off from haem is stored mainly as *ferritin* and *haemosiderin* and re-used.

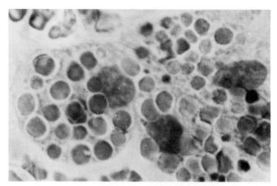

Fig. 10.7 Macrophages containing red cells in phagocytic vacuoles. From the subcutaneous tissue of a mouse six days after an injection of red cells. × 1200.

Breakdown products of Hb may accumulate in the body in the following circumstances: (*a*) local deposition results from haemorrhage into the tissues; (*b*) more generalised accumulation of bilirubin occurs when there is excessive red cell destruction, i.e. in haemolytic anaemias; (*c*) increase in bilirubin or its glucuronides occurs when there is some defect in the metabolic or excretory pathways by which the iron-free part of haem is delivered into the intestine as bilirubin glucuronide; (*d*) accumulation of iron-containing compounds occurs when the amount of iron entering the body exceeds significantly the small amount which is lost physiologically. The effects of these abnormalities are described below.

Local accumulation of pigments

When haemorrhage into tissues occurs, many of the red cells in the escaped blood undergo lysis; their Hb diffuses away and is taken up and catabolised in macrophages in the draining lymph nodes, spleen, etc. However, some of the red cells are phagocytosed locally by macrophages derived from monocytes which migrate into the lesion and bilirubin and iron compounds are produced as described above: this process is illustrated experimentally in Figs. 10.7 and 10.8: in man it is reflected in the changing colours of a 'black eye' or any other superficial bruise. Most of the bilirubin diffuses away and is eventually dealt with by the liver, but some of it may persist locally in crystalline

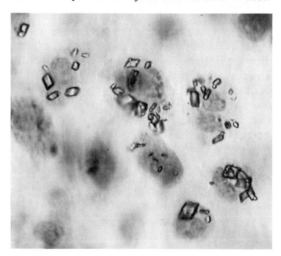

Fig. 10.8 Intracellular formation of bilirubin crystals in macrophages of mouse, 16 days after injection of haemoglobin. × 1200. (From preparations by the late Dr. Janet S. F. Niven.)

form around an old haemorrhage, particularly in the brain (Fig. 10.9): this may be due to the absence of lymphatics in brain tissue. Some of the iron released may also be retained locally as the pigment haemosiderin (see below), either within macrophages or as an incrustation of collagen and other tissue components.

Localised accumulation of haemosiderin may occur in the **lungs** as a result of haemorrhages in pulmonary venous congestion, e.g. in *mitral stenosis* (Fig. 10.10) and also in *idiopathic pulmonary haemosiderosis* where it is accompanied by fibrosis. Haemosiderin deposition also

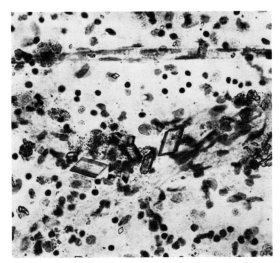

Fig. 10.9 Crystals of bilirubin and granular pigment, some of which is in phagocytes, at the site of an old cerebral haemorrhage. × 500.

occurs in the **renal tubular epithelium** when intravascular haemolysis results in release into the plasma of haemoglobin, which leaks into the glomerular filtrate and is taken up by the tubular cells (p. 525).

Bile pigments

A rise in the level of **bilirubin** in the plasma results from increased breakdown of red cells in the haemolytic anaemias, or from failure of the liver cells to remove and conjugate it with glucuronic acid. Lesions of the liver or biliary tract which prevent excretion of **bilirubin glucuronide** result in its regurgitation into the plasma. When the levels of either compound exceed 2–3 mg per 100 ml (35–50 μmol/l), **jaundice** develops, i.e. the skin, sclera and various other

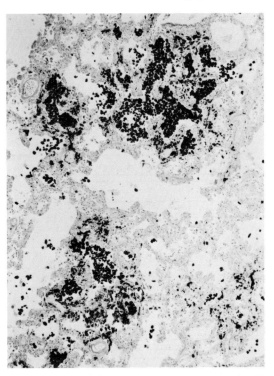

Fig. 10.10 The lung in mitral stenosis. Red cells escaping from the congested pulmonary capillaries are ingested by alveolar macrophages which became engorged with haemosiderin. The macrophages accumulate in the alveoli adjacent to respiratory bronchioles and are thus seen as aggregates. Prussian blue reaction. × 50.

tissues become distinctly yellow. In adults, jaundice itself causes little disability, but in infants a rise of (unconjugated) bilirubin in the plasma to over 15 mg per 100 ml (250 μmol/l) carries a risk of toxic brain injury. The types of jaundice and their causes and effects are, however, dealt with more fully in Chapter 19.

Iron pigments

About 70 per cent of the 3–4 g of iron in the body is incorporated in the haem of haemoglobin: 5 per cent is in myoglobin and small amounts are incorporated in cellular cytochrome, respiratory and metallo-flavo enzymes. The remainder (1–1·5 g) is mostly in storage form in macrophages of the spleen, bone marrow, etc. and in various tissue cells, but particularly hepatocytes.

Iron absorption is by way of the epithelial cells lining the gut, mainly those of the villi of the duodenum and proximal jejunum, absorption decreasing progressively more distally. Dietary iron consists of both haem (from meat and fish) which is absorbed as metalloporphyrin, and non-haem iron which is absorbed mainly as ferrous salts, ferric salts being poorly absorbed. The cells of the villi probably possess receptors for haem and for ferrous salts, both of which appear to be taken into the cells by endocytosis. The amounts of iron taken up by the epithelium depend mainly on two factors, the body's total storage iron and the amount of available iron in the diet. *The amount taken up is inversely proportional to the total storage iron in the body* (Fig. 10.11) *and*

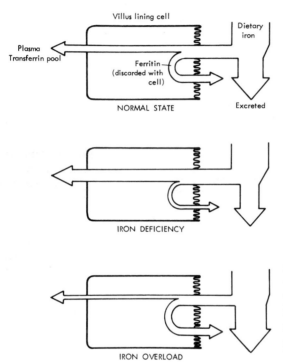

Fig. 10.11 The effect of the total iron store on absorption of dietary iron by intestinal epithelium. Only a fraction of the available dietary iron is normally taken up by the epithelium (*upper*): the fraction taken up is increased when total storage iron is depleted (*middle*) and decreased when the iron store is increased (*lower*). Of the iron taken up by the epithelium, the proportion transferred to the plasma transferrin pool is similarly affected by the total iron store.

directly proportional, within limits, to the amount available in the diet. It is not known how the storage iron influences absorption, but it seems likely that in iron deficiency states the number of iron receptors on the lining cells of the villi is increased. These observations apply to absorption of both haem iron and ferrous salts. Other dietary factors also influence iron absorption. For example, absorption of **non-haem iron** is aided by ascorbic acid, citric acid

and amino acids, all of which form monomeric complexes with iron and prevent the formation of non-absorbable polymers. Gastric HCl also favours absorption by preventing polymer formation and alcoholic drinks increase iron intake, possibly by stimulating gastric secretion but also because some drinks are rich in iron. Reduction of ferric to ferrous iron by ascorbic acid and other reducing agents also promotes absorption of non-haem iron. Formation of non-absorbable polymers is favoured by gastric achlorhydria and by the presence in the diet of certain compounds, e.g. phytate from cereals, tannates, calcium phosphate and ethylenediamine tetra-acetic acid (EDTA) used as a food preservative. These factors explain why iron deficiency is common among people living on a largely vegetable diet. **Haem** is a particularly important source of iron because, although it represents only a small part of the total dietary iron, the proportion absorbed is relatively high: its absorption is favoured by amino acids and is not inhibited by dietary factors (or achlorhydria) which inhibit absorption of non-haem iron.

Within the mucosal epithelial cells, haem iron is broken down and forms a common pool with the absorbed non-haem iron. Part of this pool is bound to a transferrin-like protein and is rapidly transferred through the epithelial cells to enter the plasma. The remainder is incorporated into intracellular ferritin (see below), much of which is lost when, within a few days, the cell exfoliates. The amount of epithelial-cell iron transferred to the plasma increases with the concentration of iron in the lumen of the gut, but the *proportion* transferred diminishes. Over a wide range of iron concentrations in the lumen, *the proportion of iron transferred is greater in subjects with iron deficiency, i.e. with depleted iron stores,* and is diminished when the iron stores are large (Fig. 10.11). How these factors influence the proportions of epithelial iron which bind to the transfer protein and to ferritin is not known.

Iron loss amounts to approximately 1 mg daily, most of it in the form of ferritin in the epithelial cells desquamated from the skin (0·2–0·3 mg) and gut (0·6 mg). Only a small proportion is lost in the bile, sweat, etc., and some of that lost by gut epithelium has been absorbed from the lumen by the cells, and incorporated into ferritin; it has never really entered the body's iron pool. In women of reproductive age, menstruation accounts for an average loss of an additional 0·6 mg daily, although there is enormous individual variation. Pregnancy, childbirth and lactation represent a rather greater loss than this.

From the above it will be apparent that *iron balance depends largely on the control of absorption from the gut: iron loss is small and subject to much less variation than is absorption.*

Plasma iron. The plasma of normal adults contains an average of about 120 μg of iron per dl, although the range is large. Over 95 per cent of this is in the form of **transferrin**, which consists of ferric iron bound to a specific transport protein, a β-globulin termed **apotransferrin**. This possesses two binding sites for iron and is normally only about 30 per cent saturated in the plasma. *Although transferrin makes up only a very small percentage of total body iron, it is very important, for it is the form in which iron is transferred from macrophages, parenchymal cells and intestinal epithelium to the erythropoietic cells.* In fact, the plasma iron is provided mainly by macrophages of the spleen, haemopoietic marrow, liver, etc., which break down red cells and synthesise apoferritin: these cells thus release transferrin, most of which is taken up by red cell precursors and used for haemoglobin synthesis.

A small proportion of plasma iron is in the form of ferritin (see below) and this is of importance because its concentration reflects the size of the total iron store of the body.

Haemoglobin synthesis. Red cell precursors have surface receptors for transferrin, which they take up avidly, probably by endocytosis. Uptake is proportional to the concentration in the plasma. Within the cell, iron is split off and used in haem synthesis, while the apotransferrin is returned to the plasma. With increasing maturity, the number of transferrin receptors on the erythroid cell diminishes, the mature red cell having none.

Storage iron. Iron is stored within cells in two forms, ferritin and haemosiderin. Most if not all cells synthesise apoferritins and store iron as **ferritin**, which consists of micelles of ferric oxide phosphate enclosed in a protein molecule which is water soluble. Ferritin is capable of incorporating approximately 5000 atoms of iron per molecule, but it is never fully saturated and provides an immediate reserve

iron storage capacity: it is not detectable by light microscopy but has a characteristic electron-microscopic appearance. The amount of iron stored as ferritin is limited and normally most of the total iron is stored in more concentrated form as **haemosiderin**. This is probably formed from ferritin and has a ferric iron content of up to 40 per cent. It is insoluble and if present in large amount is seen microscopically as golden-yellow intracytoplasmic granules, while it imparts to the tissue a brown appearance to the naked eye. Haemosiderin gives the prussian blue reaction on treatment with hydrochloric acid and potassium ferrocyanide, the intense blue colour being due to formation of ferri-ferrocyanide.

Most of the stored iron is present in the form of haemosiderin in macrophages in the spleen, marrow, etc. In parenchymal cells, notably in the liver, iron is normally stored mainly as ferritin, although there may be sufficient haemosiderin in the hepatocytes to give a faint prussian blue reaction. Absence of microscopically detectable haemosiderin in the macrophages in smears or sections of haemopoietic marrow indicates depletion of the iron stores. In states of increased storage, the proportion of iron in the form of haemosiderin increases and in gross iron overload it may be present in enormous amounts, its distribution between macrophages and parenchymal cells depending on the cause of the iron overload (see below).

In states of negative iron balance, iron is transferred from intracellular ferritin and haemosiderin to the plasma transferrin pool, most of it being provided by macrophages and hepatocytes, and anaemia does not develop until after the stores are depleted.

Iron deficiency

This is the commonest disturbance of iron metabolism. It results first in depletion of storage iron, secondly in anaemia, and lastly, and less certainly, in fall of the cytochrome content of cells. Most of the important effects of iron deficiency are due to anaemia, and accordingly the subject is dealt with in relation to the blood in Chapter 17.

Iron overload

This can result either from absorption of excessive amounts of iron from the gut or from administration of parenteral iron, for example by multiple blood transfusions.

The outstanding example of naturally occurring iron overload is provided by the disease termed **idiopathic haemochromatosis**, in which storage occurs predominantly in the parenchymal cells of the internal organs where it has serious consequences. By contrast, when multiple transfusions are administered over a period of years to patients with aplastic anaemia (due to marrow aplasia), iron accumulates mainly in macrophages, where it causes little injury. The effects of iron overload thus depend not so much on the amount of iron stored, as on its distribution between macrophages and parenchymal cells.

In iron overload due to excessive dietary iron or oral iron therapy, and in certain disorders of haemoglobin or red cell production, the distribution of stored iron, as explained later, is more complex.

States of increased iron storage are conveniently termed **haemosiderosis** or **siderosis**.

Idiopathic haemochromatosis

This is characterised by excessive absorption of dietary iron, probably from birth. The total iron of the body gradually increases until, by the age of 40 years or so, it may exceed 20 g instead of the normal 3–4 g. Erythropoiesis is normal and the excess of iron is stored as haemosiderin mainly in the parenchymal cells, particularly in the liver (Fig. 10.12), pancreas and myocardium, but also in many other organs.

The condition usually affects men, and the quantity of iron stored depends on the amount of available iron in the diet and is also increased by heavy alcohol consumption, which is common among affected individuals. Iron in excess has a cytotoxic effect: hepatocyte destruction with accompanying fibrosis leads to cirrhosis, which is often the cause of presenting symptoms. The toxic effect on the myocardial cells commonly leads to congestive heart failure and cardiac arrhythmias, while heavy deposition in the pancreas results in cell loss and fibrosis. Over 50 per cent of patients develop diabetes, probably due to a combination of liver and islet-cell injury. The liver, pancreas, etc. appear brown to the naked eye and give an intense prussian blue reaction. Microscopy shows heavy deposition of haemosiderin in the

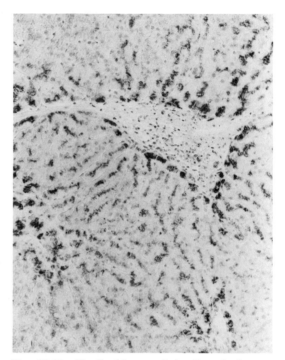

Fig. 10.12 Needle biopsy of the liver in haemochromatosis. The excess iron is stored mainly as haemosiderin in the hepatocytes, and is seen as dark granules. Prussian blue reaction. × 150.

parenchymal cells. Death of damaged cells results in release of haemosiderin, which is therefore seen also in the adjacent stroma and in macrophages in the affected organs and their draining lymph nodes. Apart from this, the amount of haemosiderin in macrophages in general, e.g. in the spleen and bone marrow, is not greatly increased. The gastric mucosal cells are rich in haemosiderin, but not the cells of the villi of the upper small intestine. The skin develops a bronzed appearance (hence the term **bronzed diabetes**) due to excess melanin production, which is unexplained; in some cases, however, the skin appears more leaden owing to iron deposition, mainly in relation to the sweat glands. Other features include the polyarthritis of pseudo-gout, due to the formation in the joint tissues and spaces of calcium pyrophosphate crystals; this may result from the inhibitory effects of iron on pyrophosphatase. Hypogonadism, probably due to injury to the adenohypophysis, is common, and also vague neurological symptoms of unknown cause.

Aetiology. The nature of the metabolic defect responsible for excessive iron absorption is unknown. The plasma transferrin is not increased but is fully saturated with iron (cf. normal 30 per cent saturation). Tests of iron absorption have given conflicting results, but if the iron stores are depleted by venesection etc., absorption can then be demonstrated to be increased. If the iron stores are allowed to reaccumulate, absorption falls, sometimes to normal. The inverse relationship between total iron store and absorption is thus maintained, but *the proportion of dietary iron absorbed at all levels of iron storage is abnormally high*: as noted by Bothwell *et al.* (1979) the 'absorbostat' is set too high.

Although the nature of the defect is unknown, it appears that macrophages are incapable of storing excess iron as haemosiderin, and that in consequence the plasma transferrin becomes saturated and so excess iron is taken up by the parenchymal cells of the liver, etc. Because transferrin is saturated, iron absorbed from the gut and transferred to the plasma may be transported by the portal circulation in a form which is readily taken up by the liver cells, thus explaining why the liver is particularly severely affected.

Inheritance of haemochromatosis has been much debated. Occasionally it affects more than one member of a family, and investigation of the relatives of patients has shown that many of them, although apparently healthy, have a sub-clinical form of the disease with lesser degrees of increased iron storage, increased saturation of plasma transferrin, and sometimes liver injury short of cirrhosis. Such individuals are believed to be particularly prone to develop the clinical picture of haemochromatosis if their alcohol consumption is high. It has been suggested that the disease is inherited as a recessive character, the homozygous state resulting in overt haemochromatosis and the heterozygous state causing sub-clinical iron overload. In both the overt and sub-clinical disease, alcohol probably acts by its toxic effect on the liver and by increasing iron absorption.

The importance of genetic factors is suggested also by the reported high incidence of HLA-A3 and B7 antigens in patients, and by the occurrence of the sub-clinical form of the disease in siblings of identical HLA types. The nature of genetic inheritance is, however, unlikely to be elucidated until a test for the defect in the presumed heterozygote becomes available.

Apart from treatment of heart failure, diabetes etc., reduction of the excess iron store, for example by repeated phlebotomy and by limiting the dietary iron, is the most effective form of therapy.

Iron overload in anaemia

Iron deficiency is a common cause of anaemia, but in certain types of anaemia due to other causes there may be greatly increased iron storage. For example, in aplastic anaemia, in which haemopoiesis fails and the marrow becomes hypocellular, life can be maintained only by regular blood transfusions and since each unit of blood contains 200–250 mg of iron, gross iron overload can develop over a number of years. In contrast to haemochromatosis, most of the iron accumulating as haemosiderin is stored in macrophages in the spleen, liver (Fig. 10.13), marrow and elsewhere. There is some increase of iron in the hepatocytes; initially it is relatively slight, but later may increase as a result of redistribution of iron.

The situation is different in patients in whom anaemia is due to defective red cell production

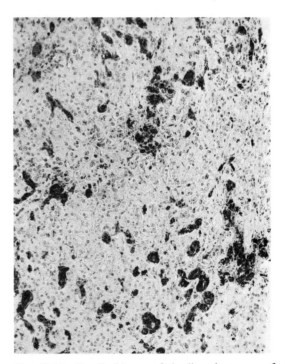

Fig. 10.13 Needle biopsy of the liver in a case of haemosiderosis resulting from multiple blood transfusions. Haemosiderin is present in groups of enlarged Kupffer cells and macrophages in the portal areas. The patient suffered from chronic renal failure and had been maintained on haemodialysis. × 150.

in spite of hyperplasia of the erythropoietic tissue, i.e. in which there is '*ineffective erythropoiesis*'. A good example is provided by thalassaemia major (p. 524) in which there is defective haemoglobin synthesis, and in the familial form of sideroblastic anaemia (p. 540) in which incorporation of iron into haemoglobin is defective. In such conditions, immature erythroid cells are destroyed in the marrow. In some unknown manner, increased but ineffective erythropoiesis increases iron absorption and thus causes overload, which, as in haemochromatosis, results in deposition in parenchymal cells. If the condition is inherited and so present from birth onwards, a picture similar to haemochromatosis may develop.

In anaemia with increased but *effective* erythropoiesis, e.g. chronic haemolytic anaemia, in which circulating red cells are destroyed abnormally rapidly, and in which compensatory increase in erythropoiesis occurs, there is little or no increase in iron absorption and overloading does not usually occur unless multiple transfusions are administered.

Dietary iron overload

It is rare for serious iron overload to occur from increased iron intake in the diet, partly because in most diets with a high iron content much of the iron is in unavailable form, and partly because any increase in iron stores inhibits absorption of dietary iron. There is, however, one outstanding example of overload resulting from dietary factors, and that is in South Africans of the Bantu tribe. Their intake of iron is very high, partly because iron pots are used in cooking, but mainly from drinking beer brewed in iron containers. Because of its low pH, the brew dissolves iron and as much as 50–100 mg of iron may be ingested daily in a few litres of the (rather weak) beer. The distribution of iron varies: in many cases, however, it accumulates both in macrophages and in the parenchymal cells in the liver and sometimes other organs, and the picture of haemochromatosis with hepatic cirrhosis and sometimes diabetes may develop. In such cases, the degree of liver injury has been shown to correlate partly with the amount of iron in the hepatocytes. A striking difference from haemochromatosis is the deposition of haemosiderin in the lamina propria of the villi of the proximal small intestine. In other individuals, storage of iron is predominantly in macrophages and without serious effects. It is not known why iron deposition is parenchymal in some and in macrophages in others, but it has been reported that, in the former, there is a high degree of saturation of plasma transferrin. With the increasing use of commercially prepared beverages, the incidence of haemosiderosis in the Bantu has declined considerably. The alcohol in the beer also doubtless contributes to the hepatic injury and in some cases the picture is that of alcoholic cirrhosis with excess of iron deposition.

The risk of serious iron overload from prolonged taking of medicinal iron by mouth appears to be slight, for although there are reports of haemochromatosis developing, in many other cases the iron stores do not appear to have been very greatly increased. Acute iron poisoning can, however, result from gross overdosage with iron.

Malarial pigmentation

In malaria the parasites within the red cells produce from the haemoglobin a dark brown pigment, haematin, in the form of very minute granules, which accumulates within the parasites. When the adult divides into young forms (merozoites), the red cell disintegrates and the pigment is released to be taken up by monocytes (Figs. 17.22, 17.24, p. 529) and by macrophages, especially in the spleen, liver and haemopoietic marrow, where it remains practically unchanged for many years. In chronic malaria these tissues appear dark brown. Malaria pigment does not give the prussian blue reaction and resembles closely the artefact pigment derived from formalin acting on blood. When there is much blood destruction, especially in severe cases of malaria, haemosiderin may be deposited in the organs in addition to the malarial pigment.

Lipofuscin: Age Pigment

In the later years of life a fine brownish-yellow pigment tends to appear in the heart muscle, smooth muscle, etc.; and in wasting diseases this accumulation of pigment is more marked. In some cases of malabsorption syndrome, for example due to coeliac disease, it is present in the smooth muscle of the small intestine and oesophagus, and in smaller amounts in that of the stomach and colon: experimental studies suggest that vitamin E deficiency may be responsible.

In the heart muscle the pigment accumulates in the central part of the cells around the poles of the nucleus, and when this is associated with wasting of the muscle, the term *brown atrophy* is applied. Similar pigment may occur in the liver cells, especially in the central parts of the lobules, in the cells of the testis, and in the nerve cells of the cortex of the brain. Heavy deposits of pigment in the cortical neurons are seen in senile dementia and allied conditions. The pigment must be distinguished from that which occurs normally in the pigmented neurons of the locus caeruleus and substantia nigra, which belongs to the melanin group. In brown atrophy the pigment is believed to be chiefly lipid, as it reduces perosmic acid and is usually coloured by the sudan stains. It is often called *lipofuscin*, but differs in its chemical and staining reactions in the various organs, some being fluorescent, doubly refracting or acid-fast in varying degree, e.g. *ceroid*, an acid-fast pigment found in the liver in certain forms of experimental cirrhosis. In electron micrographs it is seen as *residual bodies* (p. 23), which result from incorporation of cell constituents into phagosomes in the process of autophagocytosis, the lipofuscin persisting as indigestible residues of cellular lipids.

Exogenous Pigmentation

Inhaled compounds. The most important exogenous pigments are those inhaled as dust particles and entering the body through the respiratory passages. A certain amount of soot, stone dust, etc., enters and accumulates in the lungs of all individuals living in urban conditions, but the accumulation becomes excessive in those exposed occupationally to an atmosphere rich in dust. The lungs may be infiltrated by foreign particles of various kinds— coal, silica, asbestos, iron and other ores and various organic substances. The resulting pathological changes will be described later with the diseases of the lungs.

The entrance of such particles into the lungs is favoured by the presence of chronic bronchitis or other condition in which there is interference with the action of the ciliated epithelium, but even in normal health, particles of less than 5 μm gain access to the pulmonary alveoli if the amount in the inspired air is great. The dust particles are quickly taken up by macrophages in the pulmonary alveoli (Fig. 10.14). Some of the macrophages with the ingested particles are expelled *via* the bronchi, some enter

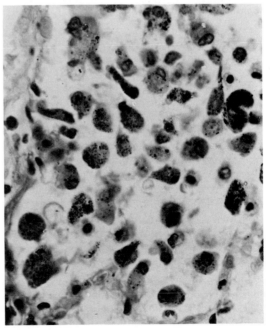

Fig. 10 14   The lung of a coal-miner showing phagocytosis of inhaled particles of coal dust by alveolar macrophages. × 520.

the interstitial tissue of the lungs, and pass into the lymphatics, while some settle in the alveoli alongside respiratory bronchioles, and the pigment is eventually incorporated into the respiratory bronchiolar walls. Much of the pigment, however, is carried into the lymphatics; most of it is deposited in the hilar nodes, but some in the pleura. The degree of irritation resulting depends on the nature of the particles. Large collections of carbonaceous particles (*anthracosis*) may provoke little or no overgrowth of connective tissue, whereas fibrosis is very marked in the case of silica-containing stone dust, the condition of *silicosis* resulting. The bronchial lymph nodes become pigmented and enlarged, the accumulation within their phagocytic cells being virtually permanent. Some of the pigment which has accumulated in the lungs may be removed by macrophages which appear in the sputum for a long time after removal of the individual from the dusty atmosphere.

Ingested compounds. Deposition of brownish granules of silver compounds (*argyria*) was a common result of taking medicines containing silver preparations. The granules are formed by reduction of silver albuminate and are seen especially in the skin (giving a dusky appearance), the gut wall, and the basement membranes of the glomeruli and renal collecting tubules. It is now rare. In *chronic lead-poisoning* an albuminate is produced in a similar way, and around the teeth hydrogen sulphide reacts with it to produce the characteristic blue line on the gums. *Melanosis coli* (p. 277) is now the commonest example of pigmentation resulting from ingestion of chemicals.

Tattooing. In tattooing, fine particles such as india ink, ultramarine, cinnabar (mercuric sulphide), etc., introduced through the epidermis, are taken up by macrophages and lodge in small spaces or clefts in the connective tissue of the cutis. Some particles are carried also by the lymph stream to the regional lymph nodes and then are conveyed by phagocytes into the lymphoid tissue. Both at the site of introduction and in the lymph nodes the pigment persists for life.

Pathological Calcification

Pathological calcification of soft tissues occurs most commonly without any general disturbance of calcium metabolism: the level of plasma calcium is normal, and deposition is due to local changes in the affected tissue. This is termed *dystrophic calcification*. Less commonly, pathological calcification is a result of an increase in the level of ionic calcium in the plasma, and occurs in normal soft tissues: this is termed *metastatic calcification*.

In both dystrophic and metastatic calcification the deposits resemble in composition the minerals of bone, but show much greater variations in the proportions of calcium to magnesium and phosphate to carbonate.

Identification of calcium salts in tissues. Calcium salts have an affinity for haematoxylin, and the earliest sign of calcification is given by the appearance of hyaline or finely granular material of a deep violet tint. Later the calcium salts form irregular and somewhat refractile masses: they are, of course, readily soluble in weak acids, and small bubbles of carbon dioxide are released from the carbonates. When treated with dilute sulphuric acid, the characteristic crystals of calcium sulphate separate out. This occurs more readily when the sections are in 50 per cent alcohol, in which the solubility of the crystals is low. When carbonate or phosphate (which are nearly always deposited as calcium salts) are treated with silver nitrate, yellow silver phosphate is formed, and this quickly undergoes reduction on exposure to light and turns black (von Kossa's method). Neither the affinity for haematoxylin nor von Kossa's method is specific for calcium. Silver nitrate is reduced by other substances, e.g. iron, and the reaction with haematoxylin is given by a substance formed before the deposition of calcium, and is positive after the tissue is decalcified. The best reagent is alizarin, the staining principle in madder, or its derivatives. Alizarin stains calcium salts red, but the reaction may not be given by very old deposits. When injected *intra vitam*, alizarin colours growing bone (but not fully formed bone) and also pathological deposits of calcium unless they are very old.

Calcification is often accompanied by diffuse or granular deposition of iron compounds which give a prussian blue reaction.

Dystrophic calcification

This consists of the irregular deposition of calcium salts in altered or necrotic tissues and formed elements such as thrombi. Deposition is irregular and may be sufficiently heavy to render the part chalky or even stony hard.

Predisposing changes. The local changes which predispose to dystrophic calcification are as follows.

(*1*) *Hyaline changes in fibrous tissue.* This occurs as an ageing change in arteries. Increase in calcium in hyalinised artery walls is usual, and it may be sufficient to convert the vessel to a rigid tube, as in Monckeberg's sclerosis (Fig. 14.19, p. 376). Calcification is also common in dense connective tissues, for example tendons, the dura mater, and the scarred heart valves following rheumatic endocarditis. It occurs in some tumours, for example in fibromas (Fig. 10.15) and in uterine myomas undergoing involution after the menopause. The 'brain-sand' bodies of some meningiomas consist of concentrically arranged cells which undergo hyaline change followed by calcification.

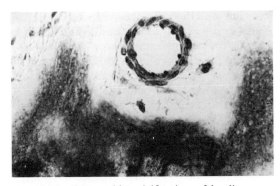

Fig. 10.15 Dystrophic calcification of hyaline connective tissue adjacent to a small blood vessel in a fibroma. The calcified tissue is stained by haematoxylin (even after decalcification), and presents a dark granular appearance. × 500.

(*2*) *Tissue death.* Calcification commonly occurs in (*a*) the necrotic lipid debris in atheromatous patches, (*b*) fat necrosis (usually around the pancreas or in the breast), (*c*) old infarcts (*d*) caseous patches in tuberculosis, necrotic foci in histoplasmosis and other chronic infections, (*e*) necrotic foci in malignant tumours, and (*f*) dead parasites (e.g. *Trichinella spiralis* and echinococcal cysts). Calcification of such dead tissue is a slow process, and occurs only when necrotic material persists for a long time without undergoing organisation.

(*3*) *Inspissated pus* and *organic material in ducts, etc.* A large collection of pus, unless discharged, may eventually become inspissated, then calcified, and even ossified. Organic material accumulating in the ducts of salivary glands, or in the appendix, may become calcified, forming 'stones' in these sites. Calcium deposition in the urinary tract, both as discrete stones and as soft, crumbling material, is caused by urinary infections, but stone formation occurs also as a result of increased calcium excretion (see below).

(*4*) *Thrombi.* Calcification occurs very commonly in old venous thrombi which have not undergone organisation: hard masses are thus formed in veins, e.g. in the legs, and show up on x-ray as *phleboliths*.

The chemical reactions involved in dystrophic calcification are not understood. Factors which may be involved include the following. (*a*) Local changes in pH of hyaline or necrotic tissue, etc.: calcium is deposited more readily from an alkaline medium. (*b*) Breakdown products of cells or tissue elements to provide a nucleus with an affinity for calcium salts. Release of phosphate from nucleoprotein breakdown is a possible example. The strong tendency for calcification of necrotic fatty tissue was formerly explained by the affinity of fatty acids for calcium, forming insoluble calcium soaps. This suggestion lacks supporting evidence, and in particular subcutaneous injection of fatty acids does not lead to calcification. (*c*) Local enzyme changes: the normal process of calcification of growing bone occurs in the presence of high local concentrations of alkaline phosphatase. In experimentally induced lesions, some correlation has been observed between high levels of alkaline phosphatase and deposition of calcium salts, but the correlation is not a very good one, and this is not a convincing factor in dystrophic calcification in man.

Calcinosis circumscripta. This is a condition in which irregular nodular dystrophic calcification occurs in the skin and subcutaneous tissues, especially of the fingers. The overlying skin becomes ulcerated and the chalky material is discharged or may be scraped out. This appears to consist chiefly of calcium carbonate, as shown by solution with effervescence in hydrochloric acid. Microscopically a mild chronic inflammatory reaction with giant cells surrounds the nodules. The causation of the lesion is obscure. The deposits are easily distinguished from gouty tophi by their dense opacity to x-rays and by histochemical tests. (See also tumoral calcinosis, p. 928).

Occasionally calcium deposition is more widespread, involving also muscles and tendons—this is known as **calcinosis universalis**.

A number of other diseases, including scleroderma and dermatomyositis, are occasionally complicated by calcification of the dermis or subcutaneous tissues.

Metastatic calcification

This occurs in the following conditions.

(1) Excessive absorption of calcium from the gut, seen most commonly in infants with hypervitaminosis D due to over-fortification of infant foods with vitamin D and calcium (p. 889). Similar experimental changes can be produced readily in the rat (Fig. 10.16).

Excessive intake can result also from taking very large amounts of calcium by mouth, for example milk and calcium carbonate by sufferers from peptic ulcer: this may lead to hypercalcaemia and alkalosis (the milk-alkali syndrome).

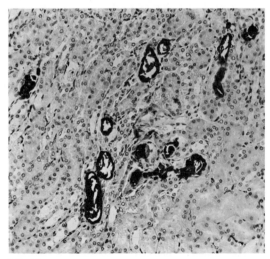

Fig. 10.16   Rat kidney in hypervitaminosis D. Note calcified small vessels and renal tubules. × 120. (From preparation kindly lent by Dr. J. R. M. Innes.)

(2) Excessive mobilisation of calcium from the bones. This occurs in patients with *widespread bone destruction*, as for example in multiple myeloma or metastatic carcinoma. *Prolonged immobilisation* in bed for any reason is also of importance, the bones undergoing disuse atrophy. Excessive mobilisation of bone calcium is also brought about by *primary hyperparathyroidism*, usually due to a parathyroid adenoma (p. 1035), but a more common cause is *secondary hyperparathyroidism* associated with parathyroid hyperplasia and resulting from chronic renal failure with retention of phosphate (p. 1036).

Metastatic calcification occurs especially in the walls of arteries and in the kidneys. It is occasionally seen in the myocardium, acid-secreting gastric mucosa and the alveolar walls of the lungs. It may be that the sites of metastatic calcification are determined by a relatively high pH, e.g. around the renal tubules and the acid-secreting gastric glands. Deposition is seen initially on the surface of elastic fibres, basement membranes and other formed elements.

The **kidneys** and **urinary tract** are the commonest and most important sites of metastatic calcification. In the kidney, deposition of calcium occurs in the tubular epithelium and may be seen by electron microscopy in relation to mitochondria. More gross calcium deposition may occur in the tubular basement membranes, the interstitial tissue, and calcified concretions may form in the tubular lumen, usually of the collecting tubules. These changes are accompanied by impaired function, and by the development of coarse scars involving segments of the cortex and medulla (possibly due to obstruction of individual collecting tubules). Chronic renal failure may result. The renal arteries may also be calcified but, as elsewhere, patency is little affected.

Another important feature of hypercalcaemia is the formation of calcium carbonate/phosphate stones in the urinary tract (p. 868).

Nephrocalcinosis and stone formation are particularly liable to occur when there is increased intake of calcium associated with alkalosis and an alkaline urine, as in the milk-alkali syndrome; they occur also in renal tubular acidosis (p. 845).

Deposition of Uric Acid and Urates

Uric acid is formed as the final breakdown product of purine bases, and is thus derived from catabolism of nucleic acids. Normal plasma urate levels depend greatly on the assay technique, but levels above 7·0 mg/100 ml (0·42 mmol/l) for men and 6·0 mg/100 ml (0·36 mmol/l) for women are abnormally high. Adults produce 400–700 mg of endogenous uric acid daily and dietary purines contribute 300–600 mg. Most of this uric acid is excreted by the renal distal convoluted tubules, which can normally increase the rate of excretion, as necessary, to maintain homoeostasis.

Hyperuricaemia is not uncommon, particularly in men over 40. It tends to be familial, but sporadic cases occur. The metabolic abnormalities concerned are not clearly understood. In some instances, increased production of uric acid results from a deficiency of the phosphoribosyl-transferase enzyme which is necessary for the re-utilisation of hypoxanthine for purine synthesis. This deficiency results in increased breakdown of hypoxanthine into uric acid. Other enzyme deficiencies with similar effect have been detected in some instances of hyperuricaemia. In others, there is a defect of unknown nature in renal excretion of uric acid. These defects account for at least some cases of *primary hyperuricaemia* in which nucleic acid breakdown is normal. *Secondary hyperuricaemia* results from increased nucleic acid breakdown, as in chronic myeloid leukaemia (p. 547).

There is considerable variation in the effects of hyperuricaemia. In most instances, there are no associated pathological changes. In others there is deposition of uric acid or urate in the collecting tubules of the kidneys, seen macroscopically as brown-yellow streaking of the medulla: this may have little or no effect, or may be followed by formation of uric acid stones (p. 868). Uric acid streaking of the medulla is a common necropsy finding, particularly in children, and appears to be associated with a state of dehydration before death. The most important complication of hyperuricaemia is **gout** (p. 923), in which crystals of monosodium urate are deposited in and around the joints, in the skin (Fig. 10.17) and elsewhere. It is always accompanied by hyperuricaemia, and yet the relatives of patients may have equally high levels of plasma uric acid without developing gout. As indicated above for hyperuricaemia in general, a number of individual abnormalities of purine metabolism can result in gout.

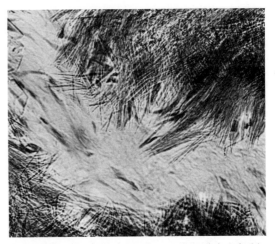

Fig. 10.17 Section through gouty nodule of skin, showing deposit of needle-like crystals of monosodium urate. × 370.

Further Reading

Bothwell, T. H., Charlton, R. W., Cook, J. W. and Finch, C. A. (1979). *Iron Metabolism in Man*, pp. 576. Blackwell Scientific, Oxford, London, Edinburgh and Melbourne. (A comprehensive review by four leading experts, with an extensive bibliography.)

Glenner, G. G. and Page, D. L. (1976). Amyloid, Amyloidosis and Amyloidogenesis. In *International Review of Experimental Pathology*, Vol. 15, pp. 1–92.

Lendrum, A. C. (1969). The Validation of Fibrin and its Significance in the Story of Hyalin. In *Trends in Clinical Pathology*, pp. 159–183. British Medical Association, London.

Scheinberg, M. A. and Cathcart, E. S. (1976). Comprehensive study of humoral and cellular immune abnormalities in 26 patients with systemic amyloidosis. *Arthritis and Rheumatism*, **19**, 173–182.

11

Tumours: 1. General Features, Causation and Host Reactions

General Features of Tumours

In previous chapters we have seen examples of cell proliferation and growth of tissues in the process of repair, in response to irritation, and as a hyperplastic response to increased workload or hormonal stimulation. Such growth is purposeful, and, up to a point, capable of explanation. In a tumour (neoplasm), however, the growth is not only excessive but apparently purposeless, progressing without regard to the surrounding tissues or the requirements of the individual as a whole. While forming a part of the body, tumour cells seem to have become largely unresponsive to the factors which control the proliferation of non-neoplastic cells. Accordingly, tumours exhibit various degrees of uncontrolled growth and in some instances uncontrolled function, e.g. the production of hormones or enzymes. Such behaviour is commonly termed *autonomous*, but a tumour is, of course, dependent on the host for its nutrition, blood supply and supporting stroma, and escape from host control factors is only relative.

Definition. A tumour, or neoplasm, is an abnormal mass of tissue, the growth of which exceeds and is unco-ordinated with that of the normal tissues and continues in the same manner after cessation of the stimuli which have initiated it. This definition covers most tumours, which form discrete lumps, but in the leukaemias, which are tumours of myeloid or lymphoid cells, the tumour cells may extend diffusely through the marrow or lymphoid tissues, and also circulate in the blood.

Origin. Tumours show an extraordinary variety of structure, but the majority retain a resemblance to some normal tissue or cell type; occasionally the resemblance is to some precursor cell or tissue rather than to the fully differentiated adult type. These resemblances are attributable to the origin of each tumour from abnormal and excessive proliferation of a cell derived from the previously normal tissue. Tumours arise most often from tissues in which the cells are normally labile (i.e. they are continually being replaced by new cells—p. 77), and which are exposed to the various noxious agents in the environment (especially the skin and the epithelium of the alimentary and respiratory tracts). Many tumours do, however, originate from the cells of organs not so exposed and normally having more stable cells, e.g. those of the liver, thyroid, adrenal, cartilage or fat. The adult neuron is probably the only type of nucleated cell in the body incapable of giving rise to a tumour.

Classification. The cell or tissue origin of a tumour is called its *histogenesis*, and provides the basis of a principal mode of classification. On this basis, nearly all tumours may be classified as *epithelial* or *connective tissue* tumours according to the cell of origin. Tumours are further classified by their naked-eye appearances, their microscopic features and by the nature of their products. *The most important mode of classification is, however, based on behaviour, and divides tumours into benign and malignant types (see below).* So little is known of the precise causal factors of most individual tumours that a classification based on aetiology is not yet widely applicable.

In this text, **tumour** or **neoplasm** is used for all lesions of this type, whether benign or malignant. **Cancer** is used for all malignant tumours, regardless of their origin. **Carcinoma** is used only for malignant tumours of epith-

elium, and **carcinogenesis** for the changes involved in the development of malignant tumours of all types.

Variations in tumour behaviour

Tumours vary considerably in their
behaviour, notably in the following important
features.

Rate of growth. There are all gradations between slowly-growing tumours that hardly
change in size from year to year and those
which grow so rapidly that differences in size
may be detected from week to week. Many
tumours consist very largely of tumour cells,
with blood vessels and supporting stroma contributing little to the total mass: their rate of
growth depends on the rate of proliferation and
the life-span of the tumour cells. Epithelial
tumours may add to their bulk by accumulation of material secreted by the tumour cells,
e.g. mucin, or they may induce a fibrous reaction, so that they come to consist largely of fibrous stroma in which lie groups of tumour
cells. The growth of some connective tissue
tumours depends largely on the production of
matrix (collagenous, cartilaginous, etc.) by the
tumour cells. Vascular congestion, oedema and
infection can all occur in tumours, as in normal
tissues, and contribute to fluctuations in their
rate of growth.

By definition, the *rate of cell production* in
tumours exceeds the rate of cell death. The rate
of cell production depends on the *growth fraction*, i.e. the proportion of cells entering the cell
cycle which culminates in mitosis (Fig. 11.1),
and the time taken to complete the cycle. The
number of mitoses seen microscopically is thus
a general indication of the rate of tumour
growth. In general, the rate of cell production
is greater in malignant than in benign tumours.
The kinetics of tumour cell proliferation are of
importance in planning certain types of therapy, for many anti-tumour drugs destroy
mainly cells undergoing mitosis. The features
determining the *life-span of tumour cells* are
complex and not fully understood. In some
tumours, for example basal cell carcinoma of
the epidermis, many cells undergo shrinkage
necrosis (*apoptosis*—p. 11), and in spite of a
high mitotic rate, growth is surprisingly slow.
In many malignant tumours *disorders of mitosis*
result in abnormalities in the number and

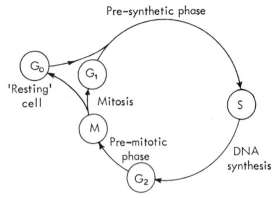

Fig. 11.1 The mitotic or cell cycle, showing the relative duration of each phase. The whole cycle normally takes from about 24 hours to several days,
depending largely on the duration of G_1, the phase
preceding the synthesis of DNA (S phase). The S
phase is followed by a brief (G_2) phase before the
cell undergoes mitosis (M). After mitosis, the cell
may leave the cycle to enter the 'resting' (G_0) stage,
in which it may remain for its whole lifespan; cells in
G_0 phase may, however, re-enter the cycle at the G_1
phase. The factors which inhibit cell division do so
by arresting cells in the G_0 or G_1 phase.

structure of the chromosomes. The cells produced are pleomorphic (Fig. 11.3) and many of
them are non-viable. *Aberrant mitoses* are thus a
feature of malignant tumours. Malignant tumours also tend to outgrow their blood supply
and the rapidly increasing number of cells compress the small blood vessels. Accordingly, *ischaemic necrosis* is a conspicuous feature of many
malignant tumours (Fig. 11.2); those involving
the skin or a mucous membrane tend to ulcerate and *bacterial infection* then results in more
extensive necrosis.

Although many malignant tumours grow
progressively and relentlessly, individual tumours may fluctuate greatly in their growth rate.
It is, for example, not uncommon for removal
of a breast cancer or a melanoma of the skin to
be followed by many years of good health: in
some patients, local or distant foci of residual
tumour eventually become apparent and grow
rapidly. Clearly, tumour has persisted since
before the time of excision of the original
tumour, but for many years has failed to grow
significantly. This suggests that host defence
mechanisms are involved, and that they may
arrest tumour growth for long periods.

Invasion and spread. *The cells of benign tumours remain at the site of origin, forming a single*

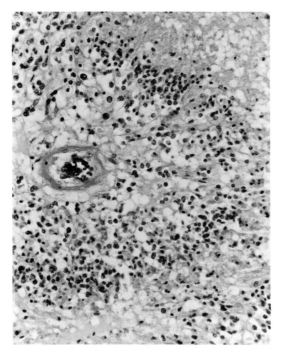

Fig. 11.2 Ischaemic necrosis in a tumour. In this example, the tumour is a rapidly growing anaplastic astrocytoma of the brain, composed of cells with a round dark nucleus. The tumour cells immediately around a small blood vessel have survived, forming a cuff which occupies most of the picture. More peripherally the tumour has undergone ischaemic necrosis with loss of nuclear staining. × 190. (Dr. A. M. Lutfy.)

mass. When growing in a solid tissue, they compress the surrounding normal cells which undergo pressure atrophy and necrosis: the tissue stroma is more resistant and may become condensed to form a fibrous *capsule* (Fig. 12,8, p. 326). The formation of a capsule has however been given too much emphasis, for in some benign tumours the capsule is incomplete, little or no stroma separating the adjacent tissue from the tumour cell mass: this is particularly the case in tissues like the adrenal which can expand readily without pressure atrophy occurring.

The cells of malignant tumours invade locally and also spread by the lymphatics, bloodstream and body cavities to form **secondary tumours** *or* **metastases** remote from the site of origin. In some instances it is difficult or impossible to determine which is the original or **primary tumour**, particularly when their cells are poorly differentiated (see below).

Differentiation. This is the degree of resemblance of a tumour to its tissue of origin and can be applied morphologically and functionally to the tumour cells. The naked eye appearances of a well differentiated tumour sometimes reveal its nature: for instance a lipoma is usually recognisable as an encapsulated mass of adipose tissue of essentially normal microscopic appearance. The less differentiated a tumour is, the more difficult it is to identify its tissue of origin and the tissue of origin of a poorly differentiated tumour may remain unknown despite naked eye, light- and electron-microscopic and biochemical examination. Partial loss of differentiation is termed **dysplasia** and complete loss, so that the tumour no longer resembles its tissue of origin, is termed **anaplasia** (Fig. 11.3).

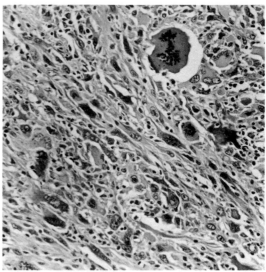

Fig. 11.3 Section of an anaplastic malignant tumour showing also great variation in shape and size of the cells and of their nuclei (pleomorphism). Note also the abnormal mitoses. × 200.

There is a general correlation between the above features; *malignant tumours are usually rapidly growing, poorly differentiated, and have a high mitotic rate with nuclear pleomorphism and abnormal mitoses (Fig. 11.3), while benign tumours are usually slow growing, well differentiated, and show infrequent mitoses and little cytological variation (Fig. 11.4, see also Figs. 12.2–20, pp. 323–32 and 13.2–15, pp. 341–7).*

Benign tumours seldom kill unless they arise near and press on vital structures or secrete ex-

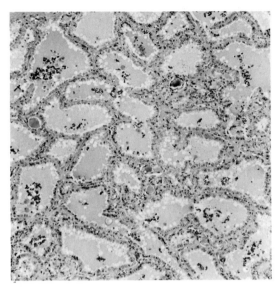

Fig. 11.4 Section of a benign tumour of the thyroid. Note the close resemblance to thyroid tissue. × 75.

Table 11.1 Contrasting features of benign and malignant tumours

	Benign	Malignant
(a) *Evidence on rate of growth*		
Mitoses	Few and normal	Numerous and often abnormal
Nuclei	Little altered	Enlarged, often irregular (pleomorphic)
Nucleoli	Little altered	Usually large
Cytoplasmic basophilia	Slight	Marked
Haemorrhage and necrosis	Inconspicuous	Often extensive
(b) *Differentiation*		
Naked-eye resemblance to tissue of origin	Often close	Variable: from close to none
Microscopic resemblance to tissue of origin	Usually very marked	Usually poor
Function, e.g. secretion	Often well maintained	May be retained, lost, or abnormal products
(c) *Evidence on transgression of normal boundaries*		
Capsule intact	Frequent	Rare (usually none)
Local invasion	Absent	Very frequent
Metastases	Never	Frequent

cessive amounts of hormone. Most fatal tumours are malignant, and death may result from local invasion, from the effects of metastases, or from a combination of both. The identification of tumours as benign or malignant is therefore crucial and is a major responsibility of the hospital histopathologist. Table 11.1 compares the characteristics of benign and malignant tumours. However, the distinction is not absolute and borderline tumours occur. Some tumours, for example, are locally invasive and yet rarely metastasise.

Progression of a benign tumour to malignancy is not common, and most malignant tumours do not arise from a benign tumour. The behaviour of the innumerable different kinds of tumours of different organs varies greatly, and it is necessary to know these variations before one can apply the criteria in Table 11.1 with safety to the individual patient.

Examples of exceptional behaviour. *Rate of growth.* Some benign tumours (especially of the female genitalia, e.g. myomas of the uterus and cystadenomas of the ovary) may grow very rapidly and reach a great size. Some malignant tumours—basal cell carcinomas of the epidermis, some breast carcinomas and in particular carcinoid tumours of the gut and 'latent' carcinoma of the prostate—grow very slowly. Incidentally, the normal fetus grows faster than any tumour.

Differentiation. Some benign tumours show a high degree of cellular specialisation and structural arrangement, but do not resemble the parent tissue. Mucinous cystadenoma of the ovary (Fig. 24.21, p. 962) is an example: it is 'well differentiated' but in a different direction from the parent tissue. Some malignant tumours (some squamous carcinomas, for instance, and well differentiated thyroid carcinomas) may closely resemble the parent tissue. Function is not always lost in malignant tumours; indeed, such normal functions as the production of keratin, mucus, melanin, and hormones, may be well maintained by malignant tumours.

Invasion is perhaps the most nearly reliable criterion of malignancy, but it is often surprisingly difficult to assess in practice, especially where the normal structures are distorted by some other pathological process such as infection, metaplasia or congenital anomaly. As already mentioned, a capsule is absent in some benign tumours, and some malignant tumours are encapsulated, including clear-cell carcinoma of kidney and some thyroid carcinomas.

Metastasis is another generally reliable criterion, but benign tumours and even normal tissue may sometimes become implanted at a distance as a result of trauma or surgical accident. The placental trophoblast not only invades the uterus but is often carried by the blood to the lungs. Also some undoubted malignant tumours practically never metastasise: basal cell carcinoma is the best example, but intracranial tumours also fail to metastasise outside the cranio-spinal cavity.

Despite these exceptions, the hallmark of the malignant tumour is its capacity to spread to, and grow progressively in, tissue remote from its site of origin. Spread may occur by lymphatic vessels as tumour cell emboli, or a column of tumour cells may grow along the vessel until a lymph node is reached. Invasion of a lymph node may be followed by further spread via the efferent lymphatic. Similar invasion and spread by blood vessels is also common. Tumour cells disseminated by the bloodstream may involve any organ, but the lungs, liver and bone marrow are specially common sites of secondary tumours. (It should be noted, however, that by no means all tumour cells which enter the bloodstream go on to establish metastases. Circulating tumour cells can be detected in the bloodstream of patients with early cancer and it seems that many such cells are destroyed). Less common but important routes of spread are across body cavities (transcoelomic spread) and intra-epithelial extension as in Paget's disease of the nipple. The spread of tumours is discussed more fully in Chapter 12.

Effect of tumours

These are various and many of them can be readily understood.

Local effects. The presence of a mass of growing tissue of whatever kind may lead to **pressure effects** on various important structures, e.g. on blood vessels (especially veins), nerves, hollow viscera and ducts and solid organs, resulting in a wide variety of complications. This is true both of benign and of malignant tumours, but in addition the latter infiltrate and destroy such structures, and are especially liable to produce obstructive effects, e.g. stenosis of pylorus, intestine or bronchi.

As mentioned earlier, extensive necrosis commonly occurs in malignant tumours: those involving the skin or mucous membranes very often ulcerate and become infected by bacteria

to which they are more susceptible than normal tissues.

Widespread replacement of organs by tumour tissue may impair their function: involvement of bones leads to fractures: direct invasion or compression of nerves causes much of the pain associated with malignant disease. Compression or infiltration of blood vessels or lymphatics leads to regional congestion, ischaemia and oedema.

General effects. Absorption of bacterial products from infected tumours and of the products of necrosis of tumour tissue contributes to the pyrexia, debility and wasting (**cachexia**) seen in some cancer patients. Where there is a large volume of tumour, a further factor in producing cachexia is the competition between tumour and normal tissues for essential nutrients, such as amino acids and vitamins. Actual reduction of food intake is important in patients nauseated from liver metastases or the effects of cytotoxic drugs, or with dysphagia resulting from neoplastic involvement of the upper alimentary tract. There is little direct evidence that tumours commonly produce toxic compounds, although some patients with cancer develop unusual types of neuropathy, etc. (see below), which are likely to be due to abnormal tumour products.

Anaemia is common in cancer patients; it can result from haemorrhage from, or infection of, an ulcerated tumour, replacement of the haemopoietic marrow by tumour, or marrow depression by cytotoxic drugs or radiotherapy.

Malignant tumours cause **depression of immunological and other defence mechanisms.** This depression, which may be increased by chemotherapy or radiation, predisposes patients with cancer to **infection** with both virulent and opportunistic pathogens.

Occasional effects of cancer include various ill-defined **neuropathies and myopathies** which interfere respectively with the functioning of the nervous system and skeletal muscles: they are most likely due to humoral products of tumours. Other remote effects include **multiple venous thromboses** (especially in pancreatic cancer) and **various skin rashes. Renal disturbances** (usually nephrotic syndrome) occasionally result from deposition of tumour-antigen/antibody complexes in the glomeruli. These and other effects of tumours will be exemplified in the accounts of individual systems and organs.

Hormonal effects. *Syndromes of hormone excess* may result from the production of large quantities of hormone by benign (and less commonly malignant) tumours of the endocrine organs. These effects may be regarded as appropriate as they reflect 'appropriate' functional differentiation of the tumour cells. Much more surprising is the increasing list of hormones shown to be produced by some tumours arising from tissues with no known relevant hormone secretion. The most commonly encountered examples are production of hormones with ACTH or ADH activity by carcinomas of the bronchi. Syndromes due to such **'inappropriate' secretion of hormones** by tumours of apparently non-endocrine origin occur in relatively few patients with cancer, but a much higher proportion of tumours can be shown to have the enzyme systems necessary for the production of such hormones. The tumours most commonly associated with the inappropriate secretion of hormones are listed in Table 11.2.

The basis of the 'inappropriate' secretion of hormones by non-endocrine tumours remains unclear. Normal somatic cells contain the whole genome of the individual, and during differentiation the genes not required by each particular cell type are suppressed. Apparently the nuclear changes in tumour cells sometimes include re-expression of suppressed genes, but the association between particular types of tumour and hormone production cannot readily be explained by random de-repression. A recent and attractive theory holds that there are widely distributed cells with an endocrine function ('apud' cells) and that tumours arising from such cells ('apudomas') amplify and make detectable their actual or potential hormonal activities (p. 1034).

By invading and destroying endocrine glands, tumours can also cause hormonal deficiencies.

Table 11.2 Examples of 'inappropriate' hormone secretion by tumours

Hormone secreted by tumour	Type of tumour
ACTH	Oat cell carcinoma of bronchus; epithelial thymomas; carcinoid tumours; islet cell tumour of pancreas.
Parathormone	Squamous carcinoma of bronchus; carcinomas of oesophagus, colon, liver, pancreas, kidney.
Antidiuretic hormone (ADH)	Oat cell carcinoma of bronchus; haemangioblastoma of cerebellum.
Insulin	Retroperitoneal fibrosarcoma; mesothelioma; hepatoma; adrenal carcinoma.
Thyroid stimulating hormone	Choriocarcinoma; hydatidiform mole; embryonal carcinoma of testis.
Erythrogenin (erythrocytosis)	Renal carcinoma; cerebellar haemangioblastoma; hepatoma; phaeochromocytoma.
Gonadotrophin (precocious puberty in males)	Hepatoma.

The Causation of Tumours

Paradoxically we know many causes for cancer, but not *the* cause of cancer. We can detect many changes in the cancer cell, but we do not know the nature of the essential change in the cell which makes it a cancer cell. We know that various chemical compounds, x-irradiation and (in animals) viruses can produce tumours but we do not know exactly how any of them renders cells neoplastic.

The process of conversion of a normal cell to malignancy is called **carcinogenesis** and agents which cause this are termed **carcinogens**. Carcinogenesis in man is nearly always a complex process, usually involving the interaction of many factors, some of which favour tumour development and others which appear to provide some protection against it. They may be divided into (1) **genetically determined factors**, which in total determine an individual's susceptibility to develop a particular cancer on exposure to (2) the **exogenous influences** encountered in the complex environment in which we live. The complexities of genetic and environmental factors and of their interactions account for many of the difficulties of the epidemiological and experimental investigation of the causes of cancer.

There is great variation in the intensity and length of exposure to individual carcinogens necessary to bring about tumour development. A subthreshold dose of a carcinogen will not produce a tumour, but subthreshold doses of two separate carcinogens given together may be effective (**syncarcinogenesis**). The combination of certain substances which are not of themselves carcinogenic (**co-carcinogens** or **promoters**) with a subthreshold dose of a carcinogen will also cause tumour development (**co-car-**cinogenesis) For example, if a chemical carcinogen such as methylcholanthrene is painted on the skin of a mouse, application of a dilute solution of croton oil (itself not carcinogenic) will hasten the development of tumours and increase the number which develop—only, however, if applied together with or after the carcinogen. The carcinogen thus appears to *initiate* an irreversible process, while the co-carcinogen (in this case croton oil) *promotes* its progress after initiation. In most experimental studies, administration of a sub-threshold dose of carcinogen and a co-carcinogen has resulted in benign tumours and the role of co-carcinogens in human cancer is uncertain.

Genetic factors

The share of genetic factors in cancer causation varies extremely widely, from almost negligible in some common cancers to practically 100% in a few rare tumours, with many intermediate positions.

Clearly there must be strong selective pressure against genes producing major cancers in childhood and young adults, and such conditions are always rare. *Polyposis coli* (p. 651) is a good example of the tumours which escape this pressure. It is determined by a Mendelian dominant factor, multiple polyps developing in the colon in half the members of affected families; cancer of the colon develops regularly in early adult life—late enough, however, to permit reproduction. No known environmental factor is involved, though it is possible that the unknown basic abnormality of the colonic epithelium involves genetically-determined susceptibility to some material present in the bowel contents. *Retinoblastoma* (p. 803) is also determined by a Mendelian dominant factor, and so are the multiple benign tumours (only occasionally becoming malignant) of *neurofibromatosis* (p. 794), and also *Peutz-Jegher's syndrome* (p. 650) in which benign tumour-like polyps develop, usually in the small intestine.

A particularly illuminating example of the interaction of a genetic factor and environment is *xeroderma pigmentosum*. Sufferers show severe sunburn on minimal exposure to sunlight, and develop multiple skin cancers, ultimately fatal, often while still in their teens. The condition has been shown to be due to a simple enzyme defect, the absence of an endonuclease that removes abnormally linked pairs of bases in the DNA chain and replaces them by normal pairs. Such linkages are produced *in normal skin* in enormous numbers by exposure to the UV light in ordinary sunlight, and require constant repair by the endonuclease. In the absence of the normal repair mechanism, many cells die and others undergo permanent genetic damage that ultimately leads to tumour growth in some of them. It can therefore be said that the cancer of xeroderma is in fact caused by the external carcinogen, UV light, the genetic defect being simply the absence of a defence mechanism against this agent. This is confirmed by the great improvement in life expectancy produced in these cases by rigorous protection from sunlight.

The relationship of *skin cancer* to skin pigmentation is also instructive. The defence mechanism just mentioned fails in normal skins if exposure to UV light is maintained at high levels for a lifetime. Races exposed to much sunlight have developed more or less heavy melanin pigmentation as a defence (its function being confirmed by its localisation as caps over the epidermal-cell nuclei). The white races evolved in high latitudes where there is much less exposure to UV, and so little danger of skin cancer. Rickets is a powerful factor selecting against dark-skinned races in high latitudes because it causes distortion of the female pelvis and so endangers mother and infant during childbirth. Recent emigrations demonstrate these factors: celtic types in Australia have a colossal incidence of basal cell carcinomas of the skin (present in 75% at the age of 75 in some areas), while in Glasgow some Pakistani children develop rickets unless their diet is supplemented by vitamin D. We have here another example of a 'normal' genetic variant which greatly influences the production of cancer by the external carcinogen, UV light.

The interspecies differences in enzyme handling of 2-naphthylamine, which influence the incidence of the urinary bladder cancer (p. 299) fall into this same category of gene-environment interaction in cancer production. Recent work suggests a similar factor in lung cancer in man. The carcinogenicity of cigarette tar hydrocarbons depends on their conversion to epoxides by an enzyme, aryl hydrocarbon hydroxylase (AHH), the concentration of which varies considerably in different individuals; some studies suggest that the incidence of lung cancer is highest in those with high AHH levels.

A more remote connection is shown by the relation of some tumours to *genetic markers*—gastric cancer with blood group A, Hodgkin's disease with the HLA antigen B5 and acute lymphoblastic leukaemia with HLA antigens A2 and B12: all that is known with certainty is the raised frequency of the tumour in bearers of the gene concerned. In all three examples the effect is small and the mechanism obscure.

A high incidence of a particular cancer, e.g. of the breast, stomach or colon, has been observed in some families, but the great majority of such cancers arise in members of families without any such predisposition. The relative importance of genetic and environmental causal factors in cancer-prone families is not known.

Chromosomal abnormalities in tumour cells

The abnormal behaviour and morphology of tumour cells seems likely to result from alterations in the numbers, arrangement or operation of genes. Morphologically, we are limited at present to seeking evidence of abnormalities in chromosomal morphology and number: we

cannot yet detect morphological changes in individual genes, even with modern chromosomal banding techniques (Fig. 2.8, p. 16).

Chromosomal abnormalities cannot be detected in most benign tumours, but in malignant tumours the number of chromosomes is often abnormal and structural chromosomal abnormalities are found. However, these changes seem to occur in random manner. As they are more marked in advanced than in early tumours, they probably merely reflect the progressively disordered nuclear behaviour consequent upon the development and evolution of cancer. Of more interest are chromosomal abnormalities which occur in some benign and malignant tumours in a non-random fashion. The outstanding example is the Philadelphia chromosomal abnormality, involving C22 and C9 (p. 549), which is demonstrable in 90% of cases of chronic myeloid leukaemia (CML). The change affects haemopoietic stem cells and is now believed to be the basic cell change leading to this form of CML. It is also of interest that many cases of CML pass into a more acute, malignant form of leukaemia, and in about 75% of such cases the acute phase is accompanied by further non-random chromosomal changes, usually involving C8 and C17. CML without the Philadelphia chromosome abnormality may well be a separate entity, for the course and response to treatment are different. Other examples of non-random chromosomal changes associated with particular forms of neoplasia are known, but apart from CML, they appear likely to develop as secondary events, for they are often absent from the tumour cells obtained by early biopsy.

Interesting observations have been made on the effects of cell hybridisation (p. 304) on malignant cells. When cancer cells are fused with normal cells, the hybrid cells are often non-malignant, as assessed by their failure to produce tumours in suitable animals or to grow progressively with loss of contact inhibition in culture (p. 302). The hybrid cell is, however, unstable, and in culture it loses chromosomes with successive divisions. Loss of particular chromosomes derived originally from the normal cell has been found to be associated with the re-emergence of malignant behaviour. It thus appears that the factors which make a cell malignant may be present but suppressed by genetically-determined factors of the normal cell: they may become operative with loss of the suppressor factors.

The development of malignancy as a result of chromosomal aberrations is suggested also by the increased incidence of cancer in rare congenital disorders characterised by chromosomal instability, e.g. Fanconi's anaemia, ataxia telangiectasia (p. 171) and Bloom's syndrome.

Chemical carcinogens

In 1775, Percivall Pott*, a London surgeon, recorded a high incidence of cancer of the scrotum in chimney sweeps (Fig. 11.5). Because they lacked facilities (and perhaps enthusiasm) for washing, sweeps retained soot in their rugose scrotal skin, where it exerted a carcinogenic effect. Another occupational cancer was reported in 1874 by Volkmann, who observed a high incidence of skin cancer in workers exposed to tar and mineral oil. Numerous other examples of chemically-related occupational cancers have since been reported.

Testing for chemical carcinogenicity. A major advance in the investigation of chemical carcinogenesis was made by Yamagiwa and Ichikawa who in 1917 reported the induction of cancers by repeated painting of rabbits' ears with tar. This provided the means to test individual chemicals for carcinogenicity, and since that time a very large number of compounds have been tested. The basic experimental design has varied little. Suspected carcinogens are administered at regular intervals, (e.g. daily, thrice weekly, etc.) by whatever route seems most appropriate, either alone or together with co-carcinogens, and with or without manipulation of the animals' hormonal, metabolic or immunological status.

A large number of chemicals has been shown to be carcinogenic, and the following principles have been established.

1. There is a latent period between the first administration of the carcinogen and the development of tumours. The latent period varies

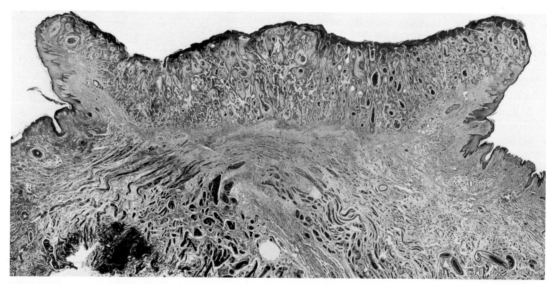

Fig. 11.5 Cancer arising from the epidermis of the scrotum in a chimney sweep. The tumour forms a raised plaque. Numerous small groups of tumour cells are seen invading the dermis. The dark fibres in the deep part of the tissue are cremasteric muscle. × 5.

* Percivall Pott's name is also commemorated by Pott's fracture and Pott's disease of the spine.

with different carcinogens and with the same carcinogen for different species and strains of animal.

2. For some carcinogens, the latent period varies inversely with the size of each dose of carcinogen over a wide range of dosage. Doubling the dose will thus half the time taken for tumours to appear. This means that the effect of each dose is irreversible and that tumours appear after a certain *total* dose of the carcinogen. There is thus a *threshold dose* for each carcinogen/strain combination.

3. For other carcinogens, the latent period is influenced by the dosage, but to a smaller degree, so that doubling the dosage does not reduce the latent period by half. In these instances, very small doses will induce tumours if the animals live long enough, and it has been concluded that, for such substances, there is no sub-threshold dose, but merely a lengthening of the latent period.

4. Following administration of the threshold dose of carcinogen, there may in some instances be no morphological changes in the target cells, but tumours will eventually develop, even without further administration of carcinogen.

5. Some carcinogens act specifically on one organ, e.g. the liver; this is usually because the carcinogen is concentrated in that organ, or because it is really a *procarcinogen* which is converted to a carcinogen in that particular organ. Other carcinogens are non-organ-specific, and induce tumours at the sites of maximal exposure, which are usually determined by the route of administration.

6. The physical properties and chemical reactivity of the carcinogen are important, for they determine whether it diffuses throughout the body or stays at the site of administration, and also whether it is concentrated in certain organs and in the urine.

Testing chemicals for carcinogenicity is a complex, exacting procedure and, as illustrated below, it may take years to establish that a substance is carcinogenic. Carcinogenicity also varies considerably with species. An example is provided by the induction of cancer of the urinary bladder by 2-naphthylamine. This substance came under suspicion because a high incidence of bladder cancer was observed in workers in the aniline dye industry and analysis of the jobs of those workers developing cancer pointed to 2-naphthylamine as the causal agent. Tests in laboratory animals of several species failed to demonstrate its carcinogenicity, but eventually it was shown to induce tumours of the bladder in dogs after *five years* oral administration. It was subsequently shown that dogs and men convert the bulk of the non-carcinogenic 2-naphthylamine to carcinogenic 1-hydroxy-2-naphthylamine in the kidney. This compound is concentrated in the urine and can induce carcinoma in the transitional epithelium lining the urinary tract, and particularly, because of its relatively large surface area, in the bladder. Most species of animals convert 2-naphthylamine to non-carcinogenic substances such as glucuronides, and this explains the initially negative studies of 2-naphthylamine carcinogenicity.

Testing for mutagenic activity. As exemplified above, carcinogenicity tests often take a long time, and even when very thorough they cannot provide an absolute guarantee that a compound is non-carcinogenic for man. More recently, tests have been devised to determine whether chemical compounds are capable of causing mutations in bacteria. By selecting suitable bacterial strains, tests for mutations of various types can be made, both with a suspected compound and with its metabolites. Such tests are rapid, and for most of the substances which have been tested there is a very good correlation between carcinogenicity and mutagenicity.

The nature of chemical carcinogens

Thousands of chemicals can induce the development of tumours. The first to be proved carcinogenic was the polycyclic hydrocarbon, 1:2, 5:6 dibenzanthracene, which was synthesised by Kennaway and his colleagues approximately 50 years ago. The first carcinogen to be identified in soot and tar was 3:4 benzpyrene. Since that time, many other **polycyclic hydrocarbons** have been proved to be carcinogenic. These compounds produce cancer at the site of local application. They are present in mineral oils and are released by combustion of most organic materials, including fossil fuels; accordingly, they are widespread atmospheric pollutants.

Other classes of compounds which are carcinogenic include **aromatic amines** used in the aniline dye industry, e.g. 2-naphthylamine (see above) and benzidine (formerly used also in the laboratory to detect blood in the faeces), which cause cancer of the urinary bladder. **Azo-dyes**, e.g. 'butter yellow' formerly used to tint margarine, cause liver cancer (see below), and **aminofluorenes**, notably 2-acetylaminofluorene, can induce cancer of the liver and of the urinary bladder. In each of these classes of compound, *carcinogenicity cannot usually be predicted from the molecular structure, and small changes in the molecule can greatly influence carcinogenicity*. It is, however, apparent that certain molecular features, for example double-bonds at certain sites in the benzene rings of the polycyclic hydrocarbons, are of importance.

Certain non-aromatic organic compounds are also carcinogenic. They include some **alkylating agents**, e.g. mustard gas and methylnitrosourea, and **nitrosamines** which may be formed from chemical action on foodstuffs in the stomach and bacterial action in the large intestine.

Various inorganic compounds also act as carcinogens; for example inhaled **asbestos** fibres cause cancer of the pleura, peritoneum and bronchus, while cancer of the bronchus can apparently be caused also by inhalation of dusts containing compounds of **arsenic, beryllium, nickel** and **chromates**. Long-continued administration of arsenical compounds or exposure to arsenical dusts can also cause skin cancers.

The mechanism of chemical carcinogenesis

This is poorly understood. All carcinogens do appear, however, to induce progressive and irreversible changes in the target cells, leading eventually to the development of a cancer cell. This is illustrated by studies of the effects of butter-yellow   (p-dimethylaminoazobenzene), the most carcinogenic of the azo-dyes, on the liver. The dye is taken up by liver cells and, like all carcinogens, it causes cell injury resulting in this case in loss of some liver cells and compensatory regeneration of surviving cells. There is thus cellular proliferation which, as mentioned earlier, is important in carcinogenesis. If slices of normal rat liver are placed in culture

medium and oxygen uptake is measured as an index of cellular metabolism, addition of butter-yellow to the medium is found to depress metabolism. Administration of butter-yellow to rats progressively diminishes the effect of butter-yellow on the uptake of oxygen by liver slices *in vitro*, and when liver tumours finally develop the oxygen consumption is found to be unaffected by butter-yellow. It may thus be concluded that the liver cells become progressively adapted to the presence of butter-yellow *in vivo*. Such adaptation could be explained either (a) by the development of increased amounts of enzymes which detoxify butter-yellow or provide metabolic pathways not affected by it, or (b) by the production of mutations by butter-yellow and growth of mutant cells which are resistant to the effects of the dye on metabolism. The fact that precancerous changes induced by carcinogens are non-reversible (see above) suggests strongly that selection of mutants is the correct explanation.

Most of the organic carcinogens are either capable of reacting with DNA (e.g. alkylating agents) or are metabolised within the cell to compounds, e.g. epoxides, which can do so. Such reactions are believed to occur between electrophilic groupings on the carcinogen and electron-rich groupings of DNA, notably in guanosine: but binding occurs at various sites within DNA, and may possibly result in the development of mutations of various types when the DNA replicates prior to mitosis. In view of the close correlation between carcinogenicity and mutagenicity (p. 299) *it seems very likely that chemicals induce cancer by causing mutations*. Such mutations can only occur in cells which undergo mitosis, and this may explain why cancer arises most commonly from labile populations of cells (p. 290), and also why mature neurons, which appear incapable of division, do not become neoplastic. In some instances where cancer arises in relatively stable cell populations, e.g. liver cells, cell loss and compensatory proliferation caused by disease, e.g. cirrhosis of the liver, or by the carcinogen itself, are probably essential for carcinogenesis.

It has also been suggested that chemical carcinogens may act by activating a latent oncogenic (tumour-producing) virus already present in the target cell (pp. 302 *et seq.*).

Physical agents in carcinogenesis

The main physical factor concerned with tumour formation is radiant energy, and much is known of this important form of carcinogenesis. Other physical factors, such as mechanical trauma, chronic irritation and the tendency for cancer to develop in scars, are difficult to study and their role in carcinogenesis is poorly understood.

Radiant energy. A detailed account of the effects of radiation on cells is included in Chapter 2. *Radiation of diverse kinds, x-rays, α, β and γ rays and ultraviolet light all induce tumours in man and animals.* They produce effects by release of energy during their passage through the tissues with resulting alteration of various cellular molecules, including the nucleic acids. The most important long-term consequence of these events is an increased rate of mutation in the irradiated cells. The degree of effect on a tissue depends largely on the total radiation dose, physical characteristics of the radiations (such as their penetrating capacity), and on features of the affected tissues, such as density, mitotic rate, and the nature of their blood supply. Thus short exposure to a high concentration of radiation, as occurred in those exposed to the atomic bomb or to accidents involving nuclear apparatus, and oft-repeated exposure to low doses of radiation, as occurred in the early radiologists, can both be carcinogenic. Tumours may arise in tissues affected by radiation necrosis (p. 38) and also in those where direct radiation injury appears to have been relatively slight.

The early **radiologists** frequently calibrated their machines by exposing their own arms. This cumulative exposure to x-rays was carcinogenic, but as the early x-rays were 'soft' and did not penetrate deeply through the skin, their tumours were accessible **squamous carcinomas of the epidermis** which could be successfully treated surgically. Later, however, despite the recognition of the hazard and introduction of safe practices, the use of 'harder', more penetrating x-rays led to a raised incidence of deeper tumours, and particularly to the development of **chronic myeloid leukaemia** originating in the haemopoietic marrow as a result of the capacity of bone matrix to impede and scatter the x-rays. Further developments in safety techniques have now virtually abolished this problem.

The effects of **radio-isotopes** depend on the dosage, and the site of absorption of the radiation produced. Inhaled radioactive dust is likely to produce lung cancers (p. 497). Radio-iodine produces thyroid tumours in experimental animals because it is concentrated within the gland: external irradiation of the neck with x-rays can produce much the same effect.

The situation with **UV light**(UV) is interesting. *Long continued exposure to UV, especially medium-wavelength UVB, such as occurs in outdoor workers, is associated with the occurrence of basal cell and squamous carcinomas, which usually arise in those areas of skin exposed to light, and less often malignant melanomas of the skin.* Those most at risk are pale skinned individuals who tan poorly, albinos, and especially those with the genetic predisposition of xeroderma pigmentosum (p. 296). Not only is there a very high frequency of skin cancers in white inhabitants of sunny Australia (p. 297) but they affect relatively young people as compared with most other cancers, with some predilection for those of higher socio-economic groups.

Much of the UV radiation in sunlight is filtered out by ozone in the stratosphere and does not reach the earth. There is current concern that the ozone is being reduced by supersonic transport and especially by fluorocarbons used as propellants in spray-containers and as refrigerants. It has been postulated that this will lead to an increase in skin cancer in sunny places, but the evidence on which this fear is based is, at present, inconclusive.

Trauma and chronic irritation. Many patients ascribe the onset of a visible (usually skin) tumour to some specific incident of trauma. It is difficult to understand how a gross mechanical injury could cause neoplasia, and it seems likely that, in most cases, an already growing tumour becomes more liable to injury and that this draws the patient's attention to the lesion—*traumatic determinism*. It is possible, however, that mechanical trauma may be important in a few cancers.

Chronic irritation, which could also be regarded as repeated minor trauma, seems important in squamous carcinomas of the mouth associated with ill-fitting dentures and in those cancers which arise in association with chronic infected sinuses opening onto the skin. Also, malignant melanoma in African negroes occurs mainly on the soles of the feet of those who go barefoot: this may not, however, be due simply to trauma, for most such tumours arise at the margin of the pale plantar skin, whereas trauma is obviously not so restricted in distribution.

Scars. Tumours do not ordinarily arise in a burn scar or surgical wound scar on a rabbit's skin. But if one paints a carcinogen evenly over an area which includes such a scar, the tumours appear first (and grow largest) in relation to the scar. 'Burn cancers' of man, or 'brand cancers' of animals, occur almost always in areas exposed to excessive sunlight or similar carcinogenic stimulus. Scars thus seem to act as 'cocarcinogens'. Although chronic peptic ulcers of the stomach and duodenum have closely similar features, only those in the stomach appear to predispose to cancer. It may be that the chronic ulceration predisposes to cancer because of the active proliferation of the surface epithelium at the ulcer margins (which is where cancer develops) and that, in addition, the gastric (but not the duodenal) mucosa is exposed to carcinogenic agents.

Induction of tumours by viruses

Both RNA and DNA viruses have been shown to be oncogenic, i.e. capable of causing tumours, in various species of vertebrates. In many instances, however, it has not been easy to establish that a particular animal tumour is caused by a virus. The only human tumours which have been proved to be caused by a virus are the common wart and some venereal warts, but many of the procedures used to establish the viral nature of tumours in experimental animals are not applicable to man, and it is not surprising that evidence is only now accumulating which suggests that some human cancers are virus-induced. The evidence is, however, particularly strong for an unusual form of lymphoid cancer, the Burkitt lymphoma, and for nasopharyngeal carcinoma and fairly strong for liver cell cancer (p. 305).

Viral integration and transformation of host cells

When a virus particle enters a host cell, two things may happen. Firstly, in so-called *permissive cells* virus can **replicate**, producing infective virus particles which are released and may enter other cells. Secondly, sequences of virus DNA may be inserted into the DNA of the host cell, a process termed **integration**. *In all instances of virus-induced tumours which have been sufficiently elucidated, the development of cancer has been found to be associated with integration of the virus*, and this phenomenon must be studied in some detail.

Many of the important advances in viral carcinogenesis have been made by investigating the effects of viruses on cell cultures, and some oncogenic viruses have been shown to be capable of **transforming** normal cells in culture into cells which behave like cultures of cancer cells. For example, cultures of normal cells proliferate only until such time as they form a continuous monolayer on the surface of the culture vessel: they then stop proliferating, a phenomenon known as **contact inhibition**. By contrast, virus-transformed cells (and cancer cells in culture*) continue to proliferate and become heaped up on one another (Fig. 11.6). Virus-transformed cells also show other features of cancer cells; for example increased motility, morphological changes and increased glycolysis, and in many instances they have been shown to develop into tumours when injected into histocompatible animal hosts: there is thus very strong evidence that certain viruses can convert normal cells into cancer cells *in vitro*.

The demonstration of integrated viral DNA in host cells has been achieved by elegant techniques, one of the most useful being *nucleic acid hybridisation*. To give an example, a suspected DNA virus is grown in a culture of permissive cells, which allow the virus to replicate,

---

*In general, cells from tumours of experimental animals grow much more readily than human cancer cells in culture, although in some instances the latter will grow continuously.

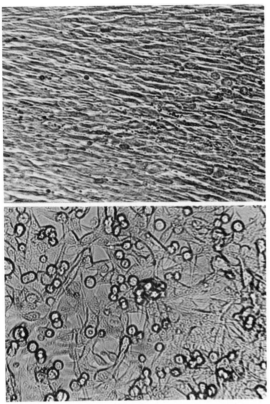

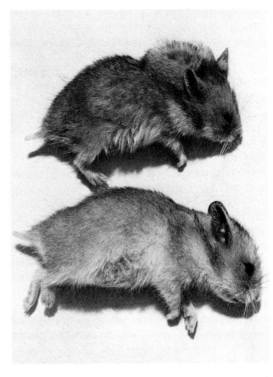

Fig. 11.6 Cultures of hamster fibroblasts (*left*). The upper culture shows formation of a regular monolayer. The lower culture is infected with polyoma virus and shows cellular pleomorphism and loss of contact inhibition, the cells being piled on top of one another. The upper hamster (*right*) was injected with the polyoma-transformed cells which have grown to form a tumour. The lower hamster was injected with the uninfected cells, and has remained healthy. (Dr. Joan McNab.)

and viral DNA is prepared in single-stranded form. Complementary strands of radioactive RNA are prepared *in vitro* by incubating the viral DNA with a mixture of suitable bases (one or more of which is labelled with a radio-isotope) and the enzyme RNA polymerase (Fig. 11.7). The labelled RNA thus produced will bind to the corresponding sequences of the viral DNA, and can be used to detect viral DNA integrated into the host cell genome. By this technique, viral DNA can be detected in various animal tumours and virus-transformed cells. The features of virus integration and its relation to tumour formation differ for DNA and RNA viruses, which are considered separately below.

Fig. 11.7 Use of the nucleic-acid hybridisation technique to detect integrated viral DNA. Note that the preparation of the RNA 'probe' requires replicating virus to provide the viral DNA genome, which is used as a template.

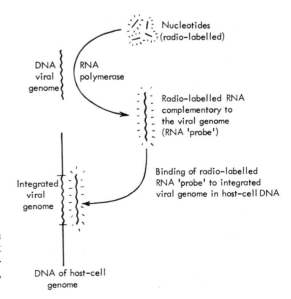

Oncogenic DNA viruses

In 1933, it was demonstrated by Shope that naturally-occuring benign epithelial tumours (papillomas or warts) of American cotton-tail rabbits could be transmitted by filtered extracts of the tumours. When scratched into the skin of cotton-tailed rabbits, benign tumours were produced. In domestic rabbits, the filtrates caused skin tumours which frequently became malignant. It is now known that oncogenic DNA viruses can *either* integrate and transform a cell, *or* replicate within it: they cannot do both in the same cell, for replication of virus kills the cell. The infectivity of the cotton-tail papillomas was due to replication of the virus (subsequently termed the *Shope papilloma virus*) in keratinised, non-dividing epithelial cells: in the proliferating tumour cells, the virus is integrated, but does not replicate. The cells of the more malignant tumours produced in domestic rabbits contain integrated, but not replicating virus, and their filtrates are non-infective. This point is important, because in other DNA virus tumours, infective virus is not produced, and integrated virus can only be detected by nucleic-acid hybridisation (see above) or by means of **cell hybridisation**. The latter consists of fusing together two cells from animals of the same or different species, forming a tetraploid cell. When a (non-permissive) cell containing an integrated DNA virus is fused with a permissive cell, complete virus particles may be formed in the hybrid cell, thus revealing the presence of the integrated virus in the non-permissive cell. Skin papillomas in other species have been shown to be caused by papilloma viruses, including the human common wart (*verruca vulgaris*) and the venereal wart (*condyloma acuminatum*); in both these human tumours, the virus replicates in some non-dividing cells, and so they are infectious.

The papilloma viruses belong to a group termed *papovaviruses*, which include also *Polyoma virus* and a virus termed *SV40*. *Polyoma virus* is unusual in that it can induce tumours of various types (hence the name) in several species: most oncogenic viruses are more specific in the type of tumour and in the species in which they induce tumours. Polyoma virus occurs naturally in mice, and when injected into neonatal mice, other rodents or rabbits, it induces a wide range of tumours. When added

to cell cultures, it integrates into and transforms some cells and replicates in others. The relative ease with which Polyoma virus produces tumours when injected into *neonatal* animals is a general feature of oncogenic viruses: when introduced into adult animals, the host immune response usually results in antibodies which inactivate free virus, and in cell-mediated immunity which destroys any transformed cells. For this reason, tumours are rare in the naturally-infected adult mouse, but tumours can be produced by introducing the virus into immunologically suppressed or congenitally immunodeficient (nude) mice. *SV40* occurs naturally in monkeys, in which it replicates but does not produce tumours, but it can cause tumours when injected into neonatal rats and can transform cells in culture. This illustrates a general feature of DNA oncogenic viruses—they usually replicate and destroy cells in the natural host and integrate into cells of the host(s) in which they are oncogenic. Perhaps because of man's close relationship to monkeys, SV40 can infect man, producing in immunosuppressed or immunodeficient patients a form of encephalitis by replicating in cells of the brain; it has not, however, been shown to produce human tumours.

Herpesviruses

Two herpes viruses are of considerable interest because there is evidence associating them with tumours in man. One, *Epstein-Barr virus*, is associated with a tumour termed the Burkitt lymphoma and also with cancer of the nasopharynx: the other, *Herpes simplex virus type 2*, has been associated with carcinoma of the uterine cervix.

Epstein-Barr virus (EBV). In certain parts of Africa where malaria is highly endemic, Burkitt noted the relatively high incidence of an otherwise rare tumour of lymphocytes which occurs in children and affects the jaw and various internal organs. Cells from this tumour, the **Burkitt lymphoma**, are lymphoblasts derived from B lymphocytes and grow continuously in cell culture. Occasional cells in such cultures produce EBV particles and this was the original source of the virus. Most of the cells in culture, and those of the tumour itself, have been shown to contain several EBV genomes in their nuclear DNA. Moreover, when added to cultures of human lymphocytes, EBV transforms them into lymphoblasts resembling those derived from the tumour. Involvement of B lymphocytes appears to depend on their possessing a surface receptor for C3d (an activation product of the third component of complement) which also binds EBV and so facilitates its entry into B lymphocytes.

EBV is widespread throughout the world. Most people develop immunity to it without clinical illness, but in some it causes the acute febrile illness known as *infectious mononucleosis*: in this, antibody to EBV appears and there is also an unusually vigorous immune response on the part of T cells, which presumably eliminate any B cells transformed by the virus. Complete recovery is the rule and there is no evidence of subsequent increased risk of developing a lymphoma. The occurrence of the Burkitt lymphoma in Africa is associated closely with endemic malaria, and the tumour incidence is low in areas where malaria has been eradicated and in Africans with the sickle-cell trait of their red cells, which protects against malaria. The most likely explanation of the association with malaria is the effect this disease has in depressing cell-mediated immunity, with consequent failure to destroy lymphocytes transformed by EBV. The suppressive role of immunity is supported by the spontaneous regression of the tumour in some cases, and by its unusually good response to low doses of anti-tumour drugs.

EB virus is also associated with poorly differentiated carcinoma of the nasopharynx, which is the commonest form of human cancer in parts of Southern China. Integrated EB virus DNA can be detected in the tumour cells. The high incidence of this otherwise rare tumour in the Southern Chinese is probably due to a genetic factor, for it occurs also in Chinese groups who have settled in other countries, and is rarely observed in Caucasians living in Southern China. Recently, a high incidence of the histocompatibility antigen HLA-A2 has been reported in patients with this cancer, and it may be that this is associated with a particular repertoire of immune response (Ir) genes (p. 167) which do not provide for a normal vigorous T-cell response to EBV-transformed epithelial cancer cells.

Herpes simplex type 2 virus (HSV2) is known to be transmitted sexually, and female genital infection is associated with sexual activity and promiscuity. These behaviour patterns are also associated with a high incidence of carcinoma of the cervix uteri, and patients with this condition have higher titres of antibody to *HSV2* than those without the disease. *HSV2* has also been detected in cells from cervical cancer. Although these findings are suggestive, it still remains entirely possible that *HSV2* infection is incidental and that the virus is simply a 'passenger' and not the cause of the tumour.

Other DNA viruses

Hepatitis B virus is associated with acute and chronic hepatitis in man. Chronic hepatitis commonly progresses to cirrhosis of the liver, which in a proportion of cases is followed by cancer of the liver cells. A factor of importance in this progression is the continuous loss and compensatory proliferation of liver cells, which are normally stable (p. 77). As mentioned earlier, such proliferative activity predisposes to cancer. There is, however, evidence that hepatitis B virus may be more directly carcinogenic, for liver cell cancer is a much less common complication of cirrhosis due to causes other than the virus, e.g. chronic alcoholism. Also, there is preliminary evidence suggesting that hepatitis B viral DNA is integrated into the genome of liver cancer cells. Experimental animal studies have proved difficult with this virus, and more evidence is needed to determine its role in human cancer. The subject is discussed more fully on pp. 701–2.

Adenoviruses are a common cause of upper respiratory infections in man. One of them (type 12) has been shown to be capable also of causing tumours in rodents and of transforming rodent cells in culture. There is, however, no evidence that they are oncogenic for man.

How do oncogenic DNA viruses cause cancer?

Integration of viral DNA into a host cell could produce the transformation to a cancer cell either by its direct effect on the host-cell DNA, i.e. by acting as or causing mutations. Alternatively, the virus might contain a gene coding for a product which transforms the host cell. Some support for the mutation theory has been provided by the demonstration that although a transformed cell may contain several genomes of the transforming virus in its DNA, transformation is associated with integration into a particular chromosome. This does not, of course, prove that a particular mutation occurs and is responsible for transformation, and indeed there is evidence that transcription produces a protein which is necessary for both integration and transformation of the host cell. This protein, termed *T-antigen*, is detectable in the nucleus of transformed cells, and may induce transformation by binding to host DNA. Antibody to the appropriate T-antigen, which is specific for each oncogenic DNA virus, is found in the serum of animals with DNA-virus induced tumours. Some of the oncogenic DNA viruses have only sufficient DNA to code for a few proteins, and elegant studies have been performed in which the small DNA strands of such viruses have been broken into several fragments by means of enzymes. The individual parts of the DNA may then be isolated and their effects tested on suitable host cells in culture. In such experiments, it has been shown that *only the part of the viral DNA which codes for T antigen is capable of integrating into and transforming host cells.*

Oncogenic RNA viruses (retraviruses)

Introduction. RNA viruses which produce tumours are commonly termed *oncornaviruses* (an abbreviation of oncogenic RNA viruses) but increasingly they are described as *retraviruses* because of their capacity to produce *reverse transcriptase* (see below).

Like the DNA oncogenic viruses, the retraviruses must become integrated into the host cell to induce transformation to a cancer cell. To do so, the retravirus, having invaded the host cell, synthesises a strand of DNA complementary to its RNA genome, by means of *reverse transcriptase* (RNA-directed DNA polymerase). The viral-coded DNA, known as a *provirus*, is then inserted into the host cell genome (Fig. 11.8) Such integration is restricted mainly to RNA viruses which have been shown to be oncogenic, and is essential for viral transformation to a cancer cell. The integrated DNA provirus can be transcribed into the RNA genome of the virus, and (unlike other RNA viruses) replication occurs only in this way. Nearly all retraviruses have a char-

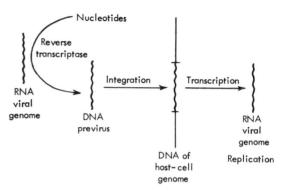

Fig. 11.8 Formation of an RNA viral provirus and integration into the host-cell genome. Viral replication is effected by transcription of the integrated provirus.

acteristic morphology: they form *C-type particles* at the host cell membrane by a process of 'budding,' and the infective virion thus includes part of the host cell membrane (Fig. 11.9). This form of replication can occur without killing the host cell and thus, unlike DNA viruses, the retraviruses can both integrate and replicate in the same cell.

The presence of an integrated oncogenic RNA virus in cells may be detected by means of nucleic acid hybridisation (p. 302), using a transcript of the viral RNA genome as a template for production of a DNA 'probe'. Strong evidence of the presence of integrated virus is provided also by the detection of reverse transcriptase, and also by the appearance of provirus-coded proteins on the surface of the host cell (p. 314).

Types of oncogenic RNA viruses

There are three main groups of oncogenic retraviruses—the *sarcoma viruses, leukaemia viruses* and *mammary tumour viruses*.

RNA sarcoma viruses

The first of these was discovered by Rous in 1911, when he showed that a sarcoma of chickens was transmissible by a filtered extract of the tumour. This agent (*Rous sarcoma virus*) and other similar avian-tumour producing viruses rapidly transform chicken fibroblasts in culture. Some strains of sarcoma viruses are *deficient* in that they can transform cells but lack some of the genetic material required for replication: they may be induced to replicate by

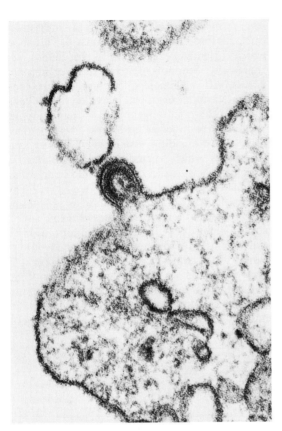

Fig. 11.9 A part of a cell from a cat infected with feline leukaemia virus, showing formation of a virion by budding from the cell surface. Note that the envelope is formed from the plasma membrane, and that the virus particle becomes coated with an outer spiky layer. The section happens to include part of another cell immediately above the virion. × 80 000. (Dr. Helen Laird.)

addition of a 'helper' virus which supplies the defective gene product, and some defective viruses will replicate in cells which already contain an *endogenous virus* (i.e. an integrated virus transmitted genetically from generation to generation by the germ cells—p. 309) which makes good the deficiency. Sarcoma viruses affecting a number of mammalian species have been described.

RNA leukaemia viruses

Viruses of this group induce various types of cancer of lymphoid cells (lymphomas), including leukaemia, in chickens, mice, cats and bovines. For convenience, this group of tumours will be referred to as *leukaemia* in this account. Chicken leukaemia virus was discovered as long ago as 1908, when chicken leukaemia was shown to be transmissible, most readily to newly-hatched chickens, by a filtrate of leukaemic cells. Mouse leukaemia virus was demonstrated in the leukaemic cells obtained from inbred strains of mice in which 'natural' leukaemia was common. Filtrates of the leukaemic cell extracts were shown to induce leukaemia when injected into neonatal mice of strains in which leukaemia was uncommon. It is noteworthy that leukaemia virus in replicating form is detectable in the cells of *all* fetal mice, and it has even been speculated that it plays a physiological role in the proliferation and differentiation of fetal cells. During maturation, replicating leukaemia virus disappears, but integrated virus persists in the cells of various tissues, and may be detected by nucleic-acid hybridisation, or by treating mice with x-rays or various chemical carcinogens, which results in replication of the virus, and also in leukaemia. In high-incidence strains the spontaneous development of leukaemia is also associated with the reappearance of replicating virus, probably because the latter impairs the T-cell immune response of the animal and so allows transformed lymphocytes to proliferate.

Feline leukaemia virus, the cause of leukaemia in cats, is of considerable interest for at least four reasons. Firstly, infection by feline leukaemia virus occurs naturally by horizontal transmission (i.e. by personal contact); secondly, the virus spreads among an *outbred* cat population; thirdly, infection of adult cats can induce leukaemia, and fourthly it has proved possible to protect cats from leukaemia by use of a vaccine which is effective even when administered *after* the animal has become infected by the virus. These findings are due largely to the work of Jarrett and his co-workers in Glasgow. They have shown that, while vertical transmission of the virus does occur, as in mice, horizontal transmission is usually responsible for leukaemia. Young animals receiving a large infecting dose of the virus are more likely to develop leukaemia, probably because these factors lead to immunosuppression, and epidemiological studies have shown that cats of a low 'social class', which roam freely, are much more likely to become infected and to develop leukaemia.

Viruses and human leukaemia. It is apparent

that there are important differences between virus-induced leukaemia in different species, and this must be taken into account in elucidating the causal factors of lymphomas and leukaemias in man. Retraviruses, including the leukaemia viruses, can replicate in cells in culture, but do not transform them. In the living animal, integrated leukaemia virus may remain latent (i.e. may give rise to no detectable products) throughout life although, as noted above, it may be activated by administration of carcinogens or x-rays. In man, such latent proviruses, if present, would be extremely difficult to detect, although the development of leukaemias in people exposed to heavy doses of ionising radiations could be explained by activation of an endogenous leukaemia virus. Antibodies to leukaemia viruses are very commonly present in human serum, and C-type virus particles have been observed in some cultures of human leukaemic cells, while nucleic-acid hybridisation techniques have revealed the presence of apparent leukaemia proviruses in such cells. There is thus some preliminary evidence that, as in a number of animal species, certain forms of leukaemia in man may be due to retraviruses. Indeed, in view of the demonstration that retraviruses cause leukaemia in several species, and that feline leukaemia virus can induce a variety of lymphomas closely resembling most of those observed in man, it would be surprising if leukaemia viruses were not the cause of some types of human lymphomas.

A major difficulty in the detection of oncogenic viruses in human lymphomas and leukaemias is the lack of a specific 'probe' for the provirus. The base sequences in feline and bovine leukaemia viruses show considerable differences, so that bovine leukaemia provirus cannot readily be detected by nucleic acid hybridisation with a probe prepared from feline leukaemia virus RNA. Accordingly, while leukaemia viruses are likely to be involved in human tumours, the detection of provirus requires the preparation of RNA from replicating virus, and this has not yet been accomplished. It must also be emphasised that, in feline and bovine leukaemia, the causal virus can be detected in only about 50% of tumours, although from epidemiological studies it is very likely that the 'virus-negative' tumours are caused by leukaemia viruses.

Mouse mammary tumour virus is responsible for breast cancer in mice. It is of interest for three reasons. Firstly, it accounts for a cancer which originally appeared to be determined genetically. Secondly, the virus causes tumours particularly in female mice, and requires oestrogen stimulation of the target epithelial cells. Thirdly, there is some evidence that a similar virus may be involved in human breast cancer. By selective breeding, strains of mice were established in which virtually all the females developed breast cancer late in life, and other strains in which this tumour was rare. This looked like a genetic effect until it was found by Bittner that female neonates of a low-cancer strain suckled by foster mothers of a high-cancer strain frequently developed breast cancer. By contrast, high-cancer strain offspring suckled on low-cancer foster mothers did not develop cancer (Fig. 11.10). Thus the carcinogenic influence was transmitted by the milk in the post-natal period and not by germ

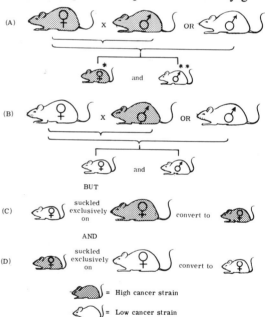

Fig. 11.10   Discovery of the Bittner milk factor. The incidence of breast cancer was high in the daughters of 'high-cancer' strain *mothers* (A), but low in the daughters of 'high-cancer' strain *fathers* (B). The strain of female on which neonates were suckled (C and D) was then found to determine the incidence of cancer, showing the importance of a milk factor, since shown to be a virus. Oophorectomy* reduces the incidence of breast cancer in virus-infected females, and oestrogen** increases the incidence in virus-infected males.

cells nor transplacentally by the mother. Investigations with filtrates of 'high-cancer strain milk', cell-free filtrates of mammary tumour, and electron microscopic studies of milk and tumour tissue, have confirmed that the active principle ('Bittner milk factor') is a virus—mouse mammary tumour virus.

Female neonates which have been infected with the virus are protected from breast cancer by removal of the ovaries, and male neonates infected with the virus only develop breast cancer if given large doses of oestrogens. Thus oestrogenic activity is a necessary co-factor for this virus-induced tumour.

How do retraviruses cause cancer?

Integration of provirus into the host cell genome is an essential feature of cancer induced by retraviruses, but this alone is not sufficient to transform the cell to a cancer cell, for it is known that in many vertebrate species integrated retraviruses are transmitted genetically via the germ cells (*endogenous viruses*) and are thus present in all nucleated cells. In some instances, it is probable that expression (i.e.

transcription) of one or more genes of the provirus, is necessary to transform the host cell. The mechanism of such activation of viral 'oncogenes' is not known, although, as noted earlier, administration of chemical carcinogens and ionising radiation may induce changes which trigger it off. In the case of the sarcoma viruses, which transform cells in culture, transformation has been shown to be effected by a single oncogene. This may be detected by nucleic-acid hybridisation, and its continued expression appears to be necessary for both transformation and maintenance of the transformed state in the host cell. Its product is a protease capable of acting on several cellular substrates, including components of the cell membrane.

Information on the mechanism of induction of cancer by leukaemia viruses is scanty. There is, however, preliminary evidence that it may depend on a proviral gene which behaves as an operator, inducing transcription of an adjacent gene of host (i.e. non-viral) origin. If this is correct, then it appears that the sarcoma and leukaemia viruses induce cancer by different mechanisms.

Hormones and carcinogenesis

In general, any induced change of hormone level which causes prolonged hyperplasia of a target organ may cause tumours of the latter, but there are many exceptions. The following are the best known experimental situations.

Oestrogens can undoubtedly cause tumours in susceptible strains of mice; their administration in high dosage leads to an increased incidence of cancer of the breast in females and to the occurrence of breast cancer in males. Reduction of natural oestrogen levels by oophorectomy abolishes cancer of the breast in susceptible female mice. It might seem that the excessive proliferation of breast ducts induced by oestrogen, carried to excess, has been the actual cause of the cancer. But, as noted above, the oestrogens appear to act effectively only in the presence of the mammary tumour virus in mice. In virus-free mice (and in other species) the effect is much harder to demonstrate. In tissues other than the breast the position

becomes somewhat anomalous. The most obvious oestrogen target cell, the endometrial glandular epithelium, rarely develops tumours in treated animals, though connective-tissue tumours of the uterus are often produced and tumours result also in organs not usually regarded as oestrogen-responsive, for example the kidney in the hamster, and the Leydig cells of the testis in the mouse. These effects appear to depend only on the oestrogen activity of the various compounds concerned, and not on their precise structure.

It now seems likely that there is an increased risk of carcinoma of the endometrium in women receiving prolonged oestrogen therapy and in patients with an oestrogen-secreting granulosa-cell tumour of the ovary. In the past the risk has been exaggerated by confusion between endometrial hyperplasia and carcinoma.

Contraceptive hormonal preparations. Considering the very large number of women taking oral contraceptive pills there is little evidence of any carcinogenic effect. There is a small increase in benign tumours of the liver, which correlates with dose and duration of therapy, while benign breast lesions are decreased. There is no obvious change in the incidence of cancer of the breast or uterus. An early type of 'pill', in which different hormones were administered sequentially, was associated with an increase in endometrial carcinoma, and has now been withdrawn.

Androgenic/anabolic steroids. These hormones, notoriously used by athletes competing in field events to increase muscle mass, may be involved in the development of cancer of the liver.

Experimental endocrine disturbances and tumours. Experimental procedures which induce an increased output of trophic hormones by the adenohypophysis have been shown to result in cancer in the target organs, although trophic hormones have not been shown to induce cancer in man.

Examples of this mechanism of tumour induction include the following. (a) If the ovaries of a rat are removed and pieces are implanted into the spleen, they continue to secrete oestrogen, but this passes via the portal vein to the liver, where it is mostly inactivated. In consequence, there is increased secretion of FSH by the adenohypophysis and a granulosa-cell cancer eventually develops in the stimulated follicular tissue of the transplanted ovaries. (b) If rats are treated with a drug such as thiouracil, which blocks the production of thyroid hormone, increased secretion of TSH by the adenohypophysis causes hyperplasia and eventually cancer of the thyroid follicular epithelium. Cancer develops more rapidly, and with more certainty, if a carcinogen, e.g. 2-acetylaminofluorene or radio-iodine (which is taken up by the thyroid epithelium) is administered to the experimental animals.

Another example of functional hyperplasia leading to neoplasia is provided by removing the thyroid gland in mice, or destroying it with a large dose of radio-iodine. In the absence of thyroid hormone, the TSH-secreting cells of the adenohypophysis undergo hyperplasia and in some strains of mice this progresses to cancer. It is of interest in relation to the following section that initially the cancer cells can be suppressed by thyroxine, but eventually they may continue to grow when transplanted serially into mice with normal thyroid function.

Hormone-dependent tumours in man. The pituitary and thyroid tumours just mentioned may both be 'hormone-dependent' in the sense that they may regress if the hormonal disturbance that invoked them is corrected. Related phenomena in man are few, but the following three carcinomas deserve mention. (1) Many **prostatic carcinomas** are sufficiently dependent on a normal male hormonal environment to be slowed down, arrested, or even to regress for long periods if oestrogens are given. (2) Some differentiated **thyroid carcinomas** are partially dependent on TSH, and their rate of growth and spread may be reduced or arrested by continued administration of thyroxine, which suppresses secretion of TSH by the pituitary. (3) Some **breast carcinomas** regress under various hormonal manipulations—treatment with male hormones or even oestrogens, oophorectomy, adrenalectomy, hypophysectomy. Treatment by these methods has been largely empirical, but the cells of some breast cancers have receptors for oestrogens or other steroid hormones, such as progesterone. When hormone binds to the receptors the hormone-receptor complex enters the cell and is passed to the nucleus where it affects nucleic acid metabolism. The clinical significance is that patients with tumours consisting of receptor-positive cells are likely to respond to hormone therapy, whereas those whose tumours are receptor-negative are unlikely to respond.

Just as the experimentally-induced hormone-dependent pituitary tumours become independent after serial transplantation (see above), hormone-sensitive tumours in man practically always ultimately resume growth, though with the thyroid and prostatic carcinomas the period of arrest or partial regression is often long.

Epidemiological considerations in cancer prevention

There are two major approaches to prevention of cancer. One is by basic biological research on the mechanisms of the cellular changes leading to the development of cancer in animals and man. The second is by detecting carcinogenic factors in the environment, i.e. in the air, soil, foods and in industrial processes, and taking steps to eliminate exposure to them.

So far, we have considered the roles of genetic factors, chemical and physical agents, viruses and hormones in the development of cancer. We must now discuss the epidemiological approach to the detection of environmental factors which, together with the genetic predisposition or resistance to particular forms of cancer, determine the incidence and types of cancer to which man is subject. This is an exceedingly complex subject, and the following account is necessarily limited to some general principles and illustrative examples.

Life expectancy. As illustrated in Fig. 11.11, the risk of cancer increases with age. In this country, the life expectancy of newborn infants has increased from 40 to 70 years in the last 100 years, and this has been accompanied by a very great increase in cancer, which is now the cause of death of just over 20% of the popula-tion. By contrast, in countries with a much shorter life expectancy (due mainly to malnutrition and infections) the incidence of cancer is much lower. One reason for this relationship between cancer and age is obvious: *the cellular changes leading to cancer progress slowly over a long period, and accordingly cancer usually develops many years after first exposure to environmental carcinogens.*

Natural environmental factors. The importance of U.V. in *sunlight* as a cause of skin cancers, particularly in pale-skinned people, has already been considered (p. 297). Other natural factors which may have an influence on the incidence of cancer include *geological features* which influence the level of *background radiation* and also the amounts of various chemicals in the soil, water and vegetable foods. Climatic and other factors also determine the presence and incidence of certain parasitic diseases which predispose to cancer, e.g. schistosomiasis (bladder cancer in Egypt) and liver flukes (biliary-duct cancer in the Far East).

Occupational factors. Some examples of cancer resulting from exposure to carcinogens used in industry have already been given (pp. 298–301): these and some others are listed in Table 11.3, but it should be emphasised that, with the ever-increasing variety of industrial processes, the number of chemical carcinogens and co-carcinogens is now enormous, and screening of compounds potentially useful in industrial processes or as drugs, food additives, cosmetics, weedkillers, insecticides, etc., is becoming an increasingly heavy task. As already pointed out (p. 299) it may take years to detect that a substance is carcinogenic in animals, and even the most careful tests on animals cannot exclude the possibility that a substance is carcinogenic to man. Nor does it always follow that a substance found to be carcinogenic in the laboratory will be a danger to man. It is therefore important that general medical practitioners and epidemiologists should be on the alert for an unusually high incidence of cancer in particular occupational groups. A good example is provided by bladder cancer in workers in the aniline-dye and rubber industries (p. 299). More recently, it has become clear that asbestos miners and workers inhaling asbestos

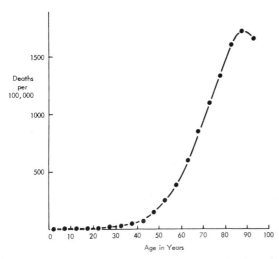

Fig. 11.11 Deaths from cancer in England and Wales during 1977, shown as the number of deaths per 100 000 for each 5-year age group. (Mortality Statistics, 1977, HMSO, London).

Table 11.3 Some Examples of Cancer Associated with Occupational Exposure to Carcinogens

Types of tumour	Occupational group	Carcinogen
Skin cancer	(a) Radiologists	(a) 'Soft' x-rays
	(b) Farmers and fishermen	(b) Ultraviolet light
Chronic myeloid leukaemia	Radiologists	'Hard' x-rays
Bladder cancer	Rubber workers	1-hydroxy-
	Aniline dye workers	2-naphthylamine
Lung cancer	(a) Miners	(a) ? Silica
	(b) Uranium miners	(b) γ-radiation
Mesothelioma of pleura or peritoneum	Asbestos miners	Asbestos
	Pipe-laggers, etc.	
Adenocarcinoma of nasopharynx	Furniture makers	Wood-dust
Angiosarcoma of liver	Polymerisation-chamber cleaners	Vinyl chloride monomer

dust, for example in the manufacture of vehicle brake linings and heat insulating material, have an unusually high risk of developing pleural or peritoneal mesotheliomas and bronchial carcinoma. In the plastics industry, an unusually high incidence of an otherwise rare tumour, haemangiosarcoma of the liver, has been observed in workers producing polyvinyl-chloride (PVC). This plastic is not itself carcinogenic, but it is manufactured by polymerisation of vinyl chloride monomer (VCM) which is carcinogenic. The risk is apparently greatest for workers who clean out the polymerisation tanks in which relatively high concentrations of residual VCM are inhaled, and safety measures have accordingly been introduced.

The risk of industrial carcinogens may spread beyond those directly involved in their use. For example, the spouses of asbestos workers have been reported to have an increased risk of asbestos-related cancers, and people living close to industrial plants emitting solvent vapours (which may contain ketones, alcohols, aromatic hydrocarbons, ethers, chlorinated hydrocarbons and nitrites), smoke or dust, are believed to have an increased incidence of lymphoid and other cancers. A recent study of the distribution of respiratory tract cancer in a Scottish town revealed a higher incidence among those living downwind from a steel foundry. Analysis of the polluted atmosphere showed relatively high concentrations of sulphur dioxide and of dusts containing compounds of iron, manganese, nickel, lead and cadmium. Similarly, quite apart from the hazard of cigarette smoking, the incidence of

lung cancer is significantly greater among those living in industrial zones than in rural communities.

Social factors. The countless ingredients of food, use of an ever-increasing number of drugs and various social habits are without doubt of importance in the causation of cancer. Dietary factors are discussed below. Two social habits known to cause cancer are cigarette smoking and betel chewing. *Cigarette smoking* is very largely responsible for the high incidence of lung cancer throughout the world: it accounts for the death, from carcinoma of the bronchus, of approximately 10% of men over 45 years old in this country (i.e. approximately 40% of male cancer deaths). The chewing of *betel leaves* mixed with tobacco leaves and slaked lime is widespread in Southern India and South East Asia, and is associated with a high incidence of cancer of the oral mucosa. It is a depressing fact that, although the consequences of these two habits have now been known for many years, they continue to be largely disregarded.

The influence of social habits is illustrated also by the incidence of *breast cancer*, which is lower in women who have borne children than in nullipara and appears to be lower in mothers who have suckled their children than in those who have used artificial infant foods (but see p. 979). A curious observation was the higher incidence of cancer in the left breast than in the right among women of the Tanka boat people in Southern China. This is possibly due to the design of the tunics they wear, which makes it easier to feed their infants from the right breast. In experimental animals, breast duct ligation or excision of the nipple is followed by an increase in cancer in the breast so treated, and it is postulated that retained breast secretions have a carcinogenic effect.

Dietary factors. The wide variations in diet, including the nature and amounts of foods eaten, methods of cooking, and the types of cooking vessels used, are all likely to influence the incidence of cancer, particularly of the alimentary tract. Additional potential sources of carcinogens in food include chemical fertilisers, insecticides, organic and inorganic chemicals fed to livestock, and chemicals used in the preservation of food. Natural diseases of plants and animals used as food may also be of importance, as exemplified by the experimental production of liver cancer by feeding aflatoxin, a product of the fungus *Aspergillus flavus* which contaminates ground nuts.

Investigations on *carcinoma of the large intestine* (colorectal cancer) illustrate how epidemiological and laboratory studies may help to elucidate causal factors in cancer (Hill, 1977). The incidence of this tumour has been shown to be relatively high in technologically advanced countries with a high standard of living. The incidence in migrant groups who have adopted the dietary habits of their new country changes from that of their country of origin to that of their country of adoption and thus genetic factors appear to be unimportant. The incidence is approximately the same in both sexes, and hormonal factors are unlikely to be involved. As regards diet, the incidence shows a positive correlation with the total caloric intake and with the amount of meat, animal fat and protein in the diet, and a negative correlation with the amount of vegetable fibre: animal foodstuffs are thus in some way responsible. Although many dietary ingredients have been suspected, current interest is centred on the production of carcinogens or co-carcinogens by bacteria in the lumen of the large intestine. It has been shown that gut bacteria can convert dietary factors to substances carcinogenic for animals, for example methylazoxymethanol from β-glucoside and N-nitrosamines from secondary amines and nitrate. Thus a diet which provides a suitable substrate and encourages the colonisation of the colon by particular species of bacteria might lead to the production of carcinogenic bacterial metabolites in the gut. A number of such possibilities exist: for example, gut bacteria can produce carcinogenic or co-carcinogenic metabolites from a variety of compounds present in food or produced by digestion in the gut, including tryptophan, tyrosine, methionine, cycasin and cholesterol. The available epidemiological and other evidence does not, however, provide strong support for an important role of these various bacterial metabolites in colorectal cancer. Nor can the geographical distribution of this tumour be explained readily by the carcinogenic activities of N-nitrosamines, aflatoxin (see above) or polycyclic aromatic hydrocarbons in the diet (although the latter may well play a causal role in gastric cancer).

At present, there is considerable interest in the possibility that *bacterial metabolites of bile acids* may be of importance. A correlation has been shown between the mean concentration of total bile acids in the faeces and the incidence of colorectal cancer in the population, and analysis of the faeces of patients with this tumour has shown a higher mean concentration than that of controls. A group of bacteria known as the nuclear dehydrogenating clostridia (NDC) are capable of desaturating the bile acid nucleus, producing unsaturated bile acids which have been shown in animal studies to act as carcinogens or co-carcinogens in the large bowel. These bacteria are commonly present in the faeces of populations with a high incidence of colorectal cancer and rare where the incidence is low: they are particularly common in the faeces of patients with colorectal cancer. The effect of diet may thus be to favour a flora which includes bacteria capable of converting bile acids to carcinogens. It is noteworthy that in communities with a high incidence of colorectal cancer most of the tumours develop in the left side of the colon and rectum, and the protective action of a diet rich in *vegetable fibre* may be attributable either to its effect on the bacterial flora or to more rapid transport of the gut contents through the lower part of the large intestine.

Host reactions in cancer

The natural history of cancer is not determined solely by the characteristics of the tumour cells, but also by the host's reaction to them. As indicated below, there is good evidence that protective host mechanisms exist, and that although these are very often unsuccessful in preventing the growth and spread of malignant tumours, and only very rarely bring about their complete destruction, they may nevertheless restrict the rate of tumour growth and spread and contribute to the degree of success achieved by various forms of treatment.

The nature of the host defences is largely unknown, but it has been shown that the cells of human and animal tumours possess surface antigens which are sufficiently foreign to the host to stimulate an immune response. This important property of tumour cells raises the possibility of immunotherapy, and in consequence there is considerable interest in the immunology of cancer, some of the major features of which are summarised below.

Experimental animal studies

Much of the experimental work has involved transplantation experiments, and before the importance of 'transplant' alloantigens was appreciated, rejection of transplanted tumours was frequently observed, but is likely to have been due to histo-incompatibility rather than to a tumour-specific reaction. Since the importance of alloantigens was demonstrated in mice by Gorer, the provision, by close inbreeding, of syngeneic strains of mice and rats has greatly facilitated experimental cancer research, not only by eliminating the 'transplant' antigens as a cause of rejection, but also by excluding other genetically-determined variables.

Specific immune responses to tumours

The elimination of cancer cells by a specific immune reaction on the part of the host requires (1) that cancer cells exhibit antigens to which the host is capable of mounting an immune response, and (2) that the products of the host immune response—antibodies and/or specifically reactive T lymphocytes—are capable of effecting destruction of the tumour cells. If these conditions are fulfilled, it must further

be asked why tumours grow and spread in spite of the host's immunity, and whether the balance can be tilted in favour of the host.

Tumour-cell antigens. To render a tumour cell susceptible to an immune reaction, the tumour cell antigens must be exposed on the cell surface, and must also be sufficiently foreign to stimulate an immune response; this excludes those surface antigens which, although present on tumour cells, occur also on the host's normal cells. Thus species- and organ-specific antigens, 'transplant' antigens (e.g. those of the H2 system in mice and of the HLA system in man) and blood-group antigens are all found (although often in reduced concentration) on tumour cells, but none of them is tumour-specific. There are, however, surface antigens on tumour cells which cannot be detected on normal cells: they are capable of eliciting immune responses and reactions and are sometimes called tumour-specific transplantation antigens (TSTA). In experimental carcinogenesis, these apparently tumour-specific surface antigens are largely dependent on the agent which has induced the tumour. *All tumours produced by any one oncogenic virus have been found to have relatively strong common surface antigens.* These include antigens which, although coded for by the viral genome, are not a structural component of the virion, and also, in the case of C-type viruses, antigens of the virus envelope which consists of modified host-cell-membrane (p. 306). It follows that antibody or primed T-lymphocytes reactive with these virus-coded antigens on a particular tumour should be reactive with the cells of all tumours produced by the same virus. By contrast, *tumours induced by chemical carcinogens or by physical agents have only weak common antigens; they develop stronger tumour-specific surface antigens, but these differ for each tumour, even when multiple tumours have been produced in the same tissue of the same animal by the same carcinogen.*

Immune responses to tumour-specific antigens. Both antibodies and cell-mediated immunity have been demonstrated, by *in-vitro* techniques, to develop in animals bearing tumours. In general, these responses are more readily demonstrable when the tumour is small, and as it enlarges and spreads they tend to diminish and disappear. They are readily demonstrable after excision of the tumour and then gradually diminish unless the tumour recurs or is re-introduced into the animal.

Effects of the immune response to tumours. Although tumours grow in spite of the host immune response, under experimental conditions a protective effect can sometimes be demonstrated. For example, when tumour cells are injected into a histocompatible animal, a certain minimal number of cells (which varies with the particular tumour and with the age of the animal) is required to produce a tumour. This alone shows that the animal can destroy a limited (sub-threshold) number of tumour cells. Moreover, in an animal already bearing a tumour, the number of tumour cells of the same type which must be injected to produce a second tumour is often considerably greater than the threshold dose for a normal animal. This apparent paradox—that the animal can destroy an oncogenic dose of injected tumour cells while its original tumour continues to grow—has not been satisfactorily explained.

There is also evidence that animals can be actively immunised against tumours, e.g. by injecting (a) a sub-threshold dose of tumour cells, (b) a larger dose of tumour cells previously rendered incapable of dividing by radiation or cytotoxic drugs, or (c) membrane preparations of tumour cells. Animals so-treated are capable of rejecting a normally oncogenic dose of cells of the corresponding tumour. Protection against virus-induced tumours can also be provided by immunising against the virus. Only partial protection is provided by these procedures: it varies from tumour to tumour and can be overcome by injecting large numbers of tumour cells.

Experimental evidence indicates that immunological defence against solid tumours is attributable mainly to cell-mediated immunity and little, if at all, to antibody. For example, when lymphocytes from an animal which has been immunised to a tumour (as described above) are transferred to a second, syngeneic animal, they afford some protection against challenge with the same tumour: antibodies give little or no protection.

As already noted, antibodies are probably capable of killing free tumour cells in the blood and in exudates in the peritoneal cavity etc. This may result from the susceptibility of antibody-sensitised cells to the lytic effect of complement, to phagocytosis and destruction by macrophages, and to the cytotoxic effect of K (antibody-dependent cytotoxic) cells (p. 152). Antibodies may thus play a role in preventing the formation of metastases by cancer cells gaining entry to the blood, serosal cavities, etc. However, as explained below, in some circumstances antibodies may actually enhance the growth of tumour cells.

The mechanism of destruction of tumour cells by specifically primed T-lymphocytes (Fig. 11.12) may be a direct cytotoxic effect requiring contact between the lymphocyte and target cell (p. 157) or may be mediated by lymphokines, including those which attract, immobilise and enhance the phagocytic and killing capacities of macrophages, and also by the specific arming of macrophages (p. 159).

Enhancement and 'blocking' factors. The injection into animals of antibody to the surface antigens of tumour cells has been observed, under certain conditions, to reduce the dose of the tumour cells necessary to cause a tumour, and to enhance the growth of a previously-implanted tumour. This **experimental enhancement of tumour growth** is antigen-specific; it is closely similar to the protection of tissue allografts by antibody (p. 167) and appears to be due to the antibody combining with antigen on the surface of the tumour cells and thus protecting them from attack by specifically primed lymphocytes. In other words, the antibody blocks the delayed hypersensitivity reaction of T lymphocytes with the tumour cells. In animals with large and progressing tumours, **blocking factors** have been detected in the serum; they have been shown to interfere with the killing of tumour cells *in vitro* by specifically-primed lymphocytes. It now seems unlikely that these are antibodies, for they disappear rapidly from the blood after excision of the tumour, at a time when the level of antibody increases. Other possibilities are that the blocking factors are free antigen molecules shed by the tumour cells as part of the normal turnover of plasma membrane constituents, or such antigens combined with antibody, i.e. immune complexes. Free antigen or immune complexes are capable of combining with the tumour-specific receptors on the surface of T lymphocytes or 'specifically armed' macrophages, thus preventing them from reacting with tumour cells: immune complexes might, in addition, bind to the Fc receptor sites of 'K'

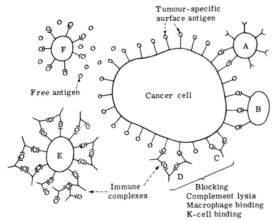

Tumour-specific
surface antigen

Cancer cell

Free antigen

Immune
complexes

Blocking
Complement lysis
Macrophage binding
K-cell binding

Fig. 11.12 Immunological cytotoxic mechanisms which may injure the cancer cell, and blocking factors which may protect the cell from immunological attack. The cancer cell may be killed by the reaction of cytotoxic T lymphocytes (A), or specially-armed macrophages (B), with tumour-specific surface antigen. Antibody (C) and antigen–antibody complexes in antibody excess (D) may protect the cancer cell from T lymphocytes and macrophages by binding to and blocking its surface antigens. Antibody and complexes may also promote cytotoxicity by complement, macrophages or K cells, but these effects seem to be of little or no importance except perhaps on free cancer cells in the circulation or in serosal exudates. Immune complexes in antigen excess (E) or free antigen (F) shed by cancer cells may block the specific binding sites on T lymphocytes or specifically-armed macrophages.

lymphocytes or macrophages, thus inhibiting their antibody-dependent cytotoxic activity for the tumour cells. These phenomena are shown diagramatically in Fig. 11.12.

Immunology of cancer in man

Once a cancer has spread beyond the possibility of excision, it usually progresses, and eventually proves fatal. This applies to most but not all types of human cancer. There are, however, considerable variations in the rate of growth, even for tumours of the same type and histological appearances. In patients with carcinoma of the breast, for example, surgical excision is sometimes followed by many years of normal health, but with subsequent reappearance and relatively rapid growth of tumour in the operation scar or of metastases: this is sometimes observed also with some other cancers. Very rarely, complete spontaneous regression of a cancer occurs. Partial regression is

more common, and it is not very unusual for patients with metastatic melanoma to have no obvious primary tumour: examination sometimes reveals an area of skin depigmentation which on histological examination shows evidence of a regressing malignant melanoma.

Observations of the sort outlined above suggest that defence mechanisms against cancer can develop in the host, and that in some instances these are partially (and rarely fully) effective. The nature of host defence in these instances is unknown, but there is circumstantial evidence that specific immune responses may influence the course of some tumours. In the rapidly growing form of breast cancer termed encephaloid cancer, for example, a favourable prognosis following excision has been reported to show some correlation with lymphocytic infiltration of the cancer, and this suggests that a delayed hypersensitivity reaction, or possibly antibody-dependent lymphocyte cytotoxic activity, is involved. Seminoma, a rapidly growing carcinoma originating in the germinal epithelium of the testis, is very commonly infiltrated with large numbers of lymphocytes and may also contain tubercle-like macrophage granulomas, both of which are consistent with a delayed hypersensitivity reaction. This may help to explain why the cure-rate is unusually high for such a rapidly progressing cancer: even when there is extensive metastasis, radiotherapy is often curative. A third example of a cancer which is often highly susceptible to therapy is choriocarcinoma arising from the placental trophoblast. Although it grows and spreads very rapidly, this rare tumour can often be destroyed by cytotoxic drug therapy. It is, however, unique among human tumours, in being a tumour of fetal tissue which grows in the mother; the tumour cells thus have HLA antigens which are inherited from the father and are foreign to the maternal host, so that allograft rejection is likely to contribute to the success of therapy.

Immune responses. *As in animal studies, antibodies and lymphocytes which react specifically with tumour cells have been demonstrated by in vitro techniques in patients with various types of cancer.* They react with the patient's own tumour cells, with the cells of other tumours of similar type, and with cell lines derived from such tumours. This sharing of common antigens by similar tumours in different individuals is consistent with, but not strong evidence of, a viral aetiology. Antibodies and cell-mediated immunity to the tumour cells are most often detectable in patients with early cancer, and tend to diminish as the tumour enlarges and spreads. Blocking factors, similar to those in animals (see above) also appear in the blood, particularly when the cancer is advanced. These observations are based on recent work, and the prognostic significance of fluctuations in the immune responses is not yet known. In a study of neuroblastoma, a malignant tumour of infancy and early childhood, which regresses completely much more often than most other cancers, Dr. Lindsay Morrison, working in Glasgow, has demonstrated the development in patients of antibody and cell-mediated immunity to the tumour, but in this instance the immune response does not appear to correlate with spontaneous regression. The antigenic preparations in such investigations have consisted of whole tumour cells or crude homogenates or extracts, and the tumour-specific cell-surface antigens have not yet been fully characterised. Like HLA antigens, they have been reported to contain a β_2-microglobulin chain.

Oncofetal antigens are so called because they were first detected as products of cancers and of fetal tissues. Sensitive radio-immunoassay techniques have, however, detected low levels of them in normal adult serum and tissues and in raised amounts in some patients with cancer or with non-neoplastic cellular proliferation. The serum level of *carcino-embryonic antigen* (*CEA*) is raised in many patients with colorectal or various other cancers and in some patients with hepatitis, chronic bronchitis or ulcerative colitis etc. Raised levels of α-*fetoprotein* (*AFP*) are *relatively* specific for liver-cell cancer and malignant teratoma but occur also in some patients with other forms of cancer or hepatitis etc. Alpha-fetoprotein assay is of value in the ante-natal detection of neural tube defects (p. 772).

Immunological surveillance

The concept of immunological surveillance was advanced by Burnet, who postulated that one function of T lymphocytes is to monitor host cells and respond immunologically against any which have developed surface antigens foreign to the host. By this means, it is conceivable that many (perhaps most) malignant cells are destroyed before they are capable of developing into a tumour. As regards **experimentally-induced tumours**, there is little evidence that this hypothesis applies to those caused by chemical carcinogens, for such tumours are produced no more readily in immunosuppressed animals, or in congenitally immunodeficient (nu nu) mice than in normal animals (Stutman, 1979) Immunological surveillance is, however of considerable importance in preventing virus-induced tumours in animals. This is illustrated by the ease with which such tumours can be induced in neonatal mice, which are immunologically immature, and in adult immunosuppressed or immunodeficient mice. Protection of neonates or immunodeficient mice is also afforded by transfer of syngeneic lymphocytes from an animal immunised against the virus-induced tumour. Indeed, immunosuppression by the oncogenic virus itself, as in the case of feline leukaemia virus, predisposes to tumour production.

As regards **cancer in man**, there is also some evidence favouring immunological surveillance, for children with certain congenital immunodeficiencies, and renal transplant recipients receiving long-term immunosuppressive therapy, have an increased incidence of cancer. However, the tumours arising in such patients do not reflect the natural incidence of cancer in the general population. The increased incidence is greatest for tumours of the lymphoreticular system (lymphomas and lymphoid leukaemias). These include tumours similar to those induced in animals by the leukaemia viruses, and it thus seems likely that such tumours in man, as in animals, are susceptible to immunological surveillance.

The most likely example of effective immunological surveillance in man is provided by infection with the Epstein-Barr virus (p. 304) which in normal individuals induces a strong immune response on the part of T cells, and does not cause cancer. In African children with chronic malaria, which depresses the immunity system, infection with EB virus is associated with the development of the Burkitt lymphoma, and in the Southern Chinese, in whom genetically-determined immunological responsiveness may play a role, the virus is associated with nasopharyngeal carcinoma.

In the past few years, there has been increasing interest in the possibility that immunological surveillance is a function of **'natural killer' (NK) lymphocytes**, which are present in the blood of normal animals, including man. NK cells can react with and kill foreign cells, including tumour cells, apparently without the need for previous immunological priming (see Herberman and Holden, 1978). The nature and importance of NK cells are not yet established. It has been claimed recently that their reaction with foreign cells depends on surface antibody bound to the NK cell by its Fc receptors (Takasugi and Akira, 1979). If this is correct, it is not clear how NK cells differ from K cells.

It may be significant that most cancers occur in old age, for there is no doubt that immune responsiveness declines in the elderly, but prolonged exposure to environmental carcinogenic factors and the long latent period of human cancers could also account for the age incidence. Tests for immune responsiveness to various antigens have not, in general, revealed immunodepression in patients with early cancer as compared with age-matched control subjects. Advanced cancer patients commonly show evidence of immunodepression, but this is most obvious in those with tumours which invade and destroy the lymphoid tissues, and is likely to *result* from the cancer.

The prospect of immunotherapy. The possibility of immunotherapy for cancer has been appreciated since the early 1900s. The advances in tumour immunology outlined above have strengthened the scientific basis of such treatment, but they have also demonstrated that, in spite of the occurrence of anticancer immune responses in many patients, their tumours still progress and cause death. It remains possible, however, that boosting the immune response might have some therapeutic effect. The administration of immunological adjuvants, such as BCG, *Corynebacterium parvum* and Levamisole, has been attempted in various neoplastic conditions, and has been claimed to have some effect in acute lymphoblastic leukaemia: in other neoplastic conditions the results have so far been disappointing. Various attempts have also been made to stimulate active specific immunity by implanting pieces of tumour which have been excised and treated with x-irradiation to prevent the cells from dividing. Such a procedure is not very hopeful, for if the patient's tumour does not stimulate effective immunity it seems unlikely that the implanted cells will do so, but it remains possible that, by increasing the antigenicity of the implanted cells, e.g. by coupling with haptens, or by using

homologous tumour with its 'foreign' transplant antigens, the immune response to the relevant tumour antigens may be augmented. Attempts have also been made to provide passive immunity by transplanting tumour to a volunteer in the hope that therapeutically effective antibody will be produced. On at least one occasion, the volunteer failed to reject the transplanted tumour, which proved to be fatal. The therapeutic value of lymphocyte products, and of interferon (p. 194), are being investigated.

Immunotherapy of cancer patients faces at least three major difficulties. Firstly, excision of an early cancer may effect a cure. It is not possible, at present, to identify those patients who will develop recurrences, and it therefore seems unjustifiable to apply to early cancer patients a form of therapy which is of unknown value. Accordingly, attempts at immunotherapy have mostly been made on patients with advanced cancer, when it is likely to be too late. Secondly, there is no guarantee that active immunisation will induce immune responses which contribute to the destruction of the tumour. There is, in fact, a risk of inducing the production of 'enhancing' antibody (p. 315) and thus increasing the rate of tumour growth. Thirdly, problems in assessing the results of any form of cancer therapy arise from the natural individual variations in the rate of growth and spread of cancer. In consequence, any trial of therapy must usually be extensive.

Attention has also been given to the possibility of vaccines to prevent cancer, and this has been achieved in feline leukaemia (p. 307). If it could be shown that some forms of human cancer are due to particular oncogenic viruses, immunisation against the virus, or against tumours induced by it, should be possible, but it would still be necessary to identify those individuals likely to develop that form of cancer unless one is prepared to immunise whole populations.

Finally, the induction of a delayed hypersensitivity reaction at the site of a tumour has been used as a method of tumour destruction. This has achieved some success in the treatment of epidermal tumours, notably basal cell carcinoma. The patient is sensitised by application to the skin of an agent which induces cell-mediated immunity, e.g. dinitrochlorobenzene (DNCB) and subsequently DNCB is applied to the tumour and surrounding skin: a delayed hypersensitivity reaction develops, and may be successful in destroying the tumour. Two mechanisms may be involved: firstly, the delayed hypersensitivity reaction, if intense, causes necrosis of normal cells (as in tuberculin skin testing—p. 157) and may similarly induce necrosis of the tumour. Secondly, macrophages accumulate and become more actively phagocytic and cytotoxic for foreign cells (including cancer cells) unrelated to the antigen which has induced the delayed hypersensitivity reaction. Similarly, attempts have been made to destroy tumours by immunising the patient with BCG (p. 209) and injecting the tumour with either BCG or tuberculoprotein.

What makes the cancer cell multiply?

Although we are aware that many agents can cause individual cancers, we know neither how they induce the essential change in the cell which makes it a cancer cell, nor indeed what is the exact nature of this change. This last section will review briefly the major theories which attempt to account for the most characteristic feature of the cancer cell—its property of multiplying regardless of the mechanisms which govern the behaviour of the normal cell.

Cell surface changes. The inherent nature of the cancer cell abnormality is reflected in its loss of contact inhibition when grown in culture (p. 302), a phenomenon which points to an abnormality of the cell membrane.

It has been shown that most types of tissue cell form *gap junctions*, through which there is continuity of the cell sap of adjacent cells. These connections may be of importance in transmitting signals from cell to cell, for cancer cells in general lack gap junctions. The surface of cancer cells also carries a higher negative charge than most normal tissue cells, and increased mutual repulsion may thus interfere with the adhesion and contact inhibition of cancer cells.

Two other cell membrane components of possible importance in the mitotic activity of cancer cells are proteins and sugar residues, e.g. N-acetylglucosamine, on the cell surface. It is known that mitosis is associated with some loss of surface protein, and normal tissue cells in culture can be induced to multiply by treatment with trypsin: after mitosis, however, the daughter cells develop surface proteins and contact inhibition is restored. By treating cancer cells in culture with compounds which bind to surface N-acetylglucosamine, contact inhibition can be restored and the cells cease to multiply. It is postulated that exposed sugar residues on the cell surface are involved in the signal which stimulates cells to multiply, and that surface protein in some way inhibits this role of the sugar residues.

The signal at the cell surface appears to be relayed within the cell by its effect on intracellular cAMP, the level of which falls during mitosis, and cGMP, which rises. Malignant cells have, in general, low concentrations of intracellular cAMP, addition of which to transformed cells in culture can inhibit their growth.

A defective response to *chalones* (p. 86) has also been postulated to account for proliferation of cancer cells, but is at present little more than speculative.

Whatever the nature of the essential change in the cancer cell, it is obviously transmitted to the daughter cells during mitosis, and this raises two possibilities. Firstly, that carcinogenesis involves *mutations*, i.e. abnormalities in the genome of the cell, and secondly that the cancer cell represents *abnormality or reversal of differentiation* (*the epigenetic theory*).

The mutational theory of carcinogenesis

This proposes that the altered behaviour of the cancer cell arises from mutation. In support of this theory, most chemical and physical carcinogenic agents are mutagenic, chromosomal anomalies are a common feature of cancer, and oncogenic viruses bring about their effects by the activity of a viral oncogene integrated into the cell DNA, which itself could be regarded as the equivalent of a mutation. However, we have seen that carcinogenesis is usually a gradual process. With the exception of some of the oncogenic viruses, carcinogenic agents bring about gradual changes in the cell, illustrated above by the effect of azo-dyes on liver cells (p.

300). If mutation is the essential change in carcinogenesis, then it is necessary to postulate a series of mutations.

Related to the mutation theory is the *oncogene theory*. As already noted, the proviruses of endogenous oncogenic retraviruses (p. 309) are demonstrable in the normal cells of various vertebrates. In such cells, the oncogene of the provirus is inactive: the oncogene theory proposes that carcinogenic agents bring about cancerous transformation by inducing changes which result in expression of the proviral oncogene. This might conceivably occur without expression of other proviral genes, in which case there would be little or no evidence of the role played by the endogenous virus. If, however, the virogene is fully expressed, then viral products are likely to be detectable in the cancer cell, and unless the provirus is deficient (p. 306), the development of cancer would be associated with viral replication, as occurs with some of the leukaemia viruses.

The epigenetic theory of carcinogenesis

Although the mutation theory of cancer is widely favoured, it must be emphasised that heritable changes in cells occur without mutations. With the exception of committed lymphocytes and their progeny (pp. 126–9), all somatic cells are believed to possess the whole genome of the individual, and this has been supported by the growth of plants from single cells and the development of a normal frog when the nucleus of a fertilised frog ovum is replaced by a frog's somatic cell nucleus. Nevertheless, during differentiation, the somatic cells develop special features which characterise them as neurons, liver cells, fibrocytes, etc., and this differentiation is retained by its descendants when the differentiated cell divides. It is thus conceivable that the special features of the cancer cell have developed as a result of reversal of the process of differentiation, or of abnormal differentiation of a primitive stem cell. While at first sight the cancer cell might appear to have gained positive properties—increased mitotic activity, motility, invasiveness, production of inappropriate and excessive amounts of hormones, etc.—these may, in fact, represent *loss* of cell components and consequent failure of normal homoeostasis. As noted above, uncontrolled growth of cancer cells appears to be closely associated with loss of a surface protein. Similarly, production of excess of hormones or of inappropriate hormones could be due to loss of the suppressor mechanism for a particular gene. Such loss of controlling factors could be explained by a particular pattern of gene expression, i.e. a form of differentiation, without the need to postulate mutations.

A number of phenomena support the epigenetic theory of cancer (Uriel, 1979). For example, some undoubtedly malignant tumours stop growing and their cells become highly differentiated. A good example is the neuroblastoma, whose cells may develop into mature neurons. This is a rare happening, but even in the common squamous carcinoma many of the tumour cells stop dividing and become highly keratinised (Fig. 12.13, p. 329). Malignant cells in culture can also, in some instances, be made to regain contact inhibition and other features of normal cells by addition to the culture medium of various chemicals, e.g. 5-bromodeoxyuridine. Of particular interest is the dedemonstration that replacement of the nucleus of a fertilised frog's ovum (see above) by the nucleus of cells from a Lucké carcinoma (a virus-induced renal cancer of the frog kidney), does not result in the growth of a tumour cell-line but of a normal tadpole. This implies that the normal fertilised ovum and its progeny contain cytoplasmic factors which can suppress the activity of an integrated viral oncogene, and that the cancer cell lacks such factors. Other important findings have arisen from the implantation of malignant cells from mouse gonadal teratomas (tumours derived from primordial germ cells of the mouse testis or from parthenogenetically activated ova) into mouse blastocyst embryos. The malignant cells divide during embryonic development, producing cells which differentiate normally and contribute to the formation of several tissues. By contrast, when the teratoma cells are implanted into adult mice, they produce a teratoma. It is thus apparent that, in this instance, the environment of the embryo induces normal behaviour in the malignant cells.

While of limited scope, experiments such as those described above indicate the need for further studies on the relative importance of nuclear and extra-nuclear changes in carcinogenesis.

In conclusion

The essential nature of carcinogenesis—mutations, epigenetic changes or oncogenes—has not been settled. It may well be that more than one type of fundamental cellular change can result in cancer. The protective host factors are really no better understood: immunological surveillance appears to play an important role in some of the human lymphomas, and by analogy with animal studies this suggests a viral aetiology for these tumours.

So far, experimental studies on the fundamental nature of cancer have contributed little to cancer prevention in man, but detection and elimination of exposure to chemical and physical carcinogenic agents has without doubt achieved considerable success. The curtailment of such habits as cigarette smoking and betel chewing could also prevent huge numbers of cancers.

In many countries, cytological screening for uterine cervical pre-malignancy appears to have reduced the incidence of invasive cancer, and the earlier detection of cancer of the breast and some other sites is being attempted by education and screening of the public.

Once cancer has developed and spread far beyond the possibility of complete removal, symptomatic relief of pain may be offered by radiotherapy and cytotoxic drugs, or in some instances by hormonal therapy; such therapy may slow down or even for a while arrest the growth of the tumour. Complete cure of advanced malignancy is, however, a rarity except in a few particular types of cancer.

References

Herberman, R. B. and Holden, H. T. (1978). Natural cell-mediated immunity. *Advances in Cancer Research* **27**, 305–77.

Hill, M. J. (1977). Bacterial Metabolism pp. 45–64. In *Topics in Gastroenterology*. Ed. by S. C. Truelove and E. Lee. Blackwell Scientific, Oxford.

Stutman, O. (1979). Chemical carcinogenesis in nude mice from heterozygous matings and homozygous matings. *Journal of the National Cancer Institute* **62**, 353–8.

Takasugi, M. and Akira, Donna (1979). Role of antibodies in specificity of natural cell-mediated immunity. *Journal of the National Cancer Institute* **62**, 1361–5.

Uriel, J. (1979). Retrodifferentiation and the fetal patterns of gene expression in cancer. *Advances in Cancer Research* **29**, 127–74.

Further Reading

Advances in Cancer Research. Academic Press Inc., New York. (Detailed reviews of oncological topics of major importance—mostly excellent. Usually one volume published annually since 1953.)

Cochran, A. J. (1978). *Man, Cancer and Immunity*, pp. 206. Academic Press, London, New York and San Francisco. (A review of immunological aspects of cancer, including some of the author's recent work.)

Neville, A. Munro, Grigor, K. M. and Heyderman, Eadie (1978). Biological markers and human neoplasia. In *Recent Advances in Histopathology*, No. 10, pp. 23–44. Edited by P. P. Anthony and N. Woolf. Churchill–Livingstone, Edinburgh, London and New York.

Symington, T. and Carter, R. L. (Eds.) (1976). *Scientific Foundations of Oncology*, pp. 690. Heinemann, London. (Authoritative reviews on many aspects of oncology.)

Taussig, M. J. (1979). Neoplasia. In *Processes in Pathology*, pp. 241–353. Blackwell Scientific, Oxford. (A more detailed account than provided in this chapter—clearly written and well illustrated.)

12

Tumours: II. Epithelial Varieties and Modes of Spread

After the introductory account of tumours in the last chapter, we turn for the next two chapters to the more practical questions of what kinds of tumour occur in man, what they look like and how they behave. There are many aspects of tumours that are best described as part of the pathology of the organs from which they are derived: these chapters are concerned with aspects of more general application, though they will be found to include also descriptions of a number of specialised tumours, usually because they illustrate some general principle.

Classification

In the introduction to the previous chapter the distinction between *benign* and *malignant* tumours was discussed in some detail. We must now use the other chief mode of classification, the *histogenetic*, which is based on the tissue of origin. We may conveniently distinguish tumours of:

(*a*) epithelium;
(*b*) connective tissues (including muscle);
(*c*) blood vessels and lymphatics;
(*d*) the nervous system;
(*e*) lymphoid and haemopoietic tissue;
(*f*) other tissues.

Of these, the epithelial tumours are overwhelmingly the commonest and are responsible for 90 per cent of all cancer deaths in this country. This first chapter will be devoted to them alone.

General features of epithelial tumours

Epithelium has two essential characteristics which are carried over into its tumours.
(*a*) It forms continuous *sheets* or *masses* of cells of similar type, which adhere together without any intervening intercellular structures (Fig. 12.1). This adherence of the cells into larger or smaller groups is retained as an indication of an epithelial origin even in tumours which have lost all the other distinctive features of epithelial cells.

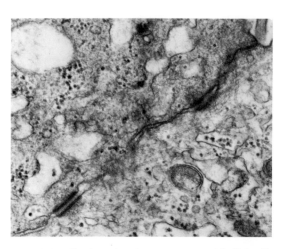

Fig. 12.1 The junction between two epithelial cells showing their close apposition. Two zones of adherence (desmosomes) are seen as double lines of increased density of the cell membranes. Desmosomes are observed in the cells of malignant epithelial tumours, but are reduced in number or defective with consequent weakening of cell adhesion. × 40 000.

(*b*) It requires a stroma of connective tissue and blood vessels for its support and nourishment. This is equally necessary for tumour epithelium, and all epithelial tumours appear to be able to stimulate the local connective tissues and blood vessels to proliferate and supply a stroma which surrounds and supports the epithelial cell groups. This '**desmoplastic reaction**', as it is called, varies in degree; it is often inadequate, so that much of the tumour dies from ischaemia, but it is sometimes excessive, so that the fibrous stroma becomes more conspicuous than the epithelium ('scirrhous' tumours, so-called). We know very little about the way in which the tumour cells influence the development of connective tissue. As so often in cancer studies, the basic problem is a much wider one: the relationship between epithelium and connective tissue is established as a convenient form of organisation in a large part of the animal kingdom, and we know little of its basic

mechanism. The cancer cells are simply exploiting a normal process.

The way in which an epithelium is organised naturally affects profoundly the structure of the tumours to which it gives rise, and this is especially marked in the case of the slow growing and well-differentiated benign tumours. Epithelia which cover surfaces generally give rise to **papillomas**; epithelia of exocrine or endocrine glands, and of solid organs like the liver and kidneys, give rise to **adenomas.**

Benign Epithelial Tumours (Papillomas and Adenomas)

Papillomas

If one considers what will happen to a sheet of epithelium such as the epidermis when its cells have begun to multiply, it is clear that the first effect will be to thicken the layer. But since this is limited by the extent to which nutriments can diffuse from the underlying blood vessels, the tumour cells must soon spread in other directions. So long as the tumour is benign, they do not spread downwards into the underlying tissue, and so the epithelium must increase in thickness or in surface area. Most often it increases in both. The effect of increase in area is most readily understood if one tries to visualise the epithelium as a sheet of cloth which is pinned down at the edges and then increased in area; it is obvious that it will be thrown into folds. If the increase is in one dimension only, the folds will be regular pleats, but since in a benign epithelial tumour it occurs in two dimensions simple folding cannot occur, and the result is an irregular mass of peaks and hollows. Where the epithelium is raised into peaks, the underlying connective tissue proliferates and accompanies it, forming a fibrous core (the 'desmoplastic reaction' in effect) and the epithelium covering it remains well nourished and continues to grow. Since each peak is compressed by the other peaks around it, it can only grow upward, producing a higher peak which may finally become a long finger-like process, or *frond*. The resulting mass of 'papillae' constitutes a papilloma.

If such a papilloma arises in a squamous epithelium the processes are naturally covered by squamous epithelium, thickened but other-

wise not grossly abnormal. They are well seen in a papilloma of the skin (Fig. 12.2), the commonest form of which is the virus-induced wart of children.

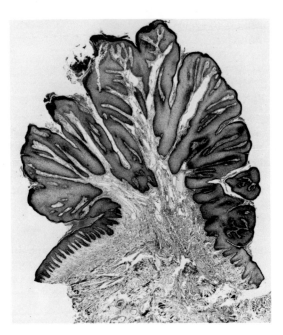

Fig. 12.2 Papilloma of muco-cutaneous junction of lip, showing branching processes of connective tissue covered by stratified epithelium. × 10.

The transitional epithelium of the urinary tract produces papillomas covered by transitional epithelium, in which the papillary processes are often very numerous, long and thin: such tumours are sometimes called **villous**

papillomas. * (Figs. 12.3 and 12.4). This is possibly due, not to any special characteristic of the epithelium, but to the environment provided by the bladder, in which the fronds of the papilloma float like seaweed in a sheltered bay: similar complexity is seen in the rare choroid plexus papillomas which float in the cerebrospinal fluid.

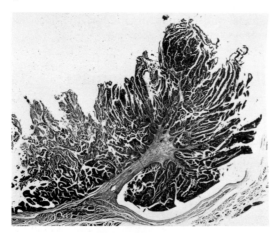

Fig. 12.3 Papilloma of bladder, showing innumerable delicate fronds, which are covered by transitional epithelium. A stalk, as seen in this case, is often absent. It is unusual for a bladder papilloma as large as this to be completely benign. × 4.

Epithelium lining ducts, e.g. of the breast, can give rise to papillomas (Fig. 12.5) and villous papillary tumours arise also from the surface epithelium of the large intestine (Fig. 12.6), although here it is commoner to find more complex tubulovillous tumours (described on p. 327).

The papillary structure of papillomas is not usually obvious to the naked eye, though the educated naked eye may recognise it. In most skin papillomas it is hidden by the thick horny layer of keratin which develops on the surface, filling up the gaps between the fronds and producing a rough dry hard surface in which only an ill-defined cauliflower pattern gives a hint of the underlying structure. The result is a well defined little lump, usually round, always projecting above the surface (except for the plantar wart on the sole of the foot, where pressure flattens it) and at times slightly polypoid—i.e. having a slight neck between it and the skin level. The villi of excised bladder papillomas

* *Villus:* a fine hair-like process.

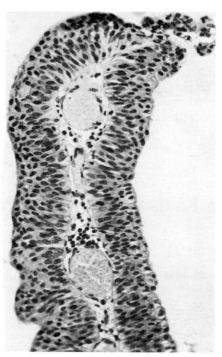

Fig. 12.4 Papilloma of bladder. Section of the tip of a single process, showing a narrow core of connective tissue, including capillaries, covered by transitional epithelium. The epithelium is rather thicker and has rather more cells than normal, but differentiation is still excellent. × 200.

are difficult to recognise by naked-eye; unless the excised tumour is submerged in fluid, they collapse against each other and leave nothing but a somewhat velvety surface to indicate their true nature. Seen *in situ* with a cystoscope, or examined with a lens under saline, the fronds will be obvious. The fronds are even harder to see in the soft velvety plaques of a villous tumour of the rectum, and a dissecting microscope may be necessary.

Adenomas

Adenomas are benign epithelial tumours of glandular origin and often retain some secretory function. They occur more commonly, in general, in the endocrine than in the exocrine glands, though the commonest of all are the tubular adenomas (adenomatous polyps) arising from the mucosa of the large intestine.

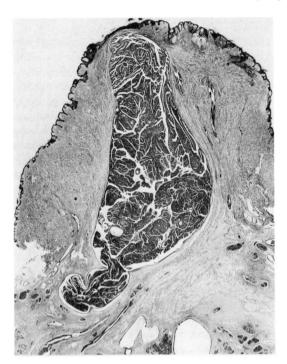

Fig. 12.5 Papilloma of the breast, growing into and distending a duct near the nipple. × 4.

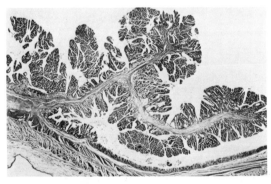

Fig. 12.6 Papillary tumour of rectum. The structure is obviously similar to that of the bladder papilloma, but a higher power would show that the covering epithelium is of columnar type. The majority of benign tumours of colorectal epithelium are of mixed papillomatous and adenomatous structure and are rather misleadingly termed adenomas. × 3.

Adenomas of endocrine glands

These are of particular importance because many are capable of excessive hormonal secretion. This is a particularly common feature of adenomas of the parathyroid, the islets of Lan-

gerhans and the adrenal medulla, all of which usually reveal their presence by excessive secretion of one or more of the appropriate hormones of the parent gland. Some adenomas of the adenohypophysis, thyroid and adrenal cortex behave in this way, although most such tumours do not function sufficiently to cause hormone imbalance. As with tumour cell function in general, the secretory activity of most endocrine adenomas is not subject to control by the normal feedback mechanisms.

In all these glandular tissues an adenoma usually appears as a rounded or lobulated nodule, generally solid and of the same colour as, or paler than, the surrounding tissue (Fig. 12.7). It is enclosed in a fibrous capsule, usually thin, and resulting from pressure atrophy of the surrounding glandular tissue and condensation of its stroma (Fig. 12.8). Adenomas range in size from the microscopic to over 10 cm in diameter, but most of those of the endocrine glands, with the exception of thyroid adenomas, are less than 2 cm in diameter.

As might be expected from their functional activities, the cells of endocrine adenomas re-

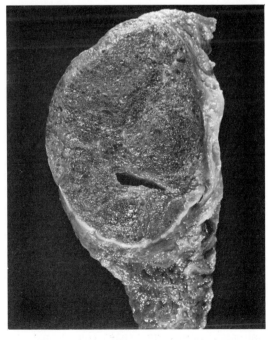

Fig. 12.7. An adenoma of the thyroid gland. The tumour is partly enclosed in normal thyroid tissue and is enclosed in a fibrous capsule, most clearly seen around the lower margin. The cut surface of the tumour resembles thyroid tissue. × 1·5.

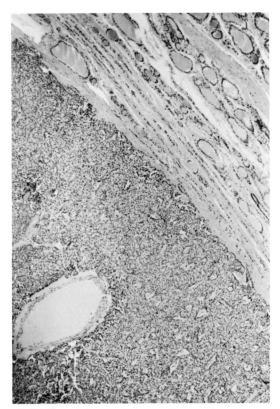

Fig. 12.8 Part of a thyroid adenoma of the 'solid' or micro-acinar type, which contrasts in appearance with normal thyroid tissue. Note the fibrous 'capsule' which is composed largely of residual stroma of compressed, atrophic thyroid surrounding the tumour. × 40.

semble closely those of their parent tissue; adenomas of those endocrine glands composed of several cell types, e.g. the adenohypophysis and pancreatic islets, may be predominantly of one particular cell type and secrete the particular hormone(s) normally secreted by that type of cell. For example, islet cell adenomas may be composed predominantly of β-cells and secrete insulin, of α-cells and secrete glucagon, or of δ-cells and secrete somatostatin.

Although endocrine adenomas are usually well differentiated, they often show great variation in nuclear and cell size, which in these tumours does not suggest malignancy unless accompanied by other features (numerous mitoses, invasiveness, etc.). The stroma may also resemble that of the parent gland, although it is often more dense, abundant and sometimes hyaline. Illustrations of endocrine adenomas can be found in Chapter 26.

Adenomas of the exocrine glands

These are uncommon, apart from the very common **fibro-adenoma of the breast** (Fig. 24.41), which is really a mixed tumour in which both the epithelium and stroma are neoplastic. Both the prostate and breast are very prone to develop multiple nodularity due to foci of proliferation of both glandular and stromal elements in various proportions, but such nodules are not sharply defined and are really examples of focal hyperplasia, perhaps due to hormonal influences, and are not true tumours. Adenomas of the **salivary glands** are not rare. They show pleomorphism of both epithelial and stromal elements (Figs. 19.14, 19.15, p. 596) and projections through the capsule make their complete removal more difficult.

Cystadenomas. Curiously, the **ovary** is a common site of an unusual type of adenoma in which the cells arrange themselves in gland-like structures resembling acini. The cells secrete copious mucous or watery secretion and as they have no ducts into which this can drain, it

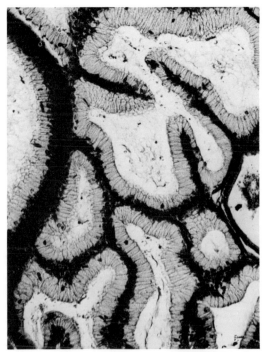

Fig. 12.9 Mucinous cystadenoma (cystic adenoma) of ovary. The cysts (small in this case) are lined by tall mucin-secreting epithelium. The nuclei, situated at the base of each cell, form a continuous line hardly distinguishable in this picture from those of the next cyst. × 150.

distends the lumen of the acinar-like structures, resulting in large cystic spaces and giving the tumour its name, **cystadenoma.** Epithelial-lined processes may project into the lumens (**papillary cystadenoma**). Such tumours, particularly those which secrete mucin (Fig. 12.9 and Fig. 24.20, p. 961), may grow enormous, and examples are on record of such tumours which outweighed the patient!

It might be expected that the pure cystadenomas, in which secretion is abundant and hence differentiation is good, are more benign than papillary cystadenomas, in which proliferation is more active: this is generally, although not always, true.

Papillary cystadenomas occur rarely in the pancreas and kidney.

Colorectal adenomas. The common **tubular adenomas of the large intestine** are composed of mucus-secreting cells arranged in tubular glands, thus resembling in structure the normal mucosal glands, and they are surrounded by a stroma similar to the lamina propria. These tumours are not embedded in the mucosa and are not encapsulated. Each consists of a rounded or lobulated mass which projects from the mucosal surface, and as it enlarges it becomes pedunculated, i.e. develops a stalk or pedicle, with a fibrovascular core and lined by normal mucosa, from which it dangles in the lumen of the bowel. Such a tumour is termed an **adenomatous polyp** * or **tubular adenoma** (Fig. 12.10). Although the glands secrete mucin, most of them drain (like the tubular glands of normal mucosa) into the lumen of the bowel and so do not become distended. As already mentioned (p. 324) papillary tumours ('villous adenomas') also arise from the large intestinal mucosa, and many epithelial tumours of this site have a complex structure in which papillary and adenomatous elements are mixed (tubulo-villous adenomas).

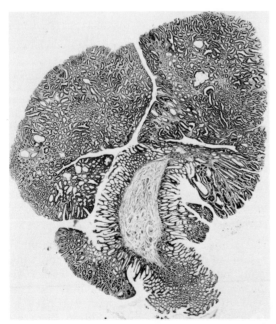

Fig. 12.10 Tubular adenoma of the colon. The rounded darker mass of the adenoma is made up of close-packed glands, less regular and more cellular than those of the normal mucosa which is seen below, covering the stalk of the polyp. (Unusually, two smaller adenomas arise from the stalk. In this case there were multiple adenomas and a carcinoma, seen in Fig. 12.14.) × 8.

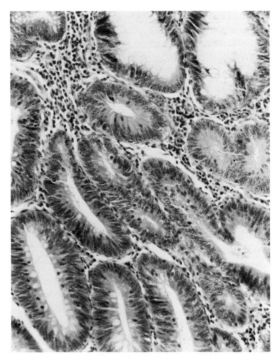

Fig. 12.11 Part of tubular adenoma of the colon, showing cellular aberration. Although the epithelium still forms crypts, these are hypercellular and irregular in size and shape. The epithelial cells show abnormal proliferative activity which has resulted in their becoming tall and narrow, and in some the nucleus has left the basal position and is undergoing mitosis. Many of the cells no longer contain the large globule of mucin characteristic of goblet cells. × 150.

*A polyp is a lump of tissue at the end of a stalk. It is not necessarily neoplastic.

Another important feature of these large intestinal tumours is that the glandular epithelium often shows marked mitotic activity and the cells become squeezed together and hence tall and narrow (Fig. 12.11): they may also become heaped up into two or more layers, or even form solid groups. Cell aberrations, such as nuclear irregularity and enlargement and cytoplasmic basophilia, are also common, and this proliferative activity and cell aberration is a warning that many of these tumours are pre-malignant: they are prone to invade the stalk and adjacent bowel wall and spread by lymphatics and blood stream. In patients with large numbers of adenomatous polyps (*polyposis coli*), the risk of malignancy is very high.

It is noteworthy that adenomas of exocrine glands do not show the high degree of specialisation and functional activity characteristic of many endocrine adenomas: they secrete a thin watery or mucoid fluid, but not the various enzymes secreted by the exocrine glands.

Adenomas occur also in the cortex of the **kidney** and rarely in the **liver**, the latter being of interest because their incidence appears to be increased in women using oral contraceptives.

Malignant Epithelial Tumours (Carcinomas)

The term **carcinoma** may be applied to any malignant tumour of epithelial origin. It may arise from one of the benign epithelial tumours just described, or directly from a non-neoplastic epithelium. In either case, it retains the two features already described as characteristic of epithelium and its tumours—the formation of sheets or masses of contiguous tumour cells, and the ability to excite a stromal reaction between and around the tumour-cell masses. In addition, the epithelial element commonly retains some resemblance to the tissue of origin, though in poorly differentiated (and usually more malignant) tumours this may be tenuous.

Naked-eye appearances

While there are many variations, it is possible to describe a typical carcinoma. It forms a firm lump, often irregularly nodular, its edge well defined in places and in others blending into the surrounding tissue (areas of invasion) so that it cannot be dissected out cleanly. On section it is predominantly whitish, as are most dense collections of young cells: there are often red patches of haemorrhage and, especially towards the centre, yellow areas of necrosis. When carcinoma arises in the epidermis or other surface epithelium it forms at first an irregularly dome-shaped swelling. The centre of this swelling however has often a poor blood supply and has lost the surface epithelium: it is exposed to trauma, infection and (in the case of lesions in the gut) digestive juices. It therefore often sloughs out, leaving a ragged ulcer. At the edges the tumour has a better blood supply and is partly protected by the surface epithelium, and so survives: the ulcer therefore commonly retains a thick irregular raised edge which is responsible for the highly characteristic appearance of the ulcerated malignant tumour (compare, for instance, Figs. 12.14, 19.36, p. 615 and 27.36, p. 1075).

Varieties of carcinoma

There are many special types of carcinoma characteristic of particular sites, though the more highly malignant 'anaplastic' ones all tend to look alike. Most malignant epithelial tumours can, however, be included in the two great classes of **squamous carcinoma** and **adenocarcinoma**.

Squamous carcinoma

This is the characteristic malignant tumour of squamous epithelia, both epidermis and squamous mucosae. (The names *squamous-cell* and *epidermoid* carcinoma are sometimes used instead of squamous carcinoma, but have no particular advantages). In addition there are some unexpected sites, where squamous carcinomas arise in organs containing no squamous epithelium: the most important of these is the bronchus, where squamous metaplasia of the bronchial epithelium is the probable explanation; similar metaplasia can account for less common sites such as the urinary tract and the gall bladder. Unstable squamo-columnar junctions such as the uterine cervix are also important sites.

Histologically, most squamous carcinomas are very readily recognisable. In early lesions, the downgrowth of the surface epithelium into the deeper tissues can be detected (Fig. 12.12). At the

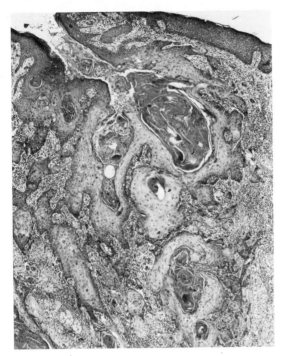

Fig. 12.12 Squamous carcinoma of the tongue, showing squamous cell masses with, in places, central keratinisation. These remain in continuity with the over-lying epithelium (*above*). Ulceration is beginning (*above left*). There is a well-marked inflammatory infiltrate in the connective tissue, which a little obscures the distinction from the infiltrating tumour. × 38.

periphery, small masses and narrow columns of cells burrow into the surrounding tissues. Behind this margin, the invading cell groups have had time to enlarge and differentiate, becoming recognisable as prickle cells and usually forming keratin: the keratin forms rounded concentric nodules in the centre of the cell groups, a very characteristic appearance called 'cell nests' or 'epithelial pearls' (Fig. 12.13). The amount of keratin formed and the proportion of cells recognisable as prickle cells both vary greatly: they are the best guides to degree of differentiation of the tumour, which, of course, affects its prognosis.

There are some variations from site to site—

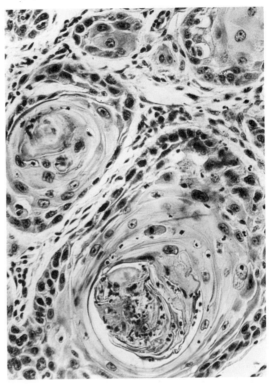

Fig. 12.13 Squamous carcinoma at higher magnification, showing cell nests. The largest shows central keratin (still with some stratum granulosum granules), then large pale prickle-cells and a periphery of darker undiffereniated cells. In the smaller cell masses at the top keratinisation has not yet begun: the mass at left centre is at an intermediate stage. × 290.

for instance, a squamous carcinoma of the bronchus or pharynx is usually less well differentiated than one of the lip or the skin. The site also naturally has a profound effect on the signs and symptoms produced by these tumours, and on their accessibility for treatment and hence on their prognosis.

Adenocarcinoma

This second group is a little less homogeneous than the last. Thus a histological section of an adenocarcinoma of the stomach can usually be distinguished from one of the colon with more confidence than a squamous carcinoma of the tongue from one of the bronchus. The grouping of adenocarcinomas together is, however, useful, for most of the malignant tumours of glands have a great deal in common with each other and with those that arise from all the ducts and surfaces lined by columnar epithelium. Important sites of origin include the stomach and colon, the pancreas, gall bladder and its ducts, breast and uterus; also the bronchi, which can give rise to both squamous and adeno-carcinomas.

Histologically, almost everything that has been said of the adenomas applies to adenocarcinomas, with two differences.

(*a*) Instead of remaining localised, the tumour cells invade the surrounding tissues (Fig. 12.14).

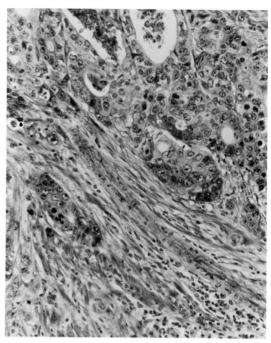

Fig. 12.15 Adenocarcinoma of bowel invading the muscle coat. *Below*, nearly solid strands of tumour are invading smooth muscle on each side of the arteriole which runs up from the bottom right corner. *Above*, the older tumour strands are developing gland-like lumens. × 160.

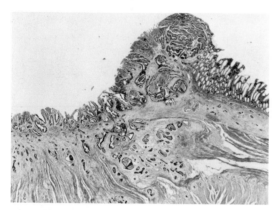

Fig. 12.14 Adenocarcinoma of colon. Ulcerated tumour to left, normal mucosa to right: between them the raised 'rolled margin' formed by a thick layer of tumour still partly protected by the normal mucosa stretched over its upper surface. Invasion of submucosa and muscularis is well seen. × 11.

(*b*) Differentiation is poorer (Fig. 12.15). In addition to all the general features of malignant tumours listed in the last chapter (p. 293) there is a marked tendency for acini to contain less secretion, to be lined not by one regular layer of epithelial cells but by a thick irregular layer, and in some tumours for most of the cell groups to form solid masses.

Several variations upon the basic pattern are common enough to be worth describing. Mixed and intermediate forms occur, and none of the following should be regarded as completely distinct entities.

(a) 'Spheroidal-cell' carcinoma, is a name commonly used for an adenocarcinoma in which most of the cell masses are solid (Fig. 12.16). This type of tumour is common in the breast, partly because of relatively poor differentia-

tion, and perhaps partly because the gland is usually in a non-secretory state.

(b) Cystadenocarcinoma, in which cysts lined by columnar or cuboidal cells are prominent. This is common in the ovary and is seen occasionally in the pancreas and kidney.

(c) Papillary adenocarcinoma, in which papillary processes project into cysts. This is seen particularly in the thyroid, ovary and biliary tract.

(d) Mucous (or mucoid) carcinoma, an adenocarcinoma in which mucus secretion is unusually marked. The term should be used only when the whole tumour looks like a mass of jelly, and under the microscope most of the tumour cells float free in lakes of mucus (Fig. 12.17). The commonest site of origin in this country is the colon, but it occurs also fairly often in the stomach and breast.

Hard and soft carcinomas

Classification of carcinomas into the two following types depends on features of the stroma

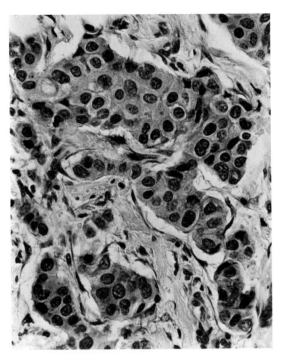

Fig. 12.16 Spheroidal-cell carcinoma of breast infiltrating tissue spaces. The tumour cells are still obviously epithelial, and nuclear changes are not gross, but there is no trace of glandular differentiation. × 300.

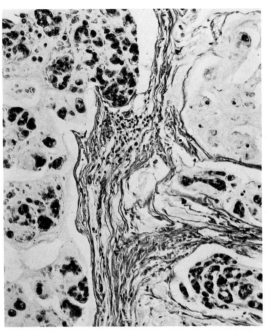

Fig. 12.17 Mucous carcinoma. The tumour cells, still in this case with some traces of glandular arrangement, lie in large pools of mucin. × 65.

and not of the tumour cells. It is thus an essentially different mode of classification. For example both spheroidal-cell carcinoma and adenocarcinoma can be either scirrhous (hard) or encephaloid (soft).

(1) Scirrhous carcinoma* is one that shows a very dense fibrous reaction (Fig. 12.18) which is responsible for its hardness. The term is used most often for breast cancer and for the curious 'signet-ring' cell carcinomas of the stomach (Fig. 19.41, p. 617).

(2) Encephaloid carcinoma (Fig. 12.19) has minimal stroma and so is soft and 'brain-like' to the touch. The term is rarely used except for the uncommon soft carcinomas of the breast.

These two types appear and feel very different, but behave in much the same way.

Special types of carcinoma

The names of some carcinomas reflect a striking appearance linked to a distinctive behaviour. Examples include clear-cell carcinoma of the

* *Scirrhus:* a hard swelling.

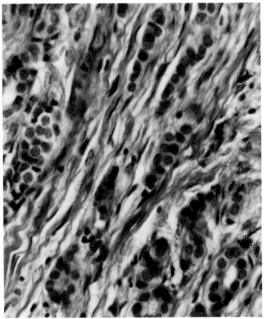

Fig. 12.18 'Scirrhous' carcinoma of breast, with dense poorly cellular collagen between the tumour cell groups. In this case, in contrast to Fig. 12.16, some of the cell groups (bottom right) show some glandular differentiation. × 240.

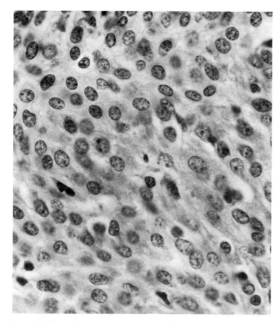

Fig. 12.19 'Encephaloid' carcinoma of breast, showing cells essentially similar to those of Figs. 12.16 and 12.18, but in large masses with very little stroma. Only part of a large mass of cells is shown here. × 525.

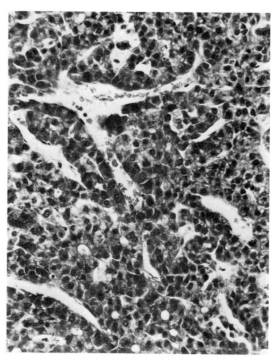

Fig. 12.20 Carcinoma arising from liver cells, showing trabecular arrangement. × 190.

kidney, hepatocellular carcinoma (Fig. 12.20), choriocarcinoma of the placenta, and rodent ulcer of the skin; these are highly distinctive lesions with very marked peculiarities of histogenesis as well as appearance and behaviour. They are described in the appropriate systematic chapters.

Spread of carcinoma

Local invasion

Local invasion by a carcinoma depends in part on the sheer expansive pressure of the mass of growing cells, but also on the active migration of motile tumour cells which penetrate the surrounding tissues and then multiply at the new site. Sometimes they appear to migrate as single cells: more often they appear to penetrate as columns of cells which extend by growth at the forward end. We know little about why cancer cells behave thus, but, as indicated in the last chapter, it may be due to increased motility, or to loss of cell adhesiveness or of other normal restraining processes.

Growth is easiest along the planes of loose connective tissue, and may be checked by dense

structures such as thick fascia, the walls of large arteries, cartilage and compact bone. Structures such as glands and muscle, once penetrated, are rapidly destroyed, partly by pressure, partly by loss of blood supply. The carcinoma itself tends to outrun its blood supply, and necrosis of the tumour which ensues includes ischaemic destruction of any normal tissues which have been invaded. Unfortunately the growing edge of the tumour is hardly ever included in the necrosis.

Local invasion, may, of course result in damage to major structures nearby. Of greater significance from the point of view of the life of the patient in most cases is the appearance of **secondary deposits** or **metastases**—new areas of growth of the tumour at a distance from the primary tumour. These result from spread of tumour cells from the primary growth, usually by the lymphatics or blood vessels, as described below.

Spread by lymphatics

This is one of the most characteristic features of carcinoma and is of prime importance from the surgical point of view. Cancer cells penetrating into the lymphatics may either float free in the lymph and be arrested in the lymph nodes, or they may (probably less often) form columns of proliferating cells filling and growing along the lymphatics (Figs. 12.21, 12.22). Small nodules of tumour may be formed along the line of the lymphatics, but the largest nodules are those which form in and replace the lymph nodes. Early node metastases usually lie in the peripheral sinus (Fig. 12.23). The lymph nodes draining the region of the carcinoma are usually first and most extensively involved. Occasionally spread may take place in a direction contrary to normal lymph flow (Fig. 12.24) as a sequel to lymphatic obstruction.

By excising a carcinoma together with the surrounding tissues, it is often possible to remove completely the local growth. But there may be extensive permeation of lymphatics by cancer cells, although often not visible to the naked eye (Fig. 12.25). Accordingly tissues

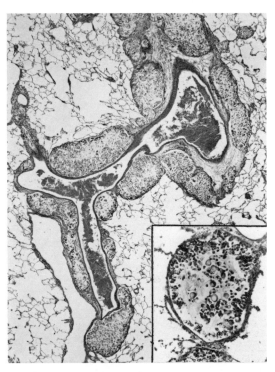

Fig. 12.22 Lymphatic spread of carcinoma. This section of lung shows gross distension of perivascular lymphatics (normally scarcely seen at this magnification) by cancer. × 12. The primary tumour was a carcinoma of stomach, seen at higher magnification (inset) to be composed of mucus-secreting 'signet-ring' cells (see p. 617).

which appear grossly normal may be extensively involved.

The presence of these minute foci of cancer cells, extending beyond the main mass of the tumour either by direct invasion or via the lymphatics, explains the local recurrence of cancer after surgical removal. **Recurrence** is nearly always the result of growth of cancer cells which have been left behind in the surrounding tissues. Such cells may remain dormant, so that years or even decades may elapse before a recognisable tumour reappears. Because carcinogens often affect a large area of epithelium, e.g. chemicals affecting the urinary tract epithelium (p. 299) or ultraviolet rays affecting the exposed skin (p. 301), successful removal of a carcinoma may be followed by the development of a second one nearby. It is usually not possible to distinguish this from recurrence, although the detection also of premalignant change (p. 337) in the epithelium concerned makes it more

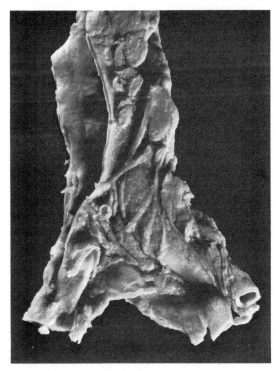

Fig. 12.21 Lymph spread of carcinoma, involving both lymphatics and lymph nodes, around the bifurcation of the aorta. Lymphatics filled with tumour are particularly well seen as they cross the left common iliac artery just below right centre of the specimen. × 0.75.

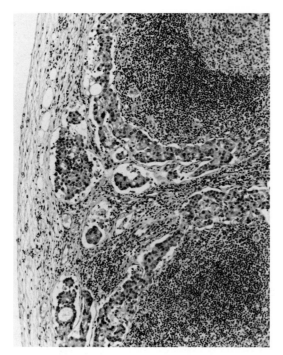

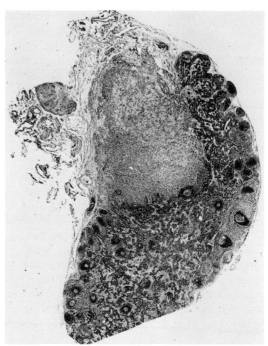

Fig. 12.23 Carcinoma invading lymph node. Carcinoma cells are seen in the lymph vessels in the capsule of the node and in the peripheral lymph sinus, from which they are extending into the radial sinuses. × 75.

Fig. 12.24 Retrograde invasion of lymph node by carcinoma. The lymphatics at the hilum of the node are filled with cancer cells, which have spread into the node against the normal direction of lymph flow. × 95.

likely that the second tumour is not a recurrence of the first.

Blood spread

With most carcinomas, the effects of blood spread are seen later than those of lymphatic spread, though the wider dissemination makes them usually of more serious immediate consequence to the patient. The small veins in and around the primary tumour are the usual route of entry to the circulation. Tumour cells are then carried away to lodge in the next capillary bed that the blood passes through, e.g. in the liver if the primary tumour is in the portal drainage area (Fig. 12.26), and in the lungs from tumours in most other sites. Thence they may spread further, from the liver to the lungs and from the lungs via the systemic circulation to any part of the body (Fig. 12.27). Blood-spread metastases in a solid organ present a very characteristic picture of multiple rounded nodules, scattered randomly throughout the organ and varying in size but usually with no single nodule conspicuously larger than the rest (Figs. 12.28 and 20.55, p. 703).

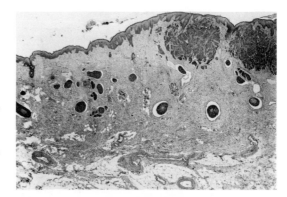

Fig. 12.25 Squamous carcinoma of vulva, showing lymphatic permeation in the dermis beyond the clinically apparent margin. The larger tumour masses (*above right*) would appear to the naked eye to be the edge of the tumour, the bulk of which lies further to the right. Lymphatic permeation can usually only be recognised with certainty in microscopic sections, though when it is as gross as that seen here it may be suspected on careful examination with the naked eye. × 15.

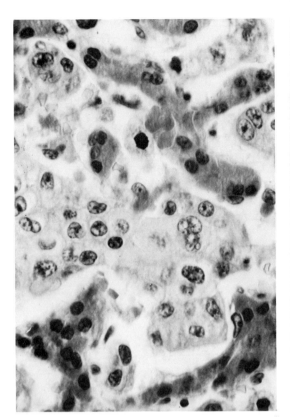

Fig. 12.26 Secondary carcinoma in the liver. Note masses of cancer cells in the sinusoids between the (darker) liver cells, without any formation of stroma. × about 200.

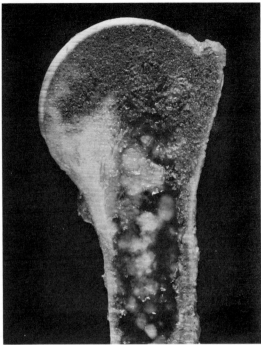

Fig. 12.28 Secondary carcinoma in bone. Multiple rounded white masses in the humerus, in a case of carcinoma of breast. × 0·75.

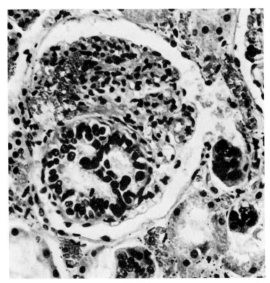

Fig. 12.27 An embolus of carcinoma cells in a glomerulus, with extension into the tubule. × 150.

There are in practice many apparent anomalies in the distribution of metastases: some may be due to confusion between blood and lymph spread—there is for instance a strong case for regarding the curious predilection of bronchial carcinoma to spread to the adrenals as a consequence of lymph spread rather than (as has been generally believed) blood spread. But even allowing for this, there must be great variations between capacities of different tissues to resist the growth of tumour cells arriving by the bloodstream. It is highly probable that in most cases the great majority of cells leaving the primary tumour by the veins fail to establish themselves.

In his old but still valuable series of necropsies on patients with carcinoma, Willis (1973) gave the following incidences of metastases in various organs:

liver	36%	brain	6%
lungs	29%	spleen	3%
bones	14%	skeletal muscles	1%
adrenals	9%	skin	1%

These incidences clearly do not correspond with blood flow, and so with the number of tumour cells likely to be arriving in the various organs. The liver and bone marrow are susceptible sites: the spleen and muscles resistant. There is experimental evidence for destruction of tumour cells by the spleen, but the nature of the defence mechanism is not known. The lung, which must receive by far the largest number of tumour cell emboli, provides an environment which is only moderately favourable to their growth. Cases of carcinoma in some organs, for instance kidney, prostate and thyroid, often have multiple systemic metastases, for example in bone, with no obvious lung lesions: in some such cases it can be shown that there are minute microscopic foci in the lung where tumour cells have lodged in the pulmonary vessels, and, while failing to grow to any substantial extent at the site, have been able to launch further tumour emboli into the systemic circulation (Fig. 12.29).

Retrograde venous spread. One type of anomaly that has a special explanation is the localisation of metastases within the axial skeleton. Carcinoma of the prostate spreads early

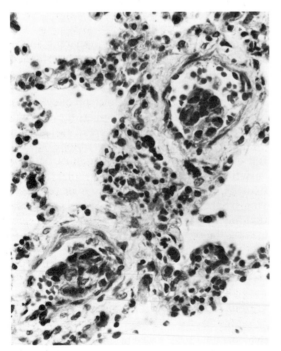

Fig. 12.29 Lung from a case of prostatic carcinoma, showing two pulmonary arterioles containing tumour cells. × 190.

to the lumbar spine and pelvis, carcinoma of the breast to the thoracic vertebral bodies, and carcinoma of the nasopharynx to the cervical spine and the base of the skull. This is not attributable to direct or lymph spread but to spread by the blood. Yet blood spread in the usual fashion via the lungs should result in uniform spread to all parts of the vertebral column. The explanation for the localised involvements of the spine appears to lie in the peculiarities of blood flow in the intra-vertebral venous plexus, in which differences of pressure above and below the diaphragm often lead to reversal of flow: the effect is to draw venous blood at times into the vertebra from neighbouring organs, and this may carry malignant cells, which find a very favourable site for multiplication within the vertebral marrow.

Intracavitary spread

When carcinoma involves a body cavity, cancer cells may be liberated into the space and graft themselves on the surface to form new foci of growth. Any cavity can be involved, and the *subarachnoid space*, for example, is of some importance in the spread of intracranial tumours, but the serous cavities are especially important for carcinoma. Involvement of the *peritoneum* results most often from carcinomas arising in the stomach or the ovary, while the *pleura* and *pericardium* are most commonly invaded by carcinomas of breast or bronchus. In most cases there is an effusion of fluid into the sac concerned, and this may be bloodstained. Malignant cells are often present in such an effusion, but very often it is difficult to distinguish them with certainty from altered serosal cells. A special example of this form of spread is seen in transperitoneal metastasis to the ovary, usually before the menopause and usually from a gastric carcinoma of the 'signet-ring' type (p. 617): the ovaries may become very large, and have the characters first described by Krukenberg, who thought that such tumours originated in the ovaries (see p. 966).

Although not everyone agrees, it is nearly certain that the rare so-called 'alveolar-cell carcinoma' of the lung (p. 498) grows by spread of carcinoma cells within the air passages of the lung.

Intra-epithelial and intracellular spread

Cancer cells may invade the epidermis, which is the only extensive epithelium in the body thick enough to withstand such invasion without disruption. Cells may spread for several centimetres in the epidermis without destroying it completely. Paget's disease of the breast (p. 983) is the only common example involving carcinoma cells (the tumour being derived from the underlying breast): rarely this occurs in the epidermis at other sites, and something similar is seen in malignant melanoma of the skin (p. 1082).

Carcinoma invading skeletal muscle may sometimes be seen under the microscope to be growing within the sarcolemma of muscle cells: this rare curiosity is the only known example of 'intracellular' spread (Fig. 12.30).

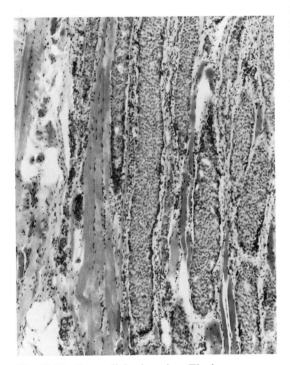

Fig. 12.30 Intracellular invasion. The long sausages of tumour cells have grown within and expanded striped muscle fibres, being still confined by the sarcolemma: compare with unaffected muscle fibres on the left. × 60.

Premalignant lesions

These are conveniently considered here, as most such lesions involve epithelium, and are precarcinomatous.

A premalignant condition is one which can be recognised by either clinician or pathologist, and which indicates that the bearer has a substantially greater than normal risk of developing a malignant tumour. The early stages of premalignant change (which presumably indicate the occurrence of the earlier mutations of a multistage conversion to malignancy) can often be recognised histologically. The signs include nuclear irregularity, increased mitotic activity, and abnormalities of differentiation, often combined with inflammatory infiltrates and stromal changes. The risk of such lesions' becoming malignant can be established only in the light of experience of their behaviour in each particular site in which they occur. The following are examples of premalignant lesions.

(a) Some benign tumours. Probably all benign tumours carry some increased risk of malignancy, but in most it is very little more than that of the normal tissue, while in others it is high. There is little obvious logic about the differences. The rare polypoid adenomas of the small intestine seldom become malignant, while the (much commoner) adenomas of the large intestine carry a much greater risk of cancer. Comparable anomalies could be quoted at other sites.

(b) Certain chronic diseases. Carcinoma may develop as a more or less common complication of some non-neoplastic diseases, such as cirrhosis of the liver, ulcerative colitis, asbestosis and a variety of skin diseases.

(c) Carcinoma-in-situ. In the most extreme degrees of premalignant change in an epithelium, all the cytological changes of malignancy are seen in its cells, but the altered cells remain in the intact layer of epithelium and do not invade the underlying tissues. The name carcinoma-in-situ is often given to this lesion: it is not strictly accurate, as no carcinoma is present until invasion begins, but it is a vivid reminder of the need for action. *Intraduct carcinoma* of the breast (p. 982) is an essentially similar lesion.

Carcinoma-in-situ of the cervix uteri is particularly important, for the cervix is accessible for examination, the lesion is relatively common, and is readily detected by cytological examination of smears and confirmed by biopsy. Also, in most cases the in-situ change persists for years without becoming invasive, allowing its detection by routine screening and prevention of cancer by excision of the affected epithelium (which varies widely in extent).

Although frank invasive cancer in many other sites is preceded by carcinoma-in-situ, detection at this stage is more difficult because of inaccessibility, etc.

The degree of risk of developing malignancy varies greatly with different premalignant lesions, and is often hard to determine with precision. In a few conditions, such as polyposis (adenomatosis) coli and xeroderma pigmentosa, it is practically 100 per cent. In carcinoma-in-situ of the cervix, the rate remains uncertain despite extensive studies, but it is believed that about 30 per cent progress to invasive carcinoma. In most other lesions the risk appears to be much lower.

Staging and grading of cancers

A quantitative measure of the factors affecting the prognosis of a particular type of tumour is often required. Sometimes it is used in deciding on the best method of treatment, but it is most useful in statistical studies. If, for instance, a surgeon claims that his new operation is curing more patients than his colleagues (or, to be more precise, raising the proportion of five-year survivals) it is necessary to be sure that he is not seeing by some accident an exceptionally favourable group of cases—e.g. smaller, earlier or better differentiated tumours. The production of completely unambiguous criteria is much more difficult than it sounds, and elaborate special systems have been developed for most of the common tumours. All agree, however, in separating two main elements, *grading* and *staging*, and these should not be confused.

Grading. This is a *histological* estimate of the degree of *differentiation*. Exact numerical systems do not work (Broder's system, depending on the percentage of differentiated cells, though still often talked of, has long been abandoned

in practice). In general, most tumours are graded for this purpose by the pathologist into well differentiated, average, and poorly differentiated: the system is most useful if the criteria used put about 25 per cent of the tumours into the good group, 50 per cent into the average and 25 per cent into the worst.

Staging. This is a *clinical* estimate of the degree of *spread*. Most systems use four stages, roughly definable as (I) confined to the organ of origin, (II) local spread not interfering with surgical excision, (III) fixation to surrounding structures and (IV) distant spread. A 'Stage O' is sometimes added for invasive tumours of microscopic size or for carcinoma-in-situ: the difference between the two is, however, important and, if used at all, 'Stage O' should be clearly defined.

How this works in practice may be seen from the usual definitions for cancer of the uterine cervix: *Stage O*—carcinoma-in-situ only: *Stage I*—confined strictly to the cervix: *Stage II*—local spread, not reaching the pelvic wall or the lower third of the vagina: *Stage III*—fixed to pelvis, or involving lower third of vagina: *Stage IV*—distant metastases, or involvement of bladder or rectum. Stage II is often subdivided, IIa including spread to the uterine body, vaginal fornices and the immediately adjacent connective tissue, Stage IIb including further spread, but short of Stage III. It will be seen that even here the position is not altogether simple. For most other tumours staging is a good deal more complicated and often controversial.

Staging must always be based primarily on the clinical examination, for the assessment at operation often differs from the clinical assessment, and to compare surgical with other forms of treatment, both groups of patients must first be 'staged' in the same way, i.e. clinically. Grading, on the other hand, requires pathological examination of at least a biopsy. The results of the two procedures are not, however, altogether independent: as one might expect, in all series the worse differentiated cases tend to be more numerous in the higher stages.

Further Reading

Ashley, D. B. (1978). *Evans' Histological Appearances of Tumours*, 3rd edn., pp. 857. Churchill-Livingstone, Edinburgh, London and New York. (An account of the behaviour and appearances of human tumours based on a considerable experience.)

Sobin, L. H., Thomas, L. B., Percy, Constance and Henson, D. E. (Eds.) (1978). *A Coded Compendium of the International Histological Classification of Tumours*, pp. 116. World Health Organisation, Geneva. (A widely accepted system of classification, coding and nomenclature of human tumours.)

Willis, R. A. (1973). *The Spread of Tumours in the Human Body*, 3rd edn., pp. 417. Butterworths, London.

Atlas of Tumour Pathology. US Armed Forces Institute of Pathology, Washington, DC. (Numerous 'Fascicles' on tumours of particular organs, tissues and regions. A valuable source of detailed information on the histology and behaviour of individual tumours.)

Cancer. A journal of the American Cancer Society. Lipincott, Philadelphia and Toronto. (A monthly publication of well-illustrated articles on human neoplasms.)

13

Tumours: III. Other Varieties

There are far more kinds of non-epithelial tissue than epithelial, and equally there are far more kinds of non-epithelial tumour. As already indicated, however, the balance between this chapter and the last reflects the practical circumstance that the carcinomas greatly outweigh all other tumours in clinical importance. Nevertheless, even the tenth of deaths that are due to non-epithelial malignant tumours is a substantial number, and no one can dismiss as unimportant a group that includes the lymphomas, gliomas, mela-nomas and bone sarcomas. There are moreover some benign tumours, e.g. the myomas, and the tumour-like angiomas, which are very common, although responsible for few deaths.

Though all the main types of non-epithelial tumours will be found mentioned here, detailed description will be given only of those varieties which are of such general distribution as not to be easily included under any one system. Length of description does not therefore always reflect importance.

Tumours of the Connective Tissues

Nomenclature

In this group it is usual to name tumours by adding **-oma** to the appropriate stem for the benign lesion, and **-sarcoma** for the malignant. Thus *fibroma* and *fibrosarcoma* are respectively benign and malignant tumours arising from fibrocytes; *chondroma* and *chondrosarcoma* are benign and malignant tumours arising from cartilage cells.

Benign tumours

These are composed chiefly of fully developed tissues, such as are found in the adult body, e.g. fibrous tissue, cartilage, muscle. They are usually rounded or lobulated and well defined, being generally enclosed within a distinct fibrous capsule. They displace the surrounding tissues and produce atrophy by pressure, but they do not usually infiltrate tissues and never metastasise. Such benign tumours are sometimes multiple, but then each tumour represents an independent focus of growth. Blood vessels grow in relation to the tumour tissue, and are usually well formed, though the arteries are often deficient in muscle fibres. The well-defined reactive fibrous tissue stroma of epithelial tumours is, however, altogether absent in most cases, the tumour relying for its support on the matrix produced by its own cells—though exceptions occur, for example in the myomas.

Malignant tumours (sarcomas)

In the corresponding malignant tumours, the activity of the cells is mainly proliferative, the tumour is more cellular, and although a certain amount of matrix is formed, this is usually scanty. Sarcomas often form large masses, usually soft and commonly with areas of haemorrhage and necrosis (Fig. 13.1). While these malignant tumours may appear to the surgeon to be encapsulated, as in Fig. 13.1, diffuse destructive infiltration of the surrounding tissue occurs at the margin of most such masses so that wide excision rather than enucleation is required in their treatment. There is an exten-

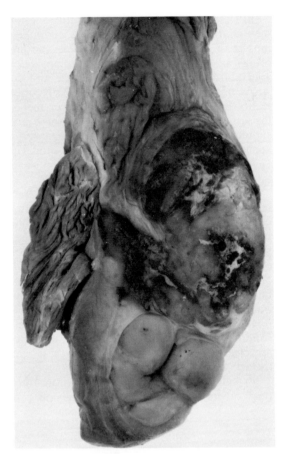

Fig. 13.1 Spindle-cell sarcoma arising in intermuscular fascia of thigh. Above and left there is normal voluntary muscle. The upper half of the ovoid tumour shows extensive necrosis and haemorrhage: the lower half is well preserved, appearing characteristically greyish-white, soft and slightly lobulated. × 0·6.

Tumours of fibrous tissue

Although it is usual to regard these as the 'typical' connective tissue tumours, they are in fact not very common and genuine benign fibromas are rare.

Fibroma

This is the name given to benign tumours of fibrous tissue. The cells of the tumour are fibrocytes; their nuclei are long and narrow and densely staining, the cytoplasm so scanty as to be hard to see, and mitoses are very rare. Bundles of dense collagen separate the cells, and the appearances, in short, may not be very different from that of fibrous tissue as seen in a thick fascia or a scar. Fibromas do, however, vary greatly in the amount of collagen and in cellularity (Figs. 13.2, 13.3).

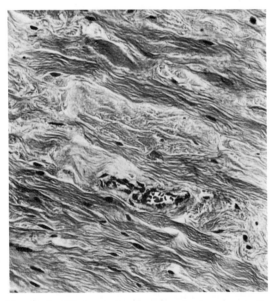

Fig. 13.2 Fibroma showing abundant mature collagen and few cells. Distinction from normal fibrous tissue can be difficult, and depends on careful examination of the whole lesion. × 240.

sive new formation of poorly formed blood vessels. Numerous capillaries, and larger channels composed mainly of a layer of endothelium, are supported by the cells of the tumour, while fibrous tissue is found only round the larger vessels. Two results follow—(*a*) the cells of the tumour readily break through the vessel walls and are conveyed in the venous blood until arrested in the smaller vessels of lungs, liver, etc., and thus **metastases** may develop, and (*b*) **haemorrhages** are common. Spread by the lymphatic vessels is unusual, except in the case of synovial sarcoma and lymphoma, and blood-borne metastases, especially in the lungs, are the usual cause of death.

Fibromas may occur in any type of connective tissue (Fig. 13.4) and may be seen with varying degrees of rarity in most of the internal organs. Special varieties occur in the sheaths of nerves (Schwannoma, etc., pp. 793–4), skin (dermatofibroma, p. 1084) and ovaries (p. 965) which have their own peculiarities of behaviour

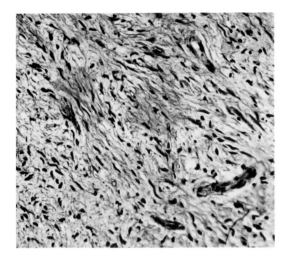

Fig. 13.3 Fibroma showing more numerous cells (which are however mature fibrocytes) and less abundant and looser collagen. × 280.

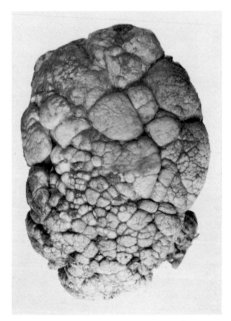

Fig. 13.4 Lobulated fibroma removed from buttock. Natural size.

and which probably do not arise from ordinary fibrocytes.

Fibromatoses

This term can be usefully applied to some fibroma-like lesions which may cause considerable difficulties of diagnosis and which may not be true tumours. They include:

(a) Desmoid tumour, which is a curious lesion seen characteristically in the rectus abdominis muscle of multiparous women. It has the histology of a fibroma, but is not encapsulated and infiltrates the surrounding muscle and destroys the muscle fibres (Fig. 13.5). It often recurs locally after excision, but never metastasises. Desmoids occur also in the thigh and shoulder, where they may be termed **musculo-aponeurotic fibromatosis** and behave similarly. Genuine fibromas are particularly rare in skeletal muscle.

(b) Palmar fibromatosis (Dupuytren's contracture) consists of a fibroma-like lesion, often quite cellular, involving the palmar fascia and producing flexion deformities of the fingers (see p. 929). A similar but much less common lesion of the plantar fascia (*plantar fibromatosis*) is often particularly cellular and sarcoma-like under the microscope but does not cause contracture. There is also a penile fibromatosis (*Peyronie's disease*). Two or even all three of these conditions may occur in one patient, and they are clearly related. Again, none of these ever metastasises.

(c) Keloid. Some people (negroes more often than others) have a curious tendency to pro-

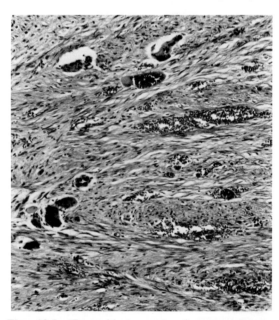

Fig. 13.5 'Desmoid tumour' of rectus sheath. Moderately cellular fibrous tissue forms the bulk of it. The large dark-staining cells are multinucleate sarcolemmal giant cells, the remains of infiltrated muscle fibres. × 120.

duce excessive amounts of dense hyalinised fibrous tissue, instead of the normal inconspicuous scars, after injury to the skin. They nearly always cease growth after a time, and are then clearly not tumours, though they may be mistaken for them histologically.

Myxoma and mesenchymoma

The rare myxomas (Fig. 13.6) are translucent tumours, usually benign, composed of 'myxoid' tissue, a kind of connective tissue with stellate cells widely separated by a ground substance rich in mucopolysaccharide (p. 247) and poor in blood vessels. They usually occur within skeletal muscles and only rarely recur; even after incomplete excision. There is a group in which a predominantly myxomatous tumour contains scattered elements of other mesenchymal tissue types, including muscle and cartilage. The name **mesenchymoma** is usually given to them, reflecting a belief, not necessarily well founded, that they represent a return to the capacity for multipotent differentiation of primitive mesenchyme. These tumours, most often seen in the subcutaneous tissues of the trunk, rarely metastasise but have a high incidence of local recurrence. The *embryonal rhabdomyosarcoma* of children (p. 346) also combines myxoid connective tissue with poorly formed striated

muscle cells but has a very different age and anatomical distribution and is much more malignant.

Fibrosarcomas

These tumours arise especially from fascia and deep connective tissues, but may occur almost anywhere in the body. Similar tumours arise from nerves—**neurofibrosarcomas** or **malignant schwannomas** (Fig. 13.7). While most fibrosarcomas are clearly malignant from the start, some progress over a period of many years from an early stage in which they may be difficult to distinguish from a benign fibroma.

Fibrosarcomas differ greatly in their degree of differentiation. *Low grade fibrosarcomas* differ little from cellular fibromas: they are firm and fibrous, produce abundant collagen, and the cells differ little from normal fibroblasts. A moderately high rate of mitosis is often the only real evidence of malignancy. Such tumours are slow growing and are often cured by adequate local excision, and recurrences tend, at least at first, to remain localised. Tumours of intermediate malignancy are often called 'spindle-cell sarcomas' (Fig. 13.8). They are softer, more rapidly growing tumours in which the cells are still recognisably fibroblast-like and regularly arranged, but collagen is relatively inconspicuous: such tumours often metastasise and are usually ultimately fatal.

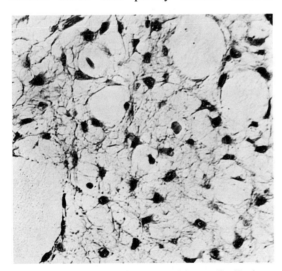

Fig. 13.6 Myxoma. The branching cells lie in a semi-fluid matrix which stains pale lilac with haematoxylin and eosin but much more deeply with stains for connective tissue mucin. The round spaces are included fat cells of the breast, in which this tumour was found. × 300.

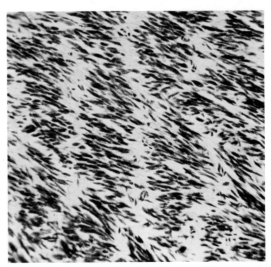

Fig. 13.7 Well-differentiated neurofibrosarcoma arising in recurrent neurofibroma. Note the very pronounced palisading of the nuclei. × 270.

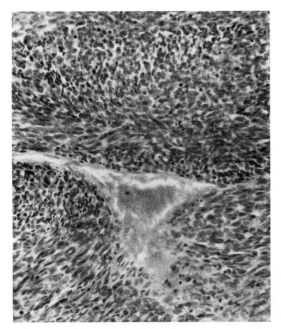

Fig. 13.8 Spindle-cell sarcoma. This is very cellular, but the cells are relatively uniform and still resemble fibroblasts. Special stains would show sparse collagen fibres. The triangular cleft is one of the poorly formed blood vessels characteristic of sarcomas. × 250.

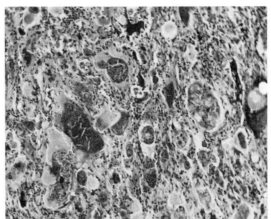

Fig. 13.9 Anaplastic sarcoma showing great variation in the size of the cells. Note the numerous enormous polyploid nuclei. × 125.

From this type, transitions occur to the anaplastic sarcoma (Fig. 13.9), a soft, rapidly growing tumour consisting of large irregular cells with large irregular nuclei, with little or no collagen and very little evidence of the tissue of origin; metastasis is usually rapid and prognosis poor. Obviously, in such tumours it may be impossible to identify the cell of origin, and indeed tumours with this kind of histology may arise from dedifferentiation of almost any kind of cell.

Fibrosarcomas, like most other sarcomas, may recur locally or metastasise by the bloodstream, especially to the lungs, but rarely spread by the lymphatics.

Tumours of adipose tissue

Lipoma

This is a common benign tumour which consists of adipose tissue. It increases in size by proliferation of fibroblast-like cells which lie around the blood vessels but are hard to see in most cases because they rapidly accumulate fat and become lipocytes. The common lipoma is a rounded, well-demarcated, subcutaneous mass. It sometimes reaches a considerable size, and may have blunt projections which pass into the tissues around. Multiple tumours may be present and occasionally they are symmetrical. They are commonest over the neck, back and shoulders and occur also in the retroperitoneum, especially in the perirenal fat. They may, however, arise almost anywhere in the body. Should the patient become emaciated, the fat in the tumour is not utilised—a good example of the failure of tumours to respond to the factors controlling the metabolism of normal tissues. In a lipoma there may be areas of fibrous or capillary angiomatous tissue—the tumour being then called a *fibrolipoma* or *angiolipoma* respectively; occasionally there are areas of calcification.

In a rare variant the fat is finely divided in droplets within the cells, which thus closely resemble brown fat. The supposed role of brown fat in hibernation of rodents led to the name '*hibernoma*' (Fig. 13.10).

Liposarcoma

This tumour is uncommon, although one of the least rare of the soft tissue sarcomas. It occurs most often in the thigh, buttocks and retroperitoneum. It varies widely in naked-eye and microscopical appearances and also in prognosis.

The best differentiated liposarcomas are

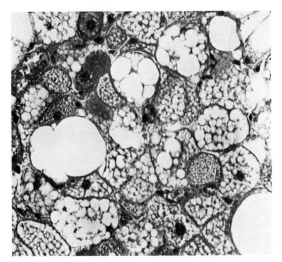

Fig. 13.10 'Hibernoma' showing the characteristic appearances of the fat-laden cells, with central nuclei. × 480.

obviously fatty, and have a marked microscopic resemblance to lipoma, but with more obvious collagenous areas and groups of cells with larger and more hyperchromatic nuclei.

The least uncommon type, the *myxoid liposarcoma*, appears gelatinous, having a mucopolysaccharide-rich matrix, with a prominent capillary network (Fig. 13.11). It has a marked

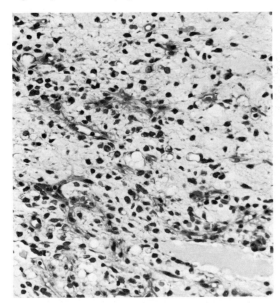

Fig. 13.11 Myxoid liposarcoma, showing the relatively small sarcoma cells, with scanty cytoplasm, lying in an abundant homogeneous matrix. Note the numerous capillaries. × 250.

tendency to repeated recurrence after successive attempts at removal, and sometimes recurs in a more malignant form, consisting of round cells containing little fat and with much less stroma. The round-cell liposarcoma and another type of liposarcoma consisting of cells containing abundant fatty droplets but showing extreme cellular pleomorphism (Fig. 13.12) are liable to metastasise.

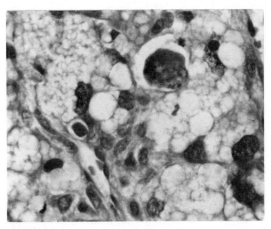

Fig. 13.12 Pleomorphic liposarcoma, consisting of very large cells with very large nuclei, and with much fat in the cytoplasm. × 450.

Alveolar soft tissue sarcoma. This rather uncommon variety of sarcoma arises in the soft tissues, usually of a limb. It is composed of large polygonal or round cells with coarsely granular cytoplasm, and arranged in a curiously alveolar pattern. In paraffin sections the appearances resemble those of liposarcoma or even carcinoma but the granules do not give the staining reactions of lipids, mucin, glycogen or other specifically stainable substances. Its origin and true nature are obscure, but some regard it as a variety of chemodectoma (p. 349).

Tumours of cartilage and bone

These are dealt with in detail in Chapter 23. The benign tumours of bone are a perplexingly varied group, and their precise histogenesis is often obscure. Most of the masses of cartilage called chondromas and many bony outgrowths (exostoses) are not true tumours but developmental defects or hamartomas (p. 358). **Osteosarcomas** particularly and **chondrosarcomas** are among the commonest sarcomas. Osteosarcoma especially exemplifies many of the most characteristic features of sarcomas generally—a high incidence in childhood, high mortality, rarity of lymphatic spread and frequent blood spread, especially to the lungs.

Fibrosarcomas may arise from bone. Conversely (though very rarely) bone-forming osteosarcomas sometimes arise from connective tissue elsewhere, and sometimes even from such organs as the breast, kidney, etc.

Bone and cartilage are sometimes seen in non-bony tumours. Both are common in teratomas (p. 355). Cartilage is often seen in the mixed tumours of the parotid and other salivary glands. Bony metaplasia of the fibrous stroma of carcinomas is a rare but striking finding, least rare in man in large-bowel cancers, and not uncommon in breast tumours in bitches.

Tumours of muscle

There are two varieties of myoma, the **leiomyoma**, composed of smooth muscle fibres, and the **rhabdomyoma** of striped muscle. The latter is so rare that the term **myoma** without qualification is often used to signify leiomyoma.

Leiomyomas are composed of smooth muscle cells orientated in a more or less parallel manner within bundles, which are arranged in a whorled pattern (Fig. 13.13). A small amount of supporting fibrous tissue runs among the individual cells, while broader bands separate the bundles. The proportion of fibrous tissue to muscle varies much in different specimens. The tumours are usually firm and rounded, and on section are pinkish with a characteristic whorled appearance due to the arrangement of the fibres (Fig. 13.14).

Leiomyomas of the *uterus* are among the commonest of tumours: their usually high content of fibrous tissue earns them their common name of '**fibroids**', though the muscle is the only true tumorous element and it is incorrect to call them fibromyomas. Of general interest is their tendency to cease growth at the menopause and subsequently regress.

Leiomyomas are probably next most common in the muscular coat of the alimentary canal, though here most are too small to be found without special search and few are large enough to cause trouble. They can occur at many other sites, all uncommon: a rare painful vascular myoma of the skin is of special interest (p. 349).

Leiomyosarcomas occasionally arise from the same sites as leiomyomas, especially the uterus

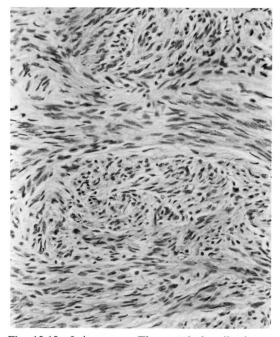

Fig. 13.13 Leiomyoma. The muscle bundles interlace irregularly, and are to be seen cut transversely, longitudinally and obliquely. The cytoplasm of the muscle cells stains somewhat indistinctly but gives a darker shade to the substance of each bundle. Occasional fibrocytes seen between the bundles have smaller darker nuclei and no obvious cytoplasm. × 185.

and the stomach. Most appear to be malignant from the start but some may arise by malignant progression in a benign myoma. The histological diagnosis of malignancy is usually easy on general cytological grounds, but the better differentiated tumours can be hard to distinguish from the more cellular benign tumours. It is a useful empirical rule, which can be applied to few other tumours, that a smooth muscle tumour in which mitoses can be found easily is liable to metastasise.

Rhabdomyosarcoma. In proportion to their bulk, the voluntary muscles are one of the rarest of sites for tumours of any kind, both primary and secondary: the reasons for this are not known. The rare tumours in which striped muscle fibres or their precursors are seen are nearly always malignant, and arise mostly in sites where no striped muscle is present normally. They are found most often in the female genital tract, characteristically in the cervix or vaginal vault in young girls, and in the lower

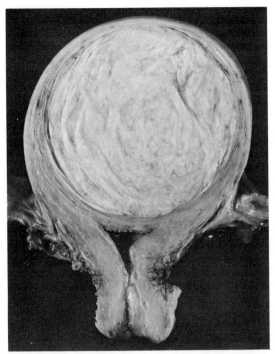

Fig. 13.14 Leiomyoma of uterus. The tumour is paler than the normal muscle because of its higher content of fibrous tissue. The pattern of the cut tumour surface is formed by brownish slightly translucent strands of muscle, here seen as an indistinct network but often whorled. Note the distorted uterine lumen. Natural size.

urinary tract in both sexes; also in the soft palate. Usually the tumours have a large myxoid element, and recognisable muscle cells (though very characteristic when found) are often scanty and difficult to find, even with special stains which accentuate their cross striations. Rounded or irregular cells with coiled myofibrils but without cross-striations are usually more readily apparent. (Fig. 13.15). When growing beneath a mucous membrane, these tumours often present with numerous blunt translucent processes—hence the name of *sarcoma botryoides* (grapelike sarcoma). These are highly malignant tumours: local recurrence after excision and blood-spread metastases are usual, and (unlike most sarcomas) lymph node metastases are common.

Rhabdomyosarcomas are also seen very rarely in the heart. Benign tumours, perhaps better regarded as hamartomas (p. 358), are seen there in children with epiloia (tuberous sclerosis): they consist of swollen muscle cells packed with glycogen and some confusion has in the past existed between these lesions and the cardiac changes of glycogen storage disease (p. 30).

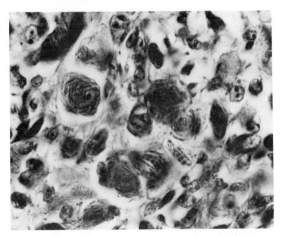

Fig. 13.15a Rhabdomyosarcoma. Large pleomorphic cells in a slightly myxoid matrix. Special stains and high magnification show coiled myofibrils (best seen in cells just below and to the right of centre).

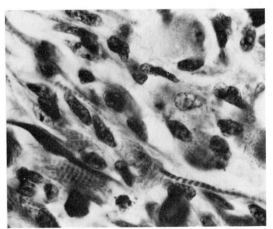

Fig. 13.15b As 13.15a. The nature of the myofibrils is more obvious when the cells are elongated 'strap cells' and the fibrils produce cross striations as seen here, especially below right, but these are usually hard to find.

Tumours and Malformations of Blood Vessels and Lymphatics

Angiomas

Haemangioma. A haemangioma consists of a mass of blood vessels, atypical or irregular in arrangement and size. A corresponding growth, **lymphangioma**, is composed of lymphatic vessels similarly altered; but, as this is rarer, the term angioma is often used as synonymous with haemangioma.

The majority of the lesions called angiomas are not true tumours, but hamartomas.* They are present at birth, even if not always visible, and their enlargement ceases with the growth of the patient. Most angiomas are well-defined masses of vascular tissue which resemble tumours sufficiently to justify their inclusion here. The two common varieties are as follows.

(*a*) *Capillary angiomas* consist of dense plexiform arrangements of vessels of capillary size (Fig. 13.16). They occur especially in the skin, where they form one of the two common types of **naevus**†or birthmark, but are also seen in the internal organs. Most are small, but larger lesions occur, e.g. the 'port-wine stains' of the face, which consist of capillary-like vessels with an abnormally large lumen. Capillary angiomas are usually well defined, and deep red or purple. The capillary vessels have a more prominent endothelial lining than normal capillaries and endothelial cells may be seen scattered or in clusters without formation of a lumen (Fig. 13.16). The stroma consists of well-formed collagen. There is no capsule, and outlying groups of capillaries in adjoining tissues often give a false appearance of invasion. The blood supply is usually clearly separated from that of the surrounding tissues, there being generally only one artery of supply.

(*b*) *Cavernous angiomas* are found in the skin, subcutaneous tissue, lips and tongue and also in the liver. They consist of relatively large interconnecting sinus-like vascular spaces (Fig. 13.17). In the liver they form deep-purple well-defined masses, usually polygonal rather than round and not raised above the surface, signs of their lack of expansile growth.

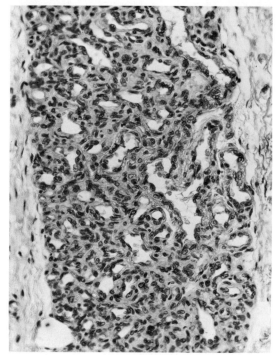

Fig. 13.16 Capillary angioma showing well-formed capillaries with prominent endothelial cells. The solid areas between capillaries include many cells which appear to be endothelial cells not related to a lumen. × 200.

Angiomas are often multiple, and are also an important component of several diseases with a strong genetic predisposition., e.g. hereditary haemorrhagic telangiectasia (multiple small angiomas in skin and mucosae with a strong tendency to haemorrhage—p. 557), Lindau's disease (cerebellar and retinal angiomas with cysts of liver and pancreas) and Sturge–Weber syndrome (facial and meningeal angiomas).

A special form of angioma of the skin, the so-called sclerosing angioma, is dealt with later (p. 1084).

Glomangioma (glomus tumour). This uncommon but interesting lesion apparently arises from the glomus bodies, small arteriovenous anastomoses with a coiled arteriole and abundant nerve supply

*A *hamartoma* is a malformation developing in early life and consisting of a tumour-like mass of cells or tissue which grows with the individual and then ceases to grow when general body growth ceases (p. 358).

†A *naevus* (mole or birthmark) is a hamartoma of the skin made conspicuous by some definite colour difference from the surrounding normal area. Angiomas and pigmented naevi (pp. 1078–81) are the two common types..

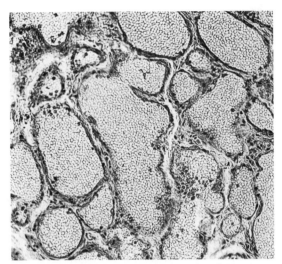

Fig. 13.17 Cavernous angioma of subcutaneous tissue, showing large intercommunicating spaces filled with blood. × 130.

which control blood flow and temperature, particularly in the fingers and toes. In its most characteristic form, the glomangioma is a small bluish nodule, usually near the end of a finger, and extraordinarily tender to even light touch. On microscopic examination the tumour is found to consist of two kinds of tissue variously interblended (Fig. 13.18). The first is angiomatous, with spaces containing blood, lined by endothelium, and separated by connective tissue containing varying amounts of smooth muscle. The other is cellular, with rounded or cuboidal cells

called 'myoid', as transitions to smooth muscle fibres can be found. The growth contains numerous medullated and non-medullated nerve fibres and the pain is apparently due to distensile pressures in the blood-containing spaces, though the painfulness is not in proportion to the neural content. A small dermal leiomyoma may likewise be painful and the two may be related in origin. Glomangiomas have been described in deeper tissues, including the gut, but the characteristic pain occurs only with those in the limbs.

Chemodectoma. Because of their close anatomical relationship with blood vessels it is convenient to consider here the tumours arising from the chemoreceptor organs, viz. the carotid body, glomus jugulare, organ of Zuckerkandl and no doubt other less clearly defined structures such as the aortic bodies. These tumours have also been called **non-chromaffin paragangliomas**; they do not appear to produce any endocrine effects.

Chemodectomas are usually benign, but their anatomical sites may render complete surgical removal difficult. Thus carotid body tumours, which are the commonest variety, closely embrace the bifurcation of the common carotid artery, and the glomus jugulare tumours involve the middle ear and present as recurrent bleeding aural polyps; they may also present intracranially. Microscopically the architectural pattern is similar to the tissue of origin, consisting of many small masses of cells of variable size, sometimes enclosed in a boxlike framework of fine fibrous tissue (Fig. 13.19). The tumour cells are usually polygonal and may be spindle-shaped in places but aberrant types with hyperchromatic nuclei are not

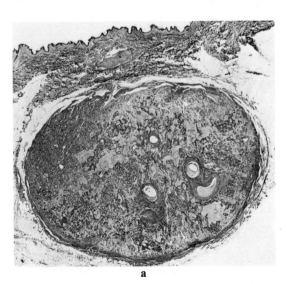

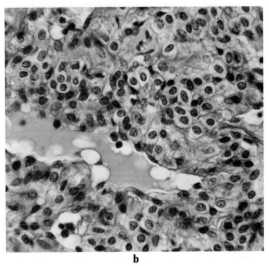

a

b

Fig. 13.18 Glomangioma.
a Small subcutaneous encapsulated growth showing the coiled arteriole. × 8.
b The clear myoid cells surrounding a vascular space. × 350.

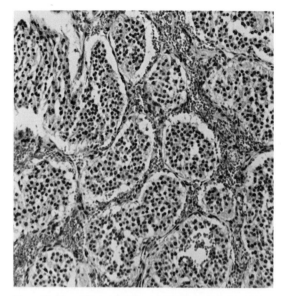

Fig. 13.19 Chemodectoma of the carotid body, showing the characteristic boxlike pattern and highly vascular stroma. × 160.

uncommon and do not indicate malignancy. The blood supply is very rich and of sinusoidal pattern.

Malignant vascular tumours

With the possible exception of Kaposi's sarcoma (see below) which is relatively common in Central Africa but is of uncertain origin, true tumours of blood vessels are rare.

Occasionally a lesion with the histological features of haemangioma grows unusually rapidly and is classed by some as a *haemangio-endothelioma*. Very rarely an apparent capillary haemangioma gives rise to metastases and thus merits the term *haemangio-endotheliosarcoma*. This latter term is also applied to malignant tumours which show the cellular abnormalities characteristic of malignancy, but in which the neoplastic cells also show, in places, the structural arrangement of endothelial cells lining a lumen.

Rare tumours also arise from vascular pericytes (*haemangio-pericytoma*), the tumour cells being separated from vascular endothelium by basement-membrane material demonstrable by silver impregnation staining techniques. Some remain localised, but others metastasise.

Exposure to vinyl chloride monomer predisposes to the otherwise very rare *haemangiosarcoma of the liver* (p. 312), but it is not certain that this tumour arises from vascular endothelium.

Kaposi's sarcoma. This remarkable disorder is rare in Britain. It is more frequent in some other parts of Europe and Africa, and relatively common in some well-defined areas of Central Africa, where it is much more frequent in males. The condition presents the syndrome of lymphoedema, multiple cutaneous tumours which later ulcerate, lymphadenopathy and ultimately visceral involvement. The skin tumours at first consist of lobulated masses of highly vascular and cellular tissue resembling granulation tissue deep within the corium and separated by fibrous trabecula (Fig. 13.20). Later there is much haemorrhage in and around the lesions, the spindle cells and vascular sprouts increase progressively, mitoses are abundant, ulceration of superficial lesions occurs and the regional lymph nodes may be replaced by similar highly vascular spindle-celled tissue. Despite their tumour-like appearance many lesions ultimately stop growing and heal with scarring, although the disease may progress elsewhere. However, in many cases (the proportion is uncertain), the lesions become progressive in internal organs, especially the intestines. This occurs more frequently in Central African cases than in those in South Africa or elsewhere. The superficial lesions respond well to radiotherapy and chemotherapy. The condition is sometimes associated with lymphomas.

It is uncertain whether this is a true neoplasm but in some cases it certainly behaves like one. Evidence from histochemistry and tissue culture indicates that the spindle cells are not fibroblasts: the lesion may

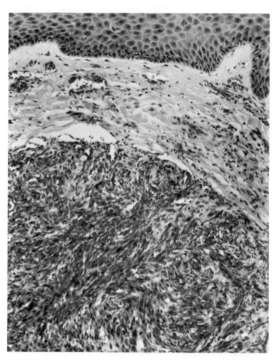

Fig. 13.20 Kaposi's sarcoma. An early lesion showing the zone of fibrous tissue between the vascular spindle-celled tumour and the epidermis. × 130.

be an angiosarcoma derived from lymphatic endothelium as the cells lack the enzymes characteristic of blood capillary endothelium.

Tumours of lymphatics

Lymphangioma. This may be composed of numerous lymphatic vessels—the *plexiform* lymphangioma—but more frequently it has a *cavernous* structure. Dilatation and diffuse growth of vessels may give rise to enlargement of a part, e.g. the tongue (*macroglossia*). In such lesions there is even less evidence than in haemangiomas of neoplastic growth, and the more diffuse lesions may be hard to distinguish from the effects of lymphatic obstruction, though in most cases it is clear from the anatomy that no such obstruction can be present, and a congenital malformation (or hamartoma—p. 358) of the lymphatics is present. It is becoming increasingly common to describe such lesions as *lymphangiectasis* rather than lymphangioma. Lesions, whether diffuse or compact, are commonest in the skin and subcutaneous tissue. Each forms a somewhat ill-defined, doughy or semi-fluctuant swelling, containing large, intercommunicating lymphatic spaces. They contain clear lymph with occasional lymphocytes. Sometimes bleeding into the spaces renders the diagnosis between haemangioma and lymphangioma difficult. Lymphangiomas occur occasionally also in mucous membranes in the wall of the bowel (Fig. 13.21), in the tissues of the orbit and mesentery, and elsewhere.

In rare cases lymphangiomas of neck, retroperitoneum or mesentery undergo great dilata-

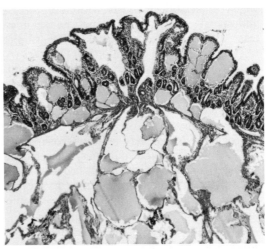

Fig. 13.21 Cavernous lymphangioma of small intestine. It is made up of large intercommunicating spaces filled with clear lymph (which has coagulated and then shrunk in processing the tissue). It occupies both mucosa and submucosa, the mucosa being much distorted but otherwise not much damaged.

tion, forming a multilocular ramifying cystic mass which may become very large. Occasionally a single cyst is formed which may be distinguished from other cysts by its endothelial lining.

Lymphangio-endothelioma (lymphangiosarcoma) is a very doubtful entity, but has been described as arising in the lymphatics of the arm, following their obstruction by mastectomy and irradiation for mammary cancer. Very similar appearances may result from a slow, diffuse permeation of the lymphatics by carcinoma and it remains undecided whether this is the real nature of the so-called lymphangiosarcoma.

Tumours of Neuro-Ectodermal Origin

From the ectodermal cells of the neural tube and crest are derived the tumours of (*a*) the neuroglia, (*b*) nerve cells and their precursors, (*c*) nerve sheaths, (*d*) peripheral neuro-receptor organs, (*e*) the melanocytes, and probably also of (*f*) the meninges. These tumours will be discussed in detail in the chapters on the nervous system and the skin. It will suffice at this stage to mention very briefly a few types and their features.

Tumours of neuroglia

These tumours, termed the **gliomas**, are the commonest primary tumours of the central nervous system. They occur mostly in the brain, but also rarely in the spinal cord. Because of their anatomical site and the pressure effects they may exercise on vital structures most gliomas eventually kill the patient. Even those of high cellularity and aberrant cellular structure, which often spread widely within the cranial and spinal cavities, do not metastasise in extracranial tissues except rarely after surgical treatment involving craniotomy. (This rarity of distant metastases applies to all intracranial tumours, and appears to be a characteristic of the intracranial site, not of the type of tumour.)

Gliomas may take origin from all types of neuroglial cells and may be slow-growing, and rich in glial fibrils, but may nevertheless undergo central necrosis and become cystic. Even these well-differentiated tumours have ill-defined margins and differ from most benign tumours in having no capsule. At the other extreme are highly pleomorphic rapidly growing cellular tumours in which necrosis and haemorrhage are conspicuous.

Tumours of nerve cells

Perhaps because mature neurones are permanent cells which do not divide, nerve cell tumours are very rare in adults.

Medulloblastoma, a rapidly growing tumour of primitive nerve cell type, occurs in children, usually in the cerebellum (p. 787).

Ganglioneuromas are rare tumours composed of mature ganglion cells and nerve fibres. They arise chiefly in the sympathetic chain and adrenal medulla (p. 789). Clinically and histologically they behave as benign tumours except when they contain foci of neuroblasts.

Neuroblastoma or **sympathicoblastoma** is a highly cellular tumour which occurs chiefly in the adrenal medulla and in the sympathetic chain, usually in children. It consists of small round or oval cells with scanty cytoplasm, in places arranged in ball-like clusters which, on section, appear as rosettes. These tumours are highly malignant and metastasise widely, especially to the skull and other bones (p. 788).

Although strikingly different in appearance, it appears that ganglioneuroma and neuroblastoma are benign and malignant variants of the same tumour. Some differentiation commonly occurs in a neuroblastoma. Rarely, it matures completely into a ganglioneuroma.

Melanocytic tumours

The cells which form melanin are of neural crest origin and are called melanocytes (p. 1078). The skin and the eye are their chief sites, and in both places they are important sources of tumours.

Skin tumours are dealt with fully in Chapter 27. The so-called **pigmented naevus** is so common that few people are free of them. It is a benign lesion, better regarded as a hamartoma than a true tumour, formed by a mass of melanocytes ('naevus cells') which accumulate in the dermis as a result of excessive proliferation of melanocytes in their normal site in the basal layer. **Malignant melanomas** are much less common, but common enough to be an important type of cancer. They arise from epidermal melanocytes, often at the site of a pigmented naevus. They are highly malignant and, unless excised at an early stage, are liable to metastasise extensively, both to lymph nodes and via the blood: since the tumours are often very dark due to melanin production, they can present a striking picture at necropsy.

Ocular melanomas. Malignant melanomas of the eye, though far from common, are the least rare of all intraocular malignant tumours (p. 802).

Melanomas at other sites. Melanocytes spill over all the mucocutaneous junctions into the adjoining mucous membranes to varying distances and in varying numbers, and melanomas occur at the corresponding sites. They are least rare in the nose, but arise also in the mouth, conjunctiva, vagina and anus and even in such deeper sites as oesophagus and rectum. The presence of melanocytes in the meninges is also reflected in the rare occurrence of meningeal melanomas, which, like other intracranial tumours, are remarkable for their inability to metastasise outside the cranial cavity.

Tumours of the Haemopoietic, Lymphoid and Mononuclear Phagocyte Systems

Classification within this group is difficult, and it is only in the last few decades that some of its most important members—the leukaemias and Hodgkin's disease for instance—have become fully accepted as neoplastic. Nomenclature still tends to be anomalous and classification disputed. The principal varieties are described in Chapters 17 and 18 and only a few general points will be made here.

The cells of these three systems are all derived from pluripotent haemopoietic stem cells which are present in the haemopoietic tissue and in small numbers in the blood (p. 116). Another common feature is the continuous production of the various cell types throughout life. Thirdly, the mature cells of these systems leave their site of origin in the haemopoietic marrow and circulate in the blood. Lymphocytes (which are produced also in the thymus) multiply in the secondary lymphoid tissues in response to antigenic stimuli and recirculate continuously between the blood, secondary lymphoid and other tissues. Monocytes settle as macrophages in nearly all tissues in the body, but especially in the spleen and lymphoid tissues, the liver, lung and haemopoietic marrow.

Immature precursors of cells of the blood do not normally escape into the blood, but may do so in various conditions of stress, and the spleen and liver can revert to their fetal role of haemopoiesis.

With all this movement and wide distribution of the normal cells of these systems, it is not surprising that neoplastic cells arising from them often do not form a single tumour mass, but spread widely from the start. The more slowly-growing, better differentiated neoplasms tend to spread particularly to the sites which normally contain the corresponding type of non-neoplastic cells. For instance, in chronic myeloid leukaemia, a well-differentiated neoplasm of the granulocyte series, very large numbers of tumour cells appear in the blood from the start, but the solid organs most involved are usually the marrow, liver and spleen, i.e.

the normal sites of haemopoiesis at various stages of life. By contrast, the poorly differentiated acute leukaemias produce far fewer mobile cells in the blood (and sometimes none at all) and tend to a more destructive infiltration of the marrow and other organs. Similarly the better differentiated lymph node tumours characteristically cause widespread moderate enlargement of multiple lymph nodes and other lymphoid structures but often do not spread very much to non-lymphoid tissues, while the less well differentiated may cause large local masses and are less discriminating in spread to other structures.

Any tissue which contains any of the cells belonging to the relevant categories (which means practically any tissue in the body) can give rise to tumours within this group, but the vast majority arise either in the bone marrow (leukaemias and myeloma*) or the lymph nodes (lymphomas, including Hodgkin's disease). As will be obvious from what has been said above, a benign tumour in the ordinary sense of the word must be exceptional, although non-progressive monoclonal proliferation of plasma cells is common in old age. Localised nodules of abnormal lymphoid tissue are sometimes found, for example in the rectum and skin, and may be called 'benign lymphoma' or 'benign lymphocytoma' but it is very doubtful whether these are tumours at all.

The immunological importance of these tissues is naturally reflected in their tumours. Immunological abnormalities are fairly commonly associated with some lymphoid tumours, the most striking example being production of immunoglobulin in large amounts by the neoplastic plasma cells of myeloma.

The viral aetiology of lymphomas and leukaemias in several animal species is now beyond doubt, and it is very likely that these human tumours are also virus-induced: so far, however, the evidence is largely indirect, except in the special case of Burkitt's lymphoma (p. 304).

---

*Myeloma is a neoplastic proliferation of plasma cells, and thus a B-cell lymphoma.

'Mixed' Tumours

A considerable number of tumours consist of two or more different kinds of tissue. The reasons for this are very diverse: the most important can be classified as follows:

(*a*) *'Collision' tumours* result when two different tumours arise close together and intermingle; the juxtaposition may be a chance event, or the result of a local carcinogenic stimulus affecting several tissues.

cinomas (*'adeno-acanthomas'*), with mixed squamous and glandular elements, which arise especially in the uterus and the bronchi.

(*d*) *Tumours with variable differentiation.* This occurs especially in carcinomas, parts of which are so poorly differentiated as to resemble sarcomas. It is almost certain that most so-called **'carcinosarcomas'**, both human and experimental, are of this type (Fig. 13.22).

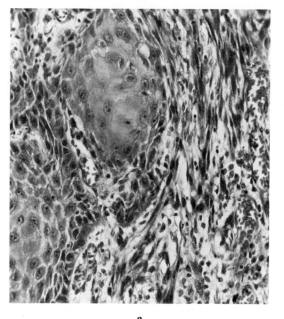 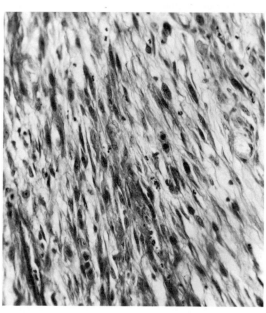

a   b

Fig. 13.22   Squamous carcinoma of tongue, showing so-called carcinosarcoma.
a On the left typical squamous carcinoma, showing continuity with spindle-shaped epithelial cells.
b On the right a purely spindle-cell area containing many mitoses. Transitions from (**a**) to (**b**) are readily found. × 200.

(*b*) *Stromal changes in epithelial tumours.* The cartilaginous metaplasia of the stroma in mixed-salivary tumours, the bony metaplasia seen in a very few carcinomas of the colon, and the lymphoid stroma of some seminomas all produce the *appearance* of a mixed tumour, though only the epithelial element is truly neoplastic.

(*c*) *'Metaplastic' tumours.* Tumours arising from tissues which readily undergo metaplasia from one type to another often reflect this characteristic. Such are the **adenosquamous car-**

(*e*) With the exception of teratoma (see below) *true mixed tumours* involving the co-ordinated neoplastic growth of two independent tissues are hard to find. The fibroadenoma of the breast is the only completely acceptable example, though some connective tissue tumours, such as the angiolipoma, may qualify.

(*f*) *'Embryonal' tumours.* There is a group of tumours, mostly highly malignant, which arise usually in infancy and appear to be derived from immature tissue. Most of these (neuroblastoma, medulloblastoma, hepatoblastoma, for

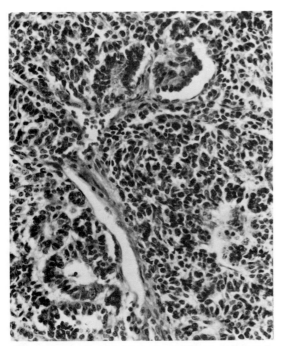

Fig. 13.23 Nephroblastoma (Wilms's tumour), showing cellular sarcoma-like tissue with indistinct differentiation of tubules in several places and a glomerulus-like structure (*at top right*). × 225.

example) are not truly mixed, but the partial differentiation of some of the elements, while others continue to resemble primitive embryonal tissue, may give rise to appearances that simulate a mixed tumour.

One of the commonest of these tumours, the renal nephroblastoma (Wilms's tumour), consists of sarcoma-like masses of short spindle cells, among which some elements differentiate to tubules and occasionally glomerulus-like structures (Fig. 13.23). More discordant tissues such as cartilage and striped muscle are occasionally present, possibly representing a derivation of the tumour cells from the myotome at an earlier stage.

(*g*) *Teratomas.* These, the most extreme examples of mixed tumours, are dealt with in the following section.

It should be emphasised that the grouping together of these tumours is not intended to indicate any special relation between them: they have nothing in common except the presence of more than one kind of tissue.

Teratoma and Choriocarcinoma

As stated above, *teratoma* is the outstanding example of a true mixed tumour; it is of sufficient importance and interest to consider more fully. *Choriocarcinoma* is not a mixed tumour: it is described here because it sometimes develops within a teratoma, but it also occurs alone, originating usually from placental trophoblast.

Teratoma

A teratoma is a tumour composed of various tissues, chaotically arranged and usually of the most diverse types, with no relation to the site of origin. They are not rare and are of practical importance. They are most common in the ovaries and testes, though they occur in other parts, such as the mediastinum, retroperitoneal tissues and pineal. They are usually single but occasionally more than one is present. There is great variation in naked-eye appearances, and

cyst formation may be a notable feature, as in the common benign ovarian teratoma ('dermoid'). There is endless variety in the tissues and in their arrangement. Cartilage, bone, epidermis, glandular epithelium, hair, teeth, etc., are common components, especially in the benign forms, but other specialised tissues e.g. hepatic, renal, nervous, ocular and haemopoietic are also found (Figs. 13.24, 13.25). While a teratoma may be of such a complicated constitution, there is no proper formation of organs, limbs, etc., and a very important fact is that there is no trace of a vertebral column and no metameric segmentation. Germ cells and germinal epithelium are also always absent.

Because of their complicated structure, teratomas were formerly believed to arise from totipotent cells, i.e. from dislocated blastomeres. However, proliferation of a blastomere gives rise to an organised embryo, in

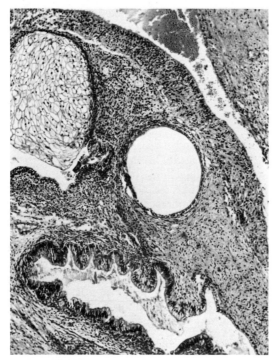

Fig. 13.24 Benign ovarian cystic teratoma or 'dermoid'. Above there is a cleft lined by squamous epithelium which is part of the main cyst. The cyst on the left is lined partly by columnar, partly by non-keratinising squamous epithelium. The lowest cyst is lined by folded columnar epithelium of alimentary type, and the resemblance to gut is heightened by an incomplete layer of smooth muscle related to it. × 72.

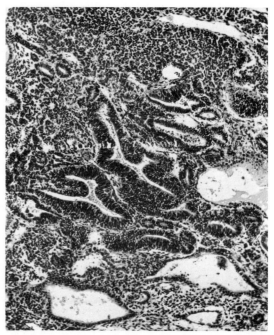

Fig. 13.25 Testicular teratoma (malignant). Because of loss of differentiation the diversity of tissue types is harder to demonstrate, but there is obviously a variety of epithelia present here, the large dark-staining tubules being of primitive neural type. × 62.

contrast to the chaotic mixture of tissues in a teratoma. Another view is that teratomas are derived from the male or female germ cells. The frequency of teratomas in the gonads supports this possibility. Something of the nature of parthenogenetic development would have to be assumed, as is known to occur in amphibian ova under the influence of certain salt solutions. In cocks the intratesticular injection of solutions of zinc salts during the breeding season or after stimulation by pituitary gonadotrophin has led to the development of highly malignant complex teratomatous tumours closely resembling those in man (Bagg, 1936) but similar results do not appear to have been achieved in mammals.

Study of the sex chromatin (p. 1002) has provided some evidence in favour of the parthenogenetic origin of teratomas. It has been found that all teratomas in women have nuclei of the right sex (i.e. are XX) but about half of those in men have female nuclei, as would be expected if they were produced by fusion of two haploid cells in the male gonad. Recent evidence from chromosome studies supports this view: the genes carried in the cells of a benign teratoma are identical with those of the host, but are redistributed between the members of each pair of chromosomes in a manner which normally occurs only during meiosis.

Teratomas are commonest in the ovary, in which site they are usually benign: elsewhere they are nearly always malignant. One type of tissue in a benign teratoma sometimes undergoes malignant change and when this happens the metastases consist of that one tissue only. In malignant teratomas of the type seen especially in the testis, all the tissues present are malignant from the start and metastases may contain any or all of them.

Benign teratomas never contain tissues of extra-fetal origin, such as trophoblast (see below) or yolk sac: their presence in a tumour, either alone or as part of a teratoma, always indicates malignancy.

Monstrosities. Any sufficiently striking congenital structural abnormality may be called a monstrosity. When identical twins develop from a single fertilised ovum a variable amount of fusion may take place. This may be of limited extent as in so-called Siamese twins, or it may affect a considerable part of the body. Partial fusion of two germinal areas is often invoked. Then there are cases where one fetus is imperfectly represented and fused with the other, growing on it in parasite-like fashion or included within its abdominal cavity—*fetus in fetu.* Many sacral teratomas and epignathi probably belong to this group. All such abnormalities, which are extremely varied, are spoken of as monstrosities. They show wide deviations from the normal, but the formation of parts and the relations of the tissues to one another are well maintained: thus, organs may be doubled, and a limb, though abnormal in size or form, is still a limb. Monstrosities are now generally thought to be a fundamentally different nature from teratomas and apparent transitions are almost certainly fallacious. A defect in the mechanism of the primary organisers at a very early stage of formation of the embryo may well be responsible for this type of abnormality.

Choriocarcinoma

This is uncommon except in the Far East. It is a highly malignant tumour which usually originates from, and retains recognisable features of, trophoblastic epithelium (Fig. 13.26). It also retains the trophoblastic property of invading blood vessels, and so metastases are usually early and widespread. Choriocarcinoma arises occasionally from trophoblastic differentiation in a teratoma of the testis, mediastinum, etc., but its usual site is in the uterus, where it origi-

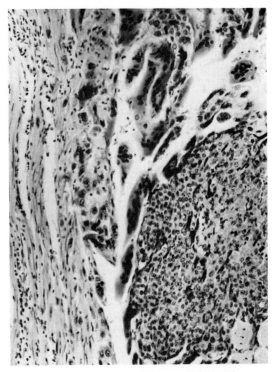

Fig. 13.26 Choriocarcinoma, showing Langhans' cells (cytotrophoblast, *bottom right*) and giant cells (syncytiotrophoblast, *centre*) invading uterine wall (*left*). × 230.

nates from the placental trophoblast of a pregnancy and is thus a fetal tumour growing in the mother. In spite of this, it grows and extends rapidly, but responds unusually well to chemotherapy, and in some instances removal of the primary tumour has been followed by apparently spontaneous disappearance of metastases. These unusual features, which apply only to the uterine (fetal) choriocarcinomas, are probably due to a homograft reaction.

Tumour-like Lesions and Cysts

There are a number of lesions which resemble tumours but have distinctive features which cast doubt on their neoplastic nature. Examples already described in this chapter include the fibromatoses (p. 342), haemangiomas (p. 348) and monstrosities. Among such tumour-like lesions the groups termed *hamartomas* merit further description. *Cysts* are not tumours and are described here for want of a better place.

Hamartoma

This is a convenient term for an ill-defined group of lesions which have some resemblance to tumours but are not neoplastic. They usually appear before or soon after birth, grow with the individual and cease to grow when general body growth ceases. They may consist of a single type of cell, e.g. pigmented naevi, composed of a collection of melanocytes (p. 1080), a particular type of tissue, e.g. haemangioma, or a mixture of tissues, e.g. cartilage, epithelial-lined clefts, adipose and fibrous tissue in the so-called adenochondroma of the lung (p. 496). Those in the internal organs form lumps which can be mistaken grossly for tumours, while in the skin they may be nodular or may present as a patch of discolouration, e.g. the capillary haemangioma (p. 348) and some pigmented naevi. Hamartomas can best be understood as arising from a localised disorder of the relationships of normal tissues leading to overproduction of one or more elements but without the property of progressive growth characteristic of tumours. There are many varieties, and some have a tendency to progress to true neoplasia, for example pigmented naevi (although the risk is small) and exostoses (bony projections with a cartilaginous cap) arising from the axial skeleton or proximal limb bones (p. 904).

Cysts

The term 'cyst' properly means a space containing fluid and lined by epithelial cells. In most cysts the epithelial lining is not neoplastic and such cysts are neither tumours nor parts of tumours: they are included here only for convenience. Nearly all cysts arise by the abnormal dilatation of pre-existing tubules, ducts or cavities, though a cyst may lose its cell lining due to inflammatory or other change, and come to be lined by granulation or denser fibrous tissue. The term is, however, often applied in a somewhat loose way to other abnormal cavities containing fluid. For example, the term 'apoplectic cyst' is applied to a space in the brain containing brownish fluid, which has resulted from haemorrhage. Some tumours, e.g. gliomas, undergo softening in their interior, so that a collection of fluid is formed, and the term 'cystic change' is often used even when no true cyst is formed.

The cysts peculiar to each organ will be described in the later chapters: we shall give here only a classification of their causes. True cysts also occur in some tumours, the lining epithelium being neoplastic, e.g. in *cystic adenomas* (p. 326) and *teratomas* (p. 355). Apart from these, cysts fall naturally into two main groups: (1) those due to congenital abnormalities, and (2) acquired cysts, i.e. those produced by lesions in post-natal life.

(1) Congenital cysts

These may also be grouped into two types:

(a) They may arise *within otherwise normal organs or tissues*, as a result of the presence of epithelium of a type not usually present at that site after birth, either as a result of some minor displacement of an embryonal tissue or (more often) the failure to disappear of some embryonic duct or cleft. The commonest site of cysts derived from vestigial ducts is the genito-urinary tract, where the disappearance of the mesonephros and its duct in both sexes, and of the Wolffian ducts in females and Müllerian ducts in males, often leaves behind a variety of persistent epithelial remnants: small cysts are very common among these, and larger ones (**parovarian cysts**) are not uncommon in the broad ligaments (p. 970).

Other embryonic ducts which may persist and give rise to cysts include the thyroglossal duct (mid-line of neck, usually near the hyoid, p. 1030) and the urachus (usually at the umbilicus). A similar mechanism operates with the branchial clefts; **branchial cysts** are produced at the side of the neck and are lined by squamous epithelium with usually a rim of lymphoid tissue.

A different mechanism produces the **sequestration dermoids** which result from imperfect fusion of embryonal skin flaps. They are lined with squamous epithelium and filled with keratin, and are found mostly in the mid-line of the chest and neck or at the angles of the eye.

The 'pearly tumour' of the meninges, etc. (actually a squamous-epithelium-lined cyst, p. 792) is an example of a simple displacement of squamous epithelium into the meninges, at the time of neural tube closure.

(b) Cysts arising as *part of a major congenital abnormality of an organ*. Examples are (i) **polycystic disease of the kidneys** (p. 860), in which a major maldevelopment of the renal tubules (of several possible types) results in the formation of cysts in great numbers; (ii) the **meningocele** and other types of cystic swelling that complicate some cases of spina bifida, failure of proper closure of the neural tube being the basic defect (p. 772).

(2) Acquired cysts

These are of several varieties, the three following being the most important:

(a) Retention cysts. These are formed by retention of secretion produced by obstruction to the outflow of secretion. A single cyst, sometimes large, may be produced by the obstruction of the main duct, e.g. of a salivary gland or of a part of the pancreas. Obstruction of the orifice of a hair follicle gives rise to a cyst-like swelling filled chiefly with breaking-down keratin—the so-called **sebaceous cyst**, seen especially in the scalp. On the other hand, numerous small cysts may result from obstruction of small ducts, an occurrence which is not uncommon in fibrosing lesions of the kidney.

(b) Distension cysts are formed from natural enclosed spaces. They occur in the thyroid from dilatation of the acini, and occasionally also in the pituitary: cystic dilatation of Graafian follicles in the ovaries is also common. Distension of spaces lined by mesothelium is also seen; for example, a bursa may enlarge to form a cystic swelling, and there is the common condition of hydrocele due to an accumulation of fluid in the tunica vaginalis.

Occasionally in the adult an **implantation cyst** occurs by the dislocation inwards of a portion of epidermis by injury. The epithelium grows and comes to line a space filled with degenerate epithelial squames (Fig. 13.27); rarely hair follicles are present in the wall. Implantation cysts may result also from wounds of the cornea.

(c) Parasitic cysts. These are cystic stages in the life cycle of cestode *parasites*. The most striking examples are the **'hydatid'** cysts produced in man, usually in the liver, by the dog tapeworm *Taenia echinococcus*, though small cysts may be produced in the brain and other parts by the cysticerci of *Taenia solium*.

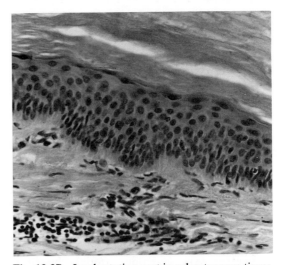

Fig. 13.27 Implantation cyst in subcutaneous tissue, showing lining of stratified squamous epithelium and keratin in the lumen. × 200.

Further Reading

Ashley, D. B. (1978). *Evans' Histological Appearances of Tumours*, 3rd edn., pp. 857. Churchill-Livingstone, Edinburgh, London and New York. (An account of the behaviour and appearances of human tumours based on a considerable experience.)

Sobin, L. H., Thomas, L. B., Percy, Constance and Henson, D. E. (Eds.) (1978) *A Coded Compendium of the International Histological Classification of Tumours*, pp. 116. World Health Organisation, Geneva. (A widely accepted system of classification, coding and nomenclature of human tumours.)

Willis, R. A. (1973). *The Spread of Tumours in the Human Body*, 3rd edn., pp. 417. Butterworths, London.

Atlas of Tumour Pathology. US Armed Forces Institute of Pathology, Washington, DC. (Numerous 'Fascicles' on tumours of particular organs, tissues and regions. A valuable source of detailed information on the histology and behaviour of individual tumours.)

Cancer. A journal of the American Cancer Society. Lipincott, Philadelphia and Toronto. (A monthly publication of well-illustrated articles on human neoplasms.)

14

Blood Vessels and Lymphatics

Arteries

Introduction

Lesions of the arteries are very important because of their frequency and serious consequences. The commonest important disease in developed countries is **atheroma (atherosclerosis)**, which consists of prolonged, slow, patchy accumulation of lipids and fibrosis, in the intima of arteries of various sizes. The patchy thickening results in narrowing of the lumen with consequent chronic ischaemia of the various organs and tissues. Acute ischaemia can result from the occlusion of an artery by local **thrombosis** or **embolism**; these processes have been dealt with in Chapter 9, but it is important to emphasise here that *arterial thrombosis is usually the result of disease of the artery wall, and atheroma is the commonest predisposing cause.*

Another very common arterial change is termed **arteriosclerosis**. This is a diffuse change in the walls of arteries, in which the muscle and elastic tissue slowly diminish and are replaced by fibrous tissue, with the result that the arteries become more firm and rigid. Like atheroma, these changes occur in various degrees with increasing age, but they are aggravated and accelerated by systemic hypertension in which the fibrous replacement is preceded, at least in some instances, by hypertrophy of muscle and elastic tissue. Arteriosclerosis alone is usually without serious consequences, but the accompanying changes in the arterioles— **arteriolosclerosis**—result in ischaemia, particularly of the kidneys.

A very common and important condition which affects the arteries and arterioles is **systemic hypertension**, a state in which the arterial blood pressure is raised. In most cases, the cause of the rise in blood pressure is not known, but it is likely that, in all instances, the rise is mediated by increased muscle tone in the arterioles. Prolonged hypertension, as mentioned above, leads to severe arteriosclerosis and arteriolosclerosis; it is by far the commonest cause of rupture of the cerebral arteries to produce haemorrhage into the brain, and is an important cause of heart failure.

Diseases of the arteries which bring about severe destruction of the muscle and elastic tissue, particularly of the media, may weaken the wall to such an extent that dilatation results, and if localised this is termed an **aneurysm**; rupture of the vessel wall may occur, with or without preceding dilatation. Severe weakening can result from various forms of *arteritis*, including that due to syphilis, but also from *atheroma* and from *degenerative changes of unknown nature in the media*. All three of these conditions can give rise to aortic aneurysm. Aneurysm formation and rupture may result also from *developmental defects*, as seen in the arteries at the base of the brain. Another effect of the various types of arteritis is to promote thrombosis, although atheroma is a much more important cause of this in certain arteries.

Effects of ageing. Throughout adult life, the walls of arteries of all sizes become gradually less resilient and more rigid; they tend to enlarge both in diameter and in length. These changes constitute **senile arteriosclerosis**: they are well illustrated by the prominence and tortuosity of the temporal arteries in older people, and are due to gradual increase in collagen and ground substance at the expense of smooth muscle and fine elastic fibres. The media is mainly affected, but also the intima which becomes appreciably thickened. Chemical analysis has shown that there is also a gradual increase in calcium salts in the artery walls. Senile arteriosclerosis has little effect on function. Similar changes, but with some thickening of the artery walls, are a feature of chronic hypertension.

Patchy thickening and hyalinisation of the walls of arterioles (**hyaline arteriolosclerosis**) also occurs with increasing age, particularly in the spleen and kidneys, but also in other viscera. When severe, it results in luminal narrowing, and may thus cause ischaemia, e.g. of the renal glomeruli. Hyaline arteriolosclerosis is exaggerated in hypertension and diabetes: it is described more fully on p. 373.

Adaptation and hypertrophy. The muscular and elastic nature of the arterial wall readily permits dilatation to provide an increased blood flow to the part supplied. If the requirement is more than transient, the lumen becomes persistently dilated and there is hypertrophy of the muscular and elastic tissue, e.g. the physiological hypertrophy of the uterine arteries during pregnancy. Similar compensatory dilation and hypertrophy occurs in collateral vessels when a main artery is obstructed.

In persistent hypertension, the tendency for the increased pressure to dilate and lengthen the arteries is partly prevented by compensatory hypertrophy of the circular muscle of the media and the intimal longitudinal muscle fibres which lie next to the internal elastic lamina (Fig. 14.1). The vascular changes in hypertension are described in more detail on pp. 371–4.

Endarteritis obliterans. Intimal thickening of arteries occurs when concentric laminae of cellular connective tissue form in the intima and obliterate or narrow the arterial lumen. New elastic tissue is laid down independently of the internal elastic lamina and may appear as a layer under the endothelium or as a number of small new laminae. This lesion is called endarteritis obliterans and is found in chronic inflammatory lesions. It is well seen in the base of chronic peptic ulcers (Fig. 14.2) and in the walls of tuberculous cavities, where it is beneficial in tending to prevent haemorrhage. It occurs also in the lesions of syphilis, in tuberculous meningitis (Fig. 21.33, p. 751) and silicosis, and in small arteries exposed to radiotherapy. Similar obliterative changes occur in the smaller arteries in severe hypertension and in progressive systemic sclerosis.

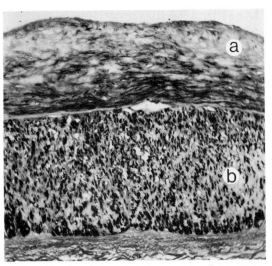

Fig. 14.1 Longitudinal section of the wall of an artery in essential hypertension, showing hypertrophic thickening of the longitudinal muscle in the intima **a** and of the circular muscle in the media **b**. (Myocytes stained black.) × 110.

When the functional requirements for blood flow through an artery are greatly reduced, the lumen is narrowed by obliterative endarteritis, which is the physiological mechanism of arterial involution. It occurs, for example, in the umbilical arteries and ductus arteriosus after birth, in the uterine and ovarian arteries after the menopause, and in the arteries supplying an area which is excised (e.g. a limb) or destroyed by disease.

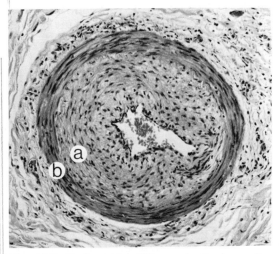

Fig. 14.2 Endarteritis obliterans in the base of a chronic peptic ulcer, **a** = intima, **b** = media.

Atheroma (Atherosclerosis)

This is one of the most important diseases of developed communities. It causes narrowing of the lumen of arteries, is often complicated by occlusive thrombosis, and is the major cause of disability and death from heart disease, cerebral infarction and ischaemia of the lower limbs. It is virtually always present in some degree in middle-aged and old people.

Definition. The lesions of atheroma consist of patches ('plaques') of intimal thickening of the walls of arteries, due mainly to deposition of lipids and formation of fibrous tissue. The alternative term **atherosclerosis** is used because the lesion has a soft, lipid-rich part (athere = porridge) and a hard (sclerotic) fibrous component.

Naked-eye appearances. The earliest deposits of lipid in the intima of the aorta and large arteries are seen predominantly in childhood and adolescence and are known as *fatty streaks*. They appear as yellow non-raised spots in the luminal surface, which enlarge and coalesce to form irregular yellow streaks. Microscopy shows them to consist of accumulations of lipid droplets in intimal cells (now known to be smooth muscle cells—see below) and in aggregates of macrophages lying beneath the endothelium (Fig. 14.3). Fatty streaks are seen in children dying from various causes, including trauma, and are apparently equally common in all communities, regardless of whether or not there is a high incidence of atheroma later in life. Because they are found mainly in children, many of the fatty streaks

must disappear, but it is not known whether some of them persist and progress to atheroma in communities with a high incidence of this disease.

The earliest recognisable atheromatous lesions are seen commonly from young adulthood onwards in atheroma-prone communities. They consist of small disc-like yellowish, slightly raised patches of intimal thickening with a smooth glistening surface. As the condition progresses, the patches enlarge and thicken by further deposition of lipid deep in the intima and by fibrosis more superficially (i.e. adjacent to the lumen): the patches become distinctly raised and when viewed from the intimal surface they may appear yellow or white depending on the amount of white fibrous tissue overlying the yellow lipid deposits. In any one individual, the patches are at various stages of development, indicating progressive formation.

Aorta. Atheroma occurs throughout the length of the aorta, but the abdominal aorta is usually more severely affected and patches often develop first around the origins of the intercostal and lumbar branches (Fig. 14.4). The

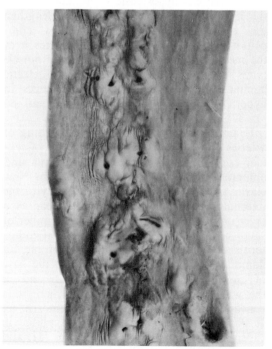

Fig. 14.4 Mild atheroma of the abdominal aorta. The lesions are seen as raised patches and are located mainly around the origins of the arterial branches. × 0·8.

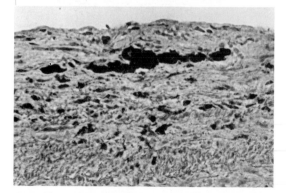

Fig. 14.3 Intimal lipid deposit in the aorta of a child aged 11 years: accidental death. (Frozen section; lipid stained black.) × 200. (Dr. Morag McCallum.)

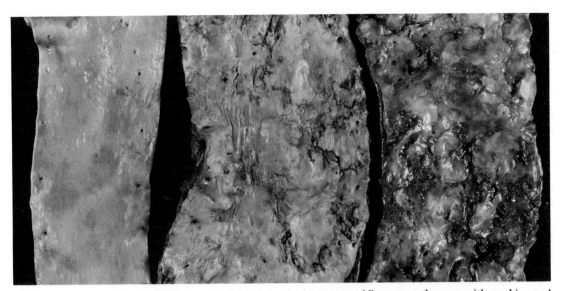

Fig. 14.5 Lengths of the abdominal aorta: *left*, minimal atheroma; *middle*, severe atheroma with cracking and early ulceration of patches; *right*, very severe atheroma with ulceration and mural thrombosis. Note also that the two atheromatous aortas have lost their elasticity and stretched: this may be due to atrophy of the media beneath the extensive atheroma, but could also be the result of arteriosclerosis.

patches vary in size up to several centimetres diameter and may in places become confluent. If a sizeable patch is cut across, lipid-rich paste-like material can be expressed from its deeper part, and fibrous thickening is seen as a white layer overlying this. The fibrous layer may break down, resulting in *ulceration* of the plaque, and *mural thrombus* is then likely to be deposited on the ulcerated surface; another common change is *deposition of calcium salts* which may convert the plaque to a hard brittle plate. Plaques showing ulceration, calcification or thrombus deposition are commonly referred to as **complicated atheroma**, and may produce great irregularity of the luminal surface of the aorta (Fig. 14.5). Other important features of aortic plaques are *thinning of the overlying media*, and in some instances *extension of the plaque into the adjacent media*: the wall is thus weakened and an *aneurysm* may develop, with the danger of rupture (p. 385).

Other arteries. Atheroma occurs in arteries of all sizes down to approximately 2 mm diameter and is seen occasionally in mild form in even smaller vessels. The general features are similar to those seen in the aorta except that the plaques are necessarily smaller, often involve the whole circumference of the intima, and can cause all degrees of *luminal narrowing* down to virtual occlusion (Figs. 14.6, 14.7,

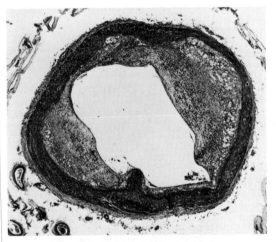

Fig. 14.6 Atheroma of a coronary artery causing moderate narrowing of the lumen. The spaces in the deep part of the plaque represent lipid accumulation. × 10.

14.8). Atheroma tends to affect especially arteries supplying the heart, brain and abdominal viscera, and also the arteries of the lower limbs. There is considerable individual variation in its distribution, in some instances the aorta being mainly affected, in others the arteries at the base of the brain and/or the coronary arteries. The coronary arteries are often severely affected and are more often involved at a relatively early age than any other arteries.

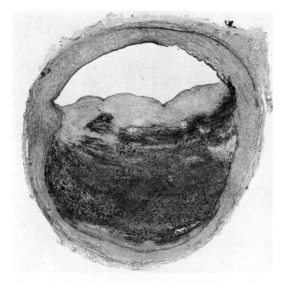

Fig. 14.7 Severe atheroma of the superior mesenteric artery, causing marked reduction of the lumen. Frozen section, stained with Scharlach R, showing the large amount of fatty material in the patch. × 15.

The cerebral arteries also are subject to severe atheroma, but this is found chiefly in elderly persons. For unknown reasons, the renal arteries are seldom severely affected except in diabetics, in whom atheroma is often widespread and very severe.

In the thin-walled arteries at the base of the brain the patches are visible from both inner and outer aspects of the vessels, and their yellow opaque appearance contrasts with the reddish translucency of the normal parts of the vessel wall (Fig. 14.9).

Complications include: (*a*) **haemorrhage into a plaque**, which increases the degree of luminal narrowing (Fig. 15.2, p. 401); (*b*) **rupture or ulceration of a plaque** (Fig. 15.12, p. 406); and (*c*) **occlusive thrombosis** (Fig. 15.6, p. 403) which is a major cause of infarction in the heart, brain and intestine, and of ischaemia of the legs.

Microscopic appearances. The early changes are due to accumulation of lipids in proliferated spindle cells, shown by electron microscopy to be smooth muscle cells, lying in the intima (Fig. 14.10). Lipids also accumulate between cells deep in the intima (i.e. close to the media), particularly in relation to elastic fibres

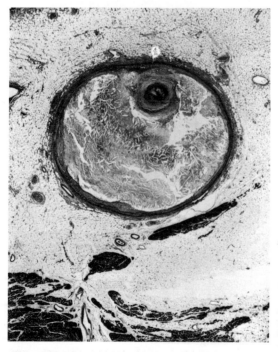

Fig. 14.8 Severe atheroma of the left coronary artery in a patient with myxoedema. The lumen has been greatly reduced by atheroma and occluded by recent superadded thrombosis. × 10.

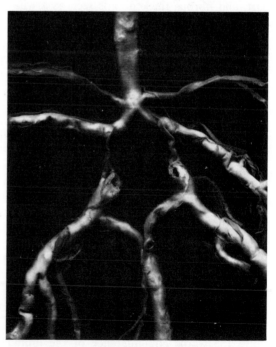

Fig. 14.9 Circle of Willis and branches, showing marked patchy atheroma.

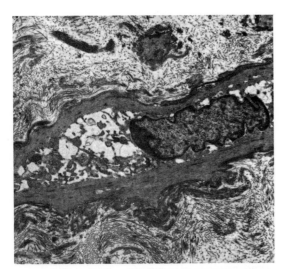

Fig. 14.10 Electron micrograph of part of a smooth muscle cell in an atheromatous plaque. The cytoplasm is made up largely of myofibrils, and contains globules of fat, shown as light spaces. The fine fibres on either side of the cell are collagen. × 7500.

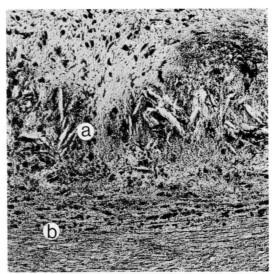

Fig. 14.11 Section showing part of an atheromatous patch of the aorta. In the deep part of the intima there is degenerate lipid-rich material **a**, the spindle-shaped spaces being due to cholesterol crystals. Lipid accumulation stops abruptly at the junction with the media **b**. × 110.

and the internal elastic lamina. As the patch develops, thin laminae of connective tissue appear in the more superficial part of the intima and form the fibrous part of the lesion. Lipid-containing cells lie among the collagen fibres in this region. Areas of necrosis then develop, converting the deep part of the patch into a structureless accumulation of lipids, tissue debris (Fig.14.11) and sometimes altered blood, and the necrosis gradually extends into the overlying fibrous tissue. Calcium deposition may be visible microscopically. Infiltration of neutrophil leukocytes and other inflammatory cells is common, and lipid-laden macrophages—'foamy cells'—may appear around the lipid deposits, which usually contain crystals of cholesterol, represented in paraffin section by the typical elongated clefts (Fig. 14.11). The internal elastic lamina deep to the plaque is usually disrupted and lipid deposition, necrosis and fibrosis may then extend into the adjacent media. Quite apart from this, the media deep to the plaque becomes thinned and atrophic (Fig. 14.12).

Small blood vessels grow into the atheromatous patch from the media of the affected vessels and sometimes also from the intimal surface. These may be the source of the haemorrhage which commonly occurs in the patch, although, as already stated, the overlying fib-

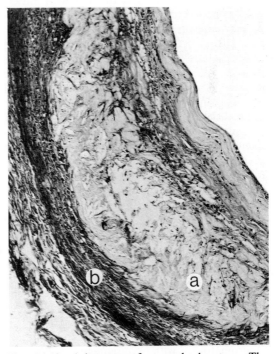

Fig. 14.12 Atheroma of a cerebral artery. The intima is greatly thickened with accumulation of lipid in its deeper part **(a)** and dense overlying fibrosis. The media **(b)** shows local atrophy over the patch. × 110.

rous patch may be very thin and may rupture, allowing blood to track in from the lumen.

Effects

Although the changes of atheroma are essentially the same in all arteries, their effects vary in arteries of different sizes.

Large arteries. Uncomplicated atheroma of large arteries, such as the aorta, very often has no clinical effect because usually it does not substantially reduce the lumen or seriously weaken the wall. In advanced cases, however, an *aneurysm* may form in the abdominal aorta (p. 385) or occasionally in a common iliac artery. *Thrombi* which form on ulcerated plaques in the aorta seldom cause complete occlusion, probably because the rapid flow limits platelet adhesion. Occasionally, however, thrombus may extend to occlude the whole aortic lumen and when this occurs at the bifurcation it can result in gangrene of the legs unless adequate collateral circulation has developed, in which case there may be merely coldness and weakness of the legs with muscle wasting and sexual impotence but without ischaemic pain or gangrene (*Leriche syndrome*). Apart from occluding the aorta, thrombi and atheromatous debris from ulcerated plaques may break away and form *emboli* in the arteries of the lower limbs and abdominal organs such as the kidneys.

Smaller arteries. By far the commonest important effects of atheroma are due to involvement of smaller arteries, the lumen of which may be progressively narrowed by an atheromatous patch or suddenly occluded by superadded thrombosis (Fig. 14.8). These effects are well seen in the coronary arteries. Atheroma is the chief cause of *ischaemic heart disease*, the largest single cause of death in Europe and North America today (p. 400). *Ischaemic brain damage* is also very common and is usually the result of atheroma of the carotid, vertebral and basilar arteries, vessels of the Circle of Willis and cerebral arteries (p. 742). Atheroma does not cause aneurysms of smaller arteries.

Arteries supplying the legs are often severely atheromatous, with consequent progressive diminution in blood supply. Eventually the collateral circulation becomes inadequate: relative muscle ischaemia can then be induced by the increased metabolic demands of exercise, which produces severe pain in the leg, relieved by rest. This is the clinical syndrome of *intermittent claudication*. In time ischaemia may be so severe as to cause *gangrene*, which usually starts in the toes (Fig. 2.6, p. 12) and spreads proximally. Examination of legs amputed for gangrene usually shows narrowing or obliteration and calcification of the main arteries of the leg. Because atheroma is often widespread, patients with severe involvement of the arteries of the lower limbs frequently suffer also from ischaemic heart disease.

The arteries of the arms are rarely severely affected by atheroma.

Aetiology

Epidemiological surveys have revealed a number of predisposing factors in atheroma, but the mechanisms involved in the development and growth of the plaque are not yet understood. Most of the available information has been provided by morphological, histochemical and biochemical studies on the atheromatous plaque, and by experimental animal studies. It seems appropriate to discuss these biomedical investigations, and then to consider how the various known risk factors may contribute.

The main features of the early lesion are accumulation of lipid, cellular proliferation and formation of fibrous tissue.

Accumulation of lipid. Studies in man with labelled cholesterol suggest that most of the cholesterol in the human aortic intima is derived from the plasma. Since the arterial vasa vasorum supply only the outer part of the wall, plasma lipid must enter the intima from the lumen via the endothelial lining, and animal studies have shown that plasma proteins and certain lipids normally pass into the intima via this route, particularly around the mouths of arterial branches. This localisation suggests increased endothelial permeability at sites where atheroma tends to occur in man, and where lesions resembling human atheroma can be induced experimentally by feeding animals on a cholesterol-rich diet. Such focal increase in permeability is associated with an increased rate of endothelial cell-turnover and it has been suggested that the endothelium at certain sites, including the vicinity of arterial branching, is subject to increased shearing stress which may account for its greater permeability and turnover rate. There is no good evidence on the route of transport of lipid across the endothelial barrier: micropinocytic vesicles or the development of gaps between cells (p. 49) are obvious possibilities. Other agents which may play a causal role in atheroma have been shown to cause endothelial-cell injury, for example inhalation of cigarette smoke by rabbits results in focal endothelial-cell loss, while the formation of circulating antigen–antibody complexes, which increase endothelial permeability by inducing gaps between endothelial cells (p. 154), has been shown to enhance the dietary-induced atheroma-like lesions of rabbits. In man, cardiac allotransplants tend to develop extensive and heavy deposition of lipids in the intima of the coronary arteries, possibly as a result of endothelial injury resulting from the reaction of host antibody with donor vascular endothelium.

Cholesterol is transported in the plasma as a component of lipoproteins (p. 24), which are now usually classified into *chylomicrons* and three other groups which differ in their composition, electrophoretic mobility and specific gravity—the α or *high density lipoproteins* (HDL), the β or *low density lipoproteins* (LDL) and the *pre-β* or *very low density lipoproteins* (VLDL). The LDL are particularly rich in cholesterol, much of which is in the form of cholesterol esters rich in linoleic acid, and a high proportion of the cholesterol in early atheromatous plaques is also in this form. When pieces of aorta are incubated in culture medium containing lipoproteins, both HDL and LDL (but not VLDL) pass through the endothelium, but LDL accumulate in the intima in much greater amounts than HDL: there appears to be some mechanism of clearing HDL from the intima which is not effective for LDL. Immunological assay of lipoproteins in the human aortic intima, and particularly in early atheromatous patches, has demonstrated disproportionately large amounts of LDL.

Findings such as those outlined above have led to the widespread belief that the lipid of atheromatous plaques is derived from the plasma, that LDL make a major contribution to it, and that injury to the endothelium probably plays an important role in allowing lipid to enter the intima.

Cellular proliferation. The intimal cells which proliferate in early atheroma, and which accumulate droplets of lipid, have been shown by electron microscopy to be modified smooth muscle cells (Fig. 14.10) which migrate from the media, through the internal elastic lamina, into the intima. Two factors have been suggested to account for their proliferation. Firstly, it has been shown that LDL promote proliferation of smooth muscle cells in aortic explants in culture. (Curiously, only LDL prepared from plasma in which the LDL level is high appear to have this effect.) Secondly, when platelets adhere to an injured vessel wall or form aggregates, they discharge their storage granules (the platelet release reaction—p. 232), and one of the stored products released is a basic protein which stimulates proliferation of smooth muscle cells in culture.

So far, we have considered accumulation of lipid in the intima by the process of insudation from the plasma (**filtration theory**), but with mention of platelets the time is opportune to introduce the **thrombogenic theory** of atheroma, which was suggested by Rokitansky in 1852, only to be forgotten and re-introduced independently by Duguid in 1946. This theory proposes that injury to arterial endothelium results in recurrent deposition of a fine layer of mural thrombus consisting of platelets and fibrin, and that the thrombus is rapidly covered by endothelium and thus incorporated into the superficial part of the intima. It is further suggested that such thrombus is the origin of the lipid of atheroma and that its recurrent deposition accounts for the gradual development and growth of the atheromatous plaque.

By use of labelled antibodies, both fibrin and platelets have been detected in approximately 40 per cent of atheromatous patches. Experimentally, injury to aortic endothelium, e.g. by abrasion, has been shown to result in adherence of platelets which soon become covered by endothelium: platelet deposition is followed by active proliferation of smooth muscle cells in the intima, with formation of a fibromuscular plaque resembling early atheroma. Depression of platelet adherence by dipyridamole or anti-platelet antibody inhibits the proliferation of smooth muscle cells in such experiments.

It may be concluded that deposition of a thin layer of platelets and fibrin on the surface of atheromatous patches is a common occurrence, and that such thrombus is rapidly incorporated into the plaque. The role of thrombus in the development and growth of the plaque is uncertain, and many workers consider that it is unlikely to be the major source of atheromatous lipid.

The fibrous tissue which forms the superficial (sub-endothelial) part of the atheromatous plaque is provided, at least in part, by the proliferated smooth muscle cells, which have been shown in tissue culture to be capable of producing collagen, elastin and the proteoglycans of ground-substance. These are curious cells, reminiscent in their properties of the myofibroblasts of healing wounds (p. 84). Another surprising observation has been provided by the study of iso-enzymic forms of glucose-6-phosphate dehydrogenase. These enzymes are encoded by X chromosomes, and many American negresses are heterozygous, so that, as a result of Lyonisation (p. 513), half of their cells produce one type (A) of iso-enzyme and the remainder produce another (B). Analysis of early cellular atheromatous plaques from such heterozygous women has shown that the smooth muscle cells of some plaques produce only iso-enzyme A, while those of other plaques (from the same individual) produce only B. This suggests that the cellular proliferation in each plaque is *monoclonal*, although there are other possible explanations. This remarkable finding may be of basic importance in atherogenesis (see Benditt, 1977).

The necrosis which occurs in the lipid-rich depth of the atheromatous plaque may be due to ischaemia, although the deeper part of the plaque is supplied by the vasa vasorum which extend into the (normally avascular) intima of affected arteries. Another possible factor is the presence in the plaque of small amounts of unusual lipids shown to be capable of inducing tissue injury.

The story of focal endothelial injury resulting in ingress of lipids by insudation and in deposition of platelets seems a reasonable explanation of the development of early atheroma. It does not, however, account for the growth of the plaque once a well-defined superficial layer of fibrous tissue has formed: neither insudation from the lumen nor mural thrombosis would account for further increase in lipid *deep* in the intimal plaque, the most likely source of which seems to be the vasa vasorum.

Predisposing or 'risk' factors

While the pathogenesis of atheroma is not fully understood, there are a number of factors which are known to predispose to its development. These are as follows.

Blood lipids. An important relationship between blood lipids and atheroma is indicated by the following observations.
(1) There is a positive correlation between the average level of the serum or plasma cholesterol (which depends mainly on diet) in a community and the incidence and severity of atheroma.
(2) Individuals with a high plasma total cholesterol level have an increased risk of atheroma, and the incidence of severe atheroma is very high in subjects with diseases accompanied by hypercholesterolaemia, for example diabetes mellitus, myxoedema, familial hyperbetalipoproteinaemia (p. 30) and the nephrotic syndrome.
(3) Lesions resembling atheroma can be produced in various animal species by a cholesterol-rich diet.

Hyperlipidaemia is now classified into the various types of hyperlipoproteinaemia, which differ in the type of lipoprotein which is increased and in their dependence on genetic and dietary factors. It is obviously important to determine whether atheroma is related to rise of a particular lipoprotein fraction and, if so, whether the hyperlipoproteinaemia can be corrected by diet. Unfortunately there is no simple method of assessing the presence, distribution and severity of atheroma during life unless it gives rise to symptoms. Accordingly, it is usual to regard ischaemic heart disease (IHD) as an indication of severe atheroma, and to seek associations between possible risk factors, e.g. hyperlipidaemia and IHD. It must be appreciated that IHD is a crude indication of atheroma, for in some patients with IHD, atheroma is limited mainly to the coronary arteries, and many people without IHD have severe atheroma. Also, IHD is commonly due to occlusive coronary artery thrombosis superimposed on atheroma, and accordingly it is not known whether risk factors implicated by such studies predispose to atheroma, to superadded thrombosis, or to both.

Nevertheless, useful information has been provided by population studies. In the Framingham investigation in Massachussets, reported by Kannel (1971), the levels of serum cholesterol, phospholipid, LDL and VLDL were determined in over 5000 individuals, who were then followed up for 16 years. Ischaemic heart disease, indicated by myocardial infarction, sudden death or angina pectoris, was shown to correlate strongly with each of these lipid fractions. Since this study was undertaken a classification or hyperlipoproteinaemias has been published by the World Health Organisation (1970). Extensive prospective studies on the relationship between the types of hyperlipoproteinaemia and atheroma have not yet been reported, but it is already apparent that there is a greatly increased risk of atheroma in individuals with high levels of LDL and VLDL. The two commonest types of hyperlipoproteinaemia (IIb and IV), both of which carry a high risk of IHD, are attributable to dietary excess, either of animal fats or of total caloric intake, and *it seems very likely that the incidence and severity of atheroma, or at least of IHD, could be greatly diminished by modification of the diet.*

The association of LDL with a high risk of IHD fits well with the biomedical studies described earlier. Many cells, including smooth muscle cells, ingest LDL by micropinocytosis and make use of its cholesterol in the production of cell membranes. As mentioned on p. 30, the cell uptake of LDL is controlled by cell receptors, etc.: the subject is more fully explained by Goldstein and Brown (1977). Defects of the control mechanisms result in the very severe atheroma of the familial hyperlipidaemias. No such defects have been demonstrated in the great majority of individuals with severe atheroma, but high levels of LDL passing from the plasma into the intima of arteries might overwhelm the normal control mechanisms, resulting in accumulation of LDL. Unsaturated vegetable oils do not raise the LDL and are not atherogenic: they may even have a protective effect.

There also appears to be an *inverse* relationship between serum HDL levels and ischaemic heart disease. A possible explanation is provided by experiments mentioned earlier in which pieces of aorta were incubated in culture medium containing lipoproteins: the presence of HDL was reported to result in transfer of cholesterol from the intima to the culture medium.

Age and sex. It is not surprising that atheroma and its complications increase with advancing age, for the plaques grow slowly. Men are more severely affected than women at all ages, and indeed severe extensive atheroma is much less common in women until after the menopause, when it progresses as in younger men. The sex difference may be due to oestrogens, which are known to influence lipid metabolism and reduce the total plasma cholesterol.

Hypertension. There is no doubt that hypertension is associated with an increased incidence and severity of atheroma. This has been established by necropsy studies. Moreover, in the Framingham and other prospective studies, a clear correlation has been demonstrated between the height of the blood pressure and the risk of IHD, particularly in older men. It is not known how hypertension contributes to atheroma; one possibility is that it might promote endothelial injury by increasing the shearing stress on the endothelium.

It is noteworthy that the pulmonary arteries, in which the pressure is low, are usually not affected by atheroma except in patients with pulmonary hypertension, e.g. in mitral stenosis.

Cigarette smoking. The incidence of IHD in cigarette smokers is at least double that in non-smokers, and the risk increases with the number of cigarettes smoked daily. The duration of the habit does not appear to be an important factor and this, together with the fact that sudden deaths from IHD are especially increased in smokers, suggests that smoking may promote coronary artery thrombosis rather than atheroma itself. As mentioned earlier, inhalation of cigarette smoke has been shown to cause vascular endothelial injury in rabbits. It has also been shown that plasma fibrinogen, clotting factor VIII and the haematocrit levels are all raised in chronic smokers and that nicotine stimulates release of noradrenaline and thus promotes vasocontraction. The role of smoking in atheroma and IHD thus appears complex.

Physical activity. The Framingham and other studies have demonstrated beyond doubt that the incidence of IHD is lower in people who are physically active than in more sedentary individuals. Exercise may be protective by using up lipids and carbohydrates for energy production, and study of the blood lipids has demonstrated relatively high levels of HDL in active subjects: as stated above, HDL appear to protect against atheroma.

Psychological factors. Emotional stress appears to predispose to IHD, perhaps by increasing the output of catecholamines. Psychological factors may also play an indirect role by influencing choice of occupation, smoking or eating habits.

Prospective studies have shown that the various risk factors are synergistic: for example, an individual who smokes and has a high blood cholesterol level, hypertension and obesity, is *especially* likely to develop IHD. The factors predisposing to IHD have been shown (e.g. by Kannel *et al.*, 1976) to contribute also, in various degrees, to the risk of developing cerebral infarction and ischaemia of the lower limbs, both of which are nearly always complications of atheroma.

Systemic hypertension

Definition

Blood pressure usually increases with age, but there is considerable individual variation in the increase, and recordings of the blood pressures in a general adult population show a wide range. Any definition of hypertension must therefore be arbitrary, and there is no general agreement on the level of blood pressure to be regarded as pathological. Indeed, there is good evidence, for example from insurance companies' statistics, of a general inverse relationship between the height of the blood pressure, including variations within the 'normal range', and the expectation of life.

Classification

In about 85 per cent of cases of hypertension the cause is not apparent and these patients are said to have **primary, essential** or **idiopathic** hypertension. In the remaining 15 per cent hypertension is **secondary** to other disease processes: nearly always diseases of the kidneys are responsible (**'renal hypertension'**) but occasional cases result from certain functioning adrenal tumours or as a feature of Cushing's syndrome (see Table 14.1). Coarctation of the aorta (p. 428) is accompanied by hypertension in the arteries arising proximal to the constriction. It is likely that, as diagnostic techniques improve,

further causes of hypertension will be identified, and the proportion of patients with so-called essential hypertension will thus become smaller. Conn's syndrome (primary hyperaldosteronism, p. 1041) is an example of a condition which has been distinguished relatively recently from essential hypertension.

Table 14.1   Classification of systemic hypertension

I. Essential { benign / malignant   *[handwritten: or idiopathic; 85%]*

II. Secondary { benign / malignant   *[handwritten: 15%; 2 nearly always]*

(*a*) of renal origin ('renal hypertension'), due to:

[handwritten: most important]
chronic pyelonephritis
glomerulonephritis
diabetes
polycystic disease of the kidneys
renal amyloidosis
connective tissue diseases, particularly polyarteritis
urinary tract obstruction (occasional cases)
renal artery disease
radiation nephritis
some renal tumours
some congenital diseases of kidney, possibly by predisposing to pyelonephritis

(*b*) adrenal-mediated hypertension.
Conns' syndrome (primary hyperaldosteronism)
Cushing's syndrome
phaeochromocytoma

(*c*) coarctation of the aorta.

Regardless of the aetiology, hypertension may be divided into **chronic** or so-called **'benign'**, and **malignant** (sometimes called **accelerated**) types. In benign hypertension the rise of blood pressure is usually moderate, although sometimes marked. Many patients with benign hypertension lead active lives for many years with few or no symptoms, and die of some independent disease. Unless the blood pressure is controlled by antihypertensive drugs, however, it frequently causes disability and death from heart failure, and also increases the risk of myocardial infarction and cerebral vascular accidents.

Malignant hypertension is characterised by a very high blood pressure, by eye changes which include retinal haemorrhages and exudates and sometimes papilloedema, by rapidly progressive renal injury terminating in uraemia, and by hypertensive encephalopathy. The pathological hallmark of this state is fibrinoid necrosis of arterioles (see later). These special features appear to depend on the rapid development of a very high blood pressure. Unless treated, patients with malignant hypertension usually die within six months or so, but frequently the blood pressure can be reduced by anti-hypertensive drugs, and the outlook is then greatly improved.

Benign and malignant hypertension should not be regarded as unrelated conditions. Malignant hypertension supervenes in a small proportion of cases of benign essential hypertension although more often it arises apparently *de novo*, i.e. without evidence of preceding benign hypertension.

Changes in the blood vessels

Changes develop in arterial vessels of all sizes as a result of hypertension. In the larger arteries, from the aorta down to vessels of about 1 mm diameter, the changes are widespread, and are termed **hypertensive arteriosclerosis**. Changes in the vessels below this size, i.e. in the smallest arteries and arterioles, tend to affect especially the small vessels of the viscera, and in particular those of the kidneys. The changes occurring in the larger arteries are of the same nature in all types of hypertension, but those in the smaller vessels, particularly the arterioles, are different in benign and malignant types of hypertension, and require separate descriptions.

Large and middle-sized arteries. The vascular changes in hypertension, uncomplicated by the arterial lesions common in the aged, are most readily studied in young patients with high blood pressure secondary to renal disease. **In the early stages** they consist mainly of hypertrophy of smooth muscle and elastic fibres. In the aorta, there is increase in both of these elements in the media. In muscular arteries the increase is mainly in the circular muscle of the media (Fig. 14.13) but also in the longitudinal muscle fibres of the intima (Fig. 14.1, p. 361); the internal elastic lamina becomes thickened, and very often new laminae are formed towards the intima (Fig. 14.14). **In longstanding hypertension**, which is usually of benign essential type, these hypertrophic changes give way to fibrous replacement of muscle and the

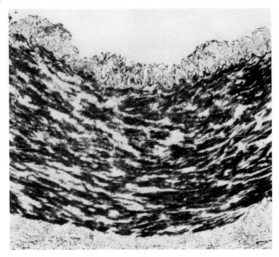

Fig. 14.13 Section of hypertrophied radial artery, from a case of chronic glomerulonephritis in a young subject, showing hypertrophy of the media. (Myocytes appear black.) × 140.

elastic tissue may break up and undergo partial absorption. The arterial walls are thickened and of increased rigidity, the lumen is dilated (Fig. 14.15) and the vessels are often elongated and tortuous. In the aorta, there is increase in the elastic and fibrous tissue of the media. In the muscular arteries, the media is thickened and fibrosed with patchy loss of smooth muscle,

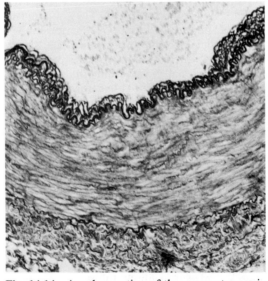

Fig. 14.14 Another section of the same artery as in Fig. 14.13, showing increase of elastic tissue formed by replication of the internal elastic lamina. (Elastic tissue appears black.) × 120.

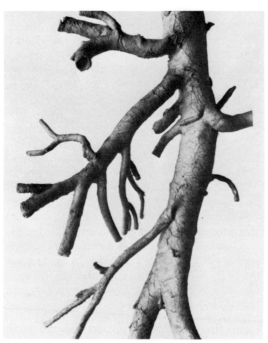

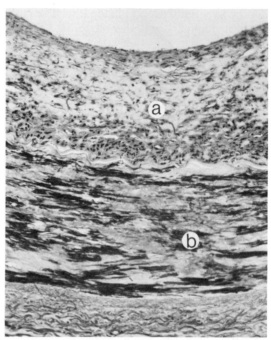

Fig. 14.15 Arteriosclerosis of the aorta and its branches in a patient with hypertension who died aged 36 from chronic renal failure. The walls of the vessels are thickened and rigid: they are also dilated, although this is not readily apparent. × 0·35.

Fig. 14.16 Part of a transverse section of an arteriosclerotic artery. The intima **(a)** is thickened, while the muscle (shown as black) of the media **(b)** is partly replaced by fibrous tissue. (Compare with Fig. 14.13.) × 200.

and there may be fibrous thickening of the intima (Fig. 14.16). These changes are widespread, and vary in degree. They are mostly without important effects. Hypertension increases the risk of rupture of the 'berry' aneurysms which develop in the arteries at the base of the brain in some individuals (p. 388), resulting in subarachnoid haemorrhage.

The arteriosclerotic changes described above are similar to those observed in normotensive elderly subjects (*senile arteriosclerosis*) but in the absence of hypertension they are usually less pronounced, and the media, although fibrosed, is often not thickened.

Atheroma tends to be particularly severe in individuals with chronic hypertension, and there is no doubt that prolonged elevation of the blood pressure aggravates this condition.

Hypertension thus results at first in hypertrophy of the arterial walls, with increase in muscle and elastic fibres, followed by arteriosclerosis and a tendency to severe atheroma. The early hypertrophic changes are usually observed only in young hypertensive subjects:

in older patients with chronic hypertension, arteriosclerosis and atheroma predominate.

Small arteries and arterioles. In arteries of 1 mm diameter or less, and in the arterioles, the changes differ from those in the larger vessels, and they differ also in benign and malignant hypertension.

(*a*) *Benign hypertension.* The small arteries show the medial thickening seen in the larger vessels, but a more pronounced degree of intimal thickening, due to concentric increase in connective tissue; in the smallest arteries the intimal change predominates, and may result in narrowing of the lumen in contrast to the dilatation seen in the larger arteries.

The *arterioles* undergo *hyaline thickening* of their walls (*hyaline arteriolosclerosis*), which consists at first of patchy deposition of hyaline material, often beneath the endothelium, but sometimes more peripherally: the hyaline change gradually extends to involve the whole circumference, and when severe it replaces the normal structures of the wall apart from the endothelium. This change occurs also apart from hypertension, and is seen especially in old age. In both normotensive and hypertensive subjects it is observed most commonly in arterioles in the spleen, then in the afferent glomerular arterioles of the kidneys (Fig. 14.17), and in

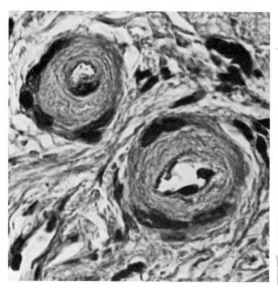

Fig. 14.17 Hyaline arteriolosclerosis of afferent glomerular arteriole in chronic systemic hypertension. The arteriole is not only thickened, but also tortuous, and so has been cut twice in cross-section in the same plane. × 1500.

the pancreas, liver and adrenal capsules. In all these sites, the change is appreciably commoner and usually more severe in hypertensives than in normotensive subjects of corresponding ages. Hyaline arteriolosclerosis is uncommon in the arterioles of the brain, gastro-intestinal tract, pituitary, thyroid, heart, skin and skeletal muscles (Smith, 1956). When severe, hyaline arteriolosclerosis results in considerable narrowing of the arteriolar lumen. This has important effects upon individual glomeruli, but does not usually cause renal failure. The nature of the change is not fully understood: initially, the hyaline material resembles fibrin in its staining properties, but later it stains like collagen. It also contains lipid material, and there is evidence that it may result from an exudative process in which plasma seeps into the arteriolar wall (p. 809). Apart from its occurrence as an ageing process and in hypertensive subjects, hyaline arteriolosclerosis is often severe and extensive in diabetes mellitus (pp. 840, 1033).

(*b*) *Malignant hypertension*. In this condition, the concentric fibrous thickening of the intima of the small arteries is often of extreme degree, particularly in the interlobular arteries of the kidneys (Fig. 22.10, p. 812). The arterioles are thickened and of hyaline appearance, as in benign hypertension, but the change is relatively acute, and consists of necrosis of the arteriolar wall, accompanied by permeation with plasma and deposition of fibrin (so-called **fibrinoid necrosis**): pyknotic nuclei, neutrophil polymorphs and red cells can often be found in the necrotic wall. The lumen is considerably narrowed, and superadded thrombosis may complete its occlusion. These changes affect especially the viscera, and the arteriolar lesions may result in haemorrhages and in ischaemic necrosis (Fig. 14.18). Focal fibrinoid necrosis may develop also in the small arteries.

In both benign and malignant hypertension, the changes in the small vessels in the kidneys cause renal damage, as described on pp. 809–12.

Cerebral haemorrhage in hypertensives is probably due to rupture of micro-aneurysms of the small arteries within the brain (p. 388).

Course of chronic and of accelerated hypertension

Chronic ('benign') essential hypertension. As already stated, this is much the commonest type of hypertension. The blood pressure rises very gradually over a period of years, in most cases to moderately high levels, e.g. 180/110 mm Hg, but occasionally much higher. The increase nearly always starts before the age of 45 years, and individuals with a resting blood pressure consistently below 140/85 at this age are very unlikely to develop essential hypertension. The diastolic pressure is less subject to physiological variations than the systolic pressure, and a diastolic pressure persistently exceeding 90 mm Hg is generally regarded, on an arbitrary basis, as abnormal. However, the disease develops very slowly, and it may be years before the rise in pressure clearly exceeds that which occurs normally with age.

The condition may be symptomless, and many cases come to light during routine medical examination for insurance or other purposes. *Common symptoms* include palpitations, audible pulsation in the head, headaches,

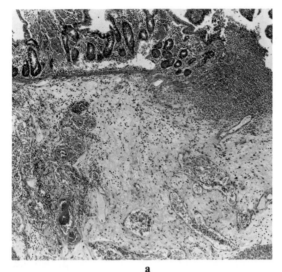
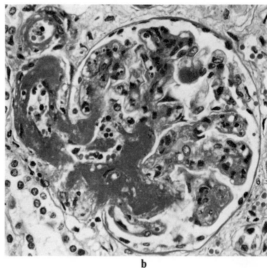

a   b

Fig. 14.18   Arteriolar lesions in malignant hypertension. **a** Ulceration of the colonic mucosa due to fibrinoid necrosis and thrombosis of arterioles: one such vessel is seen (*lower left*) in the submucosa. **b** Fibrinoid necrosis of a glomerular afferent arteriole and part of the tuft.

attacks of dizziness particularly on stooping, and reduced exercise tolerance.

About 60 per cent of deaths in those known to have 'benign' essential hypertension are from left ventricular or total heart failure; this is due to the increased work load thrown on the left ventricle and to the commonly associated severe coronary artery atheroma. About 30 per cent of patients die from cerebral haemorrhage, and the remaining 10 per cent from various causes unrelated to the hypertension. Although changes occur in the kidneys as a result of the vascular lesions, renal failure is uncommon in benign essential hypertension. When heart failure develops, however, there is usually a moderate rise in the blood urea level. In those patients who progress from chronic to malignant hypertension renal failure commonly supervenes.

Malignant ('accelerated') essential hypertension. This develops in approximately 10 per cent of cases of chronic essential hypertension. In those cases not preceded by chronic hypertension, the onset is usually between 30 and 45 years. It can result in heart failure or cerebral haemorrhage, but *without effective treatment renal injury is severe and usually causes death within a few months* (p. 811).

Eye changes are another important feature in malignant hypertension: lesions in the small arteries in the retina result in oedema, haem-

orrhages, infarcts and exudates, and blindness may ensue. Papilloedema, associated with cerebral oedema, is often present. *Hypertensive encephalopathy*, characterised by epileptiform fits and transient paralysis, is not uncommon, and is attributable to cerebral oedema, resulting from arterial spasm and focal cerebral ischaemia. This has been observed directly in rats with experimental hypertension and the fits have been shown to cease when the blood pressure is lowered and cerebral vasoconstriction ceases.

Secondary hypertension. Hypertension is a feature of **chronic renal failure**, and is more often of malignant type than is the case in essential hypertension. The superadded imposition of further renal injury from hypertensive vascular lesions, whether benign or malignant, aggravates and accelerates renal failure.

Aetiology of hypertension

In all types of hypertension, the raised blood pressure is a result of increased peripheral vascular resistance. In normal circumstances the peripheral resistance is controlled by the muscular tone in the arterioles throughout the body, and the major aetiological problem is the elucidation of the factors which, by increasing arteriolar tone, bring about the various types of hypertension. The possibility that the structural changes of arteriolosclerosis initiate the hypertensive state is unlikely, for such changes are sometimes absent, particularly in early cases, and moreover structural changes do not develop in arterioles which are protected from hypertension by occlusive changes in the larger arteries supplying them. For these reasons, it is widely believed that the observed structural changes in the arteries and arterioles are the result of hypertension, and not the cause. It is likely, however, that structural changes in the arterioles and small arteries of the kidneys impair renal blood flow, and this may play a part in *maintaining* hypertension once the vascular changes have become pronounced.

Humoral vasoconstrictive factors. In patients with hypertension due to a phaeochromocytoma, the large amounts of catecholamines released by the tumour into the blood (see p. 1047) are very likely to be the cause of the hypertension.

The vasoconstrictor substances renin and angiotensin (p. 258) are believed to be of importance in the pathogenesis of malignant hypertension secondary to renal disease: plasma concentrations of both renin and angiotensin are increased in this disorder. By contrast, their levels in most patients with benign essential hypertension are quite normal, and in patients with Conn's syndrome (primary aldosteronism, p. 1041) plasma renin concentration is actually reduced. Nevertheless, it cannot be concluded from this that renin and angiotensin do not contribute to the increased blood pressure in these conditions, as sensitivity to the pressor effects of injected angiotensin is known to be increased in hypertensive patients, and thus the normal or subnormal amounts of angiotensin in the blood might conceivably raise the blood pressure to abnormal levels.

Search for other vasoactive substances in the blood of patients with hypertension has failed.

Renal hypertension. A firm experimental basis for renal hypertension was provided in 1934 by Goldblatt and his colleagues, who showed that partial clamping of the renal arteries produced hypertension in dogs. This has been confirmed repeatedly in several species and it has been shown that hypertension can be produced in the rat by partial clamping of one renal artery. Vascular hypertensive changes have been produced by this method, and it is of interest that they do not

affect the kidney which is protected by the clamp from hypertension. Experimental hypertension of short duration produced in this manner may be abolished by removing the clamp or excising the clamped kidney, but if the clamp has been left in place for some months, the hypertension persists in spite of these manipulations, because of arteriolar changes produced in the unclamped kidney.

Renal hypertension in man is similar in many ways to the experimental condition. The diseases which cause it are listed in Table 14.1 on p. 370 and are described in Chapter 22: because of their relatively high incidence, *chronic glomerulonephritis* and *chronic pyelonephritis* are the most important ones. Release of excess renin from the abnormal kidney or kidneys may be an important factor in producing hypertension in such diseases, but the original view that the hypertension is due simply to the pressor effect of excessive renin production by the ischaemic kidney is now known to be an oversimplification. High levels of renin have usually been found only in malignant hypertension with underlying renal disease, and even in these the importance of renin is not fully established.

Secondary hyperaldosteronism in hypertension. In some cases of severe hypertension, particularly those with malignant hypertension and/or renal disease, secondary hyperaldosteronism develops. Plasma renin concentration is invariably increased and this leads to stimulation of aldosterone secretion which in turn produces potassium depletion (see p. 1038). The condition is recognised usually by a decrease in the concentration of potassium, and often of sodium, in the plasma. It must be distinguished from primary hyperaldosteronism (Conn's syndrome) in which the hypertension and hypokalaemia are associated with *increased* sodium and *decreased* plasma renin concentration (see p. 1041).

Neural factors in the pathogenesis of hypertension. The possibility that neural factors may play a role in primary hypertension deserves consideration. There is evidence that in both human and experimental hypertension the threshold of the vascular receptors is elevated, so that abnormally high pressures are necessary to initiate neurogenic anti-pressor reflexes. It may also be that variations in sensitivity to pressor agents, possibly genetically determined, are involved.

Pulmonary hypertension

In contrast to systemic hypertension, a rise in blood pressure in the pulmonary arterial system is usually explicable on the basis of disease of the lungs, heart or major vessels. These causes, and the effects of pulmonary hypertension, are described on pp. 454–7.

Calcification of the media (Mönckeberg's sclerosis)

Definition. This is a degenerative disease of unknown cause characterised by dystrophic calcification (p. 287) in the media, especially common in the major arteries of the lower limbs in elderly people. It may also affect the arteries of the upper limbs, and less commonly visceral arteries.

Naked-eye appearances. The affected vessels are generally dilated and show transverse bars of medial calcification due to deposition of calcium in the circular medial muscle layer (Fig. 14.19). At a later stage, lengths of the arteries may be converted into rigid tubes. There may be no noteworthy alteration of the intima though atheroma is sometimes present in addition.

Microscopy shows that the earliest change is hyaline degeneration of the muscle fibres and connective tissue, usually starting about the middle of the media (Fig. 14.20). Calcium salts are deposited first as fine granules, and confluent calcification follows. There may be little or no cellular reaction. Occasionally true bone may be formed in an area of calcification, and may even contain red marrow.

Aetiology. This is generally regarded as an exaggeration of the natural increase of calcium salts in the arteries with age. It sometimes

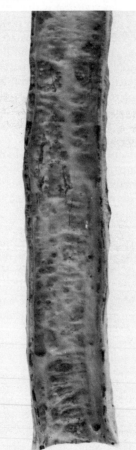

Fig. 14.19 Calcification of media of iliac artery, showing transverse markings caused by confluent calcification. × 0·8.

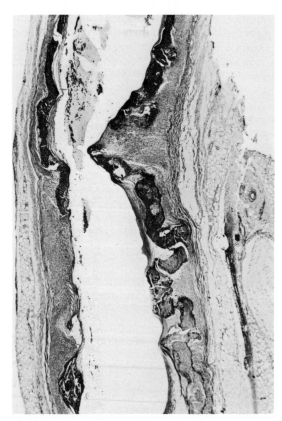

Fig. 14.20 Calcification of media. The calcified tissue is darkly stained. × 16.

occurs earlier in arteriosclerotic vessels but in man is not intimately related to high blood pressure. A similar lesion has been produced in the aorta of rabbits by injections of adrenaline.

Effects. The radiological appearance is striking but the lumens of the arteries are seldom narrowed. Ischaemic effects, if present, are usually due to co-existing atheroma and its complications.

Inflammatory lesions (arteritis)

Syphilitic arteritis

Small arteries. Wherever syphilitic lesions occur there is intimal and adventitial fibrosis of small arteries associated with infiltration of lymphocytes and plasma cells (endarteritis and periarteritis). In some cases the change is diffuse and a number of the vessels show general thickening, while in others it is of a patchy or nodular type.

Effects. Reduction of the lumens of small arteries and arterioles due to endarteritis may contribute to the necrosis in gummas. The essential change in syphilitic mesaortitis is probably involvement of the small nutrient vasa vasorum of the aortic media. Effects purely attributable to ischaemia are seen in the brain in tertiary syphilis (meningovascular syphilis) due to endarteritis obliterans of cortical vessels (Fig. 21.36, p. 753) and this may be complicated by thrombosis leading to cerebral infarction at an early age.

Syphilitic mesaortitis. This is a common manifestation of tertiary syphilis and an important cause of death in this disease. It occurs in acquired and congenital syphilis but has become increasingly rare in most developed countries.

Naked-eye appearances were formerly readily studied in untreated young subjects before the onset of arteriosclerosis and atheroma. The first visible lesions are greyish-white translucent areas of thickening in the intima, with little tendency to degenerate. Later they extend and fuse, forming areas with wrinkled 'tree bark' appearance: the intima between appears healthy (Fig. 14.21). In places, contraction of the tissue may occur with formation of stellate scars. Localised depressions which are potential aneurysms may be seen. In older subjects, yellow patches of atheroma, which is often

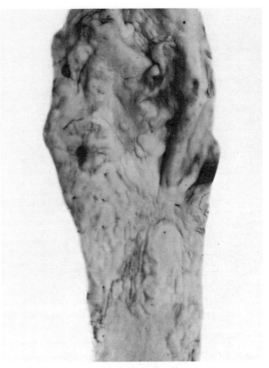

Fig. 14.21 The thoracic aorta in syphilitic aortitis. The arch of the aorta is stretched, with localised bulgings, thickened intimal patches and irregular wrinkling and scarring. In this example the changes stop abruptly below the arch. × 0·5.

severe, may be associated with the syphilitic lesions. Occasionally, on cutting through the wall of the aorta, gummatous necrosis may be seen extending inwards from the adventitia.

The part of the aorta immediately above the aortic valve is usually involved first and the aortic arch is by far the commonest and at times the only part of the aorta with syphilitic lesions. Syphilitic changes are usually limited to the thoracic aorta.

Microscopic appearances. The earliest change is periarteritis and endarteritis of the vasa vasorum in the adventitia (Fig. 14.22). These changes then extend into the aortic media, in which foci of cellular infiltration appear (Fig. 14.23), with new formation of thin-walled vessels. This leads to breaks or windows in the elastic tissue and muscle of the media, best seen in a section stained to show the elastic fibres (Fig. 14.24). The elastic tissue and muscle are replaced by fibrous tissue, but gummatous necrosis may also occur.

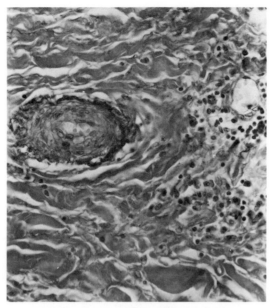

Fig. 14.22 Syphilitic aortitis, showing severe endarteritis of an arteriole in the adventitia of the aorta, and infiltration by plasma cells and lymphocytes around two small vessels (*right*). × 330.

Dense fibrous thickening of the intima occurs over the lesions of the media (Fig. 14.24), and vasa vasorum may extend into these intimal patches which account for the pearly-white raised areas seen by naked eye.

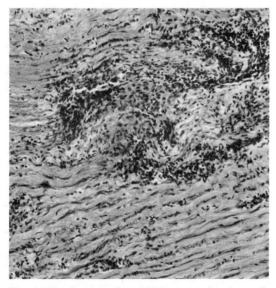

Fig. 14.23 Section of syphilitic aorta, showing cellular accumulations around the small vessels in the media, with destruction of the laminae. × 160.

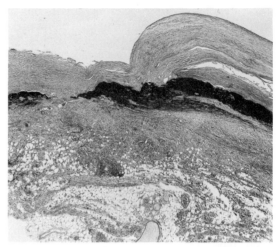

Fig. 14.24 Syphilitic aortitis; elastic tissue appears black. The section shows part of a thickened intimal plaque (*upper right*) and irregularity, thinning and interruptions in the elastic tissue of the media, which has also lost most of its muscle and is grossly thinned: the paler tissue below is the adventitia and adjacent fatty tissue. × 10.

Effects. *Aneurysm formation* is an important complication of syphilitic mesaortitis and is due to weakening of the vessel wall from loss of medial elastic and muscle tissue: the effects of aneurysm are described on p. 385.

Aortic incompetence. The dilatation of syphilitic aortitis may involve the root of the aorta, with consequent incompetence of the aortic valve. The cusps become stretched, thickened and distorted (p. 419).

Coronary artery narrowing due to involvement of their orifices by mesaortitis is now a rare cause of myocardial ischaemia.

Thromboangiitis obliterans (Buerger's disease)

Definition. Buerger's disease is an inflammatory condition of arteries and veins, with thrombosis, organisation and recanalisation of the affected vessels. It occurs almost exclusively in men, and affects mainly the vessels of the lower limbs, but sometimes also those of the upper limbs, giving rise to severe pain and progressive ischaemic changes.

Pathological changes. The early changes are not often available for histological examination. They consist of occlusion of the affected vessel by thrombus which contains foci of intense polymorph infiltration. The whole thickness of the vessel wall is also infiltrated with polymorphs. These acute changes give way to chronic inflammation, and the thrombus is replaced by granulation tissue containing lymphocytes, macrophages and multinucleated giant cells (Figs. 14.25, 14.26). The inflammatory changes eventually subside, and although the original vascular lumen has been obliterated there is often a surprising degree of recanalisation. The inflammation of the vessel wall also progresses to a chronic stage but without the degree of disruption which occurs in polyarteritis nodosa (see below). Fibrosis extends into the surrounding connective tissue, and the burned-out lesions thus consist of recanalised vessels with thickened fibrosed walls, enclosed in fibrous tissue which may envelop and compress adjacent nerves and vessels (Fig. 14.25).

The lesions affect short lengths of the small and medium sized arteries and veins of the legs and feet, but seldom the larger vessels. Similarly, when the upper limbs are affected, the lesions are mainly in the vessels of the forearms and hands. The disease is chronic, acute lesions

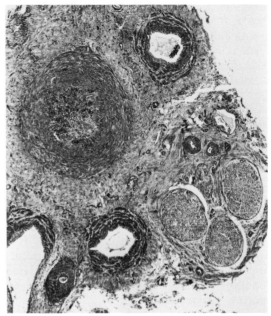

Fig. 14.25 Thromboangiitis obliterans. Occlusion of the posterior tibial artery (*upper left*) and surrounding fibrosis extending around the adjacent veins and nerves. × 32.

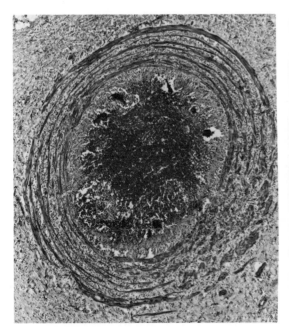
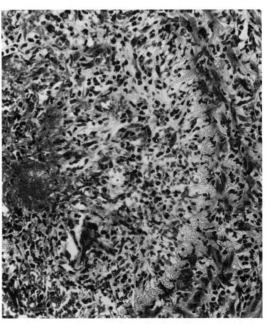

Fig. 14.26 Thrombophlebitis in Buerger's disease. *Left*, a superficial vein, showing inflammation of the wall, thrombosis and early organisation. Several multinucleated giant cells lie in and adjacent to the thrombus. × 60. *Right*, an older lesion with more advanced organisation of the thrombus: note the giant cell (*below centre*) and pleomorphic inflammatory infiltrate. × 250.

developing intermittently over a period of years. It may involve mainly either arteries or veins, but usually both. The changes of ischaemia, including gangrene of the extremities of the affected limbs, eventually result.

Aetiology. Features which distinguish Buerger's disease from atheroma with superadded thrombosis are its relatively early onset, inflammatory nature, predilection for smaller vessels, involvement of veins as well as arteries and of the upper limbs as well as the lower, and its rarity in women. Suggestions that the lesions are simply a variant of atheroma are almost certainly mistaken, and have probably arisen from the examination of limbs amputated after prolonged disease, when the lesions are burned-out and there is co-incidental atheroma. It is also a misconception that the disease occurs especially in Jews, but a high incidence of HLA antigens A9 and B5 in sufferers has been reported, suggesting a genetic predisposing factor.

The inflammatory nature of the early lesions suggests a specific causal agent (as was postulated by Buerger) but none has been detected. The single known important predisposing factor is cigarette smoking. The disease is practically confined to heavy smokers, and there is a strong clinical impression that its progress is arrested or diminished by giving up smoking. Hypersensitivity to tobacco proteins has been suggested as a causal factor.

Clinical features. The symptoms are varied and depend on the degree of arterial obstruction. The earliest are pain, paraesthesia and circulatory disturbances e.g. local redness which disappears on elevating the limbs. On walking there is often cramp-like pain and inability to progress—'*intermittent claudication*'; this is a result of ischaemia of the calf muscles and occurs in other forms of arterial disease. Later, more severe trophic changes appear, including intractable ulceration, and gangrene which is apt to spread slowly (Fig. 14.27); amputation, sometimes repeated, is often necessary but the need for surgery may be minimised by therapy which improves the collateral circulation. In view of the widespread involvement of the arteries, amputation, if required, should be performed at a high level. If the vessels of the arms are severely affected, the condition may simulate Raynaud's disease in the male.

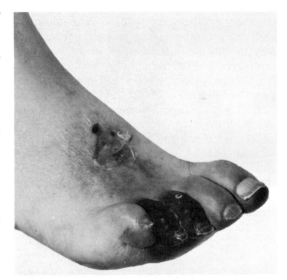

Fig. 14.27   Gangrene of part of the foot and toes in a case of thromboangiitis obliterans.

Polyarteritis nodosa (*Periarteritis nodosa*)

The lesions of this disease consist of multiple foci of necrosis, inflammation and usually thrombosis, followed by healing, in the walls of medium sized and small arteries and arterioles. Vessels in any part of the body may be affected, and there is involvement of many organs and tissues. In its most severe form, with many simultaneous acute lesions, it is rapidly fatal from haemorrhage due to rupture of a weakened artery, or more often from ischaemia of vital organs. Most cases are, however, chronic, with acute lesions developing over years, and usually causing death from ischaemic effects. The condition occurs over a wide age range, but predominantly between 20 and 40.

Pathological findings. The early lesion consists of a focus of fibrinoid necrosis of the media and intima of a small or medium sized artery (up to about 3 mm diameter) or an arteriole. Necrosis is accompanied by acute inflammation with polymorph infiltration (often including eosinophils) of the whole thickness of the vessel wall and particularly intense in the adventitia and surrounding tissue (Fig. 14.28). Lesions affect the whole circumference of smaller arteries, but often only a segment of the wall of the larger vessels (Fig. 14.29). Occlusive thrombosis is common in the acute stage, but in some cases there is severe haemorrhage. The acute changes progress to more chronic inflammation, with replacement of the necrotic vessel wall by fibrous tissue infiltrated with lymphocytes, plasma cells and macrophages, and the thrombus undergoes organisation. The weakened wall may stretch to form an aneurysm (Fig. 14.30),

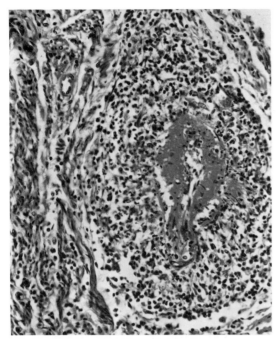

Fig. 14.28 An acute lesion of polyarteritis nodosa in a small artery in the kidney. There is fibrinoid necrosis and an intense inflammatory cellular infiltrate in and around the wall of the artery. × 100.

but even without this the healed lesion may project as a nodular thickening of the vessel wall, and microscopy then shows a sharply-defined zone of fibrous replacement of the artery wall.

The lesions are multiple; they occur in almost any small or medium-sized artery or arteriole, but are commonest in those of the kidneys, heart, gut, liver, pancreas and nervous system, and in the skeletal muscles. Their effects, apart from haemorrhage, are due to acute or chronic ischaemia, and depend on the distribution of the lesions and arterial anastomoses in particular sites. Infarcts and patches of chronic ischaemic atrophy result in the heart, kidneys, etc.

The disease may be severe and progress rapidly to death, but more often the course extends over some years, with periods of quiescence alternating with the development of new lesions. In most cases, death eventually results from lesions in the kidneys, heart or other vital organs.

Clinical features depend on the number and sites of lesions, and as these are widespread and vary greatly in their distribution, the clinical features also show great variation. In severe cases there is fever, prostration, neutrophil (and sometimes eosinophil) leukocytosis and a very high ESR. In less acute cases the disease fluctuates, with quiescent periods and exacerbations. Lesions in the peripheral nerves (Fig.

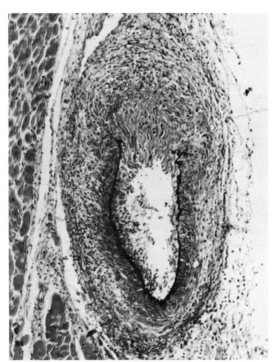

Fig. 14.29 Polyarteritis nodosa involving a coronary artery. The lesion is less acute than in the previous figure. Part of the circumference of the vessel wall (*above*) has been severely damaged, with interruption of the internal elastic lamina (stained black) and replacement of the inner part of the wall by fibrous tissue. There is more diffuse inflammatory cellular infiltrate. × 70. (The late Dr. Janet Niven.)

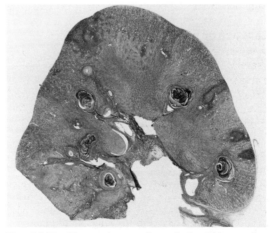

Fig. 14.30 Transverse section of the kidney of a patient who died of acute polyarteritis nodosa. In this instance, the necrotising lesions have resulted in aneurysmal dilatations, together with thrombosis. This has led to multiple infarcts. × 1·4.

21.66, p. 782) result in paraesthesias, and symptoms may arise from ischaemia of virtually any tissue. Angina, cardiac failure, renal failure and hypertension are among the commoner clinical manifestations, but infarction of the gut, etc., can also cause death.

Diagnosis depends on suspecting the disease from the clinical features, blood changes, etc., and confirmatory biopsy. The choice of tissue for biopsy depends on the clinical features, but confirmation is often obtainable from skeletal muscle biopsy, particularly if tissue is removed from a tender spot in a muscle. Inflammatory changes are much more severe than in the necrotising arteriolar lesions of malignant hypertension.

Aetiology. The arterial lesions of experimentally-induced acute immune-complex disease (p. 154) resemble those of polyarteritis nodosa. To explain the development of acute lesions over a prolonged period, as in polyarteritis nodosa, it is necessary to assume that fluctuations in the plasma levels of postulated antigen and antibody results, from time to time, in the formation of heavy concentrations of immune complexes in the circulation. In support of the disease being due to a hypersensitivity type 3 reaction, immunoglobulins and products of activation of complement have been demonstrated in the acute lesions. The disease sometimes complicates systemic lupus erythematosus and the lesions in such cases are presumably due to complexes of auto-antibodies with DNA, etc. (p. 164). Approximately 50 per cent of cases arise in chronic carriers of hepatitis B virus with circulating HBsAg-Ab complexes, and HBsAg has been demonstrated in the acute lesions in some such cases. In many cases, however, the postulated antigen has not been identified, although there is often an association with various drugs, notably sulphonamides and penicillin.

Variants of polyarteritis nodosa

A microangiopathic form of polyarteritis nodosa affects mainly arterioles and very small arteries in the kidneys and elsewhere, and gives rise to microangiopathic haemolytic anaemia (p. 531) and uraemia, sometimes without hypertension: the renal lesions include **focal** and **rapidly progressive glomerulonephritis** (p. 821). In many instances the condition appears to be a hypersensitivity reaction to drugs or micro-organisms.

Wegener's granulomatosis is a variant in which lesions in vessels in the nasopharynx result in an ulcerating granulomatous lesion, and lesions also tend to occur especially in the lungs and kidneys.

Localised polyarteritis, with lesions indistinguishable from polyarteritis nodosa, occurs in the gallbladder and appendix, and has an excellent prognosis. *Necrotising vasculitis of the skin* is a complex subject (p. 1065). The lesions of polyarteritis nodosa can remain confined to the skin for some years, but there are other, localised forms of dermal vasculitis which are distinct from polyarteritis nodosa.

Other forms of arteritis

Idiopathic aortitis in Africans. An inflammatory lesion affecting all parts of the aorta has been described in young Africans. There is infiltration of the adventitia and media with lymphocytes and plasma cells, and destruction of the elastic tissue, ending in dense collagenous fibrosis. The mouths of the renal arteries are often involved, resulting in unilateral or bilateral renal artery stenosis often leading in turn to hypertension. Micro-organisms have not been demonstrated and the aetiology of the lesion is unknown.

Tuberculosis. Marked periarteritis and endarteritis sometimes occur in relation to tuberculous lesions. They are often a prominent feature in tuberculous meningitis, especially with late or inadequate treatment (Fig. 21.33, p. 751). These changes may lead to complete obstruction of the vessel and cerebral infarction. Occasionally, however, the wall of an artery adjacent to a pulmonary tuberculous cavity may be weakened before obliteration occurs and an aneurysm may form (p. 478).

Rheumatic arteritis. Lesions similar to those found in the heart in rheumatic fever occur in the walls of large arteries. In the aorta they commence in the adventitia and consist of an infiltration of the tissues with lymphocytes and plasma cells. There may be foci of histiocytes, and typical Aschoff bodies with characteristic cells (p. 412) may form. The cellular infiltration may spread into the media and lead to absorption of elastic tissue, but this rarely extends beyond the outer third of the media. Such lesions do not weaken the wall sufficiently to produce aneurysms.

In the smaller arteries, rheumatic lesions of various distribution have been found, especially in the visceral branches. They are acute and may be accompanied by necrosis of the media as well as by leukocyte infiltration; they thus resemble the lesions of polyarteritis nodosa but thrombosis and aneurysms have not been found. Further work is required to establish the relation of rheumatism to disease of the smaller arteries. The lesions are clinically silent, but they may form the basis of the subcutaneous lesions which commonly occur in rheumatic fever and illustrate its systemic nature.

Aortitis in ankylosing spondylitis. Unexplained lesions of the aortic valve and ascending aorta, identical in appearance to syphilitic arteritis but without serological evidence of syphilis, sometimes develop in males with ankylosing spondylitis.

Giant-cell or temporal arteritis. This is a fairly uncommon condition, occurring mostly in old people of both sexes. It affects mainly arteries of the head, but is sometimes much more widespread, and the aortic arch and its major branches are occasionally involved. Diagnosis is often based on clinical examination and biopsy of the temporal artery, which is conveniently superficial and often affected.

The lesion is an inflammation of the whole thickness and whole circumference of the affected arteries, affecting either a continuous length of the vessel or appearing as multiple focal lesions along it. The vessel wall is infiltrated with leukocytes (mainly polymorphs) in the early stages, but the subsequent reaction is granulomatous, with accumulation of lymphocytes, macrophages and multinuclear cells (of both Langhans' and 'foreign-body' types) which sometimes appear to develop in relation to fragments of the disrupted internal elastic lamina. Fibrous thickening of the intima, fibrous replacement of the media, and commonly thrombosis and organisation, result in a severely scarred vessel with a narrowed or obliterated lumen (Fig. 14.31).

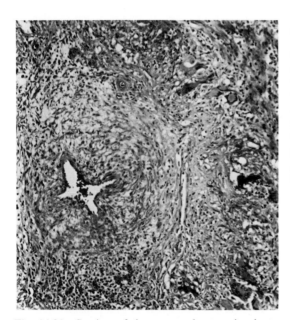

Fig. 14.31 Section of the temporal artery in giant-cell arteritis, showing multinucleated giant cells lying in relation to the internal elastic lamina (now disrupted and seen only as small fragments). There is gross intimal thickening, possibly from organisation of thrombus, and a very narrow lumen. × 120.

Clinically there may be localised reddening of the skin over an affected vessel, which is usually tender or painful and sometimes nodular. Depending on which arteries are involved, there may be headache, visual disturbances and even blindness (from involvement of the retinal arteries), facial pain, and sometimes cerebral infarction and other features resulting from more extensive arteritis. In some instances, the disease occurs in association with polymyalgia rheumatica. It is of entirely unknown aetiology and usually self-limiting.

Takayasu's disease. This is a rare condition, first reported from Japan, in which the aorta and the large arteries arising from the aortic arch are affected by an arteritis which may resemble syphilitic aortitis, caseating tuberculosis or temporal arteritis. Intimal thickening, sometimes with superadded thrombosis, severely narrows or occludes the subclavian, carotid and innominate arteries (hence the term *pulseless disease*), with resulting ischaemia of the head and arms. The disease affects mainly young women, and the aetiology is unknown. Occasional cases with vascular occlusions suggestive of Takayasu's arteriopathy are encountered in Britain, but the patients are usually older, and may be of either sex: these cases are attributable to severe atheroma or syphilitic arteritis of the major arteries.

Thrombotic microangiopathy (thrombotic thrombocytopenic purpura)

This is characterised by the deposition of homogeneous eosinophilic material, at least some of which is fibrin, in the intima and lumen of visceral arterioles, without an associated inflammatory reaction. It sometimes accompanies, and may belong to, the group of connective tissue diseases. Further details are given on p. 531.

Raynaud's disease

Nomenclature. In 1862 Maurice Raynaud described a series of cases of intermittent impairment of the circulation through the extremities, usually presenting as an abnormal response to exposure to cold. It has since become apparent that these effects can occur in subjects with or without organic vascular disease. There has been considerable confusion over nomenclature, but it is now customary to apply the term *Raynaud's disease* to cases apparently due wholly to abnormal angiospasm and to group together under the term *Raynaud's phenomenon* cases in which organic vascular changes play a major role.

Raynaud's disease occurs mainly in women, usually starting in adolescence and often continuing indefinitely. It usually affects the fingers, but occasionally the tip of the nose, ears and toes. Involvement is symmetrical, e.g. the fingers in both hands are equally susceptible. On exposure to cold the fingers become cold, white or cyanotic and may be numb or extremely painful. The circulation is restored by warmth, but trophic changes may occur in the skin and whitlows are common: ulceration and gangrene seldom occur unless exposure to cold is prolonged.

Histological reports on the condition are few, because material is not usually excised unless gangrene develops. Thickening of the digital arteries has been reported, but these vessels are normally very thick walled, and reports of thickening have usually been erroneous. In cases where gangrene develops, however, there may be thrombosis and recanalised vessels may be found (Fig. 14.32).

The condition appears to be an exaggeration of the normal response to exposure to cold. Pre-ganglionic sympathectomy is not curative.

Raynaud's phenomenon. This consists of symptoms similar to those of Raynaud's disease, but attributable to organic vascular disease. It may result from a number of different conditions, including thromboangiitis obliterans, use of vibratory power tools (e.g. pneumatic drills), acrosclerosis, systemic lupus erythematosus, cold-antibody auto-immune haemolytic anaemia and cryoglobulinaemia.

Involvement is not always symmetrical, and sympathectomy does not usually improve the condition. Both sexes are affected and, depend-

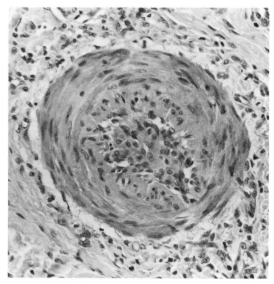

Fig. 14.32 Transverse section of a digital artery in Raynaud's disease. The lumen is obliterated by cellular fibrous tissue which has resulted from organisation of thrombus. × 250.

ing on the causal condition, gangrene may develop.

Raynaud's phenomenon can result from vasoconstriction in response to cold superimposed on organic vascular disease, from arrest of the circulation in the extremities by cryoglobulins, and from agglutination of red cells in cold-antibody auto-immune haemolytic anaemia.

Aneurysms

Definition. An aneurysm is a local enlargement of the lumen of an artery.

Classification. A *true* aneurysm is formed by local dilatation of an artery, the blood being contained by the stretched vessel wall, or, when this is no longer recognisable, the surrounding connective tissue. A *diffuse* or *fusiform* aneurysm involves the whole circumference of the wall symmetrically whereas the *saccular* type is an asymmetrical bulge communicating with the artery through an aperture which does not involve the whole circumference. These terms may not be applicable to advanced lesions, which are often very irregular in form.

The term *dissecting aneurysm* is used to describe a condition in which the wall of an artery (usually the aorta) splits, and blood tracks along the media, separating the inner from the outer layers. Some other lesions are described as aneurysms (p. 389).

Pathogenesis. The force which expands an aneurysm is the blood pressure, but for an aneurysm to form there must be an arterial lesion which weakens the media locally. Stretching usually results in further weakening, so that once an aneurysm has started it tends to expand and commonly ruptures. Occasionally thrombus forms in thick layers which fill the whole sac (Fig. 9.19, p. 239).

Atheromatous aneurysm

In Europe and N. America, atheroma is now the most common cause of true aortic aneurysm, due to the decline and early treatment of syphilis and the concurrent increase in atheroma. Atheromatous aneurysms occur usually after the age of 50, and much more commonly in men than women. They are usually fusiform (Fig. 14.33) and may rupture while still quite small. The aneurysm forms as a result of pressure atrophy of the media over atheromatous

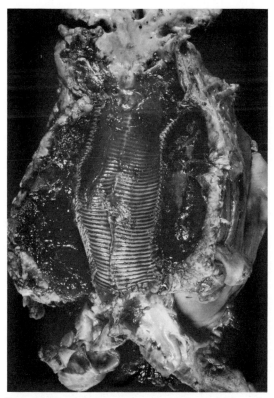

Fig. 14.33 Atheromatous aneurysm of the abdominal aorta arising below the origins of the renal arteries. The aneurysm, which is fusiform, has been repaired by a dacron tube, but death resulted from haemorrhage from rupture at the suture line.

plaques or actual extension of the plaque into the media. The microscopic changes seen at the edges of the aneurysm are those of atheroma, sometimes with a marked leukocytic reaction around the fatty debris, and there may be some lymphocytic infiltration round the vasa vasorum in the adventitia and media. These aneurysms are usually a complication of *severe* atheroma and affect especially the abdominal aorta or a common iliac artery. They usually arise below the level of the renal arteries.

Effects. Large aneurysms are very liable to rupture with retroperitoneal haemorrhage, the clinical features being those of an acute surgical abdominal emergency. In some cases thrombosis of the aneurysmal sac results in ischaemia in the legs, kidneys, etc. Pressure effects are not conspicuous.

Syphilitic aneurysm

This occurs as a complication of syphilitic aortitis, usually above the age of 40. Large aortic aneurysms were previously due in most instances to syphilis, but are now very rare as a result of successful treatment in the primary and secondary stages of the disease. The commonest site is the aortic arch, because it is the part most frequently affected by syphilitic mesaortitis (p. 377), of which aneurysm is a complication. The focal loss of elastica and muscle in the media results in weakening of the wall, and there may be diffuse dilatation of the ascending aorta and arch: more localised stretching results in a fusiform or saccular aneurysm, which is often accompanied by smaller aneurysmal bulgings, along with the stellate scars and intimal thickening characteristic of syphilitic mesaortitis. As an aneurysm forms, the elastic tissue and muscle of the artery wall soon degenerate and the sac comes to be composed of layers of fibrous tissue, on which laminated thrombus forms (Fig. 9.19, p. 239). Blood may infiltrate the wall of the aneurysm and ooze for some distance into the tissues around; accordingly the limits of the aneurysm are badly defined.

Effects. *Pressure* on surrounding structures leads to the syndrome of superior mediastinal compression; the great veins may be displaced and undergo thrombosis, resulting in congestion of the head and neck and enlargement of collateral veins. Involvement of the oesophagus may cause dysphagia, while pressure on a major bronchus may cause a chronic cough and suppurating bronchopneumonia. Aneurysms of the transverse part of the aortic arch may compress and stretch the left recurrent laryngeal nerve and cause paralysis of the left vocal cord. Rigid structures such as the bodies of vertebrae may be eroded and the bare bone come to form part of the wall of the sac; the intervertebral discs offer greater resistance to absorption and persist longer.

Rupture of an aneurysm may occur into practically any tube or cavity in its neighbourhood, and occasionally takes place externally through the chest wall.

Embolism from thrombus formed within an aneurysm is uncommon.

Cardiac hypertrophy and dilatation occur only when the syphilitic mesaortitis results in aortic-valve incompetence. Otherwise aortic aneurysms, even very large ones, do not affect the heart as there is no interference with cardiac output.

Dissecting aneurysm

This is now the commonest cause of rupture of the aorta. In most cases it results from rupture of the inner part of the wall of the aorta (Fig. 14.35) often due to degenerative changes in the media in which the elastica and muscle are replaced, in an irregular, patchy manner, by a metachromatic mucoid substance (Fig. 14.34) and the surviving elastica often appears fragmented. These changes are known as **Erdheim's medial degeneration**. Sometimes there are small areas of necrosis with softening (*medionecrosis*) but in our experience this is rare. The cause of these changes is unknown and in some cases of dissecting aneurysm they are not apparent. Dissecting aneurysm is commonest in people over 40 years old, usually with high blood pressure, but it occurs also in young people without hypertension, and is commoner in men than in women.

The event which causes dissecting aneurysm is a sudden transverse tearing of the inner part of the aortic wall, through which blood from

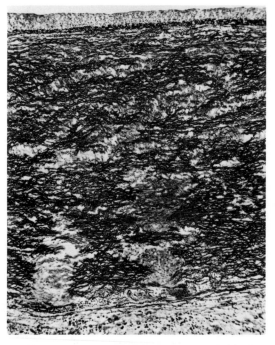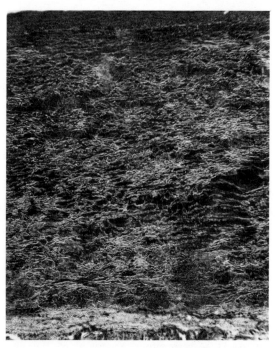

Fig. 14.34 Medial degeneration of the aorta. There are gaps in the elastic tissue of the media, which is stained black in the left illustration. In the right photomicrograph, myxoid ground substance is stained black and is patchily increased. The patient was a woman of 24 who died of spontaneous rupture of the aorta. × 50.

the lumen penetrates into the weakened media. The tear is usually in the ascending aorta and may extend around almost the whole circumference (Fig. 14.35). Much less commonly, it occurs just distal to the point of insertion of the ductus arteriosus. It tends to occur during physical exertion and is probably brought about by the frictional tractive force of the blood during systole, which thrusts the intima in the same direction as the blood flow. Because of the weakened media, the inner part of the wall slides to and fro with each heart-beat and eventually ruptures. Blood tracks between the inner two-thirds and outer third of the media, effectively dissecting the inner part of the wall from the outer part.

In some cases, the outer part of the aortic wall is ruptured almost immediately by the pressure of blood entering the media, with fatal haemorrhage. Occasionally the dissection re-

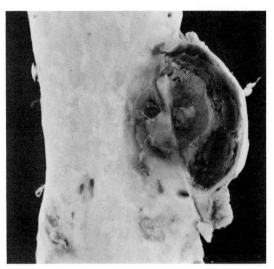

Fig. 14.36 Localised dissecting aneurysm; the space in the media is filled with dense thrombus. × 1·2.

mains localised (Fig. 14.36) and clotting and organisation of the blood in the media results in healing. In most cases, however, blood tracks proximally and distally in the media. Commonly it reaches the aortic ring and ruptures into the pericardial sac, causing death from cardiac tamponade. It may also track distally as far as the abdominal aorta and even into the iliac arteries, and rupture may result in haemorrhage into the mediastinum, pleura, retroperitoneal tissue or peritoneal cavity.

When dissecting aneurysm extends to the origins of branches of the aorta, it compresses and narrows the lumen of the branches and may extend along them: this can result in obstruction of the coronary arteries, branches of the aortic arch, mesenteric and renal arteries, etc., obviously with serious effects.

Occasionally a second tear develops, usually in the abdominal aorta, through which blood in the dissecting aneurysm re-enters the lumen. If the patient survives, the channel in the media may become lined by endothelium supported by fibrous tissue and 'double-barrelled' aorta results (Fig. 14.37).

Dissecting aneurysm is generally accompanied by severe tearing pain in the chest. If untreated, it is usually fatal within a few days, and even with surgical treatment the outlook is poor.

Marfan's syndrome. This is a disorder of connective tissue, inherited usually as an autosomal domin-

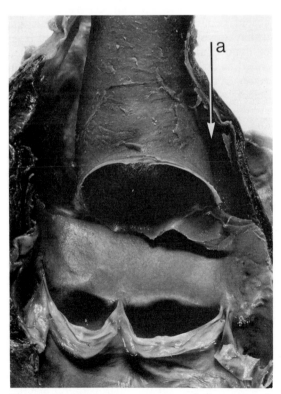

Fig. 14.35 Dissecting aneurysm of the aorta. A rupture of the inner part of the wall, above the aortic valve, extends almost around the circumference, and blood has tracked up between the inner and outer parts of the wall, producing a space, **a**, the so-called dissecting aneurysm. × 1.

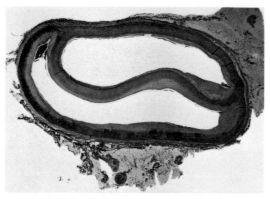

Fig. 14.37 Dissecting aneurysm of the aorta. In this case the blood burst back into the lumen through a second rupture, giving a 'double-barrelled' aorta, seen here in cross section. × 2·5.

ant, and characterised by laxity of ligaments, e.g. of joints and of the eye lens, inadequate elastic fibre formation in the aorta, tall slim build, long tapering fingers (*arachnodactyly*) and other skeletal abnormalities. Disturbances of vision result from subluxation of the lens, and there may also be deafness. The aortic media lacks elastic fibres, the appearances resembling those in Erdheim's medial degeneration. Fusiform aneurysm or dissecting aneurysm may result, and at necropsy there may be multiple healed aortic intimal tears.

Other causes of aortic rupture. Apart from aneurysm, rupture of the aorta may result from damage to its wall from outside, as by the perforation of an impacted fishbone or other sharp foreign body in the oesophagus; also from very severe injury such as crushing of the chest. In children traumatic rupture can occur without fracture of the ribs. Carcinoma of bronchus or oesophagus may invade the aortic wall and cause fatal haemorrhage.

Infective (mycotic) aneurysm

This may occur at the beginning of the aorta by direct extension of micro-organisms from vegetations in bacterial endocarditis, particularly *Staphylococcus aureus* (Fig. 15.32, p. 423). The organisms settle on the intima, an infective thrombus forms, invasion and weakening of the wall follow, and an *acute aneurysm* is produced, which may rupture; occasionally multiple aneurysms are present. In smaller arteries infective aneurysms result from lodgment of small infected emboli in the vasa vasorum, rather than from the presence of an infected embolus in the lumen of the artery. Inflammatory softening of the arterial wall results. Infective aneurysms may occur in a limb or viscus, and the effects are similar to those seen in the non-infective

aneurysms of polyarteritis nodosa (p. 380). Infected emboli in the lumen of an artery may give rise to acute inflammatory softening with rupture and cerebral haemorrhage, e.g. in staphylococcal pyaemia.

A mycotic aneurysm is sometimes seen in the wall of a tuberculous pulmonary cavity and may cause fatal haemoptysis. Usually, however, occlusion of the vessel by endarteritis obliterans or thrombosis prevents aneurysm formation.

Cerebral aneurysms

Berry aneurysms of the circle of Willis and its branches occur at all ages and appear to be due mainly to congenital weakness of the arterial wall. Evidence of this is destroyed when the aneurysm forms, but a deficiency in the medial muscle, especially in the acute angle between large branches, is demonstrable in other arteries at the base of the brain, and similar deficiencies are found in a small proportion of people without aneurysms. Probably as a result of stretching, the internal elastic lamina is absent in much of the wall of the aneurysm, which consists of a thin, often transparent layer of hypocellular fibrous tissue. Although often called *congenital*, most of these aneurysms develop from adolescence onwards. The muscle defect, which *is* congenital, and hypertension are contributory causes of aneurysm formation and rupture in older people. The aneurysms usually occur singly, but may be multiple: they are usually less than 1 cm diameter, but may be much larger. The commonest site is at the origin of the middle cerebral, followed by the anterior communicating artery (Fig. 14.38), but they may arise practically anywhere on the circle of Willis and its major branches. Rupture of these aneurysms is the principal cause of spontaneous subarachnoid haemorrhage, but in some cases the sac is buried in the cortex and they bleed into the brain. The effects of rupture are described more fully on p. 740. Quite commonly, an aneurysm becomes partly or completely occluded by thrombus (Fig. 14.39). Occasionally a fusiform aneurysm of the basilar artery develops as a result of atheroma.

Micro-aneurysms. The occurrence of multiple micro-aneurysms on the small cerebral arterial twigs in hypertensive subjects was described over a century ago, but they are difficult to find without special techniques, and only recently has their common occurrence been reaffirmed. In a painstaking study, Cole and Yates (1967)

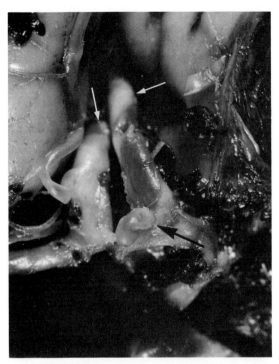

Fig. 14.38 Base of the brain showing subarachnoid haemorrhage which resulted from rupture of a berry aneurysm of the basilar artery (not shown). A second, intact berry aneurysm (*black arrow*) is seen on the anterior communicating artery. (The anterior cerebral arteries are marked by white arrows.)

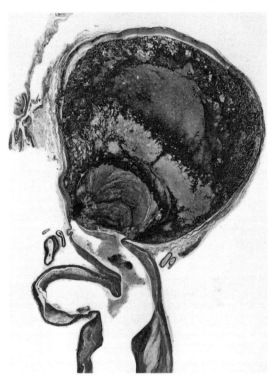

Fig. 14.39 Aneurysm of circle of Willis, almost completely filled with thrombus. × 7·5.

using a micro-angiographic necropsy technique reported the occurrence of multiple (usually 15–25) aneurysms of up to 2 mm diameter, occurring mainly on arteries of less than 250 μm diameter. They were detected in over 50 per cent of hypertensives over 50 years of age, and the incidence increased with age: in normotensives, the incidence was low, aneurysms being found only in a few subjects over 65 years old. The aneurysms were most numerous in and around the basal ganglia, and occurred usually at or near branchings of the striate arteries: they were found also in the subcortical white matter and in the mid-brain and cerebellum.

The aneurysms may be saccular or fusiform, and the adjacent artery and wall of the sac show hyaline thickening of the intima, sometimes with fibrinoid change: the internal elastic lamina is usually absent from, or fragmented in, the wall of the sac, and muscle is usually absent. Thrombus, sometimes organised, may fill the sac, and there is often evidence of old or recent leakage of blood into the surrounding tissues.

Cole and Yates detected micro-aneurysms in 18 of 20 hypertensives dying from cerebral haemorrhage, and they provide evidence which suggests strongly that rupture of such aneurysms is the usual cause of cerebral haemorrhage in hypertensive subjects (p. 740).

Other forms of aneurysm

Injury to the wall of an artery by a stab wound, etc., may result in the development of a **traumatic aneurysm**. It is difficult to understand how this can result from an injury which penetrates the whole thickness of the wall, and it seems more likely to be due to stretching of the fibrous scar resulting from healing of an incomplete laceration of the vessel wall.

Injury of an adjacent artery and vein may result in an arterio-venous fistula: in some instances the connection is by a channel with a fibrous wall, which may dilate to form an **arterio-venous aneurysm**.

A **cirsoid** or **racemose aneurysm** is a form of arterio-venous fistula which appears as a pulsatile swelling consisting of tortuous and dilated arteries and veins with multiple intercommunications. The commonest site is the scalp, and it may cause pressure atrophy of the underlying bone. The condition is sometimes congenital, but more often the result of a blow on the head; some of the allegedly congenital cases are probably the result of birth injury. Similarly a carotid-cavernous sinus aneurysm resulting from fracture of the skull base gives rise to great engorgement of the orbital veins and oedema of the orbit and conjunctiva.

Diseases of Veins

Compensatory enlargement of the veins takes place, as in the arterial system, when there is a sustained increase in blood flow, as in the uterine veins during pregnancy and in the collateral veins following obstruction of a major vein. As in the case of arteries, dilatation is followed by hypertrophy of the various elements in the wall of the vessels. Veins are, of course, not exposed to the marked variations of blood pressure which occur in arteries, but when they are subject to persistent over-distension, compensatory changes occur in their walls. There is little or no hyperplasia of the muscle, but the elastic tissue increases greatly and then undergoes degeneration; the fibrous tissue also increases and becomes hyaline (Fig. 14.40). Localised patches of thickening in the intima of veins are quite common and probably result from organisation of thrombus.

Acute thrombophlebitis

A distinction is sometimes made between *thrombophlebitis*, by which is meant a primary inflammatory condition of the vein, with secondary thrombosis, and *phlebothrombosis* (p. 239), in which a bland thrombosis of the vein occurs with, at most, mild preceding inflammatory change. In many instances the distinction is more theoretical than practical because the presence of thrombus in the lumen of the vein sets up reactive changes so that differentiation between mild thrombophlebitis and phlebothrombosis may no longer be possible. In **thromboangiitis obliterans**, however, veins are often affected and exhibit the same rather characteristic florid inflammatory lesions seen in arteries in this condition (Fig. 14.26, p. 379). The available evidence suggests that the inflammation is primary and the thrombosis a consequence of it.

Multiple venous thrombosis also occurs in **thrombophlebitis migrans** but without arterial involvement: it usually affects superficial veins, but sometimes also deeper ones, in any part of

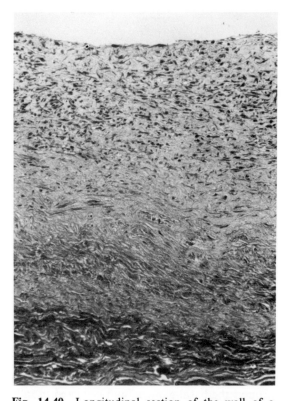

Fig. 14.40 Longitudinal section of the wall of a saphenous vein used to replace a length of an atheromatous coronary artery two years before death. The lumen is at the top and the dark fibres at the bottom are dense collagen fibres of the adventitia. The muscle coat of the media has undergone atrophy; the residual fibres are seen as an ill-defined dark layer near the periphery of the wall. Above this, the relatively acellular layer represents fibrosed and thickened media and the more cellular (inner) layer consists of greatly thickened intima which contains elastic fibres, collagen and large spindle cells. × 120.

the body. In many cases the cause is not apparent, but in others it is associated with a carcinoma, most often of the pancreas but also of breast, stomach, bronchus, ovary, etc. The thrombotic episodes may be the first clinical manifestation of the cancer. In some cases, small vegetations form on the cardiac valves.

Outbreaks of a condition known as **tropical thrombophlebitis** have been reported in Africans: thrombosis is widespread and death may result from involvement of visceral veins. The cause is unknown.

Infective thrombophlebitis used to be seen commonly in the veins of the diploë and dural sinuses in middle-ear disease, in the uterine veins in puerperal sepsis, in the veins of the bone marrow in suppurative osteomyelitis, and occasionally in the pulmonary veins in cases of bronchiectasis. Veins involved in such lesions undergo thrombosis and the thrombus becomes invaded by bacteria, and then by polymorphs: fragments may break away and produce pyaemia.

In the rare condition known as *pylephlebitis suppurativa (portal pylephlebitis)* infection, e.g. from appendicitis, involves a small tributary of the portal vein and leads to progressive ascending thrombosis and suppuration, from which multiple abscesses in the liver may result.

Thrombophlebitis may also appear as a complication of conditions in which there is a bacteraemia, notably typhoid fever, and it is presumed that organisms circulating in the blood settle in the intima and produce an acute endophlebitis with secondary thrombosis.

Chronic phlebitis

Chronic inflammatory processes may spread to the walls of the veins and lead to reactive thickening; in fact, the smallest veins are affected in this way in all chronic inflammatory conditions. Chronic phlebitis of obscure origin is occasionally observed in the large vessels, for example in the portal vein, and may lead to thrombosis; cavernous tissue develops in the portal fissure and after some time it may be impossible to say whether the changes are congenital or secondary to the thrombosis.

Endophlebitis of the hepatic veins is the basis of the veno-occlusive disease of Jamaica and certain other tropical regions (see p. 664) and involvement of the hepatic ostia with thrombosis gives rise to the Budd–Chiari syndrome (p. 664). Hepatic endophlebitis also results from infestation with liver flukes and schistosomes.

Tuberculous invasion of veins most commonly results when a caseous lesion—usually in a pulmonary hilar lymph node—involves and destroys the wall of a vein: huge numbers of tubercle bacilli then enter the bloodstream and cause generalised miliary tuberculosis.

Veins are often invaded by **malignant tumours** which may then release cells singly or in groups, with the danger of metastatic growth in the lungs, etc. Cancer may also grow along the lumen of veins, an example being clear-cell carcinoma of the kidney, which commonly extends along the renal vein and even the inferior vena cava. Such invasion is usually accompanied by thrombosis.

Varicose veins

Dilatation and tortuosity of veins is termed *varicosity*. The changes may affect a group of veins diffusely or take the form of saccular dilatations. Varicosity of veins arises from chronic continuous or recurrent increase in the pressure of the blood within them, and this results mainly either from (*a*) the effects of gravity, e.g. in the leg veins, sometimes aggravated by compression proximally, or (*b*) obstruction of a major vein, leading to increased pressure in collateral veins.

'Gravitational' varicosity occurs in the saphenous system of the legs, notably the long saphenous vein. The condition is much commoner in women and there is a distinct *hereditary predisposition. Prolonged standing* upright without much muscular movement causes marked rise in pressure and distension of the long saphenous vein, for the valves can only play their part in breaking the venous pressure gradient between the heart and the foot if assisted by the pumping action of muscular activity of the lower limbs. Eventually the veins become permanently stretched, so that the valves are now incompetent, and even muscular activity does not protect the veins from increased pressure in the upright position; in consequence, stretching tends to progress and the veins become visibly swollen and tortuous, i.e. varicose. Venous stasis occurs in the legs due to the pressure of the gravid uterus on the iliac veins and without doubt *pregnancy* is a predisposing cause of varicose veins; this probably accounts for the higher incidence in women, although *obesity* is also a predisposing factor. The venous valves and the muscle and elastic tissue of the vein walls atrophy somewhat irregularly so that thinning of the wall and pouchlike dilatations occur; finally the wall comes to be composed chiefly of fibrous tissue. The nutrition of the skin over varicose veins of the legs may be impaired. The skin becomes eczematous and pigmented, and chronic indolent '*varicose ulceration*' often follows: dilated veins involved in such ulcers may bleed severely, but this is easily stopped by raising the leg with the patient lying flat. Thrombosis is also apt to follow. Organisation of the thrombus is generally imperfect and it may become calcified.

Varicocele is another common example of 'gravitational' varicosity, in the pampiniform plexus of veins around the spermatic cord: it is commoner on the left side than on the right and various ingenious explanations have been suggested for this. The distended veins feel like a bag of worms. It often depresses spermatogenesis and impairs fertility, particularly if bilateral. This may be a temperature effect.

Haemorrhoids consist of varicosities of the haemorrhoidal venous plexuses, projecting from the surface just above or below the anorectal junction. They are common in preg-

nancy, probably due to the pressure of the uterus on pelvic veins, and also in people over 40 in whom constipation and straining at stool are causal factors. Portal hypertension, e.g. in cirrhosis, is also believed to be a predisposing factor.

Haemorrhoids may bleed and cause iron deficiency, or they may rupture into the perianal subcutaneous tissue, causing painful swellings. They may also become thrombosed or prolapse through the anal sphincter and become strangulated.

'Obstructive' varicosity. This is exemplified by chronic *obstruction to the portal venous blood flow* (due most commonly to cirrhosis or schistosomiasis of the liver), in which the vessels which form anastomoses between the portal and systemic venous systems become varicose (p. 692): the most important ones are those running longitudinally in the oesophageal and gastric submucosa (Fig. 19.22, p. 604), for they may rupture and bleed profusely. *Obstruction of the inferior vena cava* brings about dilatation of the veins of the abdominal wall, establishing a collateral circulation through the upper thoracic veins (Fig. 9.7, p. 231). *Obstruction of the superior vena cava* may occur in cases of bronchial carcinoma and leads to severe dusky cyanosis of the head, neck and arms, sometimes accompanied by pitting oedema of the hands.

Diseases of Lymphatic Vessels

The lymphatic vessels form a closed system separated by an endothelial layer from the tissue spaces. The walls of the small lymphatics are, however, extremely delicate, consisting mainly of a very thin endothelium and an incomplete basement membrane. Moreover, the junctions between endothelial cells are readily disrupted (p. 62). In consequence organisms, leukocytes and tumour cells readily pass into the lymphatic vessels; also red cells which escape from the capillaries by diapedesis may be present in large numbers in the lymphatics draining an inflamed area. The lymphatic vessels thus afford an easy means of communication between the tissues and lymph nodes. Involvement of the lymph nodes in this way occurs in two main conditions, **infections** and **tumours**, especially carcinoma. In both, the

extension may be due to transport of the organism or tumour cell by the lymph stream, i.e. metastasis in the strict sense. There may also be progressive involvement of the lymphatic vessels by the disease. In infections, this may involve either acute or chronic lymphangitis; in tumours, lymphatic permeation may occur, columns of cancer cells extending along the lymphatics (Figs. 12.21, 12.22, p. 333).

Acute lymphangitis. This is seen in pyogenic infections, and is a feature of erysipelas and infections of the hand, etc., due to haemolytic streptococci. The spread of infection along the lymphatics is sometimes accompanied by visible reddening of the overlying skin, with pain and tenderness and often swelling. Spreading lymphangitis is an important feature in puerperal sepsis and septic abortion and may be followed by cellulitis of the loose connective tissue around the uterus. In other cases of bacterial infection, the organisms are carried by the lymphatic vessels and reach the lymph nodes without causing lymphangitis. A similar striking example is seen in bubonic plague, where even at the site of infection there is usually no inflammatory reaction, the first lesion appearing in the related lymph nodes.

Chronic lymphangitis occurs in various conditions; it may follow *repeated acute attacks of erysipelas*, and is an important feature in many types of *chronic inflammation*. In various chronic infections the spread of organisms by the lymphatics is of great importance. In *tuberculosis*, a disease which in the early stages may be regarded as essentially one of the lymphatic system, the organisms may be carried to lymph nodes without causing lesions on their way. They may, however, settle in the walls of the lymphatic vessels and give rise to tubercles which thus come to form rows along the vessels. In tuberculous ulceration of the intestine, small tubercles may be found along the lymphatics passing from the floor of the ulcer (Fig. 19.60, p. 633), and also in the mesenteric lymphatics. The thoracic duct may become involved by spread of bacilli along the lymph stream and ulceration of these lesions may set free a large number of tubercle bacilli into the circulation to set up acute miliary tuberculosis (p. 212).

In *syphilis* also, chronic lymphangitis is a prominent feature in connection with the primary lesion, and induration spreading along the lymphatics leads to the characteristic bubo in the regional lymph nodes.

Lymphatic obstruction: lymphoedema. Chronic obstruction of lymphatics may give rise to interstitial accumulation of lymph (lymphoedema). When this is prolonged there is proliferation of connective tissue in the lymphoedematous area, resulting in a firm, non-pitting oedema. The most striking examples are seen in *filariasis*, in which obstruction of major lymphatics, together with recurrent inflammation in the affected region, may lead to gross thickening of the tissues known as **elephantiasis**: the lower limbs and sometimes the male external genitalia may be involved (see below) In non-tropical countries, extensive carcinomatous permeation of lymphatics is a more common cause, but surgical removal of lym-

phatics or destruction of lymphatics by radiotherapy also cause lymphoedema. This is sometimes seen following radical mastectomy and radiotherapy of the axilla for breast cancer, where the arm may be sufficiently deprived of its lymphatic drainage to develop gross lymphoedema without carcinomatous involvement of lymphatics. Several instances of tumour growth resembling lymphangiosarcoma have been observed in the lymphoedematous arm. It is not clear whether they are true sarcomas, or metastatic breast carcinoma the appearance of which is modified by the lymphoedematous environment.

Filariasis

A number of species of Filarioidae, a family of nematode worms, infest man in tropical and sub-tropical countries. Infestation results from transmission of larvae in the bite of infested mosquitoes. The larvae mature into adult worms in the human host, and the female produces *microfilariae* which are transmitted to man-biting female mosquitoes, in which the life-cycle is completed.

Bancroftian filariasis, caused by *Wuchereria bancrofti* is the most widespread and important form of filariasis. It occurs in West, Central and East Africa, Egypt, parts of Central and South America, and in South East Asia.

The adult worms are filiform, white and show wriggling movements: the female is almost 80 mm long, 0·3 mm wide, and the male is smaller and thinner with a spirally twisted tail. The adults colonise the lymphatic vessels and the sinuses of lymph nodes, particularly in the inguinal region, spermatic cord and upper arm: they may also infect the para-aortic lymph nodes and sometimes the thoracic duct.

Acute inflammatory reactions, possibly due to hypersensitivity, may develop in relation to the adult worms, involving the spermatic cord or epididymis, testis and inguinal lymph nodes. A more severe granulomatous reaction occurs when the adult worms die and disintegrate: granulation tissue containing tubercle-like follicles forms around the dead worms and extends to involve adjacent tissues and blood vessels, often with resultant venous thrombosis. This chronic inflammatory reaction results in obliteration of the lymphatics with consequent lymphoedema and permanent and sometimes enormous swelling (**elephantiasis**) which may affect the lower limb, scrotum, vulva and occasionally the arm or breast. Chronic hydrocele may also develop. The lymphatics in the lymphoedematous tissue are distended and the skin is at first tense and shiny, later scaly and rough. Secondary bacterial infection and ulceration may occur. If the thoracic duct or abdominal lymph nodes are involved, there may be chylous ascites (escape of abdominal lymph into the peritoneal cavity).

The diagnosis of infestation may be made by detecting microfilariae in the peripheral blood, bearing in mind their presence in the bloodstream mainly at night. The microfilariae are unsheathed, about 250 mm long, and are rendered conspicuous in a wet film of peripheral blood by the commotion of adjacent red cells caused by their vigorous movements. Methods for concentrating microfilariae in the blood are available. Certain differentiation from other microfilariae requires examination of a stained preparation. Microfilariae may also be detected by skin biopsy (Fig. 14.41). In chronic cases with elephantiasis, there may be no surviving adult worms and microfilariae often cannot be found. Serological and skin tests are also used in the diagnosis.

A somewhat similar form of filariasis is caused in Asia by *Brugia malayi*, in which the distribution of the adult worms and so of the lesions is different.

Loiasis, due to the filaria *Loa loa*, occurs in West and Central Africa. The adult worms live and move around in the connective tissues throughout the body and are occasionally seen wriggling in the conjunctiva! They induce superficial inflammatory lesions (fugitive or Calabar swellings) which persist for a few days and are probably due to a hypersensitivity reaction. Heavy infestation is associated with fever, vague pains, ill-health and sometimes

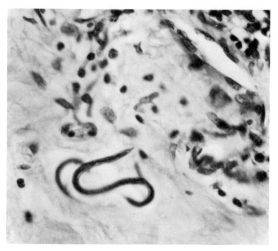

Fig. 14.41   Microfilariae of *Wuchereria bancrofti* in a skin biopsy. × 200.

intense itching. The unsheathed microfilariae appear in the blood during the daytime, presumably as an adaptation to the *Chrysops* vector mosquito which hunts man in daylight.

Onchocerciasis is caused by infection with *Onchocerca volvulus* and occurs in equatorial Africa and tropical America. It is transmitted to man by *Similium* flies which live along the banks of rivers. The adult worms are entwined in groups often ensheathed in fibrous tissue, causing subcutaneous swellings, particularly over bony projections in the lower limbs and, in tropical America, in the scalp. The female is about 500 mm long and the male is much smaller.

Microfilariae are produced from about a year after infestation, and migrate in the dermis and subcutaneous tissue. They do not circulate in the blood, but have a predilection for the conjunctiva, the chambers of the eye and optic nerve, where their presence may result in blindness.

References

Benditt, E. P. (1977). Implications of the monoclonal character of human atherosclerosis plaques. *American Journal of Pathology* **86**, 693–702.

Cole, F. M. and Yates, P. O. (1967). The occurrence and significance of intracerebral micro-aneurysms. *Journal of Pathology and Bacteriology* **93**, 393–411.

Goldstein, J. L. and Brown, M. S. (1977). The low-density lipoprotein pathway and its relation to atherosclerosis. *Annual Review of Biochemistry* **46**, 897–930.

Kannel, W. B. (1971). Serum lipid precursors of coronary heart disease. *Human Pathology* **2**, 129–51.

Kannel, W. B., McGee, D. and Gordon, T. (1976). A general cardiovascular risk profile. *American Journal of Cardiology* **38**, 46–51.

Smith, J. P. (1956). Hyaline arteriosclerosis in spleen, pancreas and other viscera. *Journal of Pathology and Bacteriology* **72**, 643–56.

World Health Organisation (1970). Classification of hyperlipidaemias and hyperlipoproteinaemias. *Bulletin of the World Health Organisation* **43**, 891–908.

Further Reading

Atherosclerosis—a new look at the problem (1977). Symposium in the *American Journal of Pathology* **86**, 655–702.

Ross, R. and Glomsett, J. A. (1977). The pathogenesis of atherosclerosis—a new look. *New England Journal of Medicine* **297**, pp. 369–77, 420–25.

Woolf, N. (1978). The pathogenesis of atherosclerosis. In *Recent Advances in Histopathology*, No. 10, pp. 45–67. Edited by P. P. Antony and N. Woolf. Churchill Livingstone, Edinburgh, London and New York.

See also Further Reading for Chapter 15, p. 430.

15

The Heart

Disease of the heart now causes more deaths in Western countries than disease of any other organ, amounting to more than a third of all deaths in England and Wales according to the Registrar General's Statistical Review for 1977. Atheroma and thrombosis of the coronary arteries account for most of these deaths by causing ischaemic heart disease in its various forms. The other frequent causes of cardiac disease include systemic arterial hypertension, chronic diseases of the lungs which cause pulmonary hypertension, rheumatic and other lesions of the heart valves, congenital abnormalities, thyrotoxicosis and anaemia. The relative importance of these conditions varies greatly throughout the world.

The work of the heart. Assuming that at rest the stroke volume of the heart is 66 ml and the rate 72 beats per minute, the left ventricle has a minute volume of about 5 litres, and a daily output of 7200 litres (about $7\frac{1}{2}$ tons). The normal heart has great reserve power, and this can be substantially increased by physical training. During exertion, there is a greater venous return to the heart with consequent increase in diastolic filling and stretching of the muscle fibres; the response is a more vigorous contraction (Starling's law) and the blood pressure is raised. The rate of contraction also increases during exertion and these two factors together can raise the minute volume to about seven times that of the resting state.

This physiological performance can be maintained only if (1) the myocardium is intrinsically healthy, (2) the valves function efficiently and (3) the conducting system of the heart co-ordinates contraction of the chambers. Disturbance of any of these requirements can cause cardiac failure.

Cardiac Failure

Definition. Cardiac failure is that state in which the ventricular myocardium fails to maintain a circulation adequate for the needs of the body despite adequate venous filling pressure. Failure of one or both atria is common, but the effect on cardiac function is relatively unimportant unless ventricular function is also deficient.

Causes

Cardiac failure is due to weakness or inefficiency of myocardial contraction, to an abnormal increase of the work required of the myocardium, or to a combination of both. These two basic causes may be further classified as follows.

(1) Intrinsic pump failure. This is most commonly due to *weakness of the ventricular contraction*, the commonest cause of which is myocardial ischaemia resulting from coronary artery disease. Other causes of myocardial weakness include myocarditis, severe toxic bacterial infections and congestive cardiomyopathy.

Systolic emptying of the affected ventricle(s) is incomplete because the force of contraction is reduced, and during diastole the chamber dilates to contain both the residual blood and that received from the atrium. The dilated chamber works at a disadvantage because the force required to provide a given pressure is greater in a large than in a small chamber. Consequently, unless the cause is reversible, dilatation and failure tend to be progressive. Moreover, left or right ventricular dilatation results in stretching and incompetence (functional incompetence) of the mitral or tricuspid valve respectively, and this, as described below, increases the work of the dilated ventricle.

A less common cause of intrinsic pump failure is *impaired compliance of the myocardium* which in plain language means that the ventricles are too stiff to relax and fill properly during diastole, as in hypertrophic cardiomyopathy and amyloid disease of the heart. The abnormal rigidity may also interfere with myocardial contraction. By restricting cardiac filling, pericardial haemorrhage or effusion and restrictive pericarditis can produce similar effects.

Disorders of cardiac rhythm, resulting from various conditions, are also included in this group. Although minor irregularities such as sinus arrhythmia and occasional extrasystoles do not significantly impair cardiac function, severe tachycardia so shortens the time for diastolic filling of the ventricles and diastolic flow in the coronary arteries that the efficiency of the heart is substantially decreased; this happens in atrial fibrillation and flutter and the paroxysmal tachycardias. The bradycardia seen in complete heart block (about 30 beats a minute) causes a marked fall in cardiac output.

(2) Increased pressure load results from any condition which increases the resistance to expulsion of blood from the ventricles. The commonest causes affecting the left ventricle are systemic hypertension and aortic valve stenosis, while resistance to emptying of the right ventricle is usually due to pulmonary hypertension resulting from various diseases of the lungs and from mitral stenosis.

If the cause is chronic, the affected chamber undergoes hypertrophy, but eventually dilatation and failure develop.

(3) Increased volume load. This arises when a ventricle is required to expel more than the normal volume of blood. It occurs when, owing to incompetence of a heart valve, some of the blood leaks backwards (e.g. through the aortic valve during diastole), and also in conditions in which the general circulation is increased, e.g. anaemia, thyrotoxicosis, and hypoxia resulting from lung disease. Other causes include shunts between the left and right sides of the circulation, and arterio-venous shunts.

(4) Coincidence of multiple factors. Each of the above aetiological groups may independently produce cardiac failure, but various factors often operate simultaneously. For example, a patient with mitral stenosis and myocardial fibrosis due to previous rheumatic fever may have only impaired exercise tolerance (i.e. diminished cardiac reserve) without evidence of cardiac failure at rest; with the onset of atrial fibrillation cardiac failure at rest may develop. An individual with systemic hypertension may develop cardiac failure as a result of occlusion of a minor coronary artery which would go virtually unnoticed but for the hypertension, or cardiac failure may be precipitated by an attack of pneumonia in a person with pulmonary hypertension due to chronic lung disease.

Manifestations of cardiac failure

In mild failure, cardiac function is adequate for the needs of the body at rest, and failure becomes apparent as undue breathlessness on exertion; this is attributable to congestion of the lungs, which stimulates respiratory reflexes. In more severe cardiac failure, cardiac output is inadequate even at rest and structural changes in various organs result. The nature of the changes depends on the duration of the cardiac failure, and on which ventricle predominantly fails.

Acute cardiac failure is due to conditions of sudden onset, e.g. coronary artery occlusion, pulmonary embolism, acute infections, the hypertension of acute glomerulonephritis, the development of an arrhythmia, or rupture of a chamber or valve cusp. When cardiac failure is acute and severe (most often due to myocardial infarction) the acute fall in cardiac output, with consequent diminished tissue perfusion, results in a reaction closely similar to that in hypovolaemic shock, with selective vasoconstriction. The term *cardiogenic shock* (p. 263) is appropriate, but the central venous pressure is raised, and the principles of treatment are quite different: the full picture of shock develops in only a small proportion of cases, but when it does occur the outlook is poor. Conversely, acute heart failure may develop as a result of severe, prolonged hypovolaemic or septic shock (pp. 262–4). In both of these circumstances, if death occurs rapidly the organs behind the failing ventricle show acute venous congestion, and the distinction between cardiogenic shock and heart failure resulting from shock may depend on the presence or absence of a causal lesion (usually a myocardial infarct) in the heart.

Chronic cardiac failure may follow acute cardiac failure if death or recovery does not occur rapidly. In cardiac disease of gradual onset, e.g. acquired valvular lesions, chronic failure is particularly common. At death the changes of generalised chronic venous congestion (see p. 228) are found, and the heart will show the features of the causative lesion, the dilatation of failure and in some instances compensatory enlargement of the chambers. These are described below.

Left ventricular failure causes 60 per cent of deaths in untreated essential hypertension, and is a common cause of death in myocardial infarction, a condition which mainly affects the left ventricle. It is also often the cause of death in patients with disease of the aortic valve. The clinical and pathological manifestations are predominantly pulmonary, for the left ventricle fails to maintain its output and, in the presence of an efficient right ventricle, blood accumulates in the pulmonary circulation causing congestion in the lungs. Severe breathlessness, cyanosis and pulmonary oedema are the outstanding clinical features. There may be no evidence of right ventricular failure, though some congestion of the neck veins is usual. Paroxysmal nocturnal attacks of dyspnoea are common in systemic hypertensive patients and are due to acute left ventricular failure, perhaps from resorption of peripheral oedema fluid when the patient is recumbent at night. At necropsy there is dilatation of the left ventricle and functional mitral incompetence: acute or chronic venous congestion of the lungs is found with pulmonary oedema and froth in the bronchi.

Right ventricular failure in its most acute form is found in cases of massive pulmonary embolism. The more chronic forms are found in pulmonary arterial hypertension due to lung disease (e.g. fibrosis or chronic bronchitis and emphysema) and to mitral stenosis. In pure right ventricular failure an excess of blood accumulates in the systemic veins, and in addition to the causal lesion there will be dilatation of the right ventricle with functional tricuspid incompetence, distension of the great veins,

e.g. in the root of the neck, and acute or chronic venous congestion of the liver, spleen and kidneys (p. 228 *et seq*). Oedema, ascites, etc., are conspicuous in untreated advanced cases. Right ventricular failure also occurs in mitral stenosis, but there is, in addition, chronic venous congestion of the lungs, with or without pulmonary oedema. The rise in pulmonary venous pressure results in pulmonary arterial hypertension due to increased tone of the pulmonary arterioles.

Total heart failure combines the features of left and right ventricular failure and is found not only in diseases which cause diffuse myocardial damage (e.g. extensive infarcts, myocarditis) but also in states requiring a persistently high cardiac output (thyrotoxicosis, etc.). In addition, when there is left ventricular failure the strain imposed on the right side of the heart by the raised pulmonary pressure sooner or later leads to right ventricular failure.

In some cases of heart failure due to lack of ventricular compliance, there may be little or no ventricular dilatation.

Hypoxic phenomena. When left ventricular output falls suddenly and markedly, the cerebral blood supply is so diminished that the patient loses consciousness. This may be momentary, as in a vaso-vagal attack (p. 260), or it may be rapidly fatal when due to occlusion of a main coronary artery, massive pulmonary embolism or rupture of a cardiac chamber. When the condition is reversible, e.g. during an attack of complete heart block, transient loss of consciousness may occur (*Stokes-Adams attack*); similar attacks occur in patients with incompetence of the aortic valve. In chronic cardiac failure, oxygen deficiency in the tissues is less marked and is seen clinically in the form of cyanosis, sometimes accompanied by mental confusion. Pathologically, the effects of stagnation hypoxia are best seen in tissues such as liver where centrilobular loss of liver cells is usually present in association with venous congestion. A compensatory increase in red cells (erythrocytosis) may occur due to hypoxia.

Cardiac oedema is dealt with on pp. 255–6.

Thrombo-embolic phenomena. Patients with cardiac failure are especially prone to develop deep venous thrombosis in the legs as a result of venous stagnation and muscular inactivity associated with lying in bed: in consequence, there is a serious risk of pulmonary embolism. Thrombus is also common in the atria and, in some forms of heart failure, in the ventricles: such cardiac thrombi, depending on their site, can give rise to pulmonary or systemic emboli. These complications are described in Chapter 9.

Compensatory enlargement of the heart

When extra work is imposed on the myocardium as a result of a chronic disease (e.g. a valvular lesion or hypertension) **compensatory myocardial hypertrophy** occurs in the walls of the affected chambers and enables them to deal more effectively with the increased work of maintaining the circulation. In conditions of increased volume load, due for example to valvular incompetence, the affected ventricle(s) dilate passively during diastole to contain an increased volume of blood, thus compensating in some degree for the blood which, instead of passing onwards, is regurgitated through the leaking valve. This occurs before the supervention of heart failure, i.e. when ventricular systolic emptying is normal, and has been termed **compensatory dilatation**. Use of the term 'compensatory' for passive over-dilatation is perhaps not well justified, but it does serve to emphasise the difference from the dilatation of ventricular failure, in which emptying is incomplete due to weakness of the myocardial contraction. Both hypertrophy and compensatory dilatation cause cardiac enlargement, which is further increased by the dilatation of cardiac failure.

The limiting factors in cardiac hypertrophy are not understood. A likely one is the difficulty in maintaining adequate myocardial perfusion and respiratory exchange when the diameter of the fibres is increased. Because of the vascular arrangements of the coronary supply, ventricular hypertrophy renders the inner part of the myocardium particularly liable to ischaemia in the presence of coronary artery disease (p. 404).

The assessment of cardiac enlargement. In left ventricular hypertrophy, the weight of the heart is increased above the normal 300–350 g often to over 500 g. Because of its smaller mass, hypertrophy of the right ventricle is only occasionally sufficient to increase markedly the total heart weight. Although hypertrophy of either ventricle is usually obvious at necropsy

from the increased thickness of its wall (Fig. 15.1), the degree of hypertrophy is not readily assessed without taking account of the volume of the chambers, i.e. the degree of dilatation. A more reliable method is to separate and weigh the individual ventricles, making allowance for epicardial fatty tissue and any gross fibrous scars, etc.

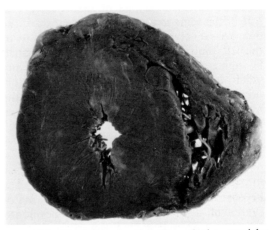

Fig. 15.1 Transverse section through the ventricles of the heart in a case of systemic hypertension, showing obvious hypertrophic thickening of the left ventricle. × 0·5.

Increase in size of the hypertrophied heart is often not readily assessed by clinical or radiological measurements unless there is also dilatation, in which case it is difficult to distinguish, from size alone, between the two processes.

Characteristic electrocardiographic changes accompany ventricular hypertrophy, especially when only one ventricle is involved.

Causes of left ventricular hypertrophy. The common causes of marked left ventricular hypertrophy are (1) systemic hypertension (essential, or secondary to renal disease, coarctation of the aorta and certain endocrine tumours); (2) stenosis of the aortic valve; (3) compensatory dilatation of the left ventricle (in aortic or mitral incompetence); (4) persistently high cardiac output (thyrotoxicosis, anaemia, arterio-venous fistula and Paget's disease of bone). Mild and focal left ventricular hypertrophy is found in the absence of hypertension or valvular lesions in certain patients with healed myocardial infarcts, and is presumably compensatory for the loss of muscle. Various cardiomyopathies (p. 408) are a less usual cause of hypertrophy.

Causes of right ventricular hypertrophy. Most examples of right ventricular hypertrophy are attributable to pulmonary arterial hyertension. The common causes are (1) chronic lung disease, especially bronchitis and widespread pulmonary fibrosis; (2) stenosis and/or incompetence of the mitral valve; (3) congenital heart disease with large shunts of blood from one side of the heart to the other; (4) stenosis of the pulmonary valve; (5) massive hypertrophy of the left ventricle, which is often accompanied by right ventricular hypertrophy without any other obvious cause. This may be due to distortion of the right ventricular lumen by the hypertrophied ventricular septum. Rarer causes of right ventricular hypertrophy include multiple small pulmonary emboli and other unusual causes of pulmonary hypertension (pp. 454–7).

Causes of compensatory dilatation. Compensatory dilatation of the left ventricle results from incompentence of the mitral or aortic valve or of both, and right ventricular dilatation from incompetence of the tricuspid and/or pulmonary valves. A lesser degree of compensatory dilatation of both ventricles occurs in patients with persistently high cardiac output, e.g. in thyrotoxicosis or arterio-venous shunts.

Compensatory dilatation is accompanied by hypertrophy of the affected ventricle, the degree of which depends on the increase in its work load.

Ischaemic Heart Disease

Myocardial ischaemia is one of the major causes of disability and death in developed countries, the outstanding cause being atheroma of the coronary arteries, often complicated by occlusive thrombosis. Practically everybody in such communities has some degree of coronary atheroma by the age of 40, and deaths even earlier than this are by no means uncommon. In recent years, however, deaths from ischaemic heart disease have apparently decreased significantly in the U.S.A., perhaps because of the factors mentioned on p. 369. In this country there has been no obvious decrease in the mortality rate, although a plateau may have been reached. Severe atheromatous narrowing, particularly of more than one major coronary artery, can give rise to (1) **angina pectoris**, severe chest pain brought on by factors which increase the work of the heart; (2) **myocardial infarction**, usually precipitated by superadded occlusive thrombosis; (3) **sudden death**; (4) **cardiac failure**; and (5) **cardiac arrhythmias**, due to ischaemic injury of the conducting system.

These last three effects may occur either with or without a history of angina pectoris or myocardial infarction.

Angina pectoris

This consists of attacks of severe, sometimes agonising chest pain of sudden onset, due to acute ischaemia of a part of the myocardium with an inadequate blood supply. The pain is brought on by factors which increase the work of the heart and is relieved by rest and by vasodilator drugs such as nitroglycerin. Physical exercise, anger, anxiety, a heavy meal and exposure to cold can all induce an attack.

Aetiology and structural changes. The primary factor in nearly all cases is atheromatous narrowing of the coronary arteries. *Coronary atheroma* shows the usual features of atheroma in other arteries (pp. 362–6). There is patchy fibrous thickening of the intima with accumulation of lipid debris (Fig. 15.2). Calcification is usually present, and confluent calcified patches of atheroma may convert lengths of the vessel into a rigid tube which cannot be cut with a knife; it is then very difficult to examine satisfactorily without decalcification. Atheroma affects all the main branches of the coronary arteries but the earliest and most severe lesions often develop in the first 2–3 cm of the left coronary artery or in its anterior descending branch. Even small distal epicardial branches may be narrowed, although branches that have penetrated into the myocardium are usually free of atheroma. At necropsy, occlusion of one or more major coronary vessels by organised thrombus can often be demonstrated, with some restoration of blood supply to the distal part of the occluded vessel by enlarged

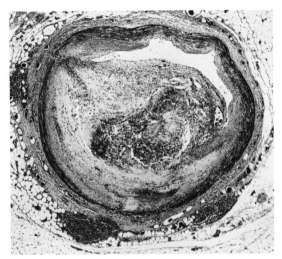

Fig. 15.2 Severe atheromatous narrowing of a coronary artery. In this instance, the lumen has been further reduced by haemorrhage into the soft lipid-rich material, seen as the dark area in the atheromatous patch. × 20.

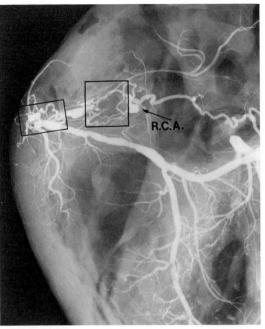

Fig. 15.3 Post-mortem radiograph of part of the right coronary artery in a case of angina. Shortly after its origin (*arrow*), a length of the artery is occluded (*square*) and adjacent vessels have enlarged to provide a collateral route, so that the artery is filled beyond the occlusion. A second occlusion (*oblong*) is present, but is partly obscured by the curving course of the artery. (Professor M. J. Davies.)

anastomotic arteries (Fig. 15.3). In most cases of angina pectoris, at the time of death there is myocardial scarring (Fig. 15.4) or recent myocardial infarction, but myocardial lesions are not invariably present.

Severe atheromatous coronary narrowing may account for the finding of areas in which the myocardium is partly replaced by scar tissue, but in which some myocardial fibres persist (Fig. 15.5), particularly around blood vessels. Old, organised coronary occlusions are, however, commonly present in such cases, and it is often not clear whether the scarring has resulted from chronic ischaemia or myocardial infarction. On the basis that the resistance to coronary blood flow is mainly in the arterioles and capillary network, it has been calculated that an atheromatous lesion of a coronary artery must reduce the sectional area by 70 per cent or more to cause a reduction in blood flow. This may be true for resting conditions, but lesser degrees of narrowing, especially if multiple, will inevitably restrict the increased flow which occurs when the arterioles relax, as in physical activity.

In most cases of angina pectoris, there is some degree of left ventricular hypertrophy, usually due to systemic hypertension: by increasing the amount of muscle supplied by the coronary arteries, this aggravates coronary

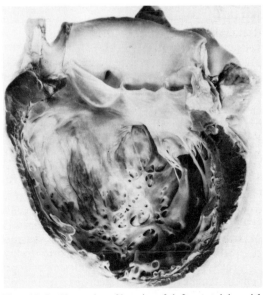

Fig. 15.4 Extensive fibrosis of left ventricle with marked thinning at places; secondary to coronary disease. × 0·5.

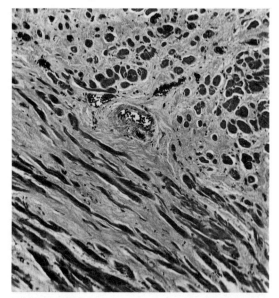

Fig. 15.5 Part of a large zone of myocardial scarring throughout which some myocardial fibres have survived.

insufficiency and acts as a predisposing cause. Ventricular hypertrophy due to lesions of the cardiac valves or to cardiomyopathy (see later) has a similar effect. Narrowing of the ostia of the coronary arteries by syphilitic aortitis is now a rare cause of angina pectoris.

Clinical course. In general, chronic coronary insufficiency can be expected to shorten life, although there are wide variations in the clinical course and some patients with angina survive more than 20 years. Many die suddenly and unexpectedly; in some this is due to sudden occlusion of a coronary artery by thrombus, but in about half the cases no recent occlusion can be demonstrated. Death in these cases is assumed to be due to the sudden onset of ventricular fibrillation, and this has been confirmed in patients being monitored by electrocardiography at the time of death.

Myocardial infarction

Myocardial infarction is the commonest cause of death in many parts of the world today. Approximately 33 per cent of males and 25 per cent of females coming to necropsy in this department have evidence of old or recent myocardial infarction. The mortality rate varies appreciably, even in different parts of the British Isles, and in the Clyde valley the rate is probably the highest in the world.

Like infarction in other tissues, it is due to acute ischaemia, usually caused by occlusive thrombosis of a coronary artery over an atheromatous patch.

Clinical course

The onset of myocardial infarction is signalled by the appearance, often abruptly, of severe persistent chest pain. Many patients already suffer from angina pectoris and they often recognise that the pain is different, being continuous for some hours and failing to respond to rest and nitroglycerin. With the onset the patient may experience profound weakness and breathlessness, and there is usually evidence of peripheral circulatory failure with hypotension, cyanosis and a cold clammy skin. Fever, leukocytosis and a raised erythrocyte sedimentation rate are commonly observed within the first 24 hours. Certain tissue enzymes are released by the dead heart muscle, with a consequent rise in blood levels, which is of diagnostic value. The serum concentration of glutamic oxaloacetic aminotransferase, for example, rises within 6 to 12 hours, and reaches a peak within 2 or 3 days. Characteristic abnormalities of the electrocardiogram are often demonstrable, but by no means always. The prognosis of myocardial infarction depends on a number of factors including the size of the infarct, its site (e.g. whether it involves the conducting system), the patient's age, and whether or not he (or she) has hypertension. Approximately 25 per cent of the patients admitted to hospital die, mostly within the first week, but this excludes a large number who die before they can reach hospital. Death is most commonly caused by ventricular fibrillation, cardiac failure or secondary embolic disease (see below).

Structural changes

The changes found in the heart at necropsy depend on how long the patient has lived since the onset of infarction.

The **coronary arteries** usually show extensive atheroma, but in some cases there will be only one or two patches causing severe narrowing. The occluding thrombus typically overlies an atheromatous patch, but may extend along a considerable length of the vessel. At first, it is usually composed mainly of red thrombus (Fig. 15.6); subsequently it becomes pale and is eventually organised, often with some recanalisation (Fig. 15.7).

Thrombosis of the anterior descending branch of the left coronary artery is particularly common and usually causes an infarct involving the anterior wall of the left ventricle together with the apex and sometimes extending to the anterior part of the interventricular septum and the adjacent part of the anterior

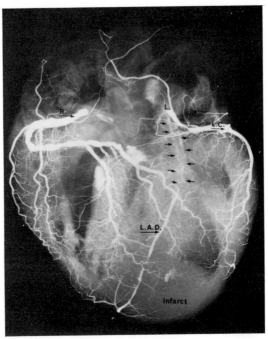

Fig. 15.8 Post-mortem angiogram in a case of recent myocardial infarction. The anterior descending artery (LAD) is occluded proximally (*arrows*), and although there was sufficient collateral supply to fill the artery distally, extensive infarction had occurred over the anterior wall and apical region. Note also the atheromatous narrowings of the right coronary artery. (Professor M. J. Davies.)

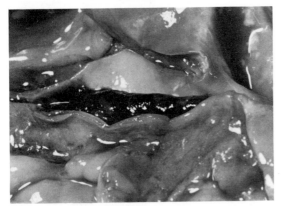

Fig. 15.6 Recent thrombotic occlusion of the right main coronary artery: death resulted 12 hours after the onset of symptoms. The artery has been opened longitudinally to reveal the thrombus.

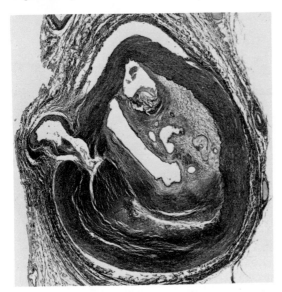

Fig. 15.7 Coronary artery recanalised after occlusion by thrombus. There was extensive healed myocardial infarction. × 25.

wall of the right ventricle (Fig. 15.8). Occlusion of the right main coronary artery is almost as frequent and is associated with infarction of the posterior wall of the *left* ventricle, sometimes involving also the posterior part of the septum and posterior wall of the right ventricle. Occlusion of the circumflex branch of the left coronary artery can cause infarction of the lateral wall of the left ventricle, but occlusion of the descending and circumflex branches of the right coronary artery are relatively rare causes of infarction. In some instances, recent thrombus is found in two major vessels, and infarction is accordingly extensive.

The extent of infarction varies considerably, depending on the severity of atheromatous narrowing and the presence or absence of previous thrombosis in other coronary arteries. There is considerable normal variation in the relative sizes of the left and right arteries, and atheromatous narrowing of a branch may result in enlargement of collateral vessels (Fig.

15.3) so that its final occlusion causes a lesser infarct than usual, or even none at all.

The detection of thrombus in coronary arteries narrowed by atheroma is not always easy. If the arteries are opened lengthwise with scissors, a small thrombus may be displaced and disrupted by the point of the blade without being noticed. A more satisfactory method of examining the vessels is by transverse section at close intervals. The presence of extensive and grossly calcified atheromatous lesions prevents satisfactory naked-eye examination of the affected parts of the vessels at necropsy, and decalcification is first necessary.

The infarct may involve the whole thickness of the myocardium, or it may be confined to the inner part of the wall. Occasionally infarction involves the deeper, subendocardial myocardium throughout most of the circumference of the left ventricle: there is usually severe atheromatous narrowing of the left and right main coronary arteries and the anterior descending branch, but without recent thrombosis. It appears that such extensive arterial narrowing renders especially precarious the blood supply to this part of the myocardium and that subendocardial ischaemic necrosis can occur without superadded occlusive arterial thrombosis (Davies, Woolf and Robertson, 1976).

Although ischaemic death of myocardium occurs within a few minutes of loss of blood supply, the visible changes of infarction in the dead muscle do not appear for 8 hours or so. Accordingly, in patients who die suddenly at the time of coronary occlusion, or within the next few hours, acute changes in the myocardium are not observed by naked-eye or ordinary light microscopy. The first changes noticed by naked eye are blotchy congestion and pallor. Although the muscle undergoes coagulative necrosis, the infarct can usually be felt after a day or so as a patch of softening, and during the next few days it becomes pale (Fig. 15.9) and its colour changes from brown to yellowish-grey. After a week or so it becomes more sharply defined by the development of a zone of vascular granulation tissue along the margin, and removal of the dead tissue by organisation gradually proceeds. When the infarct extends to the outer surface of the myocardium, the pericardial surface is often covered by a layer of fibrinous exudate with marginal haemorrhages. On the inner

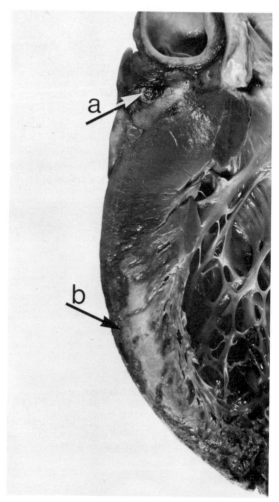

Fig. 15.9 Myocardial infarction of 11 days' duration. The anterior descending branch of the left coronary artery (**a**) is occluded by thrombus and there is extensive infarction of the wall of the left ventricle, seen as areas of pallor and surrounding congestion (**b**). Note also mural thrombus at the apex.

aspect, the endocardium and a thin layer of adjacent myocardium remain alive, nourished by blood from the lumen, but in patients surviving for several days this does not prevent thrombosis on the endocardial surface (see below).

Under the microscope the infarcted muscle shows the usual features of necrosis (Fig. 2.5, p. 11). The necrotic muscle is invaded by polymorphonuclear leukocytes and, after a few days, digestion by macrophages and organisation can be seen at the margins (Fig. 15.10).

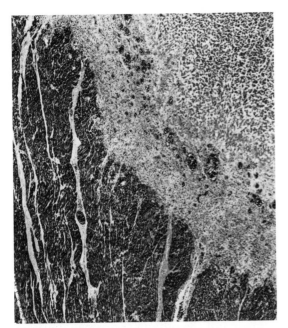

Fig. 15.10 Infarct of myocardium of 12 days' duration. The necrotic heart muscle (*upper right*) is separated from the surviving muscle by a zone of cellular and vascular granulation tissue. × 40.

Gradually, the dead muscle is replaced by fibrous tissue, the process taking some weeks or even months, depending on the size of the infarct, and eventually a pale fibrous scar remains (Fig. 15.11).

As already stated, it is sometimes not possible to determine whether myocardial fibrosis has resulted from infarction or chronic ischaemia.

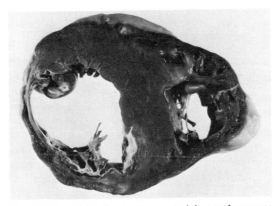

Fig. 15.11 Old infarct represented by replacement of the lateral and posterior wall of the left ventricle by a relatively thin fibrous scar.

Aetiology

The important cause of myocardial infarction is atheroma of the coronary arteries with super-added occlusive thrombosis over an atheromatous patch. The aetiology of atheroma, and the factors associated with an increased risk of myocardial infarction, have been discussed on p. 366. These include raised levels of various plasma lipids, obesity, hypertension, cigarette smoking and a sedentary occupation. These factors are all of long duration, and are likely to promote the gradual development and extension of atheroma, but they may also predispose to superadded thrombosis. Enhanced coagulability of the blood has been shown to be common in patients with ischaemic heart disease, and correlates partially with the levels of plasma lipids. It has also been shown that coronary blood flow is affected by cigarette smoking, which may also predispose to thrombosis by the mechanisms noted on p. 369.

Patients with severe coronary atheroma are particularly liable to myocardial infarction following a severe injury or major surgical operation. This may occur during a period of shock, but the risk is high for some weeks following the injury, etc. The circulatory disturbances of shock, the effect of anaesthetic agents on the heart, and the increased coagulability of the blood following injury are all probably of importance.

Relationship of coronary thrombosis to myocardial infarction. The reported incidence of recent coronary thrombosis in patients dying of acute myocardial infarction varies greatly. In some series, the incidence has been only about 50 per cent, and considerably lower in those patients dying within a few hours of the onset of symptoms. Accordingly, it has been suggested that coronary thrombosis may not be the cause of infarction, and that it occurs *after* the muscle has died. The evidence for this view depends upon the care with which the coronary arteries are examined (see above). By careful examination of the coronary arteries by close transverse section, preceded when necessary by decalcification, workers at St. Georges' Hospital, London, have found an occlusive thrombus in the expected artery in virtually all cases of myocardial infarction in patients dying 12 hours or more after the onset of clinical symptoms, and Harland's experience in this department has been similar. In patients dying within a few hours of onset, infarction cannot be identified morphologically, and the diagnosis is insecure. These findings relate to regional (transmural) infarcts occurring mainly within the territory supplied by a major coronary artery. By contrast, circumferential sub-endocardial necrosis of the myocardium (see above) is not usually associated with recent coronary thrombosis, but this lesion accounts for only about 6 per cent of all infarcts (Davies, Woolf and Robertson, 1976).

Microscopic examination of recent coronary occlusions shows that the thrombus very often forms over a *ruptured* atheromatous plaque (Fig. 15.12), and this suggests that the rupture (and not necrosis of muscle) has promoted thrombosis. It follows that, in such cases, infarction is the *result* of the occlusion. Admittedly, old organised occlusive coronary arterial

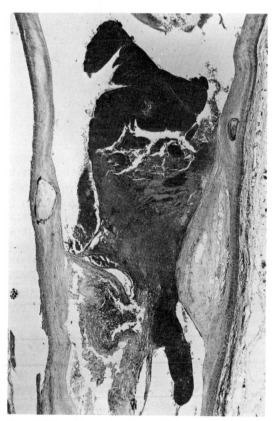

Fig. 15.12 Coronary artery in longitudinal section, showing an ulcerated atheromatous plaque (*left, lower*) with occlusion of lumen by thrombus. × 15.

thrombosis is sometimes found without evidence of previous infarction (i.e. a myocardial scar), but this is probably attributable to compensatory enlargement of anastomotic arteries due to the presence of atheroma before the thrombosis occurred.

Experimental animal studies also support the causal role of thrombosis, for occlusion of a major coronary artery results in infarction, whereas myocardial necrosis induced by other means is not followed by coronary thrombosis.

In his extensive studies on myocardial infarction, Fulton has found no evidence against the orthodox view that coronary artery thrombosis precedes and causes transmural infarction. In particular, the evidence from examination of coronary thrombi at necropsy following intravenous administration of radio-labelled fibrinogen was fully consistent with this view (see Davies, Fulton and Robertson, 1979).

Infrequent causes of myocardial infarction. Occlusion of the ostia of the coronary arteries by syphilitic aortitis is nowadays a rare cause of infarction, and so are coronary lesions due to polyarteritis nodosa or Buerger's disease. Occlusion of a coronary artery by embolus is also much less common than thrombosis, but sometimes results from bacterial endocarditis, and also from detachment of thrombus forming in relation to valve prostheses.

Effects and complications

(a) Arrhythmias. Death from myocardial infarction most frequently results from arrhythmias, particularly ventricular fibrillation. Healed infarcts may also be associated with cardiac arrhythmias and are the chief cause of heart block.

(b) Cardiac failure. Extensive infarction of left ventricular muscle can cause acute heart failure, and if severe this results in **cardiogenic shock**, the prognosis of which is poor. Loss of the infarcted muscle also predisposes to chronic heart failure, which may develop at any time after infarction.

(c) Mural thrombosis. Following acute myocardial infarction, release of tissue thromboplastin from the damaged muscle and localised eddying of blood may lead to thrombosis in the ventricular chambers (Fig. 9.16, p. 238). This is seen at necropsy in about 30 per cent of cases: in patients who survive, the thrombus is eventually organised. Systemic emboli can result from mural thrombosis, but are not very common.

(d) Venous thrombosis. Presumably because of reduced blood flow, systemic venous thrombosis is an important complication of myocardial infarction and tends to occur especially in the veins of the legs (p. 241). Detachment of such thrombus is common and consequently pulmonary embolism is not infrequently a cause of death in myocardial infarction.

(e) Rupture of the left ventricle due to myocardial softening (*myomalacia cordis*) causes 10 per cent of deaths occuring soon after myocardial infarction. It generally occurs within 14 days after infarction, when autolysis of the infarct is active, and especially when leukocytic invasion is marked and repair has not started. Rupture leads to sudden death from massive haemopericardium. When the interventricular septum is involved in infarction it may rupture, leading to sudden onset of severe cardiac failure and a loud heart murmur. Rupture of an infarcted papillary muscle in the left ventricle may also occur, leading to incompetence of the mitral valve, with a loud murmur and intractable pulmonary oedema. Persistence of hypertension and of physical activity after infarction predispose to cardiac rupture.

(f) Cardiac aneurysm. Occasionally the fibrosed wall of a healed infarct of the left ventricle may stretch to form a cardiac aneurysm. As with other aneurysms, laminated thrombus tends to form in the cavity (Fig. 15.13).

(g) Angina pectoris. Whenever myocardial infarction has occurred, the adjacent myocardium, although not infarcted, is likely to be ischaemic (and is presumably the source of the prolonged pain associated with infarction). As anastomotic channels dilate and enlarge, the blood supply to such areas of partial ischaemia will improve. However, in some patients angina pectoris dates from a myocardial infarction, and it is apparent that thrombosis of a major coronary vessel may render areas of myocardium chronically ischaemic. In some instances, angina is cured by myocardial infarction, presumably because an area of myocardium which was previously chronically ischaemic has been included in the infarct and destroyed.

(h) Recurrence of infarction. Because atheroma is generally extensive, individuals who have had a myocardial infarct are prone to recurrence.

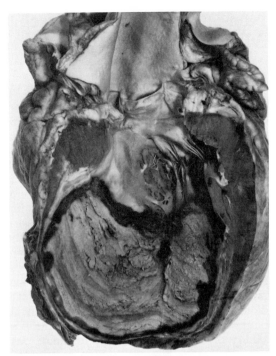

Fig. 15.13 Aneurysm of the left ventricle following ischaemic myocardial fibrosis. Much of the anterior wall (*left*) of the ventricle has been replaced by fibrous tissue, which has stretched to form an aneurysm, now largely filled with laminated thrombus. × 0·7.

Other effects of ischaemic heart disease

Ischaemic heart disease is the usual cause of **sudden death**. There may be a history of angina, previous infarction, evidence of chronic heart failure, or chest pain immediately before death, but sometimes there have been no warning symptoms. At necropsy, there is usually severe coronary atheroma, with or without old organised thrombotic occlusions. In approximately half of these cases, there is a recent occlusive thrombus or a ruptured atheromatous plaque which has apparently caused death before there has been time for the morphological changes of infarction to develop. The occasional unexpected deaths which have occurred during ECG recording suggest that ventricular fibrillation is the usual cause.

Ischaemic heart disease is also the most important cause of **chronic heart failure** and of **cardiac arrhythmias**, whether or not there has been previous myocardial infarction.

Non-inflammatory, Non-ischaemic Disorders of the Myocardium

Fatty change of the myocardium (p. 24) is an expression of impaired metabolism of the heart muscle most frequently seen in severe prolonged anaemia. *Adiposity of the heart* is a deposition of fat in the epicardium which extends between cardiac muscle fibres (Fig. 2.19, p. 28). It affects the right ventricle especially and is usually, but not always, associated with general obesity. Very rarely cardiac function is impaired by this deposition of adipose tissue. *Brown atrophy* (p. 39) is not related to the occurrence of cardiac failure. *Primary amyloid disease* (p. 272) commonly affects the heart and is a rare cause of cardiac failure. The clinical picture may be similar to that of restrictive cardiomyopathy, and diagnosis may be difficult both clinically and at necropsy unless the possibility of amyloidosis is kept in mind. *Segmentation and fragmentation of the myocardium* indicate conditions in which the heart muscle cells either separate from one another at the intercalated discs or show irregular tearing. These changes have been observed in cases of violent death. It is supposed that they result from irregular contraction at the time of death.

Cardiomyopathy

Cardiomyopathy is a convenient term for the classification of a heterogeneous group of chronic myocardial disorders which are not due to ischaemia, hypertension, valve disease or shunts, and appear non-inflammatory. Inclusion of ischaemic myocardial disease and various forms of myocarditis has also been proposed, but the term would then apply to nearly all myocardial lesions and would be of little value.

The four generally accepted types of cardiomyopathy are as follows.

1. Hypertrophic cardiomyopathy with or without obstruction. In this condition there is asymmetrical hypertrophy of the left ventricle, and especially of the septum. Function is affected by (*a*) undue rigidity of the left ventricle, which interferes with diastolic filling, and (*b*) in many, but not all cases, the bulging, hypertrophied septum obstructs the outflow of the left, and less commonly the right, ventricle.

Clinically, the condition presents from early childhood to old age, usually as heart failure or atypical angina: it also causes sudden death. It is often familial and has been detected (by echo cardiography) in some apparently healthy relatives, inheritance apparently being determined by a Mendelian dominant factor. Microscopy shows interstitial fibrosis, areas of disordered, whorled arrangement of muscle fibres and very marked thickening of the individual fibres, with enlarged, pleomorphic nuclei and increased glycogen content. These features are useful in diagnostic biopsy. The nature of the basic abnormality is unknown and current views are largely speculative.

2. Congestive cardiomyopathy. This consists of congestive heart failure which is not due to any of the known causes, and is thus diagnosed by exclusion. At necropsy all the chambers are dilated, the myocardium is pale and unduly flabby, and there is often ventricular mural thrombus and endocardial thickening. Microscopy may show gross hypertrophy of some fibres, with conspicuous nuclear enlargement, and atrophy of others. There may also be interstitial fibrosis. These changes are not diagnostic.

Congestive cardiomyopathy sometimes shows a familial tendency, and may be associated with alcoholism or follow childbirth, but the causation is entirely unknown and it occurs from childhood to old age. Congestive failure is a complication of various other conditions, e.g. dystrophy of the skeletal muscles, Friedreich's ataxia, glycogen disease of the Pompe type, beri-beri and acromegaly. Such cases are sometimes included as congestive cardiomyopathy but the cause, if known, should be specified.

3. Restrictive cardiomyopathy is also known as **endomyocardial fibro-elastosis.** It is a rare disorder, mainly of infants, characterised by a thick smooth layer of collagenous and elastic tissue between the endocardium and the myocardium. Involvement of the left ventricle, which may be hypertrophied, is most common. Cases have been attributed to fetal endocarditis, to anoxia due to origin of the left coronary artery from the pulmonary trunk, and to hypoplasia of the left ventricle associated with premature closure of the foramen ovale. Although not really a disease of the myocardium, it is a cause of heart failure of cryptic origin, and so is grouped with the cardiomyopathies.

Amyloid disease of the heart can cause a restrictive cardiomyopathy in adults.

4. Obliterative cardiomyopathy (endomyocardial fibrosis) is of unknown cause and found mainly in tropical Africa where it is one of the common forms of left or total heart failure. It occurs in many other parts of the world. In the absence of significantly narrowed coronary arteries there is dense fibrosis of the endocardium affecting usually the apex and posterior walls of one or both ventricles. Sometimes the fibrosis partially obliterates the ventricular cavity and, by enveloping the posterior papillary muscles and chordae tendineae, distorts the posterior cusps of the mitral and tricuspid valves with resulting incompetence. Mural thrombus overlying the fibrotic endocardium is common though embolism seldom occurs. The fibrosis is dense and acellular on the surface but more loose with some inflammatory reaction in the deeper layers. Fibrous tissue bands may spread through the inner third of the myocardial wall and there may be atrophy of myocardial fibres with loss of sarcoplasm. Bacterial endocarditis is recorded in about 10 per cent of fatal cases.

Inflammatory Lesions of the Heart

Myocarditis

The term myocarditis is used loosely to cover various lesions of diverse nature, some of which are due to bacterial and viral infections, others to the effects of bacterial toxins. Rheumatic myocarditis appears to be a hypersensitivity reaction to streptococcal antigens. The subject is difficult because of the impossibility of confirming myocarditis in suspected cases which recover, and the poor correlation between pathological lesions in the myocardium and clinical evidence of heart disease. The possibility of serious metabolic disorder with no histological change in the myocardium, and the difficulty of interpreting the results of bacteriological cultures of necropsy material, further complicate the subject.

In fatal cases of acute myocarditis, the heart is flabby, usually pale, the ventricles are dilated and there may be mural thrombosis.

Toxic myocarditis is a major feature of diphtheria. Similar appearances, presumed to be toxic in origin, may be seen in pneumococcal pneumonia, typhoid fever, septicaemia and other extensive septic conditions.

Morphological changes. The gross changes, mentioned above, are not diagnostic. Microscopically there is a parenchymatous lesion with numerous small foci of coagulative necrosis in the muscle. The affected fibres appear swollen and glassy, with loss of striations and nuclei, and around them there is infiltration, mostly of macrophages and lymphocytes, but polymorphs also may be present. The necrotic fibres afterwards undergo absorption (Fig. 7.1, p. 178), while the supporting cells in the areas of infiltration proliferate, and small fibrous patches ultimately result. The nature of the infection cannot be deduced from the appearances of the cardiac lesions. In some cases of toxic myocarditis due to diphtheria, the conducting system is severely affected (Fig. 15.14), with resultant heart block.

Clinically toxic myocarditis is recognised by the onset of cardiac arrhythmia or acute cardiac failure in a patient with diphtheria, pneumonia or other toxic infection. It may cause sudden death. Peripheral circulatory failure may also be present in severe cases.

Suppurative myocarditis is due to direct extension of pyogenic organisms from an adjacent valve in bacterial endocarditis, or to infection by the bloodstream. The myocardium is a common site of multiple abscess formation in septicaemia or pyaemia, particularly when due to *Staph. aureus*. In pyaemia, the abscesses have the usual haemorrhagic margin, and their presence is suggested at necropsy by small epicardial haemorrhages, incision of which may reveal underlying abscesses. Septic emboli may be found in coronary branches (Fig. 15.15).

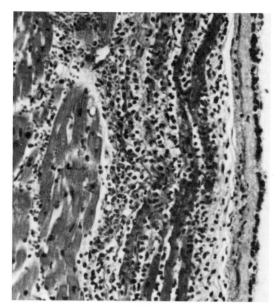

Fig. 15.14 Necrosis of the fibres of the left bundle branch, with an inflammatory reaction, in a fatal case of diphtheria. × 225. (Professor A. C. Lendrum.)

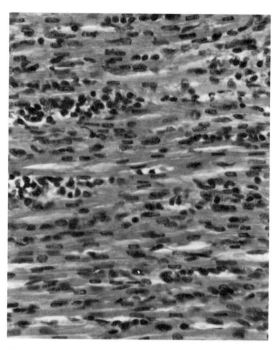

Fig. 15.16 Myocarditis due to Coxsackie B virus from a child of 11 months. The field illustrates the extensive focal infiltration with macrophages, lymphocytes, etc. × 320. (Dr. J. F. Boyd.)

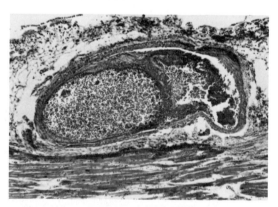

Fig. 15.15 Septic embolus in coronary artery in acute infective endocarditis. × 36.

Involvement of the myocardium in acute infective endocarditis is described on p. 423.

Virus myocarditis. Coxsackie viruses of Groups A and B cause myocarditis and pericarditis: men are most often affected but outbreaks in infant nurseries have been described. The myocardium shows widespread damage of the muscle fibres with abundant macrophages, lymphocytes, plasma cells and eosinophils in the interstitial tissue (Fig. 15.16).

Isolated myocarditis. Various forms of subacute and chronic myocarditis without con-

comitant endocarditis or pericarditis have been described, and although the appearances resemble those in Coxsackie infection in the newborn, nothing is known of their causes or relationships. In one variety, known as *interstitial* or *Fiedler's myocarditis*, the heart is dilated and hypertrophied and mural thrombi are common. Yellowish-white foci of necrosis may be visible and microscopically these show conspicuous infiltration of the interstitial tissue around the necrotic muscle fibres with macrophages, lymphocytes, plasma cells, eosinophils and also multinucleated giant cells apparently derived from the damaged muscle fibres. Figure 15.17 is from a boy aged 14 who characteristically died suddenly after a brief illness.

Clinically the disease presents with cardiac arrhythmias, chest pain and embolic phenomena, progressing in a few weeks or months to cardiac failure without obvious cause.

Sarcoidosis may involve the heart, granulomas developing in the myocardium. The endocardium and pericardium are not usually involved.

Syphilis was formerly a frequent cause of

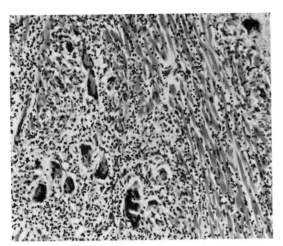

Fig. 15.17 Acute interstitial myocarditis. The heart muscle fibres are replaced by a granulomatous reaction, in which there are many giant cells derived from the muscle fibres. × 85. (Professor Sir Tom Symington.)

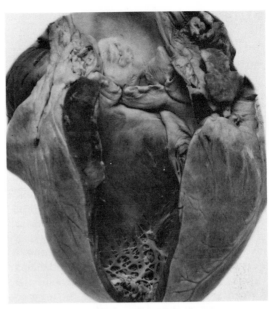

Fig. 15.18 Syphilitic aortitis, affecting the origin of the aorta. Stretching of the aortic ring has resulted in sagging and thickening of the cusps: dilatation and hypertrophy of the left ventricle are secondary to aortic incompetence. × 0·5.

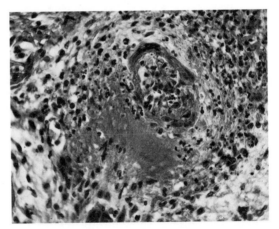

Fig. 15.19 A miliary gumma in the myocardium of a child with congenital syphilis. There is a patch of necrosis adjacent to a small thrombosed artery, and the usual surrounding infiltrate of lymphocytes, plasma cells and macrophages. × 300. (The late Professor J. W. S. Blacklock.)

serious heart disease. It may affect the heart in four ways. *Incompetence of the aortic valve* is the commonest form and is due to stretching of the valve ring as a result of its involvement in syphilitic mesaortitis. Because they do not meet, the cusps lose their mutual support during diastole and so become elongated and tend to sag (Fig. 15.18). The effects on the chambers of the heart are similar to those resulting from any other variety of aortic incompetence (see p. 419).

Myocardial ischaemia may follow narrowing of the orifices of the coronary arteries by intimal fibrous plaques formed over areas of mesaortitis or by cicatricial contraction of healing lesions. Angina pectoris, myocardial infarction and sudden death are, however, very rarely due to syphilis nowadays.

Gumma of the heart is very rare. It may involve the conducting system and cause heart-block. In *congenital syphilis*, there may be miliary gummas (Fig. 15.19) or interstitial fibrosis of the myocardium.

Rheumatic heart disease

Acute rheumatic fever

This is an acute febrile illness in which lesions occur in the heart, the joints and the subcutaneous tissue. It follows an attack of streptococcal pharyngitis and occurs mainly in children and young adults. Its incidence has fallen greatly in developed countries as a result of improved living conditions and use of antibiotics, but it is common in some tropical countries, including parts of Africa and India.

The function of the myocardium is seriously affected in the acute illness, but recovery of the myocardium is usually complete and any residual effects are due to damage to the heart valves, which may become permanently deformed with consequent increase in the workload of the heart and eventually chronic heart failure. Rheumatic fever shows a marked tendency to recur with subsequent attacks of pharyngitis, and increasingly severe valvular disease may result.

Changes in the heart

Most patients recover from acute rheumatic fever but occasionally it causes death from acute myocardial failure. This is sometimes precipitated by the additional load of acute pericarditis on the weakened myocardium, particularly if there is much pericardial effusion.

The **pericarditis** is exudative, with effusion of fluid and deposition of fibrin on both visceral and parietal layers: the surfaces have a roughened appearance (Fig. 3.21, p. 66) which has been likened to that produced by pulling apart two pieces of buttered bread. Unless very scanty, the fibrin is subsequently removed by organisation, which results in fibrous thickening of the pericardium and often adhesion between the two layers with partial or complete obliteration of the sac.

In fatal acute cases, the **myocardium** is flabby and the ventricles, particularly the left, are dilated. Apart from this, there are no obvious naked-eye myocardial changes, but sometimes tiny pale foci may be just visible: these are the **Aschoff bodies** which are pathognomonic of rheumatic carditis. They are scattered throughout the myocardium (Fig. 15.20), being par-

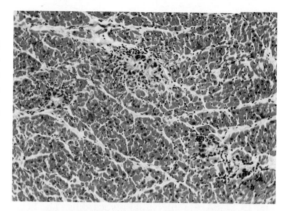

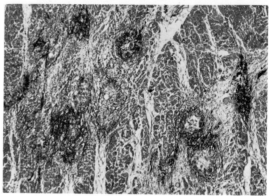

Fig. 15.20 Rheumatic myocarditis. *Above,* the acute stage, showing several Aschoff bodies. × 80. *Below,* later stage, showing fibrosis around the Aschoff bodies (Masson's trichrome stain: collagen appears dark). × 48.

ticularly numerous in the left atrium and ventricle. The Aschoff body appears to be centred on the strands of connective tissue which run through the myocardium, and microscopy reveals a focus of eosinophilic hyaline change in collagen fibres, surrounded by an aggregate of lymphocytes, macrophages, occasional polymorphs, and larger cells with two or three nuclei or a single convoluted nucleus (Fig. 15.21). In time, the Aschoff bodies subside and healing occurs with fibrosis, leaving minute focal scarring in the connective tissue of the myocardium.

Although the function of the myocardium is seriously impaired in rheumatic fever, diffuse myocardial changes in fatal cases are neither characteristic nor impressive. There is some

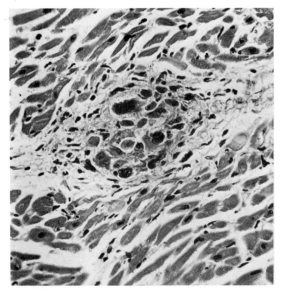

Fig. 15.21 Aschoff body in the myocardium of a child who died of heart failure during an attack of acute rheumatic fever. Central hyaline material is surrounded by macrophages, some with large or multiple nuclei, and by lymphocytes, etc. × 220.

inflammatory oedema and a slight scattering of lymphocytes and occasional polymorphs. The functional disturbance appears to be due to an immunological reaction (see below).

The **endocardium** (like the myocardium) shows diffuse inflammatory oedema and light cellular infiltration. Aschoff bodies also de-velop in the endocardium and are particularly numerous in the posterior wall of the left atrium just above the insertion of the posterior mitral cusp (McCallum's area); their healing may result in thickening and irregularity of the endocardium in this area. In the acute fever, however, the most prominent endocardial lesion is seen on the heart valves and consists of small **thrombotic vegetations**, forming an inter-rupted or continuous line of fine grey-pink nodular deposits on the surface of the valve cusps. The vegetations consist at first mainly of platelets, on which fibrin is later deposited (Fig. 9.14, p. 237). They form on that part of each valve cusp which comes into contact with the opposing cusp when the valves close, and are thus seen near the free margins of the cusps, on the atrial surface of the mitral (Fig. 15.22) and the ventricular surface of the aortic valve. Vegetations develop most commonly on both these valves, but quite often on the mitral valve alone and less commonly on the aortic valve alone. The tricuspid also is occasionally affected, but very rarely the pulmonary valve.

Microscopically, the vegetations appear eosinophilic and refractile (Fig. 15.23): the underlying tissue of the cusp shows inflammatory oedema, superficial ulceration, infiltration with lymphocytes, plasma cells, macrophages and polymorphs and prolifera-tion of fibroblasts. In their inflamed oedemat-ous condition, the impact of closure and

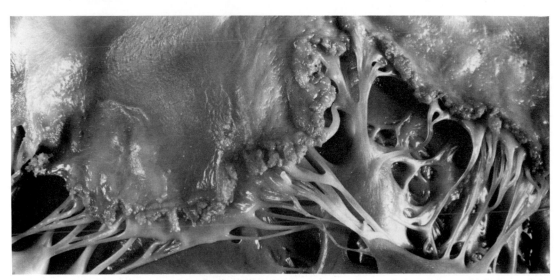

Fig. 15.22 Mitral valve in acute rheumatic endocarditis, showing the small vegetations which form along the line of apposition of the cusps. × 2.

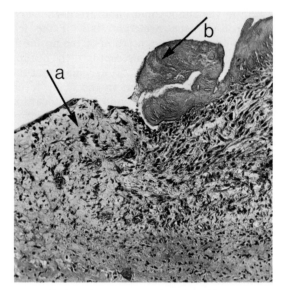

Fig. 15.23 Section of the mitral valve in acute rheumatic endocarditis. The cusp shows inflammatory oedema (**a**) and cellular infiltration, and appears to be vascularised. Where the cusps meet, the oedematous tissue has ulcerated and platelets have been deposited on the ulcerated surface to form the early vegetation (**b**). Subsequently, fibrin also is deposited (see also Fig. 9.14, p. 237). × 80. (Professor A. C. Lendrum.)

mutual pressure during the closed state appears to injure the cusps sufficiently to result in loss of endothelium and damage to the underlying connective tissue: in consequence, platelets and fibrin are deposited on the injured surface. The vegetations do not seriously impair valvular function at this stage, although they tend to glue together the margins of adjacent cusps close to the commissures. They are firmly adherent to the cusps and do not produce emboli. Vegetations may form also on the chordae tendineae, particularly of the mitral valve, and in McCallum's area of the left atrium. The tissue at the base of the mitral and aortic valve cusps is often infiltrated heavily with lymphocytes, macrophages, etc., but without the focal arrangement of the Aschoff body.

These changes are followed by vascularisation of the (normally almost avascular) cusps of the affected valves. Blood vessels around the base extend up into the cusps towards the free margin, and the vegetations are removed by the process of organisation, resulting in fibrous thickening and adherence of the cusps near the free margin. Vascularisation is also accom-

panied by more general fibrosis, so that the cusps are irregularly thickened and distorted. Fibrosis occurs also in the papillary muscles and chordae: the latter become thicker and shorter and sometimes bound together by fibrous tissue resulting from organisation of vegetations on them. With recurrent attacks, the acute changes are superimposed on the damaged tissues and distortion of the valves, described more fully on p. 417, becomes progressively more severe.

Micro-organisms are not detected in the heart in rheumatic fever.

Changes in other tissues

In patients dying of acute rheumatic fever, the **lungs** are congested, heavy, and feel firm and rubbery. Microscopy shows acute congestion, accumulation of oedema fluid containing some macrophages and desquamated pneumocytes, and lining of the alveolar ducts by a dense layer of fibrin ('hyaline-membrane disease', Fig. 15.24). These changes were formerly regarded

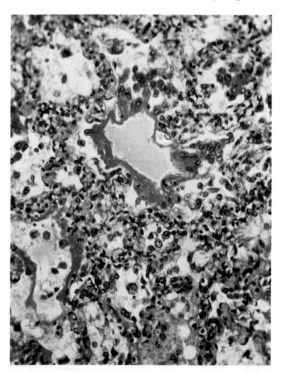

Fig. 15.24 The lung in a case of cardiac failure due to acute rheumatic myocarditis. The lung shows hyaline membranes lining alveolar ducts and mononuclear cells in the alveolar walls and lying free in the alveoli. × 220.

as a specific rheumatic pneumonia, but they appear to result from fairly acute left ventricular failure and are sometimes seen when this occurs from causes other than rheumatic fever. The **joints** show mild inflammatory changes in the synovium with cellular infiltrates resembling Aschoff bodies but more diffuse; the tendons and their sheaths may show similar changes.

In some cases, **subcutaneous nodules** develop over bony prominences of the arms and legs, the commonest sites being the extensor surface of the elbow and overlying the ulna. The nodules are usually between 1 and 2 cm in diameter, painless, and consist of a patch of eosinophilic hyaline swelling of collagen surrounded by a granulomatous reaction in which the cells are mainly lymphocytes, plasma cells, macrophages and fibroblasts. In both the subcutaneous nodule and Aschoff body, the hyaline change in collagen appears to be due to permeation by plasma proteins exuded from the small vessels. Various erythematous skin rashes may occur, the commonest being *erythema marginatum*, and in some cases there may be a mild *encephalitis*.

Clinical features

Rheumatic fever develops usually 2 to 4 weeks after a streptococcal sore throat. Symptoms may be mild, but there is usually fever, tachycardia, malaise and arthralgia flitting from joint to joint; the affected joints are sometimes swollen. The subsequent course depends on the degree of cardiac involvement: the most serious effect at this stage is on the myocardium, and various degrees of acute heart failure are observed. Signs of acute pericarditis usually appear later in the acute illness, and the valvular lesions are undetectable at this stage, although there may be evidence of secondary mitral incompetence due to dilatation of the left ventricle, or valvular abnormalities resulting from previous attacks. Involuntary movements (*chorea*) attributable to involvement of the brain may occur during or apart from the acute illness, as may the skin rashes and subcutaneous nodules.

There is no specific test for rheumatic fever. A raised erythrocyte sedimentation rate, anaemia, slight leukocytosis and high titres of streptococcal antibodies are usually present. C-reactive protein, one of the so-called 'acute-phase reactants', appears in the serum at an early stage but is found in many other acute illnesses.

Subclinical rheumatic fever

In some patients with a clinical history of rheumatic fever, valve lesions develop after many subsequent years of apparent good health. Examination of atrial material obtained at operation for chronic valvular disease reveals florid sub-endocardial Aschoff bodies in about 50 per cent of such cases under 50 years old, and since the Aschoff body is regarded as an indication of active rheumatism, it is clear that the disease can smoulder on subclinically for many years. In some cases, there is no history of an illness suggestive of acute rheumatic fever.

Aetiology. Most attacks of rheumatic fever occur 2 to 4 weeks after infection of the throat by β-haemolytic streptococci of Lancefield group A. There is no doubt that such throat infection is a major aetiological factor since prolonged administration of penicillin to patients who have had an attack of rheumatic fever greatly reduces the incidence of further attacks of this notably recurrent disease. Presumably the high incidence of rheumatic fever in the economically poor is due to increased likelihood of streptococcal infection.

It is far from clear how preceding infection of the throat leads to the cardiac and other lesions of rheumatic fever. The 2 to 4 weeks' delay in onset speaks against a direct infection of the heart, etc., or a direct effect of exotoxin. Streptococci have not been demonstrated convincingly in the cardiac lesions, and the failure of antibiotics to prevent the disease when first administered during the interval between the sore throat and the onset of rheumatic fever is not in keeping with simple spread of infection.

There is strong evidence that the disease has an immunological basis. Compared with those who make an uncomplicated recovery from streptococcal sore throat, patients who develop rheumatic fever have unusually high antibody levels against various streptococcal antigens, including antistreptolysin O (ASO) titre, which is widely used as a diagnostic aid. It is of particular interest that Kaplan (1961) has shown that certain antigens are shared by some types of group A streptococci and by myocardial fibres. The serum of many patients contains auto-antibodies which react *in vitro* with myocardial fibres and in fatal cases immunoglobulin and reaction-products of complement have been shown to be bound to the surface of the myocardial cells. It thus appears that throat infection by streptococci leads, in certain susceptible individuals, to strong immunity against various streptococcal antigens; the response includes the production of antibodies which cross-react with myocardial cells, resulting in activation of complement and consequently a cytotoxic effect on the myocardium. The full explanation is, however, likely to be more complex, for rheumatic fever may follow infection by streptococci which do not appear to contain the shared antigens; nor does auto-antibody to myocardium explain the Aschoff body, which does not contain fixed immunoglobulin and is widely regarded as a lesion of connective tissue rather than of myocardial fibres. The pericarditis and endocarditis are also unexplained and it is also not known why streptococcal infections of the skin and elsewhere are not followed by rheumatic fever. Furthermore some unexplained factor must render the cardiac tissues abnormally permeable to permit the union of antibody and complement with cardiac muscle sarcoplasm, for antibody to myocardium induced experimentally in animals does not become bound to the myocardium *in vivo*.

Chronic rheumatic heart disease

Chronic rheumatic heart disease is a common sequel to acute rheumatic fever and is characterised mainly by chronic endocarditis in which overgrowth of connective tissue and irregular shrinkage leads to valvular deformities. Compensatory dilatation and hypertrophy of the chambers are found, depending on the nature of the valvular lesions. In many cases Aschoff bodies are present together with minute foci of myocardial fibrosis representing healed Aschoff bodies. Pericardial adhesions are common but

these impede cardiac action only when the fibrous thickening is unusually severe and especially when the pericardium is adherent to other mediastinal structures.

Pathogenesis of lesions. The lesions result from the healing of acute rheumatic endocarditis and fibrosis may occur in all the sites previously inflamed in the acute stage. Thus the valves affected are the mitral, aortic and tricuspid in that order of frequency, and the chordae tendineae are much thickened and shortened. Fusion of the cusps along their contiguous edges by organisation of vegetations and fibrosis leads to permanent *stenosis* of the valves. The chronic inflammatory process leads to thickening and retraction of the valve cusps which prevents efficient closure and valvular *incompetence* thus results. Both effects are frequently present.

Effects

(1) Cardiac failure is common, mainly as a result of the mechanical problems created by stenosed and incompetent valves. These are considered in detail below.

(2) Thrombi frequently form in the atrial appendages, especially in patients with mitral or tricuspid stenosis and atrial fibrillation, and may cause emboli in the lungs and systemic arteries, e.g. in the brain, with serious consequences. A rare occurrence is the formation in the left atrium of a so-called ball thrombus which lies free in the cavity and which may reach several centimetres in diameter.

(3) Angina pectoris occurs when the cardiac output is so reduced that coronary blood flow to the hypertrophied myocardium is inadequate.

(4) Cardiac arrhythmias, especially atrial fibrillation, are a common consequence and may be due to myocardial and subendocardial scar tissue.

(5) Infective endocarditis is particularly prone to develop on valves even slightly damaged by rheumatic fever.

Deformities of the valves of the heart

Mitral stenosis

This is nearly always due to rheumatic endocarditis. The orifice may be reduced, by fusion of the cusps, occasionally to a diameter as small as 5 mm (normal 25–30 mm), but reduction to about 10 mm is more common in patients coming to operation. The fused cusps may form a thin fibrous diaphragm which is pliable and mobile; closure of the orifice during ventricular systole can then be adequately· brought about by the constriction of the annulus fibrosus, approximation of the nodular ridge, and ballooning of the cusps towards the atrium. In such cases of pure stenosis, surgical relief is often successful, but unfortunately recurrence is common. In other cases the cusps are much shortened, thickened and rigid, as well as fused at the commissures, and a dense fibrous diaphragm with a slit-like aperture results (Fig. 15.25). There may be marked thickening and shortening of the chordae tendineae, and also fibrous induration of the apices of the papillary muscles so that the valve comes to form a funnel-shaped structure with a small oval aperture. Calcification of the cusps and valve ring

may be present. The endocardium of the left atrium is thickened and opaque in most cases.

Effects. The left ventricle can receive a normal volume in the diastolic interval only if the blood is propelled more forcibly through the narrowed mitral orifice; commonly it gets less blood than normally, can easily pass it on and therefore does not undergo hypertrophy; indeed it is often slightly atrophied. The left atrium hypertrophies and readily dilates (Fig. 15.25), often to 120 ml or so (normal, 30–40 ml), but sometimes to over 500 ml. The lungs and pulmonary veins become chronically congested and the pulmonary arterioles become hypertrophied and hypertonic, resulting in pulmonary arterial hypertension. In consequence, the right ventricle becomes greatly hypertrophied (Fig. 15.26). The pressure rises in the pulmonary veins to a level at which it is sufficient, in conjunction with atrial systole, to drive an adequate volume of blood through the narrowed mitral valve during diastole. The stroke volume of the left ventricle may thus be normal—or very nearly so—even in quite severe mitral stenosis, and the patient may be very little incapacitated at rest. *This is an extremely dangerous situation, because if the tricuspid valve is competent then the relatively healthy and powerful right ventricle may, in response to physical exercise, raise the pulmonary*

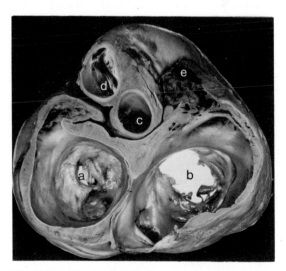

Fig. 15.25 Horizontal section through the atria in a case of mitral and tricuspid stenosis, as seen from above. **a**, mitral valve, severely stenosed; **b**, tricuspid valve, moderately stenosed; **c**, aorta; **d**, pulmonary artery; **e**, right atrial appendage containing thrombus. × 0·6.

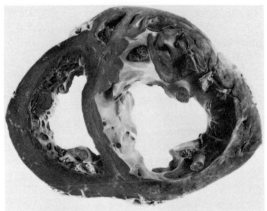

Fig. 15.26 Transverse section of the ventricles in a case of mitral stenosis, showing the comparatively small left ventricle and the greatly enlarged and hypertrophied right ventricle (on the right). × 0·75.

capillary pressure to levels which produce pulmonary oedema.

In patients with mitral stenosis and tricuspid incompetence, any severe rise of pulmonary arterial pressure is prevented by regurgitation into the easily distensible systemic venous system via the right side of the heart; this has the effect of decompressing the pulmonary circuit and bringing on right heart failure (p. 398), which is the common mode of death in mitral stenosis.

The venous congestion of the lungs in mitral stenosis cannot be alleviated by any compensatory process. The changes (p. 230) often cause slight haemoptysis, to be distinguished from the more severe haemoptysis which results from pulmonary infarction when the heart is failing. The changes in the pulmonary vessels due to pulmonary hypertension, and the factors involved in pulmonary oedema, are dealt with on pp. 451-7.

In mitral stenosis the heart comes to have a quadrangular form, but its weight is not greatly increased. There is usually a distinct presystolic murmur over the precordium and sometimes a palpable thrill during atrial systole.

Mitral incompetence

Competence of the mitral valve depends on a complexity of factors, including the size and flexibility of the annulus and cusps, and the state of the chordae tendineae, papillary muscles and left ventricle. In consequence, the diagnosis of incompetence at necropsy is far more difficult than that of mitral stenosis.

Causes. Mitral incompetence results from the following.

1. Rheumatic endocarditis, where it is due to retraction of the cusps and shortening of the chordae tendineae. Pure incompetence from this cause is now quite rare; combined stenosis and incompetence is more common, and is sometimes a result of the surgical treatment of mitral stenosis.

2. Myocardial ischaemia. Mitral incompetence from this cause is now relatively common. It may develop suddenly and in severe form from rupture of papillary muscles involved in myocardial infarction, or insidiously from ischaemic fibrosis of the papillary muscles.

3. Myxoid degeneration of the cusps, causing a 'floppy' mitral valve, occurs usually in old people. Disintegration of the collagen of the valve cusps, accompanied by increase in basophilic ground substance (p. 275), results in weakness and stretching of the cusps. Minor degrees are common but without effect: if the changes are severe, the cusps are liable to prolapse during ventricular systole with consequent regurgitation of blood.

Similar changes occur rarely in young people, sometimes as a complication of Marfan's syndrome.

4. Changes in the annulus. Closure of the mitral valve is dependent on the size and shape of the mitral ring during ventricular systole. Regurgitation due to stretching of the ring is a regular feature of the dilatation of the failing left ventricle, and occurs also in some cases of Marfan's syndrome. Senile calcification of the ring can also cause incompetence.

Effects. Mitral incompetence results in compensatory dilatation and hypertrophy of the left ventricle. From the outset, the left atrium is dilated and the pulmonary circulation congested. Increased work is thus thrown on the right ventricle, which also becomes hypertrophied. The subsequent effects are similar to those occurring in mitral stenosis. Mitral incompetence is associated with an apical murmur throughout, or late in, ventricular systole.

Aortic stenosis

Except in countries where rheumatic heart disease is still prevalent, aortic stenosis alone is probably as common as isolated mitral stenosis, and most cases are probably non-rheumatic. The commonest form is **calcific aortic stenosis** without evidence of rheumatism, and many cases appear to result from the chronic fibrous thickening and calcification of a congenitally bicuspid valve (Fig. 15.27), so that aortic stenosis develops in middle age. The condition occurs also in old age, but usually without the underlying bicuspid abnormality (Fig. 15.28).

Fibrosis and calcification occur in the connective tissue of the cusps, which become hard and rigid. Irregular calcified nodules commonly project from the upper surface of the thickened cusps. Stenosis is often very severe and, as with mitral stenosis, it is surprising how small an orifice is compatible with life.

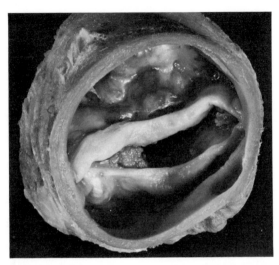

Fig. 15.27 Calcific aortic stenosis arising in a congenitally bicuspid valve. × 1·8.

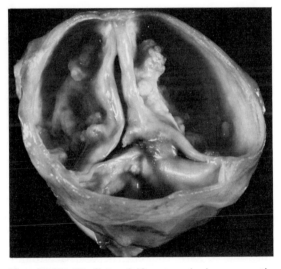

Fig. 15.28 'Senile' calcific stenosis in an aortic valve without obvious predisposing abnormality. × 2.

Turbulence of blood flow may account for those cases with a bicuspid aortic valve, but the aetiology in other cases is unknown.

Congenital aortic stenosis usually becomes apparent in infancy. The valve cusps are replaced by a single diaphragm-like membrane with a central or eccentric hole. Obstruction of the left ventricular outflow by a sub-valvular membrane is another rare abnormality.

Effects. Pure aortic stenosis produces hypertrophy of the left ventricle. When the valve is both stenotic and incompetent, the ventricle dilates and hypertrophies; the cavity becomes lengthened and more pointed. Later, the hypertropied muscle may fail and then dilatation is the prominent feature. The passage of the blood during systole through the narrow aortic orifice produces a loud ventricular systolic murmur audible over the base of the heart, and a systolic thrill. The pulse pressure is characteristically low, and some patients die suddenly.

Aortic incompetence

This results from dilatation or distortion of the root of the aorta, from contraction or stretching of the cusps, or from a combination of both types of change. In rheumatic aortic incompetence, the cusps are thickened and contracted. In syphilitic aortitis, dilatation of the root of the aorta prevents complete closure of the valve cusps, and the resulting haemodynamic disturbance probably explains the stretching, thickening and distortion of the cusps (Fig. 15.18). Aortic incompetence occurs in some cases of Marfan's syndrome, due to weakness and stretching of the root of the aorta, and rarely to myxoid degeneration of the cusps. Another rare cause is the aortitis of ankylosing spondylitis: the aortic root is distorted and there is also damage to the cusps. Congenitally bicuspid aortic valves may also be incompetent.

Effects. Aortic incompetence is associated, from the outset, with compensatory dilatation of the cavity of the left ventricle, accompanied by hypertrophy of the wall. The internal length of the cavity may reach 12 cm or more (normal 8–9 cm), resulting in twice the normal capacity. This indicates a very gross regurgitation. Thick white collagenous patches often develop on the mural endocardium beneath the incompetent valve and are known as 'jet lesions', being attributed to forceful reflux of blood during diastole. So long as the mitral valve is competent the effects of the aortic lesion may not extend backwards to the lungs and venous system. But as the enlargement of the left ventricle progresses, and especially as the muscle fails, the muscular ring round the mitral orifice becomes stretched and secondary mitral incompetence results; the effects of the latter lesion then become superadded. Incompetence of the mitral valve from rheumatic endocarditis may be present as a concomitant lesion, and such a combination causes most striking enlargement of the heart—the so-called *cor bovinum*, which may weigh more than a kilogram. The pulse in aortic incompetence is characteristic: there is a large systolic wave owing to the increased output by the left ventricle, and this is followed by a rapid fall. The pulse has a bounding and collapsing character—the so-called 'water-hammer pulse'. A ventricular diastolic murmur, corresponding with the regurgitation, is usually audible over the base of the heart. There is a risk of sudden death in cases of aortic incompetence.

Tricuspid valve

Tricuspid stenosis is usually due to rheumatic endocarditis, and nearly always accompanied by mitral and aortic valve lesions. It is usually less severe than mitral stenosis (Fig. 15.25).

Tricuspid incompetence, most often secondary to cardiac failure, produces enlargement of both right atrium and right ventricle, while tricuspid stenosis affects mainly the atrium.

Effects of valvular lesions on right side of heart. Tricuspid stenosis restricts right ventricular filling and this diminishes the likelihood of developing pulmonary oedema from the mitral stenosis, which is almost invariably present. **Pulmonary stenosis** causes hypertrophy of the right ventricle. It is very rare, but occurs as a congenital abnormality, or in the carcinoid syndrome (Fig. 15.33, also p. 649).

Infective endocarditis

In this condition, thrombi containing micro-organisms form on the endocardium, usually on the heart valves, and cause damage to the valve cusps, embolic phenomena, toxaemia and sometimes glomerulonephritis. If untreated, it is virtually always fatal, but antibiotic therapy has greatly reduced the mortality.

Traditionally, infective endocarditis is classified into *acute* and *subacute* types, the latter being a prolonged illness due to organisms of relatively low virulence and the former acute and due to virulent pyogenic bacteria. Because of the differences in the clinical pictures, the distinction between the two conditions is still valid and important, but the pattern has been somewhat altered by the widespread use of antibiotics and of drugs which depress the resistance to infection. Cases now occur which are intermediate between the two conditions, and moreover the use of the latter drugs, the development of cardiac surgery and self-administration of drugs intravenously by addicts have resulted in cases of endocarditis due to a wider range of 'opportunistic' micro-organisms, including fungi.

Aetiology

The factors which predispose to infective endocarditis are the occurrence of bacteraemia, lesions of the heart which favour the settling and survival of bacteria, and depression of the general defences against infection.

Bacteraemia commonly occurs transiently and silently following tooth extractions, tonsillectomy or even vigorous chewing in the presence of periodontal infection. In bacterial endocarditis arising from such causes the bacteria responsible are usually various non-haemolytic streptococci, normally of low virulence, which colonise the mouth and were formerly classified as *Streptococcus viridans*. Bacteraemia results also from operations on the gastro-intestinal or infected urinary tracts, or even from such minor urological procedures as catheterisation and cystoscopy, and endocarditis due to *Esch. coli*, enterococci, bacteroides, anaerobic streptococci, pseudomonas, gonococcus, etc., can occasionally result.

Obvious septic lesions, such as boils, carbuncles, bacterial pneumonias and infections of the urinary, gastro-intestinal or biliary tract, are associated with occult bacteraemia, septicaemia and pyaemia. Drug addicts who use intravenous injections are also prone to infective endocarditis due to various organisms, including particularly *Staphylococcus aureus*, *Staph. epidermidis* and fungi (usually candida or aspergillus). There is also a risk of bacteraemia from indwelling venous catheters and cardiovascular surgery.

Predisposing cardiac lesions. Permanent

structural abnormalities of the valves of the heart predispose to infective endocarditis. Rheumatic and syphilitic valvular disease were formerly common precursors, but their incidence has declined in many countries, and congenital defects, such as bicuspid aortic valve have become relatively important, as also have calcific aortic stenosis and minor degrees of fibrous thickening and distortion of the valve cusps of uncertain aetiology.

It is likely that distorted valves are subject to recurrent minor trauma with loss of endothelium and that circulating bacteria stick to platelets and fibrin deposited on such lesions and become incorporated into small mural thrombi. It had been shown experimentally that when minor vascular lesions are caused by abrasion of the endothelium, intravenously-injected bacteria settle and persist in the small thrombi forming on such lesions. It appears that thrombi protect bacteria from the host's defence mechanisms, for in subacute infective endocarditis the micro-organisms survive and multiply in spite of the presence of antibodies capable of destroying any which escape into the bloodstream.

Infective endocarditis tends to develop in endocardial abnormalities at sites where the flow of blood is rapid: in addition to the heart valves, it develops also on the walls of interventricular septal defects, and the only common site in the atria is on the posterior wall of the left atrium in cases of mitral incompetence, where a jet of blood from the leaking valve impinges during ventricular systole. Similarly, it may develop on the chordae and papillary muscles of a stenotic mitral valve and on the interventricular septum below an incompetent aortic valve. In these instances, it is likely that continuous minor physical trauma of the endothelium and consequent platelet deposition is caused where a rapid jet of blood strikes the endocardial surface. Infected thrombi similar to those of bacterial endocarditis occur also in the aorta above a stenotic aortic valve, in patent ductus arteriosus and in coarctation of the aorta, and it may be that localisation of bacteria depends on the recurrent deposition of platelets over a long period, sooner or later providing opportunity for colonisation by bacteria which have gained entrance to the bloodstream.

It should be added that in approximately 50 per cent of cases of infective endocarditis of the heart valves no predisposing local lesion can be detected, and this is particularly common in cases caused by *Staph. aureus* and other highly pathogenic bacteria.

Impaired defence mechanisms. Cytotoxic drugs used in the treatment of patients with cancer, renal transplant recipients, etc., result in depression of immune responsiveness and of production of polymorphs and monocytes, and thus predispose to infections of various sorts. Such therapy increases the risk of infective endocarditis, and the range of micro-organisms responsible includes opportunistic pathogens which are normally of low virulence, as well as virulent bacteria. Such therapy also alters the course of infective endocarditis, which tends to progress rapidly, even when organisms of low virulence are responsible.

Subacute infective endocarditis

This is usually caused by organisms of relatively low virulence, the most common being non-haemolytic streptococci from the mouth (see above), *Staph. epidermidis*, enterococci, *Haemophilus influenzae*, *Esch. coli*, fungi and *Coxiella burneti*. Periodontal infection is the commonest source of the bacteraemia, but in many cases the portal of entry is not apparent. In well over half the cases there is a preceding valvular abnormality. The condition was formerly seen most commonly in children and young adults with chronic rheumatic valvular disease, but the age incidence in developed countries has risen and the mean age is now approximately 50 years.

Naked-eye appearances. *The affected valve(s)* may show evidence of chronic rheumatic endocarditis or other acquired or congenital abnormality. The vegetations are much larger, softer and more crumbling than those in rheumatic fever (Fig. 15.29). In post-rheumatic cases the mitral valve alone, or both the mitral and aortic valves, are usually involved: the aortic valve alone is involved in about 10 per cent of cases. The vegetations tend to spread on the endocardial surface and very frequently develop on McCallum's area in the left atrium, which frequently is the site of previous rheumatic lesions (Fig. 15.29). The lesions are not so rapidly destructive as in acute infective endocarditis (see below), but nevertheless cause

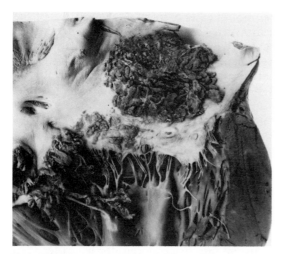

Fig. 15.29 Infective endocarditis of the mitral valve. The vegetations on the valve cusps are much larger than those in rheumatic endocarditis (cf. Fig. 15.22). In this instance, vegetations have formed also on the posterior wall of the left atrium. × 0·8.

gross valvular injury leading eventually to heart failure. Fragments of the vegetations also break away and produce embolic lesions.

Other organs. The skin often has a brownish colour and clubbing of the fingers is usual. Large emboli cause infarction in various organs, including the brain, kidneys, spleen and intestine. The emboli seldom cause suppurating infarcts, probably owing to the high titres of antibodies which develop in the blood in the course of the prolonged infection. Petechiae found in the skin, beneath the nails and in the conjunctiva and retina, may be due to embolism (Fig. 15.30). The renal complications are described on p. 831. They include focal glomerulonephritis, which is common in cases of some months duration and is responsible for haematuria, and also diffuse glomerulonephritis which may bring about renal failure. As a rule the spleen is enlarged, sometimes markedly so.

Microscopic appearances. The vegetations consist mostly of fibrin and platelets and contain colonies of bacteria (Fig. 15.31). Polymorphs are usually scanty. The underlying cusp may be vascularised: it is oedematous, often infiltrated with polymorphs and macrophages, and there are usually foci of necrosis.

The myocardium, though grossly normal, often shows microscopic areas of infarction and inflammation, due to small coronary emboli.

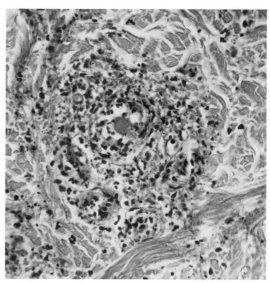

Fig. 15.30 Section through haemorrhagic spot in dermis in subacute infective endocarditis. Note small thrombosed and degenerate arteriole surrounded by leukocytes—the result of infective embolism. × 160.

Clinical features. Early diagnosis of subacute infective endocarditis is very important because antibiotic therapy has reduced the mortality from virtually 100 per cent to about 30 per cent. The longer it continues, the greater the

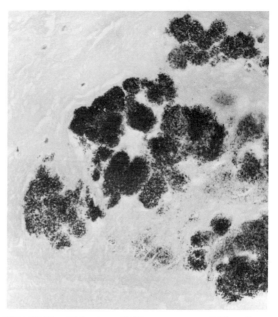

Fig. 15.31 Colonies of *Streptococcus viridans* in a section of a vegetation in subacute infective endocarditis. (Eosin, methylene blue.) × 320.

valve injury and the danger of embolic effects, etc. An irregular fever, with splenomegaly and haematuria (often only microscopic) are usually present. There may be evidence of previous valvular heart disease, and cardiac murmurs which, as the vegetations grow, alter from week to week. Various clinical effects also arise from multiple emboli, including petechial haemorrhages in the skin.

Diagnosis depends on the isolation of the causal organism by blood culture. This is often difficult, perhaps because of a high level of serum antibody, and repeated cultures may be necessary. In the absence of antibiotic therapy, persistently negative blood cultures should suggest *Coxiella burneti* endocarditis (see below). The decision on when to stop searching for bacteria and start therapy on suspicion is often a difficult one.

Healing of the valvular lesions occurs when the organisms are eliminated by prolonged antibiotic therapy. The vegetations are removed by organisation and, depending on their size and distribution, and on the extent of valve injury, various degrees of scarring and distortion of the cusps result, with subsequent danger of heart failure.

Coxiella burneti endocarditis complicating Q fever or subclinical *Coxiella* infection is clinically and pathologically closely similar to subacute bacterial endocarditis. It should be suspected when blood cultures are persistently negative and the leucocyte count is normal.

Acute infective endocarditis

This progresses much more rapidly than subacute infective endocarditis. In untreated cases, death may occur within days from overwhelming infection or the valve lesions may cause fatal heart failure within a few weeks. In classical form, it is now caused most commonly by *Staphylococcus aureus*, and often arises as a complication of an obvious septic lesion of the skin or elsewhere. However, as explained above, it occurs also in drug addicts and various factors have resulted in conditions intermediate between subacute and acute infective endocarditis: in immunodepressed patients organisms of relatively low virulence, including fungi, can cause endocarditis of either type or of intermediate severity. The condition may supervene in patients already seriously ill with

septicaemia, and in well over half the fatal cases predisposing valvular disease cannot be detected at necropsy.

Pathological appearances. The vegetations are large and tend to break down, and the valve cusps may be largely covered by crumbling masses, which consist of layers of fibrin containing clumps of bacteria, enclosed by a zone of leukocytes, macrophages and granulation tissue. The substance of the cusps may be extensively destroyed by suppuration (Fig. 15.32): rupture, especially of an aortic cusp, may occur, leading to severe incompetence. Aneurysm of a cusp is common, the organisms causing suppuration of one side of the curtain, so that the thin tissue is stretched by the blood pressure and forms an aneurysmal bulging. The vegetations may spread also to the chordae tendineae, which may rupture. Infection may extend to the intima at the commencement of the aorta and an acute mycotic aneurysm may be formed (Fig. 15.32). The organisms may also pass directly into the adjacent heart wall, and lead to ulceration or to abscess formation. The valves most often affected are those on the left side of the heart. Involvement of the tricuspid is not uncommon, but vegetations on the pulmonary valve are rare.

The lesions are more often localised to one part of a valve or are more irregularly disposed

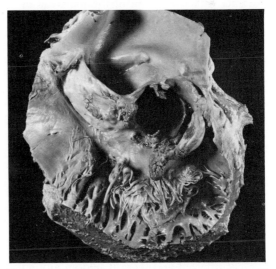

Fig. 15.32 Chronic rheumatic and superimposed acute bacterial endocarditis of aortic valve. The vegetations are large and irregular and there is severe damage to one of the cusps. Involvement of the root of the aorta has resulted in an acute aneurysm. × 0·5.

than in the other forms of endocarditis; for example, there may be massive vegetations at the junction of two aortic cusps, the rest of the valve being free. In spite of these features, in many cases it is not possible to distinguish between acute and subacute infective endocarditis from the lesions in the heart alone.

The clinical features are those of a severe acute bacterial infection often with evidence of pyaemia or embolic phenomena, together with rapidly changing heart murmurs and the development of heart failure. In the absence of antibiotics, blood cultures are usually positive.

Other valvular lesions

Non-infective thrombotic endocarditis consists of the formation of sterile thrombotic vegetations on the heart valves, usually in a patchy fashion along the lines of closure of the cusps of the mitral and aortic valves. The vegetations are usually smaller than those in infective endocarditis and softer, more friable and less regular than those in rheumatic endocarditis. They are composed of mixed thrombus, fragments of which may break off and cause systemic embolism and infarction. In most instances, this condition is discovered at necropsy on patients who have died of cancer or other wasting diseases, and it is sometimes called *marantic* or *terminal endocarditis*. It may be associated with the venous thrombosis which occurs in some patients with carcinoma of the pancreas or of other internal organs (p. 241).

Libman–Sacks endocarditis occurs in many patients with systemic lupus erythematosus. The vegetations are sterile and are softer and more friable and usually larger than those of rheumatic endocarditis. They are also more widely dispersed on the cusps, usually affect the mitral and tricuspid valves, and may extend onto the adjacent mural endocardium or over the ventricular surface of the valve cusps (i.e. the surface away from the bloodstream).

Atheroma-like degeneration of mitral valve. Yellowish patches of thickening and degeneration similar in structure to atheroma are fairly common in the mitral valve and may be attended by fibrosis and calcification, especially at the base of the cusps. The chordae tendineae are not affected and there is seldom any effect on cardiac function.

Valvular lesions in the carcinoid syndrome. Patients with secondary carcinoid tumours in the liver may develop stenosis of the pulmonary

and, less often, the tricuspid valve. The cusps show marked fibrous thickening, have a rolled edge and are adherent along the lines of the commissures. Fibrosis may extend over the adjacent endocardium both in the right ventricle and in the wall of the right atrium (Fig. 15.33). Only trivial lesions are found in the left side of the heart, probably because of destruction of 5-hydroxytryptamine, etc., by amine oxidases in the lungs (pp. 446–7).

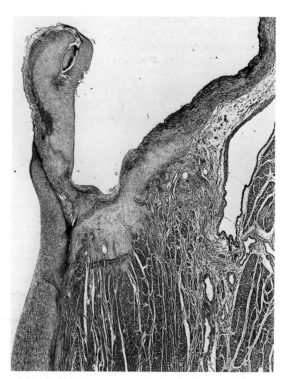

Fig. 15.33 Pulmonary valve in carcinoid syndrome showing great fibrous thickening of the cusp and of the subendocardial connective tissue. × 12.

Disorders of the conducting system

As indicated in preceding sections of this chapter, disturbances of cardiac rhythm commonly complicate various types of heart disease. Many of them, e.g. extrasystoles, paroxysmal tachycardia and atrial fibrillation, are not usually attributable to changes in the conducting system.

The most vulnerable part of the system is the A–V bundle and its right and left branches: injury may result from the various types of myocarditis (see Fig. 15.14, p. 410), chronic myocardial ischaemia or myocardial infarction, trauma during cardiac surgery, and invasion by metastatic tumours. Bundle branch fibrosis may also arise from unknown cause. The various grades of heart block can often be ex-

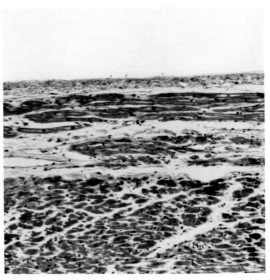

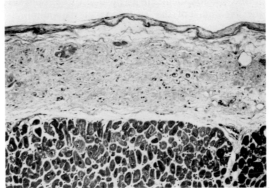

Fig. 15.35 'Idiopathic' bundle branch fibrosis. *Above*, normal left bundle branch from the heart of a young man, consisting of groups of fibres lying between the ventricular myocardium and endocardial surface. *Below*, almost complete loss of left bundle branch in a case of heart block. (Some loss of fibres occurs as a normal feature of ageing.) (Professor M. J. Davies.)

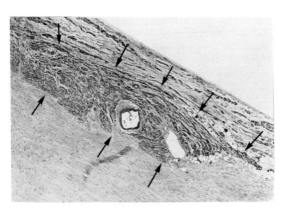

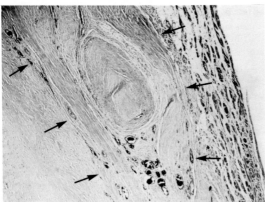

Fig. 15.34 Ischaemic fibrosis of A–V node. *Above*, normal A–V node (*outlined by arrows*), lying between the endocardium and central fibrous body. *Below*, ischaemic fibrosis of A–V node from a patient with heart block. (Professor M. J. Davies.)

plained by such injuries (Figs. 15.34, 15.35), but in some instances lesions have been sought in vain, while in others the finding of lesions has been associated with normal ECG patterns during life. This lack of close correlation probably reflects the large amount of work involved in thorough histological examination of the conducting system and the difficulties which arise from various artefactual changes.

Congenital Abnormalities

Little is known of the causation of congenital abnormalities, but the part played by rubella infection of the mother in the first three months of pregnancy is well established. About 10–20 per cent of the infants show serious abnormalities, of which heart disease constitutes about 50 per cent.

Normal development

A high proportion of congenital abnormalities of the heart result from defects or variations in the formation of the septa in the primitive heart. For details the student must consult a work on embryology and the classical studies of Maude Abbott and Helen Taussig, but it may be recalled that the heart at an early stage of development consists essentially of three chambers or parts, an atrial, a ventricular and the aortic bulb; division of each of these into two takes place separately. Of special importance in this connection is the relation of the ventricular septum to the division of the distal portion of the bulb into the beginning of the aorta and of the pulmonary artery. The ventricular septum grows upwards from the apex, with a curved margin resulting from the growing folds on the anterior and posterior walls, until ultimately there is a relatively small aperture at the base. The aortic bulb undergoes division into two nearly equal parts by the formation and fusion of two longitudinal folds in its wall, and the two vessels formed must rotate spirally in order to establish their normal continuity with the ventricles. The septum of the bulb ultimately fuses with the upgrowing ventricular septum, the last portion to close being represented by the membranous part of the septum. Important abnormalities occur in connection with the growth of these two septa. It is to be borne in mind that the positions of the semilunar valves do not correspond exactly with the junction of the primitive ventricle and the aortic bulb. This is especially the case on the right side, where the lower part of the bulb becomes the upper part of the right ventricle or conus, and, as we shall see, this part is sometimes abnormally narrow.

While some of the anomalies are incompatible with extra-uterine life, in many the circulatory dynamics are such that the patients may survive birth for varying periods of time. With the diagnostic methods of cardiac catheterisation and angiocardiography, successful surgical cure or alleviation of many of the conditions can be effected. It is convenient to divide the anomalies into those which produce *cyanosis* and those which do not. The cyanosis is produced by admixture of a relatively large amount of reduced haemoglobin from the systemic venous blood, with the oxygenated blood leaving the heart, i.e. a venous-arterial shunt exists. The resulting unsaturation of the arterial blood leaving the heart leads to *compensatory* rise in the red cell count, which makes cyanosis more prominent. Later, changes in the pulmonary vessels occur (p. 455) and the heart begins to fail. Cyanosis may then increase owing to impaired oxygenation of the blood by the lungs.

Cyanotic group

Malformations in connection with the aortic bulb—pulmonary and aortic stenosis. The commonest of these result from an unequal division of the bulb. Most frequently the septum is pushed to the right, so that the aorta is abnormally large and arises partly from left and partly from the right ventricle, there being usually also a defect in the ventricular septum. The result is pulmonary stenosis or obstruction, but the site of the narrowing varies. Sometimes the pulmonary artery is small, the division of the bulb being markedly unequal and occasionally the small pulmonary artery is completely obliterated. In other cases the narrowing is mainly at the valve, the cusps sometimes being partly fused to form a thickened diaphragm with an aperture of varying size. More rarely, there is a narrowing of the part of the right ventricle below the valve, that is, the part which is derived from the bulb. All these abnormalities interfere with the flow of blood into the pulmonary artery, and lead to a varying degree of hypertrophy of the right ventricle. Part of the blood from the right ventricle passes through the aperture in the interventricular septum and then into the aorta, and after birth the ductus arteriosus usually remains open and the lungs receive part of their blood supply through it. The foramen ovale also remains open and may be very large.

The commonest anomaly of this group and one which is amenable to surgery is the **tetrad of Fallot**. In this there is obstruction in the outflow tract of the right ventricle, usually from stenosis of the pulmonary valve, though the obstruction may be in the infundibular part of the right ventricle. This results in right ventricular hypertrophy and the pressure in this chamber is raised so that some of the reduced blood in the chamber is shunted through a high interventricular septal defect into the aorta, which, in addition to receiving the oxygenated blood from the left ventricle, partially overrides the septal defect and is thus in communication with the cavity of the right ventricle. All degrees of severity exist in the stenosis of the right ventricular outflow, the size of the septal defect and the dextraposition of the aortic root. In extreme cases the pulmonary orifice and artery may be atretic and blood reaches the lungs from the aorta through a patent ductus arteriosus.

In about 25 per cent of cases of Fallot's tetrad, there is a right aortic arch.

Eisenmenger's complex. In this there is a strong resemblance in the gross morphology of the heart to that just described, but there is no obstruction to the outflow from the right ventricle. The pressure gradients across the high interventricular septal defect are such that little right-to-left shunting of blood, and hence little cyanosis, occurs at first. Later, with the onset of pulmonary hypertension and changes in the pulmonary vessels, overt cyanosis occurs, partly from admixture cyanosis and partly from faulty oxygenation of the blood by the lungs.

Transposition of the great vessels. A curious anomaly results from failure of the proximal aorta and pulmonary artery, formed by division of the aortic bulb, to undergo the rotation necessary for the establishment of their correct relationships with the ventricles. In consequence, the aorta arises from the right ventricle and the pulmonary artery from the left. While such a condition alone is incompatible with extra-uterine life, it may sometimes be compensated, for a time, by persistence of the ductus arteriosus, patent foramen ovale or a defect of the interatrial or interventricular septum; often these defects are present in combination. In this condition, the chief difficulty is not the volume of blood reaching the lungs but the effectiveness of the mechanism allowing oxygenated blood to reach the systemic circulation. Hence the greater the volume of the shunt, the better the admixture of arterial blood to venous blood and the less marked is the cyanosis.

Truncus arteriosus. In this the arrangement of the heart and emergent arteries resembles that in elasmobranch fishes in which the aorta and the pulmonary arteries arise from a common stem vessel. The pulmonary arteries may be replaced by enlarged bronchial arteries. The truncus arises from both ventricles, overriding a ventricular septal defect. Sometimes the septum may be missing so that a single ventricular cavity exists. Defects of the interatrial septum are also common.

Single ventricle with a rudimentary outlet chamber. In this condition, a single ventricle provides blood to both the aorta and pulmonary artery, which may arise separately or from a rudimentary outlet chamber. The interatrial septum may or may not develop normally, resulting in cor binatrium triloculare or cor biloculare respectively.

Tricuspid atresia. This is associated with defective development of the right ventricle which in extreme cases is virtually absent. Blood passes from the right to the left atrium through a defect in the interatrial septum. The pulmonary artery is small, arising from the underdeveloped right ventricle. In some cases the vessel is atretic or occupies an abnormal position. Usually blood reaches the lungs from the aorta by a patent ductus arteriosus.

Aortic atresia. In this rare condition the aortic orifice is hypoplastic, the ascending aorta hypoplastic or atretic and the left ventricle poorly developed or absent. Circulation of blood is maintained by shunting of oxygenated blood from the left atrium into the right atrium and thence to the right ventricle and pulmonary artery. From this the aorta is filled via a patent ductus arteriosus.

Pure pulmonary stenosis. Here the course of the circulation is essentially normal but sometimes there is a patent interatrial septum. The lesion is a stenosis of either the pulmonary valve or the infundibulum of the right ventricle. The right ventricular myocardium is hypertrophied and able to force the blood to the lungs past the obstruction. If the interatrial septum is intact, cyanosis is not necessarily present; if there is interatrial communication a right-to-left shunt may be established with consequent cyanosis.

Anomalies of the venous return. These may involve the systemic or the pulmonary veins and vary greatly in detail. The superior and/or the inferior vena cava may open into the left atrium, thus shunting reduced systemic venous blood into the arterial side of the systemic circulation. In other cases, some of the pulmonary veins open into the right atrium: this results simply in an excessive amount of oxygenated blood being pumped around the pulmonary circulation and cyanosis will not occur.

Acyanotic group

Aortic valve stenosis and subaortic stenosis. Apart from these localised abnormalities, the heart is normal. Another isolated abnormality here is **bicuspid aortic valve**, which may later become the site of infective endocarditis or calcific stenosis.

Patent ductus arteriosus. While it will be appreciated from the foregoing description that this may coexist with many other anomalies, patency of the ductus may be the only abnormality present and closure by surgery restores the circulation to complete normality. Failure to close the ductus leads eventually to heart failure or the development of infective 'endocarditis' (endarteritis) at the site of the ductus. In a few cases there is associated pulmonary hypertension and in some the direction of blood flow in the ductus may be reversed so that unoxygenated blood passes from the pulmonary artery into the ductus and aorta distal to the ductus, usually immediately beyond the origin of the left subclavian artery. Such a patient may thus have a cyanotic tinge in the nailbeds of the toes but not in those of the hands.

Interatrial septal defect. This is one of the commonest congenital malformations of the heart. Even when the defect is large, it appears to have little effect on the circulation. Rarely a piece of detached thrombus, e.g. from the leg veins, passes from the right atrium through the defect to reach the left atrium and cause *crossed* or *paradoxical embolism*. While probe patency of the foramen ovale is very common in normal hearts (25 per cent approximately), the important malformations are of three main types: persistent ostium primum, ostium secundum and persistent atrio-ventricularis communis. In this last condition, there is often fusion of the tricuspid and mitral valves to form a common atrioventricular valve. Lutembacher's disease consists of an interatrial septal defect with mitral stenosis.

Interventricular septal defect. A high septal defect is frequently part of another congenital anomaly, e.g. tetrad of Fallot, but an isolated high interventricular septal defect is not uncommon. Maladie de Roger is the name sometimes applied to an isolated defect in the interventricular septum; the size and location of the aperture varies.

Anomalies of the aortic arch. As shown by Blalock, these are common in association with tetrad of Fallot (see above), but as isolated anomalies they rarely cause symptoms. When, however, a vascular ring is formed around the trachea and oesophagus by a right aortic arch and left descending aorta together with a persistent ductus arteriosus, ligamentum arteriosum or an anomalous left subclavian artery, pressure effects, mainly on the trachea, may result. A double aortic arch may give similar symptoms.

Coarctation (stenosis) of the aorta. Slight narrowing of the aorta between the left subclavian artery and the orifice of the ductus arteriosus, i.e. in the interval where the two main streams of the fetal circulation cross, is not very uncommon. The stenosis is rarely marked, but it may be severe and all degrees of narrowing up to complete atresia of the aorta at this point have been recorded. With major narrowing, an extensive collateral system from the carotids and subclavians links the aorta above and below the narrowed segment. The pulses in the lower limbs are poor as compared with those of the upper. Hypertension develops and death is likely to ensue from cardiac failure, cerebral haemorrhage or less commonly from local complications associated with the coarcted site, e.g. aneurysm or rupture of the aorta. Coarctation of the aorta may be associated with other congenital abnormalities, but frequently it is the only abnormality present and, moreover, it is one that can be cured by surgery. The condition is distinctly commoner in the male sex.

Ebstein's disease. In this condition there is downward displacement of the tricuspid valve so that the upper part of the right ventricle comes to be a functional part of the right atrium. The course of the circulation is normal.

Other abnormalities of the valves. Sometimes there is excess or deficiency in the number of the cusps of the semilunar valves; occasionally there are four cusps, usually somewhat unequal in size, but, as a rule, there is no interference with the efficiency of the valve. There may, however, be only two cusps, usually in the aortic valve. One cusp is usually larger than the other and often shows evidence of fusion of two cusps. Such bicuspid valves tend to develop calcific aortic stenosis (p. 418) and also bacterial endocarditis. Very rarely cases have been recorded in which two mitral valves have been present.

Diseases of the Pericardium

Pericarditis

Inflammation of the pericardium can result from bacterial and viral infections, or as a complication of myocardial infarction, and is also a feature of acute rheumatic fever and of uraemia.

Classification. Pericarditis may be classified according to its cause and may be acute or chronic. Acute cases are usually fibrinous and are divided into those with effusion (which may be serous, haemorrhagic or purulent), and those without. Some chronic cases are classified according to their effects on cardiac function (e.g. chronic constrictive pericarditis).

Causes

Pyogenic infection. Acute pericarditis may be the result of invasion by organisms from a lesion in the vicinity, such as empyema, suppurating mediastinitis, or any ulcerating tumour, e.g. of the oesophagus. In some cases, however, infection is by the bloodstream in the course of septicaemias. Suppurative pericarditis is produced chiefly by pneumococci, streptococci and staphylococci; and infection by the last may be secondary to small abscesses in the heart wall.

Tuberculosis. The pericardium is sometimes infected by lymphatic spread from an upper mediastinal lymph node in primary tuberculosis, or by direct spread from the pleura or lung in reinfection tuberculosis.

Coxsackie virus pericarditis, sometimes accompanied by myocarditis, occurs in outbreaks among infants and also affects adults (p. 410).

Non-infective. A sterile pericarditis commonly occurs in the later stages of an acute attack of rheumatic fever and may gravely impair the heart's action. In uraemia, pericarditis is a common late event, and appears to be due to vascular or metabolic disturbances. Acute fibrinous pericarditis usually accompanies myocardial infarction and is often more extensive than the infarct. Pericarditis is a feature of polyserositis (Pick's or Concato's disease, p. 658), in which great thickening of the subserous fibrous tissue occurs.

Naked-eye appearances

Fibrinous pericarditis is found in rheumatism, uraemia, myocardial infarcts and some infective cases. The exudate usually appears first posteriorly round the large vessels at the base of the heart as an opaque, dull and roughened layer, and when it becomes abundant it forms a rough covering to the heart with irregular projections (Fig. 3.21, p. 66), giving the so-called 'bread and butter' appearance.

Pericardial effusion, sometimes exceeding a litre, is usually accompanied by fibrinous pericarditis. The effusion may be serous in rheumatic fever or myocardial infarction, haemorrhagic in tuberculosis, uraemia, myocardial infarction and infiltration by carcinoma, and purulent following invasion by pyogenic bacteria.

The ordinary sequel to pericarditis is organisation of the deposited fibrin, and adhesions ultimately form with partial or complete obliteration of the pericardial sac. Sometimes, especially in rheumatic cases, there may be repeated attacks, and great thickening of the pericardium may result. Adherent pericardium may contribute to the development of cardiac hypertrophy. Pericardial adhesions are commonly found at necropsy and often the cause is not apparent.

Slightly thickened patches of opaque and whitish appearance in the epicardium are known as 'milk spots'. They occur especially over the anterior surface of the right ventricle and the apex of the left ventricle, and occasionally a large area of opacity is present. They are common in hypertrophied hearts and occasionally fibrous adhesions are present over an area of thickening. Milk spots are of no clinical significance.

Tuberculous pericarditis. At an early stage the changes may resemble an ordinary fibrinous pericarditis and its real nature may be discovered only on microscopic examination. In other cases the pleura may contain caseous material and this is usually followed by much thickening of the layers of the pericardium, and sometimes by calcification. In some cases at an early stage there is an abundant exudate, both fibrinous and fluid, and it may be heavily bloodstained. Ultimately the sac may be enormously distended. Tubercle bacilli are sometimes present in very large numbers in the exudate.

Chronic constrictive pericarditis is a rare condition of dense fibrous adhesions around the heart, usually commencing in childhood with a febrile illness and pericarditis clinically resembling rheumatism. Pericardial effusion is often followed by pleural effusion and later by absorption and healing with very dense fibrous tissue and sometimes calcification. The effect is to constrict the chambers of the heart and vena caval openings, which interferes with diastolic filling; a marked rise of venous pressure occurs and so the effects resemble those of cardiac failure. Most cases are either of tuberculous or unknown origin. Surgical resection of the visceral and parietal layers of the pericardium gives relief of symptoms and for most patients the long-term prognosis is then good.

Effects of pericarditis

Many examples of pericarditis are not recognised during life. In acute pericarditis there may be pain in the chest or neck, and pericardial friction. Signs of pericardial effusion include enlargement of the 'heart' on percussion and radiologically, with a feeble apex beat in the normal position. Chronic constrictive pericarditis may be associated with systolic retraction of the chest wall and with increased venous pressure and ascites due to interference with filling of the heart; the pulse pressure is low and decreases on inspiration (pulsus paradoxus).

Pericardial haemorrhage

Haemorrhage into the pericardial sac, giving rise to *haemopericardium*, may be due to rupture of the heart itself following infarction, to rupture of an aortic aneurysm, most often an acute dissecting aneurysm which strips open the aortic wall to the base of the heart (p. 386), or to a stab wound involving the heart or a large vessel. When the bleeding is rapid, the pressure of the blood in the pericardial sac interferes with the diastolic filling of the chambers. The output of blood from the left ventricle is greatly diminished, the blood pressure rapidly falls and death from heart failure results—this is known as **cardiac tamponade**.

Multiple minute haemorrhages occur into the layers of the pericardium in the various purpuric conditions. They are sometimes a prominent feature also in cases of death by suffocation.

Tumours of the Heart and Pericardium

Primary tumours of the heart are rare. *Fibroma, myxoma, lipoma, haemangioma* and *lymphangioma* are occasionally encountered, especially in the left atrium, the commonest being a myxomatous mass of considerable size, the so-called **cardiac myxoma**, projecting into the cavity from the margin of the foramen ovale: the commonly-associated mitral valve lesions may be due to haemodynamic or traumatic effects of the tumour. Cardiac myxoma sometimes has various unexplained effects, including weight loss, anaemia, a high ESR, serum protein disturbances, Raynaud's phenomenon and arthralgia. *Rhabdomyoma* of congenital origin occurs especially in the ventricles as multiple rounded nodules of pale and somewhat translucent tissue. It consists of large branching cells in which striped myofibrils are found; the cells have a somewhat vacuolated cytoplasm and contain much glycogen. In a number of cases, the tumour has been associated with multiple discrete gliomatous growths in the cerebral hemispheres—*tuberous sclerosis* (p. 772); in some cases there have also been malformations of the kidneys and liver, and adenoma sebaceum on the face (Bourneville's disease).

Metastatic tumours in the heart and pericardium are less uncommon than is generally realised, occurring in about 10 per cent of all fatal malignancies, secondary melanotic tumours being disproportionately numerous in relation to their total incidence. Primary carcinoma of the bronchi spreads to involve the heart more frequently than any other neoplasm (31 per cent of cases); no doubt the proximity of the primary growth is a factor in this high incidence, as direct extension readily occurs to the base of the heart and pericardium.

Neoplastic invasion of the pericardium often causes a haemorrhagic inflammatory exudate. Spread of tumour into the wall of the right atrium is liable to cause arrhythmias.

References

Davies, M. J., Fulton, W. F. M. and Robertson, W. B. (1979). The relation of coronary thrombosis to ischaemic myocardial necrosis. *Journal of Pathology* **86**, 99–110.

Davies, M. J., Woolf, N. and Robertson, W. B. (1976). Pathology of acute myocardial infarction with particular reference to occlusive coronary thrombi. *British Heart Journal* **38**, 658–64.

Kaplan, M. H. (1961). Immunopathological studies in rheumatic heart disease: concept of autoantibodies to heart in rheumatic fever and post-commisurotomy syndrome. In *Inflammation and Diseases of Connective Tissue*, pp.108–18. Edited by L. C. Mills and J. H. Moyer. Saunders, Philadelphia and London.

Lyampert. I. M. and Danilova, T. A. (1975). Immunological phenomena associated with cross-reactive antigens of micro-organisms and mammalian tissues. *Progress in Allergy* **18**, 423.

Further Reading

Abbott, M. E. S. (1954). *Atlas of Congenital Cardiac Disease*, pp. 62. American Heart Association, New York.

Crawford, Sir Theo. (1977). *Pathology of Ischaemic Heart Disease*, pp.170. Butterworth, London and Boston.

Hudson, R. E. B. (1965–71). *Cardiovascular Pathology*, Vols. 1–3. Edward Arnold, London.

Paul Wood's Diseases of the Heart and Circulation (1968). Various Authors. 3rd end., pp. 1164. Eyre and Spottiswoode, London.

Pomerance, Ariela and Davies, M. J. (Eds.) (1975). *The Pathology of the Heart*. Blackwell Scientific, Oxford and Melbourne.

Taussig, H. B. (1960). *Congenital Malformations of the Heart*. 3rd edn, pp. 204 and 1049. Harvard University Press, Cambridge.

16

Respiratory System

Introduction

The primary function of the respiratory system—oxygenation of the blood and removal of carbon dioxide—requires that air be brought into close approximation with blood. Accordingly, **the respiratory tract is particularly exposed to infection,** both by microbes in the inspired air and by spread downwards of the bacteria which commonly colonise the nose and throat. Another important hazard is presented by **inhalation of pollutants** contributed to the air we breathe in the form of dusts, smokes and fumes, a particularly important example being cigarette smoke. These pollutants are responsible for the high incidence of chronic bronchitis and chronic lung disease and also bronchial carcinoma in many parts of the world. Thirdly, the lungs are the only organs, apart from the heart, through which all the blood passes during each circulation: accordingly, cardiovascular diseases which disturb pulmonary haemodynamics are likely to have serious secondary effects on the lungs, such as pulmonary oedema, and conversely diseases of the lungs which interfere with pulmonary blood flow have important effects on the heart and systemic circulation. In short, *normal cardiac and pulmonary function are closely interdependent.*

Apart from infections, injury due to inhaled pollutants and the effects of cardiovascular disease, the respiratory tract is remarkably trouble-free, and most of this chapter will be devoted to the effects of these three hazards.

Although the respiratory tract, like other systems, is best considered on a regional basis, the continuity of the mucous membranes from nose to alveolus, and the microbial contamination of inspired air, allow ready spread of infection, and accordingly it seems appropriate to give a brief general account of the main factors concerned in respiratory tract infections before proceeding on a regional basis.

Respiratory infections

The defences of the respiratory tract against infection have been described in Chapter 7: they include upward flow of the surface film of mucus which coats the air passages and is impelled by ciliated epithelium; the cough reflex; the secretion of IgA antibodies; and the phagocytic activity of alveolar macrophages.

Bacterial infections of the respiratory tract may be primary (i.e. occur in healthy individuals), or secondary to a large number of conditions which depress resistance. **Primary infections** are now relatively rare in many parts of the world: they include laryngeal or nasal diphtheria, bacterial pneumonia due usually to *Strep. pneumoniae,* and pulmonary tuberculosis. Other examples include pneumonic plague and anthrax pneumonia. *Primary pneumonia due to various pyogenic bacteria is, however, relatively common in infants and old people.* **Secondary bacterial infections** occur especially when the local resistance of the respiratory mucosa is lowered by various virus infections, e.g. the common cold, influenza and measles: in these conditions, bacteria growing in the nose and throat extend downwards, usually giving a mixed infection, but in hospitals and other institutions, outbreaks of respiratory virus infections may be complicated by spread of virulent pathogenic bacteria from patient to patient. Chronic liability to bacterial infections also results from persistent abnormalities of the bronchi, especially chronic bronchitis and bronchiectasis, from various debilitating and wasting diseases, and from congenital and acquired immunodeficiencies.

Virus infections. *Most acute respiratory disease seen in general medical practice every* *winter is caused by viruses.* Over 150 different viruses have been isolated and antibody acquired against one virus rarely gives any cross-protection against any of the others. Many virus infections of the respiratory tract such as 'viral sore throat' and the common cold are frequent and comparatively trivial. Others, like bronchiolitis in infants due to the respiratory syncytial virus, may be fatal.

Most of the respiratory virus pathogens fall into a few well-defined major groups which replicate readily in tissue culture (Table 16.1).

The clinical syndromes due to acute respiratory virus infections depend to some extent on the age of the patient and the depth to which the respiratory tract is invaded. These syndromes are not sharply defined and may be produced by many different viruses. Nevertheless, recognisable clinical syndromes produced by viruses in the respiratory tract are the common cold (coryza), viral sore-throat, influenza and febrile catarrh, infantile croup, infantile acute bronchiolitis and 'atypical pneumonia'.

The common cold occurs throughout the world, including tropical countries, and exposure to low temperature does not appear to be a predisposing factor. The main cause is the group of *rhinoviruses* composed of more than a hundred serologically distinct picornaviruses (pico = small, RNA viruses). There is no cross immunity so that repeated infections are common. Other viruses causing common colds are the parainfluenza, respiratory syncytial, and more rarely some coxsackie and echo viruses.

Adenoviruses give rise to ill-defined syndromes of 'viral sore-throat' in which pharyngitis and conjunctivitis are prominent. They may cause epidemics of acute respiratory disease or endemic pharyngitis and follicular conjunctivitis. There are about thirty serological types of these DNA viruses.

The *parainfluenza viruses* cause a febrile catarrh that is intermediate in severity between the common cold and influenza. They are the major cause of acute laryngo-tracheo-bronchitis (succinctly termed 'croup') in young children. There are four serological types of these large RNA viruses.

Respiratory syncytial virus infection is common in young children, generally giving rise to trivial signs and symptoms. However, *it is highly virulent for children under two years of age and especially in infants less than one year old. It accounts for most of the young children*

Table 16.1 The respiratory viruses

Virus group	No. of serotypes	Disease
Influenza viruses	3*	Influenza
Parainfluenza viruses	4	Croup, colds, lower respiratory infections in children
Respiratory syncytial virus	1	Bronchiolitis and pneumonia in infants, colds in older children
Rhinoviruses	> 100	Colds
Adenoviruses	33	Pharyngitis, conjunctivitis
Coronaviruses	3	Colds
Coxsackieviruses	Types A21, B3	Colds
Echoviruses	Types 11, 20	Colds
'Virus pneumonia agents' (not true viruses)	A heterogeneous group	Atypical pneumonia

* There is considerable antigenic variation within the three major types (A, B and C) of influenza virus.

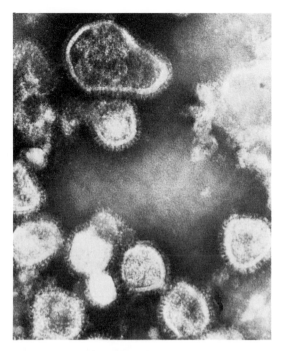

Fig. 16.1 Individual virus particles of the influenza H3N2 Hong Kong strain showing spikes of haemaglutinin by which the particle attaches itself to susceptible cells in the respiratory mucosa. Electron micrograph. × 128 000. (Dr. D. Hobson.)

admitted to hospital each winter with acute bronchiolitis and pneumonia.

The most serious disease of the upper respiratory tract caused by a virus is **influenza**. This is an acute febrile illness attended by malaise, often followed by lassitude and depression. In a minority of cases this may progress to influenzal pneumonia, which is commonly fatal. From time to time new antigenic strains arise and cause world-wide pandemics in the population having no immunity to the new strain. Three major types of this RNA myxovirus exist, called A, B and C in decreasing order of virulence (Fig. 16.1). The first influenza A virus, H0N1, was isolated in 1933. Strain H1N1 emerged in 1947 and H2N2, causing 'Asian flu', appeared ten years later. When a new virus variant appears, as in 1918 or 1957, world-wide pandemics usually ensue, in which rapidly fatal virus pneumonia with extreme cyanosis may occur in previously fit young people. However, in most epidemics bacterial complications are the chief cause of pneumonia. During influenza epidemics it is important to protect those who are at special risk, such as chronic bronchitics. The pathology of influenza and viral pneumonias is considered later in this chapter. **Measles**, and in lesser degree the other viral exanthemata of childhood, may be followed by acute tracheobronchitis, which is commonly associated with bacterial infection sometimes progressing to pneumonia.

Nose, Nasal Sinuses and Nasopharynx

Inflammatory conditions

Acute rhinitis is the common inflammatory disorder of the nasal mucosa. The familiar clinical form, **the common cold** (**acute coryza**), is caused by any one of a group of rhinoviruses or sometimes by parainfluenza virus and may be followed closely by secondary bacterial infection. The specific infectious fevers, such as measles, are often preceded by acute rhinitis. Nasal diphtheria is another cause but is now a rarity in many countries.

Another common clinical disorder is **hay fever**, or *acute allergic* or *atopic rhinitis*, which occurs as a result of sensitisation to certain pollens, such as the pollen of Timothy grass, or to house dust, animal dandruff, feathers or other specific antigens (p. 146). Atopic hypersensitivity is also a factor in some cases of nasal polyposis.

Acute sinusitis is generally a complication of acute infection of the nose, less commonly of dental sepsis. Gram + ve cocci such as *Streptococcus pyogenes, Streptococcus pneumoniae* or *Staphylococcus aureus* are the usual causal organisms.

Acute nasopharyngitis usually accompanies either acute rhinitis or acute tonsillitis in which *Streptococcus pyogenes* is the common pathogen.

The histopathology of acute inflammation of the nose, sinuses and nasopharynx is similar. There is hyperaemia and oedema of the mucosa, and the mucosal glands are hyperactive. In **virus infections,** neutrophil polymorphs are generally sparse in both the mucosa and the exudate until secondary bacterial infection supervenes, but thereafter increasing numbers of neutrophils migrate through the mucosa and the exudate becomes mucopurulent in character. There is a variable degree of loss of the superficial ciliated epithelium. In **atopic inflammation,** oedema of the submucosa is a prominent feature, giving rise to polypoid thickening of the mucosa. The mucosal glands are often enlarged and distended and the oedematous stroma is characteristically infiltrated by numerous eosinophil polymorphs.

Chronic rhinitis, sinusitis and nasopharyngitis may follow an acute inflammatory episode which has failed to resolve. Inadequate drainage of the sinuses, nasal obstruction due to polypi, or enlargement of the nasopharyngeal lymphoid tissue (adenoids), may be underlying factors.

Nasal polyps. Chronic inflammation of the nose may lead to polypoid thickening of the mucosa. Polyps are rounded or elongated masses commonly arising from the region of the middle turbinate. They are often bilateral, a point of distinction from nasal tumours. Nasal polypi are usually gelatinous in consistency with a smooth, shiny surface. Their microscopic structure consists of a core of loose oedematous connective tissue containing occasional mucous glands and covered by normal ciliated respiratory type of epithelium (Fig. 16.2), but squamous metaplasia is common. Lymphocytes, plasma cells and eosinophils infiltrate the submucosa to a variable degree. Polyps in which eosinophils predominate are considered to have an atopic basis.

Chronic granulomatous rhinitis. In contrast to acute infection, specific forms of chronic infection of the nose are rare in most communities. Chronic granulomas may be due to tuberculosis, tertiary syphilis, leprosy, scleroma or fungal infections such as aspergillosis or rhinosporidiosis.

Two rare forms of necrotising granuloma of uncertain nature occur in the upper respiratory tract. In one form, **Wegener's granuloma,** a necrotising lesion with giant cells develops usually in the nose or the maxillary sinuses, followed by necrotic lesions in the lung and associated with disseminated lesions of polyarteritis, particularly in the lungs and kidneys. The

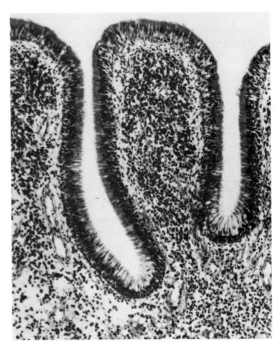

Fig. 16.2 Section through the margin of a nasal polyp, showing the respiratory epithelial lining and the loose oedematous stroma infiltrated with chronic inflammatory cells. × 100.

other, so-called **malignant granuloma of the nose,** presents as an ulcerated lesion which spreads progressively to erode the soft tissues and bones around the nose. Histologically the lesion consists of proliferating lymphocytes and macrophages: some authorities consider it to be a lymphoid neoplasm.

Tumours

Benign tumours. The common benign lesions of the nose are **haemangioma** of the septum and **squamous papilloma** of the vestibule. A much less common tumour is the **juvenile angiofibroma** which usually occurs in the nasopharynx. It appears in childhood, almost exclusively in boys, and tends to become quiescent by the end of the second decade. It is an enlarging vascular tumour which may cause bone erosion and destruction by pressure atrophy. Microscopically, it is seen to consist of small vascular spaces set in poorly cellular fibrous tissue. The histogenesis of the lesion is uncertain and, like haemangiomas, it may be a hamartoma of the nasal erectile tissue rather than a true neoplasm. Angioma may also occasionally present as a nasal polypoid lesion, but this form does not occur particularly in boys.

Malignant tumours. *Transitional-cell epithelial tumours* are common in the nasal passages. Some of these do not recur, and may be termed *transitional cell papillomas*: some recur in the same form, and some show a rapid change to *squamous carcinoma*. Transitional cell tumours are found mainly in the nasal cavity itself, probably because most of those in the nasal sinuses remain undiscovered unless they become squamous carcinomas. **Squamous carcinomas** are common in the nose and nasal sinuses, but anaplastic carcinoma and adenocarcinoma also occur. The so-called lymphoepithelioma of the nasopharynx is now generally accepted as a highly anaplastic carcinoma invading the normal non-neoplastic lymphoid tissue of the region.

Nasopharyngeal carcinoma, usually squamous, often poorly differentiated or of lymphoepitheliomatous (i.e. anaplastic) type, is particularly common in China, Malaysia, Indonesia and East Africa, where there is some evidence that the anaplastic forms of this tumour are associated with the same (EB) virus as Burkitt's lymphoma (p. 304). There is also an association with certain tissue antigens, e.g. HLR-A2. *Adenocarcinoma of the nose and nasal sinuses*, especially in the ethmoid, has been found to be unduly frequent in woodworkers in the furniture industry in Southern England. It arises after a very long latent period, sometimes of forty years or more.

Larynx and Trachea

Inflammatory conditions

Acute inflammation

Mild *acute laryngitis and tracheitis* are commonplace in the conditions of modern urban life with its atmospheric pollution with cigarette smoke, car exhaust fumes, industrial and domestic smoke, etc. While these factors in themselves are rarely the cause of significant clinical laryngeal disease, they may be of importance in predisposing to viral and bacterial infections. The viruses concerned have been considered above. The bacteria commonly involved are *Streptococcus pneumoniae*, *Streptococcus pyogenes* and *Neisseria catarrhalis*. Once secondary bacterial invasion occurs it may progress to bronchitis. Acute laryngo-tracheitis commonly complicates acute febrile states such as measles, influenza and typhoid. It usually subsides but it may pass into the chronic stage.

Pseudomembranous inflammation may be due to diphtheria (see below) or may be associated with secondary infection by *Streptococcus pyogenes*, *Staphylococcus aureus* or *Streptococcus pneumoniae* following infection with parainfluenza virus. Frequently such infections spread to involve the bronchial tree as laryngotracheo-bronchitis. In this condition there is necrosis of epithelium and the formation of an extensive fibrinous membrane in the trachea and main bronchi. There may be pronounced oedema of the subglottic area, resulting in stridor. In a minority of cases *Haemophilus influenzae* is the secondary invader, with severe sore throat, fever, tender lymph nodes and swelling of the epiglottis. In laryngo-tracheo-bronchitis the danger of laryngeal obstruction is, in general, greater than that of toxaemia or lung infection but bronchopneumonia and lung abscess are recognised complications. Pseudomembranous inflammation may result also from the action of corrosive substances or from the inhalation of irritating gases, notably ammonia.

Diphtheria is an acute pseudomembranous inflammation which is now very rare in countries where prophylactic immunisation is carried out. It usually affects the fauces, soft palate and tonsils but may also involve the nose, larynx, trachea and bronchi. The local lesions are characterised by the formation on the affected surface of a false membrane composed of fibrin, neutrophil polymorphs and necrotic epithelium and containing clumps of *Corynebacterium diphtheriae*. In the lower larynx and trachea the epithelium is columnar and the coagulated exudate rests on the basement membrane from which it separates easily and is coughed up. Over the vocal cords, where the mucosa consists of squamous epithelium, the membrane is firmly adherent. When it is coughed up from the trachea, it may remain attached to the vocal cords and may then impact in the larynx and cause death from suffocation. In nasal diphtheria the infection is often unilateral and the child may appear to have a cold with discharge from one nostril. This type may be overlooked until the appearance of such toxic manifestations as palatal paralysis or myocardial failure.

Acute epiglottitis. This condition, which is caused by *Haemophilus influenzae* type b, is a disease of early childhood which may lead to death within a few hours of onset. Histological examination shows swelling of the tissues due to acute inflammatory oedema and infiltration by neutrophil polymorphs. There is no mucosal ulceration.

In typhoid fever there may be laryngitis and bronchitis. Typhoid bacilli may be recovered from such lesions but more commonly the inflammatory reaction is produced by infection by other bacteria. Occasionally ulceration involves the perichondrium of the laryngeal cartilage, sometimes followed by necrosis and suppuration.

In smallpox, in addition to catarrhal or membranous inflammation, nodular inflammatory foci, similar to those in the skin, may form in the larynx and especially in the trachea. They are accompanied by intense congestion and haemorrhage but have less tendency to necrosis than those in the skin. Sometimes, however, they break down and form ulcers.

Endotracheal intubation. Sore throat, hoarseness, subglottic oedema and non-specific arytenoid granuloma may follow brief endotracheal intubation during general anaesthesia for a surgical operation. Endotracheal intubation exceeding forty eight hours, using a tube with an inflatable cuff, may lead to pressure injury and abrasion of the trachea with production of large ulcers which expose the underlying cartilaginous rings. Such ulcers, which may be oval or linear transverse lesions, are often located on the antero-lateral surface of the trachea: they may become infected by organisms such as *Pseudomonas aeruginosa* and *Candida albicans* and may be covered by a pseudomembrane. Occasionally, prolonged intubation is complicated by the development of tracheo-oesophageal fistula or tracheal stenosis.

Oedema of the glottis. This is an acute inflammatory oedema of the loose tissue of the upper part of the larynx and not of the vocal cords. The aryepiglottic folds and the tissues around the epiglottis become greatly swollen and tense. The false cords also are affected. This is an important lesion as *the swelling may lead to obstruction and death by suffocation.* It should be noted that after death the tissues become less swollen and tense than they were during life. Oedema of the glottis may occur in cardiac and renal diseases but rarely to such an extent as to cause serious results. The severe type occurs as a complication of other lesions of the larynx such as diphtheria or the deep-seated ulceration and perichondritis seen in tuberculosis and syphilis and sometimes in typhoid. It may result also from erysipelas or from the spread of inflammation from tonsillitis and suppurative conditions in the neighbourhood, or from agranulocytic angina. Oedema of the glottis is also caused by the trauma following impaction of a foreign body in the larynx and may be produced by irritating gases or scalding fluids. It occurs in angio-oedema (p. 254) and in some cases this form has proved fatal.

Chronic laryngitis

Chronic catarrhal inflammation of the larynx and trachea is frequently associated with excessive smoking. The mucous glands are swollen and give the surface a granular aspect. Heavy smoking also leads to extension of squamous epithelium beyond its normal distribution in the larynx.

Watt, Gregory and Stell (1975) have shown that the normal adult larynx is lined by squamous epithelium over the true cords, posterior glottis, a variable rim at the lateral margins and tip of the epiglottis on its posterior surface. Respiratory epithelium covers the central parts of the posterior surface of the epiglottis, the false cords, the ventricles and the subglottis. Squamous metaplasia is common among city dwellers, chronic bronchitics and smokers. Among heavy smokers, the entire larynx, including the subglottis and upper trachea, may be lined by squamous epithelium, thus interfering with clearance of mucus. Extensive squamous metaplasia is almost invariably present in association with carcinoma of the larynx.

Tuberculous laryngitis occurs secondary to

pulmonary tuberculosis, the tubercle bacilli being carried directly to the larynx in the sputum: they enter the mucosa and give rise to tubercles which caseate and form small ulcers with a tendency to spread. Any part of the larynx, or less commonly the trachea, may be affected but the disease usually starts first, and is most pronounced, in the arytenoid region and on the vocal cords. Occasionally small papillary outgrowths form at the margins of the tuberculous ulcers, and epithelial hyperplasia in biopsy material may be mistaken for carcinoma. Tuberculosis may spread deeply and involve the perichondrium of the arytenoid cartilages, there being chronic thickening with caseation and ulceration from which portions of dead cartilage may be separated and discharged. These various changes are often accompanied by great pain and considerable inflammatory swelling. Sometimes oedema of the glottis is superadded.

Syphilis. In the secondary stage there may be a catarrhal laryngitis, white 'mucous' patches of hyperkeratinisation or 'snail-track' ulcers (p. 218). The most important effects, however, are in the tertiary stage: the lesions usually start in the submucosa of the larynx or trachea, or in the perichondrium as a diffuse but irregular thickening and stiffening which often leads to immobility of the cartilage. Gummatous change follows. The epiglottis and affected cartilages may be extensively ulcerated and the latter may become necrotic and separated. There is a pronounced tendency to extensive scarring, with stenosis and deformity of the larynx.

Tumours

Benign tumours. Small inflammatory polyps are common and may contain amyloid or show myxoid degeneration. They may simulate neoplasms. The *squamous papilloma* is the commonest benign tumour of the larynx. It occurs usually on the vocal cords and especially at the commissure. In adults, it is generally single, but in children less than five years old it may be multiple and arise anywhere within the larynx. *Papillomas in children* are mostly of viral origin and they regress spontaneously at puberty, sometimes with great rapidity. *In the adult*, a papilloma may recur after removal, but seldom undergoes malignant change. The *laryngeal fib-*

roma is less common. It is usually small, rounded, and sometimes pedunculated. Like the papilloma, it is common on the vocal cords, and both are apt to occur in singers and others who use their voices a lot. Angioma, myxoma and lipoma are all very rare.

Granular cell myoblastoma sometimes arises in the larynx.

Malignant tumours. *Carcinoma* is the commonest malignant tumour of the larynx: it is usually squamous, and occurs most often in men over fifty years old. The incidence in Britain has declined steadily over the past twenty years and an association with pipe smoking has been postulated. When the tumour is on the true or false vocal cords, it is usually less invasive and has a better prognosis, after removal, than when it arises in the upper part of the larynx or in the subglottic region. Carcinoma of a vocal cord appears first as a small indurated patch, sometimes with a papillary surface, and subsequently ulcerates (Fig. 16.3). In the latter case, diagnosis will be unsatisfactory if only a superficial part is removed for

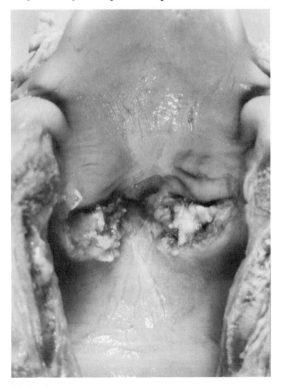

Fig. 16.3 Carcinoma of the larynx, causing extensive ulceration of the vocal cords. The false cords are intact. × 2. (Dr. J. Watt.)

microscopic examination. A carcinoma of the larynx infiltrates and destroys the surrounding parts by ulceration. This may be accompanied by septic infection from which the discharge passes down the bronchi into the lungs and causes aspiration pneumonia.

In contrast to the larynx and bronchi, **the trachea** is a rare site of tumours.

The Bronchi

The cells of the bronchial epithelium in health and disease

As explained in Chapter 7, the ciliated and mucus-secreting cells of the bronchial epithelium are intimately concerned in the defence of the airways and lungs against microbes and foreign material. Certain viruses may damage the ciliary mechanism of the respiratory epithelium, thus facilitating invasion of the deeper parts of the bronchial tree and lung by bacteria. Chronic irritation of the bronchi by polluted air and particularly by cigarette smoke may lead to the hyperplasia and hypertrophy of goblet cells and mucous glands which is an important feature in chronic bronchitis. Other, less familiar cells are present in the bronchial epithelium and subserve functions which are not yet well understood. The role of these cells in pulmonary pathology is at present not clear but we consider them briefly here in anticipation of a fuller understanding of them in the near future.

Within the bronchial epithelium there are argyrophilic cells, termed *Feyrter cells* (Fig. 16.4), which have the cytological and ultrastructural features of the chief cells of the carotid body. They appear to belong to the group of 'apud' cells, many of which are associated with the secretion of polypeptide hormones (p. 1034). Feyrter cells may possibly have an endocrine function and may be responsible for the hormonal effects of some types of bronchial carcinoma. On exposure to chronic hypoxia, these bronchial argyrophilic cells show the same fine structural changes in their intracytoplasmic vesicles as those shown in the chief cells of the carotid body. They may act as airway chemoreceptors. It has been postulated that bronchial argyrophilic cells may produce histamine and catecholamines which may be of importance in dilating the pulmonary arterial musculature of the fetus, thus aiding adaptation to neonatal life.

Scattered among the ciliated respiratory epithelial cells in the bronchi and especially in the respiratory bronchioles are the non-ciliated *Clara cells* (Fig. 16.5). These have all the features of apocrine secretory cells; the secretory product accumulates within smooth cisternae at the apex of the cell, and the apical region is then extruded into the bronchiolar lumen. Administration of chlorphentermine to

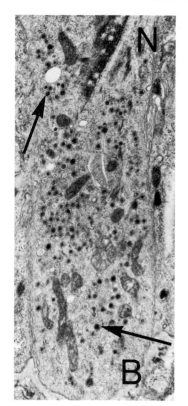

Fig. 16.4 Feyrter cell. Electron micrograph of bronchial epithelium from a neonatal rat showing a Feyrter cell lying on the basement membrane (B). The cell contains characteristic round osmiophilic bodies (arrows) and elongated mitochondria. Only part of the nucleus (N) is shown in the figure. × 12 500.

rats induces hyperplasia of Clara cells with accumulations of phospholipid within them and in the alveolar spaces. On evidence of this sort, it is possible that these cells may be one source of pulmonary surfactant.

Brush cells are also found in the epithelium of the conducting airways. They resemble alveolar brush cells, or type III pneumocytes. Their most striking feature is the large regular microvilli which cover their relatively small free surface. Their function is as

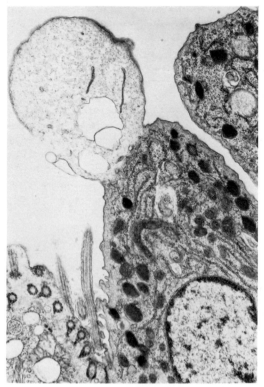

Fig. 16.5 Clara cell. Electron micrograph of bronchiolar epithelium from a neonatal rat showing the apex of the cell caught in the process of extrusion into the bronchiolar lumen. It contains little smooth endoplasmic reticulum. The main body of the cell contains rough endoplasmic reticulum and mitochondria. × 12 500.

yet unknown but they may be some type of receptor because their fine structural features are similar to those of the chemoreceptor cell in taste buds.

Acute bronchitis

A distinction must be made between acute inflammation of the larger bronchi which lie outside the lung lobules (**acute bronchitis**) and of the small, intralobular bronchi and bronchioles (**acute bronchiolitis**). These different anatomical sites influence the likely consequences and hence seriousness of the inflammatory reaction. *The common acute bronchitis of the adult affects the large and medium-sized bronchi.* It is usually mild but may be the cause of much disability when it aggravates an established chronic bronchitis, especially in aged or debilitated subjects. *Except as a complication of influenza, acute bronchiolitis is rare in healthy adults,* because

bacteria do not readily spread so far down the bronchial tree. It does, however, occur in children, old people and in states of debility: it is a serious condition owing to the liability of the organisms to spread to the adjacent acini and cause bronchopneumonia. Accordingly, acute bronchiolitis is dealt with in relation to pneumonia on p. 467 *et seq.*

The larger bronchi have mucous glands in their walls so that their involvement in acute inflammation is characterised by excessive production of mucus. Acute bronchitis may be catarrhal, membranous or putrid.

Catarrhal bronchitis is characterised by excessive secretion of mucus together with inflammatory exudation. If the inflammatory stimulus (usually bacterial infection) persists, neutrophil polymorphs appear and the sputum changes from a mucoid secretion to yellow muco-pus. In very severe cases the superficial part of the bronchial wall may be shed with exposure of deeper tissues—the so-called ulcerative bronchitis. *Much acute bronchitis is probably initiated by viruses or mycoplasma which impair local defence mechanisms and allow secondary bacterial invasion by the more pathogenic bacteria present in the upper respiratory tract at the time.* Of these, *Haemophilus influenzae* and *Streptococcus pneumoniae* are the commonest, being found in the upper respiratory tract in half the adult population and in an even higher proportion of children. *Staphylococcus aureus* and *Streptococcus pyogenes* can produce a severe purulent bronchitis in infants. Sometimes catarrhal bronchitis is an early symptom of typhoid. A much rarer cause of acute bronchitis is the inhalation of smoke or irritant gases such as sulphur dioxide or chlorine.

Pseudo-membranous bronchitis sometimes occurs in diphtheria, which has been described above. Rarely it may be produced by severe infections due to *Staphylococcus aureus* and parainfluenza viruses.

Putrid bronchitis commonly occurs in dilated bronchi or bronchiectatic cavities as a result of decomposition of stagnating bronchial secretions by putrefactive bacteria, such as *Borrelia vincenti* and anaerobic streptococci. It is also associated with aspiration pneumonia following inhalation of infected fluids during narcosis or coma, and is a common result of ulceration of malignant tumours growing into the trachea or bronchi.

The bronchi become covered with necrotic debris consisting of fibrin, dead tissue and the various bacteria concerned, and the sputum is abundant and foul-smelling.

Chronic bronchitis

In spite of its name, *chronic bronchitis is not primarily an inflammatory disease but consists of metaplastic and other changes resulting from chronic irritation of the bronchial epithelium.* The two main irritants responsible are cigarette smoke and atmospheric pollution, aggravated by dampness and fog. Accordingly, it is exceptionally common in heavy smokers and in industrialised areas. It is especially prone to occur in middle-aged men and is a major cause of absenteeism from work, of great economic and sociological importance. Under certain atmospheric conditions, sulphur dioxide and other pollutants accumulate in the air and give rise to the lethal aerosol called smog which will kill sufferers from the disease. *One serious aspect of chronic bronchitis is that it frequently becomes associated with the condition of pulmonary emphysema, which is described later* (p. 460).

The chronic irritation of the bronchial epithelium leads to a pronounced hypertrophy and hyperplasia of mucous glands within the bronchial wall and an increase in the number and proportion of goblet cells, at the expense of ciliated cells, in the lining epithelium. Goblet cells appear also in the terminal bronchioles, where they are normally absent. The hypertrophy and hyperplasia of mucous glands can be detected and assessed by quantitative histological techniques, such as point counting, or less accurately by comparing the thickness of the mucous gland layer, which is in fact very irregular, with that of the bronchial wall. These changes are persistent and lead to an excessive production of mucus, which is the hallmark of both the histological and the clinical pictures. In fact chronic bronchitis has been defined by the British Medical Research Council as a clinical entity characterised by a cough productive of sputum, in the absence of cardiac or other pulmonary disease: to fulfil the definition sputum must be produced on most days for a period of at least three months of the year, during at least two consecutive years. Areas of squamous metaplasia of the bronchial epithelium are common in chronic bronchitis, especially in heavy cigarette smokers.

Excessive production of mucus, combined with the loss of ciliated epithelium, results in accumulation of mucus which penetrates even into the alveolar spaces. There is a tendency for colonisation of the retained secretion by bacteria, although they are of little importance in the primary causation of the disease. The bacteria usually found are *Haemophilus influenzae* and *Streptococcus pneumoniae*. Thus in chronic bronchitis the lower respiratory tract, which is normally sterile, is very liable to be infected, and an episode of virus infection or of irritation by atmospheric pollution, fog or cigarette smoke could be sufficient to precipitate an acute exacerbation, with more extensive invasion of tissues by bacteria already present in the bronchial tree.

When such secondary pyogenic infection occurs, the sputum changes in character from a glairy mucus to a frankly yellow pus. Bouts of acute infection of this type may occur several times during the course of a year, especially during winter.

It is important to distinguish between chronic bronchitis, which is based on a chronic irritation of the bronchial tree, and emphysema, which is a destructive disease of the lung substance. The two conditions commonly exist together but they are quite distinct. Chronic bronchitis must also be distinguished from bronchial asthma. Clinicians and respiratory physiologists are inclined to refer to chronic bronchitis and emphysema together as '*chronic obstructive airways disease*' but this is not a pathological diagnosis. Organic obstruction to airways may, in fact, occur in cases of chronic bronchitis without emphysema. The episodes of mucopurulent inflammation may give rise to ulceration, scarring and destruction of the walls of bronchioles and this may lead to multiple stenoses and airway obstruction. This should be contrasted with the much rarer condition of *bronchiolitis obliterans* where bronchiolar epithelium may be destroyed by irritant gases such as ammonia or by a severe infection, and replaced by polypoid masses of granulation tissue.

Bronchial asthma

In bronchial asthma there is widespread bronchial obstruction due to muscular spasm and plugging by thick mucus.

Aetiology and types. Bronchial asthma may be classified into extrinsic and intrinsic types. **Extrinsic asthma** usually starts in childhood or early adult life and may be preceded by infantile eczema or hypersensitivity to foodstuffs in childhood. It is due mainly to atopic (type I) hypersensitivity (p. 146) to one or more extrinsic antigenic substances ('allergens') and inhalation of the offending allergen brings on an attack within a few minutes. As already explained, such hypersensitivity occurs in individuals who have a genetically-determined predisposition to develop reaginic antibodies of IgE class, and skin tests or provocative inhalation tests with the allergen(s) responsible typically produce an immediate (type I) reaction. The allergens commonly responsible include various pollens, animal dandruff, house dust and various fungi.

The most important allergen in house dust is provided by house-dust mites, notably *Dermatophagoides pteronyssinus* (Fig. 16.6) which infests mattresses and lives on human squames. This mite is commonly found in house dust, and inhaled excreta or fragments of the mite produce an asthmatic reaction in sensitised individuals. *The prognosis in extrinsic asthma is good, although deaths may result from overmedication or from sudden withdrawal of corticosteroids.*

Intrinsic asthma usually develops later in adult life in subjects without an individual or family history of previous atopic diseases. In contrast to extrinsic asthma, skin tests or provocative inhalation tests fail to reveal a responsible allergen. Nasal polypi are common, and microscopic examination of them shows infiltration with eosinophils. The prognosis is less good than in extrinsic asthma. Patients tend to develop drug hypersensitivities, particularly to aspirin and penicillin, and administration of these drugs may then be followed by a generalised atopic reaction which is sometimes fatal. *Intrinsic asthma is commonly associated with chronic bronchitis,* and atopic hypersensitivity to allergens provided by bacteria in the infected bronchi has been suggested, although this has seldom been established.

Psychological factors are of importance in asthma and in many patients the attacks are more likely to occur during periods of anxiety or emotional disturbance.

Clinical features. Asthmatic patients usually

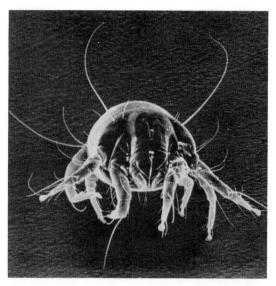

Fig. 16.6 The house-dust mite, *Dermatophagoides pteronyssinus.* × 300. (By courtesy of Bencard.)

suffer from acute attacks characterised by a feeling of tightness in the chest, difficulty in breathing, and particularly in exhaling, which is accompanied by loud wheezing, and often coughing which, during the attack, tends to be non-productive. As the attack subsides, thick viscid sputum, which contains eosinophils, is coughed up. An attack may last from a few minutes to days and may vary in severity from mild dyspnoea to wheezing with severe respiratory distress. Attacks may occur almost continuously, the so-called *status asthmaticus.* Some years ago there was a striking increase in mortality in Britain associated with the use of pressurised aerosols of sympathomimetic drugs. This declined following the issue of warnings against excessive use of such aerosols.

During attacks the lungs become overdistended with air, but such distension should not be confused with pulmonary emphysema (p. 460), which is only likely to complicate bronchial asthma when there is associated chronic bronchitis. *Right ventricular hypertrophy does not result from uncomplicated bronchial asthma.*

Pathology. When death has occurred during an acute attack, at necropsy the lungs appear overdistended with air and fail to collapse. Their cut surfaces show occlusion of many segmental bronchi by plugs of tough mucoid material (Fig. 16.7). Occasional areas of bron-

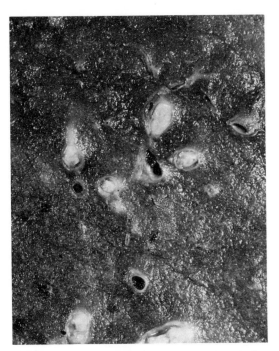

Fig. 16.7 The cut surface of a lung from a patient who died during an acute attack of bronchial asthma. The bronchi are distended by plugs of tough white mucoid material. × 2. (Dr. P. S. Hasleton.)

chiectasis (see below) may be present but chronic emphysema (p. 460) is slight or absent. The outstanding feature in sections of asthmatic lung during an attack is the plugging of the bronchial lumen by mucinous material containing eosinophils and normal or degenerate columnar respiratory epithelial cells. The cellular elements tend to form twisted strips, known as Curschmann's spirals, which are sometimes found in asthmatic sputum. The bronchial epithelium is shed into the lumen, exposing the basal layer of cells overlying the basement membrane which shows a characteristic hyaline thickening. The submucosa shows vascular congestion, oedema and infiltration by eosinophils from which Charcot's crystals are derived. There have been claims that the number of mast cells is increased. There is hypertrophy of the smooth muscle of the small bronchi, clearly associated with the repeated spasm of these airways (Fig. 16.8). Eventually the changes of chronic bronchitis may supervene, i.e. hypertrophy and hyperplasia of the mucous glands in the bronchial walls and extensive replacement of ciliated epithelium by goblet cells.

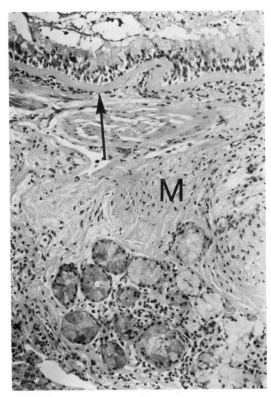

Fig. 16.8 Bronchial asthma. The bronchial lumen (top) contains mucinous material and is lined by intact respiratory epithelium. The basement membrane shows a characteristic hyaline thickening (arrow). The layer of bronchial smooth muscle (M) is hypertrophied and there is a proliferation of mucous glands (bottom). × 130.

Bronchiectasis

Definition and classification. *Bronchiectasis means an abnormal and irreversible dilatation of the bronchi, which may be generalised or localised, and may result in the formation of multiple large spaces or cavities.* It is said to be *cylindrical* when the bronchi are affected over most of their length; this is most pronounced in the lower lobes. In the *saccular* form the dilatation is more localised and severe. *Congenital bronchiectasis* results from failure of development (agenesis) of pulmonary alveolar tissue or failure of large portions of a lobe or lobes to expand at birth (atelectasis): the affected lobe is small and shrunken and dilated bronchi form cyst-like spaces which extend almost to the pleural surface, there being virtually no trace of lung substance between them.

Structural changes. In chronic bronchitis the transverse markings of the bronchial lining are often increased and depressions are present between the ridges; from this condition all degrees of generalised dilatation are seen up to fully established cylindrical bronchiectasis. Saccular bronchiectasis (Fig. 16.9) is usually due to fibrosis of the surrounding lung tissue with obliteration and destruction of the smaller bronchi and bronchioles. The dilated sacs so clearly displayed in a bronchogram appear to be the expanded terminations of the first few branches of the segmental bronchi. The lining of the bronchiectatic spaces resembles an irregularly swollen and vascular bronchial mucosa and is often congested. For a time the cavities are almost dry, but later secretion accumulates, becomes purulent, and ulceration of the wall occurs. Bilateral saccular bronchiectasis is seen in the upper lobes in the more fibrotic varieties

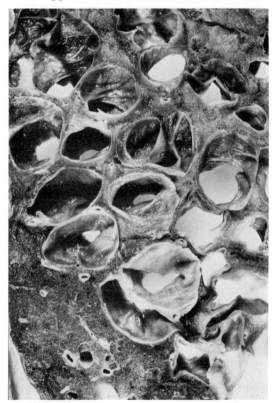

Fig. 16.9 Bronchiectasis. There is pronounced dilatation of bronchi which appear crowded together with obliteration of intervening lung substance. The dilated bronchi have thick white fibrous walls and their lumens are tortuous and lined by congested mucosa.

of chronic tuberculosis, where the true nature of the lesion may be difficult to prove; such cases are now becoming rare in countries where tuberculosis has declined. Apart from tuberculous infection, saccular bronchiectasis is usually unilateral and is commonest in the lower lobes of the lung, especially in the left posterior basal segment.

On microscopic examination of the bronchiectatic cavities an epithelial lining may be present to a varying extent, the cells being columnar, rounded or flattened. They may occur in single or several layers; sometimes there is squamous metaplasia. In specimens removed surgically at an early stage, the walls of the larger affected bronchi often show surprisingly good preservation of their structural elements, the chief change being dilatation of the lumen, with collapse and obliteration of their terminal divisions and fibrosis of the lung tissue. In the later stages the epithelium disappears, the surface being formed by a thinned basement membrane beneath which there is granulation tissue. Deeper ulceration also may be present. The various structures of the bronchial wall such as muscle, elastic tissue and glands become atrophied and may disappear. This is the usual state found in necropsy specimens.

Effects. Ultimately an abundant purulent secretion accumulates within the bronchiectatic cavities and this tends to stagnate and undergo decomposition. Accordingly, patients suffering from bronchiectasis often have halitosis and abundant foul-smelling sputum. Organisms may spread from the bronchiectatic cavities to the alveolar tissue, either by the air passages or by direct ulceration, and cause pneumonia or a lung abscess. In such conditions the wall of a vein may become involved, with the formation of septic emboli and the development of secondary abscesses, particularly in the brain. The abundant putrid secretion from the bronchi may lead to infection of the nasal sinuses.

In chronic bronchiectasis pulmonary haemodynamic changes may occur. There is usually considerable enlargement of the bronchial arteries (Fig. 16.10) with the development of bronchopulmonary anastomoses so that the bronchial blood flow is substantially increased. This may be a factor in raising pulmonary arterial pressure and increasing the degree of right ventricular hypertrophy that results. Left ventricular hypertrophy may also occur.

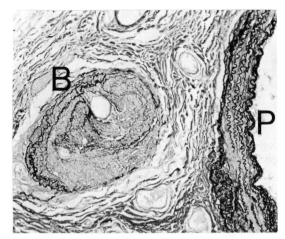

Fig. 16.10 Arteries in the wall of a dilated bronchus in a case of bronchiectasis. An elastic pulmonary artery (P) is seen to the right. Alongside it is a hypertrophied bronchial artery (B). × 132.

Aetiology. In the production of bronchiectasis three main factors may be concerned:

(a) loss of aerated lung substance so that the force of inspiratory expansion of the chest falls, in the affected part of the lung, on the bronchial walls alone, **(b)** weakening of the supporting tissue of the bronchial wall caused by inflammatory changes, and **(c)** contraction of fibrous bands connecting the bronchial wall with the fibrosed and adherent pleura.

In long-established cases these factors are variously combined and usually all three are present, but it is important to ascertain which is of primary importance in the pathogenesis of the condition.

Bronchiectasis is usually a sequel of bronchiolitis and bronchopneumonia in childhood with partial collapse and imperfect resolution; it may also follow congenital atelectasis of a portion of the lung. In children the bronchopneumonia may be primary or it may complicate whooping cough or measles. In adults, influenza may have similar effects. Some cases of juvenile bronchiectasis were shown by Macfarlane and Somerville (1957) to be associated with adenovirus infection; the bronchi show pronounced irregularity and narrowing of the lumen by hyperplastic submucosal lymphoid tissue. The condition closely resembles that seen in certain virus infections of the lung in cattle ('cuffing pneumonia'), and is called *follicular bronchiectasis*.

There has been much uncertainty about the relative parts played by infection with consequent weakening of the bronchial walls and by collapse of lung tissue with subsequent fibrosis. Radiological investigations clearly indicate that any major degree of pulmonary collapse with negative intrapleural pressure is followed almost at once by dilatation of the bronchi supplying the collapsed zone; this dilatation may subsequently disappear when the lung becomes re-expanded. Permanent collapse is, however, followed by fibrosis and the bronchi remain dilated. Radiographic examination indicates that this state is commoner than had been supposed and that it may exist for long periods without the clinical symptomatology associated with bronchiectasis. The dilated bronchi are relatively dry, and if lobectomy is performed at this stage, remarkably little structural change in the larger bronchial walls may be seen. Infection, with destruction of the specialised elements and consequent weakening of the wall cannot, therefore, be the primary change in these cases, and *it is probable that pulmonary collapse is the all-important initial causal lesion*. No doubt bronchial dilatation is hastened by the forced inspiration which follows the act of coughing. A vicious circle is thus set up, the effects of which become more severe when the accumulation of infected secretions has produced inflammatory damage to the bronchial walls with loss of the cartilage, muscle and elastic tissue.

Undoubtedly *the bronchopneumonias of childhood* are the most important antecedent to bronchiectasis, but any extensive pulmonary fibrosis may have this effect. In *chronic pulmonary tuberculosis* with fibrotic change, saccular bronchiectatic cavities are common in association with tuberculous cavities, and they also occur in silicosis and fibrotic conditions generally. In infants a few months old suffering from *fibrocystic disease of the pancreas*, the trachea and bronchi are lined by tough mucoid secretion which soon becomes purulent; bronchopneumonia follows, and, if the infant survives, bronchiectasis is a common sequel (p. 721).

Bronchial obstruction

Various degrees of obstruction may occur up to complete occlusion and either large or small bronchi may be affected, the causation being different in the two cases. Progressive obstruction of a **large bronchus** is most frequently produced by a primary carcinoma infiltrating the wall and growing into the lumen, or by pressure of massively enlarged lymph nodes. A rare cause of progressive bronchial obstruction is pressure on a main bronchus by an aneurysm of the aortic arch. Sudden obstruction may be produced by a foreign body lodging in a large bronchus. This may obstruct the bronchus completely, whereupon the air in the related part of the lung is absorbed rapidly and pulmonary collapse follows. Usually, however, obstruction is partial at first, resulting in the accumulation of oedema fluid and secretions with some degree of bronchial dilatation. Bacterial infection in the part beyond the obstruction follows, leading to a purulent bronchitis which by further extension may bring about suppurative bronchopneumonia. This is the usual sequence of events when a major bronchus is invaded by a neoplasm or is otherwise progressively obstructed.

Obstruction of individual **small bronchi** does not lead to collapse of the segment of lung supplied, because collateral ventilation from adjacent lobules through the pores of Kohn and canals of Lambert, connecting bronchioles to distal air passages, supplies enough air to expand the obstructed segment. It is more likely to become distended.

Obstruction of **bronchioles** is usually produced by inflammatory exudate, such as purulent plugs of bronchopneumonia, or by fibrinous exudate. In bronchial asthma the obstruction is due to the spasmodic contraction of the walls of the bronchioles, aided by the presence of tough secretion. If the obstruction is such that air can be sucked in and cannot be expelled, as may occur in bronchiolitis and in asthma, then hyperinflation may occur in the area supplied by the obstructed bronchioles. Such hyperinflation is at first reversible when the obstruction is removed. When the bronchiolitis is repeated, destruction of the wall of the respiratory bronchiole may occur, leading to centrilobular emphysema (p. 462).

The Lungs

Functions

The essential function of respiration is to provide oxygen to the cells of the body and to remove excess carbon dioxide from them. In large animals such as man, *respiration in its broader physiological context involves four processes*. The first act of respiration is **ventilation** which is the exchange of gases between the alveolar spaces and external atmosphere. Then in the lungs the blood gases exchange with alveolar air by **diffusion** across the alveolar walls. Finally the blood circulatory system is used to **transport** gases to and from the tissues, while **exchange** between blood and tissue cells occurs in the systemic capillaries. *Respiration in its clinical sense is generally restricted to those aspects which concern the major airways and lungs.* The primary function of the lungs is, therefore, to oxygenate mixed venous blood. This involves the controlled absorption of oxygen and the elimination of carbon dioxide so that the blood gas tensions are maintained within normal limits.

Although primarily involved in gas exchange, the lungs also have important non-respiratory functions: they act as a filter for the blood passing through them and are also concerned in the metabolism of certain vasoactive substances. Their anatomical situation is ideal for these roles for, apart from the heart, the lungs are the only organs through which all the blood passes in a single circulation. The pulmonary capillary bed is a huge network, the average diameter of the capillaries being about 8 μm. Particles ranging in diameter from 10 to 75 μm tend to be delayed in passing through the pulmonary circulation. Small emboli such as fibrinous clots, bone marrow, fat, placental tissue and particulate matter contaminating intravenous infusions, are trapped in the lungs and may be cleared by the action of proteolytic enzymes and phagocytosis. The lung, therefore, plays an important role as a sieve in protecting organs such as the brain and kidney.

The lungs also have the ability to clear certain vasoactive substances from the blood and to synthesise or activate others. Thus significant proportions of the 5-hydroxytryptamine, bradykinin and noradrenaline present in the blood are removed during its passage through the lungs. The lung is probably the main site for the conversion of the relatively inactive decapeptide angiotensin I to the potent systemic vasoconstrictive octapeptide angiotensin II. The enzyme mechanisms responsible for the clearing and activation of these vasoactive substances are probably localised in the endothelial cells lining the pulmonary arteries, capillaries and veins.

Respiratory failure

The primary function of the lungs is to maintain the blood gas tensions at normal levels. *Respiratory failure exists when a patient is unable to maintain his blood gas tensions within normal limits* and it is usually said to be present when the systemic arterial oxygen tension (Pa_{O_2}) falls below 60 mm Hg or when the carbon dioxide tension (Pa_{CO_2}) exceeds 50 mm Hg, while the patient is breathing air. Figures such as these imply that the patient's respiratory function is impaired, but it should be emphasised that many people are able to live comparatively unrestricted lives with blood gas tensions at least as abnormal as these.

The maintenance of normal gas tensions depends on the following factors.

1. Adequate ventilation of the alveolar spaces.
2. Unimpaired diffusion across the alveolar-capillary wall.
3. An even distribution of ventilation to the alveoli relative to the pulmonary capillary blood flow (perfusion).

The causes of respiratory failure may, therefore, be divided into three groups: *hypoventilation, impaired diffusion* and *uneven ventilation and perfusion.*

Hypoventilation

Ventilation of the lung is the volume of gas inspired in unit time and is 7 litres per minute in a normal adult breathing a tidal volume of 500 ml at a respiratory rate of 14 breaths per minute. This quantity of gas does not reach the alveoli because part of each breath merely fills the large conducting airways and takes no part in gaseous exchange. This is the *anatomical dead space* which amounts to about 150 ml. *Alveolar ventilation* in a normal adult, therefore, amounts to $(500 - 150) \times 14 = 4900$ ml per minute. Alveolar ventilation is achieved not only by the mass movement of gases caused by the rhythmic expansion and deflation of the lungs, but also by diffusion of gas molecules within the airways. The total cross sectional area of the airways at the level of alveolar ducts and spaces is many times greater than that at the levels of the bronchi and bronchioles. This means that the mass flow of gas which is the major transport mechanism in the relatively narrow bronchi and bronchioles suddenly drops to zero as the airways abruptly widen into the alveolar ducts and spaces. Thus, transport of gas over the few millimetres between the respiratory bronchioles and alveolar-capillary wall is achieved by molecular diffusion. An important adverse effect of airways obstruction is to impede the mass transport of gases and consequently increase the distance over which molecular diffusion has to take place, so giving rise to a state of alveolar hypoventilation.

Causes of alveolar hypoventilation. In its broadest sense the term alveolar hypoventilation means that the volume of gas reaching the alveolar gas-exchanging interface is inadequate to maintain the normal systemic arterial tensions of oxygen and carbon dioxide. However, *alveolar hypoventilation in the clinical sense is usually applied to those patients with evidence of respiratory failure without underlying disease of the lungs.* Ventilation is a complex process which requires intact airways and involves the co-ordinated action of the respiratory centre, peripheral nerves, respiratory muscles and thoracic cage. Hypoventilation may, therefore, be caused by depression of the respiratory centre, neurological disease, muscular disorders and disorders of the chest wall and pleura.

Respiratory centre depression. Alveolar hypoventilation, leading to cyanosis and carbon dioxide retention, is a common complication of overdosage or poisoning with narcotic drugs such as the barbiturates and morphine. The action of the medullary respiratory centre may also be impaired by the direct or indirect effects of cerebral infarcts, cerebral haemorrhage and intracranial neoplasms.

Neurological disease. Conditions such as poliomyelitis, acute polyneuritis and spinal cord lesions at or above the origin of the phrenic nerve (C3, 4, 5) may cause hypoventilation due to paralysis of the respiratory muscles. Tetanus, botulism and neuromuscular block produced by curare or by ganglion-blocking agents may produce a similar effect.

Muscular disorders. These include conditions such as myasthenia gravis, dermatomyositis and muscular dystrophy which may affect the intercostal muscles and diaphragm.

Chest wall disorders. Multiple fractures of the ribs may produce a 'flail chest' in which the affected part of the chest wall collapses inwards on inspiration, so reducing effective ventilation of the alveoli. Severe kyphoscoliosis can interfere with the respiratory excursions of the thoracic cage and produce hypoventilation.

Pleural disease. Large pleural effusions and pneumothorax induce hypoventilation by causing compression collapse of the adjacent lung.

Excessive obesity (*Pickwickian syndrome*). Some excessively obese people develop hypoventilation although objective tests of pulmonary function are normal. They are liable to episodes of somnolence and develop cyanosis with secondary polycythaemia, hypercapnia and often pulmonary hypertension leading to right ventricular failure. Numerous factors have been suggested to account for the ventilatory disorders in these subjects, including mechanical impairment of respiration due to fatty infiltration of the respiratory muscles, excessive elevation of the diaphragm in the supine posture, and decreased compliance of the thoracic cage.

Effects of hypoventilation. Alveolar gas differs from the inspired air because carbon dioxide is being continually added to it, and oxygen removed from it, by the blood perfusing the alveolar capillaries. Its composition depends on a balance between ventilation and blood flow. Hypoventilation causes a fall in alveolar oxygen tension and an increase in the carbon dioxide tension. This is accompanied by an elevation in the systemic arterial carbon dioxide tension (*hypercapnia*) and an arithmetically equivalent depression of the oxygen tension. *The main effects of hypoventilation are attributable to hypercapnia.* Oxygen desaturation with cyanosis are late events. The symptoms and signs of hypercapnia are a rapid bounding pulse, moist warm hands, constricted pupils and elevation of the systemic blood pressure. Dyspnoea is often absent. Severe carbon dioxide retention leads to confusion, drowsiness, coarse tremors and eventual coma. The tendon reflexes are depressed and the plantar response is extensor. An important feature of hypoventilation as a cause of respiratory failure is that the lungs are normal and the prognosis is excellent if the precipitating cause can be removed.

Impaired diffusion

In the normal lung, alveolar gas is separated from capillary blood by the alveolar-capillary membrane which is $0.2 \mu m$ wide at its thinnest points and is composed of three distinct anatomical layers: alveolar epithelium; a narrow interstitial zone; and capillary endothelium (Fig. 16.11). The exchange of respiratory gases between the alveolar space and capillaries is by diffusion, the gases flowing from a region of high partial pressure to one of low partial pressure. Blood entering the alveolar capillaries is mixed venous blood having a relatively high carbon dioxide tension and a low oxygen tension. It gives off carbon dioxide and takes up oxygen from the alveolar gas. In a healthy individual at rest, equilibration between alveolar gas and capillary blood is virtually complete. Lung disease may impede the diffusion of gases if the thickness of the alveolar-capillary membrane is increased, or if there is a decrease of the anatomical surface area available for diffusion due to excision of lung tissue or its destruction by disease such as emphysema. There are conditions such as diffuse fibrosing alveolitis, sarcoidosis, asbestosis and alveolar cell carcinoma where microscopically the alveolar-capillary wall appears to be thickened and it is probable that some of the systemic arterial

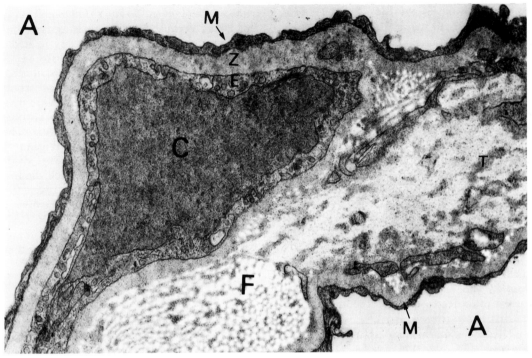

Fig. 16.11 Alveolar wall in normal human lung. The capillary lumen (C) is lined by endothelial cells (E). The alveolar spaces (A) are lined by membranous pneumocytes (M). In the thinnest portion of the blood-air pathway the endothelial cell is separated from the membranous pneumocyte by a granular amorphous zone (Z) consisting of their fused basement membranes. Elsewhere, the endothelial and epithelial cells are separated by an interstitial space containing collagen (F) and elastic fibres (T). Electron micrograph. × 25 000.

hypoxaemia in these conditions is caused by defective diffusion. The term 'alveolar-capillary block' was coined for this condition but it should be used with caution because the diffusion of oxygen through tissues is very rapid and calculations have suggested that the observed degree of thickening of the alveolar-capillary wall is insufficient to impair oxygen diffusion seriously. The hypoxaemia in such patients is now known to be due mainly to a disturbed ratio of ventilation/perfusion (see below) rather than to impaired diffusion.

The functional effect of impaired alveolar-capillary gas exchange is interference with oxygen uptake and the development of systemic arterial desaturation. Patients with impaired diffusion are particularly liable to develop sudden systemic arterial desaturation with cyanosis on exercise or if alveolar hypoxia occurs. The effect of exercise is to reduce the time spent by the blood in the pulmonary capillaries and thus reduce the time available for diffusion and

equilibration. In alveolar hypoxia the difference between the oxygen tension of alveolar gas and mixed venous blood is reduced, so decreasing the diffusion gradient across the alveolar-capillary wall and slowing the rate of diffusion of oxygen. Carbon dioxide is much more soluble than oxygen and diffuses twenty times more readily through the tissues, so that thickening of the alveolar-capillary wall has no effect on the exchange of carbon dioxide between alveolar gas and capillary blood.

Uneven ventilation and perfusion

A factor of fundamental importance in gas exchange in the lungs is the ventilation/perfusion ratio, usually signified by the formula $\dot{V}A/\dot{Q}$. That is, the distribution of alveolar ventilation ($\dot{V}A$) relative to the pulmonary capillary blood flow ($\dot{Q}$). The dots indicate that the volumes are expressed in unit time, e.g. ml per min. When the lung is considered as a whole under normal circumstances the overall $\dot{V}A/\dot{Q}$ ratio approximates to unity:

$$\frac{\dot{V}A}{\dot{Q}} = \frac{\text{Alveolar ventilation}}{\text{Pulmonary capillary blood flow}}$$
$$= \frac{4900 \text{ ml per min}}{5000 \text{ ml per min}}$$

The situation in an 'ideal' lung is shown diagrammatically in simplified form in Fig. 16.12. In each of the two alveolar units, ventilation is closely matched by perfusion. In practice, the situation is more complicated because gravity affects the distribution of ventilation and perfusion. In a normal healthy individual who is upright, the alveoli at the apex of the lung have almost no blood flow and a moderate ventilation, while at the base the blood flow is much larger, but the ventilation only slightly increased. The result is that the ventilation/perfusion ratio decreases down the lung.

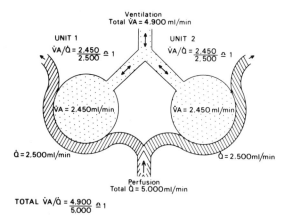

Fig. 16.12 The ideal distribution of ventilation ($\dot{V}A$) and perfusion ($\dot{Q}$) in a lung composed of 2 alveolar units. Both ventilation and perfusion are evenly distributed to all parts of the lung. Ventilation and perfusion are almost precisely matched to give a $\dot{V}A/\dot{Q}$ ratio of approximately one.

The anatomical organisation and physiological regulation of the lungs, which are composed of three hundred million functioning alveolar units, allow a large volume of gas and blood to be brought into close proximity over an enormous area (about 70 m²). The efficiency of gas exchange is largely dependent upon the precision with which appropriate proportions of the total ventilation and total pulmonary blood flow are conveyed to each alveolus. *Uneven distribution of ventilation and perfusion is the most*

common cause of respiratory failure. It may arise either because ventilation is uneven but perfusion is normally distributed, as in acute bronchial asthma, or because perfusion is uneven but ventilation is normally distributed, as in multiple pulmonary emboli. More commonly, both ventilation and perfusion are irregularly and unevenly distributed as in chronic bronchitis and diffuse fibrosing alveolitis. The effects of irregular and uneven distribution of ventilation and perfusion are illustrated diagrammatically in Fig. 16.13, from which the following three points should be noted:

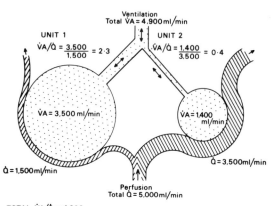

Fig. 16.13 Uneven ventilation ($\dot{V}A$) and perfusion ($\dot{Q}$). Unit 1 is excessively ventilated but underperfused ($\dot{V}A/\dot{Q} = 2\cdot3$). Unit 2 is underventilated and overperfused ($\dot{V}A/\dot{Q} = 0\cdot4$). The blood leaving unit 1 has a normal oxygen tension. The blood leaving unit 2 has a reduced oxygen tension due to hypoventilation. Thus, although the overall ventilation and perfusion of the lung are the same as in the ideal lung (Fig. 16.12), the effect of unevenness is to reduce the systemic arterial oxygen tension.

1. The excessive ventilation of unit 1 cannot materially increase the oxygen tension of the blood perfusing that alveolus. This excessive ventilation which is superfluous to the respiratory capacity of the perfusing blood is wasted. The *physiological dead-space* is wasted alveolar ventilation added to the anatomical dead space.
2. The mixed venous blood reaching unit 2 is unable to be fully saturated with oxygen because of the hypoventilation. The blood flow which is superfluous to the ventilatory capacity is wasted.
3. Although the overall blood flow and ventilation of the lung are the same as in the ideal

lung (Fig. 16.12), the effect of the uneven distribution of ventilation and perfusion is to produce a decrease in the oxygen tension of arterial blood.

Although inequalities of both ventilation and perfusion commonly occur together in the same patient, it is easier to consider the pathological causes of each separately.

Uneven distribution of ventilation. This may be caused by narrowings and dilatations of airways, by variations in the distensibility of airways, and by the presence of oedema fluid and exudate.

Narrowing of airways. This occurs in acute bronchial asthma, chronic bronchitis and acute bronchiolitis.

Dilatation of terminal airways. If the terminal airways such as the respiratory bronchioles are dilated, as occurs in bronchiolar emphysema, ventilation of the alveoli diminishes because part of every inspired breath is used to fill these abnormal airspaces. The distance over which gas molecules have to travel by diffusion is increased.

Variation in distensibility of different airways leads to uneven ventilation because those with stiff, inelastic walls expand to a smaller extent for a given intrathoracic pressure change than those which are compliant and easily distensible. This type of uneven ventilation is probably the major cause of impaired gaseous exchange in patients with diffuse pulmonary fibrosing diseases.

Alveolar exudates. In pneumonia, the alveolar capillaries are perfused but the alveolar gas is replaced by inflammatory exudate.

Uneven distribution of perfusion. This may be due to conditions leading to obstruction of the pulmonary vascular bed such as multiple pulmonary emboli, fibrous obliteration secondary to pneumoconiosis or diffuse fibrosing alveolitis, the occlusive lesions of severe hypertensive pulmonary vascular disease, and pulmonary vasoconstriction resulting from hypoxia. This last mechanism may have a compensatory effect by reducing perfusion of poorly ventilated alveoli and thus improving the ventilation/perfusion ratio.

Pulmonary oedema

This condition may be defined as an excessive extravascular accumulation of fluid within the lung. It can result from (1) an *imbalance of hydrodynamic forces* across the alveolar-capillary wall which causes more fluid to leave the capillaries than can be removed from the tissues, and (2) *increased permeability* of the endothelial layer of the pulmonary capillaries.

The fine structural appearance of the alveolar septum is shown in Fig. 16.11. Capillary blood is separated from alveolar air by three distinct anatomical layers: capillary endothelium; a narrow interstitial zone; and alveolar epithelium. The alveolar capillaries are lined by the thin cytoplasmic extensions of endothelial cells which contain few organelles apart from numerous small pinocytotic vesicles. Normal alveolar capillary endothelial cells are not fenestrated. They are joined by 'tight junctions' containing narrow constrictions (p. 49). Sandwiched between the capillary endothelium and alveolar epithelium is an interstitial zone of variable width. Over the convexities of the

capillaries protruding into the alveoli, there is no true interstitial space because the contact surface between the endothelium and epithelium is formed exclusively by the fused basement membranes of these two cell layers. In other regions, the epithelial and endothelial basement membranes are separated by an interstitial space containing fine elastic fibres, bundles of collagen fibrils, fibroblasts and macrophages. The alveolar septa are devoid of lymphatics, which first appear in the interstitial space surrounding terminal bronchioles, small arteries and veins. Over 95 per cent of the area of the alveolar walls is lined by the thin, extensive membranous pneumocytes. The cytoplasm of these epithelial cells closely resembles that of the subjacent endothelial cells. The margins of adjacent membranous or granular pneumocytes (p. 482) abut bluntly or overlap with the formation of narrow clefts. However, unlike the endothelial cell junctions, which allow exchange of fluid between intravascular and extravascular spaces, the clefts between adjacent epithelial cells are actually obliterated by fusion of opposing cell membranes. Escape of fluid through the inter-endothelial junctions is dependent, as elsewhere, on capillary intraluminal pressure: a rise in intravascular pressure results in an increase in the amount of fluid entering the interstitial space of the alveolar septum.

Accumulation of fluid in the alveolar spaces is a late and not an inevitable manifestation of pulmonary oedema. Flooding of the alveolar spaces is preceded by a sequence of changes which is largely independent of the cause of the oedema. If the quantity of fluid escaping from the pulmonary capillaries increases, the excess fluid is carried away by lymphatics. These have a considerable reserve capacity and the volume of lymph draining from the lung may increase several-fold without any detectable increase in the fluid content of the pulmonary interstitial tissue. When the capacity of the lymphatic system is exceeded, fluid begins to accumulate in the lung. It first accumulates in the loose, readily distensible connective tissues around the bronchi and larger vessels and next distends the thick, collagen-containing portions of the alveolar wall. Fluid does not accumulate in the thinnest portions of the blood–air pathway, i.e. over the convexities of the alveolar capillaries, until a very late stage because, as mentioned above, the membranous pneumocytes and capillary endothelial cells in this zone share a common basement membrane, and relatively high pressure is necessary to separate them. The final stage of pulmonary oedema is accumulation of fluid within the alveolar spaces. The route whereby fluid escapes from the interstitial tissues to the alveolar spaces has not been clearly defined although it is usually assumed that it is related to the opening, perhaps temporarily, of some of the intercellular junctions between membranous pneumocytes (Hurley, 1978). A striking fine structural feature, not observed in systemic capillaries, may be seen in the alveolar capillaries in pulmonary oedema: the thin layer of endothelium lining the alveolar capillary may lift away from the underlying basement membrane to form a bleb or vesicle which protrudes into the lumen of the capillary (Fig. 16.14). It has been suggested that the thin endothelium is floated off its basement membrane by oedema fluid and projects into the lumen because of the low pressure within the

capillaries. This hypothesis could account for the absence of endothelial vesicles in patients with pulmonary oedema due to mitral stenosis, where the capillary intraluminal blood pressure is increased. There is no evidence that the vesicles, although morphologically striking, have any significant effect upon the flow of blood through the affected capillaries.

Pulmonary oedema may occur in patients with *left ventricular failure* or *mitral stenosis* who develop elevation of the pulmonary venous pressure. Pulmonary oedema which follows overloading of the circulation with *intravenous infusions* is probably also due to failure of the left ventricle. The acute pulmonary oedema which may follow *sudden withdrawal of a pleural effusion* is generally attributed to a sudden increase in the negative intrathoracic pressure. Pulmonary oedema may occasionally occur in patients with *raised intracranial pressure* resulting from head injuries, neurosurgical operations, intracerebral haemorrhage and neoplasms. The mechanism of production of this oedema is not clear. *High altitude pulmonary oedema* is a rare complication following ascent to altitudes over 3000 metres. It is unusual in that it occurs in otherwise healthy individuals, such as mountain climbers and military personnel. The mechanism of its production is unknown. Susceptibility to high altitude pulmonary oedema is not limited to men from low altitude, for if a high-altitude dweller spends a few weeks at sea level, he may develop pulmonary oedema soon after returning to his usual altitude of residence. *Toxic gases and fumes* such as nitrogen dioxide, chlorine and phosgene may damage the alveolar wall and produce pulmonary oedema.

Hyaline membrane disease. The respiratory distress syndrome is a serious disorder of newborn infants with a mortality rate of between 20 and 40 per cent. It is most common in premature infants and 10–15 per cent of those with a birth weight of 2500 g or less develop the syndrome. Infants born by Caesarian section and those born of mothers with diabetes mellitus are also particularly susceptible. The disorder is characterised by increasing respiratory difficulty which starts a few minutes to a few hours after birth. There is hypoxaemia and cyanosis despite high concentrations of inspired oxygen. Physiologically, the babies have large functional right-to-left shunts and very low

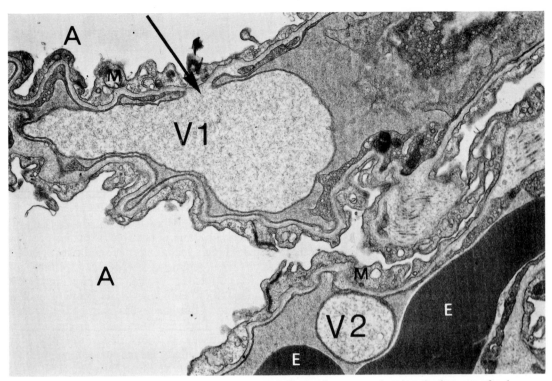

Fig. 16.14 Electron micrograph of two pulmonary capillaries from a rat showing the features of pulmonary oedema caused by acute exposure to simulated high altitude corresponding to the summit of Mount Everest (elevation 8850 metres; atmospheric pressure 250 torr.). The lower capillary contains two erythrocytes. Two endothelial vesicles, V1 and V2 are seen. The upper has been cut in longitudinal section and assumes the shape of the capillary into which it projects. Its pedicle is indicated by an arrow. The lower vesicle, V2, has been cut in transverse section and gives the spurious appearance of lying free in the capillary. The alveolar spaces (A) are lined by membranous pneumocytes (M). × 12 500.

lung compliance. At necropsy the lungs are collapsed, firm, and resemble liver in appearance and consistency. Microscopically, the alveoli are collapsed while the terminal and respiratory bronchioles are distended and lined by thick, eosinophilic 'hyaline membranes' of variable composition: they may contain fibrin, necrotic epithelial cell debris, and keratinised cells presumably derived from inhaled amniotic fluid. If the infants survive the first few days, they seem to recover completely, although pulmonary fibrosis may ensue in a small minority.

The aetiology of this disorder remains obscure. Important factors seem to be high pulmonary vascular resistance, impaired or deficient surfactant activity, increased permeability of the alveolar capillaries, and inhalation of amniotic fluid. The lungs of infants dying at the height of the disease invariably have a deficiency of pulmonary surfactant, which normally lowers the surface tension of the alveoli.

Although this deficiency is regarded as a crucial factor by some workers, whether it is a cause or effect of the disease remains unsettled.

Massive pulmonary haemorrhage in the newborn. Sometimes infants thought clinically to have died from hyaline membrane disease are found at necropsy to have massive haemorrhage involving two or more lobes of the lungs. The condition may arise from about half an hour to two weeks after birth. Sometimes the condition becomes apparent in a baby already being treated for respiratory insufficiency in a respirator, when bloodstained fluid is discovered in the endotracheal tube. Evidence of disseminated intravascular coagulation has been found in some babies. Haemorrhage into the subarachnoid space or cerebral ventricles is sometimes also found at necropsy. At present, it is impossible to ascribe a single common cause for massive pulmonary haemorrhage. Some believe that it may be due to oxygen toxicity or to the insertion of a catheter too far down the endotracheal tubes.

Uraemic lung. This term is used to describe a chronic form of pulmonary oedema long known to radiologists on account of the butterfly-shaped shadow that extends outwards from the hilum of both lungs. At necropsy, the lungs are voluminous and rubbery and, on squeezing, a frothy fluid exudes from the cut surface. Microscopically the reluctance of the oedema fluid to drain out of the cut surface is seen to be due to a fine fibrin network in the alveoli, and hyaline membranes may be formed. In longstanding cases organisation of the exudate may take place in some areas.

Shock lung and adult respiratory distress syndrome. It has been known for some years that respiratory failure is the cause of death in many patients who have suffered major trauma, haemorrhage or other catastrophe associated with hypotension. With improved techniques of resuscitation and blood transfusion, *the syndrome of post-traumatic pulmonary insufficiency or 'shock lung' has emerged as one of the most frequent and life-threatening complications to occur in both civilian and military casualties.* Shock lung occurs within one or two days of the trau-matic episode, following the initial resuscitation procedures. The patient gradually becomes hypoxic with acidosis despite oxygen therapy, and mortality is high. Initially, the chest radiograph shows patchy opacities attributed to pulmonary oedema and collapse, which progress to almost totally opaque lung fields in the severely affected patient. At necropsy, the lungs are heavy, beefy and oedematous. Microscopically, in early cases there is intra-alveolar oedema with extravasation of erythrocytes. Fibrinous exudate and hyaline membranes which line the alveolar walls develop later. In longstanding cases, pulmonary fibrosis ensues, and the alveolar walls become lined by metaplastic cuboidal epithelium.

There are many possible explanations for shock lung, including fat embolism, overtransfusion, pulmonary oedema, aspiration of gastric contents, oxygen toxicity and pulmonary micro-embolism. It is probably not a single entity, but has several causes. It has been suggested that micro-emboli originating in damaged tissue, in transfused whole blood or reconstituted dried plasma, may be responsible for the pulmonary changes. Disseminated intravascular coagulation and endotoxaemia have been recognised in some cases.

Pulmonary vascular disease

Diseases of the heart affect the lungs and diseases of the lungs affect the heart. The anatomical basis of this interrelationship is the pulmonary vasculature. Normally the blood pressure in the pulmonary arterial tree is only one sixth of that in the systemic. This is reflected in the fact that the right ventricle is thinner than the left. The pulmonary arteries are also thinner than the systemic and consist of a layer of circularly orientated smooth muscle sandwiched between elastic laminae. The pulmonary arterioles, unlike the systemic ones, do not have a muscular media but instead have a wall composed of a single elastic lamina. Normal pulmonary arterioles are thus incapable of exerting significant resistance to the flow of blood through the lungs. The main way in which diseases of the heart and lung affect each other is through the production of pulmonary arterial hypertension and associated hypertensive pulmonary vascular disease.

Pulmonary hypertension

There are many diseases which will cause pulmonary arterial hypertension and associated pulmonary vascular disease (Table 16.2). Pulmonary hypertension may be arbitrarily defined as a systolic blood pressure in the pulmonary circulation exceeding 30 mm Hg. There are various forms of hypertensive pulmonary vascular disease, and one cannot predict what vascular lesions are present from a knowledge of the level of the pulmonary arterial pressure. Rather the form of the hypertensive pulmonary vascular disease depends upon the nature of the underlying disease process. This is of considerable practical importance, since the different

Table 16.2 The causes of pulmonary arterial hypertension and hypertensive pulmonary vascular disease

Disease group	Examples
Pre-tricuspid congenital cardiac septal shunts.	Atrial septal defect.
Post-tricuspid congenital cardiac septal shunts.	Ventricular septal defect. Patent ductus arteriosus.
Elevation of left atrial pressure.	Mitral stenosis. Chronic left ventricular failure. Left atrial myxoma.
Massive pulmonary fibrosis.	Silicosis.
Fibrosing alveolitis.	Rheumatoid disease. Progressive systemic sclerosis. Berylliosis.
Chronic hypoxia.	Normal subjects living at high altitude. Chronic bronchitis and emphysema. Kyphoscoliosis. Pickwickian syndrome.
Liver disease.	Cirrhosis. Portal vein thrombosis.
Pulmonary thrombo-embolism.	Secondary to thrombosis in deep veins of limbs.
Primary pulmonary hypertension.	Classical variety. Pulmonary veno-occlusive disease.
Diet.	Crotalaria alkaloids. Some anorexigens suspected.

forms of pulmonary vascular disease are reflected in different levels of pressure, flow and resistance in the pulmonary circulation, which, in turn, have an important effect on the clinical picture and course. The causes of pulmonary hypertension and the various forms of hypertensive pulmonary vascular disease that they are associated with are as follows:

Congenital cardiac shunts. A large congenital cardiac defect between the right and left ventricles or between the aorta and the pulmonary trunk will lead to pulmonary arterial hypertension from birth, due to direct transmission of systemic arterial pressure and flow into the pulmonary circulation. Examples of such **post-tricuspid shunts** are ventricular septal defect, patent ductus arteriosus, persistent truncus arteriosus and aorto-pulmonary septal defect. **Pre-tricuspid shunts**, such as atrial septal defects, produce pulmonary hypertension in adolescence or adult life as a result of the effect of a prolonged excessive blood flow on the pulmonary vasculature.

Provided the defect is large enough, a characteristic form of pulmonary vascular disease occurs in association with the raised pulmonary arterial pressure. The form of disease produced by pre- and post-tricuspid congenital cardiac

shunts is identical. Initially there is increased thickness of the medial coat of the small pulmonary arteries. The pulmonary arterioles develop a distinct muscular media and resemble systemic arterioles. This is followed by intimal thickening of the pulmonary arteries and arterioles, at first cellular, then fibrous, and finally fibro-elastic. *These intimal changes lead to organic occlusion of pulmonary arteries.* This is followed by dilatation of the pulmonary vasculature which may be generalised or localised. Localised 'dilatation lesions' develop. These are clusters of thin-walled branches of small pulmonary arteries arising proximal to the sites of occlusion. They form a collateral circulation to maintain a flow of blood to the pulmonary capillary bed, and may be termed '**angiomatoid lesions**'. Sometimes a characteristic proliferation of myofibroblasts and fibrillary cells takes place within them in a plexiform pattern to give the structure its name of '**plexiform lesion**' (Fig. 16.15). These thin-walled branches rupture to give rise to **pulmonary haemosiderosis**. Finally, **fibrinoid necrosis** of the small pulmonary arteries may occur if the pulmonary arterial pressure rises rapidly or severely.

This form of pulmonary vascular disease offers a good example of how pathological

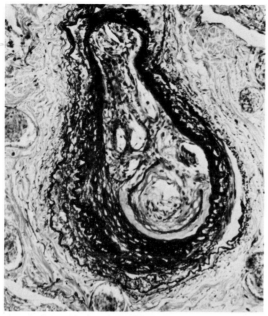

Fig. 16.15 Transverse section of a muscular pulmonary artery from a young woman with severe pulmonary hypertension secondary to a large ventricular septal defect. Internal to the hypertrophied media is a thick zone of elastic tissue (appears black). The lumen of the parent artery contains a proliferation of myofibroblasts and fibrillary cells which extend into the branch (above). This is a plexiform lesion. (Elastica and Van Gieson stain.) × 150.

changes in the pulmonary circulation may exert a profound effect on the clinical picture and course. It illustrates too how these effects may change according to the stage of the pulmonary vascular disease. Thus the early stages of medial hypertrophy and intimal fibrosis are associated with pulmonary arterial hypertension with a high pulmonary flow, and a moderate increase in pulmonary vascular resistance which is largely reversible. The later dilatation lesions and necrotising arteritis are associated with severe pulmonary hypertension, a reduced pulmonary blood flow, and a severely and irreversibly increased pulmonary vascular resistance. Hence, *the early phase of the clinical picture of a large congenital cardiac shunt is dominated by signs of left ventricular hypertrophy, increased pulmonary blood flow, and left-to-right shunting of blood with no cyanosis. The later phase, however, is dominated by clinical signs of right ventricular hypertrophy, diminished pulmonary blood flow, and right-to-left shunting of blood with cyanosis.* In the early stages of

hypertensive pulmonary vascular disease, surgical correction of septal defects is usually followed by the reversal of the associated pulmonary hypertension. In the later stages, however, the pulmonary hypertension is irreversible and this is considered by some to contraindicate attempts at corrective surgical treatment.

This florid form of hypertensive pulmonary vascular disease is characteristic of **congenital cardiac septal defects** but is not exclusively produced by them. It can also complicate an **acquired ventricular septal defect** such as septal rupture following infarction, or the rare cases of cirrhosis of the liver associated with pulmonary hypertension. It is also found in **primary pulmonary hypertension** which is a rare disease occurring in young women with no underlying disease of the heart or lungs.

Hypoxia. *Any state of chronic hypoxia will induce pulmonary arterial hypertension and associated changes in the pulmonary arteries.* Thus pulmonary hypertension occurs in anyone living at high altitude and is consistent with a healthy and active life. It also complicates chronic bronchitis and emphysema when there is associated chronic hypoxia. Kyphoscoliosis, Monge's disease (so-called 'chronic mountain sickness') and the Pickwickian syndrome are all likely to become complicated by hypoxic hypertensive pulmonary vascular disease, which also occurs occasionally in individuals with enlarged adenoids.

The hallmark of this variety is muscularisation of the terminal portions of the pulmonary vascular tree, which increases pulmonary vascular resistance. There is insignificant intimal fibrosis and the important functional implication of this is that *the pulmonary hypertension and associated pulmonary vascular disease of chronic hypoxia are largely and rapidly reversible.* This may be readily confirmed by subjecting rats to a diminished barometric pressure in a vacuum chamber, when they develop muscularisation of their pulmonary arterioles. After removing them from the chamber to ambient room air for a month or so, both the pulmonary hypertension and muscularisation regress virtually completely. Another effect of hypoxia is the development of longitudinal muscle in the intima of pulmonary arteries and arterioles, usually ascribed to longitudinal stretching of these vessels.

Elevation of left atrial pressure. *Any disease*

that brings about a sustained significant elevation of blood pressure in the left atrium is complicated by pulmonary hypertension and associated hypertensive pulmonary vascular disease. This is characerised in its early stages by medial hypertrophy and intimal fibrosis of pulmonary arteries and muscularisation of pulmonary arterioles. Rarely in the later stages there is fibrinoid necrosis of pulmonary arteries. Plexiform and other dilatation lesions do not occur in this group. The pulmonary hypertension associated with the early vascular changes is reversible whereas that associated with fibrinoid necrosis is not. Diseases which lead to chronic left atrial hypertension include mitral stenosis and incompetence (acquired or congenital), myxoma of the left atrium and any cause of chronic left ventricular failure. The interesting association of pulmonary capillary hypertension and normal left atrial blood pressure occurs in pulmonary veno-occlusive disease which is a rare form of primary pulmonary hypertension.

Pulmonary venous hypertension produces a collection of pathological effects which have been traditionally referred to as *chronic venous congestion of the lung*. As the blood pressure rises in the pulmonary venules and capillaries, they become congested with blood. This may become associated with pulmonary oedema in which, in addition to the presence of oedema fluid in the alveolar spaces, there may be collections of fluid in the interlobular septa of the lung and in the distended peri-arterial and peribronchial lymphatics. Such collections of oedema fluid may present radiographically as *basal horizontal lines* (Kerley B lines), which indicate that the pulmonary venous blood pressure exceeds a mean level of 25 mm Hg.

Persistent pulmonary congestion and oedema are associated with a hyperplasia of granular pneumocytes (p. 482) and the development of interstitial fibrosis of the lung. Red blood cells may be extruded from the distended pulmonary capillaries into the alveolar walls and spaces (Fig. 16.16). Their phagocytosis and destruction in macrophages results in collections of haemosiderin-laden macrophages within the alveoli, giving rise to the condition of *pulmonary haemosiderosis* (Fig. 10.10, p. 279) which may present to the radiologist as a 'snow storm effect' on chest radiographs. The liberated ferric iron salts may also be deposited on re-

ticulin and elastic fibres in the walls of alveoli and in pulmonary arteries and veins where it may provoke a giant cell reaction. The combination of rusty discolouration of the lung due to this deposition of ferric salts, and firmness of the pulmonary parenchyma due to increase in fibrous tissue in the alveolar walls, accounts for the classical term of *brown induration.*

Other mineral deposits may occur in states associated with chronic pulmonary venous hypertension. They include nodules of osseous metaplasia which present a characteristic radiological picture. A much rarer manifestation is the deposition in the alveolar spaces of myriads of microliths composed of laminated concretions of calcium phosphate bound within an organic envelope containing ferric salts. This condition, which may transform the lung into a rock-hard mass that may require sawing for dissection, is called *microlithiasis alveolaris pulmonum.*

The pulmonary veins themselves show the effects of increased pressure within them by the formation of a distinct muscular media so that they may resemble small muscular pulmonary arteries. They also show intimal fibrosis.

Pulmonary fibrosis. Both massive and interstitial pulmonary fibrosis may become complicated by pulmonary hypertension and pulmonary vascular changes which are initially muscular in type and reversible. Later there is obliterative fibrosis of pulmonary arteries and arterioles with an irreversible increase in pulmonary vascular resistance.

'Cor pulmonale'. The term 'cor pulmonale' has been used in a general sense to mean involvement of the heart secondary to lung disease. Unfortunately it is used equally to describe either hypertrophy or failure of the right ventricle, brought about by involvement of the pulmonary circulation by lung disease. Since this term has no precise meaning its use is best avoided.

Pulmonary hypotension

Diminished pulmonary arterial pressure is usually associated with reduction of pulmonary blood flow. This may occur in pulmonary stenosis, which may be isolated or associated with cardiac septal defects as in Fallot's tetrad. In patients with pulmonary stenosis and reversed flow (from right to left) through a congenital

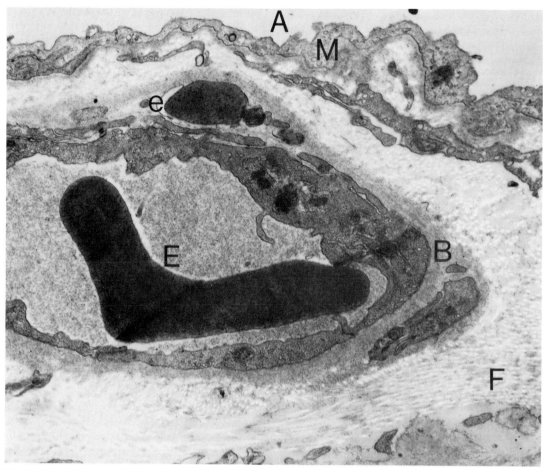

Fig. 16.16 Alveolar wall in mitral stenosis. The alveolar capillary contains an erythrocyte (E) and is surrounded by dense fibrous tissue (F) which displaces it inwards from its normal superficial position beneath the membranous pneumocyte (M) lining the alveolar space (A). The capillary basement membrane (B) is thickened and contains a disintegrating extravasated erythrocyte (e). Electron micrograph. × 16 500.

cardiac septal defect there is pronounced cyanosis. This leads to compensatory polycythaemia. The net result is the circulation of viscous blood at diminished pressure and flow through the pulmonary vessels. This leads to atrophy of the media of the pulmonary arteries with thrombosis, subsequent organisation, and recanalisation of these vessels. The media of the pulmonary trunk shows atrophy with clumping of its elastic tissue. This is in contrast to states of pulmonary arterial hypertension where there is thickening of the media even to the extent of the pulmonary trunk becoming as thick as the aorta. In states of pulmonary hypotension with an inadequate flow of blood to the pulmonary capillary bed, there is compensatory enlargement of the bronchial arteries.

Pulmonary embolism

Thrombo-embolism

By far the commonest sites of origin of thrombi leading to pulmonary embolism are the deep veins of the legs, especially in the calf. In vivo studies using intravenous injections of fibrinogen labelled with ^{131}I have confirmed this. Pulmonary thrombo-embolism is very rare in children but opinion is divided as to whether age or sex affects its incidence in adults. Predisposing factors are described on p. 240.

There is no doubt that pulmonary thrombo-embolism is very common indeed. In one study, carried out in hospitals in Oxford, its incidence, as determined by examination of the left lung in a routine necropsy service, was 12 per cent. A detailed histological examination of the right lung from the same cases revealed an incidence of 52 per cent. Morrell and Dunnill (1968) believe that pulmonary thrombo-embolism is even commoner than indicated by their results and that it is almost ubiquitous in hospital patients coming to necropsy.

The lungs have an astonishing capacity to dispose of thrombo-emboli. Even large fresh thrombi are absorbed by the lungs in dogs in six weeks and small ones much more rapidly. Two main groups of processes are involved, chemical and cellular. Chemical disposal is by *fibrinolysis* and predominates in the disposal of small thrombi. Lung tissue has a high content of fibrinolysins, which have been shown to be present in the intima of both pulmonary and systemic arteries. Cellular processes of *organisation* and *recanalisation* seem to be more important in the disposal of larger thrombo-emboli. In a few days fibroblasts and capillaries grow into the emboli, which are gradually reduced to patches of intimal fibrosis.

The clinical effects of pulmonary thrombo-emboli depend upon the size of the pulmonary artery involved and on the speed with which the occlusion occurs. Sudden blocking of the pulmonary trunk or a large pulmonary artery may be rapidly fatal owing to the inability of the right ventricle to maintain the circulation. Under certain conditions, blockage of smaller pulmonary arteries will give rise to pulmonary infarction. In the third and rarest groups of patients, multiple small thrombo-emboli lodge in the smaller branches of the pulmonary arterial tree over a period of time and give rise to severe pulmonary hypertension.

Massive pulmonary thrombo-embolism. Massive pulmonary embolism is a classical clinical emergency brought about by sudden occlusion of the pulmonary trunk (Fig. 9.25, p. 244) or one of its main branches by a large embolus (Fig. 16.17). In the normal human lung, rather more than half the pulmonary arterial bed must be occluded before the clinical syndrome of acute massive embolism will appear. In the presence of pre-existing pulmonary hypertension, however, occlusion of one primary branch of the pulmonary trunk has important haemodynamic effects. The increased pulmonary vascular resistance which occurs in pulmonary embolism in man is more likely a mechanical

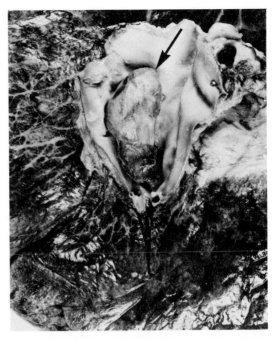

Fig. 16.17 Pulmonary thrombo-embolism. The main pulmonary artery at the hilum of the lung has been opened to reveal a pale thrombo-embolus (arrow) lying free in its lumen.

effect of blockage of pulmonary arteries rather than due to the effect of serotonin liberated from pulmonary emboli: the latter has a greater effect on the pulmonary circulation of dogs and cats than on that of man.

Pulmonary infarction. The pathogenesis of pulmonary infarction is something of an enigma, for pulmonary arterial occlusion alone fails to produce it. An additional important requirement appears to be an increased pulmonary venous pressure and infarction is therefore common in patients with mitral stenosis. In experimental studies, the presence or absence of the bronchial arterial supply seems to make no difference to the development of infarction. Pulmonary infarction occurs more often in the lower lobes, where the pulmonary venous pressure is likely to be higher. In addition, the lung bases are more prone to be affected by bronchial occlusion, pleural effusion and infection, all factors shown experimentally to favour infarction. The appearances of pulmonary infarcts are described on p. 247.

Recurrent pulmonary embolism. In this condition there is a gradual occlusion of the pulmonary arterial bed over a period of time which may extend to several years. Infarction is not a feature but *there is a progressive increase in the pulmonary vascular resistance, leading to severe pulmonary hypertension, right ventricular hypertrophy and failure.* The muscular pulmonary arteries show medial hypertrophy and excentric nodular fibro-elastic thickening of the intima due to organisation of the thrombo-emboli. The larger elastic pulmonary arteries may show lattices, due to recanalisation of thromboemboli. Smooth muscle develops in the walls of pulmonary arterioles.

In many patients with recurrent pulmonary thrombo-embolism the source of venous thrombi is not found. As already explained, the recurrent impaction of small thrombo-emboli in the pulmonary circulation is a normal phenomenon. Hence it may well be that chronic pulmonary thrombo-embolism is not caused by the production of an excessive number of thrombo-emboli, but by the intrinsic inability of the pulmonary circulation to deal with them. So far, no evidence has been found of inadequate fibrinolytic activity in the blood of these patients. The abnormality may lie in the pulmonary vascular endothelium.

Non-thrombotic pulmonary embolism

The pulmonary capillary bed is a most effective filter of particulate matter in the blood and all manner of fragments may be found impacted in it. The commonest and most important clinical form is pulmonary thrombo-embolism, but fragments of various materials other than thrombus can cause pulmonary embolism, as described below.

Bone marrow embolism may follow accidents with bone fractures, thoracic operations involving cleavage of the sternum, rib fractures due to external cardiac massage, or spontaneous fracture due to tumour metastases in bones. Masses of megakaryocytes may be found impacted in the pulmonary capillaries, especially after surgical operations and in cases of pulmonary thrombo-embolism. **Fat embolism** commonly occurs after accidents involving fractures of bones or contusion of adipose tissue (p. 244). It is detected as oily patches in the blood and can be readily demonstrated by the usual stains for fat. Fat embolism in the lungs is very common: it rarely causes significant symptoms, unless very extensive, when it can even be fatal. **Amniotic fluid embolism** to the lung is a clinical and pathological entity which may occur in women during or shortly after childbirth. It causes a sudden onset of dyspnoea, cyanosis and shock, and may be fatal. It is also possible that non-fatal amniotic fluid embolism is a cause of primary pulmonary hypertension. By contrast, small fragments of trophoblast are frequently found in the lungs of pregnant women dying from various causes, but rarely give rise to symptoms. *Cancer cells* are trapped in the pulmonary capillary bed like other particulate matter: they may degenerate or grow to form metastases. Recurrent emboli from the right atrium in cases of cardiac myxoma may lead to pulmonary hypertension. **Air embolism** to the lung may arise from many causes, including various surgical and diagnostic procedures such as intravenous injections and infusions, abortions, and the induction of a pneumothorax. The air turns into a frothy mass inside the pulmonary artery but will not easily pass the capillary bed. At necropsy, the pulmonary trunk must be opened under water to reveal air embolism. Other materials entering the pulmonary circulation include cotton wool fibres and materials injected by drug addicts.

Pulmonary emphysema

Pulmonary emphysema is a permanent enlargement of the respiratory passages or air spaces distal to the terminal bronchiole. By using this anatomical definition it is possible to avoid the use of words such as 'destructive' or 'distensive emphysema' which depend on the assumption of mechanisms of causation, the evidence for which is by no means clear. Under certain circumstances air may escape into the interstitial connective tissues of the lung. This condition is called *interstitial emphysema* and should not be confused with pulmonary emphysema as defined above. It will be considered briefly later.

Bronchi and bronchioles. To understand emphysema it is necessary to be familiar with the micro-anatomy of the terminal air passages. Large bronchi have complete rings of cartilage in their walls. They divide into small bronchi with cartilage in the form of plates which do not completely surround the lumen of the bronchus. With further division, the airways increase in number and decrease in size, and the point at which the cartilage disappears is taken as the dividing line between the small bronchus and the bronchiole. Small bronchi still have a few mucous glands left in their wall, whereas in the bronchioles the only mucin-secreting cells are goblet cells in the lining epithelium. The terminal bronchiole is the last small air passage not to bear alveoli and the respiratory bronchiole is the first in which they appear.

The cut surface of distended lung shows hexagonal areas of parenchyma, some 1 or 2 cm across, delineated by fibrous septa (Fig. 16.18). Each hexagonal area is a section of a **secondary lung lobule**; it contains the lung tissue supplied by the three to five terminal bronchioles, which radiate from the centre, accompanied by muscular pulmonary arteries. This is the unit referred to subsequently in this account as '*the lobule*'.

The respiratory acinus. The structure of the respiratory acinus is central to our understanding of the pathology of pulmonary emphysema. The acinus (previously termed a 'primary lobule') is that portion of lung tissue formed by the branching from a single terminal bronchiole (Fig. 16.19a). Hence one lung lobule (see above) consists of three to five respiratory acini. The respiratory bronchioles may branch three or as many as five times. The first order of respiratory bronchioles have only a few alveoli but they increase in number with each division. The walls of the alveolar ducts are lined entirely by alveoli, the dividing walls between the spaces ending in small knots of smooth muscle.

The varieties of pulmonary emphysema

There are complicated and detailed classifications of all the possible localised and generalised forms of pulmonary emphysema but a simple classification of the **generalised form**, which may cause death from respiratory or car-

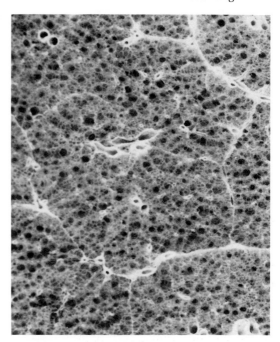

Fig. 16.18 Normal adult lung. Note the hexagonal lobule in the centre of the field with the terminal bronchioles in its centre. (Barium sulphate impregnation.) × 4. (Professor W. R. Lee.)

diac failure, follows from the micro-anatomy of the lung that we have just considered. The respiratory acinus consists of respiratory bronchioles, alveolar ducts and alveoli (Fig. 16.19a). *There are two main forms of pulmonary emphysema. One is characterised by permanent dilatation of the respiratory bronchioles, the other by permanent dilatation of the alveolar ducts and alveoli.*

Bronchiolar emphysema. In this type, the enlarged terminal air spaces are respiratory bronchioles (Fig. 16.19b). In the early stages of the disease the alveolar ducts and alveoli distal to the dilated bronchioles are normal. The disease is readily recognised by naked-eye examination of slices of fixed distended or inflated lungs, as the enlarged airspaces are seen in clusters, at the centres of the secondary lung lobules, surrounded by normal lung tissue (Fig. 16.20a). In histological sections, the emphysematous spaces appear to be derived from respiratory bronchioles, but it may be difficult to be certain of this unless many lesions or serial sections of a single lesion are examined. There is a great contrast between the greatly enlarged respiratory bronchioles and the normal alveolar ducts

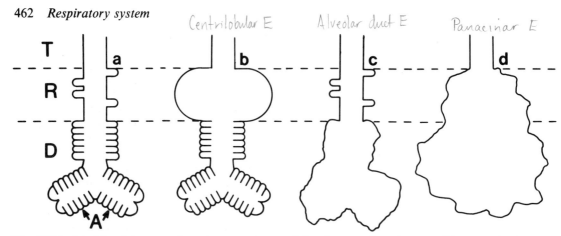

Centrilobular E   Alveolar duct E   Panacinar E

Fig. 16.19   Models of the normal respiratory acinus and the changes of emphysema. The normal acinus (**a**) consists of a terminal bronchiole (T), leading into respiratory bronchioles (R) and alveolar ducts (D) from both of which alveoli (A) arise. (For clarity, only one respiratory bronchiole is shown arising from the terminal bronchiole.) Dilatation of air spaces is confined initially to the respiratory bronchioles in centrilobular and focal duct emphysema (**b**), and to the alveolar ducts and spaces in alveolar duct emphysema (**c**). In panacinar emphysema (**d**) dilatation of the alveolar ducts and spaces extends to the respiratory bronchioles.

and alveoli distal to the emphysematous spaces. There are two varieties of bronchiolar emphysema. The first is **focal dust emphysema** which is virtually confined to coal workers (Fig. 16.21). (A minor form, which has been termed 'soot emphysema', occurs in the general population.) The second, more serious and commoner form, is found in the general population and is called **centrilobular emphysema** (Fig. 16.20a). (Because the respiratory bronchioles lie centrally in the

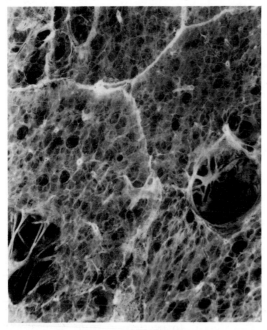

Fig. 16.20a Section of lung impregnated with barium sulphate, showing centrilobular emphysema. Note the punched out centrilobular spaces containing fibrous strands and blood vessels and the relatively normal parenchyma at the periphery of the lobules. × 7. (Professor W. R. Lee.)

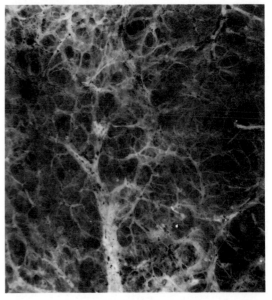

Fig. 16.20b Severe panacinar emphysema. Parts of two secondary lobules are shown, with a thickened interlobular septum (lower central). The alveolar walls throughout the lobules have been largely destroyed, with formation of emphysematous spaces. Atrophic lung tissue and some surviving small vessels are seen as fine strands. Barium sulphate preparation, × 8. (Professor W. R. Lee.)

The respiratory bronchioles are normal. In the second stage of alveolar emphysema, the enlargement of air spaces extends from the alveolar ducts proximally in the respiratory acinus to involve the respiratory bronchioles and so the entire acinus (Fig. 16.19d). This is called **panacinar emphysema**: in lung slices it is readily recognised by areas of grossly abnormal air spaces (Fig. 16.20b) scattered irregularly throughout the lung: macroscopically the lungs appear voluminous, the anterior surface of the heart is covered and the diaphragm pressed downwards. The edges of the emphysematous lung are raised above the surface, rounding off the sharp edges. The emphysematous tissue is paler than the rest of the lung as less carbon pigment is present: it contains little blood and pits on pressure owing to lack of elasticity. Emphysema is most pronounced at the apices of the lungs and along the margins, especially the anterior borders, but in extreme cases practically the whole of the lung substance may be affected, although the condition is usually slight on the posterior aspect. In severe panacinar emphysema, the involved areas frequently merge with one another so that there is little or no intervening normal lung tissue. Some of the enlarged abnormal air spaces in the lung may become cystic and project from the pleural surface; these are called *bullae*. In histological sections the alveoli are few and greatly enlarged. In some cases of centrilobular emphysema the dilatation of the respiratory bronchioles may be so pronounced that it becomes impossible to distinguish them from cases of panacinar emphysema.

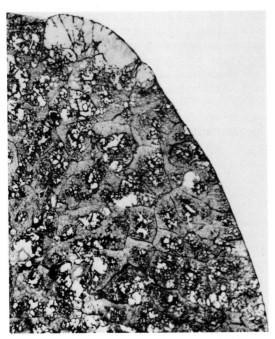

Fig. 16.21 Focal dust emphysema in coal-worker's pneumoconiosis. × 1.

lobule, the dilated spaces are, in fact, centrilobular in both focal dust and centrilobular emphysema.)

The distinction between focal dust emphysema and centrilobular emphysema depends to some extent on the occupational history but there are also micro-anatomical differences. In the focal variety, there is a fusiform dilatation of all orders of respiratory bronchioles and they are surrounded by coal dust. In centrilobular emphysema, the distal orders of respiratory bronchioles are first affected and there is little surrounding dust but evidence of chronic bronchiolitis. *Right ventricular failure is common in centrilobular but not in focal dust emphysema*, which is discussed in the later section on pneumoconioses.

Alveolar emphysema. In this type, there is permanent enlargement initially of alveolar ducts and alveoli and subsequently of respiratory bronchioles. The first stage is called **alveolar duct emphysema** (Fig. 16.19c), although it has also been called the *vesicular* variety. In slices of distended or inflated lung it may be recognised as diffuse areas of abnormally large air spaces. Histological sections show enlarged alveolar ducts and alveoli, the latter becoming wider at their mouths and shallower in depth.

The demonstration of emphysema at necropsy

Adequate fixation is very important for the demonstration of emphysema. The usual practice of cutting lungs at necropsy results in collapse and could hardly be better designed to obscure the appearances of the air spaces. Careful examination or 'point-counting', as described below, requires that the whole lungs should be distended with formol-saline until the pleural surfaces are smooth and then left for two to three days before cutting. Impregnation of slices of fixed lung with barium sulphate will allow the relationship of the abnormal air spaces and their connections to be assessed in three dimensions with the dissecting microscope (Fig. 16.20). Sections of an adequately fixed lung can be used for 'point-counting' to estimate the distribution and severity of emphysema. This may be carried out by placing over the slice of lung a perspex sheet divided into equilateral triangles with 1 cm sides, at the corners of which are small punched-out points. This enables one to determine the percentage of emphysema present by counting the number of points lying over air spaces. Such quantitative studies have not revealed any simple relation between the amount of lung destroyed by pulmonary emphysema and the weight of the right ventricle (see below). Another technique for the demonstration of emphysema is the preparation of sections, approximately 300 μm thick, of gelatin-embedded lungs. Such sections may be mounted on paper and preserved as dry specimens. If morphometric studies on histological sections are to be carried out, the lung should be inflated with formalin vapour in a vacuum chamber.

Clinicopathological correlations. There are two main clinical syndromes associated with what physicians call **'chronic obstructive airways disease',** the pathology of which is chronic bronchitis and emphysema. The 'type A' patient is characterised by obvious radiological evidence of emphysema, reduced diffusing capacity; Pa_{O_2} and Pa_{CO_2} are both normal at rest, and there is little tendency to develop congestive cardiac failure. This patient is the 'pink puffer' and his main disability is breathlessness. He has emphysema without significant hypoxia and the emphysema is commonly but not invariably of the panacinar type. The 'type B' patient does not have much radiological evidence of emphysema; diffusing capacity is normal; at rest, Pa_{O_2} is low and Pa_{CO_2} raised. This is the 'blue bloater' who has significant hypoxia and is likely to die in congestive (right ventricular) cardiac failure. The emphysema is commonly of centrilobular type. Chronic hypoxia causes pulmonary hypertension and the hypoxic form of pulmonary hypertensive vascular disease (p. 455).

Morphometry in emphysema. Quantitative methods have proved useful in the study of pulmonary emphysema. It is quite inadequate now to talk of 'severe' or 'moderately severe' emphysema. The application of histological morphometric techniques derived from principles

used by geologists for a century in the study of rocks enables one to establish fairly easily the internal surface area of the lung and the number of surviving alveolar spaces. In one study the normal internal surface area of both lungs together was 70 m². The corresponding area in centrilobular emphysema was reduced to 61 m² and in alveolar emphysema to 46 m². The total number of alveolar spaces in the normal left and right lungs together was 273×10^6, while in centrilobular emphysema it was 215×10^6, and in panacinar emphysema 63×10^6. *There is no relation between the reduction in internal surface area in pulmonary emphysema and the weight of the right ventricle, suggesting that the classical concept that right ventricular hypertrophy in emphysema is due to loss of pulmonary capillary bed is incorrect.* In fact, right ventricular hypertrophy appears to be commoner in centrilobular emphysema in which the reduction in internal surface area, and so presumably in capillary bed, is smaller.

The pathogenesis of emphysema

There is evidence to suggest that certain proteolytic enzymes can cause emphysema. It can be induced in animals by aerosols of papain, a proteolytic enzyme which attacks elastin. Emphysema can also be produced in dogs by aerosol homogenates of human leukocytes which are thought to contain an elastase capable of damaging the lung. Alpha₁-antitrypsin, which is an inhibitor of such enzymes, is synthesised in the liver and is a normal constituent of the α_1-globulin fraction of the plasma proteins. Some people have an inherited deficiency of this inhibitor in their blood. In the rare homozygous state, the deficiency is severe and there is a high frequency of emphysema. It is not generally accepted that heterozygotes are more prone to emphysema, but deterioration in lung function in cigarette smokers, and the loss of elastic recoil with increasing age, proceed more rapidly in heterozygotes than in the normal population. It is now possible to measure the serum trypsin inhibitory capacity. The emphysema associated with α_1-antitrypsin deficiency in man is panacinar in type and is mainly basal in situation. This has been attributed to the fact that in the upright posture basal perfusion exceeds that of the apex and that the proteolytic enzyme presumed to be the causative agent is blood-borne.

By contrast, *the known air-borne factors predisposing to emphysema, including cigarette smoke and coal dust, tend to induce centrilobular or focal dust emphysema*, most severe in the apices of the lung. Such apical predominance may relate to the lung apex being subject to greater inflationary stresses and having a higher ratio of ventilation to perfusion than the base. *Centrilobular emphysema is associated with chronic bronchitis* leading to post-inflammatory weakening and dilatation of the respiratory bronchioles. In focal dust emphysema the accumulation of dust in and around the walls of respiratory bronchioles leads to rigidity and loss of the smooth muscle, so that the affected segments are progressively dilated under the pressure of inspired air.

Once the initial damage to the lung tissue has occurred, the force which expands the damaged portions into emphysematous spaces is the atmospheric pressure of the inspired air. The force required to distend an elastic sphere is inversely related to the radius and therefore becomes progressively less as the sphere enlarges. A vicious circle is initiated as soon as a weakness develops in the air passages, and continuing dilatation and destruction is inevitable, particularly if the emphysematous lung is subject to the powerful inspiratory effort of the coughing which is associated with chronic bronchitis.

Other types of emphysema

'**Compensatory emphysema**' is a term sometimes used to describe the overdistension of alveoli which may occur around areas of collapsed lung tissue and during acute attacks of bronchial asthma.

With increasing age there is a concomitant increase in the size of the alveolar spaces and a decrease in the internal surface area of the lungs. In some elderly subjects these changes are of sufficient magnitude to suggest to some pathologists that they constitute '**senile emphysema**'.

'**Interstitial emphysema**'. This condition follows laceration of the lung substance. It may be produced by overdistension of the alveolar spaces as may occur with severe coughing or in dyspnoea with forced inspiration. It may also follow traumatic laceration of the lung tissue by a fractured rib or by a perforating wound. Interstitial emphysema due to rupture of alveolar walls from over-distension is much commoner in children than adults and occurs in such conditions as whooping cough, bronchiolitis, and in diphtheria of the larynx and trachea. The alveolar walls rupture as the result of over-expansion during forced inspiration, and air, in the form of small bead-like collections or blebs, extends along the lines of junction of the interlobular septa with the pleura, thus producing a reticulated appearance on the pleural surface. When the air is abundant, it passes by the lymphatics to the rest of the lungs, and in some cases it extends to the tissues at the root of the neck and gives rise to subcutaneous emphysema.

Collapse of lung tissue

Atelectasis and collapse. There is a distinction to be made between these two conditions. The term atelectasis is derived from the Greek for 'imperfect expansion' and it should be restricted to denote failure of the lungs to expand properly at birth. *Atelectasis*, which is thus congenital, should be distinguished from acquired *collapse* of a previously expanded lung. A lung may collapse because something presses on it from without; this is *pressure collapse*, or because there is obstruction of a bronchus with resulting absorption of air in the correspond-ing area of lung tissue; this is *absorption collapse*.

Pressure collapse. The lung may be compressed from without by a pleural effusion, haemothorax, empyema or pneumothorax. Spencer points out that the pulmonary changes which follow this type of collapse differ from those which follow absorption collapse because the absence of bronchial obstruction leaves the secretions from lung and bronchi free to drain in the normal fashion up the bronchial tree. Thus the changes that eventually occur within the lung parenchyma do not result from infection, but from the haemodynamic alterations and associated vascular changes. Collapse due to pyothorax (empyema) may be considerable so that the lung becomes very small and lies posteriorly against the side of the vertebral column. When the exudate on the pleural surface becomes organised, pleural thickening results and prevents re-expansion of the lung even when the infection is overcome. Accordingly it is important to drain the pleural cavity and obtain re-expansion of the lung before this happens. In pressure collapse also, the lung volume may be greatly reduced.

Absorption collapse. This is a commoner condition than pressure collapse and follows *acute and complete obstruction* of a large bronchus. Following such obstruction, collateral air ventilation may for a time keep the obstructed segment of lung filled with air provided the surrounding lung is free from pulmonary oedema, haemorrhage or pneumonia. However, as the air gradually disappears it is largely replaced by secretion and oedema fluid so that the lung does not change very much in size. Acute absorption collapse follows inhaled foreign bodies and collections of mucus occurring in terminal illnesses, after tracheostomy, during and after anaesthetics or in lung infections. *Chronic bronchial obstruction* may be caused by tumours growing in the wall of the affected bronchus or pressing on it from without. Other lesions which may press on bronchi and obstruct them are aneurysms and enlarged lymph nodes. In absorption collapse, bronchial secretions beyond the obstruction are very likely to become infected and suppuration may extend through the collapsed segment of lung tissue.

In collapse of the lung the pleural surfaces are wrinkled and the cut surface is airless. Portions of the collapsed tissue sink in water. As explained above, the reduction in volume is often much greater in pressure than in absorption collapse. The alveolar walls are pushed together. There is no respiratory movement of air in the bronchial tree in the collapsed area of lung so that the haemoglobin in its dilated alveolar capillaries is largely in a reduced state. As a result the affected lung appears purple. When the collapse has lasted for some time, there is a proliferation of granular pneumocytes, associated with progressive pulmonary fibrosis. This permanently prevents re-expansion and a return to normal. In the early stages there is a constriction of the pulmonary arteries but later they show intimal fibroelastosis.

Massive collapse, affecting most of one or both lungs, is rare and is usually caused by wounds or injuries of the chest wall. It may also follow the use of lipiodol for bronchography, and may complicate laryngeal paralysis in diphtheria.

Atelectasis. Incomplete expansion of the neonatal lung may be caused by failure of the respiratory centre or, in premature infants, because the lung is insufficiently developed. It may follow hyaline membrane disease (p. 452), or may result from laryngeal dysfunction and obstruction of the air passages. Finally, congenital lung disease may prevent expansion of the lung. All these causes are, however, responsible for only a small proportion of atelectatic neonatal lungs. In many infants with severe atelectasis, no cause can be demonstrated at necropsy.

Acute bacterial infections

The most common acute inflammatory disorders of the lung are the various types of **pneumonia**, which is defined as an inflammatory disorder of the lung characterised by consolidation due to the presence of exudate in the alveolar spaces.

The pneumonias may be classified anatomically into lobar pneumonia and bronchopneumonia. In **lobar pneumonia**, the causative bacteria lead to the production of a watery inflammatory exudate in the alveoli. This flows directly into bronchioles and related alveoli, filling them and spilling over into adjacent lobules and segments of the lung. Damage to the bronchiolar walls, although present, is relatively unimportant. The exudate and bacteria spread through the lumens rather than the walls of the terminal airways. The consolidation is sharply confined to the affected lobe, which is diffusely affected. In **bronchopneumonia**, the inflammation occurs primarily in the terminal and respiratory bronchioles. The walls are damaged so that infection and exudation extend into the surrounding peribronchiolar alveoli and into the acinus supplied by the affected terminal bronchiole (Fig. 16.22). The resulting pneumonia consists of numerous discrete foci of consolidation centred around inflamed terminal bronchioles.

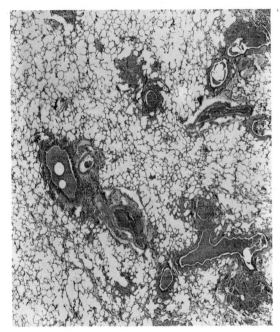

Fig. 16.22 Acute bronchiolitis and early bronchopneumonia. The bronchioles are filled with exudate which is extending into the associated respiratory acini and peribronchiolar alveoli. × 10.

The anatomical type of pneumonia (lobar or bronchopneumonia) and the subsequent liability to develop complications depend on the aetiological agent responsible. Hence the older anatomical classification is being superseded by a classification based on the causative agent.

Pneumococcal lobar pneumonia

Since the widespread use of antibiotics the fully-developed picture of classical lobar pneumonia is not often seen in Britain. However, fatal untreated cases may still be encountered in those who lie neglected at home, in those who decline medical aid, in vagrants and in alcoholics who become exposed to cold. Classical lobar pneumonia is still a common disease in many areas of the world where medical services are poorly developed. Thus it is still a very frequent and an important cause of death in many parts of Africa. The disease predominates in males and occurs at all ages, although it is uncommon below the age of one year. It is still most commonly seen between the ages of thirty and fifty years.

The causative agent is *Streptococcus pneumoniae*, a Gram +ve diplococcus which can be serologically typed according to the antigenic properties of its polysaccharide capsule. About 90 per cent of cases are caused by the following types in descending order of frequency: I, III, II, V, VII, VIII and IV. The first three types are responsible for 70 per cent of cases. Types I and II cause pneumonia mainly in younger persons who were previously healthy, and type III mainly in patients over the age of fifty suffering from some other form of chronic disease. Type III has always been known as a particularly lethal strain and it is still likely to cause high mortality in spite of the use of antibiotics and modern supportive measures.

Structural changes. Infection is acquired by inhalation of pneumococci. If the organisms are virulent and the resistance of the patient low, a disease process commences which, if untreated, runs a fairly well-defined course, usually terminating in resolution. It has been customary to recognise the following four stages in the progress of untreated pneumococcal lobar pneumonia: acute congestion; red hepatisation; grey hepatisation; and resolution. It must be emphasised that these stages occur in untreated cases in adults. The use of sulphonamides and antibiotics profoundly alters the classical clinical and pathological picture.

Acute congestion. This initial phase, which lasts for one or two days, is one of acute congestion and oedema. Macroscopically the affected lobe is heavy, dark red and firm: abundant frothy red fluid can be squeezed from it. Large numbers of pneumococci are seen in stained smears made from the cut surface. Microscopically, the alveolar capillaries are engorged with erythrocytes. There is venular margination of neutrophil polymorphs which can be seen to be migrating into the alveolar spaces. These are filled with eosinophilic oedema fluid which contains many Gram +ve diplococci.

Red hepatisation. This phase lasts from the second to the fourth days of the disease. The pleural surface of the affected lobe is covered by greyish-white friable tags of fibrin. The cut surface appears dry, firm, red and granular and feels like liver. Affected lung tissue is airless and sinks in water. Microscopically, the capillary engorgement persists, but the exudate occupying the alveolar spaces now contains a fine network of fibrin (Figs. 16.24 and 3.5, p. 48), large numbers of extravasated red cells and increasing numbers of emigrated neutrophil polymorphs.

Grey hepatisation. In this stage of late consolidation (four to eight days) the affected lung may weigh up to 1500 g. Fibrinous pleurisy is present and the cut surface is dry, granular and grey (Fig. 16.23). The affected lobe still feels like liver and slices of it retain straight, sharp edges. Microscopically, the alveolar spaces are distended and consolidated by a denser network of inspissated fibrin containing neutrophil poly-

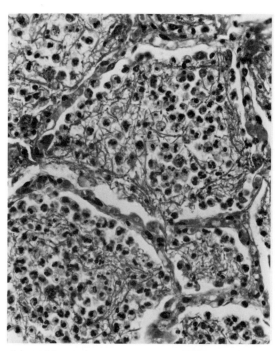

Fig. 16.24. Lobar pneumonia. The alveolar spaces are filled with exudate containing a fibrin network and many neutrophil polymorphs. × 235.

morphs, many dead and disintegrating, and occasional degenerating erythrocytes (Fig. 16.24). During this stage, antibodies to pneumococci appear in the blood, pneumococci are eliminated, and the fever subsides by crisis.

Resolution begins on the eighth day with the migration of macrophages from the alveolar septa into the exudate, which is gradually liquefied by fibrinolytic enzymes and absorbed or coughed up. The cut surface of the affected lung is at first friable and mottled red and grey in colour. Complete resolution and re-aeration take from one to three weeks. Since there is virtually no tissue destruction in lobar pneumonia, the lung parenchyma returns to normal, but the pleural exudate is commonly organised with the formation of fibrous adhesions between the two surfaces.

As already mentioned, the above account refers to cases not receiving antibacterial therapy. Sulphonamide or antibiotic therapy rapidly eliminates the pneumococci and resolution follows.

Clinical features. The onset is sudden and the patient has a fever with rigors and sharp pleuritic pain on respiration. When a lower lobe is

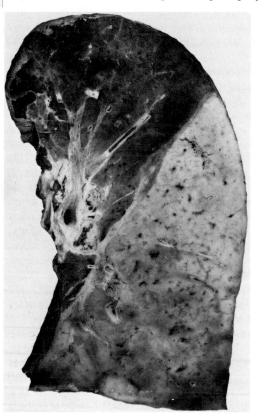

Fig. 16.23 Acute lobar pneumonia with grey hepatisation in lower lobe and red hepatisation in part of upper lobe. × ⅓.

involved, diaphragmatic pleural pain may be referred to the tip of the shoulder. Partly because of the pain, breathing is shallow and rapid, and there is usually a cough productive of brown or blood-stained sputum. There is a well-marked neutrophil polymorphonuclear leucocytosis from an early stage. Bacteraemia is common, blood cultures being positive in about 65 per cent of cases. Usually the systemic arterial oxygen saturation is only slightly reduced. As in acute inflammation in general, blood flow through the consolidated lobe(s) is at first rapid, but soon slows down, and becomes very low, although the total pulmonary blood flow is increased, as in any infective fever.

Complications. The principal complications of pneumococcal lobar pneumonia are as follows:

Organisation of exudate. In about three per cent of cases resolution does not occur and the fibrinous exudate occupying the alveoli becomes organised (Fig. 16.25). The fibrin is slowly digested by macrophages, while fibroblasts grow in from the alveolar septa, and the

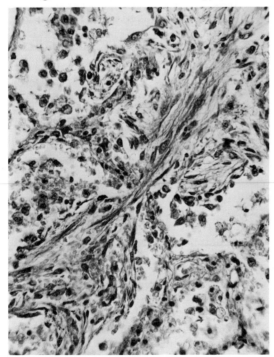

Fig. 16.25 Organisation of alveolar exudate in the lung. The inflammatory exudate has been replaced by cellular fibrous tissue which can be seen passing from one alveolus to another through the pore of Kohn in the centre of the picture. × 390.

tissue becomes fibrosed, tough, airless, leathery and grey. There is an impression that the incidence of organising pneumonia has increased since the introduction of antibiotics. Possibly these drugs cut down the inflammatory response and reduce the numbers of emigrating polymorphs, which are important in digestion of the fibrin.

Pleural effusion occurs in about five per cent of treated cases.

Empyema occurs in less than 1 per cent of treated cases.

Lung abscess is a complication which has practically disappeared since the introduction of antibiotics.

Cardiac complications include suppurative pericarditis, acute bacterial endocarditis and various degrees of acute failure from toxic myocarditis.

Bacteraemic complications include bacterial endocarditis, suppurative meningitis, acute otitis media and arthritis.

Acute bronchopneumonia

Bronchopneumonia is an inflammatory condition of the lung that occurs when micro-organisms colonise the bronchioles and extend into the surrounding alveoli, leading to numerous discrete foci of consolidation (Fig. 16.22). Many types of bacteria can cause it, including *Strep. pneumoniae*, *Staph. aureus*, *Strep. pyogenes*, *Klebsiella* and *Haemophilus influenzae*. It occurs most commonly in infancy, in old age, and in patients with some debilitating condition such as cancer, uraemia or a stroke. Acute respiratory virus infections, and chronic diseases such as chronic bronchitis, bronchiectasis and cystic fibrosis predispose to bronchopneumonia. It may develop in patients with congestive cardiac failure and after surgical operations under general anaesthesia, due to the adverse effect of narcotic drugs on respiration and ciliary activity.

At necropsy, bronchopneumonia is commonly found in the lower lobes of the lungs, where it appears as focal dark red or grey areas of about 1 cm diameter, which are firmer than the surrounding lung, and appear to be centred around a bronchiole from which a bead of pale yellow pus can be expressed. If progressive, the focal areas of consolidation become larger and eventually coalesce to simulate lobar pneumonia.

The microscopic lesions of bronchopneumonia are an acute bronchiolitis with filling of the surrounding peribronchiolar alveoli with inflammatory exudate rich in neutrophil polymorphs.

Complete resolution is uncommon in bronchopneumonia because, except in mild cases, there is usually a variable amount of damage to, and destruction of, the walls of bronchioles. In consequence, the lesions usually result in the development of small foci of fibrosis. If fibrosis of the lung is extensive, bronchiectasis may develop.

Staphylococcal pneumonia. *Staphylococcus aureus* rarely causes pneumonia as a primary event; it is usually encountered as a secondary infection in patients debilitated by chronic lung disease, such as cystic fibrosis, where antibiotics have been used for long periods. Its incidence rises sharply during epidemics of influenza, measles and pertussis, when it may be responsible for an acute, short-lived, lethal pneumonia in children and adults. In acute cases, staphylococci invade the lungs about thirty-six hours after the onset of influenza. At necropsy, the lungs appear purple and are heavy due to haemorrhagic pulmonary oedema. The bronchi are filled with blood-stained fluid which drains away to reveal an inflamed mucosa, sometimes covered by a grey membrane of fibrin. There is no pleural reaction. Microscopically there is an acute ulcerative bronchitis and bronchiolitis: the alveolar spaces are filled with oedema fluid containing fibrin coagulum, much extravasated blood, scanty neutrophil polymorphs and abundant clusters of Gram +ve cocci.

In older children and adults who survive this acute phase, multiple foci of greyish-white consolidation develop which break down to form abscess cavities containing sticky yellow pus. There is much lung destruction and the pleura at this stage is thickly coated with fibrinous or fibrino-purulent exudate. Empyema and pneumothorax may occur from rupture of pulmonary abscesses into the pleural cavity. In children, a valvular obstruction may occur at the junction of an abscess cavity and bronchus to produce a rapidly-expanding air-filled *tension cyst* or *pneumatocele*. Such lesions also occur rarely in tuberculosis treated with drugs but are otherwise a complication peculiar to staphylococcal pneumonia in children. The cyst, which can be several centimetres in diameter, may rupture into the pleural cavity to produce a *tension pneumothorax*. Usually the air is absorbed after the infection is overcome.

Klebsiellar pneumonia. *Klebsiella pneumoniae* (Friedlander's bacillus) is a Gram −ve bacillus with a very thick mucoid capsule. It is an infrequent cause of pneumonia but important because the infection is destructive, with a mortality rate of about 40 per cent and a high incidence of complications. The organism is a commensal in the upper respiratory tract in about 5 per cent of normal individuals, but more frequently in people with advanced dental caries and periodontal disease. Klebsiellar pneumonia tends to occur especially in men over the age of fifty who are chronic alcoholics, diabetics or have oral sepsis. It is about thirty times commoner in men than women. About 75 per cent of infections commence in the right lung, usually in the posterior segment of the upper lobe. Clinically, the onset is acute with severe prostration and a cough with blood-stained gelatinous sputum resembling red currant jelly. Pathologically, red-grey areas of consolidation become confluent, leading to involvement of the entire right upper lobe. The cut surface of the affected lung is mucoid. Destruction of lung tissue leads to the formation of a large apical abscess in about 80 per cent of cases, and this may be mistakenly diagnosed as tuberculosis. The infection may become chronic with severe progressive destruction of lung tissue so that the patient becomes a permanent respiratory cripple.

Streptococcal pneumonia. Cases of pneumonia due to *Strep. pyogenes* are rare and usually secondary to influenza or measles. In severe cases, death occurs within thirty-six to seventy-two hours and at necropsy the lungs appear purple with a fibrinous pleurisy. In cases dying after a week, yellow areas of consolidation are present in the lungs. These consolidated foci may cavitate, with the formation of abscesses leading to empyema and bronchopleural fistulas.

Pseudomonas pneumonia. Following the introduction and combined use of antibiotic and corticosteroid drugs, Gram −ve organisms in general, and *Pseudomonas aeruginosa* in particular, have become of greater importance as causes of bacterial pneumonia. Another factor is the increased use of tracheostomy and mechanical ventilation. Both the tracheostomy wounds and ventilation apparatus commonly become colonised by *Pseudomonas aeruginosa*, which spreads rapidly to infect neighbouring patients. It is most important to sterilise respiratory equipment properly after use to prevent the spread of infection. Unfortunately, *Pseudomonas aeruginosa* may survive and proliferate in water, soap solution, stored blood, infusion fluids and in some antiseptics. In pseudomonas pneumonia, the air spaces in the affected lung are filled with blood, oedema fluid, scanty neutrophil polymorphs and innumerable causative organisms which can be demonstrated by appropriate staining methods. A characteristic feature of pseudomonas pneumonia is bacterial invasion of pulmonary arteries, leading to necrosis of the vessel with subsequent haemorrhage or thrombosis and then pulmonary infarction.

Legionnaires' disease. An outbreak of severe pneumonia affected 180 of about 4400 persons attending the Annual Convention of American Legionnaires in Philadelphia, U.S.A. during July 1976, causing twenty-nine deaths. Investigation revealed that the pneumonia was caused by a hitherto unknown Gram —ve coccobacillus which has been named *Legionella pneumophila*. Pathological examination of the lungs shows a lobar pneumonia indistinguishable from that caused by other infecting organisms (Fig. 16.26). However, *Legionella pneumophila* can be demonstrated histologically using the Dieterle's silver staining method (Blackmon, Hicklin and Chandler, 1978). The organism can also be identified by immunofluorescence microscopy. Culture is extremely difficult. Since the original description of the disease, some 400 cases have been reported in North America and Europe.

Aspiration pneumonia results from the inhalation of food, gastric contents, or infected material from the oropharyngeal region. It may follow anaesthesia administered on a full stomach for an obstetric or other emergency. It may complicate pyloric stenosis, hiatus hernia, oesophageal obstruction and any condition associated with persistent vomiting. The likelihood of food or gastric contents being inhaled is increased in unconscious patients, drunkenness, epilepsy and neurological disorders affecting swallowing.

Massive inhalation of gastric contents may lead to rapid death from asphyxia. The aspiration of smaller amounts of sterile acid gastric contents produces pulmonary oedema due to chemical irritation of the alveolar walls: a few hours after aspiration the patient dramatically develops cyanosis, dyspnoea and shock, with bloodstained sputum. If the acute episode is survived, secondary bacterial infection is likely to follow. Non-sterile aspirate rapidly causes widespread bronchopneumonia, which becomes confluent with multiple areas of necrosis. The microscopic picture is of a suppurative bronchopneumonia with destruction of alveolar walls and abscess formation. Foreign-body giant cells may be seen surrounding vegetable matter from food, giving rise to a granulomatous reaction.

Aspiration pneumonia with suppuration may also result from partial drowning, particularly in dirty water.

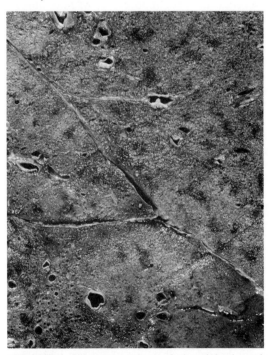

Fig. 16.26 The cut surface of the right lung in legionnaire's disease, showing the adjacent parts of upper, middle and lower lobes, all of which are diffusely consolidated by inflammatory exudate. ×0·7 (Dr. J. F. Boyd.)

Lung abscess

Lung abscess presents clinical and radiological features which must be distinguished from those of necrosis in a malignant tumour or cavitation due to tuberculosis; these two diagnoses must be considered automatically whenever there is a clinical suspicion of lung abscess.

Causes. The commonest cause of a lung abscess is *inhalation of infected material* during unconsciousness and sleep. Such material may be food, gastric contents, decaying teeth or necrotic tissue derived from lesions in the mouth, upper respiratory tract and nasopharynx. An abscess may form beyond an *obstructed bronchus* and this may be the first sign of a bronchial carcinoma or impacted foreign body. Pyogenic infection of *bronchiectatic* or *tuberculous cavities* results in abscess formation, and another important group of lung abscesses is that arising as a complication of *bacterial pneumonia*. The organisms most likely to be concerned are the type III *Strep. pneumoniae*, *Klebsiella pneumoniae*, *Staph. aureus* and *Strep. pyogenes*. Less common causes of lung abscess include infection of a pulmonary infarct, septic emboli in the lung as in pyaemia due to acute osteomyelitis or acute infective endocarditis, amoebic 'abscesses' due to *Entamoeba histolytica*, trauma to the lung, or direct extension from a suppurating focus in the oesophagus, mediastinum, subphrenic area or vertebral column.

Localisation. Abscesses due to inhalation of infected foreign material are likely to be located in the lower part of the right upper lobe or at the apex of the right lower lobe. The right bronchus is more in line with the trachea than the left and is thus more receptive to aspirated foreign material. An abscess resulting from inhalation of a large foreign body will develop beyond where the body is impacted. Small foreign particles are able to travel further into the lung and may evoke inflammation in the alveoli to produce an abscess just beneath the pleura. An abscess arising as a result of bronchiectasis tends to be centred around the affected bronchus, while an abscess complicating pneumonia has no primary relationship to a major bronchus. Pyaemic abscesses, which are usually staphylococcal or streptococcal in nature, are scattered widely throughout the lungs, although they are likely to be small and mainly subpleural.

Complications. It is possible for a small lung abscess to heal completely, leaving a fibrous scar with a small central sterile cavity. An abscess located near the pleura induces a fibrin-ous or purulent pleurisy which may progress to *empyema*. An abscess communicating with a bronchus may rupture into the pleural cavity to give a *bronchopleural fistula* and *pyopneumothorax*. Serious *haemorrhage* may occur if an abscess erodes a pulmonary or bronchial artery. A distant complication of lung abscess is dissemination of infection to the brain which occurs in 5 to 10 per cent of cases, with the development of *meningitis* or *cerebral abscess*. Abscess formation in staphylococcal pneumonia may result in *tension cysts* or *pneumatoceles* (p. 470).

Gangrene of the lung

In some cases of aspiration pneumonia (p. 471) the extent of necrosis and degree of putrefaction warrant the term gangrene or gangrenous bronchopneumonia. There is development of rapidly progressive multiple abscesses in which anaerobic organisms such as bacterioides, streptococci, clostridia and fusiform bacteria, in addition to aerobic organisms, play an active role. These abscesses are not walled-off and lung destruction is very extensive. There are irregular cavities containing foul-smelling pus surrounded by soft, friable, moist, green or black necrotic tissue.

Virus pneumonia

In viral respiratory infections there may be proliferation of bronchial, bronchiolar and alveolar epithelium, which may form multinucleated giant cells, followed by necrosis. The bronchial, bronchiolar and alveolar walls are infiltrated by lymphocytes and mononuclear cells. Neutrophil polymorphs are few or absent in the inflammatory cell infiltrate, which is mainly interstitial except in influenza. Inclusion bodies are unusual in pulmonary viral infections, and unless specific tests are performed, the viral nature can often only be inferred from the above histological features. Moreover, as previously implied, *many viral infections of the lung predispose the respiratory tissues to secondary bacterial invasion and when this occurs the distinctive histological appearances of viral pneumonia are lost. Much of the mortality attributed to viral pneumonia is, in fact, due to secondary bacterial infection.*

The nature of a viral pneumonia can be confirmed by identifying the infecting organism by isolation of the virus or by demonstrating a rising or high titre of specific antibodies in the patient's serum. In spite of their varied pathogenesis, viral pneumonias mostly present a broadly similar clinical picture which is commonly referred to as **atypical pneumonia**.

Influenza

Influenza occurs endemically in most countries, but about every three years it causes an epidemic. Every forty years or so a major epidemic or worldwide pandemic appears, as in 1918 when a large percentage of the world's population was affected. Infection is probably spread by droplets of infected secretions reaching the respiratory tract of susceptible subjects.

Influenza virus produces its effects within the epithelial cells lining the respiratory tract. It has been suggested that the susceptibility to influenza of patients with chronic heart failure is due to the proliferation of granular pneumocytes in the alveoli in this condition, thus providing more cells suitable for virus growth. The whole respiratory tract is commonly invaded. The trachea and large bronchi usually show signs of intense inflammation, which may be accompanied by haemorrhage and occasionally, in very severe cases, also by some superficial necrosis of the mucosa and fibrinous exudate. There is leukopenia, and neutrophil polymorphs are absent from the lesions. In most cases the disease progresses no further, but during epidemics, when the virulence of the virus may have become enhanced, extension of the disease to involve the bronchioles and lung parenchyma (Fig. 16.27) is much more common, although it also occurs in severe endemic cases.

In **primary influenzal pneumonia**, which is almost always fatal, the alveoli are filled with a mixture of oedema fluid, fibrin, red blood cells and mononuclear cells (lymphocytes and macrophages). These changes are accompanied by an interstitial mononuclear cell infiltrate in half the cases. In the most severely affected parts of the lung there may be focal necrosis of the alveolar walls, which are lined by hyaline membranes. At necropsy, the lungs are heavy, bulky and purple-red. The cut surfaces exude blood-stained frothy fluid from the bronchi and lung parenchyma: the latter shows extensive dark areas of haemorrhage, particularly in the lower lobes.

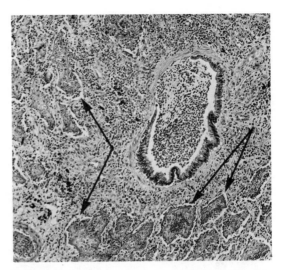

Fig. 16.27 Influenzal bronchopneumonia. There is acute inflammatory exudate in the bronchiole and in the surrounding alveolar spaces (arrows): the exudate in the alveoli is rich in fibrin and appears dark. × 60.

The lowering of the resistance of the respiratory tract to secondary bacterial infection is a striking and characteristic feature of influenza. The development of **secondary bacterial pneumonia**, also a serious complication of influenza, is usually due to *Staphylococcus aureus*, *Haemophilus influenzae* or *Streptococcus pneumoniae*.

Other viral pneumonias

Giant-cell pneumonia. In patients with measles dying early in the disease, notably in children with a deficiency in cell-mediated immunity, the epithelium of the bronchioles may be hyperplastic (Fig. 16.28) but does not usually show giant-cell formation. The alveoli may show many giant cells derived from the lining epithelium by fusion, and they, too, contain inclusion bodies. There is good evidence that this form of giant-cell pneumonia is due to the measles virus and that it represents a deficient immune response to the virus. In cases developing a secondary bacterial pneumonia the characteristic changes are lost.

Cytomegalovirus lung disease. Cytomegalovirus causes opportunistic infections in man, notably in the fetus, in premature infants, and in subjects with immunodeficiency diseases or whose immunity is depressed by corticosteroid therapy, immunosuppressive drugs, irradiation or cytotoxic drugs. In the adult form of disease, the lungs are usually involved as part of a serious widespread infection, the salivary glands and kidneys being affected more frequently

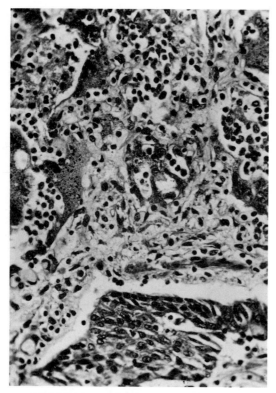

Fig. 16.28 Giant cell pneumonia in measles. There is hyperplasia of the bronchiolar epithelium and numerous giant cells in the alveolar spaces. × 240.

than the lungs. The changes occur in both bronchiolar and alveolar epithelium. Cells enlarge so that they are five to six times the size of their uninvolved neighbours (Fig. 22.66, p. 859). *Pneumocystis carinii* is often present in addition (see below).

Other types of pneumonia

Psittacosis and ornithosis. Infection with various species of *Chlamydiae* (p. 223) is very common in birds. Infection in man is acquired by inhalation of elementary bodies derived from the excreta of infected birds. Cross infection from human patients to healthy attendants may occur by droplet spread. The infection should be suspected in any patient who presents with atypical pneumonia where there is a history of contact with birds, especially parrots, budgerigars and pigeons. If the disease is acquired from parrots and budgerigars, it is termed **psittacosis** while **ornithosis** is used to describe the disease acquired from other birds. Infection produces a haemorrhagic consolidation of the lungs.

Q fever. This condition is caused by *Coxiella burneti* which primarily infects cattle, sheep and goats. Cases of human disease usually originate from the handling of carcasses of infected cattle and sheep, the inhalation of dust from infected barns and straw, or from the drinking of raw milk containing the organisms. Stockyard workers, farmers, shepherds and medical laboratory staff may be exposed to infection during the course of their work. The disease most commonly presents as an atypical pneumonia, with headache and muscle pains as prominent symptoms. The course of the illness is usually short (up to eight days) and benign, but chronic infection can occur. Endocarditis is a rare complication and is frequently fatal.

Mycoplasma pneumonia. This is caused by *Mycoplasma pneumoniae* (p. 222). The lesions consist of a low-grade inflammation of focal character centred on the bronchioles, the walls of which are thickened by interstitial mononuclear cell infiltration, while the lumina contain mucopurulent material. In some alveoli there is fibrinous exudate tending to undergo organisation, in others oedema and haemorrhage. The onset is usually gradual and the mortality is low but resolution is often somewhat delayed.

Pneumocystis pneumonia. This usually occurs as an opportunistic infection in premature and debilitated babies, in older children with hypogammaglobulinaemia, and in patients with immunological deficiency due to lymphoid neoplasms or to the administration of cytotoxic or immunosuppressive drugs. Microscopically, the alveoli are filled with a foamy, pale eosinophilic substance containing innumerable minute haematoxylinophilic dots, 1 μm in diameter, representing the trophozoites of the protozoal parasite *Pneumocystis carinii*. Cystic forms, 8–12 μm in diameter, may also be present and are best demonstrated by methenamine silver staining. The alveolar septa are distended with an infiltrate of plasma cells, lymphocytes and macrophages, but in cases of hypogammaglobulinaemia plasma cells may be absent. Pneumocystis pneumonia is sometimes accompanied by cytomegalovirus disease.

Unusual causes of pulmonary consolidation

Lymphoid interstitial pneumonia is characterised by a chronic cough, dyspnoea and pyrexia, together with enlargement of the spleen and liver. Many patients have hypergammaglobulinaemia. The disease, which is of unknown cause, affects persons of all ages, including infants. It is a slowly progressive condition and the diagnosis is usually made following lung biopsy. Histologically, the alveolar septa are distended with masses of mature lymphocytes intermingled with large pale macrophages and plasma cells. Large lymphoid follicles may be present. Differentiation from a malignant lymphoma may be difficult.

Eosinophilic pneumonia. This may occur in acute and chronic forms, both of which may be accompanied by peripheral blood eosinophilia. Acute eosinophilic pneumonia is a brief, mild, self-limiting illness commonly referred to as *Löffler's syndrome*. In chronic eosinophilic pneumonia, which may last for several months or years, the alveolar spaces contain proteinaceous exudate mixed with eosinophils and mononuclear cells. The alveolar septa and pulmonary interstitial tissues are heavily infiltrated with plasma cells, lymphocytes, eosinophils and macrophages. Most cases of eosinophilic pneumonia are of unknown cause but some are related to adverse drug reactions, or infection by helminths, *Aspergillus*, *Filaria* and *Dirofilaria* (Morrissey, Gaensler, Carrington and Turner, 1975).

'Desquamative interstitial pneumonia' is now regarded as a cellular form of diffuse fibrosing alveolitis and is discussed in the section on pulmonary fibrosis (p. 482).

Pulmonary alveolar proteinosis. This is a rare chronic disease of unknown cause, which can affect persons of all ages from infancy to old age. It is manifested clinically by dyspnoea, a cough often productive of yellow sputum, increasing fatigue and loss of weight. Some patients recover spontaneously but the disease is fatal in about one third of cases. At necropsy, confluent grey areas of consolidation are found in the lungs. A little milky or pale yellow fluid may be squeezed from the cut surface. Histologically, the alveolar spaces are distended by granular eosinophilic material, and lined by prominent granular pneumocytes. The granular eosinophilic intra-alveolar material contains lipid and protein and is apparently derived from the cytoplasm of granular pneumocytes which have degenerated, become necrotic and detached from the alveolar walls. The alveolar septa are devoid of inflammatory cells and fibrosis is usually absent. The nature of pulmonary alveolar proteinosis is obscure. It may represent a stereotyped reaction of the lung to different types of injury, rather than being a single disease entity.

Pulmonary granulomatosis. The lungs are sometimes the principal site of involvement by a number of distinctive types of focal destructive and infiltrative vascular disease and granulomatosis not produced by known infectious agents, nor associated with rheumatoid arthritis. By granulomatosis is meant necrosis of tissue with a peripheral, chronic, cellular inflammatory reaction, not ascribable to occlusive lesions of the blood vessels. The necrotic lesions are surrounded by granulation tissue rich in plasma cells, lymphocytes, large macrophages and multinuclear giant cells. Several forms of granulomatosis have been identified and classified by Liebow (1973) according to their histological picture, location within the lung and behaviour. They include Wegener's granulomatosis, lymphomatoid granulomatosis and bronchocentric granulomatosis.

Lipid pneumonia. The inhalation of oily material into the lungs may cause a lipid pneumonia. This is associated with the long-term use of oily drops or sprays taken for rhinitis. Mineral oil (liquid paraffin) taken regularly at bedtime is readily aspirated during sleep in small amounts which fail to excite the cough reflex. There is a danger of aspiration when oily vitamin preparations are given to reluctant young children or debilitated elderly persons. Occasionally, radio-opaque contrast medium used for bronchography may be retained in the lungs with a resulting lipid pneumonia. Olive oil and neutral vegetable oils are the least irritant. They stimulate slight fibrosis but are slowly absorbed. Mineral oil, although chemically inert, is much more irritant and evokes a granulomatous reaction with considerable fibrosis.

Lipid pneumonia tends to be symptomless and is usually revealed by chance during radiographic examination or at necropsy. The lesions are commonly located in the middle or lower lobes of the right lung or in the left lower lobe. There may be diffuse fibrosis of the affected lung or the formation of a well-circumscribed *oleogranuloma*. This latter firm tumour-like mass may be mistakenly diagnosed as carcinoma in a chest radiograph or during thoracotomy. The histological picture of lipid pneumonia is the presence of oil, either free or in foamy macrophages, and multinucleate giant cells with accompanying lymphocytic infiltration and fibrosis.

Chronic bacterial and fungal infections

Tuberculosis

The general features of tuberculosis have already been discussed (p. 207). The causative organism, *Mycobacterium tuberculosis*, is a slender, straight or slightly curved rod, 1 to 4 μm long, which is stained red by the Ziehl-Neelsen method. In most communities, the lungs are more commonly affected by tuberculosis than any other organ, partly because inhalation is now the commonest mode of infection, but also because lung tissue provides a favourable environment for the growth of the organism. Certain diseases and occupations predispose to the development of tuberculosis. Thus it occurs with increased frequency in chronic alcoholics and in workers with silicosis. It is an occupational hazard for all hospital personnel, particularly those who work in pathology laboratories and necropsy rooms. Corticosteroid therapy, diabetes mellitus and partial gastrectomy are associated with an increased liability to develop the disease. In all developed countries where treatment and prevention of tuberculosis is actively undertaken, there has been a tendency for the incidence of the disease and its mortality to decline steeply among the younger age groups of both sexes during the past twenty years. However, this decline in incidence and mortality has been much less pronounced among the elderly, particularly men. Thus, in countries with a low case rate, tuberculosis now tends to be a disease of older people.

Pulmonary tuberculous lesions vary widely in appearance and behaviour. In communities with a high infection rate, tuberculosis is usually contracted during infancy and childhood, and the resulting *primary* lesions may either heal or prove fatal. During this primary infection, a state of cell-mediated immunity to tuberculoprotein develops. Subsequent infection may occur in adult life, giving rise to *re-infection* or *post-primary* tuberculosis, which may either heal or produce chronic pulmonary disease. In communities with a low rate of tuberculous infection, primary lesions may occur in adult life. Thus it is no longer appropriate to refer to primary and re-infection tuberculosis as the childhood and adult types respectively. The basic features of delayed hypersensitivity reactions, which are necessary for the full understanding of this account, have been given in pp. 156-60.

Primary pulmonary tuberculosis

In patients who have not previously had tuberculosis, inhalation of tubercle bacilli and subsequent infection gives rise to a primary lesion, also termed the *Ghon focus*. This is usually single, 1 to 2 cm in diameter, and situated just beneath the pleura, usually in the mid-zone of either lung. Microscopic examination of the early Ghon focus shows central caseation and peripheral tubercles; the lesion enlarges by spread of mycobacteria, which are taken up and carried by macrophages, so that tubercles form in the adjacent lung tissue, replacing alveolar walls and filling air spaces, and as they enlarge these peripheral tubercles become incorporated in the central caseous area.

Lymphatic spread of *Myco. tuberculosis* takes place in the primary infection; tubercles are frequently seen along the line of the lymphatics between the Ghon focus and the hilar lymph nodes, and both the tracheobronchial and adjacent mediastinal nodes often become extensively involved (Fig. 16.29). Tubercles are found in large numbers in these nodes, which undergo caseation and coalesce, finally converting the nodes into large caseous masses with marginal tubercle follicles. The combination of the Ghon focus and tuberculous lymphadenitis is termed the **primary complex**. In children, the affected hilar and tracheobronchial lymph nodes form a caseous mass which is much larger than the peripheral Ghon focus. In some adults, the reverse is the case.

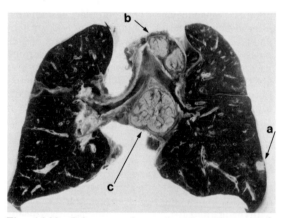

Fig. 16.29 Primary pulmonary tuberculous complex. Lung of child with primary lesion (a) in right lower lobe and enlarged tracheobronchial lymph nodes (b and c).

In most instances, the Ghon focus undergoes healing: if small, it may be replaced completely by fibrous tissue but, if larger, the caseous centre usually persists and is converted into a hard calcified nodule, often partly ossified and enclosed in fibrous tissue: such a healed lesion is readily visible in chest radiographs. The affected hilar and tracheobronchial lymph nodes usually heal and may become heavily calcified.

Progressive primary pulmonary tuberculosis. Healing of the primary tuberculous complex with a favourable outcome is usual but not invariable. Sometimes infection may spread from the Ghon focus to the pleural cavity causing *pleural effusion* or even occasionally *tuberculous empyema.** Hilar lymphadenopathy may cause bronchial obstruction by pressure and lead to segmental or lobar *consolidation or collapse.* Spread of the disease along the submucosal lymphatics of the bronchi produces a series of tubercles and sometimes ulceration of the bronchial mucosa. Involvement of the bronchial blood vessels has been said to impair the blood supply to the bronchial walls, resulting in destructive changes and subsequently *bronchiectasis.* The disease may progress to *tuberculous bronchopneumonia* or to *blood-borne* spread which gives rise to innumerable disseminated lesions in various organs (*generalised miliary tuberculosis*), to smaller numbers of disseminated foci, or to one or two metastatic foci.

Acute tuberculous bronchopneumonia can develop from the primary infection by aspiration of infected caseous material throughout the bronchial tree, either from the Ghon focus or, more commonly, from caseous lymph nodes at the hilum or in the mediastinum. In the former case, the Ghon focus continues to enlarge until eventually it incorporates a bronchus in the caseous process. Caseous material is then discharged into the lumen, from where it may be aspirated through adjacent and more distant parts of the bronchial tree. Bronchial dissemination results similarly when a caseating lesion in the hilar or mediastinal lymph nodes ulcerates into a major bronchus. The resulting tuberculous bronchopneumonia is relatively acute, and usually affects both lungs, although one is often involved more extensively than the other. The lung tissue is studded with numerous small pneumonic patches (Fig. 8.17, p. 211), which are arranged in groups or clusters around the terminal bronchi. The tubercle bacilli, after reaching a bronchiole, produce bronchopneumonic consolidation followed by caseation. The microscopic features are described on p. 211.

There may be considerable fibrinous exudate in and around the lesions, which advance too rapidly for tubercle formation or the development of granulation or fibrous tissue. As the condition progresses, the lesions may become confluent in the lower parts of the lungs, where they are most numerous. The enlarging caseous patches may also soften and discharge into bronchi, with dissemination of more mycobacteria and aggravation of the condition. The cavities resulting from discharge of caseous material have ragged caseating walls and, unlike chronic tuberculous cavities, no surrounding fibrosis. Tuberculous pleurisy usually develops in tuberculous bronchopneumonia. A small cavity opening into a bronchus may rupture also into the pleura, resulting in pneumothorax. Extensive tuberculous bronchopneumonia is associated with fever, severe debility and rapid weight loss. Unless treated early and effectively it is rapidly fatal. As stated below, acute tuberculous bronchopneumonia can occur also in patients with reinfection pulmonary tuberculosis.

Re-infection (post-primary) tuberculosis

During the primary tuberculous infection, or following BCG immunisation, the patient develops cell-mediated immunity to antigens of the tubercle bacillus: this is demonstrable by a positive tuberculin skin test (a delayed hypersensitivity reaction to tuberculoprotein) which is associated with increased resistance to subsequent infection.

Post-primary infection can be endogenous, resulting from re-activation of a dormant primary or post-primary lesion, or it may be exogenous, i.e. caused by organisms inhaled from the external environment. The causes of re-activation of a dormant primary lesion include malnutrition, the development of other severe illness, intercurrent lung infection, and systemic corticosteroid therapy, but in many instances, none of these factors is responsible.

The common sites for post-primary pulmonary tuberculosis are the posterior segment of the upper lobe and the apical segment of the lower lobe. The anatomical location of the lesion is attributed to the good ventilation but

---

* Unless there is superadded pyogenic bacterial infection, tuberculous lesions do not usually suppurate, but tuberculous lesions of the kidney, bones and pleura sometimes do so.

relatively low blood flow in these areas. The re-infection lesion results from proliferation of *Myco. tuberculosis* in the wall of a bronchiole or of an alveolus. The usual reaction takes place, with formation of tubercle follicles, and the lesion enlarges by formation of new tubercles at the margin and in the adjacent lung tissue. The infection spreads by the lymphatics, but, as it induces a delayed hypersensitivity reaction from the onset, lymphatic spread is not usually extensive, and the hilar lymph nodes are not usually affected. The developing re-infection lesion thus comes to consist of a cluster of follicles which, as they enlarge and caseate, tend to become confluent, producing one or more larger lesions. Because of the partial state of immunity which exists, progress of the lesions is slow, the tubercles are well developed and there is conspicuous formation of fibrous tissue at their periphery. The caseous material is yellowish or sometimes greyish due to inclusion of carbon pigment, which is often abundant in the fibrous tissue. If healing does not now occur, some of the nodules will spread to involve the wall of a bronchus in caseous necrosis and blockage of the lumen follows. The lesion may become encapsulated by fibrous tissue or the caseous material may be gradually discharged along the bronchus leaving a small cavity. Bronchial spread to the upper parts of other lobes and to the other lung may occur, and chronic pulmonary tuberculosis is frequently bilateral.

The cavities may coalesce and can become very large (Fig. 16.30). Even with cavitation, enlargement of the tuberculous lesions is usually slow: there is considerable overgrowth of fibrous tissue, not only around the cavities, but also in a diffusely spreading manner. In this way the lung shrinks and bronchiectasis may be superadded. Ultimately a cavity may become very large and occupy a considerable portion of the upper lobe. The walls of the chronic cavities are somewhat irregular and contain raised bands, which represent obliterated blood vessels and other structures with more resistance than the rest of the tissue. The surface is usually lined by caseous material or by pus and debris sometimes mixed with blood: if the disease becomes inactive, the lining of the cavities becomes smooth. The contents of the cavities do not usually have a putrid odour, and the organisms present along with the

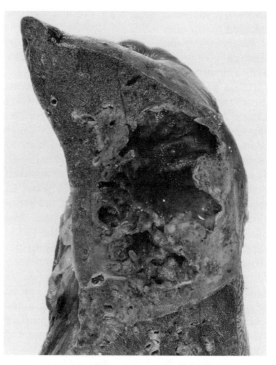

Fig. 16.30 Cavitating post-primary tuberculosis. Much of the upper lobe is occupied by a large irregular cavity with a necrotic lining and a fibrous wall in which paler caseous patches are seen. Fibrosis is most extensive below and lateral to the cavity, where it extends to the pleura. Irregularity of the cavity is due to persistence of fibrosed remnants of bronchi and blood vessels involved in the lesion.

tubercle bacilli are chiefly pyogenic cocci. Pulmonary and bronchial blood vessels involved in the wall of a cavity usually become occluded by endarteritis obliterans (p. 361). Sometimes, however, the wall of an artery may be weakened and rupture; this may be preceded by aneurysm formation. Serious and sometimes fatal haemorrhage results. This is to be distinguished from the coughing up of blood-stained sputum, or the slight bleeding which commonly occurs from small vessels in the wall of a cavity.

If at any time there should occur a rapid diffusion of large numbers of bacilli by the air passages, as may happen when a caseous focus suddenly discharges into a bronchus, the patient's resistance may be overcome and acute *rapidly spreading tuberculous bronchopneumonia* supervenes. It is not uncommon to find the latter in the lower parts of the lungs, while chronic cavity formation is present in the upper lobes (Fig. 8.18, p. 212). This is likely to occur if the patient is debilitated by intercurrent disease such as influenza or diabetes, or by overwork, malnutrition and unfavourable environmental conditions.

In patients dying from chronic pulmonary tuberculosis, and particularly when there has been breakdown of resistance and extensive bronchopneumonia, blood dissemination with *acute miliary tuberculosis* may occur, but this is much less common than in primary tuberculosis in young children.

Tuberculous ulcers may develop in the intestine from infection by bacilli in swallowed sputum (p. 633). *Tuberculosis of the larynx* (p. 437), likewise produced by direct infection from the sputum, is a serious complication.

Secondary amyloidosis is a common complication of chronic tuberculosis.

The effects of specific chemotherapy. The above account refers essentially to the disease unmodified by chemotherapy. The general changes produced in tuberculous lesions by a combination of drugs, usually rifampicin, ethambutol and isoniazid have been discussed on p. 214. In pulmonary tuberculosis, combined therapy is imperative in order to render the patient non-infective and to reduce quickly the risk of producing antiobiotic-resistant strains. If adequately carried out in the early stages of the apical lesion, chemotherapy leads to rapid healing with minimal fibrosis. In excavated lesions, the caseous lining disappears and is replaced by a layer of vascular granulation tissue which, in turn, is converted to a thin smooth fibrous layer, over which an epithelial lining may eventually grow, leaving a persistent cavity which may or may not communicate with a bronchus. The epithelial lining is rarely complete except in very small lesions. If small, fibrocaseous lesions may be almost completely absorbed; if larger, they may become hyalinised and acellular with a thin fibrous capsule. In favourable cases even actively caseating bronchopneumonia may cease to progress, the caseous material becoming liquefied and absorbed or discharged. The cavities become walled off by granulation tissue, which eventually becomes fibrosed and re-lined to some extent by epithelium. A notable feature is the lack of the dense fibrosis which characterises healing under natural conditions. Large open cavities

may become epithelialised and inactive, but since there is always a danger of subsequent aspergillosis, secondary pyogenic infection and re-activation, surgical removal is frequently performed. Patches of active disease may persist for long periods and tubercle bacilli may be isolated from such resected cavities despite long-continued chemotherapy, so that it is advisable to regard the disease process as arrested, rather than cured, by specific therapy. The naked-eye appearance of the treated lesions is an unreliable guide to the bacteriological state. Infection also commonly persists in lesions healing naturally, i.e. without chemotherapy.

Generalised miliary tuberculosis

The pulmonary lesions in this condition are part of an acute generalised tuberculosis, which occurs when a considerable number of mycobacteria gain entrance to the bloodstream. The ways by which this is brought about have already been considered (p. 212). In miliary tuberculosis, lesions are usually more numerous in the lungs than in any other organ. They consist of grey tubercles which may be too small to be visible by the naked eye or up to 3 mm in diameter (Fig. 16.31). Commonly, they are

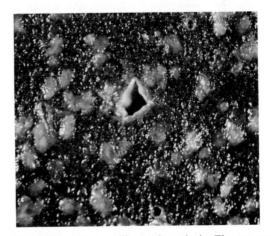

Fig. 16.31 Acute miliary tuberculosis. The cut surface of the lung shows numerous discrete grey tubercles. × 5.

more numerous and rather larger in the upper lobes than in the lower.

Microscopically the early tubercles are seen to be in the peribronchial connective tissue, fibrous septa, and in the alveolar walls but they enlarge by consolidation of the surrounding alveoli. Necrosis then occurs in the centre of the tubercle. In very acute cases the tubercle follicles are poorly formed and giant cells are virtually absent. In miliary tuberculosis there is no cavitation of the lesions, and *Myco. tuberculosis* is rarely found in the sputum.

The pleura in pulmonary tuberculosis

At a very early stage of localised lung disease, tubercles may form in the visceral pleura, and this may be followed by an extensive effusion into the affected pleural sac. Tuberculosis is a frequent cause of the apparently idiopathic pleurisy of young adults. The fluid is usually clear and the cells in it are scanty and mainly lymphocytes. A large proportion of desquamated serosal cells, as is seen in the centrifuged deposit of the serous transudate of cardiac failure, is quite exceptional in tuberculosis. In many cases tubercle bacilli cannot be found. Sometimes the exudate is serofibrinous and there may be some admixture of blood. The lesion usually resolves and the fluid is absorbed, leaving only scanty adhesions to mark its previous existence. In chronic tuberculous lung lesions there is fibrous thickening and adhesion of the overlying pleural layers, and in longstanding cases this may be pronounced. Owing to such adhesions, perforation of an underlying cavity into the pleural sac is uncommon. As mentioned on p. 477, pulmonary tuberculosis sometimes causes empyema, and secondary pyogenic infection cannot always be incriminated.

Sarcoidosis

Sarcoidosis is a systemic disease of unknown aetiology in which non-caseating epithelioid cell follicles are scattered throughout several organs. The general features of the condition are described on pp. 216–17.

The lungs are involved more frequently than any other organ. In Europe the commonest presentation of the disease is an abnormal routine chest radiograph. The four following patterns of radiological abnormality can be distinguished. (1) Hilar node enlargement with normal lung fields (38 per cent). (2) Hilar node enlargement with pulmonary infiltration (50 per cent). (3) Pulmonary infiltration without hilar node enlargement (7 per cent). (4) Pulmonary fibrosis with honeycomb lung (5 per cent).

In most cases the patients have no physical disability and the radiological changes regress within two to three years. About 13 per cent of patients develop chronic progressive pulmonary sarcoidosis, which is frequently associated with crippling dyspnoea, respiratory failure and pulmonary hypertension. Right ventricular failure may also ensue. About half the patients with chronic progressive pulmonary sarcoidosis die within ten to fifteen years of the disease being recognised.

Pathological examination of the lungs at an early stage of the disease reveals typical non-caseating epithelioid cell granulomas in the alveolar walls and fibrous septa. These lesions usually heal with minimal fibrosis. If the disease becomes progressive with extensive involvement of the lung, an interstitial fibrosis develops which leads eventually to honeycomb change (p. 484): in this late stage, no trace of the original sarcoid granulomas can usually be found.

Syphilis

Pulmonary syphilis occurs in congenital and acquired forms, both of which are extremely rare in most medically advanced countries. The majority of infants with *congenital* pulmonary syphilitic lesions are stillborn. The lungs are enlarged, pale and firm due to diffuse fibrosis of the alveolar septa and peribronchial and perivascular tissue. The interstitial fibrous tissue is diffusely infiltrated by lymphocytes and plasma cells and contains abundant *Treponema pallidum*. In *acquired* syphilis, gummas may rarely develop in the lung.

Actinomycosis and nocardiosis

Actinomycosis is caused by *Actinomyces israelii* (p. 221) which produces a chronic granulomatous reaction with pus formation. About 20 per cent of actinomycotic infections involve the lungs and thorax. Pulmonary actinomycosis may be primary or secondary, the latter usually resulting from the spread of disease from below the diaphragm, particularly from the liver. About 75 per cent of pulmonary cases are primary and the disease commonly occurs in the lower lobes, where it forms a dense fibrotic lesion honeycombed with small abscess cavities. The pus contains 'sulphur granules' which are colonies of *Actinomyces israelii.*

Nocardia asteroides is an aerobic, branching filamentous organism similar in some respects to *Actinomyces israelii.* The lungs are involved in about 60 per cent of cases of nocardiosis. The incidence of infection appears to be increasing, and to be associated with diseases or therapy that impair the patient's immune mechanisms. At necropsy the lungs show a suppurative pneumonia that may be lobular in distribution. The organism does not form colonies, but occurs as branching filaments which are not stained with haematoxylin and eosin. It is Gram +ve and appears black using the silver methenamine stain.

Fungal infections

Most pulmonary fungal infections are *opportunistic*, arising as a result of breakdown in cellular and humoral defence mechanisms (p. 169), and from the sustained use of antibiotics, which may so alter the normal human bacterial flora that fungi which are normally non-pathogenic may grow and invade the tissues. Until recent years, many of the pulmonary fungal diseases (mycoses) were little known and constituted an unimportant group of conditions. However, *since the introduction of the therapeutic immunosuppressive agents and antibiotics, the importance of fungal diseases has changed dramatically.*

The pulmonary mycoses usually encountered in Britain are aspergillosis, candidiasis and cryptococcosis, but increasing foreign travel has also brought occasional cases of histoplasmosis (p. 224), coccidiomycosis and blastomycosis from overseas.

Aspergillosis. This is the commonest pulmonary mycosis in the British Isles and it is usually due to infection by *Aspergillus fumigatus.* The hyphae are 3–4 μm in diameter, show frequent transverse septa, and exhibit dichotomous branching at acute angles (Fig. 16.32). It may give rise to four types of lung disease in man. Firstly, atopic subjects may develop reaginic antibodies to antigenic constituents of *Aspergillus*, and as a result suffer from attacks of **bronchial asthma** following heavy exposure to the spores. Secondly, some patients develop precipitating antibodies, and on further exposure to the spores may have attacks of **extrinsic allergic alveolitis** (p. 494). Thirdly, *Aspergillus* can colonise tuberculous or bronchiectatic cavities in the lung producing a rounded mass of

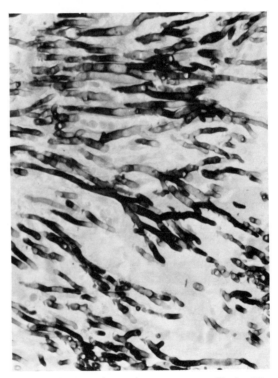

Fig. 16.32 Invasive pulmonary aspergillosis. The hyphae of *Aspergillus fumigatus* show frequent transverse septa and exhibit dichotomous branching at acute angles. From a patient who received cytotoxic therapy for Hodgkin's disease. Methenamine silver stain. × 375.

fungus (**mycetoma**) with a characteristic radiographic appearance. The chest radiograph shows an opaque spherical mass which almost completely fills the cavity, leaving a crescentic 'halo' of air between the mycelial mass and the cavity wall. Fourthly, in immunosuppressed patients, and in patients with Hodgkin's disease or leukaemia, aspergillus infection may produce nodules of **haemorrhagic consolidation and necrosis** scattered throughout the lungs. Such consolidated areas contain ramifying hyphae of *Aspergillus fumigatus* which may invade pulmonary arteries and veins leading to thrombosis and metastatic foci in other organs.

Candidiasis. *Candida albicans* (p. 223) is a normal commensal in the pharynx, where it can give rise to the lesion of **thrush**. Bronchopulmonary infection with *Candida* is rare, occurring as a result of severe underlying disease, immunological deficiency, or because of long-term treatment with antibiotic or corticosteroid drugs. Sometimes the trachea and bronchi are lined by a mass of fungus and sections show hyphae growing down through the mucosa. The lungs may show pneumonic consolidation with areas of necrosis and infiltration by neutrophil polymorphs.

Cryptococcosis (torulosis). *Cryptococcus neoformans* (p. 224) tends to cause disease in patients whose resistance to infection is diminished by leukaemia, Hodgkin's disease or by systemic corticosteroid therapy. Although rare, the incidence of infection is increasing. The most usual presentation is a meningoencephalitis, but respiratory tract infection can occur with the production of an atypical pneumonia. At necropsy, the lungs contain firm rubbery areas of consolidation which are devoid of necrosis but show a mucoid cut surface.

Pulmonary fibrosis

Pulmonary fibrosis is a result or complication of many of the diseases described in this chapter. Localised fibrosis, for example, may result from organisation of acute pneumonias, from tuberculosis and from inhalation of silica. More diffuse fibrosis may result from chronic interstitial oedema and haemorrhage secondary to pulmonary hypertension complicating mitral stenosis or chronic left ventricular failure. Chronic diffuse pulmonary fibrosis may be caused by inhalation of toxic dusts or fumes, certain connective tissue diseases, ionising radiation, sarcoidosis and as an adverse reaction to certain drugs.

We shall consider first the cells lining the alveolar walls and their role in the development of pulmonary fibrosis.

Alveolar lining cells (pneumocytes)

The alveolar walls consist of a meshwork of capillaries covered in the main by the ultrathin cytoplasmic extensions of **membranous (type I) pneumocytes**. These extensions have a large area but possess few organelles so that they are probably metabolically dependent upon the central perinuclear portion of the cells which lie in the corners and angles of alveoli. This may explain why membranous pneumocytes are vulnerable to a variety of injuries. They appear to be involved in one of two ways in pathological processes. Firstly they may be destroyed by toxic substances such as paraquat. This herbicide will cause membranous pneumocytes to develop a grossly cystic, oedematous cytoplasm which bulges into the alveolar space. Secondly, they may show intracytoplasmic pinocytotic vesicles due to haemodynamic disturbances in the lung, e.g. in mitral stenosis or high-altitude pulmonary oedema.

In striking contrast to the relatively quiescent membranous pneumocytes are the **granular (type II) pneumocytes**, which undergo pronounced hyperplasia and shedding into the alveolar spaces in various conditions. They are interposed between the flat membranous pneumocytes and unlike them do not have flat cytoplasmic extensions. The basal portion of the cell is attached to the underlying basement membrane of the blood–air barrier while the free convex surface of the cell projects into the alveolar space (Fig. 16.33). This free, curved surface of the granular pneumocyte is covered by microvilli which are short, straight and fairly regular. Within the abundant cytoplasm are prominent lamellar bodies which are thought to be the source of pulmonary surfactant (Fig. 16.33). Granular pneumocytes have a much greater capacity for division and a shorter turnover time than membranous pneumocytes and prob-

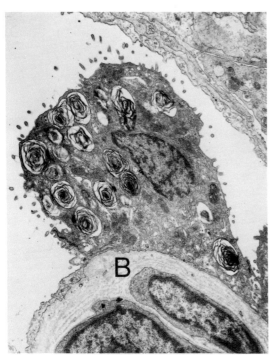

Fig. 16.33 Granular pneumocyte. The cell rests on the basement membrane (B) and projects into the alveolar space. Its surface is covered by microvilli and within its cytoplasm are lamellar bodies, considered by many to be the source of pulmonary surfactant. Electron micrograph. × 7500.

ably represent the reserve cells of the alveolar lining epithelium. They proliferate and replace membranous pneumocytes when the latter are destroyed. Thus, hyperplasia of granular pneumocytes can occur in a wide variety of circumstances and appears to be a basic mechanism of repair. Hyperplasia of granular pneumocytes assumes importance in the primary cellular and desquamative stage of fibrosing alveolitis, which subsequently proceeds to the mural stage of interstitial pulmonary fibrosis. This is considered in greater detail below.

Brush cells are common in the bronchial tree and may be demonstrated elegantly by scanning electron microscopy. They also occur rarely in the alveolar walls, where they are sometimes called **type III pneumocytes**. They are shaped like a truncated pyramid, the base being situated on the basement membrane and the tip protruding above the surrounding epithelial surface. Their most striking feature is the large regular microvilli which clothe their relatively small free surface. These thick microvilli contain fine filaments which extend down into the cell body to the basement membrane. The fine structural features of the alveolar brush cell are similar to those of the chemoreceptor cell in taste buds.

Diffuse fibrosing alveolitis

This term describes a group of diseases characterised by inflammatory changes in the lung parenchyma beyond the terminal bronchioles, with two main histological features.

1. Cellular fibrous thickening of the alveolar walls.

2. Proliferation in the alveolar spaces of large cells, the nature of which is discussed below.

The relative predominance of each of these two features varies from case to case but a study of lung biopsy specimens has revealed that there appears to be an inverse relationship between the degree of alveolar wall fibrosis and the number of proliferated intra-alveolar cells. Thus there is a histological spectrum ranging between a *desquamative pattern* with masses of large cells filling the alveolar spaces, accompanied by only scanty alveolar wall fibrosis (Fig. 16.34), and a *mural pattern* characterised by pronounced fibrous thickening of the alveolar walls combined with only occasional cells in the alveolar spaces (Fig. 16.35). The condition **desquamative interstitial pneumonia** is now believed by most workers to be identical to the cellular desquamative phase of diffuse fibrosing alveolitis. Electron microscopy has revealed that the proliferated alveolar cells consist mainly of granular (type II) pneumocytes and macrophages. The histological pattern observed at lung biopsy seems to be unrelated to the duration of the clinical symptoms. The prognosis of desquamative interstitial pneumonia is better than for the mural pattern and the response to steroids is better because desquamative interstitial pneumonia is cellular and occurs *before* the onset of fibrosis.

Diffuse fibrosing alveolitis may be associated with several types of extrapulmonary disease. Thus about one eighth of cases also have rheumatoid arthritis. Some patients with progressive systemic sclerosis develop an indolent fibrosing alveolitis of mural pattern. The prolonged administration of busulphan, hexamethonium, bleomycin or high concentrations of

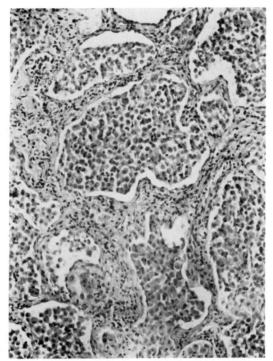

Fig. 16.34 'Desquamative interstitial pneumonia', regarded by most as an early cellular stage of fibrosing alveolitis. The alveolar spaces are filled with a mixture of macrophages and granular pneumocytes. There is only slight fibrous thickening of the alveolar walls. × 130. (From a section kindly donated by Professor D. B. Brewer.)

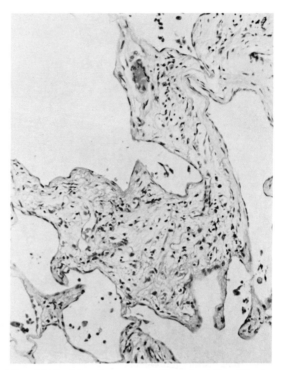

Fig. 16.35 Mural stage of fibrosing alveolitis in which the alveolar walls are greatly thickened by fibrous tissue. There are no cells in the alveolar spaces. × 130.

oxygen may induce a fibrosing alveolitis. The inhalation of cadmium fumes and excessive exposure of the lungs to ionising radiation are among other cases of this condition. However, in more than half the cases conforming to the description of diffuse fibrosing alveolitis, no cause can be found and these are commonly called *cryptogenic fibrosing alveolitis.*

Cryptogenic fibrosing alveolitis. This condition, which used to be known as *idiopathic diffuse interstitial pulmonary fibrosis* or the *Hamman-Rich syndrome,* is an uncommon disease that affects both sexes equally, usually after middle age, although it occasionally occurs in young people. In most cases, the cause of death is right ventricular failure or respiratory failure precipitated by a superimposed respiratory tract infection. There is an increased tendency to develop bronchial carcinoma.

The aetiology of cryptogenic fibrosing alveolitis is, by definition, unknown. About one third of patients have antinuclear antibodies in the serum and about one third have rheumatoid factor, although only a few have both. The titres are usually low. These serum changes and the association of fibrosing alveolitis with connective tissue diseases like rheumatoid arthritis and progressive systemic sclerosis led to speculation that the pulmonary lesions have an autoimmune basis. It has been suggested that the lung disease may depend on the combination of circulating auto-antibodies and an external provoking agent, such as inhaled dust particles, or viral or bacterial infection. Since some drugs may induce fibrosing alveolitis, the possibility must be borne in mind that ingested substances, as yet unidentified, may be concerned in the causation of some cases at present classified as cryptogenic.

Honeycomb lung

Honeycomb lung describes the naked-eye appearance of an acquired condition in which a large number of small cystic spaces develop in fibrotic lungs. Honeycomb lung is the non-specific final end-stage of many disease processes of diverse aetiology including asbestosis, beryllium and cadmium intoxication, extrinsic allergic alveolitis, cryptogenic diffuse fibrosing alveolitis, sarcoidosis, rheumatoid disease, progressive systemic sclerosis and Hand-Schüller-Christian disease. The cysts are up to 1 or 2 cm in diameter, have smooth grey-white walls, and the surrounding lung is pale, firm and fibrous. The cystic change is usually most pronounced in the sub-pleural regions on the anterior borders of the upper and lower lobes (Fig. 16.36). The presence of cysts beneath the visceral pleura gives the external surface of the lungs a nodular appearance which simulates that of the liver in macronodular cirrhosis. The essential change in honeycomb lung is obliteration by fibrosis or granuloma of some of the bronchioles and alveolar spaces with compensatory dilatation of unaffected neighbouring bronchioles. Thus the cysts are lined by columnar or

cuboidal epithelium which may be ciliated or mucin-secreting. The interstitial and pericystic tissue is composed of young fibroblasts and collagen infiltrated by scanty lymphocytes, plasma cells and macrophages. There may be an interstitial hyperplasia of smooth muscle cells probably derived from obliterated bronchioles and pulmonary blood vessels. Right ventricular hypertrophy is present in more than half the cases at necropsy. Pulmonary hypertension in honeycomb lung is attributed to a combination of chronic hypoxia, fibrous obliteration of the pulmonary vascular bed, and the development of bronchopulmonary anastomoses.

The causes of impaired gas exchange in pulmonary fibrosis are discussed in the section on respiratory failure on p. 447.

The effects of drugs and toxic compounds on the lung

A wide range of drugs and toxic compounds may give rise to clinical signs and symptoms which may resemble those of naturally occurring disease. Thus bronchial asthma may result from hypersensitivity to a wide variety of drugs, including aspirin. Some drugs, herbal substances and poisons, however, may give rise to other organic diseases in the lungs and we shall consider a few of them now.

Paraquat. This is the widely used weed-killer, 1,1-dimethyl-4, 4-bipyridylium chloride. When ingested, it may produce ulceration of the mouth within two days. Acute renal failure may result from tubular epithelial injury, but renal function usually returns, sometimes with the help of haemodialysis. The most serious effect of paraquat, however, is on the lung. Within hours of ingestion there is an initial destructive effect on the alveolar epithelium. The membranous pneumocytes become swollen and vacuolated and project into the alveolar spaces. The granular pneumocytes also show vacuolation of their lamellar bodies and disruption of their endoplasmic reticulum. Two days after administration of paraquat, many alveolar walls are denuded of their epithelial lining and there is commonly pulmonary oedema and the formation of hyaline membranes. This destructive phase is followed by a proliferative phase.

Three days after a single injection of paraquat into rats, mononuclear cells are found in

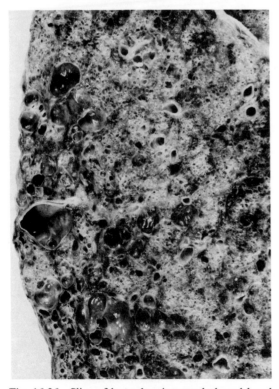

Fig. 16.36 Slice of lung showing a subpleural band of honeycomb change brought about by dilatation of terminal bronchioles. The condition is quite distinct from pulmonary emphysema.

the alveolar spaces. They resemble macrophages, but mature into fibroblasts (Fig. 16.37) and accordingly may be termed profibroblasts. They form collagen in the alveolar spaces and thus paraquat produces intra-alveolar rather than interstitial fibrosis. There may be some associated dilatation of respiratory bronchioles. Paraquat appears to kill plants by entering the chloroplasts and then taking part in an oxidation-reduction cycle in which hydrogen peroxide is liberated. A similar type of catalytic activity may occur in animal tissue, in which a small concentration of paraquat can lead to the synthesis of a high concentration of toxic by-products.

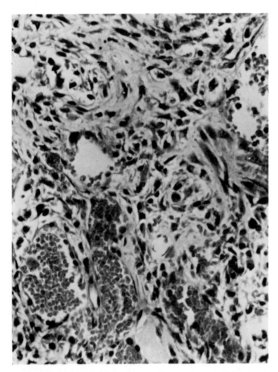

Fig. 16.37 Lung of a rat ten days after an intraperitoneal injection of paraquat. The lung architecture is obliterated by a dense mass of fibroblasts and small quantities of collagen. × 330.

Busulphan. This drug is widely used in the treatment of chronic myeloid leukaemia. In a minority of patients heavy and prolonged dosage of the drug may induce interstitial pulmonary fibrosis which impairs oxygen diffusion and causes dyspnoea. Chest radiographs show peri-hilar infiltrates and subsequently diffuse mottling throughout both lungs. Lung function tests often show considerable impairment of oxygen diffusion. A striking proliferation of granular pneumocytes, many of which disintegrate to produce intra-alveolar debris, precedes the fibrosis of the alveolar walls. Electron microscopy confirms that the desquamated alveolar cells are granular pneumocytes with characteristic lamellar bodies which break down to form phospholipid myelin figures and lattices (Fig. 16.38). Busulphan is, however, a valuable drug in the palliation of chronic myeloid leukaemia and there is no case for withholding its use because of this possible complication. Pulmonary fibrosis may also occur as a result of administration of bleomycin, salazopyrin, hexamethonium and methotrexate.

Pyrrolizidine alkaloids and anorexigens. Addition of the seeds or foliage of certain plant species of *Crotalaria* or *Senecio* to the diet of

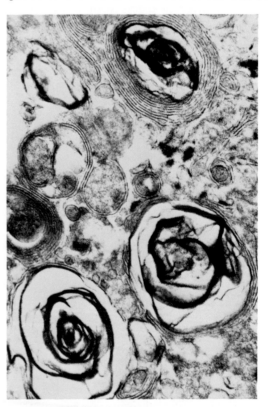

Fig. 16.38 Electron micrograph of intra-alveolar debris from a case of busulphan lung occurring in a man of sixty one years who received a prolonged course of the drug for chronic myeloid leukaemia. The apparently amorphous debris is seen to consist of lamellar bodies and myelin figures. × 28 000.

rats causes pulmonary hypertension and associated vascular disease of the lungs, with death from right ventricular failure in one to two months. The plants in question are *Crotalaria spectabilis*, a cover crop grown in the United States, *Crotalaria fulva*, used to prepare bush-tea in Jamaica and a cause of veno-occlusive disease of the liver, and *Senecio jacobaea*, the common 'ragwort' of British hedgerows. The effects of these plants are due to the pyrrolizidine alkaloids they contain.

A recent epidemic of primary pulmonary hypertension in Germany, Switzerland and Austria has been ascribed to the anorexigen, aminorex fumarate. There is as yet no proof of the association, as hypertensive pulmonary vascular disease has not been produced in laboratory animals fed on the drug. Administration to rats of chlorphentermine hydrochloride, an anorexigen formerly available in Britain, induces the accumulation of numerous prominent foamy macrophages in the alveolar spaces after prolonged dosage, this pulmonary histiocytosis does not progress to interstitial fibrosis but ends in disintegration of the cells to produce a picture mimicking alveolar proteinosis. The alveoli become packed with lamellar bodies and phospholipid lattices.

Pulmonary oxygen toxicity. One of the commonest therapeutic agents used in intensive treatment units is oxygen. The prolonged use of high concentrations of inspired oxygen can cause lung damage which may be irreversible and is potentially fatal. There is controversy as to the concentration of oxygen and the length of administration necessary to produce lung injury. Examples of pulmonary damage have been described in patients who breathed 40 per cent oxygen at atmospheric pressure for several days. There are conflicting views on the possible protective effect of pre-existing cyanosis with hypoxia on the lungs of patients receiving oxygen. The initial damage in pulmonary oxygen poisoning seems to be an increased permeability, followed by disintegration, of capillary endothelial cells and alveolar epithelium. The alveoli become filled with oedema fluid, fibrinous exudate and extravasated blood. Hyaline membranes line the alveolar walls. If the patient survives, there may be replacement of the intra-alveolar exudate by fibroblastic tissue which becomes incorporated into the alveolar walls. The thickened alveolar walls become lined by proliferated granular pneumocytes. It is of interest to note that some of the changes induced in the lung by oxygen toxicity are similar to those produced by the weed-killer, paraquat.

Pneumoconiosis and industrial lung diseases

Pneumoconiosis is a comprehensive term covering a group of lung diseases resulting from the inhalation of dust. This group of conditions grows continuously as fresh industrial hazards are created. The type of lung disease varies according to the nature of the inhaled dust. Some dusts are apparently inert and cause little or no damage, whereas others may cause widespread lung destruction and fibrosis. Certain dusts are antigenic and cause damage through immunological reactions, while others may predispose to tuberculosis or to neoplasia. The factors which determine the extent of damage caused by an inhaled dust include its physical state, its chemical composition, its concentration, the duration of exposure, and the co-existence of other lung diseases.

The size of the inhaled dust particles is of great importance as it is this factor which largely determines whether particles will reach the alveoli and whether they will adhere to the alveolar wall. Particle size is also important in determining whether dust will penetrate the thin alveolar epithelium or remain within the alveolar lumen. Practically all inhaled non-filamentous particles of more than 10 μm diameter are trapped in the nasopharynx, trachea and major bronchi, from where they are swept upwards, entangled in mucus, by the action of cilia. Many inhaled particles of 5 μm diameter or less gain access to the alveolar spaces, where they tend to collect in the lower halves of the upper lobes, the upper halves of the lower lobes, and the right middle lobe.

When particles measuring from 0·5 to 5 μm reach the alveolar walls, they adhere to the surface film of fluid and within minutes are ingested by macrophages. Ultra-fine particles, less than 0·02 μm in diameter, rapidly penetrate the alveolar epithelium. Coarse filamentous particles 30–60 μm in length, such as asbestos fibres, can reach the alveoli, but they tend to slip down and lodge in the bronchi and the resulting lesions are found mainly in the lower lobes of the lungs.

The pneumoconioses may be classified according to whether the dusts inhaled are inorganic or organic.

Mineral dusts

The principal varieties are anthracosis, coal worker's pneumoconiosis, silicosis and asbestosis.

Anthracosis

This is a pneumoconiosis caused by the inhalation of atmospheric soot particles: it is found in some degree in all adults, and is more marked in those who live in the highly polluted atmosphere of industrial areas. Most of the inhaled carbon particles are dealt with by the normal mechanisms for ridding the lungs of dust (p. 176) and are expectorated, but some are engulfed by macrophages and retained within the relatively immobile alveoli adjacent to bronchioles, blood vessels, fibrous septa, beneath the pleura and at the edges of lung scars. Some soot particles reach the lymphatic channels of the lung and are carried to the hilar lymph nodes. Thus anthracosis is the innocuous, well-known blackening seen in virtually every adult lung at necropsy.

Coal-workers' pneumoconiosis

This condition is due to the inhalation of coal dust and occurs in persons who handle soft bituminous coal with a low silica content, either in mines or by shovelling it in large quantities, as in the holds of ships. It occurs in two forms or stages: **simple coal worker's pneumoconiosis** in which the lungs become impregnated with dust, leading to a minor degree of fibrosis and causing few if any symptoms; and **progressive massive fibrosis (complicated pneumoconiosis)** which develops in a small proportion of patients with simple pneumoconiosis.

Simple coal workers' pneumoconiosis. This is due to the inhalation of coal dust particles measuring less than 5 μm in diameter. Silicosis is not involved. The inhaled dust is fairly evenly distributed within the lungs but maximal changes occur in the upper two thirds of each lung. The particles are ingested by macrophages which are then carried to the alveolar spaces surrounding the respiratory bronchioles. These dust-laden macrophages tend to be retained and adhere to the relatively immobile walls of the peribronchiolar alveoli in the centres of the lobules. Thus the respiratory bronchioles become surrounded by a sleeve of alveoli which are consolidated due to the accumulation of dust-laden phagocytes. The phagocytes eventually die and a network of fine collagen fibres develops in between the liberated dust particles; the aggregates also become covered by alveolar epithelial cells and thus incorporated into the alveolar walls. The upper two thirds of an affected lung contain numerous black, firm, spidery nodules and streaks measuring a few millimetres in diameter which produce a radiographic appearance known as **dust reticulation.** After several years there is fibrous obliteration of the peribronchiolar alveoli and atrophy of bronchiolar smooth muscle. The collagenous tissue then shrinks but the lung as a whole is not reduced in size, because the respiratory bronchioles dilate to produce **focal dust emphysema**, characterised by abnormal clusters of dust-blackened centrilobular air spaces (Figs. 16.39, 16.21, p. 463).

Simple pneumoconiosis may be seen in the chest radiographs of coal workers who are free from symptoms. It appears to have no adverse effect on pulmonary function and does not significantly alter life expectancy. Coincidental chronic bronchitis in such patients may, however, cause great concern in men who are aware that their chest radiograph is abnormal.

Progressive massive fibrosis. After ten to twenty years at the coal face a small proportion of workers with simple pneumoconiosis may develop massive confluent areas of fibrosis in one or both upper lobes, which may ultimately involve an entire lobe. Irregular masses of jet-black rubbery fibrous tissue with well-defined margins are present in the affected lobe, which is commonly adherent to the chest wall (Fig. 16.40). Sometimes the fibrous tissue contains cavities filled with black fluid resembling India ink. These cavities result either from tuberculous infection or ischaemic necrosis consequent

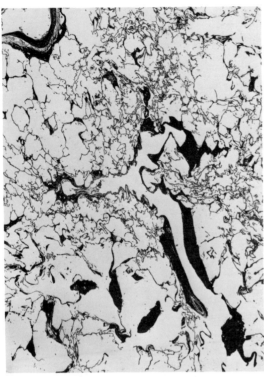

Fig. 16.39 Simple coal-workers' pneumoconiosis with focal dust emphysema, showing localisation of dust accumulation in the walls of the second order of respiratory bronchioles. × 7.

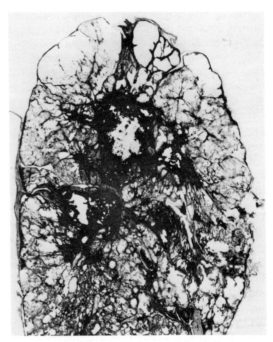

Fig. 16.40 Thick section of the lung of a coalminer, showing very severe emphysema and two foci of progressive massive fibrosis, seen as solid black areas with, in this instance, central cavitation. × 0.5.

upon fibrous obliteration of branches of the pulmonary artery in the affected lobe. Histological examination shows that the fibrous lesions are composed almost entirely of dense collagenous tissue arranged in bundles. Between the bundles are collections of coal dust and scattered lymphocytes. There has been considerable debate about the nature of progressive massive fibrosis and the factors which promote its development in a small proportion of cases of simple pneumoconiosis. Concomitant silicosis does not appear to be a factor. Careful examination of the lungs at necropsy, including culture and guinea-pig inoculation, yields evidence of tuberculous infection in about 40 per cent of cases, and many people accept that concomitant tuberculosis leads to the development of massive fibrosis in workers with simple pneumoconiosis. Progressive massive fibrosis is a serious and incapacitating disease. It may develop after exposure to coal dust has ended, and nothing can be done to halt its course once it is established; eventually death results from

respiratory failure, tuberculosis or right ventricular failure secondary to pulmonary hypertension. The pulmonary hypertension is probably due to a combination of chronic hypoxia and fibrous obliteration of a significant proportion of the pulmonary vascular bed.

Caplan's syndrome (rheumatoid pneumoconiosis)

This is characterised by rounded nodules, up to 5 cm in diameter, scattered fairly evenly throughout the lungs of workers who are exposed to inhaled dusts, including coal dust, silica and asbestos. *Rheumatoid arthritis* is usually present but occasionally the nodules develop several years before the arthritic manifestations. Rheumatoid factor is present in the blood. Cavitation and calcification of the nodules is common and clinically they may be mistaken for tuberculosis, bronchial carcinoma and secondary carcinoma. Not all patients with rheumatoid disease and pneumoconiosis develop Caplan's syndrome. The central parts of the nodules show concentric black and pale yellow rings, the pale zones frequently being liquefied. Histologically, the lesions are modified rheumatoid nodules with a central zone of dust-laden fibrinoid necrosis, separated by a cleft from an outer layer of palisaded fibroblasts and mononuclear cells.

Silicosis

The changes of silicosis are seen in the lungs of workers who inhale fine particles of silica (SiO_2) for many years. Silica and silicosis have a world-wide distribution. Wherever rock is cut, as in granite, sandstone and slate quarries or in the mining of coal, gold, tin or copper, silica dust is likely to fill the air. In the case of coal, it is the hard anthracite variety which is accompanied by significant quantities of silica. Other workers also face the hazard, particularly stonemasons, sandblasters, boiler scalers and those involved in glass and pottery manufacture. Inhaled particles of less than 5 μm in diameter are liable to cause silicosis: they reach the alveoli, where they are phagocytosed by macrophages which tend to congregate in the relatively immobile alveolar spaces adjacent to respiratory bronchioles, blood vessels, fibrous interlobular septa, and beneath the pleura. The characteristic lesions therefore develop in these sites. Silica induces production of relatively acellular collagenous fibrous tissue which is often hyaline and arranged in a concentric laminated fashion (Fig. 16.41). These silicotic nodules measure up to 5 mm in diameter and are pathognomonic of the disease. The fine silica particles are birefringent and are readily detected within the fibrous nodules on examination by polarising microscopy. The fibrosis obliterates the lumen of bronchioles and pulmonary blood vessels. As nodules increase in size beneath the pleura, adhesions form and in advanced cases the pleural cavity may be obliterated. At necropsy the pleura is thickened and adherent and the lungs feel gritty on cutting and palpation due to the presence of innumerable discrete fibrous nodules. Some of these may coalesce to form large confluent masses of fibrous tissue. In a severe case the lungs may be largely solid. The silicotic nodules are well circumscribed and greyish-black in colour. Silica dust is carried to the hilar lymph nodes, which become enlarged, fibrous and nodular.

The cause of lung fibrosis in silicosis is un-

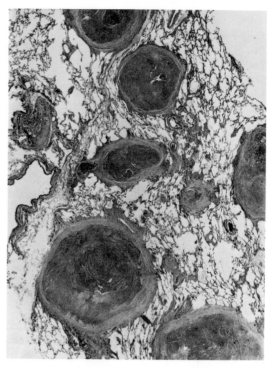

Fig. 16.41 Silicosis. The lung contains multiple nodules consisting of laminated fibrous tissue. There is no inflammatory cellular infiltrate. × 7.

certain. The solubility theory postulated that silica particles slowly dissolve to form silicic acid, which in turn stimulates fibrogenesis: this has become unacceptable because there is no relation between the severity of fibrosis and the solubility of different forms of silica. Two alternative but unproven biological theories are that silica is antigenic and provokes fibrosis through an immunological mechanism, and that collagen formation is stimulated by the release of lysosomal enzymes by macrophages which have ingested silica particles (p. 68).

Silicosis leads to progressive respiratory impairment, although twenty years exposure may have occurred before symptoms appear. Death may be due to *respiratory failure*. Progressive fibrous obliteration of the pulmonary vasculature, together with chronic hypoxia, may induce *pulmonary hypertension* with the development of right ventricular hypertrophy and eventual failure. There appears to be a synergism between silica and tuberculosis and the reported incidence of *tuberculosis* in patients with silicosis varies between 10 and 75 per cent. Tuberculosis tends to progress rapidly in silicotic patients and may terminate in tuberculous bronchopneumonia and miliary tuberculosis. It may also lead to the development of progressive massive fibrosis.

The effects of asbestos

Asbestos is a general term embracing a number of complicated fibrous silicates of magnesium of differing chemical composition and morphology. It is imported into Britain mainly from mines in South Africa and Canada. The three types of asbestos which are most important commercially are *chrysotile* (white asbestos), *crocidolite* (blue asbestos) and *amosite* (brown asbestos) which is rich in iron. Chrysotile consists of soft, curly pliable fibres which tend to split progressively into finer fibrils. Amosite and crocidolite fibres are in general rigid and harsh even when fine. The physical properties of the fibres determine the industrial use of various types of asbestos, and to some extent the depth to which they travel along the airways during inspiration and thus perhaps their differing pathological effects. The behaviour of inhaled particles is determined by their aerodynamic properties as well as their size. Chrysotile fibres are apparently more likely to be retained higher up the small airways, particularly at bifurcations, while the rigid fibres of crocidolite and amosite travel readily in the airstream and so reach the periphery of the lung. It has been suggested that these properties may explain why chrysotile has rarely been associated with pleural mesothelioma (see below) though often with asbestosis. All forms of asbestos are fire-resistant and are good acoustic and thermal insulators. Chrysotile can be spun into yarn and incorporated into textiles. Crocidolite and amosite are noted for their resistance to acids and alkalis. Large amounts of asbestos (mostly chrysotile) are used in asbestos-cement products for corrugated roofing, pipes, gutters, chimneys and tiles. Chrysotile is also used in the manufacture of floor tiles, brake linings, clutch facings, plastics, paint, and in asbestos-paper products including engine gaskets, roofing felts and wall coverings. Both crocidolite and chrysotile have been used for pipe and boiler lagging and as a spray with synthetic resins for thermal and acoustic insulation of buildings and ships.

Occupational exposure to asbestos occurs to a small extent in miners who obtain the mineral but is potentially high in the crushing and extraction processes which follow. Bagging of the fibre used to be a dusty process and before the introduction of modern methods and leak-proof bags, dockers and warehouse personnel were exposed to hazard. The asbestos textile and insulation industries have produced the highest incidence of asbestosis. There is little risk associated with cutting, sawing and trimming asbestos-cement products because the fibres are trapped within the cement matrix. In Britain, rigorous standards came into force in May 1970. The most stringent rules apply to crocidolite because of its association with mesothelioma; the use of this fibre has latterly been discouraged and much reduced in many countries.

Exposure to asbestos dust may be associated with the development of the following lesions: **pleural fibrous plaques, asbestosis** and **mesothelioma of the pleura or peritoneum**. Mesothelioma is considered on p. 501.

Pleural fibrous plaques. These are distinct from the fibrous thickening of the visceral pleura which accompanies asbestosis, in that they are located in the parietal pleura on the postero-lateral aspects of the lower chest wall, mainly over the ribs, and on the diaphragm. They are bilateral, well-circumscribed, irregularly-shaped white raised patches of hyaline fibrosis. The surface may be nodular, or smooth and polished resembling articular cartilage. Histologically the plaques consist of hyaline acellular collagenous lamellae. Extensive foci of calcification may be present. Asbestos bodies (see below) are not found in the plaques but may be detected in the lungs. Calcified parietal pleural plaques may be visible in chest radiographs but they do not produce symptoms and are free from complications. At present there is no evidence that pleural plaque formation is a precursor of malignant mesothelioma.

Asbestosis. This term means fibrosis of the lungs due to inhaled asbestos dust (Fig. 16.42). It is specific and excludes pleural fibrous plaques and mesothelioma. Chrysotile, crocidolite and amosite are all capable of producing pulmonary fibrosis, though of differing degrees of severity, probably due to differences in their penetration and retention in the lungs as a result of their aerodynamic and physical properties. The most important factors in the

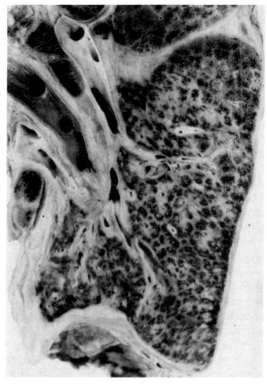

Fig. 16.42 Pulmonary asbestosis showing pronounced fibrosis and shrinkage of the lower lobe and gross pleural thickening. × ¾.

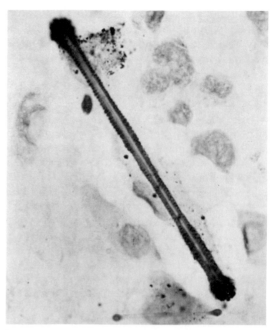

Fig. 16.43 An asbestos body in the lung. The needle-like asbestos fibre is enclosed in a crenellated protein-deposit with club-shaped ends. The body is partly enveloped by two macrophages (which also contain dust pigment), and a smaller asbestos body (below) is almost completely engulfed within a macrophage. × 900.

development of asbestosis are the concentration of dust to which an individual is exposed and the duration of exposure. Heavy exposure for a few years and exposure to fairly low concentrations over many years are equally likely to result in asbestosis. As will be seen later, this contrasts with the exposure levels associated with the development of malignant mesothelioma. The chief symptom of asbestosis is dyspnoea on effort and this usually takes more than ten years to develop. Occasionally the onset of symptoms may be delayed up to even forty years after exposure.

Inhaled asbestos fibres (50 μm long and 0·5 μm in diameter) are mostly retained in the respiratory bronchioles of the lower lobes. In time a number of them pass into the alveolar ducts and spaces. Experimental evidence suggests that short fibres or fragments less than 10 μm long are engulfed by macrophages, whereas larger fibres cannot be properly ingested but become surrounded by macrophages. In time, the asbestos fibres become coated with endoge-

nous iron and protein to produce the characteristic **asbestos body** (Fig. 16.43). When well formed, these are long (50 μm), golden-yellow or brown structures consisting of an asbestos fibre coated with layers of iron-containing protein which gives the prussian blue reaction for ferric iron (p. 281). The proteinaceous coat is usually segmented along the length of the fibre and bulbous at its ends, producing a 'dumbbell' or 'drumstick' appearance. It should be emphasised that *the finding of asbestos bodies in the sputum or lung is only an indication of past exposure to asbestos and is* not *proof of the presence of disease due to asbestos.* Asbestos bodies have been found at necropsy in the lungs of 20 to 60 per cent of otherwise normal urban dwellers with no known industrial exposure to asbestos. There is a tendency for these bodies to fragment. The mechanism by which asbestos causes pulmonary fibrosis is not understood. It has been suggested that, like silica (see above), asbestos stimulates macrophages to secrete fibrogenic lysosomal enzymes. Immunological factors may play a part: this is suggested by the finding of a high prevalence of circulating anti-nuclear antibody (25 per cent) and rheumatoid factor (23 per cent) in cases of asbestosis. Fibrosis is first evident around respiratory bronchioles and then spreads to involve alveolar ducts, atria and alveolar walls. There is progressive obliteration of alveolar spaces with compensatory dilatation of unaffected bronchioles which may progress to honeycomb lung. Asbestos bodies are found free in alveolar spaces and also enmeshed in fibrous tissue. The disease commences in the sub-pleural region of the lower lobes and then progresses inwards and upwards so that eventually the middle lobe and lower parts of the upper lobes may be affected.

Patients with asbestosis may develop *respiratory failure* and also secondary *pulmonary hypertension*, which may in turn lead to right ventricular hypertrophy and failure. Asbestosis does not predispose to pulmonary tuberculosis.

Asbestosis is the only form of pneumoconiosis with a high risk of **bronchial carcinoma**. Approximately half of British male asbestos workers with asbestosis die of bronchial carcinoma, which arises in the vicinity of the fibrosis and is, therefore, most commonly found in the lower lobe. The neoplasm may be of any cell type but it is usually an adenocarcinoma. There is no evidence that an excess of bronchial carcinoma is related to asbestos exposure in the absence of asbestosis.

Other inorganic dust diseases

Pulmonary siderosis. This occurs in silver polishers (who use rouge containing iron oxide), arc-welders and haematite miners. Iron oxide itself appears to be almost innocuous, and does not cause fibrosis or chest symptoms, but frequently in the case of haematite miners a quantity of silica accompanies it. The result is a modified silicosis. The haematite lung is rusty brown and may be extensively fibrosed. Macroscopically, free haematite pigment is brownish-yellow and does not give a prussian blue reaction: after ingestion by macrophages, however, it reacts positively.

Berylliosis. This affects workers who extract beryllium from ores or who handle it in industry, as in the making of alloys. Heavy concentrations of dust produce an acute chemical pneumonitis. Less intense but prolonged exposure, such as formerly occurred in the fluorescent lighting industry, induces a chronic granulomatous reaction histologically similar to sarcoidosis, sometimes with similar lesions in the liver and other organs. The pulmonary lesions progress to generalised fibrosis and sometimes honeycomb lung.

Cadmium fumes, in high concentration, cause an acute pneumonitis with hyaline membranes and a proliferation of alveolar cells. This condition may progress to pulmonary fibrosis and honeycomb lung. Pulmonary emphysema has been described in the lungs of workers chronically exposed to cadmium fumes. The risk from cadmium arises during the manufacture of alloys for use in the electrical industry and nuclear reactors, and in the cutting of scrap metal by welders.

Aluminium is a rare cause of pulmonary fibrosis among workers in the fireworks industry.

Tin causes a simple pneumoconiosis (stannosis) without fibrosis or functional disability.

Other metals encountered in industry may be very harmful and, when inhaled as fine dust or fumes, may cause an acute chemical pneumonitis. These include manganese, osmium, vanadium and zinc.

Biological dusts

Inhaled organic dusts may affect the bronchi, as in the case of byssinosis, or may produce an *extrinsic allergic alveolitis*.

Byssinosis. This is an occupational disease of the cotton, flax and hemp industries. The illness comes on after many years of exposure. The early stage presents as the syndrome of 'Monday fever': following the weekend break, the worker returns to the dusty atmosphere and after a few hours develops a characteristic tightness of the chest with a cough productive of scanty sputum. The symptoms persist during the day but regress for the remainder of the week. As time goes by, the symptoms persist for longer and finally progress to permanent dyspnoea with cough and sputum, and there may be severe disability. Respiratory failure, pulmonary hypertension and right ventricular failure occur in the late stages of the disease. The disease is thought to be due to broncho-constriction induced by cotton dust or associated bacteria from the cotton bales. In most

Table 16.3 Examples of extrinsic allergic alveolitis

Disease	Occupation	Dust Exposure	Circulating Precipitating Antibodies Against
Farmer's lung	Dairy farmers, cattle breeders	Mouldy hay	Thermophilic actinomycetes, usually *Micropolyspora faeni*
Bagassosis	Manufacture of paper and cardboard from sugar-cane bagasse	Mouldy sugar-cane bagasse	Thermophilic actinomycetes, usually *Micropolyspora faeni*
Mushroom worker's lung	Cultivation of mushrooms	Mushroom compost dust	Mushroom spores and/or *Micropolyspora faeni*
Maple-bark stripper's disease	Maple-bark stripping	Mouldy maple bark	*Cryptostroma corticale*
Suberosis	Cork workers	Mouldy oak-bark and cork dust	Mouldy cork dust
Malt worker's lung	Distillery or brewery workers	Mouldy barley, malt dust	*Aspergillus fumigatus*
Bird fancier's lung	Pigeon breeders, parrot and budgerigar fanciers, chicken farmers	Pigeon, parrot, budgerigar and hen droppings	Serum proteins and droppings
Pituitary snuff-taker's lung	Patients with diabetes insipidus	Porcine and bovine pituitary powder	Serum proteins and pituitary antigens

cases the pathological changes are those of chronic bronchitis, but very rarely pulmonary fibrosis has been reported around inhaled cotton fibre particles.

Extrinsic allergic alveolitis. In addition to their causal role in asthma, inhaled organic dusts can induce in the alveoli an Arthus (type III) reaction (p. 153) in which circulating precipitating antibodies react with inhaled antigen. The clinical syndromes produced by this latter reaction are known collectively as *extrinsic allergic alveolitis*. Their symptoms and pathological manifestations are similar but their origins diverse. The individual diseases are generally recognised by names descriptive of their occupational or antigenic origin (Table 16.3). The inhaled organic material may be antigenic moulds, bird droppings, fungus in dead wood or heterogeneic pituitary powder. The clinical features consist of acute episodes of fever, headache and malaise with cough, dyspnoea and basal pulmonary crepitations, arising four or five hours after exposure to dust and persisting for twenty four hours. There is seldom opportunity to examine the lung tissue during the acute stage of the Arthus reaction, with polymorphonuclear infiltration, acute exudation, etc. Subsequently, the alveolar walls are thickened by an infiltrate of lymphocytes, plasma cells and mononuclear cells and by sarcoid-like granulomas. Repeated exposure, as commonly occurs with bird fanciers, is associated with chronic ill health, weight loss, etc, rather than acute episodes, and leads to the development of a diffuse interstitial fibrosis which may progress to honeycomb lung. Of all the forms of extrinsic allergic alveolitis so far known, the most acute and severe is **farmer's lung** (which also occurs in cows). However, new sources of environmental contamination are constantly being found, and consequently new types of the disease emerge every year.

The Pleura

Pleural effusions

The passage of fluid in and out of capillaries is mainly dependent upon a balance between the colloid osmotic pressure exerted by the plasma proteins and the hydrostatic pressure within the capillary lumen (p. 49). In the systemic circulation the averages of these two forces in capillaries and venules are normally approximately equal. In the pulmonary circulation, however, the intracapillary hydrostatic pressure is only about one-third of that in the systemic capillaries, so that it is normally exceeded by the colloid osmotic pressure. The pleural surface is an interface between the pulmonary and systemic circulations. There is a pressure gradient from the interstitial tissue beneath the parietal pleura to the pulmonary interstitial tissue beneath the visceral pleura, producing a net absorptive force of about 13 mm Hg into the visceral pleura.

Causes. Pleural effusions can be caused by diseases which interfere with the mechanisms that maintain the normal balance of entry and removal of water, electrolytes and protein into and out of the pleural cavity. The following are the more important causes.

Increased intracapillary pressure may cause a pleural effusion in patients with either left or right ventricular heart failure or an increased blood volume.

Increased capillary permeability is responsible for effusions complicating pleural inflammation which may be due to pneumonia, pulmonary tuberculosis, pulmonary infarction, connective tissue diseases, bronchial carcinoma, mesothelioma, subphrenic abscess and acute pancreatitis.

Hypoproteinaemia may cause pleural effusions in patients with the nephrotic syndrome or cirrhosis of the liver.

Impaired lymphatic drainage of the lung may occur in lymphangitic carcinomatosis and in neoplasms involving the hilum of the lung.

As with oedema fluid in general, pleural effusions may be rich in plasma proteins when they are due to increased capillary permeability, i.e. **inflammatory exudates**, or of low protein content when due to haemodynamic or osmotic disturbances or lymphatic obstruction, i.e. **transudates**. As elsewhere, inflammatory exudates may be serous, serofibrinous, purulent or haemorrhagic. A haemorrhagic exudate should always raise the suspicion of tuberculosis, neoplastic infiltration or pulmonary infarction.

Empyema or pyothorax is a collection of purulent exudate or pus in a pleural cavity. It may be due to infection of the pleura from the lung or occasionally from penetrating injuries of the chest wall. Less commonly infection of the pleura may arise from the bloodstream or

through the diaphragm from abdominal disease such as a subphrenic abscess. In lung abscess, bronchiectasis and bronchial cancer, infection of the lung may extend into the pleural cavity and cause empyema. A post-pneumonic lung abscess may discharge both into a bronchus and into the pleural cavity, resulting in a **bronchopleural fistula** and **pyopneumothorax**. Empyema may also result from perforation of the oesophagus and mediastinitis, and may arise as a complication of thoracic surgery. A large empyema compresses the lung, which becomes collapsed against the side of the vertebral column: a layer of granulation tissue then forms on the pleural surfaces and matures to dense fibrous tissue. This is followed by fibrosis in the collapsed lung. These changes prevent the proper expansion of the lung and hence *it is of great importance that pus in the pleural cavity should be evacuated without undue delay*. If the empyema is small, its contents may be absorbed or changed into inspissated material. Great pleural thickening, sometimes followed by calcification, is apt to occur.

Haemothorax is a collection of blood in a pleural cavity. It may be due to trauma to the chest wall and lung, or result from rupture of an aortic aneurysm. The pleural cavity may be distended with fluid and clotted blood, with associated compression-collapse of the lung on that side.

Chylothorax is the accumulation of an opalescent creamy fluid in the pleural cavity due to obstruction of, or injury to, the thoracic duct. Obstruction is commonly due to pressure exerted by enlarged mediastinal lymph nodes, while trauma may be accidental or a complication of thoracic surgery. The fluid is an emulsion of fat globules which may separate into an upper fatty layer on standing. It is odourless and alkaline, can be cleared by adding fat solvents, and stained with dyes such as Sudan III.

Pleural fibrosis

This condition, often with pleural adhesions, and sometimes with obliteration of the cavity, may follow acute pleurisy, or may be the result of chronic pulmonary lesions such as silicosis and tuberculosis, as already described. The presence of some pleural adhesions is common after middle adult life. Hyaline fibrous plaques may develop on the diaphragmatic and posterior costal portions of the parietal pleura in people exposed to asbestos.

Pneumothorax

Pneumothorax is the presence of air in a pleural cavity. It causes the lung on that side to collapse to an extent depending on the volume of air admitted. Pneumothorax may be therapeutic or traumatic, or it may arise spontaneously due to the escape of air from the lung through a hole in the visceral pleura. Traumatic pneumothorax may be due to a penetrating injury of the chest wall or it may occur accidentally during the withdrawal of pleural fluid.

Primary spontaneous pneumothorax occurs in the absence of any clinical evidence of underlying disease, most commonly in young males between the ages of twenty and forty years. In some cases it is recurrent and rarely bilateral. Occasionally thoracotomy has revealed a tear in the visceral pleura at the site of attachment of a fibrous adhesion. The association of spontaneous pneumothorax with the Ehlers-Danlos syndrome and Marfan's syndrome (p. 387) is attributed to the rupture of gas-filled cystic spaces beneath the visceral pleura, formed as a result of the inherited defect of connective tissue.

Secondary spontaneous pneumothorax occurs in patients who have evidence of underlying lung disease—most commonly emphysema or active pulmonary tuberculosis. Other causes include sarcoidosis, honeycomb lung, pneumoconiosis, bronchial asthma, lung abscess, bronchiectasis and bronchial carcinoma.

Once rupture of the lung surface has occurred, air continues to escape into the pleural cavity until the pressure gradient reaches zero or until the aperture is sealed by collapsing lung tissue. Occasionally, a valve-like mechanism occurs so that air enters the pleural cavity during inspiration but cannot escape during expiration: the pressure within the affected pleural cavity then steadily increases to produce a **tension pneumothorax** leading to mediastinal shift and compression also of the opposite lung. In uncomplicated cases, air in the pleural cavity is gradually absorbed, a 50 per cent pneumothorax taking about six weeks to re-expand fully. Possible complications include pleural effusion, haemorrhage and infection.

Tumours of the Bronchi, Lungs and Pleura

Benign tumours

The so-called *chondroma* or *adenochondroma* of the lung forms an ovoid, largely cartilaginous mass. It usually presents as a chance finding on radiological examination as a discrete rounded shadow which requires surgical intervention to exclude a bronchial carcinoma. These tumours consist entirely of mature cartilage with clefts lined by flattened or respiratory type epithelium and with collections of adipose and fibrous tissue (Fig. 16.44). They are best regarded as hamartomas. The so-called *bronchial adenomas* are described in the following section on malignant tumours.

Fibromas and lipomas occur in the lung but they are very rare.

Malignant tumours

Bronchial carcinoma

This is the commonest primary tumour of the lung. At the turn of the century it was seen infrequently but since that time it has become a major health problem in most parts of the world. The reports of the Registrar-General for England and Wales show a rise in the number of deaths registered as due to cancer of the lung from 6500 in 1944 to over 30 000 in 1969. Bronchial carcinoma is considerably commoner in men than women. Like other carcinomas, the incidence increases with age, but it is now not exceptional for it to cause the death of young men in their thirties.

Aetiology. There is now little doubt that the most important factor in this dramatic rise in the incidence of bronchial carcinoma is the habit of **smoking, particularly cigarettes**. There is good statistical evidence that the risk increases proportionately to the consumption of cigarettes and inversely to the length of the cigarette stub left. The smoking of cigars appears to be safer and the smoking of pipes safer

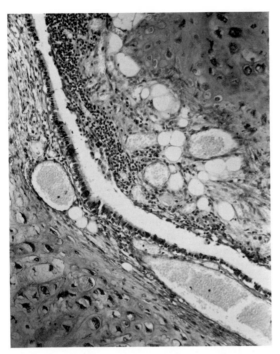

Fig. 16.44 Section of a cartilaginous hamartoma ('adenochondroma') of lung. This field shows an epithelial-lined space with cartilage on either side, some adipose tissue and blood vessels × 50.

still, although here the risk of carcinoma of the tongue is apparently increased. In spite of reports from the World Health Organisation and the Royal College of Physicians on the relationship between cigarette smoking and bronchial carcinoma, this lethal habit still maintains a grip on modern society. The risks have been clearly indicated by retrospective statistical studies and confirmed in a prospective study of the causes of death of medical practitioners. In this country, the habitual smoking of twenty-five cigarettes or more a day has been shown to be associated with a 12 per cent risk of dying from bronchial carcinoma. *In ex-cigarette smokers the risk gradually diminishes and after ten years of abstinence it is not much greater than in non-smokers.* The mode of action of cigarette smoke is uncertain. There is about 1 μg of 3:4 benzpyrene in the smoke of 100 cigarettes. This is not much (see below) and it is by no means certain that benzpyrene is the only carcinogen involved; it may be more important that the tar from cigarette smoke has been found to be a powerful co-carcinogen. Accordingly, the relationship of bronchial carcinoma

with smoking may represent the summation of the effects of a number of different substances, including carcinogens and co-carcinogens.

Another important source of smoke, apart from tobacco, is **atmospheric pollution**. Statistical evidence shows that bronchial carcinoma is commoner in towns than in rural districts and that its incidence is closely correlated with the degree of atmospheric pollution. It is commonest in large towns with an atmosphere heavily polluted by industrial and domestic smoke and by the fumes from internal combustion engines. The carcinogenic agents liberated in the combustion of coal include benzpyrene and arsenic and the concentration of the former in the air of large towns, up to 5 μg per 100 cubic metres of air, is such that under normal weather conditions about 0·5 μg may be inhaled in twelve hours. The amount is greater in winter than in summer and may be increased almost tenfold in foggy weather.

There are much rarer but established causes of bronchial carcinoma. Thus workers in the chromate industry have an abnormally high death rate from bronchial carcinoma. Other industrial workers at risk are those engaged in nickel refining, workers with asbestos and haematite miners. A much quoted example of industrial lung cancer, now of little practical importance, is that of the workers in the Schneeberg cobalt mines in Saxony. It is almost certain that radioactive substances were concerned. In these miners, as in cigarette smokers, the tumours were largely of oat-cell and squamous type (see below).

Naked-eye appearances. Bronchial carcinoma presents a variety of appearances depending upon the site of origin, the extent of local spread, and the degree of bronchial obstruction produced.

Hilar type. Usually the tumour forms a mass surrounding the main bronchus to the lung or to one lobe (Fig. 16.45). The bronchial mucosa may be ulcerated or may be merely roughened and nodular. Lymphatic spread often produces further nodules in the mucosa towards the bifurcation of the trachea. The carcinoma narrows the lumen of the affected bronchus, causing obstruction. Retention of secretions then occurs and is followed by infection with consequent bronchopneumonia and abscess formation. The tumour soon spreads by the lymphatics, giving rise to massive metastases in the

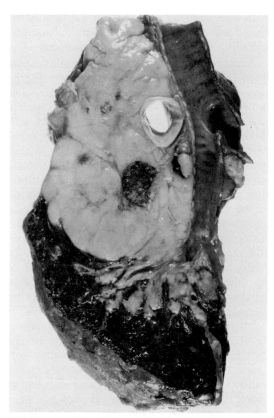

Fig. 16.45 Bronchial carcinoma. The main mass of tumour is at the hilum and has compressed and displaced the lung tissue. An enlarged lymph node, showing dust pigmentation and white flecks of tumour, lies within the mass. The major bronchi and pulmonary vessels are extensively infiltrated by tumour and appear thickened. The point of origin cannot be determined at this stage.

mediastinal nodes, which are often enveloped in the tumour mass and cannot easily be distinguished. Extension upwards into the lymph nodes of the neck is often seen. Retrograde spread also occurs along the peribronchial and perivascular lymphatics so that even the smaller bronchi and vessels may be ensheathed by whitish collars of tumour. Permeation of lymphatics just beneath the visceral pleura produces a delicate white lacework pattern, visible on the external surface of the lung ('*lymphangitis carcinomatosis*'). Invasion of the pericardial sac occurs by direct extension along the lymphatics around the walls of the pulmonary veins and the carcinoma may compress and occlude the superior vena cava, causing marked cyanosis. Infiltration of the heart is sometimes obvious on gross examination, and on careful

histological examination of necropsy material it is found to be frequent.

Peripheral type. Less frequently the tumour originates from a peripheral bronchus and sometimes apparently arises in such a small bronchus that the exact site of origin is uncertain. Some workers claim to recognise a form arising in the pulmonary alveoli. However, the histological appearances are deceptive and both carcinomas of unequivocally bronchial origin and metastatic tumours may use the alveolar walls as a convenient stroma and thus simulate an alveolar origin. Tumours behaving thus are usually, but not invariably, mucus-secreting adenocarcinomas and they may produce consolidation of large areas of the lung resembling pneumonia, the cut surface presenting a greyish, mucoid appearance. A variant of this neoplasm appears to arise in the respiratory bronchioles and may spread by way of the air passages producing a characteristic type of pulmonary invasion to which the name *pulmonary alveolar adenomatosis* has been applied (Fig. 16.46).

The spread of lung cancer. The early and

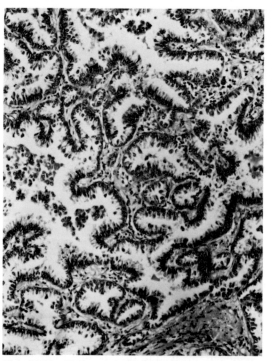

Fig. 16.46 Pulmonary adenomatosis. The alveolar walls are lined by tall columnar neoplastic cells. × 125. (From a section kindly loaned by Dr. F. Whitwell.)

widespread invasion of the lymphatics has been emphasised and this may involve the pleura, forming a thick ensheathment of the surfaces or taking the form of multiple discrete nodules. Pleurisy with effusion, often haemorrhagic in character, is common. When the tumour is at the apex of the lung, extension to the adjacent thoracic cage may involve the lower cords of the brachial plexus and the sympathetic chain, so that pain and sensory disturbances occur. This is the so-called *'Pancoast's syndrome'*. Owing to the peripheral situation of the lung cancer, symptoms and signs referable to the lung may appear only late in the disease.

Metastases. Metastases are widespread and may involve virtually any organ in the body. Spread may occur to the lymph nodes of the neck, axilla or groin, before the primary tumour presents localising signs. Ipsilateral spread to the adrenals is common and this favours the lymphatics rather than the blood-stream as the route of spread. The kidneys, with a much larger arterial supply, are less often involved by metastases. Ipsilateral spread also tends to predominate in the liver and kidneys.

There is a special tendency to the formation of secondary tumours in the brain, which may overshadow the primary bronchial tumour clinically. Surgical exploration for a cerebral neoplasm should always be preceded by a careful survey of the lungs to exclude primary bronchial carcinoma. Metastases in the bones are common, the thoracic vertebrae being especially frequently involved, possibly by the retrograde venous route. It should be kept in mind that *widespread metastasis may have occurred from a small and clinically silent bronchial carcinoma. Even at necropsy the primary tumour of lung may be very difficult to find.*

Associated clinical phenomena. Bronchial carcinoma is sometimes associated with neuropathy and myopathy mediated by humoral factors of the tumour. Cushing's syndrome with adrenal cortical hyperplasia is due to secretion of ACTH by the tumour, which is almost always of the oat cell type. Other rare systemic effects of bronchial carcinoma are the carcinoid syndrome, hypercalcaemia, hyponatraemia, encephalopathies, neuropathies, hypertrophic osteoarthropathy and gynaecomastia. Migrating phlebitis and gross lymphoedema may also occur and may cause the initial symptoms.

Histological types. There are four main his-tological types of bronchial carcinoma. They are the squamous cell carcinoma, oat cell carcinoma, adenocarcinoma and undifferentiated carcinoma. The structure may be mixed. Thus there may be gland-like structures in the oat cell type and some degree of squamous metaplasia in the adenocarcinoma. Squamous cell, oat cell, and undifferentiated carcinomas comprise over 90 per cent of bronchial cancers in countries where the incidence is high, and are the histological forms related to the smoking of cigarettes. Their increased frequency accounts for the striking male predominance of bronchial carcinoma.

Squamous cell carcinoma is the most common form of bronchial cancer (Fig. 16.47), and presents macroscopically as a dense whitish hilar mass, often with a flaky surface. It arises from bronchial epithelium which has undergone squamous metaplasia, areas of which are frequently seen in the bronchial mucosa of cigarette smokers and patients with chronic bronchitis.

Oat cell carcinoma. (Fig. 16.48) commonly arises near the hilum of the lung. The cells are

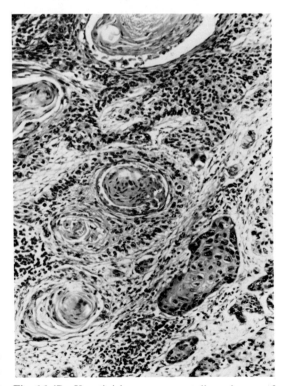

Fig. 16.47 Keratinising squamous cell carcinoma of bronchus with well-developed cell nests. × 130. (From a section kindly loaned by Dr. F. Whitwell.)

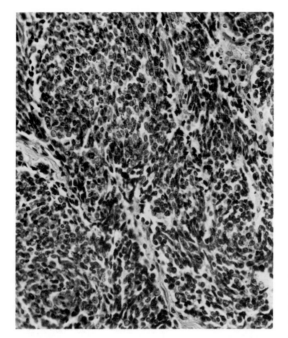

Fig. 16.48   Oat cell carcinoma of bronchus. This neoplasm is composed of small, uniform, darkly-staining ovoid cells, with scanty supporting stroma. × 115.

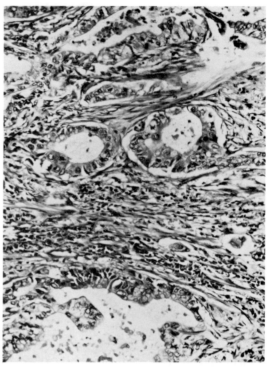

Fig. 16.49   Adenocarcinoma of bronchus. The neoplasm is composed of columnar cells which form acini situated in a dense fibrous stroma. × 130. (From a section kindly loaned by Dr. F. Whitwell.)

very short darkly-staining spindle cells and may appear oval or round, depending upon the plane of section. They are usually arranged in solid masses or anastomosing trabeculae. On electron microscopy the tumour cells are found to contain neurosecretory granules and it has been postulated that oat cell carcinomas are derived from argyrophilic cells ('apud' cells—p. 1034) in the bronchial mucosa. Perhaps this is why most endocrine syndromes caused by lung cancer are associated with the oat cell variety.

Adenocarcinoma. (Fig. 16.49) is the least common of the four main types and is composed of cubical or columnar cells which are usually mucus-secreting in places. Sometimes the tumour has a distinctly papillary structure or it may be more scirrhous. Adenocarcinomas account for 5–10 per cent of primary lung cancers and more than half arise in the more peripheral intrapulmonary sites. It is not possible to distinguish an adenocarcinoma from the other types merely by its site and naked-eye appearance. In striking contrast to the other types, adenocarcinoma occurs with equal frequency in the two sexes.

'Bronchial adenoma'

This term should mean a benign glandular tumour of bronchial epithelium. However, in practice it is used to designate a group of slowly growing malignant tumours which not uncommonly metastasise to regional lymph nodes and other organs such as the liver. A disturbing feature is that it is not possible to predict their prognosis on the basis of their histological appearance. 'Bronchial adenomas' form some 3 to 10 per cent of surgically excised tumours of the lung and they occur most commonly in people under the age of forty years and with equal frequency in the sexes. Macroscopically the tumour forms a 'dumb-bell' lesion, intraluminal growth being connected by a relatively narrow neck to invasive growth in the adjacent lung tissue. Endoscopic resection is therefore not practicable. The tumour sometimes causes haemoptysis and usually partial bronchial obstruction, with bronchiectasis beyond. Histologically, most 'bronchial adenomas' resemble the carcinoid tumours of the alimentary canal. They rarely show the argentaffin reaction but occasionally give rise to the carcinoid syndrome (p. 649) and excretion of 5-hydroxy-indole-acetic acid in the urine. On electron microscopy, they show characteristic intracytoplasmic secretory vesicles (Fig. 16.50). The remaining adenomas show a glandular histological pattern rather like tumours of the salivary glands: this suggests that they arise from the bronchial submucosal glands. These glandular variants are designated cribriform (adenoid cystic) and muco-epidermoid carcinomas.

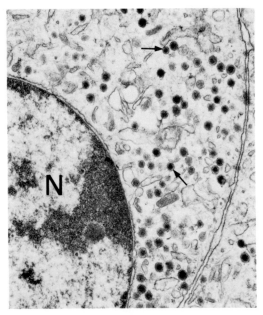

Fig. 16.50 Bronchial carcinoid tumour. Part of a neoplastic cell containing a nucleus (N) and numerous small electron-dense neurosecretory granules (arrows). × 18 750. (Dr. W. Taylor.)

Secondary tumours in the lung

The lung is the great filter of the bloodstream so it is not surprising that a wide variety of tumours may give rise to pulmonary metastases. Sarcomas of all types commonly metastasise to the lung by the bloodstream. Spread of carcinoma to the lungs is also common both by the lymphatics and by the bloodstream. **Spread by lymphatics** is common in *breast carcinoma*, the tumour cells of which may spread to the pleural lymphatics and thence to the lungs. *Abdominal carcinomas* may spread to hilar lymph nodes and thus extend into the lung (Fig. 12.22, p. 333). When the lymphatics

of the lung are involved, extensive cuffing of blood vessels and bronchi may result. *Malignant lymphomas* may involve the bronchial lymph nodes, primarily or secondarily, and show a tendency to extend along peribronchial lymphatics, forming an encasing sheath to the bronchi. Some **blood-borne metastases** may be very large. Such is the case with the 'cannon-ball' metastases which may originate from a renal carcinoma or from testicular tumours.

Pleural mesothelioma

Until recently this neoplasm was considered to be very rare. In 1960 a relation was noted between mesothelioma and occupational and environmental exposure to asbestos in South Africa. Since then the number of recorded pleural and peritoneal mesotheliomas has been steadily increasing in many countries. Only about 10 to 15 per cent of the cases recorded in Britain appear to be unrelated to asbestos. On the other hand the incidence of the tumour in people with industrial exposure to asbestos is very low. In cases of pleural mesothelioma, the duration of exposure to asbestos varies from as little as three months to sixty years. The degree of exposure is, however, likely to have been intense for at least part of the time. The latent period which elapses between exposure to asbestos and the development of mesothelioma is very long, usually more than twenty years and sometimes more than forty. Because of this long delay an increasing number of mesotheliomas can be expected to occur until well into the twenty-first century. The fibre type which has been most associated with mesothelioma is **crocidolite**. The source of exposure has usually been occupational but cases have occured in people exposed to air pollution in the vicinity of asbestos mines and factories. The tumour affects both the visceral and parietal layers of the pleura, leading to the formation of a layer of grey-white tissue 0·5 to 3 cm in thickness, which obliterates the pleural cavity, ensheaths and compresses the lung, and extends into the interlobar fissures. Areas of necrosis within the tumour give rise to large cystic spaces containing mucinous fluid. The histological picture presents a variable pattern with either carcinomatous or sarcomatous features or a mixture of the two. The carcinomatous pattern usually consists of tubular and papillary structures in a loose stroma. The sarcomatous pattern consists of spindle cells. Asbestos bodies are seen in the lungs but not in the mesothelioma tumour tissue. The neoplasm is thought to be derived from the mesothelial lining of the pleura. Metastasis to hilar and abdominal lymph nodes

is fairly common. A few years ago it was believed that distant metastasis did not occur: recent studies have, however, shown that secondary deposits can arise in the contralateral lung, liver, thyroid, adrenals, bone, skeletal muscle and brain.

Congenital anomalies

Unilateral agenesis of a lung does not in itself endanger life but other serious malformations often accompany it. Sometimes one lobe or an entire lung may be **hypoplastic**. It is not uncommon to find an excessive or diminished number of lobes in a lung and this rarely has an effect on pulmonary function. A **sequestered pulmonary segment** is one which is totally or partially separated from the normal lung. It is usually intralobar but an extralobar variety also occurs. Intralobar sequestration is observed in young adults in whom a large mass is found, usually in the lower lobe of the left lung. The sequestrated segment does not communicate with the bronchial tree and is supplied with blood from an artery which arises from the aorta above or below the diaphragm. In extralobar sequestration, which is usually encountered in infancy, the lesion is usually basal and on the left side either in the pleural cavity or within the substance of the diaphragm. It is covered by its own pleura and does not communicate with the bronchial tree. Its arterial blood supply is derived from the aorta and its veins drain into the azygos system. Rarely, a sequestration of either variety is served by a bronchus growing directly out of the oesophagus or gastric fundus.

Congenital cysts occur and may or may not communicate with the bronchial tree. In older children

and adults, congenital *pulmonary cysts* may be so altered by inflammation and fibrosis that distinction from acquired bronchiectasis and honey comb lung may be difficult. Cysts arising near the hilum of the lung may be bronchial or derived from the foregut. *Bronchial cysts* are lined by bronchial epithelium and their walls contain cartilage, smooth muscle and bronchial glands. Some bronchial cysts may arise near to or within the wall of the oesophagus. *Enterogenous cysts* derived from the foregut are lined by gastric or intestinal epithelium. Multiple small cysts in the periphery of the lung may be congenital anomalies of the distal bronchi or may be derivatives of the visceral pleura. Multiple lung cysts may be present in patients with Marfan's syndrome.

Congenital cystic adenomatoid malformation is a rare form of diffuse hamartoma usually found in the lungs of premature or stillborn infants. The lesion is generally confined to one lobe which is greatly enlarged to form a firm, white fibrous mass containing small cysts. There is commonly mediastinal displacement to the opposite side and compression of normal lung. Microscopically, the hamartoma consists of an intercommunicating mass of tubules and spaces resembling fetal bronchioles and alveoli. Mucous glands and cartilage may be present.

References

Blackmon, J. A., Hicklin, M. D. and Chandler, F. W. (1978). Legionnaires' disease. *Archives of Pathology and Laboratory Medicine* 102, 337–43.

Hurley, J. V. (1978). Current views on the mechanisms of pulmonary oedema. *Journal of Pathology* 125, 59–79.

Liebow, A. A. (1973). Pulmonary angiitis and granulo-

matosis. *American Review of Respiratory Disease* 108, 1–18.

Macfarlane, P. S. and Somerville, R. G. (1957). Non-tuberculous juvenile bronchiectasis: a virus disease? *Lancet* 1, 770–71.

Morrell, M. T. and Dunnill, M. S. (1968). The postmortem incidence of pulmonary embolism in a hospital population. *British Journal of Surgery* **55**, 347–52.

Morrissey, W. L., Gaensler, E. A., Carrington, C. B. and Turner, H. G. (1975). Chronic eosinophilic pneumonia. *Respiration* **32**, 453–68.

Smoking and Health. (1977). A Report of the Royal College of Physicians. p. 128. Pitman, London.

Smoking and its Effects on Health. (1975). Technical Report Series of the World Health Organization, No. 568, p. 100. Geneva.

Watt, J., Gregory, I. and Stell, P. M. (1975). An alcian blue-phloxine method for the gross demonstration of squamous metaplasia in the larynx. *Journal of Pathology* **116**, 31–6.

Further Reading

Cole, R. B. (1975). *Essentials of Respiratory Disease*, 2nd edn. pp. 297. Pitman Medical, London.

Harris, P. and Heath, D. (1977). *The Human Pulmonary Circulation*, 2nd edn. pp. 689. Churchill Livingstone, Edinburgh.

Heath, D. and Williams, D. R. (1977). *Man at high altitude*, pp. 292. Churchill Livingstone, Edinburgh.

Spencer, H. (1977). *Pathology of the Lung*, 3rd edn. pp. 1100. Pergamon Press, Oxford.

17

The Blood and Bone Marrow

Introduction

This chapter describes abnormalities of the red cells, leukocytes and platelets of the blood. All of these cellular elements (with the exception of most lymphocytes) are produced in the haemopoietic bone marrow, and very commonly changes in the blood reflect abnormalities of cell production in the bone marrow. It is also important to appreciate that, while the cells of the blood and their precursors are subject to their own, apparently intrinsic abnormalities, more often than not quantitative and qualitative abnormalities of the cells of the blood and marrow are the result of pathological changes elsewhere. An obvious example is the leukocytosis accompanying pyogenic infection, but the connection between the primary disease and the blood changes may sometimes be so obscure that the haematological abnormality may be mistakenly regarded as the primary pathology. Severe anaemia is, for instance, observed in some forms of renal failure, while the opposite condition, erythrocytosis, may result from chronic pulmonary or congenital heart disease (or, rarely, from a renal tumour or cyst).

Disorders of lymphocytes are considered mainly in the following chapter on the lymphoid tissues, and in Chapter 6, but lymphoid leukaemia is included with other forms of leukaemia in this chapter.

Development of the cells of the blood

Haemopoietic stem cells appear first in the embryonic yolk sac and subsequently in the primitive blood and fetal liver; in the adult, this stem cell population is maintained in the haemopoietic marrow, and from it the supply of red cells, granulocytes and platelets is provided by proliferation and differentiation. Some stem cells pass into the blood and supply the thymus,

where they differentiate into T lymphocytes. They also differentiate, probably in the marrow itself, into B lymphocytes. The haemopoietic stem cell (p. 118) is pluripotent and capable of differentiating into restricted precursors of red cells, platelets, granulocytes, monocytes and lymphocytes.

The evidence for this is based mainly on experimental work in which mice exposed to whole body x-irradiation sufficient to destroy their own haemopoietic cells are injected with small numbers of haemopoietic cells from a normal donor mouse. Some of the donor cells settle in the spleen and marrow and produce clones in the form of discrete colonies, each of which consists initially of cells which differentiate in one direction, i.e. towards production of red cells, granulocytes or platelets. If the cells obtained from a single colony (i.e. the descendants of one stem cell) are injected into a second irradiated mouse, colonies of all three types are formed from stem cells in the donor colony. These findings have been interpreted as indicating that the mouse haemopoietic stem cell is pluripotent and that the direction in which it differentiates is influenced by the micro-environment provided by the tissue in which it settles. The effect of the micro-environmental factors is to produce progenitor cells of restricted potential.

The existence of pluripotent stem cells in man is suggested by studies of chronic myeloid leukaemia (CML) in which the abnormal 22 (Philadelphia) chromosome, produced by a somatic mutation, is found not only in the leukaemic granulocytes but also in red cell, platelet and monocyte precursors (p. 544). Recently it has also been shown that, during the blast-cell crisis that may complicate CML, the predominant cell may be the precursor of both haemopoietic cells and T lymphocytes (Janossy *et al.*, 1976; p. 546), suggesting that the normal stem cell has equally wide potential. Normally, differentiation proceeds so rapidly that stem cells are scanty in marrow samples and cannot be identified morphologically, the great majority of the primitive cells present being recognisable as belonging to either the red or white cell series. Granulocytes have a much shorter life-span in the circulation than erythrocytes and their precursors outnumber erythroblasts in the marrow in a ratio of about 3 : 1.

Erythrocyte production. The developing erythrocyte passes through successive changes which involve (1) progressive diminution in cell size; (2) progressive reduction of nuclear size with condensation of the chromatin, culminating in pyknosis and ultimate disintegration or extrusion of the nuclear remnant; (3) progressive loss of the basophilic RNA of the cytoplasm and concurrent production of haemoglobin. This process of development must be

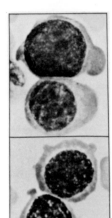

Early erythroblast with finely dispersed chromatin and basophil cytoplasm.

Pronormoblast: basophil cytoplasm, early condensation of nuclear chromatin.

Early normoblast with basophil cytoplasm and coarse well-marked condensation of the nuclear chromatin.

A slightly later normoblast with commencing haemoglobinisation.

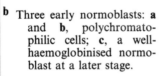

Three early normoblasts: **a** and **b**, polychromatophilic cells; **c**, a well-haemoglobinised normoblast at a later stage.

Late normoblast showing marked nuclear condensation.

Late normoblasts showing early pyknosis and more haemoglobinisation.

Late normoblasts—the lower showing complete pyknosis. The cytoplasm in a Leishman-stained film would still be polychromatophilic.

Fig. 17.1 Normoblast series. × 1000.

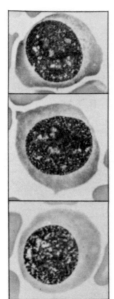

Early erythroblast: note the basophil cytoplasm and evenly dispersed nuclear chromatin containing several nucleoli.

Promegaloblast: nucleoli persist, nuclear chromatin shows commencing fine reticular condensation, cytoplasm basophilic. Note contrast to the coarse aggregation of nuclear chromatin in the normoblast series.

Early megaloblast: nuclear chromatin is finely reticulate, cytoplasm shows diminished basophilia and early haemoglobinisation.

Polychromatophilic megaloblast with haemoglobinisation in advance of nuclear maturation.

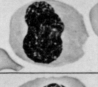

Later polychromatophilic megaloblast.

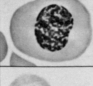

Late megaloblast with some nuclear condensation.

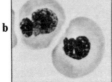

Two late megaloblasts, one showing nuclear pyknosis (**a**) and the other nuclear fragmentation (**b**).

Fig. 17.2 Megaloblast series. × 1000.

seen as a continuum, although it is convenient to define cells at various stages of maturation as in Fig. 17.1. Progressive differentiation and proliferation appear to be under the control of **erythropoietin**, a hormone derived from a plasma α_1-globulin by the action of *erythrogenin*, which is produced by the kidneys and possibly other organs. When erythropoietin production is acutely stimulated by hypoxia from any cause, including anaemia and haemorrhage, there is a resultant increase in red cell production. Normally, only late reticulocytes and mature erythrocytes appear in the peripheral blood, but in states of erythropoietin-induced increase in red-cell production, early reticulocytes and even normoblasts may enter the circulation.

The production of an abnormal series of red cell precursors—megaloblasts (Fig. 17.2)—is usually due to deficiency of either vitamin B$_{12}$ or folic acid, both of which are essential for normal haemopoiesis. Megaloblastic erythropoiesis is inefficient and anaemia (lowered haemoglobin concentration in the blood) results; the red cells also tend to be abnormally large. Pernicious anaemia and other megaloblastic anaemias are described later but this introduction to megaloblastic erythropoiesis is provided here because the disorder is referred to in several places before the main account on pp. 531–8.

After release from the marrow, the normal red cell survives for about 120 days; at the end of this time the cell is phagocytosed by macrophages, and haemoglobin release and breakdown occur (p. 278). About 1 per cent of the total red cells are destroyed and replaced each day as shown in Table 17.1.

Table 17.1 Circulating mass and turnover of red cells and iron compounds

	Circulating mass	Daily turnover
Red cells	2000 g	17 g
Haemoglobin	680 g	5·7 g
Porphyrin pigment	23 g	200 mg
Iron	2·3 g	19 mg

(Values for a normal 70 kg man)

Granulocyte production. The development of granulocytes in the bone marrow has been described on p. 185, in relation to leukocytosis.

Platelet production. Platelets are produced by mature megakaryocytes in the bone marrow (Fig. 17.3) and released into the blood. The

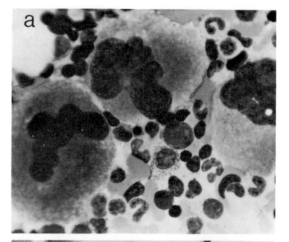
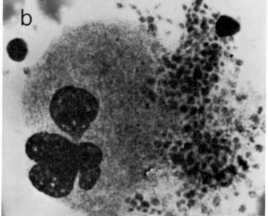
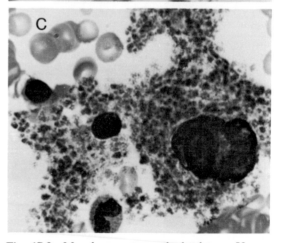

Fig. 17.3 Megakaryocytes and platelets. **a** Young megakaryocytes with commencing granulation. × 900. **b** More advanced cell showing partial conversion of the cytoplasm to platelets. × 600. **c** Mature megakaryocyte with platelet formation throughout the cytoplasm. × 600.

megakaryocyte arises from the haemopoietic stem cell by an unknown number of cell divisions, followed by repeated divisions of its nucleus in a common cytoplasm. Thereafter the cytoplasm differentiates into platelets. There is approximately one megakaryocyte per 500 nucleated red cells in the bone marrow. It is probable that platelet production is regulated by a humoral factor, rather as erythropoiesis is regulated by erythropoietin.

Extramedullary haemopoiesis. If the bone marrow has been replaced by tumour, fibrous transformation or osteosclerosis (pp. 553–4), or if there is gross hyperplasia of the haemopoietic tissue as in haemolytic anaemia, haemopoiesis may reappear in the primitive fetal sites, notably in the liver, lymph nodes and spleen, and may cause enlargement of these organs. Extramedullary haemopoiesis is often accompanied by the presence of primitive red and white cells in the peripheral blood **(leuko-erythroblastic reaction)** suggesting that in extramedullary sites there is imperfect control over the entry of immature cells into the circulation.

Physical features of blood

Blood volume. The volume of circulating blood in a normal adult male is about 5 litres and slightly lower values are found in women. There is a relationship between the blood volume and body weight, but a closer correlation is found with lean body mass. Blood volume can also be estimated from height^3/body weight. Centrifuging a column of venous blood in a glass tube shows that about 44 per cent by volume consists of cells (**packed cell volume** or **haematocrit value**), and the remaining 56 per cent of plasma; this gives a rough estimate of the proportion of cells to plasma in the blood as a whole. A rise in the haematocrit value will result either from an increase in red cell mass **(erythrocytosis)** or a decrease in plasma volume **(haemoconcentration)**. Conversely, a fall in the haematocrit value may result from a reduction in red cell mass **(anaemia)** or a rise in plasma volume **(haemodilution)**. Other haematological measurements dependent on concentration (e.g. red cell count, haemoglobin level) will vary in a similar way.

Specific gravity and viscosity of the blood are dependent largely on the concentration of red cells and the protein content of the plasma. Important increases in specific gravity and viscosity may thus occur in erythrocytosis and in conditions such as myeloma where there is a high concentration of globulin in the plasma; similar increases may be associated with very high leukocyte counts in leukaemia. This increased viscosity may slow the circulation and contribute to the thrombotic episodes sometimes found in these conditions.

Erythrocyte sedimentation rate. This is determined by placing the blood, to which anticoagulant has been added, in an upright calibrated tube and observing the rate of sedimentation of the red cells, as indicated by the length of the column of plasma after a given period of time. The range of normality depends on the details of technique, and is greater for women than men. Abnormal variations are chiefly in the direction of increased rapidity of sedimentation and are associated with increased concentrations of fibrinogen and various globulins in the plasma. The test has no specific value but has been found useful as an aid to detection of organic disease in the absence of physical signs, and notably as a prognostic aid in a particular condition, e.g. in tuberculosis or rheumatoid arthritis in which approximation of the rate to normal is taken as a favourable sign.

The Red Cell

Examination of the blood is essential in any disease affecting the haemopoietic tissues; this should include haemoglobin estimation, packed red cell volume and red cell count. From these may be derived the **absolute values** described below. Since the advent of automatic cell counters, the red cell count and also the mean red cell volume can be estimated directly, and calculation of the absolute values based on these measurements is now more dependable than formerly.

The haemoglobin concentration is usually expressed as gm/decilitre of blood (males 13·5–18·0; females 11·5–16·5) and **the red cell count** in millions per μl (4·5–6·6 depending on age and sex). **The packed red-cell volume** or

haematocrit represents the proportion by volume of whole blood occupied by the red cells and is expressed as a percentage (40–54 per cent in males and 35–47 per cent in females). Formerly it was measured by centrifugation of whole blood in a haematocrit tube: using automatic cell counters, it is derived from the product of the red-cell count and mean red cell volume.

The absolute values*

Mean corpuscular volume (MCV) (normal 76–96 femtolitres, average 86) is derived from the formula:

$$\frac{\text{volume of red cells in ml/l}}{\text{no. of red cells in millions per } \mu\text{l}}$$

As already mentioned, the MCV can now be measured directly in a cell counter.

Mean corpuscular haemoglobin (MCH) (normal 27–32 picograms/cell) is given by the formula:

$$\frac{\text{grams of Hb/dl} \times 10}{\text{no. of millions of red cells/}\mu\text{l}}$$

This indicates the average amount of haemoglobin per red cell.

Mean corpuscular haemoglobin concentration (MCHC) (normal 32–36 g/dl) relates to the degree of saturation of the red cells with haemoglobin and when lowered (hypochromia) suggests that inadequate formation of haemoglobin is a factor in the development of an anaemia. It is given by the formula:

$$\frac{\text{grams of Hb/dl} \times 100}{\text{packed cell volume}}$$

The main purpose in determining the absolute values is to classify states of **anaemia** (*usually defined clinically* as *a reduction in the haemoglobin level of the blood*) according to the average size of the red cells and their degree of haemoglobin saturation. The terms used in such classification depend upon the appearances of the red cells in a stained blood film and the three main groups are as follows:

Type of anaemia	Absolute values		
	MCV	MCHC	MCH
normochromic/normocytic	normal	normal	normal
hypochromic/microcytic	low	low	low
normochromic/macrocytic	high	normal	high

The absolute values are usually more reliable than the microscopic appearances of the red cells in the classification of anaemia, on which diagnosis and therapy usually depend. In particular, the term *hypochromia* arose from the pallor of haemoglobin-deficient red cells in a stained blood smear. However, such an appearance is now known to be due in many instances to small (*microcytic*) red cells (with a normal MCHC) rather than to a reduction in the haemoglobin concentration within the cells. Accordingly, the term has been over-used in the past.

Erythropoietin-induced erythrocytosis

Chronic hypoxia from any cause—chronic respiratory or heart failure, congenital heart disease, living at high altitudes, etc. (p. 226)—is likely to result in increased formation of erythropoietin and so in red cell production (p. 506). This may increase the red cell mass sufficiently to raise the red cell count above the normal range (*erythrocytosis*). The condition is sometimes termed *secondary polycythaemia*, a term which is inappropriate for it denotes increase also in granulocytes and platelets, as in *primary polycythaemia* (*polycythaemia vera* p. 552) which is a neoplastic-like condition of the haemopoietic tissue. Only the red cells are increased in erythrocytosis, and when due to hypoxia it can be regarded as a compensatory effect.

Rarely erythrocytosis results from increased formation of erythropoietin due to secretion of erythrogenin by certain tumours—most commonly renal carcinoma—or by cystic lesions or ischaemia of the kidney.

Morphological changes in red cells

Changes in size and shape. Anaemia is frequently associated with variations in erythrocyte size—**anisocytosis**—and irregularities in shape—**poikilocytosis**. Abnormally large red

---

* Haematological measurements are now expressed in Standard International (SI) Units in many countries. For convenience, both SI and traditional units are usually given in this text.

cells, termed **macrocytes** (see p. 506), are numerous in pernicious anaemia and some related anaemias; in air-dried blood films they may measure 10–12 μm in diameter. Although undersized cells are also usually present in pernicious anaemia, the *average size* of the red cells is usually greater than the normal, and the anaemia is thus termed **macrocytic**. Abnormally small red cells, or **microcytes**, occur in all forms of anaemia, but in certain types they preponderate so that the average size of the cells is diminished; the anaemia is then called **microcytic**.

Small poikilocytes may occur in any severe anaemia (Fig. 17.26, p. 532). While their presence is of no absolute diagnostic importance, they are usually prominent in pernicious anaemia and may appear even before the anaemia is pronounced. In certain disorders of -small blood vessels, e.g. micro-angiopathic haemolytic anaemia (Fig. 17.25, p. 531), triangular helmet-shaped or **burr cells** may be numerous in the circulation; these irregularly contracted cells result from mechanical damage in the abnormal vessels, and are frequently found along with obvious red cell fragments (**schistocytes**).

The term **spherocyte** is applied to red cells which have assumed a globular shape and so are reduced in diameter and appear densely stained. Characteristically spherocytosis is associated with red cell membrane abnormality and a reduced red cell life span. Other morphological changes are associated with genetic errors of haemoglobin structure, e.g. the sickle shape assumed by de-oxygenated cells containing Hb-S (p. 523) and the abnormally thin cells which sometimes have a central area of thickening (**target cells**) found in thalassaemia and other haemoglobinopathies. In *hereditary elliptocytosis* the majority of the erythrocytes are oval, but in most instances this is a harmless trait.

Variations in haemoglobin content. Reduction in the amount of circulating haemoglobin may be the result of diminution in the *numbers* of circulating red cells, in the *size* of the cells, their *concentration* of haemoglobin, or any combination of these. For example, in pernicious anaemia, reduction in the numbers of red cells is the cause of the anaemia; the increase in size of the individual cells does not compensate for this. By contrast, the anaemia of iron-de-

ficiency states is due initially to a reduction in cell size, and so in MCH, but a reduction in cell number and eventually in the MCHC also contribute to the anaemia. When the MCHC is greatly reduced, the cells in films show red staining only at the periphery, giving the so-called *ring-staining*, but there are so many artefacts that this feature is unreliable and should not be used as an indication of the haemoglobin content of the cells.

Polychromasia and reticulocytes. If a film of normal blood is stained with a Romanowsky stain, practically all the erythrocytes are purely eosinophilic. In certain conditions, however, in addition to the eosinophilia, a proportion of the erythrocytes show a slight bluish-violet tinge and the term **polychromasia** is applied to this double staining. These are young cells which have recently lost their nuclei but still retain enough ribosomal RNA to give a basophilic tinge to the otherwise eosinophilic haemoglobin-rich cytoplasm: hence the polychromasia. As the young cells mature in the circulation, the polychromasia gradually disappears and they become normochromic. The young erythrocytes tend also to be slightly larger than those which are older.

By supravital staining with certain dyes, cresyl blue being most frequently used, any RNA remaining in the erythrocytes is precipitated or condensed within the cells as a sharply-stained skein or reticulum, and such young cells are called **reticulocytes** (Fig. 17.4). They are normally present in a proportion of less than 1 per cent in males, but may rise to 2 per cent in females after menstrual loss. The total number of reticulocytes should not normally exceed $100 \times 10^9/l$ ($100\,000/\mu l$).

Polychromatic cells and reticulocytes appear in the blood in increased numbers when erythropoiesis in the marrow is stimulated, as after haemorrhage, in haemolytic states and during response to specific therapy in a deficiency anaemia, e.g. after injection of vitamin B_{12} in pernicious anaemia or iron therapy in iron-deficiency anaemia.

Red cell inclusions. Various inclusions may occur in erythrocytes; some are vestiges of cell elements usually lost during maturation, while others are due to pathological changes in the cells. A normal function of the spleen is to remove such inclusions from the erythrocytes without destroying the cells themselves; this is

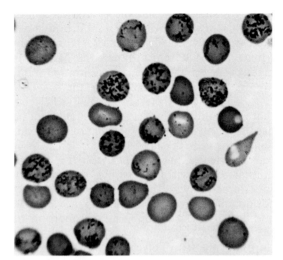

Fig. 17.4 Blood smear in haemolytic anaemia, showing numerous reticulocytes containing various amounts of reticulum. Supravital staining with cresyl blue. × 1100.

achieved in the red pulp and is known as the 'pitting' function of the spleen. If the spleen has been removed, is atrophied or is congenitally absent, cells with such inclusions may be present in large numbers in the circulation without necessarily indicating any blood disorder.

Pappenheimer bodies are small, deeply basophilic granules, usually solitary and less than 1 μm in diameter, which give a positive prussian blue reaction for ferric iron. Red cells containing them appear most abundantly in the blood of adults after splenectomy, but are present in some erythroblasts in normal marrow (*sideroblasts*).

Howell–Jolly bodies are granules of nuclear chromatin, 1–2 μm or more in diameter (Fig. 17.27, p. 532). If very small they resemble Pappenheimer bodies, but they are *iron-negative*. They are most common in the red cells in macrocytic anaemias but are found also in various other blood diseases or following splenectomy in haematologically normal individuals.

Heinz bodies appear in wet unstained preparations as irregularly shaped, highly refractile granules, which often aggregate or coalesce under the red cell membrane. Not visible in Romanowsky-stained films, they are readily demonstrated in supravital methyl violet preparations (Fig. 17.15, p. 522) or when stained by brilliant cresyl blue. They consist of granules of denatured globin, and are numerous in many forms of chemical haemolytic anaemia,

especially those induced by oxidant drugs (p. 530). Evidence of oxidative change of the iron in the haem moiety (methaemoglobin) often co-exists. A few Heinz bodies are seen after splenectomy.

In *punctate basophilia*, some of the red cells contain clumps of RNA, seen as minute blue granules in smears stained with Romanowsky dyes (Fig. 17.5). This is seen in chronic lead poisoning and red cell injury by haemolytic chemicals, but can also occur in other types of anaemia. It is not seen in splenectomised but otherwise normal individuals.

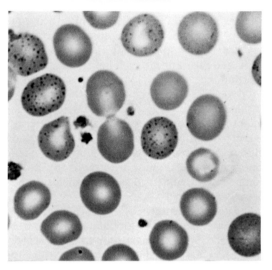

Fig. 17.5 Blood smear showing punctate basophilia. × 1250.

The red cell inclusions of *malaria* are described on p. 529.

Presence of erythroblasts. The term **erythroblast** is used throughout to mean nucleated red blood cells of all types; normally in the adult they are present only in the marrow, but they appear in the blood in various conditions.

Normoblasts are about the size of an ordinary red cell or a little larger, and have a single spherical nucleus which is condensed and thus stains very deeply. The nucleus shows a coarse network of deeply staining chromatin, or it may appear very dense and practically homogeneous in the pyknotic nuclei of the more mature normoblasts (Fig. 17.1). The presence of normoblasts in the blood is a characteristic feature in extramedullary haemopoiesis (p. 507) but may develop suddenly in acute anoxic states, e.g. in acute cardiorespiratory failure, or during the active marrow response to haemorrhage or haemolysis.

Megaloblasts. When megaloblastic change takes place in the marrow (p. 506), *megaloblasts* may appear in the blood and are most easily found in *buffy coat smears* (a smear of the top layer of cells, including most of the leukocytes, in a centrifuged preparation of blood). These cells are described on pp. 533–4.

Fragility of the erythrocytes

Osmotic fragility. When red cells are placed in a hypotonic salt solution they become swollen and finally rupture, the haemoglobin diffusing out. With normal blood, the first trace of lysis is usually seen in a concentration of 0·42–0·46 per cent NaCl; initial lysis occurring below 0·4 or above 0·5 per cent may be taken as abnormal, indicating diminished or increased fragility respectively; in some cases the abnormality may be detected only by careful quantitative methods. There is a close parallel between the volume/surface-area ratio of red cells and their osmotic fragility: cells with an increased ratio, for example in hereditary spherocytosis, are abnormally fragile, and cells with a reduced ratio, e.g. the thin cells in thalassaemia and other haemoglobinopathies, have an abnormal resistance.

Mechanical fragility of erythrocytes (susceptibility to trauma) is much increased in auto-immune haemolytic anaemia of 'cold antibody' type (p. 526) and sometimes in lead poisoning and in patients with prosthetic heart valves.

The Leukocytes

Introduction

The three classes of leukocytes in the blood—polymorphs (granulocytes), monocytes and lymphocytes—differ in their precursor cells, their morphology, and in their function. The three types of **polymorphs**—neutrophil, eosinophil and basophil—originate in the bone marrow (p. 185). The neutrophil polymorphs, as already explained in Chapter 3, are concerned in inflammatory reactions, and their chief function is the phagocytosis and digestion of micro-organisms and other foreign materials, damaged tissue elements, dead cells and immune complexes. The **monocytes** of the blood are also phagocytic; they belong to the mononuclear phagocyte system (p. 72) and provide most of the macrophages in inflammatory lesions. Disturbance of the functions of neutrophil polymorphs and monocytes, with consequent tissue injury, is a feature of certain types of hypersensitivity reaction (Chapter 6). The eosinophil polymorphs increase in the blood, and appear in the lesions, of patients with atopic hypersensitivity (p. 148) and in parasitic infestations, in which they play a defensive role. The origins of **lymphocytes**, and their essential functions in immune responses and reactions, have been considered in Chapters 5 and 6.

Increase or decrease of the leukocytes in disease can affect any or all of the different types. In practice, increase in the number of leukocytes above $11 \times 10^9/1$ (11 000/μl) is termed **leukocytosis,** while diminution below $4 \times 10^9/1$ is termed **leukopenia**: to determine the *absolute numbers* of different types of leukocytes, it is necessary to determine the total number and also the proportion of different types by performing a *differential leukocyte count* on a stained film. The normal range of numbers of the leukocytes in adults is given in Table 17.2.

Table 17.2 The normal numbers of leukocytes

	No. per μl blood	No. per litre $\times 10^9$
Polymorphs		
neutrophil	2500–7500	2·5–7·5
eosinophil	40–440	0·04–0·44
basophil	0–100	0–0·1
Lymphocytes	1500–3500	1·5–3·5
Monocytes	200–800	0·2–0·8
Total approx	4000–11 000	4–11

Changes in disease states

Neutrophil polymorphs

Neutrophil leukocytosis (neutrophilia). An account of the production of neutrophil polymorphs, and of neutrophil leukocytosis, with its accompanying myeloid hyperplasia of the haemopoietic marrow, is given on pp. 184–8. The commonest cause is bacterial infection, which should always be suspected, particularly in a neutrophil leukocytosis of over 20×10^9 per l, and may cause an increase to 50×10^9 per l. Moderate rises may accompany tissue necrosis without infection, such as myocardial infarction, and occur in burns and crush injuries: leukocytosis also develops within a few hours after a large haemorrhage, passing off after a day or two; acute haemolysis (destruction of red cells) is also accompanied by a neutrophil leukocytosis, and drug reactions, e.g. to steroids, sometimes promote a leukocytosis.

In any acute neutrophil leukocytosis, the proportion of young neutrophils in the blood increases (Fig. 17.6), and myelocytes or

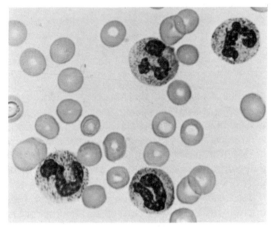

Fig. 17.6 Blood smear in neutrophil leukocytosis. × 850. (Dr. I. Evans.)

metamyelocytes may be found. Another change is a moderate increase in neutrophil alkaline phosphatase. In severe infections and toxic states the young polymorphs entering the circulation may show morphological evidence of damage; their cytoplasm contains deeply-staining granules showing abnormal variations in size, and giving a poor oxidase reaction ('*toxic granulation*'), and their nuclei fail to undergo the normal degree of segmentation. Toxic injury of greater degree results in failure of production of polymorphs, and leukopenia is thus a grave sign when associated with severe infection by pyogenic bacteria.

Reactive neutrophilia as described above may be regarded as a physiological reaction on the part of the myelopoietic (i.e. granulopoietic) marrow. By contrast, the neutrophil leukocytosis which occurs in myeloid leukaemia

(p. 545) is not a controlled response to a known stimulus, but is of neoplastic nature.

Neutrophil Leukopenia (neutropenia) occurs both as an isolated haematological feature and also as part of a reduction of all cell types in the blood (**pancytopenia**). Severe diminution or total absence of circulating neutrophils is termed **agranulocytosis.**

Neutropenia can result either from failure of the marrow to produce adequate numbers of neutrophils, or from excessive peripheral destruction or consumption of these cells. Examples of the former include bone marrow aplasia (p. 540), bone marrow replacement with secondary tumour, leukaemia or myeloma, or severe megaloblastic anaemia (p. 532). Marrow production may also be severely depressed in overwhelming infections such as septicaemias and disseminated tuberculosis, and neutropenia in such conditions is a bad prognostic sign. Many acute virus infections cause a temporary neutropenia but the mechanism is uncertain. A large number of different drugs can cause agranulocytosis, the most important being phenylbutazone, chlorpromazine and other phenothiazines, sulphonamides and related compounds, e.g. cotrimoxazole and sulphasalazine, frusemide and anti-thyroid drugs. In large doses, many compounds may depress the marrow, but neutropenia is more often the result of the development of an idiosyncrasy towards a particular compound, subsequent administration of even a small dose being capable of inducing the condition. Such idiosyncrasy is usually unpredictable, although the risk is probably greater in people prone to hypersensitivity reactions. *In every case of severe neutropenia the possibility that it is drug-induced must be thoroughly investigated.*

The mechanisms underlying idiosyncrasy towards a particular drug are not completely understood. In all probability an immunological mechanism of one kind or another is involved in most instances. Possibly a drug, in binding to the leukocyte surface, acts as a hapten to form an antigenic complex, the resulting antibodies being capable of destroying or damaging the circulating leukocytes and their more mature precursors in the marrow, on re-exposure to the drug. In other instances, leukocytes may be damaged when drug-induced antigen–antibody complexes bind to their plasma membrane. Red cells and platelets may also be destroyed by such mechanisms (p. 160). With so many new synthetic drugs being introduced, the dangers of sensitisation of this kind must always be kept in mind, since *the haemopoietic system, and in particular its granulocytic component, is often the first to exhibit signs of unwelcome toxicity.*

Immune reactions may also be involved in the neutropenia of primary atypical pneumonia, glandular fever, disseminated lupus erythematosus and cyclical agranulocytosis. In anaphylactic shock (p. 146), marked leukopenia may develop very rapidly, due apparently to aggregation of leukocytes in the capillaries of the lungs and other internal organs: this occurs also in endotoxic shock (p. 178). The syndrome of **hypersplenism** (p. 565), in which leukocytes, erythrocytes and platelets each or all undergo excessive sequestration in an enlarged spleen, is another example of neutropenia due to 'peripheral' mechanisms.

Severe neutropenia has a high mortality, especially where the absolute neutrophil count falls below $0.5 \times 10^9/l$ ($500/\mu l$). There is an increased likelihood of major infection by pathogenic organisms, and opportunistic infection with organisms normally of commensal type (e.g. gut coliforms, fungi) may become a major factor. There is often a severe inflammation of fauces and gums, which can progress to local gangrene—**agranulocytic angina.**

Defects of neutrophil function. An abnormal susceptibility to infection can be produced not only by a reduction in circulating neutrophils, but also by defective neutrophil function, even when their number is normal. The capacity of the neutrophil to combat infection by pathogenic micro-organisms is dependent upon its ability to respond to chemotactic stimuli, to phagocytose the offending micro-organisms, and to bring about their subsequent destruction intracellularly (p. 181). Defects in all three of these components of neutrophil function have been described and in some of these the abnormality appears to be intrinsic. Perhaps the most important of these is **chronic granulomatous disease of childhood**, in which the neutrophils and monocytes have an undefined enzyme defect, and as a result lack the capacity to destroy phagocytosed bacteria, especially staphylococci, Gram − ve bacteria and certain fungi. The disease is transmitted by a gene defect on the X chromosome and so, like haemophilia, affects males; female carriers can be shown to have a mixture of normal and defective neutrophils in their blood, which supports the Lyon hypothesis.* From early childhood, affected males suffer from protracted infections, with extensive suppuration and granulation tissue formation, even from bacteria of low pathogenicity. The enzyme defect can be demonstrated *in vitro* by the failure of neutrophils and monocytes to reduce the yellow dye nitroblue tetrazolium (NBT) to an insoluble precipitate of blue-black formazan.

Another example is the *Chediak–Higashi syndrome*, a rare condition in which there is a lysosomal abnormality affecting many cell types. The neutrophils possess characteristically large cytoplasmic granules, which are of lysosomal origin and fail to disrupt following the phagocytosis of bacteria: as a result there is an impaired capacity to destroy bacteria intracellularly. The condition, transmitted as an autosomal recessive character, thus gives rise to recurrent infections. Other variable features include leukopenia, defective skin pigmentation, neuropathies, lymph-node enlargement and hepatosplenomegaly: malignant lymphoma sometimes supervenes. Of the other neutrophil function defects, which are more common than was previously thought, mention should be made of the *lazy leukocyte syndrome*, in which there is a defect of neutrophil motility. There are also conditions of impaired chemotactic response and phagocytic capacity secondary to an absence of plasma factors, especially immunoglobulins and components of complement, or to drugs and toxic substances, e.g. alcohol.

The presence of myelocytes. The appearance of these cells in the blood has an important clinical significance. In addition to chronic myeloid leukaemia, where their presence in large numbers along with myeloblasts is a prominent feature, they are found occasionally in pernicious anaemia in small numbers. In the leukoerythroblastic anaemia accompanying secondary carcinoma of the bone marrow and in myelofibrosis, myelocytes may be found in relatively large numbers, as may also nucleated red cells (p. 507), and the term **leukoerythroblastosis** is then applied. A few myelocytes may be found also in some very severe infections, particularly if there is a marked neutrophilia.

Eosinophil leukocytes

These differ from neutrophil polymorphs in having larger, brightly eosinophilic cytoplasmic granules, which often appear closely packed. Also, the nucleus usually has only two lobes (Fig. 17.7).

---

*This postulates that the inactive X chromosome represented by the sex-chromatin of females' cells (p. 1002) can be *either* of the X chromosomes, selection being random in each individual cell in the early embryo.

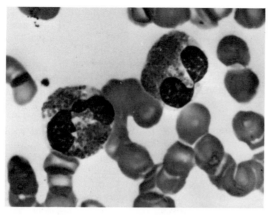

Fig. 17.7 Blood smear showing two eosinophil polymorphs. × 1250. (Dr. J. Browning.)

Eosinophil leukocytosis. Just as neutrophil leukocytosis occurs in pyogenic infections, so eosinophil leukocytosis is observed in those conditions which are characterised by infiltration of the tissues with eosinophils. The factors responsible for this local and general increase in eosinophils are not understood, but there is experimental evidence that, in hypersensitivity reactions, they are dependent on a T-lymphocyte response. Eosinophilia occurs in the following conditions.

(*a*) *Parasitic infestation* by various kinds of worm, e.g. *Trichinella spiralis*, ankylostomes and schistosomes. The eosinophil level sometimes exceeds $3 \times 10^9/l$ (3000/μl).

(*b*) *Hypersensitivity reactions.* In atopic hypersensitivity reactions (p. 146) such as asthma and hay fever, eosinophilia is usually present, and is related to the local emigration of eosinophils in the tissues. Eosinophilia may also be found in angio-oedema, food sensitivity, and in hypersensitivity reactions to certain drugs. An increase in eosinophils may also occur in polyarteritis nodosa.

(*c*) *Chronic skin disease*, such as dermatitis herpetiformis, psoriasis, etc. In some generalised skin conditions, a hypersensitivity mechanism may be present, e.g. in eczema or urticaria. Eosinophilia also occurs early in scarlet fever.

(*d*) *Malignant tumours.* The eosinophil count rises in some patients with cancer involving the bone marrow. In chronic myeloid leukaemia eosinophils may be increased along with the other granulocyte cells. In certain forms of Hodgkin's disease, the lymph nodes are infil- trated with eosinophils, and about 10 per cent of cases show an eosinophilia in the blood.

Eosinophil leukopenia. Diminution in the eosinophils is a practically constant response to increased secretion or therapeutic administration of steroids or adrenocorticotrophic hormone.

The functions of eosinophils are still obscure. There is, however, evidence that they are protective against metazoan parasites and they appear to modulate atopic reactions (p. 148).

Basophil leukocytes

The granules of these cells usually give a purplish metachromatic reaction. They resemble, but present certain differences from, the tissue mast cells, which have a role in atopic hypersensitivity (p. 147), and basophils have also been shown to be involved in hypersensitivity reactions, at least in animal studies. In chronic myeloid leukaemia, basophils sometimes contribute to the leukocyte increase and basophil myelocytes may also appear. In various chronic wasting diseases an increase of basophils in the blood may be present occasionally, but there is no condition known which regularly induces a basophil leukocytosis.

Lymphocytes

Recent advances in our understanding of the life cycle and immunological functions of the lymphocyte have been described in Chapters 5 and 6. The picture is far from complete, but it is apparent that the lymphocytes in the blood represent at least two functionally different populations, each being concerned with immune responses and reactions. Like many other cells, they are known to be capable of producing interferon (p. 194).

Lymphocytosis. Normally the proportion of lymphocytes in the child is higher than in the adult. The number is highest shortly after birth, probably because of the build-up of antigenic experience at this time, and gradually falls in subsequent years. In most patients with leukopenia the fall in total count is attributable to granulocytopenia, and there is thus an increase in the proportion of lymphocytes; a *true lymphocytosis*, that is an increase in the number of lymphocytes per μl, is less common. It usually accompanies specific infective fevers and is a useful diagnostic feature in mild cases of **whoop-**

ing cough, in which it occasionally rises to $100 \times 10^9/l$. Lymphocytosis also occurs **in glandular fever**, many of the cells being large and of abnormal appearance. **Other infections** in which lymphocytosis may be seen include typhoid and paratyphoid fever, brucellosis, influenza, secondary syphilis, toxoplasmosis and *Cytomegalovirus* infection. High lymphocyte counts are also seen in the acute infective lymphocytosis of young children. The outstanding cause of gross lymphocytosis is, however, **chronic lymphocytic leukaemia** (p. 547), and an increased proportion of lymphocytes may sometimes be observed by a differential count to precede the actual rise in the leukocyte count.

Lymphopenia occurs irregularly in various conditions. In infancy, it is a cardinal feature of some rare major immunological deficiency syndromes (p. 169). It has also been reported in intestinal lymphangiectasia (p. 640) and in coeliac disease, especially when there is splenic atrophy (p. 642). Severe lymphopenia results also from x-irradiation and use of cytotoxic drugs, including steroids, for immunosuppressive therapy or treatment of neoplasia.

Monocytes

The monocytes (Fig. 17.8) are circulating cells of the mononuclear phagocyte system (p. 72). When stimulated they enlarge, increase in motility and metabolic activity, becoming macrophages. The release of lymphokines which influence monocytes and macrophages in delayed hypersensitivity reactions is discussed on p. 157.

Like the neutrophil polymorphs, monocytes migrate into inflammatory foci and phagocytose bacteria, damaged tissue elements, dead cells, etc., but they leave the blood later than the polymorphs, and are seen in increasing numbers in the late stages of pyogenic infections in the outer part of the wall of persistent abscesses (Fig. 8.26, p. 221), and in chronic inflammations of various types and causes. **Monocytosis** is commonly present in subacute infective endocarditis, in undulant fever, and sometimes in systemic lupus erythematosus. In

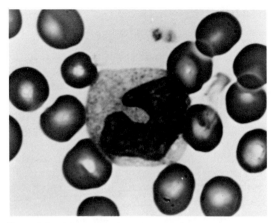

Fig. 17.8 Monocyte in a blood smear. × 1250. (Dr. I. Evans.)

tuberculosis, serial studies on individual cases have shown that the numbers of lymphocytes and monocytes in the blood tend to be inversely proportional to one another, and there is some evidence that a high ratio accompanies healing and that a low ratio is associated with extension of the lesions. The monocytes are increased also in typhus and some other rickettsial diseases, and in certain protozoal infections, e.g. malaria, trypanosomiasis and kala-azar, in which diseases there is no increase of the neutrophils. In chronic malaria, the presence of numerous monocytes is often a striking feature, and some of them may contain small granules of pigment (Fig. 17.24, p. 529). In *tetrachlorethane poisoning* there is sometimes a progressive increase in the monocytes up to $3–4 \times 10^9/l$ (3000–4000/μl).

The abnormal cells which appear in the blood in large numbers in some cases of *infectious mononucleosis* (glandular fever) resemble monocytes, but are really stimulated T lymphocytes (p. 570).

Monocytic leukaemia must always be considered in patients with monocytosis (p. 544).

Some of the functional defects of neutrophil polymorphs, e.g. that in chronic granulomatous disease (p. 513) are shared by monocytes, which are also functionally impaired in carcinomatosis and some other conditions.

Blood Platelets

Platelets are capable of releasing some histamine and 5-hydroxytryptamine, and are weakly phagocytic, but their major functions are in aggregating to form a haemostatic plug when a small blood vessel is severed, and in promoting clotting of fibrinogen by taking part in the cascade reaction described on pp. 231–5. Accordingly, diminution in the number of circulating platelets, or disordered platelet function, can result in a state of *purpura*, in which spontaneous haemorrhages occur.

The number of platelets in the blood is normally between $150–400 \times 10^9/l$ ($150\,000–400\,000/\mu l$). A temporary **increase in platelets (thrombocytosis)** occurs after injury, haemorrhage and particularly after removal of the spleen, which is the major site of normal platelet sequestration and destruction. The increase in numbers in these conditions is also accompanied by an increase in adhesiveness and a tendency to thrombosis. Thrombocytosis also accompanies a prolonged neutrophil leukocytosis, and is commonly seen in the early stages of chronic myeloid leukaemia.

Reduction in the number of platelets (thrombocytopenia) is commonly associated with depression of red cells and leukocytes, e.g. in aplastic anaemia or acute leukaemia.

The most important and commonest primary disease causing serious thrombocytopenia is *idiopathic thrombocytopenic purpura* which, in spite of its name, is due to an auto-antibody which causes excessive platelet destruction, mainly in the spleen. Excessive destruction in the spleen also occurs in *hypersplenism*, and may be accompanied by abnormal destruction of red cells and leukocytes. Drugs may also cause thrombocytopenia by inducing a hypersensitivity reaction or by a cytotoxic effect on the marrow. Rarely, thrombocytopenia alone, i.e. without reduction of red or white cells, results from marrow failure.

These and other platelet abnormalities are described in the section on abnormal haemorrhagic states (pp. 554–8).

Anaemia

Definition and types of anaemia

Anaemia is defined as a reduction in the concentration of haemoglobin in the blood below the normal range, and is usually but not invariably accompanied by reduction in the number of red cells. Anaemia develops when the rate of red cell production by the bone marrow fails to keep pace with destruction of red cells or with any losses from haemorrhage. Accordingly the anaemias can be classified simply as follows:

(1) Excessive loss or destruction of red cells
    (*a*) loss—*post-haemorrhagic anaemia*
    (*b*) destruction—*haemolytic anaemia*.

(2) Failure of production of red cells
    (*a*) diminished production with marrow hyperplasia—*dyshaemopoietic anaemia*
    (*b*) diminished production with marrow hypoplasia or aplasia—*hypoplastic* or *aplastic anaemia*.

In some types of anaemia more than one of the above mechanisms are involved; for example in pernicious anaemia (p. 535), there is not only insufficient output of red cells by the marrow, but those cells which are produced wear out too quickly, i.e. there is also excessive destruction.

Effects of anaemia

The main effect of anaemia is a reduction in the oxygen-carrying capacity of the blood, with resulting **tissue hypoxia.** The patient may complain of tiredness, dizziness, paraesthesia of the extremities, anginal chest pain and breathlessness on exertion.

Certain **compensatory adjustments** to the circulation occur in anaemia; there is a reduction in arteriolar tone, while the stroke volume and to a lesser extent the heart rate increase. Cardiac output thus rises, circulation time falls, and tissue perfusion is increased. These changes may be reflected clinically in a bounding pulse with a high pulse pressure, palpitation, cardiac enlargement and haemic murmurs; if the condition continues or the anaemia worsens, *cardiac failure* is a serious risk, especially if the load on the heart is increased by injudicious blood transfusion. These effects do not depend only on the severity of the anaemia; if anaemia develops rapidly the symptoms are correspondingly severe, whereas remarkable tolerance is often seen when the haemoglobin has fallen slowly. Co-existing vascular disease, as in the elderly, also enhances the effects of anaemia. Pallor, mild pyrexia and slight splenomegaly may be attributable to anaemia *per se*.

Tissue hypoxia resulting from anaemia stimulates the production of erythropoietin, which in turn leads to *marrow hyperplasia*; the yellow fatty marrow of the long bones becomes progressively replaced by dark red cellular marrow, and in extreme cases resorption of bone trabeculae may occur. In haemolytic and post-haemorrhage anaemias, this will lead to a useful output of new red cells from the marrow (*effective erythropoiesis*); in the dyshaemopoietic states, however, although marrow hyperplasia occurs, disordered haemopoiesis usually prevents a useful output of new red cells (*ineffective erythropoiesis*). In an aplastic marrow, compensatory hyperplasia cannot occur despite erythropoietin stimulation.

Fatty change, especially in the liver and heart, is the most constant pathological change in patients dying of anaemia (p. 25).

Post-haemorrhagic anaemia

The restoration of the fluid part of the blood after haemorrhage (p. 260) causes a temporary dilution of the blood with accompanying fall in the red cell count. The first evidence of regeneration of red cells after a large haemorrhage is a progressive increase in the number of reticulocytes in the blood (p. 509), and the degree of increase is an indication of haemopoietic

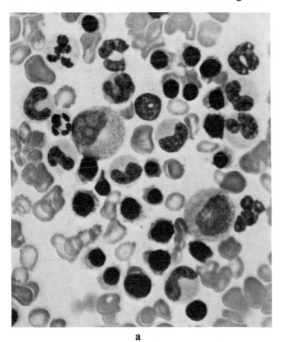   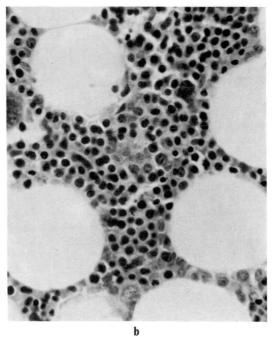

a   b

Fig. 17.9   The haemopoietic marrow, showing an erythroblastic reaction following haemorrhage. **a** Marrow smear: there is an increased proportion of normoblasts, at various stages of maturity, as compared with myelocytes. × 850. **b** Marrow section: the cellular haemopoietic tissue has increased at the expense of the fat cells. × 500.

activity. Occasional normoblasts may also be seen and after repeated haemorrhage they may be numerous. As regeneration becomes complete the reticulocytes gradually return to their normal level and normoblasts disappear. These changes are the results of proliferation of erythroblasts in the bone marrow, in which they form a larger proportion of the cells than normally (Fig. 17.9). A polymorphonuclear leukocytosis and thrombocytosis, both of moderate degree, appear within a few hours after haemorrhage; they pass off in two or three days, unless the haemorrhage is repeated.

Chronic loss of small amounts of blood does not produce anaemia due to a fall in circulating red cells because the number lost is readily replaced. Iron deficiency may, however, develop, and *chronic haemorrhage is the most important cause of iron deficiency anaemia*, a dyshaemopoietic state (p. 538). In such states the circulating platelets may also rise.

Haemolytic anaemias

General features

The haemolytic disorders comprise a group of conditions characterised by an increase in the rate of red cell destruction, and thus a reduction in the normal lifespan of the erythrocyte (100–120 days). There is a compensatory increase in the rate of red cell production, and anaemia will develop only when the rate of destruction exceeds that of production. These processes are common to all haemolytic disorders, irrespective of cause, and these general features will be described more fully before considering the various types of haemolytic anaemia.

Sites of red cell destruction. Red cells may undergo premature destruction either by phagocytosis by macrophages, or by intravascular lysis. In most haemolytic conditions, red cell destruction occurs in macrophages mainly in the spleen, liver and bone marrow. These cells are capable of destroying as much as 20 per cent of the total red cell mass each day. Mildly or moderately damaged red cells are phagocytosed mainly in the spleen, probably because circulation of red cells through the red pulp is very slow and the diminished availability of oxygen, glucose, etc. further impairs the damaged cells, rendering them more liable to haemolysis and phagocytosis. More severely damaged cells, however, undergo phagocytosis in all tissues containing vascular channels lined by macrophages (notably the liver, spleen and bone marrow).

Intravascular destruction is due mainly to severe red cell membrane damage by antibody and complement, toxic chemicals or mechanical trauma.

Changes resulting from increased destruction of red cells. Following *phagocytosis of red cells* by macrophages, haemoglobin is broken down to iron and globin, both of which undergo reutilisation, and the haem is degraded to bilirubin (see p. 278). In haemolytic disease, the production of bilirubin may exceed the capacity of the liver to remove it, and plasma levels rise; clinical jaundice results when the level exceeds about 3 mg/100 ml (50 µmol/litre). The bilirubin is bound to plasma albumin and does not pass into the urine (**acholuric jaundice**). The increased excretion of conjugated bilirubin by the liver leads to excessive formation of stercobilinogen in the gut, so that the faeces are dark. There is increased absorption of stercobilinogen which often cannot all be dealt with by the liver and so appears in the urine as urobilinogen; measurement of faecal stercobilinogen and urinary urobilinogen are helpful in diagnosing haemolysis, although time-consuming and not very accurate. The high bilirubin content of the bile may predispose to the formation of pigment gallstones in chronic haemolytic anaemias, and the high levels of bilirubin found in haemolytic disease of the newborn may cause toxic damage to the brain (p. 527).

Intravascular lysis leads to the appearance of free haemoglobin in the plasma; a proportion of this is bound at once to plasma haptoglobin and the haemoglobin/haptoglobin complex is phagocytosed by the macrophages. If the haemolysis is severe, this process is easily overwhelmed; some free haemoglobin is then converted to methaemalbumin, and the remainder is excreted free in the urine. Intravascular lysis of red cells can thus be recognised by haemoglobinaemia, haemoglobinuria, methaemalbuminaemia and by disappearance of plasma haptoglobins. Haemosiderin granules in epithelial cells in the urine are also a sensitive indication of intravascular lysis.

Changes associated with compensatory erythropoiesis. In haemolytic states, erythropoietin stimulation of the marrow induces compensatory hyperplasia of red cell precursors; kinetic studies show that the marrow is capable of increasing red cell production to a maximum of 8–10 times normal. There is thus an increased number of young red cells in the blood: in a Leishman-stained film, many of the erythrocytes show polychromasia, and there may be both early and late normoblasts. Reticulocytes are always increased, often exceeding 20 per cent (Fig. 17.4). In any untreated case of anaemia, such a reticulocytosis is strong evidence of a haemolytic process provided blood loss can be excluded. The anaemia is usually normocytic but may be mildly macrocytic (see below).

The marrow shows erythroblastic hyperplasia (Fig. 17.10) and the fat cells are partly or even completely replaced by haemopoietic tissue, which may also extend down the shafts of the long bones; eventually the medullary cavity may become widened with loss of bony

trabeculae and thinning of the cortical bone. The greatly increased erythropoiesis may result in enlargement of erythroblasts ('macronormoblastic change') and production of macrocytic red cells. Megaloblastic change due to folic acid deficiency may also develop (p. 536). In severe chronic cases extramedullary haemopoiesis occurs in the spleen and other extramedullary sites.

Measurement of red cell lifespan. A sample of the patient's red cells can be labelled *in vitro* with radiochromium (^{51}Cr) and returned to the circulation where their fate can be closely followed and the chief sites of destruction found. The rate of disappearance of radioactivity from the circulation can be estimated by serial blood samples, and is proportional to the rate of red cell destruction. If haemorrhage can be excluded, the red cell lifespan can be estimated from these data. In addition, by placing an external scintillation counter over the liver, spleen and bone marrow, the sites of red cell sequestration and destruction can be ascertained.

Types of haemolytic anaemia

Although recent advances in our understanding of the metabolism of glucose by red cells has helped to clarify the modes of red cell destruction, the causation of the different types of haemolytic anaemia is by no means fully understood, and classification is therefore tentative. Reduced red cell survival time is the essential feature of haemolytic anaemia; it may be the result either of an intrinsic abnormality in the red cells, or of an extrinsic haemolytic mechanism. The distinction was originally based on red cell survival times in cross transfusion experiments (Fig. 17.11). Such methods are not usually required for routine diagnosis as the various forms of the disease present other distinctive characteristics.

CLASSIFICATION OF HAEMOLYTIC ANAEMIA

(I) Intrinsic defects in the red cells

   A. Genetically determined defects
     (1) Hereditary spherocytosis (familial acholuric jaundice).
     (2) Hereditary elliptocytosis.
     (3) Red cell enzyme defects
       (*a*) in the Embden–Meyerhof pathway
       (*b*) in the hexose monophosphate shunt.
     (4) The haemoglobinopathies.

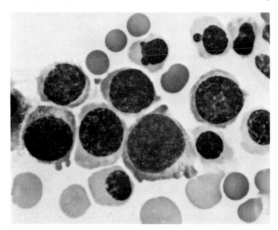

Fig. 17.10 Marrow smear in haemolytic anaemia due to hereditary spherocytosis, illustrating normoblastic hyperplasia: the cluster of erythroblasts includes all stages from early basophilic cells to late normoblasts. × 1100.

B. Acquired defects
(1) Paroxysmal nocturnal haemoglobinuria.
(2) Dyshaemopoietic anaemias.

(II) Abnormal haemolytic mechanisms.

A. Auto-immune haemolytic anaemia
(1) 'Warm antibody' type.
(2) 'Cold antibody' type.

B. Iso-antibodies to red cells
(1) Haemolytic disease of the newborn.
(2) Transfusion reactions.

C. Parasitic invasion of red cells
(1) Malaria.
(2) Oroya fever.

D. Haemolytic toxins and chemicals
(1) Bacterial toxins, e.g. *Cl. welchii, Strep. pyogenes.*
(2) Drugs and chemicals, e.g. phenacetin, dapsone, sulphonamides, phenylhydrazine, lead.
(3) Vegetable poisons, e.g. favism.

E. Mechanical damage to red cells
(1) March haemoglobinuria.
(2) Microangiopathic haemolytic anaemia.

NOTE: The groups and types of haemolytic anaemia listed above are not entirely independent. For example, subjects with glucose-6-phosphate dehydrogenase deficiency are abnormally susceptible to haemolysis by various chemicals.

I.   Intrinsic red cell defects

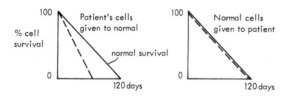

II. Abnormal haemolytic mechanisms

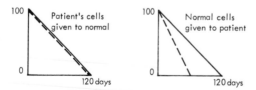

Fig. 17.11 The survival of red cells in cross-transfusion experiments in haemolytic anaemia. The continuous lines indicate the rate of disappearance of transfused red cells from normal donors to normal recipients. The interrupted lines show the rates of disappearance of transfused red cells in the stated circumstances.

I.A. Genetically determined red cell defects

(1) Hereditary spherocytosis

This common type of chronic haemolytic anaemia, occurring in most parts of the world, is caused by a red cell membrane defect of uncertain nature and inherited as an autosomal dominant trait with incomplete penetrance. In about 25 per cent of patients, however, there is no family history, and the defect presumably arises as a spontaneous genetic mutation in such cases. The membrane defect results in excessive permeability to sodium ions, and red cell integrity can only be maintained by increased glycolytic activity, required to 'pump' sodium ions out of the cell. This metabolic activity is associated with an increased turnover of membrane lipid, some of which is inevitably lost. Membrane loss is responsible for the tendency of the red cells to assume the microspherocytic form, a process which is greatly accelerated in the red pulp of the spleen where the availability of glucose is diminished. Microspherocytic red cells are trapped in the red pulp and subsequently lysed, since they lack the pliability necessary to enable them to pass through the clefts between the endothelial cells in the venous sinusoids and return to the circulation. The spleen thus occupies a critical role in the disease process, and following splenectomy the survival of the red cells returns to normal.

Clinically the disease is characterised by acholuric jaundice, often mild and fluctuating, and usually dating from early childhood. Anaemia may be mild and even absent although episodes of severe anaemia ('crises') are sometimes experienced. These crises are due either to an increase in red cell destruction, sometimes related to infections or pregnancy and associated with deepening jaundice, fever and leucocytosis, or to reduction in erythropoietic activity in the marrow, when increasing anaemia is accompanied by a fall in the reticulocyte count (hypoplastic crisis). Splenomegaly is invariable, and some patients develop chronic leg ulceration. The diagnosis is suspected when signs of haemolysis, such as persistent reticulocytosis and urobilinogenuria, are associated with the presence in the peripheral blood of microspherocytes, which are small, intensely stained spheroidal red cells (Fig. 17.12). Demonstration of

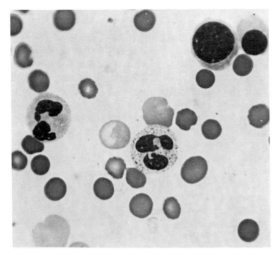

Fig. 17.12 Blood film in hereditary spherocytosis. Note the small, densely staining spherocytes. × 780.

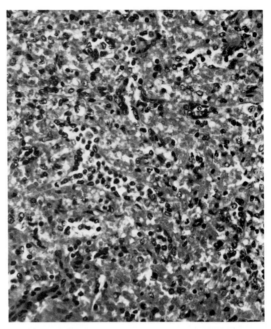

Fig. 17.13 Spleen in hereditary spherocytosis. The pulp is intensely congested and the sinuses are inconspicuous. × 230.

increased osmotic fragility of the red cells (p. 511) helps to confirm the diagnosis. The haemolytic state is cured by removal of the spleen, which is always enlarged, usually weighing about 500 g or more. Histologically, the red pulp is distended with red cells, while the venous sinusoids are compressed (Fig. 17.13). Although splenectomy relieves the haemolysis, microspherocytosis and increased osmotic fragility of the red cells persist.

(2) Hereditary elliptocytosis

This causes a much less pronounced sequestration of cells in the spleen pulp and the anaemia is usually mild. This defect exhibits genetic linkage with the Rh blood group genes.

(3) Red cell enzyme defects

Normal red cell survival is dependent upon the integrity of the two enzyme systems concerned in glucose metabolism, namely the Embden–Meyerhof pathway and the hexose monophosphate shunt (Fig. 17.14). Enzyme deficiencies in either system are usually genetically determined and can lead directly or indirectly to haemolytic anaemia. Microspherocytosis is not a feature of these defects, which are usually included in the group of conditions described as heredi-

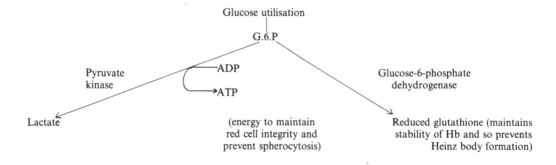

Glucose utilisation

G.6.P

Pyruvate kinase — ADP / ATP

Glucose-6-phosphate dehydrogenase

Lactate

(energy to maintain red cell integrity and prevent spherocytosis)

Reduced glutathione (maintains stability of Hb and so prevents Heinz body formation)

EMBDEN—MEYERHOF PATHWAY (90% glucose metabolism)

HEXOSE MONOPHOSPHATE SHUNT (10% glucose metabolism)

Fig. 17.14 Two enzyme systems of importance in determining the lifespan of the red cells.

tary nonspherocytic haemolytic anaemia (HNSHA).

Pyruvate kinase deficiency, although rare, is the commonest defect in the Embden–Meyerhof pathway. It is inherited as an autosomal recessive trait and produces a mild haemolytic state in individuals homozygous for the abnormal gene. The red cells show minimal morphological abnormality, despite the paradoxically high reticulocyte counts which have been recorded. Trapping of red cells in the spleen is not a prominent feature, and splenectomy confers only minimal benefit.

Glucose-6-phosphate dehydrogenase deficiency is by far the most common defect in the hexose monophosphate shunt and is, moreover, one of the commonest of all genetic defects, affecting as many as 50 per cent of individuals of Negro or Mediterranean ancestry in some parts of the world. Several allotypes of the enzyme (isoenzymes) are known, and various grades of deficiency are encountered. Inheritance of the defect is sex-linked, and so males are most often affected. *The principal effect of deficiency is a decrease in reduced glutathione: in consequence, the haemoglobin is readily oxidised and ultimately*

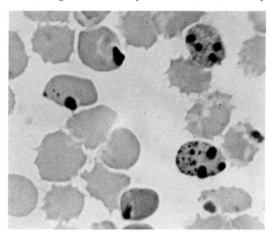

Fig. 17.15 Blood film in sodium chlorate poisoning, stained with methyl violet to show Heinz bodies. × 1400.

masses of denatured haemoglobin (Heinz bodies) are deposited on the cell membranes (Fig. 17.15). Spontaneous haemolysis has only been described in the rare Caucasian form of the disease, which presents as a form of HNSHA in neonates. Much more often haemolysis only develops following exposure to chemical agents with oxidative potential. In Mediterranean people, even the mild oxidant found in beans, or bean pollen, is sufficient to produce haemolysis—*favism* (p. 531). In negroes, however, oxidative drugs such as phenacetin or the antimalarial primaquine are required to expose the enzyme defect, although the subsequent haemolysis may be severe. The diagnosis is established by enzyme assay techniques or more simply by observing the number of Heinz bodies produced by exposing the red cells to phenylhydrazine *in vitro*.

(4) Haemoglobinopathies

Haemoglobin is a globular protein of molecular weight 68 000, consisting of two pairs of coiled polypeptide chains, a single prosthetic haem group being attached to each of the four chains. The type of haemoglobin is determined by the amino-acid sequence in the polypeptide chains. Four different chains occur normally in adults, termed α, β, γ and δ. The normal haemoglobins consist of a pair of alpha chains combined with a pair of one of the other three chains, as illustrated in Fig. 17.16. Haemoglobins differ in their electrophoretic mobility (Fig. 17.19), solubility and resistance of alkali denaturation; these features, together with chromatography, are used in their identification. Replacement of Hb-F by Hb-A starts before birth, and Hb-A and Hb-A$_2$ account for over 99 per cent of the haemoglobin normally present by one year of age. In the adult, less than 2 per cent is Hb-F. Haemoglobinopathies result from abnormalities in the synthesis of the globin fraction, due to gene mutation, deletion, etc., the haem groups being normal. Mutations are of two main varieties. The first causes *an abnormality in the amino-acid sequence of the polypeptide chain* so that an abnormal haemoglobin is produced. Over one hundred such abnormal haemoglobins have been

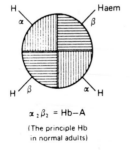

$\alpha_2\beta_2$ = Hb–A

(The principle Hb in normal adults)

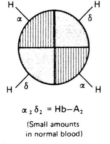

$\alpha_2\delta_2$ = Hb–A$_2$

(Small amounts in normal blood)

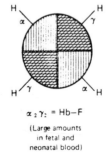

$\alpha_2\gamma_2$ = Hb–F

(Large amounts in fetal and neonatal blood)

Fig. 17.16   The structure of the normal haemoglobins.

globin. There is also a tendency to *venous thrombosis*, the cause of which is not clear. Transfusion is dangerous owing to the risk of a haemolytic crisis. Repeated haemolytic episodes cause a marked degree of anaemia with reticulocytosis, marrow hyperplasia and siderosis of the organs, especially the kidneys (Fig. 17.21); granules of haemosiderin are abundant in the urine both day and night. After a few years death results from thrombosis in the portal or cerebral veins, but milder forms occur and spontaneous permanent remissions have been observed.

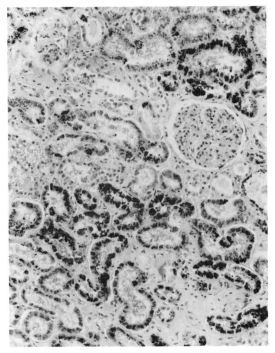

Fig. 17.21 The kidney in paroxysmal nocturnal haemoglobinuria, stained by the prussian blue reaction, showing accumulation of haemosiderin in the convoluted tubules due to prolonged haemoglobinuria. × 100.

Lysis is due to a defect (of unknown nature) which renders the red cell membrane unduly susceptible to the lytic action of complement. The normal level of complement activity by the alternative pathway (p. 143) is apparently sufficient to cause lysis, but only a proportion of the red cells are susceptible and the proportion fluctuates, accounting for exacerbations and remissions. Laboratory tests are based on demonstrating lysis on slight activation of complement, e.g. by acidification of serum (**Ham's test**). It is not known why lysis is sometimes mainly nocturnal. Occasional patients present with hypoplastic anaemia, the marrow being hypocellular, and it may be that PNH arises as an acquired red cell abnormality following an aplastic episode.

(2) Dyshaemopoietic anaemias. In many anaemias due primarily to underproduction of red cells, there is also a haemolytic element, the average life span of the red cells being shortened. This occurs in the macrocytic anaemias, iron-deficiency anaemia, in some cases of aplastic anaemia, and in leukaemia. Apart from the macrocytic anaemias, in which the mechanical injury to abnormally large cells during their passage through capillaries may be a factor, the nature of the defect in the red cells in the above conditions is unknown.

II. Abnormal extra-erythrocytic haemolytic mechanisms

There are several conditions in which excessive blood destruction results from the presence of an abnormal antibody which combines with the red cells, rendering them susceptible either to phagocytosis by macrophages or to the lytic action of complement.

II.A Auto-immune haemolytic anaemia

One of the commonest causes of acquired haemolytic anaemia is the development of an auto-antibody capable of binding to and damaging the individual's own red cells (cytotoxic antibody, or type II, hypersensitivity, p. 150). Red cells coated with **antibodies of IgG class**, which generally react at 37 °C ('*warm antibodies*'), commonly become microspherocytic and undergo phagocytosis following sequestration in the spleen, liver or bone marrow, i.e. *extravascular haemolysis*. The clinical picture thus closely resembles hereditary spherocytosis. **IgM antibodies** react at temperatures below 37 °C ('*cold antibodies*') and produce their effects in different ways. Firstly, they may lead to red cell auto-agglutination which produces microvascular occlusion and *Raynaud's phenomenon* (p. 384). Secondly, complement-binding, with consequent haemolysis, is a notable feature and the phenomena associated with *intravascular haemolysis* (p. 518) often dominate the clinical picture. The severity of these effects depends upon the thermal amplitude of the antibody; the higher the temperature at which it can react, the more severe is the disease likely to be.

The mechanism of auto-antibody formation is uncertain. In most instances, however, it seems likely that suppressor T-lymphocyte function has become defective, allowing the development of reactive clones of lymphocytes (p. 134). In other cases, exogenous agents, such as drugs or micro-organisms, may stimulate the formation of antibodies which cross-react with red cell surface antigens.

(1) 'Warm antibody' type. Although this condition can develop at any age and in both sexes, it is commonest in women of over forty. Almost half of all cases are primary, while the remainder complicate other diseases, especially systemic lupus erythematosus, rheumatoid arthritis and other putative auto-immune disorders and malignant lymphomas such as chronic lymphocytic leukaemia. Some cases are attributable to drug therapy, α-methyldopa being the most common offender. The clinical picture is that of a chronic, usually fluctuating haemolytic state. Splenomegaly is common. The red cells may show microspherocytosis and increased osmotic fragility, particularly during severe exacerbations. The presence of antibody attached to the red cell surface is the diagnostic feature. The antibody is 'incomplete', i.e., does not agglutinate red cells in saline suspension, and is detected by the direct antiglobulin test (p. 111). Antibody is sometimes present in the serum, and it can be eluted from the red cells. Occasionally it has been found to react with antigens of the Rh system, usually antigen e (p. 267). This might be important in the selection of blood for transfusion. In most cases, the haemolytic process can be controlled by corticosteroids and azathioprine although splenectomy may be beneficial in cases where the spleen is specifically sequestering antibody-coated red cells (p. 518): this may be detected by radio-labelling a sample of the patient's red cells and following their fate *in vivo* by surface scanning (p. 519).

(2) 'Cold antibody' type. In this group of conditions, the auto-antibodies are usually of IgM class and react only at temperatures below 37 °C. They are often present in the serum in high titre, of the order of 1 in 1000, and give rise to two fairly distinct clinical syndromes. Firstly, **paroxysmal cold haemoglobinuria**, which consists of attacks of haemolysis following exposure to cold, due to union of the antibody with the red cells, and subsequent fixation of complement, causing intravascular haemolysis. Secondly, **cold haemagglutinin disease**, in which the antibody also causes strong haemag-glutination, resulting in attacks of cyanosis and Raynaud's phenomenon on exposure to cold, and also chronic haemolytic anaemia in cold weather, due to complement fixation and also to increased mechanical fragility of the agglutinated red cells.

Paroxysmal cold haemoglobinuria. The classical chronic form of this condition occurred in association with congenital syphilis, and is now rare. It is seen occasionally as an acute, usually transient complication of acute virus infections *and is often accompanied by a false positive Wassermann reaction.* The cold antibody is unusual in being of IgG class; it reacts with antigens of the P system, present in the red cells of nearly all individuals and is capable of strong complement fixation and causes *intravascular haemolysis.* The mechanism of haemolysis was elucidated by Donath and Landsteiner, who demonstrated haemolysis *in vitro* by first chilling the blood to allow the cold antibody to react with the red cells, followed by warming to allow complement activity. This was the first demonstration of an auto-immune disease mechanism, and the test is still used, although paroxysmal cold haemoglobinuria must now be extremely rare as a complication of syphilis, at least in this country.

Cold haemagglutinin disease. This occurs as a chronic condition, usually in middle-aged or older individuals. It is sometimes idiopathic, but more commonly secondary to various diseases, especially lymphomas and connective tissue diseases. An acute, self-limiting form follows certain infections, especially *primary atypical pneumonia* due to infection with *Mycoplasma pneumoniae.* The antibody is of IgM class and commonly reacts with the antigen I, which is present in the red cells of nearly all individuals. In the chronic disease the antibody is a product of a clone of lymphoid cells so is homogeneous (p. 125): there may be sufficient in the serum to be seen as an 'M' band on electrophoresis (p. 549). The thermal amplitude of antibodies of this type varies, and the disease occurs only in those subjects with antibody reacting at temperatures up to about 30 °C. The direct antiglobulin test is usually positive using anti-IgM or antibody to complement, but negative with class-specific anti-IgG. The haemagglutinin titre of the serum is usually 2000–64 000 when tested at 2°C. When the condition follows primary atypical pneumonia it is self-limiting and usually mild, the antibody disappearing within a few months.

II.B. Iso-antibodies to red cells

(1) Haemolytic disease of the newborn (HDN). Fetal red cells commonly enter the maternal circulation during labour and sometimes they provoke the formation of antibodies to blood group antigens foreign to the mother. Such immune iso-antibodies tend to belong to the IgG class and are thus capable of crossing the placental barrier in subsequent pregnancies, with the result that the fetal red cells will be damaged should they possess the appropriate antigen (Fig. 6.5, p. 151). Since at least twenty common blood group systems are known to exist, some degree of fetal maternal incompatibility is inevitable, but in practice the Rh system (p. 267), and in particular the antigen D, is responsible for most of the severe cases of HDN. The disease only occurs in a small proportion of those at risk (i.e. of those with an Rh −ve mother and an Rh +ve father). This is because: (*a*) the first born child, for reasons already given, is not affected unless the mother has been previously immunised by a blood transfusion or previous abortion; (*b*) the father is sometimes heterozygous (Dd), in which case the fetus has a 50 per cent chance of being Rh −ve; (*c*) ABO incompatibility between mother and fetus often prevents immunisation of the mother with fetal (e.g. D) antigen. Incompatible fetal red cells (say Group A) entering the maternal circulation are destroyed by maternal natural (anti-A) iso-antibody before they can stimulate production of Rh antibodies. ABO incompatibility itself rarely causes severe HDN because the antibodies are usually of the IgM class and incapable of crossing the placenta, although occasionally IgG antibody is present and causes a relatively mild form of the disease.

HDN varies considerably in severity. In milder forms there may only be transient jaundice and anaemia—**congenital haemolytic anaemia**—and treatment is often unnecessary, or simple blood transfusion alone is sufficient. A more dangerous form, known as **icterus gravis neonatorum**, is of extreme importance, for urgent treatment is required and is often successful. In this condition jaundice develops shortly after birth, and if the level of unconjug-

ated serum bilirubin is allowed to exceed 15 mg per ml (250 μmol per litre) there is a serious danger of permanent brain damage—*kernicterus* (p. 746). The infant is usually anaemic, with reticulocytosis and many normoblasts and primitive erythroblasts in the blood. Marked hepatosplenomegaly is usual and in fatal cases there is widespread liver cell necrosis, together with extensive extramedullary haemopoiesis in the spleen, liver, kidneys and adrenals. The only effective treatment of this condition is exchange transfusion, that is the removal of red cells from the fetus and their replacement by compatible red cells (e.g. lacking D antigen). When very severe, HDN causes intrauterine death due to marked anaemia and congestive cardiac failure—**hydrops fetalis.**

The possibility of HDN should become known from blood grouping early in pregnancy, if necessary also on the husband. The mother's serum should be examined during pregnancy for incomplete Rh and other antibodies. Confirmation of HDN can be obtained by detecting a raised level of bilirubin in samples of aspirated amniotic fluid. Early delivery may save some infants, but with others intrauterine fetal transfusion with Rh −ve blood is indicated. Once the infant is born, the diagnosis and treatment are based on the detection of IgG antibody on its red cells by the direct antiglobulin test (p. 111), and assessment of the blood changes and clinical features outlined above.

There have been most significant advances in the prevention of HDN. Trials initiated by Clarke (1973) demonstrated conclusively that intravenous injection of Rh antibody (anti-D) of IgG class into the mother, shortly after delivery, greatly reduces the chance of her developing anti-D antibody herself and lessens the risk of HDN in subsequent pregnancies. Such prophylactic injections are now widely used. It is, of course, most important to avoid Rh-incompatible blood transfusions, which were formerly an important cause of iso-immunisation.

Incompatibilities in other blood group systems, e.g. Kell and Duffy, may also cause HDN.

(2) Transfusion reactions. When incompatible blood is transfused into a recipient in whose circulation the appropriate antibodies are already present, a haemolytic transfusion reaction results and the transfused cells are rapidly destroyed. The results of an incompatible transfusion depend to some extent on the speed of destruction of the transfused red cells and this is likely to be greater when abundant iso-antibody is present, e.g. in ABO incompatibility, especially transfusion of Group A blood into a Group O recipient, or of Rh positive blood into an Rh negative *immunised* recipient. These are not the only incompatibilities encountered, but are so much the most common that stringent precautions must be taken to avoid them. The patient is likely to suffer a rigor, pain in the back and pyrexia; shortly thereafter haemoglobinuria appears, followed by jaundice. In a severe reaction death from shock may occur within a few minutes. If the patient survives, haemostatic failure may develop, or acute renal failure may ensue (p. 848).

Similar clinical effects may result from the transfusion of blood that is too old, or contaminated by micro-organisms, some of which are cryophilic and grow freely at refrigerator temperature.

II.C. Parasitic invasion of red cells

In malaria and oroya fever the parasites invade and destroy large numbers of red cells, thus producing an anaemia.

(1) Malaria. This is still one of the most important infectious diseases in the world. In spite of the development of effective drug therapy it remains a major contributory cause of deaths, particularly in children, and of chronic ill-health in the many parts of the world where it is endemic. It presents as severe bouts of fever, of sudden onset and with headache, muscle pains and haemolytic anaemia. Classically, such bouts occur at regular intervals, depending on the life cycle of the parasite in man, but in chronic cases and in those on inadequate drug suppression the fever is often irregular. With increasing world travel and mass migration, malaria is one of the tropical diseases now being encountered in temperate zones where its diagnosis presents particular problems.

There are three classical types of malaria caused by four different parasites. These are **tertian**, with paroxysms of fever every *second* day, caused by *Plasmodium vivax* and by *Plasmodium ovale*, **quartan**, with paroxysms at 72 hour intervals, caused by *Plasmodium malariae* and

subtertian or **malignant** malaria caused by *Plasmodium falciparum*, in which the fever is irregular. These parasites belong to the *Haemosporidia*, a sub-class of the *Sporozoa*. The first three are closely allied, being of the same genus, and the gametocytes or sexual cells are spherical; in the fourth the gametocytes are crescentic. Each parasite passes through two cycles of development—an asexual one of *schizogony* in man, and a sexual one of *sporogony* in the mosquito. In man the gametocytes are formed, but their development into gametes and conjugation occur only in the mosquito. For each species of plasmodium several species of mosquito of the genus *Anopheles* are capable of carrying infection. The onset of a febrile attack of malaria coincides with the setting free of a new brood of young parasites (merozoites), produced by the division of the adult forms within the red cells (Fig. 17.22), and the periodicity of fever depends on the time taken for the full cycle of development. Multiple infection occurs when parasites are introduced by mosquitoes on more than one occasion, so that parasites at different stages of development are present. Sometimes also mixed infection occurs, e.g. by the tertian and subtertian parasites.

Cycle of development in man. When man is bitten by infected mosquitoes, sporozoites are injected and are carried to the liver, where they undergo a stage of development within the hepatic cells (Fig. 17.23). This culminates after 6–9 days in the liberation of merozoites in large numbers into the blood, where they enter the red cells. This pre-erythrocytic development constitutes the incubation period of the disease of about 6–9 days. Within the red cells the parasites go through successive cycles of schizogony which cause the paroxysms of fever. It is highly probable that there are persistent exoerythrocytic forms of *P. vivax* and *P. malariae*, from which the relapses so characteristic of these infections are derived.

Malarial anaemia. With each bout of fever a large number of red cells are destroyed by the parasites, and the dark brown pigment formed from the haemoglobin is taken up by monocytes and by macrophages in the spleen, liver, etc. It is accordingly not surprising that in chronic malaria anaemia may be severe. It is generally of the normochromic or mildly microcytic type and there is an early reticulocytosis, but in chronic cases deficient formation of red cells may be present. A few normoblasts may sometimes be found. When severe, mal-

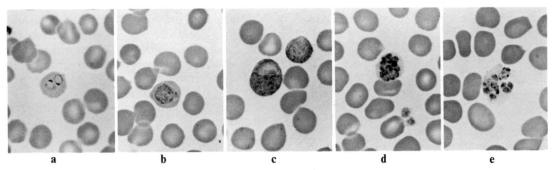

a b c d e

Fig. 17.22 Malaria, showing the various stages of *Plasmodium vivax* in the red cells. Merozoites formed in the liver, etc., enter the red cells and develop into trophozoites which in the early stage are ring-shaped **(a)**. As the trophozoite grows, chromatin increases and this, together with malaria pigment, gives the cytoplasm a granular appearance **(b)**. The fully grown trophozoite (schizont) almost fills and enlarges the red cell **(c)**. Division into merozoites then occurs **(d)** and these are released, with lysis of the red cell **(e)** and fever. The merozoites then enter other red cells. × 800. (The late Dr. H. E. Hutchinson.)

arial anaemia may become macrocytic, especially in falciparum infections. This may, in some cases at least, be due to excessive demands for folic acid. There is usually a mild leukopenia, but with an increase in monocytes, some of which may contain malarial pigment (Fig. 17.24). In chronic cases the serum level of IgM is often abnormally high. The certain **diagnosis** of malaria depends on detecting the parasites in thick or thin blood film preparations; thin films are better for species identification.

Blackwater fever is an acute attack of intravascular haemolysis, occurring usually in Europeans who have or have had subtertian malaria. There is haemoglobinaemia and methaem-albuminaemia and the urine is dark from the presence of haemoglobin and methaemoglobin. It is accompanied by fever, vomiting, shock, and sometimes convulsions and coma, and is often fatal. Acute renal failure with anuria is common. The haemolytic mechanism is not known: the condition was often associated with inadequate prophylaxis with quinine and is much less common when modern synthetic anti-malarial drugs are used.

Other effects. Quartan malaria is an important cause of glomerulonephritis in children (p. 827) and probable accounts for some cases of tropical splenomegaly (p. 564). Subtertian malaria can give rise to a wide variety of conditions,

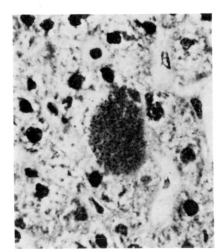

Fig. 17.23 Malaria: development of merozoites within a liver cell × 600. (Preparation kindly lent by Professor P. C. Garnham.)

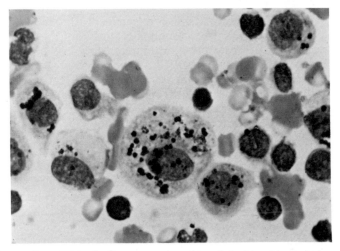

Fig. 17.24 Buffy coat preparation of the blood in malaria, showing monocytes containing pigment. × 680.

some of which are apparently due to blockage of the small vessels of internal organs by aggregated parasitised red cells: the changes may affect mainly the brain (*cerebral malaria*), or the lungs, producing a haemorrhagic pulmonary oedema, or an acute shock syndrome (*algid malaria*) may develop, but the manifestations are many and varied. In chronic malaria there is defective antibody production and various *secondary bacterial infections* are common.

The possible relationship between malaria and *Burkitt's lymphoma* (p. 305) is of considerable interest. The geographical distributions of the two conditions in Africa coincide fairly closely, and it seems likely that either malaria in childhood, or an infective oncogenic agent transmitted by insects, plays a carcinogenic role.

(2) Oroya fever. This is caused by infection with a small Gram-ve bacillus—*Bartonella bacilliformis*—which colonises the red cells and macrophages. Infection is transmitted by certain species of sandfly (*Phlebotomus*) and is limited to the slopes of the Andes. The infected red cells show increased mechanical fragility and become sequestered in the liver and spleen, haemolytic anaemia resulting. The organisms can be seen in Romanowsky-stained blood films. Fever, joint and muscle pains, and enlarged lymph nodes are followed by a papular skin eruption.

II.D. Haemolytic toxins and chemicals

Bacterial toxins. Extensive infections with bacteria which secrete haemolytic toxins can result in acute haemolysis. Examples are *Cl. welchii* and *Strep. pyogenes*.

Haemolytic chemicals are numerous. Phenylhydrazine, lead, arseniuretted hydrogen, saponin, potassium chlorate are a few examples which have been extensively investigated. In *chronic lead poisoning* the effect of lead is upon the red cell surface, rendering the cells brittle and increasing the mechanical but diminishing the osmotic fragility: they are short-lived, and mild anaemia results. Lead also interferes with haemoglobin synthesis and the utilisation of iron and in consequence *sideroblasts* (p. 510 and Fig. 2.15, p. 22) are seen in the marrow and the mature red cells tend to be *microcytic* although the patient is not iron deficient. Lead also precipitates the RNA of young polychromatophilic erythrocytes in the form of *punctate*

basophilia (p. 510), seen as 'stippled' cells which are most easily detected in smears from the buffy coat. Diagnosis can, however, be achieved earlier and with more certainty by estimating the concentration of lead in the blood. The disorder in haemoglobin synthesis induced by lead is reflected in the high levels of erythrocyte protoporphyrin, urinary coproporphyrin and δ-aminolaevulinic acid, the estimation of which can also be valuable in diagnosis.

Drugs. These are an important cause of haemolysis, involving various mechanisms. Most common is the *Heinz body type of haemolytic anaemia*, in which there is oxidative denaturation of the haemoglobin molecule (p. 510 sometimes preceded by methaemoglobinaemia. Many drugs with oxidative potential have been incriminated, including phenacetin, sulphonamides, salazopyrin, dapsone and primaquine. *Individuals with a defective hexose monophosphate shunt mechanism, usually as a result of glucose-6-phosphate dehydrogenase deficiency (p. 522), are particularly susceptible*, although if drugs of this kind are taken in large enough amounts even normal individuals are affected. Haemolysis is usually only moderate and tends to be self-limiting since reticulocytes are more resistant to this kind of drug-induced damage. Withdrawal of the drug is curative. Occasionally drugs produce haemolysis by an *antibody-mediated mechanism*. Such drugs act as haptens and stimulate the production of antibodies. In two instances (*penicillin* and *cephalosporin*) metabolites of the drug bind firmly to the red cells, destruction of which is then brought about by the reaction of antibody with the cell-bound hapten. Other haptenic drugs form immune complexes in the plasma and these bind to the red cells and mediate their destruction. Thirdly, the anti-hypertensive drug α-*methyldopa* induces formation of auto-antibodies which are identical with those of the warm antibody type of auto-immune haemolytic anaemia, but gradually disappear on stopping the drug. These drug-induced immunologically-mediated conditions are described more fully on p. 160.

Vegetable poisons. The term 'alimentary haemolysis' is used to describe haemolytic states arising as a result of the ingestion of various fruits and vegetables. Usually this only happens in individuals affected by the more severe Mediterranean type of glucose-6-phosphate dehydrogenase deficiency. The best-known example is **favism**, caused by the ingestion of broad beans (*Vicia faba*). The chemical component in beans responsible for haemolysis is uncertain, although it known to induce oxidative denaturation of haemoglobin with the formation of Heinz bodies (p. 510). Similar haemolysis can result from inhalation of certain pollens.

II.E Mechanical damage to red cells

March haemoglobinuria. This consists of acute haemoglobinuria, usually mild, resulting from long marches. The haemolysis is now believed to be due to mechanical injury to the red cells sustained in the circulation through the soft tissues of the plantar aspect of the feet and brought on by the prolonged mild trauma of long walks, particularly on hard surfaces and carrying heavy loads. Haemoglobinuria has also been reported from mechanical trauma of red cells in the soft tissues of the hands in over-enthusiastic exponents of **karate**.

Microangiopathic haemolytic anaemia is a haemolytic state of varying severity, associated with red-cell fragmentation (Fig. 17.25) and thrombocytopenia; it is observed in various clinical situations, including obstetric complications such as ante-partum haemorrhage and pre-eclampsia, malignant hypertension, thrombotic thrombocytopenic purpura (Moschcowitz syndrome), the 'haemolytic-uraemic' syndrome of childhood (p. 852), carcinomatosis, especially if the tumour is of mucin-secreting type, and in septic shock (p. 264). A common factor in all these conditions is the presence of

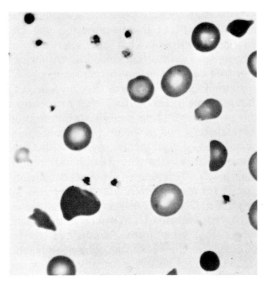

Fig. 17.25 Fragmentation of red cells in microangiopathic haemolytic anaemia. × 1000.

widespread fibrin deposition in small blood vessels due either to intravascular activation of the blood-clotting mechanism or to vascular damage (microangiopathy). It is thought that the red cells are fragmented when they become enmeshed in fibrin strands or adhere to damaged endothelium. A similar form of red-cell fragmentation has also been observed in patients with prosthetic heart valves, which invariably produce some degree of red cell damage, occasionally resulting in overt intravascular haemolysis with haemosiderinuria and even iron deficiency.

Dyshaemopoietic anaemias

The essential feature of this type of anaemia is the failure to deliver to the blood sufficient numbers of normal red cells despite the presence of adequate precursors in the marrow. Indeed, under the influence of erythropoietin, there is often grossly increased marrow cellularity in dyshaemopoietic anaemias, which contrasts strikingly with the paucity of red cells in the circulating blood. This implies that many of the red cell precursors fail to produce red cells, either because maturation is arrested or because they are destroyed. Both phenomena occur, and

much of the erythropoietic activity is ineffective (p. 517). Anaemias of this type are usually due to failure of the marrow to obtain substrates which it requires for normal red cell maturation. The most important examples are the megaloblastic anaemias and iron-deficiency anaemia.

Megaloblastic anaemia

This form of anaemia is characterised by the presence in the bone marrow of a distinct abnor-

mality of haemopoiesis known as **megaloblastic change.** This affects granulocytes and platelets as well as red cells, but the alteration in erythropoiesis is most conspicuous. *By far the commonest cause of megaloblastic haemopoiesis is deficiency of either vitamin B$_{12}$ or folic acid* although, much less often, similar changes occur in cytotoxic drug therapy, rare inherited enzyme defects, and in the uncommon neoplastic condition of erythraemic myelosis (di Guglielmo's disease). In the peripheral blood, megaloblastic anaemia is typified by an increase in the mean corpuscular volume (MCV) of the red cells and is the commonest cause of 'macrocytic' anaemia. It must be emphasised, however, that other forms of anaemia can be macrocytic in the absence of megaloblastic marrow change. This is especially true of the anaemia of alcoholic liver disease, but anaemia following severe haemorrhage or haemolysis or with extramedullary haemopoiesis is occasionally macrocytic, presumably because of a high reticulocyte count, although some forms of aplastic or refractory anaemia also show this change.

The effects of vitamin B$_{12}$ and folic acid deficiencies

Of the many tissues affected by deficiency of these two substances, those in which there is a high rate of cell replacement or nucleic acid synthesis are particularly susceptible. This explains the predominant involvement of the haemopoietic system, in which the haemopoietic changes are identical in vitamin B$_{12}$ and folic acid deficiency. In some other tissues, however, the effects differ; spinal cord changes, for example, are only obvious in B$_{12}$ deficiency.

   (1) Peripheral blood. In fully developed cases the red cells, granulocytes and platelets are all reduced in number, i.e. there is a **pancytopenia**. The red cells usually show an increase in MCV and since the MCHC is normal, the MCH rises in direct proportion to the MCV. These changes may all be evident before anaemia becomes apparent. As anaemia develops, the red cells show increasing variation in size (anisocytosis) with many small cells or cell fragments as well as macrocytes over 10 μm in diameter. Red cells of grossly abnormal shape (poikilocytes) are also conspicuous in advanced cases (Fig. 17.26). Nucleated red cells, often with megalo-

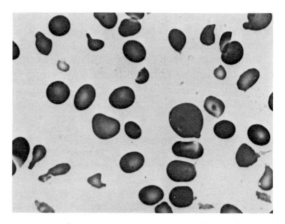

Fig. 17.26   Red cells in pernicious anaemia, prepared from below the buffy coat, showing gross anisopoikilocytosis. × 650.

blastic features (see below), can almost always be detected in severe cases (Fig. 17.27), especially in smears prepared from the buffy coat (p. 511) in centrifuged whole blood. This technique may be diagnostically useful should marrow examination prove to be impracticable. The reticulocyte count is usually less than 2 per cent, although sometimes there is a slight increase in serum bilirubin. This latter may, however, result from breakdown of red cell precursors in the marrow (see below). There is often significant neutropenia, associated with the presence of large hypersegmented neutrophils with six or more lobes (macropolycytes), often detectable at an early stage of the disease. Conversely, occasional myelocytes are seen in severe cases. Platelets are moderately reduced,

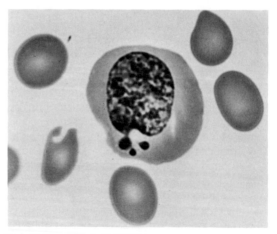

Fig. 17.27   Blood in pernicious anaemia showing a megaloblast with Howell–Jolly bodies. × 1300.

but may fall below $50 \times 10^9/l$ ($50\,000/\mu l$) and purpura may then result (p. 557).

(2) Bone marrow. Diagnostic changes are observed in marrow aspirated from sites in the axial skeleton, such as the sternum or iliac crest. The cellularity in such aspirates is maximal, with complete loss of the fat spaces (Fig. 17.28), even when anaemia is minimal. Necropsy studies further reveal the marked expansion in haemopoietic tissue, which may ultimately extend throughout the entire length of the long bones (Fig. 17.29). Cytologically all the haemopoietic elements are affected to some extent. Erythropoiesis undergoes a profound alteration, described as **megaloblastic change** nearly 100 years ago by Ehrlich, who noted its resemblance to the form of erythropoiesis predominating in fetal life. *The essential feature of this change is a delay in nuclear maturation, with the accumulation of many cells in an early stage of development* (Fig. 17.30). *Not only is there maturation arrest but many of the immature cells die in the marrow. This is called* **ineffective erythropoiesis** *and is the hallmark of a dyshaemopoietic anaemia.* Morphologically, nuclear immaturity is expressed by an increase in nuclear size with a characteristically stippled chromatin pattern. A variety of other 'dyserythropoietic' abnormalities, including polyploidy and

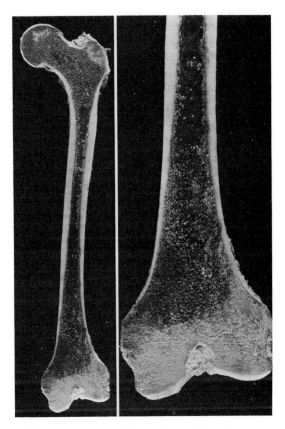

Fig. 17.29 Section of femur in pernicious anaemia, showing the dark red marrow throughout the shaft. *Left,* $\times 0.3$. *Right,* lower end, $\times 0.7$.

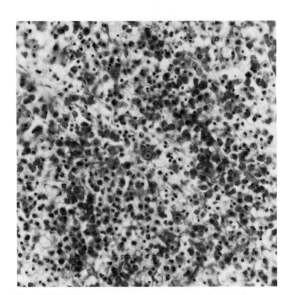

Fig. 17.28 Bone marrow from femoral shaft in pernicious anaemia, showing an extreme degree of megaloblastic hyperplasia with complete loss of fat and absorption of the bony trabeculae. $\times 250$.

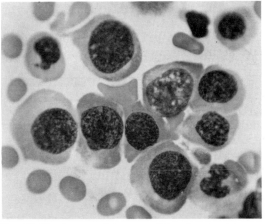

Fig. 17.30 Smear of bone marrow from a case of pernicious anaemia, showing large megaloblasts. $\times 1100$.

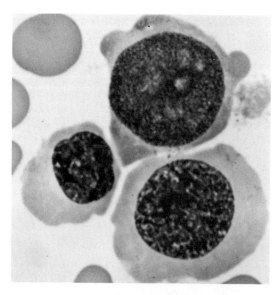

Fig. 17.31 Smear of bone marrow in pernicious anaemia, showing a promegaloblast (*above*) and two typical haemoglobinised megaloblasts. × 1700.

nuclear fragmentation with Howell–Jolly body formation (Fig. 17.27), can also be found. Haemoglobinisation of the cytoplasm of developing erythroblasts is much less seriously affected, and the asynchrony between nuclear and cytoplasmic maturation leads to the appearance of the most distinctive manifestation of megaloblastic erythropoiesis in the marrow, the '**haemoglobinised megaloblast**', a cell which, although fully haemoglobinised, possesses an immature nucleus (Fig. 17.31). The various stages of normoblastic and megaloblastic erythropoiesis are compared in Figs. 17.1 and 17.2 (p. 505). Interference with granulocytic development is most readily identified by the presence of abnormality at the metamyelocyte stage. This cell is greatly enlarged, and possesses a large horseshoe-shaped unsegmented nucleus (the giant metamyelocyte). Megakaryocytes are often difficult to find, possibly as a result of a defect in the maturation of precursors.

(3) **Neurological changes.** These are only conspicuous in B_{12} deficiency, and it is important to note that *they may be present when anaemia is mild or even absent*. The principal lesion is referred to as **subacute combined degeneration** of the spinal cord, characterised by a discontinuous demyelination of the long pyramidal tracts and posterior columns in the mid-thoracic region. There is in addition a **peripheral neuropathy**, and foci of demyelination are sometimes found in the cerebral hemispheres. These changes are fully described on pp. 778–81. Early clinical recognition of subacute combined degeneration is extremely important because, although it can be arrested by treatment, it is disabling and not completely reversible. Further, *the administration of folic acid alone can exacerbate the condition. Should urgent treatment of a megaloblastic anaemia be required before the cause can be established, it is essential to give both B_{12} and folic acid.*

(4) **Other tissue effects.** Epithelial changes can be detected in both B_{12} and folic acid deficiency. Atrophy of the epithelium of the tongue, sometimes associated with glossitis and focal ulceration, is a common feature of B_{12} deficiency, and megalocytic epithelial cells have also been detected in smears from the cervix uteri. In both B_{12} and folic acid deficiency mild villous atrophy may be found in the small intestine (p. 642) and 'megaloblastic' nuclear changes have been observed in the crypts of Lieberkuhn. Sterility, presumably due to disturbed maturation of germ cells in the gonads, has been described both in males and females suffering from B_{12} deficiency and can be reversed by specific therapy. Marked haemosiderin deposition in the renal tubules is observed in untreated cases of megaloblastic anaemia, probably a result of the haemolytic element mentioned above. Slight to moderate splenic enlargement, due to increased red cell destruction or to extramedullary haemopoiesis, is often present.

Causes of vitamin B_{12} deficiency

Although existing in several forms, B_{12} is basically a cobalamin which consists of a cobalt-containing porphyrin linked to a ribonucleoside. It is derived mainly from animal sources, such as glandular meats, muscle and eggs, although produced commercially from bacteria and moulds. The minimal daily requirement is approximately 1 μg and the normal serum level as assayed by microbiological techniques is between 160 and 1000 ng/litre (=pg/ml). Normally the liver stores sufficient vitamin to provide the total needs for 3 to 7 years. Absorption from the gut is dependent on the binding of dietary B_{12} to a gastric mucoprotein known as intrinsic factor (IF), the existence of which was demonstrated by

Castle in 1929. In man, IF is produced by the parietal cells of the gastric fundus and the IF-B_{12} complex formed in the stomach traverses the greater part of the small bowel before the vitamin is absorbed in the terminal ileum. The causes of B_{12} deficiency are as follows.

(1) **Dietary deficiency.** Diets deficient in B_{12} are quite common in, and largely restricted to, underdeveloped parts of the world. Strict vegetarians would theoretically be expected to develop B_{12} deficiency, but this is observed only occasionally.

(2) **Intrinsic factor (IF) deficiency.** This is by far the commonest cause of B_{12} deficiency. The classical example is **pernicious anaemia**, recognition of which is usually attributed to Addison in 1855. This disease, described in detail below, results from a diffuse atrophic gastritis, in which there is almost complete destruction of the specialised fundal cells, including the all-important parietal cells, by an inflammatory process now thought to be auto-immune in origin.* Total gastrectomy also eliminates IF secretion, but overt signs of B_{12} deficiency may be delayed as long as 10 years if the liver stores are normal. A small proportion of patients also develops B_{12} deficiency following partial gastrectomy, usually due to chronic gastritis in the remaining portion of the stomach. Rarely, B_{12} deficiency is due to a congenital deficiency of, or functionally defective, IF secretion, although the stomach is morphologically normal.

(3) **The 'blind-loop' syndrome.** There are several conditions in which the IF-B_{12} complex formed normally in the stomach fails to reach its absorptive site in the distal ileum. Uptake of B_{12} by bacteria proliferating abnormally in the more proximal parts of the small bowel is the usual cause. Almost any form of intestinal stasis, if sufficiently prolonged, can cause such colonisation, although surgical blind loops, jejunal diverticula and chronic obstruction are most often responsible, and co-existent malabsorption of fat can usually be demonstrated. Stasis in the afferent jejunal loop might be involved in some cases following partial gastrectomy of the Polya type. Infestation with the tapeworm *Diphyllobothrium latum* which absorbs B_{12} (free and bound to IF) is a rare cause of megaloblastic anaemia in Finland and

probably occurs only in individuals who also have atrophic gastritis and thus impaired IF production.

(4) **Malabsorption.** Extensive disease of the distal ileum interferes with the final stage of B_{12} absorption. This occurs invariably in tropical sprue (p. 642) but in only 30 per cent of cases of adult coeliac disease, in which the mucosal lesions tend to be mild or even absent in the distal ileum (p. 641). In Crohn's disease (p. 620) in which the terminal ileum is frequently involved, B_{12} deficiency is a recognised complication, and of course surgical resection of the ileum inevitably eliminates B_{12} absorption. A rare congenital condition in which there is an isolated defect of B_{12} absorption in the ileum has also been described.

Pernicious anaemia

This disease was the first cause of B_{12} deficiency to be described and is still the most important. It is particularly prevalent in individuals of North European stock and is predominantly a disease of the elderly, being uncommon under the age of 40 years. There is a strong familial tendency, relatives of patients being at much greater risk of developing it than the general population. Relatives also have a high incidence of auto-immune thyroiditis, and there is convincing evidence that pernicious anaemia belongs to the group of organ-specific auto-immune disturbances (p. 163). The basic lesion is a diffuse atrophic gastritis (p. 605), involving the fundal portion of the stomach and leading ultimately to histamine-fast achlorhydria and grossly impaired IF secretion. Antibodies to parietal cells are found in the serum in 90 per cent of cases, and in 60 per cent antibodies to IF itself can also be demonstrated. Perhaps more significantly, IF antibodies have been found in the gastric juice in about 50 per cent of cases and in the majority the antibodies block the B_{12} binding site of IF, thus inactivating what little IF is secreted by the atrophic gastric mucosa. Appearance of IF antibody in the gastric juice is often the final event precipitating frank B_{12} deficiency. In the few young patients with pernicious anaemia, IF antibody is more frequently found and there

---

*It is a curious coincidence that both of Addison's diseases should have turned out to be in the organ-specific auto-immune group (p. 162).

are often associated auto-immune disturbances such as adrenal insufficiency, hypoparathyroidism and malabsorption ('juvenile pernicious anaemia'). The role of auto-immunity in these diseases, including atrophic gastritis, is discussed on pp. 163 and 606. Symptoms directly referable to the stomach are seldom evident, and the effects of B_{12} deficiency, especially anaemia and neurological disturbance, dominate the clinical picture. There is, however, an increased risk of gastric carcinoma in patients with pernicious anaemia. The anaemia is usually insidious and many patients are severely anaemic before they seek medical advice.

The diagnosis of vitamin B_{12} deficiency states

Once evidence of a megaloblastic anaemia has been obtained, usually by marrow examination, B_{12} deficiency is established by the demonstration of a reduced level of the vitamin in the serum, which is assayed by radioimmunoassay (p. 112) or by a microbiological technique. The marrow reverts to normoblastic erythropoiesis within 24 hours of parenteral administration of B_{12} and confirmation of the diagnosis is provided by a reticulocytosis in the blood within 10 days. It is now standard practice to identify the cause of B_{12} deficiency by the use of radioisotopic techniques, especially the *Schilling test*. In this test, a small dose of B_{12} labelled with ^{58}Co is administered orally, followed by a parenteral loading dose of 1000 μg of unlabelled vitamin to prevent cellular uptake of any of the labelled B_{12} absorbed from the gut. The degree of absorption is assessed by measuring either the urinary excretion of labelled vitamin over a 24-hour period, or the serum level after 36 hours. If dietary deficiency is responsible, absorption is normal, whereas in IF deficiency, as in pernicious anaemia, there is subnormal absorption which is corrected when IF is given orally together with labelled B_{12}. In the blind loop syndrome, IF does not improve absorption, although broad-spectrum antibiotics usually do so. More specific therapy is, however, required to improve B_{12} absorption in malabsorptive states, e.g. the gluten-free diet in coeliac disease (p. 640). Although the demonstration of IF deficiency is necessary for certain diagnosis of pernicious anaemia, the demonstration either of histamine-fast achlorhydria or

of antibody to IF establishes the diagnosis beyond reasonable doubt. Antibody to parietal cells is not so helpful, for it is common in people with less severe gastritis, without pernicious anaemia.

Causes of folic acid deficiency

Folic acid (pteroyl-glutamic acid) consists of pteridine and para-aminobenzoic acid coupled to glutamic acid. The main dietary sources are fresh green vegetables, e.g. spinach and lettuce, cereals, meat, fish and eggs. The estimated minimum daily requirement is 50 μg, but much more is needed in pregnancy and in some pathological states (see below). The storage capacity of the body is sufficient for about 80–100 days. Absorption of folic acid takes place predominantly in the upper small bowel. The causes of folic acid deficiency are as follows.

(1) Dietary deficiency. This is a common contributory factor in many folic acid deficiency states, and is of particular importance in elderly people on a poor diet and in infancy when weaning is delayed; dried milk is also a poor source of folic acid. Any condition in which there is anorexia and poor dietary intake, e.g. alcoholism or chronic gastrointestinal disease, predisposes to folic acid deficiency.

(2) Malabsorption. Only two conditions are known with certainty to cause malabsorption of folic acid, namely coeliac disease (p. 640) in which folic acid deficiency is invariable, and tropical sprue (p. 642). In both these diseases there are extensive pathological changes in the upper small bowel. Few other intestinal diseases produce such extensive chronic lesions and folic acid deficiency arising in conditions such as Crohn's disease (p. 620) or following partial gastrectomy, are more likely to be due to impaired dietary intake. There is, however, a rare condition known as *congenital malabsorption of folate*, which is thought to be due to an inherited defect in the intestinal mucosal transport system for folic acid.

(3) Increased requirements. The most important condition in which the requirement for folic acid is increased is pregnancy, the haematological complications of which discussed below. Diseases in which there is greatly increased haemopoietic activity, such as haemolytic states, leukaemia or the myeloproliferative disorders (p. 552), or rapid proliferation (usually neoplastic) of other tissues, can similarly predispose to folic acid deficiency.

(4) Drugs. It cannot be over-emphasised that therapeutic agents can produce an astonishing variety of haematological disturbances, and one of the most notable examples of this is the megaloblastic anaemia associated with **anticonvulsant drugs such as phenytoin**. The mechanism involved is uncertain, but these drugs probably interfere with folic acid absorption. It is also suspected that oral contraceptives can lead to folate deficiency. Some drugs are **folic acid antagonists** and are given deliberately to induce folate deficiency in dividing tumour cells (e.g. methotrexate, cytosine arabinoside) or to combat infection (e.g. cotrimoxazole—Septrin): some degree of megaloblastic change in the marrow is thus inevitable.

The diagnosis of folic acid deficiency

Anaemia with megaloblastic haemopoiesis in the absence of B_{12} deficiency strongly suggests deficiency of folic acid. The microbiological assay of the serum folate level, using *Lactobacillus casei* as the test organism, has some diagnostic value if the result is less than 3 μg/litre, although the more time-consuming assay of the red cell folate content is more reliable, especially in deficiency of some duration, but a low red-cell folate, less than 100 μg/litre, may be found in B_{12} deficiency. Whole blood folate assays by radioimmunoassay are being increasingly used, but they too have drawbacks, and the *haematological response to folic acid remains the most convincing evidence of deficiency.*

The biological actions of B_{12} and folic acid

These two substances are important for normal cell function, and in particular for normal cell division. Their activities are clearly interrelated, although the nature of this relationship has yet to be fully clarified. Certainly both act as co-enzymes in a number of biochemical reactions. The main co-enzymic function of folic acid is the transfer of single carbon units in such reactions as the breakdown of histidine, the synthesis of methionine and, of particular relevance to the pathogenesis of megaloblastic haemopoiesis, the synthesis of DNA and RNA. It now seems likely that folic acid is only active biologically in the polyglutamate form, and that B_{12} is required for the intracellular conversion of the transport form of folic acid, 5-methyl-tetrahydrofolate, to the polyglutamate form. This would explain why B_{12} deficiency leads to megaloblastic haemopoiesis, which is largely due to a failure of DNA synthesis, and to neurological disturbance, thought to be a result of impaired RNA synthesis in nerve cells (Chanarin, 1979). It would also account for the observation that biochemical tests of folic acid deficiency, such as the urinary excretion of formimino-glutamic acid (FIGLU) following a loading oral dose of histidine, are often positive in B_{12} deficiency. B_{12}, however, has other co-enzymic functions, including a critical part in the catablolism of methyl-malonic acid, an intermediate product of valine and propionic acid metabolism: B_{12} deficiency thus leads to the appearance of this metabolite in the urine following a loading dose of valine, a test of potential diagnostic value.

Anaemias of pregnancy

It is well recognised that the haemoglobin level tends to fall during normal pregnancy. This so-called 'physiological anaemia' is probably due to an expansion of plasma volume rather than to any fall in the total haemoglobin content of the blood. Nevertheless, true anaemia is common, mainly because of the demands of the developing fetus on iron and folic acid. These demands are greatest during the later months of pregnancy. An adequate diet will normally meet the increasing requirements imposed on the mother, but haematinic deficiency is especially liable to develop when a woman is in negative haematinic balance at the onset of pregnancy.

Iron deficiency is common enough in non-pregnant women of reproductive age (p. 538) and not surprisingly is the commonest cause of anaemia during pregnancy: although debilitating, it is seldom severe. **Megaloblastic anaemia**, often severe, is not uncommon in the last third of pregnancy. It is due to deficiency of folic acid and so the traditional term 'pernicious anaemia of pregnancy' is inappropriate and should be discarded. Since it is potentially dangerous for a woman to begin labour in an anaemic state, supplementation of the diet with both iron and folic acid is now a routine part of ante-natal care, and it is recommended that the daily intake of folic acid should be not less than 200 μg during pregnancy. Rarely other forms of anaemia, such as aplastic anaemia, arise during pregnancy, although almost any form of blood disorder can complicate pregnancy as a fortuitous event.

Congenital dyserythropoietic anaemia (CDA)

In this group of rare congenital conditions varying degrees of anaemia are associated with ineffective erythropoiesis and morphological abnormalities in red cell precursors unrelated to B_{12} or folate deficiency. There is hereditary erythroblastic multinuclearity together with a positive acid serum test for haemolysis (p. 525), hence the name HEMPAS. In other types 'megaloblastoid' and giant erythroblasts have been described.

Iron-deficiency anaemia

Since there is no excretory mechanism for iron, body iron content is controlled entirely by absorption from the gut. The mechanism of control of absorption, and the distribution, control and forms of storage of iron are discussed on p. 279 *et seq.*

Less than 1 mg of iron is lost passively from the body every day, and this is easily balanced by absorption of a similar amount of iron from food. In menstruating females, however, the average daily losses are increased to around 1·6 mg daily, and in the second and third trimesters of pregnancy the loss includes fetal requirements and is about 3·0 mg daily; iron balance is thus more precarious in women in the child-bearing era, and iron-deficiency anaemia occurs commonly in this group.

Negative iron balance results from excessive losses of iron from the body, or from impaired intake or absorption of iron relative to physiological requirements. In some patients both factors are involved. Negative iron balance is compensated for, for a time, by mobilisation of the iron stores and by enhanced absorption from the gut, allowing the haemoglobin to be maintained at normal levels. Eventually, however, the stores become depleted and the characteristic changes of iron deficiency begin to appear in the blood.

Causes of iron deficiency

(1) Low dietary intake of iron is an important factor in iron deficiency, especially in underdeveloped countries, and in infants before the onset of mixed feeding. Dietary deficiency of iron is, however, often not the sole cause of anaemia.

(2) Chronic blood loss. This is the only way by which large amounts of iron can be lost from the body. Heavy menstrual bleeding is important, but any source of chronic or recurrent blood loss will have the same effect. Of particular importance diagnostically is occult bleeding from unsuspected gastro-intestinal tract lesions, especially peptic ulceration, since iron-deficiency anaemia may be the only indication of such underlying conditions. Infestation with hookworm (ankylostomiasis), which causes considerable gastro-intestinal bleeding, is probably the most common cause of iron deficiency in the world, and an important cause of chronic morbidity in tropical areas.

(3) Malabsorption of iron. Iron is absorbed mainly in the duodenum and diseases affecting it may cause iron deficiency, e.g. coeliac disease. Normal gastric function is also important for iron absorption, and gastrectomy or achlorhydria predispose to iron deficiency.

(4) Increased requirement of iron due to expanding red cell mass occurs especially in actively growing infants and adolescents and in pregnancy (in which there are, in addition, the fetal requirements). Accordingly these groups, but particularly pregnant women, are prone to iron deficiency.

The blood picture

The anaemia is predominantly of the *microcytic type*, the cells being of smaller diameter than normal and of reduced volume, e.g. 50–70 fl (μm³). The MCH is reduced to 27 pg or less. In severe cases the MCHC also falls and the red cells may show ring-staining owing to deficiency in haemoglobin but this is not a reliable diagnostic feature, and can appear as an artefact in smears of normal blood. A more useful feature is the presence of poikilocytes, including rod-shaped cells (Fig. 17.32). The

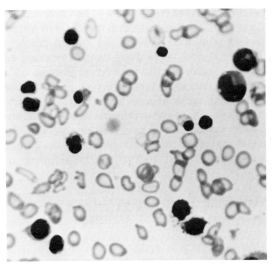

Fig. 17.33 Sternal marrow in severe microcytic anaemia, illustrating the increased proportion of erythroblasts, many of which are poorly haemoglobinised normoblasts. × 1000.

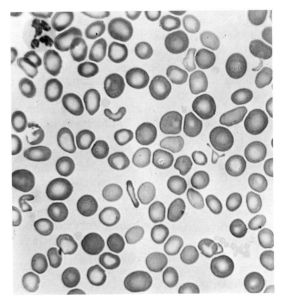

Fig. 17.32 Blood smear in iron-deficiency anaemia, showing some variation in the size of red cells and some rod cells: note that ring-staining is not conspicuous and certainly not diagnostic. × 800.

fall in the number of red cells is usually slight or moderate, and erythroblasts are rarely found. The leukocyte count is usually normal. The platelet count is also normal but in long-standing cases it may be increased. If blood loss is an important factor there may be a reticulocytosis. There may also be a very mild degree of haemolysis. The serum iron is low and the total iron-binding capacity is increased. **The marrow** is hyperplastic due to erythropoietin stimulation, but because of lack of iron, production of haemoglobin, and therefore of red cells, is inadequate: cytologically there is an increased number of early forms and of small, poorly haemoglobinised pyknotic normoblasts (Fig. 17.33). Sections of marrow stained by the prussian blue reaction show an absence of stainable iron in the macrophages, confirming that all storage iron has been used up.

Associated conditions

In iron deficiency, the haematological effects are the most obvious, but other signs of tissue iron depletion may be found. The nails become striated and brittle and may eventually become spoon-shaped (*koilonychia*). Atrophic glossitis and angular cheilosis with fissuring of the angles of the mouth also occur. A minority of patients suffer from dysphagia (difficulty in swallowing), which may be purely functional, but is sometimes related to a folding of lax mucosa in the upper oesophagus. Such an 'oesophageal web' may disappear with successful treatment of the anaemia. The association of anaemia, glossitis and dysphagia was first recorded by Brown-Kelly and Patterson in 1919, but is more usually known as the Plummer-Vinson syndrome; it may predispose to the later development of post-cricoid carcinoma of the oesophagus. A high proportion of iron-deficient patients have achlorhydria and there may be various degrees of gastric mucosal change ranging from superficial gastritis to gastric atrophy as severe as that found in pernicious anaemia. In most patients, however, it is likely that the achlorhydria is the result of iron deficiency, analogous to the other tissue changes mentioned above: only in a minority does it appear to precede and predispose to the anaemia by interfering with iron absorption. Once achlorhydria has developed, it will nevertheless tend to aggravate the iron deficiency. The oral and nail changes usually respond to iron, but achlorhydria may be permanent.

Iron deficiency is much the commonest cause of hypochromic microcytic anaemia, but any condition characterised by failure of haemoglobin synthesis will have the same effect. In some patients the fault may lie in globin synthesis (p. 524) and in others a failure to synthesise adequate amounts of haem.

Anaemia from disturbances of iron metabolism

Iron deficiency is a disorder of iron balance, but other anaemias are characterised by abnormalities in internal iron exchange. Iron derived from haemoglobin catabolism by macrophages is usually bound to plasma transferrin and returned to the bone marrow for haemoglobin synthesis; such iron is donated to the developing normoblasts by transferrin, and is later inserted into protoporphyrin to form haem. This pathway may be compromised in two situations:

(a) 'Secondary anaemia' in infections, fevers and wasting diseases. In chronic infections, rheumatic fever, rheumatoid disease and systemic lupus erythematosus, renal failure with uraemia, extensive carcinoma and other wasting diseases, there is often a mildly microcytic anaemia due partly to a block in release of iron by macrophages: the level of plasma iron is low and the erythroblasts are deficient in iron. In addition, there is often a depression of erythropoiesis in these conditions and often a mild reduction in red-cell lifespan. So long as the causal condition persists, treatment by oral iron therapy is usually ineffective.

(b) Sideroblastic anaemia. This is a heterogeneous group of disorders which have in common the presence of prussian blue +ve staining granules in the normoblasts, usually arranged around the nucleus in a ring fashion. granules are iron-laden mitochondria (Fig. 2.15, p. 22), and result from impairment of iron utilisation within the cell; since iron is not being inserted into the porphyrin precursors, haem cannot be formed and there is thus poor haemoglobinisation of the red cells. Sideroblastic anaemia may occur in a familial form, or be secondary to various conditions including carcinomas, leukaemia and exposure to drugs and toxins, notably lead and certain antituberculous drugs. Some cases respond to pyridoxine therapy.

Hypoplastic and aplastic anaemias

Anaemia due to diminution in the volume of haemopoietic marrow is termed *aplastic* when little or no cellular marrow exists, and *hypoplastic* when the marrow is merely of reduced cellularity, as is more commonly the case. Aplasia restricted to red cell precursors is rare and it is more usual for all the haemopoietic cell lines to be affected, resulting in pancytopenia in the peripheral blood; the blood picture is thus attributable to marrow failure to produce cellular elements in sufficient numbers to replace natural wastage from ageing or destruction. Pure red cell aplasia and pancytopenia may each occur in a congenital or acquired form:

(a) Pure red cell aplasia
   Congenital—Blackfan–Diamond   anaemia ('erythrogenesis imperfecta').

   Acquired—usually in adults, often associated with thymic tumours.
(b) Pancytopenia
   Congenital—Fanconi anaemia, usually associated with other mesenchymal, e.g. skeletal, abnormalities.
   Acquired—see below.
   All these forms are rare apart from acquired pancytopenia and this will be considered in greater detail below.

Aplastic anaemia with pancytopenia

The characteristic blood findings are normochromic, normocytic anaemia, granulocytopenia and thrombocytopenia; this produces anaemic manifestations which may be severe, increased liability to infection, which is often fatal, and thrombocytopenic bleeding. The bone marrow is hypocellular and fatty (Fig. 17.34) and most of the few cells left are lymphocytes and plasma cells. There may be small haemopoietic foci or, in cases of very rapid onset, patches of cell debris lying between the fat cells.

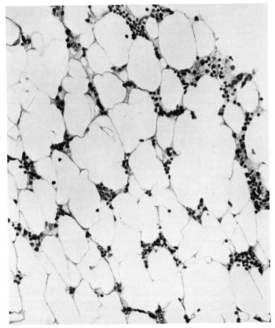

Fig. 17.34 Sternal marrow biopsy in aplastic anaemia due to chloramphenicol. There is great reduction in the numbers of all cell types. × 250.

Aplastic anaemia may be apparently spontaneous or may result from the administration of agents toxic to the bone marrow. *Cytotoxic drugs or x-rays used in the treatment of malignant disease regularly produce marrow depression in proportion to the dosage*; usually it is possible to avoid severe damage by careful monitoring of the blood and adjustment of dosage. In some patients, however, marrow aplasia results from an *idiosyncratic reaction* to certain drugs,

particularly chloramphenicol, sulphonamides, phenylbutazone and other antirheumatic agents, and antithyroid drugs; such drug reactions are now a major problem and are not infrequently fatal. However, some cases are reversible on stopping the drug. Some hair dyes and many industrial organic chemicals can also cause aplastic anaemia. When (as is usual) there is pancytopenia, the causal agent probably affects the haemopoietic stem cells and there may also be lymphopenia. In other instances the effect is mainly on committed precursor cells (p. 504) and there may then be red cell aplasia, agranulocytosis or thrombocytopenia. Sometimes, however, the drug affects more than one type of cell. On occasion, the marrow may be found to be hypercellular, e.g. in some cases of benzene poisoning, but this group of conditions is poorly understood; the anaemia in such cases is attributed to failure of red cell maturation and release from the bone marrow, rather than diminished precursors.

In some cases there appears to be an inborn defect of haemopoietic cells which renders them susceptible to injury by the drug. In others, immunological reactions may be involved.

About 50 per cent of cases of aplastic anaemia are 'idiopathic' and a virus aetiology has been suspected, but the only virus infection so far incriminated is infectious hepatitis. The aplastic anaemia is usually severe and often fatal; it appears within 10 weeks of an (often mild) attack of hepatitis.

It is important to distinguish pancytopenia attributable to aplastic anaemia from the other pancytopenias, e.g. in marrow replacement, leukaemia, megaloblastic anaemia and hypersplenism.

Agranulocytosis and thrombocytopenia, due to failure of marrow production, may each occur in pure form and are considered respectively on pages 512 and 557.

Neoplasia of the Haemopoietic Tissues

Introduction

All precursor cells of the erythroid, myeloid, lymphoid and megakaryocyte series may undergo physiological proliferation in response to appropriate stimuli. Each cell line may also

undergo purposeless proliferation, giving rise to conditions which can be regarded as neoplastic, although in some features they differ from typical tumours of other tissues (see below). The grouping together of neoplasms of such a wide range of cell types has received support from the wide acceptance of the pluri-potency of the haemopoietic stem cell (p. 504), from which all the haemopoietic and lymphoid cells are now considered to originate.

By far the most important group of conditions arising in the haemopoietic marrow are the **leukaemias**, which may be of myeloid, lymphoid or monocytic cell type (see below). Then there are a large number of ill-defined conditions of which the least uncommon are *polycythaemia vera*, a proliferation mainly of the erythroid series, and *myelofibrosis*, a related condition in which there is also fibrosis, probably of reactive nature, of the marrow: a third and rare member of this group is *haemorrhagic thrombocythaemia* in which megakaryocytic proliferation predominates. These three conditions have overlapping features and transformations between them are sometimes observed. They are often referred to as **the myeloproliferative disorders** and are described on p. 552 along with secondary tumours of the marrow.

Neoplasms of lymphoid cells pose a problem of classification, for they include the *lymphoid leukaemias and plasma-cell tumours*, most of which appear to originate in the marrow, and also the *solid lymphomas of the lymphoid and other tissues.* We have included the former lymphoid neoplasms in this account and deal with the solid lymphomas in the following chapter on the lymphoid tissues.

General features

Although, as indicated above, the haemopoietic neoplasias are classified by cell type, there may be proliferation of two or more lines. For example megakaryocytic proliferation and thrombocytosis are common features in chronic myeloid leukaemia, while erythroid, myeloid and megakaryocytic cells all proliferate in poly-cythaemia vera. There is, moreover, a tendency for one condition to transform into another during the course of the disease.

Most of the haemopoietic neoplasias differ from those of other tissues in that they infiltrate the marrow extensively, and usually diffusely, rather than forming tumour masses. They thus replace the normal haemopoietic elements, often with consequent reduction in the production of red and white cells and platelets.

As with other neoplasms, a high degree of cell differentiation is associated with a rela-tively chronic course and poor differentiation with more aggressive behaviour, but there is no division into benign and malignant, for these neoplastic conditions are all likely to be fatal in the untreated patient. They occur mostly in chronic forms, but can also take a more aggressive course.

The leukaemias

Leukaemia is a neoplastic proliferation of leu-kocyte precursors in the bone marrow. Like normal leukocytes, the neoplastic cells escape into the blood where they may be very numerous (hence 'leukaemia'). They usually infiltrate into various other tissues, producing general organ enlargement or less commonly tumour masses. Most of the clinical effects of leukaemia are due to tissue infiltration or to interference with normal marrow function by the proliferation of neoplastic leukocytes.

Precursors of each of the three main types of leukocyte—granulocytes, lymphocytes and monocytes—can become leukaemic, and each type of leukaemia may be either acute or chronic. The acute forms are characterised by a rapid clinical course and the predominance of primitive cells (myeloblasts, lymphoblasts or monoblasts), both in the marrow and the blood, whereas the chronic forms run a longer course and the neoplastic cells are mostly more mature. Monocytic leukaemia, the least common of the three major types, is usually acute or subacute. Certain rare forms of marrow neoplasia closely resemble acute leukaemia clinically; these include megakaryocytic leukaemia, erythraemic myelosis (di Guglielmo's disease) and promyelocytic leukaemia (often accompanied by a haemorrhagic tendency).

Acute leukaemia

Leukaemia occurring in childhood or adolescence is most often one of the acute types. Acute lymphoblastic leukaemia (**ALL**) tends to occur most frequently in the young, whereas acute myeloblastic leukaemia (**AML**) predominates in adults. *The clinical features of acute leukaemia are attributable mainly to haemopoietic failure, with the characteristic triad of anaemia, infection and thrombocytopenic bleeding.* The disease appears abruptly with fever, weakness, pallor, bleeding from the gums and petechial haemorrhages in the skin. Intercurrent infections are very common and the whole course from onset to death may be only a few weeks. In adults the disease may be more insidious, but the clinical features are similar.

Blood picture. The leukocyte **count** is usually raised, often to $20-50 \times 10^9/l$. Most of these cells are primitive, with nucleoli and a high nuclear/cytoplasmic ratio (Figs. 17.35, 17.37, 17.38). In over one-third of cases, however, the total white cell count is normal or even reduced—so-called *aleukaemic leukaemia*—although primitive cells can almost always be demonstrated.

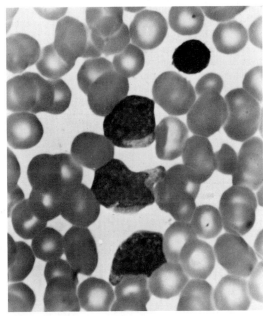

Fig. 17.35 Blood smear in acute lymphoblastic leukaemia, showing three large, primitive leukaemic cells with dispersed chromatin and basophilic cytoplasm. The cell at upper right is a mature lymphocyte. × 1000.

Bone marrow. In marrow aspirates, a marked increase in cellularity is usual and most of the cells are primitive 'blasts' (Fig. 17.36). Sections of the marrow show replacement of the fat spaces by the primitive leukaemic cells. Normal haemopoietic elements, especially neutrophils and megakaryocytes, are sparse. At necropsy in untreated cases, there is variable degree of extension of cellular leukaemic marrow along the shafts of the long bones, replacing the fatty tissue: it often has a reddish-grey or green hue and a firm consistency.

Other organs. Splenic enlargement is common, but is seldom gross. Lymphadenopathy is unusual in AML but can sometimes be detected in ALL. In some instances a thymic lymphoid tumour (Sternberg's tumour) precedes the onset of ALL in childhood (p. 584). Rarely AML, especially in children, is preceded by the

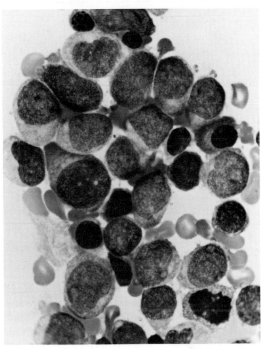

Fig. 17.36 Smear of sternal marrow in acute leukaemia. Nearly all the cells are primitive 'blasts', with a large nucleus containing one or more nucleoli, and with scanty basophilic cytoplasm. × 750. (Dr. Annette Mallinson.)

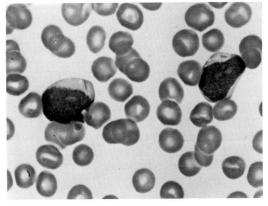

Fig. 17.37 Blood in acute myeloid leukaemia, showing two large myeloblasts containing Auer rods. × 900. (Dr. Annette Mallinson.)

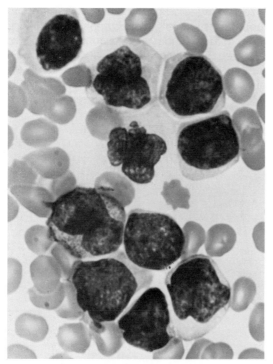

Fig. 17.38 Acute monocytic leukaemia (Schilling type). × 1000.

discovery of a myeloblastic tumour, usually arising under the periosteum of the facial bones; this kind of tumour is called a *granulocytic sarcoma* or *chloroma*, since it has a curious green colour which fades rapidly on exposure to air.

More diffuse tissue infiltration occurs during the course of acute leukaemia and almost any organ can be affected. Meningeal infiltration occurs most frequently in ALL under treatment; leukaemic cells in the subarachnoid space evade destruction by intravenous cytotoxic agents which fail to cross the blood–brain barrier and provide a nidus of malignant cells from which relapse may develop. Similarly leukaemic cells in the gonads, especially the testis, may escape destruction and be a source of relapse.

The effects on blood viscosity of high leukocyte counts have already been referred to (p. 507) and occlusion of small blood vessels in the brain by leukocyte thrombi may cause extensive haemorrhagic infarctions.

Identification of cell type. Before effective treatment became available, identification of the cell type involved in acute leukaemia was mainly of academic interest. Nowadays, although sometimes difficult, such identification is critically important from the

therapeutic viewpoint and must always be attempted. It is helpful if the primitive blast cells show some degree of differentiation into later forms; thus the association of blast cells with promyelocytes suggests acute myeloid leukaemia, whereas the presence of mature lymphocytes in appreciable numbers would favour acute lymphoblastic leukaemia. The blast cells themselves occasionally show distinctive features; thus myeloblasts tend to have more nucleoli (2–5) than lymphoblasts and sometimes contain crystalline structures known as Auer rods (Fig. 17.37). Certain cytochemical tests have also proved useful. The Sudan Black B or peroxidase stains can detect the early phases of granulation in myeloblasts, whereas lymphoblasts never show such staining. The periodic acid–Schiff (PAS) reaction for glycogen can demonstrate a distinctive pattern in different blast cells; lymphoblasts commonly show coarse cytoplasmic clumps of PAS +ve material under the cell membrane, whereas myeloblasts are usually negative. It has been shown that high serum or urine levels of lysozyme (muramidase) are characteristic of acute myeloid or myelomonocytic types of leukaemia (see below). In most cases of ALL, especially in childhood, the tumour cells lack T- and B-cell markers (p. 117) and this is associated with a relatively good response to chemotherapy. The less common forms of ALL, including those with a Sternberg tumour (see above) have T-cell markers and a poorer prognosis. The rare cases of ALL of B-cell type are highly aggressive: the cells resemble those in Burkitt's lymphoma (p. 584).

Monocytic leukaemia

This relatively uncommon variety of leukaemia is usually acute or subacute and thus presents clinically with increasing anaemia, pyrexia associated with infective mucocutaneous lesions, and thrombocytopenic purpura. Bleeding, swollen gums and nodular infiltrative skin lesions are characteristic. The total white cell count is not usually very high but in occasional patients may reach 250×10^9/l. Most of these cells are monocytes or monoblasts (Fig. 17.39), which may exhibit pseudopodial cytoplasmic projections, a fine peripheral cytoplasmic PAS +ve granularity and lysozyme production (see above). In addition to this purely monocytic form of leukaemia (*Schilling type*), an acute myelomonocytic form of leukaemia in which there is an admixture of myeloid cells and monoblasts (Fig. 17.39) is known as the *Naegeli type*: presumably the leukaemic cells, like the normal myeloid progenitor cell (p. 187), retain the capacity to differentiate into either type of cell line.

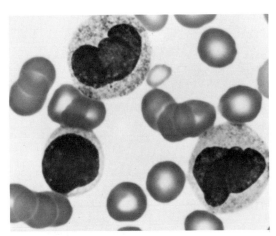

Fig. 17.39 Blood smear in monocytic leukaemia of Naegeli type, showing a myelocyte (*above*) and a promonocyte (*lower right*). The third cell is a lymphocyte. × 1300.

Chronic myeloid leukaemia (CML)

While commonest in middle-aged and elderly people this disease can occur at any age from birth onwards. The clinical picture tends to be dominated initially by gross hepatic and splenic enlargement. Signs of impaired marrow function such as anaemia and thrombocytopenia are usually inconspicuous until late in the course of the disease. After a variable period, usually of some years, acute leukaemia of myeloblastic (AML) or lymphoblastic (ALL) type commonly supervenes (see below).

Blood picture. The outstanding feature is the huge number of circulating leukocytes which may exceed $300 \times 10^9/l$ ($300\,000/\mu l$). Most of them are mature neutrophil polymorphs (Fig. 17.40) although metamyelocytes and myelocytes are almost always present and in more rapidly progressing cases myelocytes may predominate (Fig. 17.41). Occasionally eosinophils are numerous and a significant increase in basophils is a useful diagnostic feature in the blood film. Anaemia is only moderate and indeed a polycythaemic state has been observed initially in some cases.

Transformation to the aggressive phase mentioned above is indicated by increasing anaemia usually with an increase in promyelocytes and

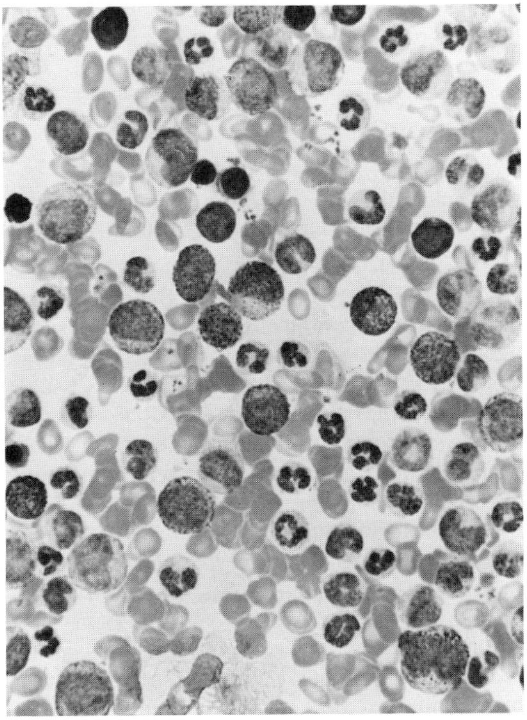

Fig. 17.40 Blood in chronic myeloid leukaemia, showing myelocytes, polymorphonuclear leukocytes and intermediate forms; two erythroblasts are seen above centre of field. × 500.

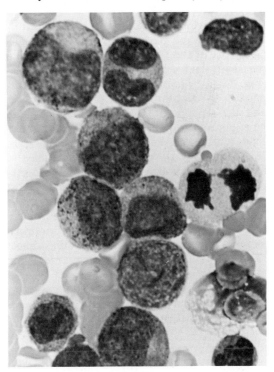

Fig. 17.41 Blood in chronic myeloid leukaemia, showing finely granular myelocytes and polymorphonuclear leukocytes. One cell is in mitosis. × 1000.

myeloblasts in the blood (*myeloblastic transformation*). Sometimes, however, the blast cells in this phase resemble closely those in the common type of *lymphoblastic* leukaemia of childhood (p. 544) and it has been suggested that this is because the cell initially undergoing neoplastic change is the stem cell common to both lymphocytes and haemopoietic cells (Janossy, Roberts and Greaves, 1976).

Diagnosis is usually easy but rarely a pronounced reactive neutrophilia associated particularly with infections, especially haematogenous tuberculosis, can produce a blood picture closely resembling that of chronic myeloid leukaemia, myelocytes and even less mature cells being observed. Features which help to confirm the diagnosis of chronic myeloid leukaemia include (1) an unusually high proportion of myelocytes, (2) the presence of an absolute basophilia, (3) the presence of the Philadelphia chromosome in proliferating marrow cells in 90% of cases (p. 549), (4) the markedly reduced level of alkaline phosphatase in leukaemic neutrophils in contrast to the elevated levels observed in reactive leukocytosis, and (5) elevation of the serum vitamin B_{12} thought to be due to an increase in vitamin B_{12}-binding protein.

Bone marrow. The red marrow is replaced by soft pale pink or greenish tissue, which usually also replaces the fatty marrow, extending into the shafts and distal ends of the long bones (Fig. 17.42). The marrow cavities are also expanded by reabsorption of bone trabeculae, and the expanded marrow can be cut out in large portions, although at necropsy it is sometimes almost fluid and may even resemble pus. Microscopically there is seen to be a massive increase in the marrow cells; granulocyte precursors predominate, myelocytes being most numerous except in the acute terminal stage. In some cases megakaryocytes are also conspicuous, while in others there may be a pronounced increase in red cell precursors, the appearances resembling those of polycythaemia vera (p. 552).

Other organs. The **spleen** is usually massively enlarged and may exceed 3 kg; it often causes great discomfort. It is moderately firm and the cut surface has a pale red mottled appearance, often with even paler patches of infarction. Microscopically the red pulp is packed with myeloid leukaemic cells, but there is probably also non-leukaemic extramedullary haemopoiesis, for erythroid precursors and megakaryocytes are usually conspicuous. The Malphighian

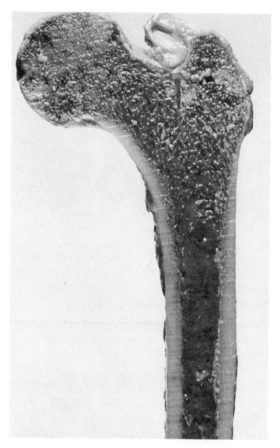

Fig. 17.42   Upper end of the femur in chronic myeloid leukaemia. Pale cellular marrow occupied the whole shaft. The marrow cavity is also widened by resorption of bone trabeculae.

bodies are largely obscured by the massive cellular infiltration of the red pulp. In cases in which the disease progresses rapidly, splenic enlargement is usually not so great. The **liver** is usually markedly enlarged and microscopy shows extensive sinusoidal infiltration with myeloid cells. Diffuse infiltration of **any other organ**, including the central nervous system, may occur and accounts for the varied symptomatology.

Other features include *fatty change* of the organs due to anaemia; widespread *petechial haemorrhages* due mainly to thrombocytopenia or defective platelet function; occasionally *more extensive haemorrhage*, especially in the brain, due to diffuse microvascular occlusion by aggregates of leukocytes, and *haemorrhagic infarcts* in various organs. There is usually a rise in the level of serum uric acid derived from the breakdown of nucleic acids from large numbers of leukaemic cells, especially during cytotoxic drug therapy. Unless prevented by appropriate treatment, for example xanthine oxidase inhibitors, the large uric acid load may lead to formation of *urate crystals in the renal tubules* and impairment of kidney function.

Chronic lymphocytic leukaemia (CLL)

This is a disease of middle and old age. It may cause little disability for several or even many years, death commonly resulting from anaemia and infections.

Blood picture. The outstanding feature is a marked increase in leukocytes, commonly to around $100 \times 10^9/l$ ($100\,000/\mu l$); nearly all are lymphocytes, mainly with the appearance of normal mature small lymphocytes (Fig. 17.43), but with a small proportion of larger, more primitive cells. Although the disease appears to originate in the bone marrow, anaemia, granulocytopenia and thrombocytopenia due to marrow replacement are late features. Auto-immune haemolytic anaemia and mild thrombo-cytopenia, possibly also of auto-immune nature, are however complications which some-

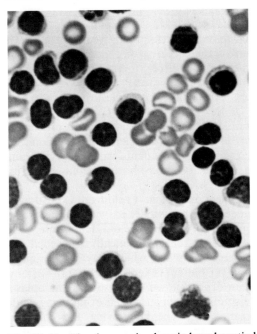

Fig. 17.43 Blood smear in chronic lymphocytic leukaemia. Most of the leukaemic cells have the appearances of normal small lymphocytes, a narrow ring of pale cytoplasm enclosing a round, dense nucleus of about the diameter of a red cell. × 750.

times occur quite early in the course of the disease.

Commonly there is a reduction in the normal plasma immunoglobulins with *decreased resistance to bacterial infections* and sometimes a monoclonal gammopathy (p. 551) due to secretion of Ig by the leukaemic cells. In most cases the leukaemic lymphocytes can be shown to possess readily demonstrable surface immunoglobulin, and sometimes other surface markers, characteristic of B cells. Occasional cases, however, appear to be of T-lymphocyte type.

Bone marrow. From an early stage the bone marrow shows abnormal lymphocytic infiltration which may initially be focal but later becomes diffuse and gradually replaces the haemopoietic cells. Eventually the fatty marrow is also replaced and the shafts of the long bones become filled with pale leukaemic marrow resembling that of chronic myeloid leukaemia but usually of firmer consistency.

Other organs. Generalised enlargement of the **lymph nodes** is a conspicuous feature and commonly the presenting sign of the disease. The nodes are soft and rubbery and appear homogeneous and pinkish-grey on cutting. Large nodes may cause clinical effects by compressing important structures such as the common bile duct. Microscopically, the nodal architecture is lost and replaced by massive lymphocytic infiltration, the appearances being those of lymphocytic lymphoma (p. 581). The **spleen** is greatly enlarged but not often as massive as in chronic myeloid leukaemia. It usually weighs between 1 and 2 kg and microscopy shows extensive infiltration by mature lymphocytes which fill the red pulp and obscure the Malpighian bodies.

Involvement of the **other organs** is usually extensive, although it tends to be more patchy than in myeloid leukaemia. The **liver** is usually enlarged due to infiltration of the portal and periportal areas by leukaemic cells (Fig. 17.44). The **kidneys** are also usually enlarged, either diffusely or with nodules of leukaemic infiltration. As with chronic myeloid leukaemia the extent of infiltration of the various other organs varies greatly. The risk of renal damage by urate crystals is not as great as in chronic myeloid leukaemia.

Other features include *fatty change* due to the anaemia, which develops late in the disease,

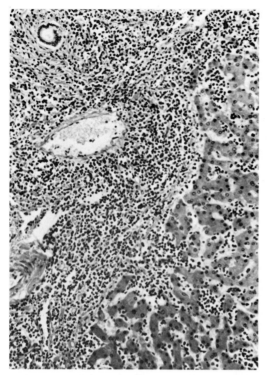

Fig. 17.44 Section of liver in chronic lymphocytic leukaemia, showing infiltration of lymphocytes around the portal tracts. × 60.

and *bacterial infection*, especially bronchopneumonia, which is often the immediate cause of death.

Leukaemic states resembling CLL. The term **prolymphocytic leukaemia** is applied to a leukaemic state of either B or T lymphocyte lineage in which the tumour cells resemble small lymphocytes but have prominent nucleoli and much more abundant cytoplasm. Typically the white count is very high. Splenomegaly is more pronounced and the disease progresses more rapidly than classical CLL. In **hairy cell leukaemia** (leukaemic reticuloendotheliosis) splenic enlargement is also marked and there is evidence of hypersplenism. The leukaemic cells, which may be sparse in the blood, show prominent cytoplasmic projections (hence the name) and ovoid nuclei with homogeneous finely dispersed chromatin. It is now known to be of B lymphocyte origin. In the **Sézary syndrome** there is a primary lymphocytic tumour of the skin resembling mycosis fungoides (p. 1070) and the tumour cells, which are of T-cell origin, show a characteristic cerebriform nuclear morphology: they exfoliate into the blood. The unfortunate term *lymphosarcoma cell leukaemia* is used when cells from a solid lymphoma (especially follicular lymphoma) likewise exfoliate into the blood, where they may exhibit the 'cleaved' or irregular nuclear outline characteristic of small follicle centre cells (p. 582).

The aetiology of leukaemia

The cause of leukaemia in man is still unknown but much has been learned recently about factors that may be involved. The mortality in England and Wales attributed to leukaemia increased from 17 per million in 1931 to 54 per million in 1957. Subsequently, this rate of increase has not been maintained (65 per million in 1977) and this suggests that the increase was due, at least partly, to improved diagnosis.

X-irradiation. An undoubted association with ionising radiation has been revealed by: (*a*) an increased risk of both acute and chronic myeloid leukaemia following deep x-ray therapy of the spine for ankylosing spondylitis; (*b*) a high incidence of CML in radiologists before precautions were taken; (*c*) a high incidence of myeloid leukaemia among survivors of the atomic explosions at Hiroshima and Nagasaki. The incubation period between exposure to irradiation and the appearance of the disease is from 6 to over 20 years, and it has been shown that any considerable exposure to x-irradiation produces recognisable chromosome damage which may persist for many years. In all these examples there is a strong indication that the leukaemogenic effect is proportional to the total dose of irradiation.

Less certain are the suggestions that exposure of the fetus *in utero* to diagnostic x-ray examination in the late stages of pregnancy increases the risk of leukaemia in childhood, or that treatment of patients with polycythaemia with radioactive phosphorus increases the incidence of AML.

Chemical induction. Prolonged exposure to benzene may be associated with the later development of acute myeloid leukaemia. The leukaemia is characteristically preceded by bone marrow aplasia which may last for many years if the patient is kept alive by transfusions. Certain drugs known to cause marrow aplasia have similarly been suspected of inducing acute leukaemia, e.g. phenylbutazone and chloramphenicol, although this has not been proved; it has also been suggested that cytotoxic agents, e.g. phenylalanine mustard (Melphalan), used in the treatment of multiple myeloma, have been responsible for inducing acute myeloid leukaemia.

The role of viruses. It has long been known that viruses are implicated in the causation of leukaemia and related forms of haematological neoplasia in experimental animals such as mice and fowls. Recent work has also shown that cat leukaemia is due to infection with a retravirus (p. 307). Of particular interest is the integration into the host genome of DNA produced through the action of virus-derived reverse transcriptase on the template of viral RNA. Such virus-directed enzymes have been reported in human leukaemic cells, indicating the presence of an integrated virus, but a causal role has not been established. In view of the demonstration of a viral aetiology in leukaemias and lymphomas in several animal species, it would, however, be surprising if such neoplasias in man were not virus-induced.

Genetic factors. There is no good evidence of an increase in the incidence of leukaemia among the relatives of affected patients; a high rate of concordance for leukaemia has, however, been reported for monozygotic twins. Certain genetic diseases appear to predispose to leukaemia, e.g. Fanconi anaemia, and Down's syndrome, and these are associated with a high frequency of chromosomal abnormalities. In 90% of cases of CML there is an **abnormal ('Philadelphia') 22 chromosome**, resulting from a reciprocal translocation between chromosomes 9 and 22 (Fig. 17.45). This is due to a somatic

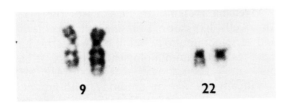

Fig. 17.45 The Philadelphia chromosome anomaly. This shows the classical anomaly, in which there is reciprocal translocation between chromosomes 9 and 22, with breakpoints in the long arms of the chromosomes: the right chromosome of each pair is the anomalous one. (Professor M. A. Ferguson Smith.)

mutation in a haemopoietic stem cell and can be detected not only in the leukaemic cells but also among the red-cell and monocyte precursors, megakaryocytes and lymphocytes. Additional chromosomal abnormalities often precede the development of the terminal, acute phase of CML.

Plasma cell tumours

Plasma cells are derived from B lymphocytes (p. 107) and are responsible for the synthesis and secretion of antibodies. It is therefore not surprising that those lymphomas which show plasma-cell differentiation commonly produce large amounts of immunoglobulin. Analysis of these so-called *myeloma* or *'M' proteins* has shown molecular homogeneity for each tumour, and this has important implications relating both to the nature of tumours and also to the basis of antibody production and specificity (see below).

The most important and best defined of the plasma-cell neoplasms is *multiple myeloma*, which differs from other lymphomas in affecting predominantly the bone marrow. Other members of the group are rare: they include *Waldenström's macroglobulinaemia* and *heavy-chain disease*, the morphological and other features of which are intermediate between myelomatosis and the other lymphomas.

Multiple myeloma (myelomatosis; myeloma)

Plasma cells are normally present in the bone marrow and may be increased in chronic infections, connective tissue diseases, etc. The proportion in such reactive states, however, rarely exceeds 10 per cent.

Multiple myeloma is a neoplastic proliferation of plasma cells or their precursors, usually confined to the bone marrow, and occurring in elderly subjects, more commonly in men than women. Death results within 2–3 years, mainly from anaemia, infection, renal failure or skeletal lesions.

Although not a common disease, multiple myeloma is of considerable interest because investigation of the myeloma proteins produced by the neoplastic cells has contributed significantly to our understanding of both antibody production and neoplasia.

Pathological changes. The neoplastic tissue occurs sometimes in the form of numerous reddish nodules throughout the marrow of bones which normally contain haemopoietic tissue (Fig. 17.46). The nodules are osteolytic so that absorption and rarefaction of the affected bones take place and *spontaneous fractures* are common, especially in the ribs. The lesions may be seen radiologically as sharply punched-out

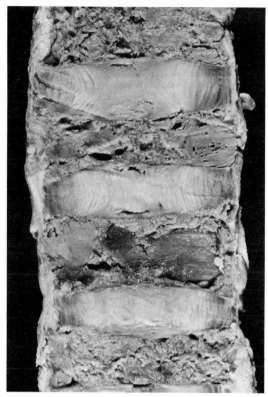

Fig. 17.46 Multiple nodules of myeloma in vertebral column. The vertebral bodies show compression collapse.

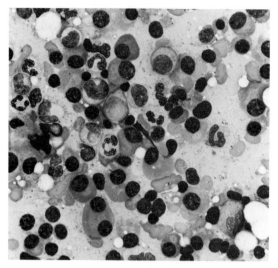

Fig. 17.47 Smear of sternal marrow aspirate in multiple myeloma, showing large numbers of plasma cells. × 600. (Dr. Annette Mallinson.)

defects in the bone, for example in the skull. More often, widespread plasma cell proliferation in the marrow produces a diffuse osteoporosis without the formation of discrete nodules, and *vertebral collapse* may occur. Rarely a **solitary plasmacytoma** may develop, usually in a long bone, but in most cases multiple myeloma develops sooner or later. Excision is therefore unlikely to effect cure, though a few successful cases have been recorded. A solitary plasmacytoma may occur in various other tissues, e.g. the nasopharynx, or stomach, and its relation to multiple myeloma is uncertain.

Microscopic appearances. The nodules or diffuse infiltrates of myelomatosis are highly cellular and vascular. The appearance of the cells is variable, but most commonly many of them are recognisable as plasma cells (Fig. 17.47), having the typical eccentric cartwheel nucleus,

and cytoplasm of various grades of basophilia and pyroninophilia due to a high content of RNA. As in normal plasma cells, the golgi zone may be seen as a crescent of pale-staining cytoplasm beside the nucleus, and bi- and tri-nucleate cells are often seen. More primitive cells—plasmablasts—are also present in various proportions. Cells of intermediate appearance between small lymphocytes and plasma cells may occasionally predominate. There is usually little or no fibrous stroma.

Myeloma proteins. In most cases the myeloma cells, like normal plasma cells, synthesise and secrete immunoglobulin, but when this has been tested for immunological reactivity, it has only rarely been shown to react strongly and specifically, i.e. like an antibody, with any one of a large number of antigens; nor is there any other evidence to indicate that myeloma cells have proliferated as a result of an antigenic stimulus. In most cases, the level of serum immunoglobulins is raised, in some instances exceeding 100 g/litre.

A remarkable feature is the homogeneity of the myeloma protein in each particular case: it is usually all of one or other immunoglobulin class, usually IgG, less commonly IgA, rarely IgD and almost never IgE.* Invariably, its light chains are of one type, either kappa or lambda

---

* The frequencies of these Ig classes of myeloma proteins correlate with the levels of the classes of Ig in normal serum, and so presumably with the numbers of plasma cells normally producing each class.

(p. 106). Its uniformity is most readily shown by electrophoresis, when it appears as a narrow dense 'M' band, contrasting with the broader less well-defined bands of each class of normal serum immunoglobulins. Moreover, chemical analysis has shown that the individual molecules are identical in the amino-acid sequences of the variable regions of their polypeptide chains (p. 106). These findings indicate that myeloma originates from a single plasma cell or plasma-cell precursor—hence the term **monoclonal gammopathy**. This conclusion supports the view that neoplasms in general arise from single cells, and also provides strong evidence for Burnet's clonal selection theory of antibody production (p. 128). Comparison of myeloma immunoglobulins of the same class (e.g. IgG) from a number of cases shows that, in contrast to the homogeneity of the protein in each case, the proteins from different cases all differ from one another in their amino-acid sequences.

Another feature of myeloma cells is that they may produce an excess of immunoglobulin light chains in addition to whole Ig molecules. In 50 per cent of cases light chains in the form of monomers and dimers, of molecular weights 22 000 and 44 000 respectively, are demonstrable in the urine, where they are known after their discoverer as **Bence–Jones proteins**. Adjustment of the pH of the urine to 4–6 and heating results in precipitation of the light chain molecules at about 50 °C, and they redissolve at about 80 °C. This test is useful in diagnosis, and especially so in 15 per cent of cases in which only light chains are produced—**light chain myeloma**.

Production of myeloma proteins is usually accompanied by a fall in the plasma level of normal immunoglobulins, and it has been suggested that myeloma cells produce a factor which suppresses normal plasma cell function.

Associated changes. *Skeleton.* Myelomatosis causes pronounced bone resorption with focal or generalised osteoporosis, hypercalcaemia, and increased excretion of calcium and phosphorus in the urine; the serum alkaline phosphatase is usually not much raised.

Blood. The increased level of immunoglobulin in the plasma results in a tendency to unusually strong *rouleaux formation* and sludging of red cells, and a *high ESR*; it accounts also for increased background staining in blood films. *Anaemia* results from extensive infiltration of the marrow by myeloma cells, and is usually of normochromic normocytic type, although blood loss from haemorrhage may bring about an iron-deficiency anaemia. The tendency to *haemorrhage* may be due to formation of complexes between myeloma immunoglobulin and several of the clotting factors, but there may also be thrombocytopenia. Another factor is increased viscosity of the blood due to hyperglobulinaemia and sludging of red cells: this may result in Raynaud's phenomenon (p. 384), and occasionally gangrene of the extremities, particularly in patients with a myeloma protein which gels on cooling (cryoglobulin).

Rarely the neoplastic plasma cells appear in the blood in numbers which warrant the term *plasma cell leukaemia*. Infiltration of various organs may also occur.

Renal changes are common, and result from precipitation of Bence–Jones protein in the lumen of the renal tubules to form dense hyaline casts. These cause tubular obstruction and also stimulate a foreign-body giant-cell reaction, and consequent tubular destruction may bring about renal failure. Nephrocalcinosis resulting from hypercalciuria may also be a contributory factor.

Immunological deficiency results from the casual reduction of normal immunoglobulins mentioned above. There is an increased susceptibility to infections and death often results from bronchopneumonia.

Amyloid deposition is a common complication of myelomatosis, and usually presents the pattern of 'primary' amyloidosis (AIO–p. 272); it occurs particularly in the light-chain and IgA varieties of the disease and only rarely in IgG myelomas.

Waldenström's macroglobulinaemia

This uncommon condition occurs in individuals over 50 years of age, more often in men than women. The primary form of the disease, which is described below, runs a prolonged course; it is basically a monoclonal gammopathy of IgM class, and may be regarded as a low-grade neoplasm of lymphoid cells. In some cases, however, the syndrome is associated with a frankly malignant lymphoid neoplasm, and the outlook is then poor.

The clinical features include weakness and tiredness; spontaneous haemorrhage from the respiratory, urinary or alimentary tracts and in the periphery of the retinae, susceptibility to bacterial infections, and a variable degree of enlargement of the liver, spleen and lymph nodes. The plasma protein level is usually raised to 80 g/litre or more due to a gross increase of (monoclonal) IgM detectable as an M band on serum electrophoresis. It is insoluble in water, and precipitates when the plasma is diluted with water (Sia test).

Of particular importance is the *increase in plasma viscosity* due to the high level of IgM: this produces extensive microcirculatory stasis with varied symptoms, including blurring of vision, neurological disturbances and haemorrhagic phenomena. This last may also result from the IgM coating the platelets, and preventing release of platelet factor III, but the macroglobulin also interferes with the polymerisation of fibrin.

The macroglobulin also commonly behaves as a cryoglobulin (see above) so that exposure of the patient to cold may result in ischaemia, and even gangrene, of the extremities. The red cells often show a strong tendency to aggregate *in vitro* which renders cell counting difficult, and the ESR is raised.

All these effects are rapidly reversed by the removal of the protein from the patient's circulation by plasma exchange. The peripheral blood usually shows some degree of anaemia, leukopenia and thrombocytopenia as a result of impaired marrow function, although there is a lymphocytosis in some cases.

Histological changes. There is a diffuse pleomorphic infiltration of the marrow by small lymphocytes, plasma cells and mast cells, although the most characteristic cell has a morphology intermediate between the lymphocyte and the plasma cell ('*plasmacytoid lymphocyte*') and may have PAS +ve intranuclear inclusions. There are, however, no focal lesions in the bones, which are either normal radiologically or show diffuse osteoporosis. The **lymph nodes** are moderately enlarged and are overrun by the pleomorphic lymphoid infiltrate, although the architecture is not usually destroyed. Similar infiltration is also noted in the portal tracts of the **liver** and the Malpighian bodies of the **spleen**, and has even been observed in the brain—Bing-Neel syndrome. The pathological picture somewhat resembles chronic lymphocytic leukaemia and represents a link between the plasma cell tumours and the other malignant lymphomas (p. 582).

Heavy-chain disease

This term is used to describe a group of rare neoplastic conditions in which infiltration of the tissues by lymphoid cells is associated with the presence in the serum of a protein identifiable as the Fc fragment of the immunoglobulin heavy chains (see p. 106). In the most remarkable member of the group, the heavy chain is derived from IgA and lymphoid infiltration of the same pleomorphic nature as that noted in Waldenström's disease is largely confined to the mucosa of the small intestine. This unusual type of lymphoma, known as **'alpha-chain disease'**, is mainly found in young adults of eastern Mediterranean origin.

The myeloproliferative disorders

As explained on p. 542, there are a number of ill-defined neoplastic-like conditions of the haemopoietic tissue which differ from the leukaemias and plasma cell tumours. The least rare are *polycythaemia vera* and *myelofibrosis*. A third member of the group, *haemorrhagic thrombocythaemia*, is much less common. These three conditions are interrelated: intermediate forms occur and polycythaemia vera and haemorrhagic thrombocythaemia may both progress to myelofibrosis.

Polycythaemia vera (primary polycythaemia)

This is characterised by neoplastic hyperplasia of the haemopoietic tissue with excessive production, particularly of red cells, but also of leukocytes and platelets, resulting in polycythaemia.

The neoplastic cells replace the fat cells of the red marrow and extend to occupy the whole of the marrow cavities of the long bones. The marrow appears uniformly red and although there is an increase in all haemopoietic cell lines, erythropoiesis predominates. Megakaryocytes may also be numerous and some are abnormally large.

Blood picture. The outstanding feature is a marked increase in red cell mass, reflected in a rise in blood volume and in a red-cell count usually over $7 \times 10^{12}/l$ (7 million/μl), a Hb level over 18 g/dl and a packed cell volume over 60 per cent. The production of so many red cells and the frequent occurrence of haemorrhages (see below) may result in iron deficiency, with consequent microcytosis. The leukocyte count is increased, sometimes to over $20 \times 10^9/l$ (20 000/μl) and the platelets are also increased and irregular in size with some giant forms.

Other features. The increase in the blood volume results in engorgement of the microcirculation which, together with the erythrocytosis, produces a florid appearance, particularly of the face. The blood viscosity is also increased with consequent hypertension and a tendency to vascular thrombosis, notably in the cerebral vessels. In spite of the increase in platelets (which may be functionally deficient), there is also a bleeding tendency, and recurrent haemorrhage from the gastro-intestinal tract is a common complication which is only partly explained by the increased incidence of peptic ulceration in this condition.

The spleen is usually palpably enlarged, firm, engorged with red cells, and is a common site of infarction. The increased cell turnover may be reflected by a raised blood uric acid and may lead to secondary gout or renal injury (p. 289).

Course. The disease is often advanced when first detected and may run a long course. However, death may result from the effects of hypertension or from thrombotic episodes. It may progress to myelofibrosis (see below) or acute myeloid leukaemia. Venesection supplemented by radioactive phosphorous (^{32}P) or cytotoxic drugs is often effective in reducing the polycythaemia, at least for a time.

Erythropoietin-induced erythrocytosis, sometimes inappropriately termed **secondary polycythaemia** is discussed on p. 508.

Myelofibrosis

The essential feature of this condition, which occurs in elderly people, is increased fibroblastic activity in the haemopoietic marrow, resulting in a great increase in reticulin fibres and sometimes in thicker collagen strands (Fig. 17.48). This change extends also to replace the fatty marrow in the long bones and there is evidence that it is reactive rather than part of the neoplastic process. Needle aspiration of the marrow is unsuccessful ('dry tap') and trephine or open biopsy is necessary for its examination. In some cases there is an increase in the bony trabeculae (**myelosclerosis**). The haemopoietic elements in the marrow may be increased diffusely or focally or diminished, and abnormal megakaryocytes may be seen.

The spleen is enlarged, often enormous, and this may give abdominal discomfort and pain due to splenic infarcts, which may be the presenting symptoms. The liver also may be enlarged and there is extensive extramedullary haemopoiesis in both organs; the microscopic appearances resemble those in the marrow, including the increase in reticulin or fibrous tissue.

Blood picture. There is a progressive anaemia

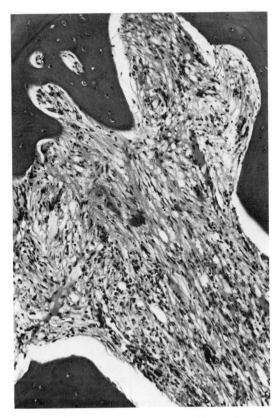

Fig. 17.48 Myelofibrosis. Section of bone showing replacement of the haemopoietic marrow by fibrous tissue.

with poikilocytosis, and some normoblasts are seen. The number of granulocytes may be low, normal or increased and they include some myelocytes and occasional myeloblasts. The picture is thus one of **leuko-erythroblastic anaemia** (p. 507). Platelets may be increased, but as the disease progresses all the formed elements in the blood tend to decrease, due to impaired haemopoiesis and sometimes also to hypersplenism (p. 565). Infections are common.

The condition can be distinguished from carcinomatosis of the marrow (see below) by marrow biopsy.

Haemorrhagic thrombocythaemia (megakaryocytic myelosis)

This resembles polycythaemia vera in being characterised by a neoplastic hyperplasia of all the haemopoietic cell lines, but in this condition megakaryocytic hyperplasia and platelet production predominate.

The platelet count is usually over $1000 \times 10^9/l$ ($10^6/\mu l$) but they are functionally inadequate and haemorrhage from the gastro-intestinal tract and elsewhere is common. Although the red-cell count may be raised initially, microcytic anaemia commonly develops. There may be a moderate increase in granulocytes. Thrombotic episodes with infarction of the internal organs are common, particularly in the spleen, which is usually enlarged initially but may become atrophic from repeated infarction.

Cases intermediate between this condition and polycythaemia vera are observed and, as in the latter, myelofibrosis develops in some cases.

Secondary tumours of bone marrow

The bone marrow is a common site of metastases of various carcinomas and sarcomas. In malignant melanoma and carcinoma of certain organs, especially the breast, bronchus, prostate and thyroid, the nodules may be very numerous and widespread. They occur especially in the red marrow and are sometimes detectable in histological sections of marrow aspirates (Fig. 17.49) or by bone scanning. When the marrow of the short bones is extensively invaded, there is often a compensatory

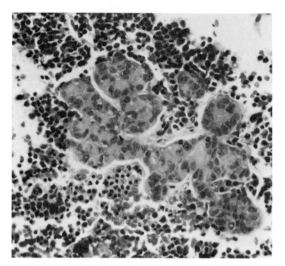

Fig. 17.49   Section of sternal marrow aspirate showing metastatic breast carcinoma. $\times$ 250.

hyperplasia of red marrow in the long bones. Leuko-erythroblastic anaemia (p. 507) may result, particularly when metastases are numerous and widespread, or when they stimulate an osteosclerotic reaction, a common feature of prostatic cancer metastases.

Haemorrhagic States

Under this heading we have grouped together a number of conditions of different aetiology, which have in common the liability to haemorrhage into the tissues or from mucous membranes. They fall into two broad classes, the **coagulation defects** and the **purpuras**. In coagulation defects, haemorrhage is usually initiated by trauma and is characterised by its persistence rather than by its severity. In purpura, the bleeding is chiefly in the skin and from the surface of mucous membranes and is spontaneous.

Before reading the following account of haemorrhagic disorders, it is essential to have a basic understanding of the physiological mechanisms and the various factors involved in haemostasis and coagulation of the blood (pp. 231–5).

Defects of coagulation

Coagulation defects may be **genetically determined** or **acquired**. The only common examples of the former are haemophilia (deficiency of factor VIII or anti-haemophilic globulin) and Christmas disease (deficiency of factor IX). Genetically-determined defects are due to a defect of an individual gene controlling the production of the corresponding clotting factor; thus only single defects occur, affecting one coagulation factor. By contrast, acquired defects of coagulation more often show multiple deficiencies affecting several factors, most frequently II, VII, IX and X.

Congenital defects

Haemophilia is characterised by genetically-determined production of an abnormal, ineffectual factor VIII. This interferes with the intrinsic system of blood coagulation and results in poor formation of thromboplastin. The severity varies widely, but is likely to be the same in affected members, and in different generations, of the same family. The coagulation time of whole blood is greatly prolonged, although it may approach normal after a major haemorrhage. The bleeding time, estimated from a small prick wound, is usually normal, since capillary haemostasis is largely dependent on vasoconstriction and the formation of a platelet plug: for the same reason, venepuncture is usually safe in haemophilic patients.

Excessive bleeding on minimal injury is usually apparent in the first year of life. Operations such as circumcision, tonsillectomy or dental extractions may cause very severe or fatal bleeding. Recurrent haemorrhage into joints is characteristic and leads to erosion of cartilage, fibrous adhesions resulting in ankylosis, and eventual crippling. Bleeding can, however, occur from any site, including the nose, gastro-intestinal and urinary tracts; haemorrhages into the tissues around the floor of the mouth may cause respiratory obstruction and death by suffocation. Skin petechiae characteristic of the purpuric diseases do not occur.

Haemophilia nearly always affects males. It results from a defect in a gene in the X chromosome coding for Factor VIII, the anti-haemophilic globulin normally present in the plasma. The chromosome (X') containing the abnormal gene does not cause haemophilia in heterozygous females (X'X) because the normal X is sufficient to prevent the bleeding tendency; such females do, however, have an abnormally low plasma level of Factor VIII, a feature which is explicable on the Lyon hypothesis (p. 513).

The Y chromosome does not compensate for the X' chromosome, and so X'Y males are haemophiliacs: their sons do not inherit the defect, but all their daughters are carriers (Fig. 17.50). Half the sons of a female carrier are haemophiliacs and half her daughters are carriers. Theoretically, half of the daughters of a carrier (XX') mother and a haemophiliac (X'Y) father would be X'X' female haemophiliacs, but in the past such matings were rare.

The abnormal factor VIII reacts with antibodies to normal factor VIII and so immunological assays suggest normal levels in haemophiliacs. The defect is, however, readily demonstrated by functional tests. Similarly in the female carrier the immunological assay indicates a level approximately twice that of the functional assay.

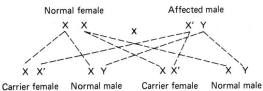

Fig. 17.50 The genetic transmission of the abnormal X chromosome (X') responsible for haemophilia.

The deficiency can be corrected temporarily by the transfusion of fresh blood or fresh plasma, or more efficiently by the intravenous administration of factor VIII concentrates. After repeated transfusions, a refractory state occasionally develops, possibly indicating immunisation of the recipient against donor antihaemophilic globulin. It appears that there are subtle individual antigenic differences in factor VIII.

Christmas Disease* is due to congenital deficiency of factor IX, which leads to deficient formation of thromboplastin from the intrinsic system. It shows a similar sex-linked inheritance to classical haemophilia, and the clinical pattern of bleeding is identical. Treatment is by the administration of factor IX concentrates.

Von Willebrand's disease. This condition is characterised by various genetically-determined defects of factor VIII, resulting in defective coagulation and impaired platelet function: there is a tendency to bleed from minor trauma, but not usually purpura.

Acquired defects

Combined deficiency of factors II, VII, IX and X in various combinations is seen most commonly in **patients on anticoagulant therapy**, but occurs also in the following conditions.

(1) *Haemorrhagic disease of the newborn.* This condition, characterised by spontaneous haemorrhages from the umbilicus and mucous membranes, often causes severe melaena (the presence of altered blood in the faeces); it occurs in about 0·3 per cent of neonates and may be due to inadequate supplies of

* Christmas disease was named after the patients in whom it was first described (in the Christmas issue of the British Medical Journal, 1952).

vitamin K before the intestinal bacterial flora is established. Lack of vitamin K results in the above combined deficiency and its administration to the infant rapidly restores the coagulation time to normal and bleeding ceases. Administration of 5 mg of the vitamin to the mother in the 24 hours before labour raises the plasma prothrombin of the infant above the danger level. However, if given direct to a premature infant, the dose must be carefully regulated because it may increase physiological haemolysis and thus raise the load of bilirubin which the immature liver cannot conjugate and excrete: the risk of kernicterus is thus increased.

(2) *Malabsorption.* In prolonged obstructive jaundice, or malabsorption from other causes, impairment of absorption of vitamin K may be sufficiently severe to result in combined deficiency of clotting factors; tests for impaired coagulation are therefore of importance before surgical procedures in these conditions.

(3) *Liver failure.* The liver is responsible for production of factor II and other clotting factors. Severe liver insufficiency may thus result in a combined defect, and also in deficiency of fibrinogen (factor I). Needle biopsy of the liver may, in the circumstances, result in severe and even fatal haemorrhage.

Disseminated intravascular coagulation (DIC) and the defibrination syndrome. In some conditions intravascular activation of the clotting system results in the deposition of fibrin thrombi in the small vessels, particularly in the internal organs.

In addition to obstruction of the microcirculation, which may result in ischaemic injury to the kidneys (p. 851), liver, adrenals, etc., fibrinogen may virtually disappear from the blood, partly because it is used up and partly because the fibrinolytic system is activated (probably by Hageman factor—p. 55) and the plasmin produced digests both fibrin and fibrinogen. Plasmin also destroys some other clotting factors, while fibrin degradation products (FDP) also interfere with clotting. All these factors, and sometimes also acute thrombocytopenia, result in a **haemorrhagic state** and bleeding occurs into the internal organs, from mucous membranes, etc.

DIC occurs in conditions of shock, particularly when associated with sepsis, in which injury to the neutrophil polymorphs by bacterial endotoxin releases factors which trigger the clotting system (p. 264). The circulatory collapse is aggravated and in some cases acute adrenocortical insufficiency develops (p. 1043).

Another important cause is premature separation of the placenta, in which release of tissue thromboplastin (factor III) may trigger the clotting system. DIC may also be a complication of surgical operations, certain tumours, the viral haemorrhagic fevers, anaphylaxis and circulating immune-complex disease (p. 154). Treatment of DIC is difficult. Heparin may be helpful in preventing further clotting, but aggravates the bleeding state: fibrinolytic inhibitors such as ε-aminocaproic acid may also be indicated.

Afibrinogenaemia also occurs as a rare congenital defect with recessive inheritance.

Purpura

This term is applied to various conditions in which small haemorrhages occur from *capillaries* throughout the body, resulting in haemorrhagic spots (petechiae) in the skin, mucous membranes and serous surfaces, while more gross bleeding may occur from the mucous membranes of the alimentary, respiratory and genito-urinary tracts; the pattern of bleeding differs from that of coagulation defects, in that haemorrhage from larger blood vessels into tissue spaces is uncommon. In many cases of purpura the bleeding is due to direct damage to the capillaries by an underlying systemic disorder, and the platelets are normal—**non-thrombocytopenic purpura**. Platelets themselves, however, contribute to the integrity of small vessel walls, possibly by continually forming plugs at sites of minimal injury; reduced numbers of circulating platelets may therefore cause abnormal capillary fragility, leading in turn to purpuric bleeding—**thrombocytopenic purpura**. Accordingly it is customary to classify purpura into non-thrombocytopenic and thrombocytopenic types; in each case however the characteristic bleeding occurs from abnormally fragile or permeable capillaries.

Non-thrombocytopenic purpura

(a) 'Toxic' damage to the capillaries may occur in severe acute bacterial infections. The purpura found in acute meningococcal septicaemia (Fig. 21.27, p. 747) and subacute bacterial endocarditis may be caused by septic micro-emboli or by toxaemia.

(b) Drugs. Many severe cutaneous drug reactions are purpuric, in particular those due to antibiotics and sulphonamides; such vascular reactions must be distinguished from those due to drug-induced thrombocytopenia.

(c) Poor supporting tissues. The common senile or cachectic purpura of the backs of the hands and arms is probably attributable to poor capillary support from collagen, as is the purpura associated with corticosteroid therapy and Cushing's syndrome. Ascorbic acid is concerned, together with the phosphatase of fibroblasts, in the synthesis of collagen by promoting the polymerisation of mucopolysaccharide. It may also have a role in the formation of intercellular cement substance; thus haemorrhage from capillaries, most characteristically from the gums around carious teeth, and under the periosteum, but also from other sites as well, is common in **scurvy**. The anaemia of scurvy usually results from haemorrhage but has a mild haemolytic component; since ascorbic acid is concerned also in the conversion of folic acid to active folinic acid, megaloblastic anaemia occasionally results. Important changes in the bones also occur (p. 889).

(d) Anaphylactoid (Henoch–Schönlein) purpura. Damage to capillaries may have an *allergic* basis, especially in children. The purpuric rash may develop explosively 2 to 3 weeks after a streptococcal respiratory infection, but the high titres of anti-streptolysin O found in rheumatic fever are not present. Common accompaniments are acute polyarthritis similar to that of rheumatic fever, colicky abdominal pain, haemorrhage and serosanguineous effusion into the gut, and an acute focal glomerulonephritis (p. 832), which sometimes progresses to renal failure. The preceding streptococcal infection and the lesions resembling rheumatic fever and glomerulonephritis all suggest that this type of purpura is the result of hypersensitivity. Drugs and common articles of food, e.g. chocolate, may similarly be responsible for sensitisation.

(e) Congenital abnormalities. Although itself rare, the commonest of these is *hereditary haemorrhagic telangiectasia*. This disease is transmitted as a simple dominant trait. Symptoms vary greatly in severity and time of onset, but epistaxis is usually a prominent feature. Multiple small telangiectatic spots, which are, in fact, arteriolar-venular anastomoses, occur in the skin and mucous membranes; they are a source of recurrent haemorrhage and

severe anaemia may result. In the lungs similar lesions may give rise to profuse haemoptysis.

Thrombocytopenic purpura

Thrombocytopenia may be said to occur when the platelet count is less than $150 \times 10^9/l$ ($150\,000/\mu l$). Bleeding is, however, unusual when the count is greater than $60 \times 10^9/l$ and spontaneous haemorrhage does not usually occur until the count has fallen to less than $20 \times 10^9/l$. Thrombocytopenia may result from impaired marrow production of platelets, as in aplastic anaemias (p. 540), marrow replacement syndromes of all types, and in megaloblastic anaemias (p. 533). Thrombocytopenia may also be caused by damage to platelets in the circulation or by their consumption or trapping in excessive numbers. Such damage may have an immunological basis as in idiopathic thrombocytopenic purpura, the thrombocytopenia of systemic lupus erythematosus, in some cases of chronic lymphatic leukaemia, and in certain drug reactions. Excessive consumption or trapping may occur in disseminated intravascular coagulation, in micro-angiopathic haemolytic anaemia (p. 531) or in hypersplenism. In cases where the thrombocytopenia is due to excessive consumption or destruction of platelets in the circulation, normal or increased numbers of megakaryocytes are present in the bone marrow (Fig. 17.51); this is an important point

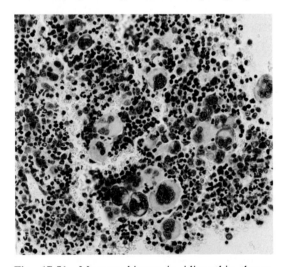

Fig. 17.51 Marrow biopsy in idiopathic thrombocytopenic purpura, showing increased numbers of megakaryocytes, many of which are immature. × 205.

of distinction from thrombocytopenias due to impaired marrow function.

Idiopathic thrombocytopenic purpura occurs chiefly in children and young adults. It is often a self-limiting disease which disappears spontaneously within 3 months of onset and does not recur, but chronic relapsing cases also occur. Sometimes the onset is acute and follows an upper respiratory infection, and fulminating cases may occur during pregnancy. The clinical pattern of bleeding may vary from mild cutaneous purpura to gross uterine, renal or gastrointestinal haemorrhage. In severe cases, intracerebral bleeding is a particular danger. As in other causes of thrombocytopenic bleeding, the whole-blood clotting time is normal, but the bleeding time is prolonged and clot retraction impaired.

The evidence for an immunological causation for the disease includes: (*a*) the presence of transient thrombocytopenia in neonates born to mothers suffering from the disease, probably due to the transplacental transfer of a maternal antibody; (*b*) the production of temporary thrombocytopenic purpura in a normal individual following the transfusion of plasma from an affected patient; (*c*) the response of many patients to corticosteroids or ACTH; (*d*) the recent demonstration of specific anti-platelet auto-antibodies in many cases; and (*e*) the strong resemblance clinically to the thrombocytopenia complicating systemic lupus erythematosus (SLE): idiopathic thrombocytopenic purpura may precede by months or even years the development of other features of SLE.

Many patients respond to immunosuppressive drugs, failing which splenectomy may be beneficial; this operation presumably does not affect the degree of platelet sensitisation by antibody, but simply removes the site of their destruction. Following splenectomy there may be a remarkable overswing in the platelet count which can exceed $1000 \times 10^9/l$; there is thus a temporary danger of thrombosis, but in such cases the platelet count usually falls to normal again in a week or two.

Immunological drug purpura. Although drugs may produce non-thrombocytopenic purpura by direct capillary damage, and may also cause thrombocytopenia by bone marrow toxicity, some thrombocytopenic drug purpuras are due to immune damage to platelets, the drug form-ing immune complexes in the plasma, which bind to the platelets and effect their destruction, or, less probably by binding directly to the platelets (p. 151). Such drugs include digoxin, chlorothiazides, quinine, quinidine, rifampicin and sulphonamides

Other thrombocytopenic states due to excessive platelet consumption or destruction. In disseminated intravascular coagulation (p. 556) and micro-angiopathic haemolytic anaemia (p. 531), platelet trapping by widespread intravascular fibrin deposition may induce thrombocytopenia, with the paradoxical combination of abnormal bleeding and excessive coagulation. Increased platelet sequestration or destruction in the spleen can occur in splenomegaly of any type, e.g. portal hypertension, tropical splenomegaly, myelofibrosis, and this may respond to splenectomy (p. 565). Thrombocytopenia may also result from massive blood transfusion, since stored blood is itself poor in platelets.

Qualitative platelet abnormalities

Aspirin and related drugs inhibit the production of thromboxane and interfere with platelet aggregation. This may be significant in promoting haemorrhage from aspirin-induced haemorrhagic erosions in the gastric mucosa (p. 604).

In certain rare conditions, the platelets may be present in normal numbers but are qualitatively abnormal, resulting in haemorrhage. An example of this is *Glanzmann's disease*, in which the features characteristic of thrombocytopenic bleeding are present although the platelet count is normal. Poor platelet function may also occur in the thrombocytoses associated with some myeloproliferative disorders (e.g. polycythaemia vera), and in conditions of increased intravascular fibrinolysis, e.g. DIC (p. 556).

References and Further Reading

Chanarin, I. (1979). *The Megaloblastic Anaemias*, 2nd edn., pp. 880. Blackwell Scientific, Oxford.

Clarke, C. A. (1970). The prevention of rhesus iso-immunisation. *Clinical Genetics* 1, 183–215.

Clinics in Haematology. Saunders, Philadelphia, London and Toronto. (An excellent series of reviews on haematological topics, from 1972 onwards.)

Dacie, J. V. and Lewis, S. M. (1975). *Practical Haematology*, 5th edn., pp. 629. Churchill-Livingstone, Edinburgh.

Hoffbrand, A. V. and Lewis, S. M. (1972). *Haematology*, pp. 652. Heinemann Medical, London. (Volume 2 in the series *Tutorials in Postgraduate Medicine*.) New edition in preparation.

Janossy, G. *et al.* (1976). Blast crisis in chronic myeloid leukaemia (CML). *British Journal of Haematology* 34, 179–92.

Janossy, G., Roberts, M. and Greaves, M. F. (1976). Target cell in chronic myeloid leukaemia and its relationship to acute lymphoid leukaemia. *Lancet* ii, 1058–61.

McDonald, G. A., Dodds, T. C. and Cruickshank, Bruce (1978). *Atlas of Haematology*, 4th edn., pp. 309. Churchill-Livingstone, Edinburgh, London and New York.

Thomson, R. B. (1977). *Disorders of the Blood: a Textbook of Clinical Haematology*, pp. 851. Churchill-Livingstone, Edinburgh, London and New York.

Williams, W. J., Bentler, E., Ersler, A. J. and Rundles, R. Wayne (1977). *Haematology*, pp. 1977. McGraw Hill, New York.

Woodliff, H. J. and Herrmann, R. P. (1979). *Concise Haematology*, 2nd edn., pp. 208. Edward Arnold, London.

18

The Lympho-Reticular Tissues

The lymphoid tissues subserve two major functions. First, they are responsible for specific immune responses to antigenic stimulation: this function has been described in Chapter 5 and its harmful and protective effects in the two subsequent chapters. Second, the **lymph nodes** and **spleen** also monitor the tissue fluid and blood respectively for abnormal constituents. To perform this second function they contain sponge-like areas of *reticular tissue* and *sinuses* rich in macrophages, through which the fluid filters. Such tissue, together with vascular sinusoids rich in lining macrophages in various non-lymphoid tissues, e.g. the liver and bone marrow, is traditionally grouped together as the *reticulo-endothelial system*. The characteristic feature of such tissue is its richness in macrophages. It also contains fibroblasts and other, possibly heterogeneous, cells termed *reticulum cells*, the nature of which is uncertain. Because the macrophage is the only specialised cell of

the reticulo-endothelial system whose origin and functions have both been well established, we have preferred the term mononuclear-phagocyte system (p. 72). The lymph nodes and spleen are thus subject to abnormalities of the lymphoid cells proper and also of macrophages and cells associated with them in the reticular tissue and sinuses. **The thymus** differs from other mammalian lymphoid tissues in being a 'primary' lymphoid organ, concerned not with immune responses but with antigen-independent lymphopoiesis (p. 116), and it lacks also the filtering tissue of the lymph nodes and spleen. The **tonsils** and **Peyer's patches**, etc., are not sites of filtration of body fluids but are strategically placed in the wall of the alimentary tract to encounter micro-organisms or their products which penetrate the epithelium (p. 138) or are transported across it by phagocytes, and to mount the appropriate immune responses.

The Spleen

Functions

As indicated above, the spleen is a composite organ consisting of: (*a*) units of **lymphoid tissue** termed *lymphoid follicles* or *Malpighian bodies* or collectively the *white pulp*, and (*b*) the vascular network and sinuses termed the **red pulp**, which makes up most of the organ.

The spleen is not an essential organ, but its removal, especially in childhood, greatly increases the risk of septicaemia and meningitis by pneumococci and other pyogenic bacteria (Chilcote *et al.*, 1976). This is probably attributable in part to the capacity of the spleen to phagocytose micro-organisms in the blood

before there has been time for the development of a specific immune response with production of protective antibody. Splenectomised animals, e.g. sheep, are abnormally susceptible to various parasitic infections. In both animals and man, the spleen is an important site of formation of antibodies in response to *intravascular* injection of antigens, and considerably less antibody is produced by splenectomised individuals. The spleen is of less importance than the lymph nodes in the response to antigens injected into the tissues. The drainage of the spleen into the portal venous system allows antibodies produced in the spleen to encounter antigenic material absorbed from the gut, and this may facilitate phagocytosis of such material by the Kupffer cells.

There is also evidence that a tetrapeptide termed *tuftsin* is derived from a protein produced in the spleen. Tuftsin has the property of stimulating the phagocytic activity of neutrophil polymorphs, although its importance in defence against micro-organisms *in vivo* is uncertain (Constantopoulos, Najjar and Smith, 1972).

The spleen plays an important physiological role in the removal from the blood of old or injured red cells, which are phagocytosed and digested by macrophages in the cords of the red pulp. The bilirubin formed from the breakdown of haemoglobin is secreted into the blood, to be extracted, conjugated and excreted by the liver cells, while the iron is re-utilised in haemoglobin synthesis in the marrow. The average life of the red cells and the number in the blood are not increased following splenectomy, and it is apparent that the phagocytic cells in the liver, marrow and other tissues also destroy old red cells. However, the macrophages in the red pulp of the spleen have a special function in extracting from the red cells various cytoplasmic inclusions, and also in removing the nuclei of any normoblasts which have gained entrance to the circulation, the cells then being returned to the blood. Loss of this function, which is known as 'pitting', is observed following splenectomy, when normoblasts and red cells containing Howell–Jolly bodies and siderotic granules, etc., may be found in blood films (p. 509).

It is less certain that the spleen is an important site of physiological destruction of leukocytes and platelets, but splenectomy is commonly followed by a polymorphonuclear-leukocytosis of up to $30 \times 10^9/l$ (30 000 per μl), a monocytosis, and a thrombocytosis of up to 10^{12} per litre ($10^6/\mu$l). The polymorphs reach a peak level during the few days following splenectomy, the platelets 2–3 weeks later. The levels decline thereafter, but monocytes and platelets may remain above the normal ranges for months or even years.

Structure

The vascular arrangements of the spleen are of particular importance in relation to its two major functions. The larger arteries branch within the trabeculae, and give off arterioles of approx. 200 μm diameter which leave the trabecula and become ensheathed in a cuff of lymphoid tissue—the Malpighian bodies—to which they supply capillaries. At the periphery of the lymphoid tissue, each central arteriole divides into several penicillar arterioles, which enter the red pulp. They show a fusiform swelling of the wall, termed an ellipsoid; this consists of an inner layer of prominent capillary endothelium surrounded by layers of large pale cells and a basement membrane. The red pulp consists of a spongework of vascular channels which are richly endowed with cells of the mononuclear phagocytic system and are sometimes referred to as the *splenic* cords. Lying within the red pulp are larger vascular channels which are known as *sinuses* and represent the radicles of the splenic vein. The sinuses are lined by elongated endothelial cells between which are fenestrations about 3μm in maximum diameter. While it is possible that some of the blood from the penicillar arterioles passes directly into the sinuses, thus bypassing the red pulp (the 'closed' circulation), most enters the splenic cords of the red pulp (the 'open' circulation) and in order to reach the venous system the blood cells and especially the erythrocytes must pass through the narrow endothelial fenestration of the sinuses. The red cells must therefore retain elasticity or deformability and cells lacking these properties, e.g. spherocytes, are trapped in the cords and may undergo premature destruction (p. 520). The process of 'pitting', by which rigid inclusions are removed from the red cells (see above), also takes place as the red cells pass between the endothelial cells of the sinuses, the inclusions being extracted by macrophages in the adjacent red pulp. The 'open' circulation through the splenic cords clearly provides opportunity for phagocytic removal of abnormal materials or cells from the blood, whereas the 'closed' circuit is a more direct route. In man, the spleen normally contains only 20–30 ml of blood although it can become enlarged and engorged with blood in various diseases.

Shrinkage of the spleen

Atrophy of the spleen occurs in old age, affecting both red and white pulp, and is sometimes a feature of wasting diseases. Hyaline thickening of the walls of the small arteries and arterioles of the spleen is very common and increases in incidence and severity with increasing age; it is by no means confined to subjects with chronic hypertension or generalised arteriosclerosis. The resulting ischaemia brings about splenic atrophy with some increase in reticulin. Splenic ischaemia is also a feature of *sickle-cell disease* (p. 523) and is due to blockage of sinuses by hypoxic sickle cells; infarcts

and atrophy result, and eventually the spleen may be converted into a small fibrous remnant, often heavily pigmented by haemosiderin derived from phagocytosed red cells. Loss of splenic function may explain the predisposition to bacterial infections in sickle-cell disease. Severe splenic atrophy is also a feature of some cases of *coeliac disease* (p. 640), the mechanism being obscure.

Splenomegaly

As already stated, the two known major functions of the spleen are the production of specific immune responses and phagocytosis of abnormal materials in the blood. Accordingly, increased functional activity of the spleen, with hyperplasia of the lymphoid or macrophage cells, or of both, commonly results from antigenic stimulation or the presence of abnormal materials, for example micro-organisms, toxins or abnormal cells, in the blood. Splenomegaly is therefore a very common secondary phenomenon in a great many diseases. Apart from neoplastic conditions, splenomegaly is, in general, attributable to enlargement of the red pulp due, for example, to venous congestion or to increase in the number and size of phagocytes (as in various storage diseases). Hyperplasia of the Malpighian bodies, with development of large germinal centres, occurs as an immune response in many diseases, and especially in infections. Another feature of the immune response in many diseases, particularly infections, is the development of large numbers of plasma cells, both in relation to the Malpighian bodies and throughout the red pulp, but these immunological changes alone are seldom sufficiently marked to give rise to significant splenic enlargement.

Because of its vascular nature and phagocytic role, the spleen is prone to *blood-borne infection*: it has, however, strong defences against pyogenic bacteria, and abscess formation is uncommon except for septic infarcts in pyaemia. However, bacteria are commonly arrested in the spleen and may be recovered from it in non-pyogenic generalised infections, as in typhoid fever, brucellosis and generalised tuberculosis. Significant splenomegaly is not usual in

acute viral infections, but an exception is infectious mononucleosis, in which it is often palpable. Colonisation of the spleen with great enlargement is brought about also by trypanosomes, and by micro-organisms which are capable of survival and multiplication within macrophages, as in leishmaniasis and histoplasmosis.

Congestive splenomegaly occurs in systemic venous congestion, usually due to right ventricular failure, but is usually slight. Greater enlargement is usually seen in chronic portal venous hypertension, as in cirrhosis of the liver or hepatic schistosomiasis.

In *diseases of the blood*, splenomegaly may result from accumulation and phagocytosis of abnormal cells or platelets; also the spleen may re-assume its fetal role of haemopoiesis, as in anaemia resulting from replacement of the haemopoietic marrow by fibrous tissue (myelofibrosis) or by neoplastic deposits. There is evidence also that splenic enlargement from various causes is sometimes accompanied by increased phagocytic activity (*hypersplenism*) leading to anaemia, leukopenia and thrombocytopenia (*splenic anaemia*). This is dealt with more fully on p. 565.

Like most other organs, the spleen may be the site of deposits of *amyloid*. Splenic involvement is common in *sarcoidosis*, and in the various types of *lymphoid and myeloid neoplasias*—the leukaemias, Hodgkin's disease, etc.

Infections

Acute pyogenic infections

The earliest change in the spleen is congestion of the cords of the red pulp. As the number of circulating polymorphs increases, they accumulate progressively in the red pulp of the spleen, and in septicaemia, or severe localised pyogenic infections with a high leukocytosis, they may be present in the spleen in huge numbers. At post-mortem examination in such a case, the spleen is slightly enlarged (200–300 g), acutely congested and the splenic tissue is so softened that it looks and feels almost like a bag of fluid; the cut surface is pinkish or deep red, and the tissue is semi-fluid. These changes, sometimes termed '*septic spleen*', are due to congestion, accumulation of polymorphs and marked terminal and post-mortem autolysis by the digestive enzymes released from degenerate polymorphs.

In fatal septicaemia, the bacteria may be recovered from the spleen, as from other organs, and the macrophages in the red pulp may contain bacteria, red cells, degenerate polymorphs and cell debris. However, microscopic examination of the septic spleen is seldom satisfactory owing to severe autolytic changes.

As already stated, abscess formation in the spleen is uncommon except when brought about by septic infarction in pyaemia. Involvement of the capsule produces perisplenitis, which may progress to perisplenic abscess.

Non-pyogenic bacterial infections

Moderate degrees of splenic enlargement commonly accompany generalised non-pyogenic bacterial infections, and are due to hyperplasia of both the lymphoid tissue and red pulp of the organ, together with granulomatous lesions brought about by arrest and proliferation of bacteria in the red pulp. As enlargement is due mainly to accumulation and local proliferation of macrophages, lymphocytes and plasma cells, together with increase in reticulin, the spleen is usually firm, and post-mortem autolysis is not nearly so marked as in pyogenic infections. Some examples are given below.

In **typhoid fever** splenic enlargement is an important feature, the weight sometimes reaching 500 g; it is usually deep red from congestion and not particularly soft: as elsewhere in typhoid, there is a virtual absence of polymorphs and accumulation of macrophages (many of which contain ingested red cells), lymphocytes and plasma cells. Typhoid bacilli usually occur in clumps in the red pulp. There may be no

sign of damage in their neighbourhood, but sometimes there is necrosis around them.

Undulant fever is due to infection with small Gram −ve bacilli, the *brucellae*. There are three important species, *Br. abortus*, *Br. melitensis* and *Br. suis*, which commonly infect cows, goats and pigs respectively. Traditionally, infection in man results from drinking the milk of infected cattle or goats. A combination of pasteurisation and elimination of infection from dairy herds has considerably reduced the incidence in many countries. In this country, infection with *Brucella abortus* still occurs and is an occupational hazard of those who handle infected cattle, particularly in the veterinary profession: infection is also occasionally acquired in medical bacteriology laboratories.

The organisms, which are not easy to isolate in culture, colonise the macrophage system and cause lesions closely resembling tubercle follicles, sometimes with central necrosis (Fig. 18.1): these occur in the lymph nodes, spleen

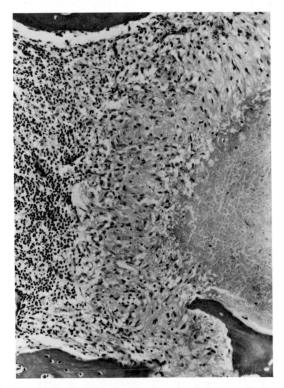

Fig. 18.1 Biopsy of a vertebral body in brucellosis. The lesion consists of an epithelioid macrophage granuloma with central necrosis (*right*) and peripheral aggregation of lymphocytes and plasma cells (*left*). × 130.

and liver, all of which may be enlarged, although the spleen becomes palpable in only a small proportion of cases. Other organs may be affected, and in some cases there is a transient polyarthropathy. The clinical features vary greatly; there is usually fever, either acute or low grade with vague symptoms, malaise and weight loss. Bacteraemia commonly occurs, but is irregular and multiple blood cultures may be negative. Without treatment the condition usually subsides spontaneously but it may continue for months or even years. Diagnosis is dependent usually on either positive blood culture or demonstrating a high or rising titre of antibodies in the serum. Individuals with occupational exposure to brucellae frequently have antibodies but no symptoms, and diagnosis, particularly of chronic brucellosis, is accordingly difficult.

Tuberculosis. In acute miliary tuberculosis the tubercles are specially numerous in the spleen. They generally appear as minute grey points of about the size of Malpighian bodies, from which they may be distinguished by appearing to project slightly from the cut surface when viewed by oblique lighting. In less acute generalised tuberculosis in children, the spleen is occasionally studded with yellowish tubercles of 3–5 mm diameter. In chronic pulmonary and other forms of tuberculosis, a few tubercles of various sizes, and occasionally larger nodules, may be present in the spleen. Rarely the blood may present a very striking leukaemoid reaction difficult to distinguish from true leukaemia.

Protozoal infections

Massive splenic enlargement is seen in malaria and in kala-azar. In **malaria**, the spleen swells acutely during each attack of pyrexia, from acute congestion due to the accumulation of red cells containing the parasites. After repeated attacks, thickening of the stroma with induration may ultimately occur and in chronic cases the organ becomes firm, brownish-grey owing to accumulation of malarial pigment, and may weigh 1–1·5 kg. Some cases of so-called *tropical splenomegaly* (see below) are now thought to be due to chronic quartan malaria.

Kala-azar is the generalised type of leishmaniasis, in which there is widespread colonis-ation of macrophages by the leishmanial form of the protozoan *Leishmania donovani*. The vectors are various species of sandflies: in Indian kala-azar, man appears to be the only host and sandflies are infected by feeding on cutaneous lesions. In other affected areas of the world, canines and rodents act as reservoirs of infection. In the sandfly and in cultures, the parasite assumes a flagellate (leptomonad) form. *L. donovani* and other species of leishmania also cause localised cutaneous or muco-cutaneous infections in which the parasites are relatively few and the histology is similar to that of tuberculous lesions. The cell-mediated immune response appears to be of importance in determining whether the infection remains localised or becomes generalised.

In kala-azar there is anaemia, leukopenia and usually thrombocytopenia. The spleen is greatly enlarged, often exceeding 1·5 kg. It is firm and the red pulp is largely occupied by collections of macrophages which contain the leishmanial forms of *L. donovani*, known as *Leishman–Donovan bodies*. These occur also in the bone marrow and in the liver, and diagnosis can be made by sternal puncture, but if this fails, liver biopsy or splenic puncture may be required. The parasites are rounded or oval intracellular bodies of $2 \times 3 \ \mu m$. Each contains a nucleus and a rod-like kinetoplast.

Haematological disorders

The normal function of the spleen in destroying effete red cells, and probably also polymorphs and platelets, has been described on p. 561. Numerous abnormalities of the red cells, as for example in various types of haemolytic and macrocytic anaemias, are accompanied by an increased rate of their destruction in the spleen, and as a consequence there is a great increase in the number of macrophages in the red pulp. The degree of splenomegaly depends on the severity and duration of the process, and is due mainly to engorgement of the red pulp with red cells. Similarly in idiopathic thrombocytopenic purpura there is increased splenic destruction of the antibody-coated platelets, although splenomegaly is usually absent or slight. In contrast to these conditions, in all of which splenic hyperfunction is secondary to an abnormality of the blood cells concerned, splenomegaly from various causes may be accompanied by an increased rate of destruction of normal red cells, leukocytes and platelets. This is termed *hypersplenism*, or *splenic anaemia*, and is described below.

The haematological disorders accompanied by **great splenomegaly**, i.e. to about 2 kg, are chronic myeloid leukaemia, extramedullary haemopoiesis (p. 507) and sometimes chronic lymphocytic leukaemia. **Moderate splenomegaly**, to about 1 kg, occurs in acute leukaemia, various haemolytic anaemias and polycythaemia vera. The changes in the spleen in these conditions have been described in the previous chapter.

Splenic anaemia and hypersplenism

The concept that certain disorders of the blood might be attributable to overactivity of the spleen was based on the observation that splenectomy is sometimes followed by improvement in the anaemia, leukopenia and thrombocytopenia (either singly or in any combination) commonly associated with splenomegaly. While it is possible that instances of primary hypersplenism occur in which there is no underlying disorder to account for the splenomegaly, most cases are secondary to splenomegaly due to various disease processes. The commonest of these is *portal hypertension* from hepatic cirrhosis or hepatic schistosomiasis, leading to congestive splenomegaly and sometimes splenic anaemia (the *Banti syndrome*). The anaemia is at first normocytic but after severe or repeated haemorrhage from oesophageal varices it may become markedly microcytic as a result of iron deficiency. Reticulocytes are scanty and the anaemia responds only slowly to iron. The leukocyte count is generally low, often 2000–3000 per μl (2–3 $\times$ 10^9/litre), and usually all types of white cell are proportionately affected. The platelets in some cases are about normal in number, in others distinctly decreased. Radio-isotope studies indicate excessive sequestration and destruction of red cells by the spleen, and imprints of the cut surface of the spleen sometimes show evidence of phagocytosis of both red and white cells.

In splenic anaemia the marrow shows a normoblastic hyperplasia and primitive cells tend to predominate.

The spleen in portal hypertension. The degree of splenic enlargement is usually much greater than in systemic venous congestion (p. 229); it is commonly about 500 g but occasionally as much as 1·5 kg. The capsule is thickened and often adherent to surrounding tissues. In some cases the organ is congested and blood readily flows out of the excised spleen, leaving the organ somewhat collapsed. In longer-standing cases the spleen is firm, and the Malpighian bodies are usually fibrotic and ill-defined, but may be quite distinct. In many cases siderotic nodules, the so-called Gandy–Gamna bodies, are present. These are organised haemorrhages of from 1 to several mm in diameter: they often have a yellowish centre surrounded by a brown zone due to deposition of haemosiderin.

Microscopy shows increase in reticulin fibres in the walls of the sinuses and in the reticulum of the red pulp, which may eventually progress to fibrosis. There is also an increase in the numbers of macrophages and fibroblasts in the red pulp and the venous sinuses are not as uniformly nor as greatly engorged and distended as might be expected. The trabeculae are thickened and prominent and recent haemorrhages or older haemosiderin-rich scars (see above) may be seen.

The walls of the dilated splenic and portal veins are often thickened and similar splenic changes, sometimes accompanied by hypersplenism, may result from portal vein thrombosis without cirrhosis. It remains unexplained why hypersplenism occurs in some cases of chronic portal hypertension and not in others.

Splenomegaly with extramedullary haemopoiesis. Great enlargement of the spleen may occur when the bone marrow is extensively destroyed by fibrosis, osteosclerosis or secondary carcinoma, especially of the prostate. The increase is due to the development of haemopoietic tissue in the red pulp. All the elements of marrow are represented, but in some cases megakaryocytes are present in marked excess. No doubt such extramedullary haemopoiesis is sometimes compensatory for marrow destruction but in cases of myelofibrosis the splenic abnormality is regarded by some authorities essentially as part of a myelo-proliferative disorder. The spleen may reach a huge size—e.g. 2·5 kg and may contain all the remaining haemopoietic tissue. The organ is of deep red or pinkish red colour but sometimes there are discrete somewhat firm red nodules of 10 mm or more in diameter in which the haemopoietic tissue is more abundant. The Malpighian bodies are indistinct, infarcts are usually absent and as a rule there are no adhesions.

In some cases the spleen is overactive in destroying red cells, and splenectomy may then be beneficial. It is, however, important to determine, for example by double isotope techniques, how much the spleen is contributing to red cell production and destruction.

As usual with extramedullary haemopoiesis, the blood picture is that of leuko-erythroblastosis (p. 507).

Other causes of splenomegaly

Amyloid disease. The spleen is commonly involved in generalised amyloidosis. Deposition may be mainly in the Malpighian bodies, which are changed to translucent rounded patches (Fig. 10.5, p. 271)—*Sago spleen*—or there may be diffuse involvement of the red pulp, in which case the spleen is most often enlarged, sometimes to over 1 kg. The occurrence of the two forms is unexplained, but diffuse involvement is said to be a feature of amyloidosis complicating syphilis.

Sarcoidosis. The spleen is commonly involved in sarcoidosis, although it is not usually enlarged, and frequently the lesions are not visible macroscopically; their histological features are the same as in sarcoidosis elsewhere in the body (Fig. 18.10 and p. 216), i.e. follicles resembling those of tuberculosis, but showing little or no necrosis, and with multinucleate giant cells which often contain curious stellate and laminated inclusions. In some cases the spleen is extensively affected and moderately enlarged; the coalescent lesions are then visible macroscopically. Splenic anaemia may complicate the condition.

Disorders involving lipid storage

Storage of lipids in macrophages occurs in human disease in two groups of conditions.

(a) **The hyperlipidaemias** (pp. 29–30), which include the familial forms of hyperchylomicronaemia, alpha-lipoprotein deficiency (in which unstable beta-lipoproteins are formed in excess) and hyperbetalipoproteinaemia. In these conditions and also in poorly controlled diabetes mellitus, in hypothyroidism, prolonged obstructive jaundice and in dietary hypercholesterolaemia, various grades of accumulation of cholesterol or its esters occur in macro-

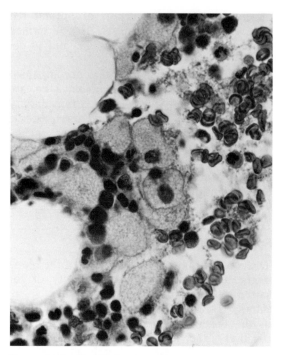

Fig. 18.2 Familial hyperbetalipoproteinaemia. Bone marrow biopsy showing foamy cells. × 540.

phages (Fig. 18.2), not only in the spleen, lymph nodes, liver, bone marrow, etc., but also in the form of xanthomas in the skin and elsewhere. The increased incidence and severity of atheroma in these conditions is discussed on p. 368. Accumulation of sufficient lipid to cause splenic enlargement occurs only occasionally. Macrophages in the red pulp increase in number and in size and excess lipid is present either as cytoplasmic globules which react variously with fat stains, or in a masked state apparently combined with protein. For example, cholesterol may be present in the spleen in increased amount without birefringent esters being detectable in the cells. Although the deposit occurs secondarily to hypercholesterolaemia it is not known what actually determines the extent of deposition.

(b) **Various rare hereditary lipid storage diseases**, such as Gaucher's disease and Niemann–Pick disease, in which the lipid storage becomes excessive in various tissues and the enlargement of the spleen is very great. These conditions result from inborn abnormalities of lipid metabolism (p. 28). The composition of the lipids varies in different types.

Gaucher's disease. This uncommon condition was described by Gaucher in 1882. In its least rare form it becomes apparent in adult life, usually as slowly increasing and eventually extreme enlargement of the spleen and liver. This is due to accumulation of glucocerebrosides in macrophages which increase in number and size in the affected organs. Spleen weight may exceed 5 kg and microscopy shows huge numbers of macrophages termed **Gaucher cells**: they mostly have a single nucleus (but occasional cells have two or three) and abundant cytoplasm which shows a characteristic streaky or irregularly vacuolated appearance (Fig. 18.3). Stains for fat are only weakly positive but the Gaucher cells are rich in acid phosphatase, the level of which may be raised in the plasma. The liver also is much enlarged by aggregation of Gaucher cells in the sinusoids. Involvement of the haemopoietic marrow may result in resorption of bone with widening of the marrow cavity, thinning of the cortex, and a tendency to pathological fractures. Displacement of haemopoietic elements by Gaucher cells may lead to a pancytopenia, but this may arise also from hypersplenism. Enlargement of lymph nodes, especially in the abdomen and mediastinum, is usual. In late cases Gaucher cells may form visible aggregates in the skin and also in the conjunctiva where they may be seen as wedge-shaped yellow-brown patches, termed *pingueculae*.

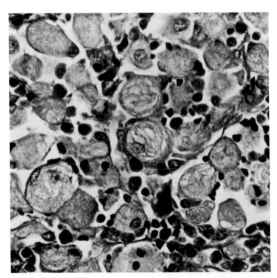

Fig. 18.3 Section of spleen in Gaucher's disease, showing the characteristic large cells with striated and vacuolated cytoplasm. × 440.

The adult form of Gaucher's disease described above is due to a deficiency of a lysosomal beta-glucosidase, resulting in accumulation of glucocerebroside derived from normal breakdown of red cells. The defect is consistent with long life, and death may eventually result from the effects of marrow replacement. It is transmitted as a Mendelian recessive factor and diagnosis of both the disease and the heterozygous carrier state, by the demonstration of beta-glucosidase deficiency in leucocytes, has been described and provides the possibility of prenatal diagnosis from a sample of fetal blood or fibroblasts.

At least one other form of Gaucher's disease exists and becomes apparent in infancy. Glucocerebrosides accumulate not only in macrophages but also in neurones and death occurs in infancy or childhood from the effects on the central nervous system.

Niemann–Pick disease. This condition is an example of abnormal storage, chiefly of the phospholipid sphingomyelin, but also of cholesterol and other lipids. It is a very rare condition of early childhood which causes mental deficiency and is usually rapidly fatal. The storage of the lipid is very extensive, occurring in the specialised cells in the brain, intestinal mucosa, adrenals, lungs, pancreas, etc., as well as in macrophages in the spleen, liver, lymph nodes, bone marrow, etc. The accumulation of lipid enlarges the cells and gives their cytoplasm a foamy appearance. The lipid stains more readily with fat stains than in Gaucher's disease. The biochemical defect is probably an autosomal recessive trait and in some cases appears to be a deficiency of an enzyme involved in the breakdown of myelin. Occasionally similar lipid-storage diseases occur in which a different phosphatide accumulates, e.g. a cephalin, and it seems likely they are all founded on defects in the enzyme systems controlling lipid metabolism.

The histiocytoses

This term is applied to conditions in which macrophages (histiocytes) proliferate in a manner suggestive of neoplasia. It should not be used to describe reactive hyperplasia.

Histiocytosis X. This term is applied collectively to three uncommon conditions—Letterer–Siwe disease, Hand–Schüller–Christian disease and eosinophil granuloma of bone—of unknown aetiology, and characterised by apparently neoplastic proliferation of cells derived from the macrophage series.

These conditions are not related to any known abnormality in lipid metabolism, and plasma lipids are not raised. Lipids are, however, present in excess in the proliferated macrophages in longstanding cases, and particularly in Hand–Schüller–Christian disease and eosinophil granuloma.

Letterer–Siwe disease (non-lipid histiocytosis) develops most commonly in infants and usually runs a rapid and fatal course. It is characterised by hepatosplenomegaly, lymph-node enlargement and multiple nodules in the skin and bone marrow. There is usually fever, anaemia and sometimes leukopenia. The affected organs show massive replacement by proliferated macrophage-like cells. Plasma cells, fibroblasts, eosinophil polymorphs and giant cells may also be present, but usually in relatively small numbers. There is usually no storage of lipid in the macrophages, but this is sometimes observed in atypical cases running a more prolonged course.

Hand–Schüller–Christian disease occurs at all ages, but most frequently in children. The proliferated macrophages accumulate lipids, mainly cholesterol esters, and this is conspicuous in long-standing cases. The lesions are commonly infiltrated with eosinophils, lymphocytes, plasma cells and fibroblasts, and may eventually become extensively scarred: they occur particularly in the bones, but also in the skin, liver, lymph nodes, spleen and lungs. Exophthalmos or diabetes insipidus may result from lesions of the skull adjacent to the orbit or hypothalamus respectively.

In general, the course is much more prolonged than in Letterer–Siwe's disease, many patients surviving for 10 or more years, but in some instances, particularly when onset is in childhood, it is more acute.

Eosinophil granuloma of bone (p. 897), the third member of this group, is usually a solitary lesion arising most commonly in adolescents or adults, and is composed of a mixture of cells including lipid-laden macrophages, multinucleated giant cells and eosinophil polymorphs. It is not a cause of splenomegaly, and has a good prognosis, although progression to Hand–Schüller–Christian disease has been described in rare instances.

Although these conditions differ greatly in their behaviour, they are regarded by many as being closely related, and as forming a series in which eosinophil granuloma is the benign counterpart of the usually rapidly fatal Letterer–Siwe's disease, while Hand–Schüller–Christian disease lies intermediate. The aetiology is unknown, but accumulation of lipids appears to follow histiocytic proliferation, and is not the primary change.

Histiocytic medullary reticulosis is a diffuse neoplastic proliferation of macrophages in which the neoplastic cells phagocytose red cells, leucocytes and platelets, resulting in a fatal pancytopenia (p. 585).

Tumours

As in the lymph nodes, the commonest forms of primary neoplasia in the spleen are the various malignant lymphomas (p. 575). It is often not possible to determine the site of origin of a lymphoma, for many lymph nodes and sometimes the spleen, bone marrow, etc., are commonly involved when the patient is first seen. Occasional early cases do seem, however, to have originated in the spleen.

Benign tumours of the spleen, including fibroma, myoma, haemangioma and lymphangioma have been described, but all are rarities. *Cysts* of the spleen are occasionally seen. They are usually small and multiple, though one may reach a large size and form a fluctuant swelling on the surface. They contain a clear serous fluid, but there may be an admixture of altered blood. They are regarded as usually of lymphangiomatous origin.

Splenic metastases occur more frequently in sarcoma than in carcinoma, but even in the former they are not common. The spleen contrasts with the bone marrow and lymph nodes in its low frequency of secondary carcinoma, and in some cases of widespread carcinoma, microscopic haematogenous foci of cancer cells undergoing degenerative change have been observed in the spleen. Direct invasion may, however, occur from cancer of the pancreas, etc.

Lymph Nodes

A brief description of the structure of the lymph nodes has been given in Chapter 5. They consist essentially of two parts. First, the lymphoid tissue proper with its follicles and deep cortex (paracortex), which are responsible for mounting immune responses (pp. 137–8). Second, the lymph sinuses and medullary reticulum which not only house antibody-producing plasma cells, but are also involved in the phagocytosis and destruction of organisms or damaged cells carried from the tissues in the lymph. In fact, the lymph node medulla and sinuses have much the same relation to the lymph as the splenic red pulp has to the blood. The macrophages in both react similarly. In addition to being active phagocytes for particulate material, they exhibit a great capacity for uptake and storage of substances present in solution.

These two functions of lymph nodes are not entirely independent, for the antigenic constituents of bacteria etc., phagocytosed by macrophages are presented to responsive lymphocytes in highly immunogenic form (p. 135), and antibodies released locally by plasma cells in the medullary cords of lymph nodes opsonise bacteria etc., thus promoting their phagocytosis and destruction.

Acute lymphadenitis

Experimental studies have shown that in normal circumstances lymph nodes are not very efficient in removing particulate elements from the lymph passing through them: for example, bacteria and similar-sized inert particles have been shown to pass rapidly from the peripheral lymphatics, through the regional nodes, and to reach the blood stream. However, within less than an hour of the establishment of an acute infection, the sinuses of the draining lymph nodes are dilated by the increased flow of lymph, the node becomes acutely inflamed (see below), and neutrophil polymorphs migrate into the sinuses from the adjacent small blood vessels and aggregate particularly in the medulla where they provide a filter by actively phagocytosing bacteria in the draining lymph: the efficiency of the nodes in preventing spread of infection to the bloodstream is thus greatly increased. Unless the infection is rapidly overcome, the numbers of macrophages in the sinuses and medulla increase and they also participate in the phagocytosis of bacteria, degenerate polymorphs, cell fragments, etc., in the lymph.

In addition to the migration of polymorphs and monocytes, the lymph nodes draining a focus of acute infection show the other features of acute inflammation, including dilatation of the small blood vessels and inflammatory oedema: these changes are due to the local effects of bacteria or their toxins, and possibly endogenous mediators, carried in the lymph from the focus of infection. Polymorphs are also carried in the lymph, and supplement those which have accumulated in the nodes by local migration. These inflammatory changes result in swollen, tender and sometimes painful lymph nodes, a common example being in the axillary nodes in pyogenic infection of a finger, e.g. a *whitlow*.

Other changes in the lymph nodes in acute infections include those associated with immune responses, i.e. the formation of cortical germinal centres, 'blast' cell transformation and proliferation of lymphocytes in the deep cortex (p. 137).

Organisms that have invaded a lymph node are often destroyed by the leukocytes and the inflammation then resolves. They may, however, continue to multiply, with consequent suppuration which may spread to the surrounding tissues and, if superficial, discharge on the skin surface. Such changes may occur in the drainage area of infected wounds of various kinds, particularly when caused by streptococci, and sometimes by staphylococci.

In **lymphogranuloma inguinale**, a macrophage-granulomatous reaction with central necrosis and suppuration occurs in the inguinal lymph nodes (Fig. 18.4), and a closely similar lesion is seen in the draining lymph nodes in **cat-scratch disease**. Lymphogranuloma (p. 988) is caused by a chlamydia, but the cause of cat-scratch disease is uncertain.

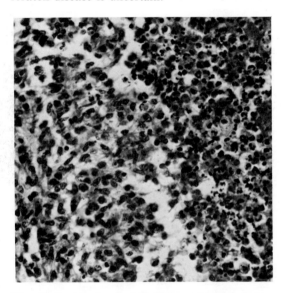

Fig. 18.4 An inguinal lymph node in lymphogranuloma inguinale, showing part of the macrophage granuloma (*left*) with central suppuration (*right*). × 320.

Another infection which involves the lymph nodes in a suppurating and epithelioid-cell granulomatous reaction is **tularaemia**, due to *Francisella tularensis*, which infects many species of animals. It occurs in various parts of the Americas and Asia, but not in Western Europe.

In **bubonic plague** there is a severe inflammation with infiltration of polymorphonuclears, brought about by *Yersinia pestis* which is present in enormous numbers; there is much haemorrhage and oedema in the nodes and in the tissue between them, and often considerable necrosis. The so-called bubo is simply an inflammatory mass consisting both of lymph nodes and the infected, inflamed surrounding tissues. In **anthrax** the lesion is mainly an inflammatory oedema with a varying amount of haemorrhage (Fig. 8.12, p. 206).

In **typhoid fever**, large numbers of macrophages accumulate in the sinuses and medullary cords of the lymph nodes draining the intestinal lesions (Fig. 18.5). The macrophages contain ingested cell debris and often erythrocytes. The nodes also contain plasma cells: haemorrhage, necrosis and autolytic softening may follow (Fig. 2.4, p. 10). As in other typhoid lesions, polymorphonuclear leukocytes are few or absent.

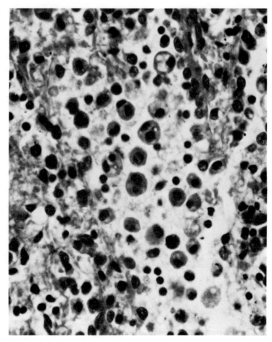

Fig. 18.5   A lymph node in typhoid fever, showing numerous macrophages in a sinus. Some of the macrophages contain ingested erythrocytes. × 520.

Infectious mononucleosis (glandular fever) is a virus infection which occurs sporadically and in small epidemics and affects chiefly children and young adults. It is characterised by swelling and tenderness of cervical lymph nodes, fever lasting a week or two and atypical lymphoid cells in the blood. The posterior cervical nodes are usually affected first, but other groups may

be involved; splenic enlargement is not uncommon and rupture may follow a trivial injury. The disease is rarely fatal, and recovery usually occurs after 1 to 3 weeks. In some cases sore throat is a prominent clinical feature: it is due to a pharyngitis with mixed secondary infection, often including candida, and may cause necrosis and ulceration of the mucosa. In others there is severe headache and a skin rash. At first there may be a neutrophil leukocytosis, but soon the characteristic blood picture appears, namely a leukocyte count usually of 10 000–20 000 per μl (10–20 × 10⁹ per litre), of which 50 per cent or more are enlarged atypical lymphoid cells with an enlarged irregular, sometimes convoluted nucleus and an increased amount of basophilic cytoplasm (Fig. 18.6). The lymph nodes show prominence of the germinal centres, but the most striking change is accumulation of huge numbers of blast cells in the deep cortex and sinuses. Mitoses are frequent and the appearances are highly suggestive of a malignant lymphoma (Fig. 18.7). The architecture of the nodes is, however, preserved. In many cases liver function tests are abnormal, indicating a degree of hepatitis, and some patients develop jaundice: liver biopsy in such cases reveals changes closely resembling those

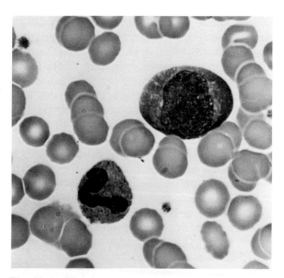

Fig. 18.6   Blood smear in infectious mononucleosis, showing an atypical lymphoid cell with enlarged irregular nucleus and abundant basophilic cytoplasm. It has the features of a lymphoblast, and is much larger than the adjacent polymorph. Leishman's stain. × 1400.

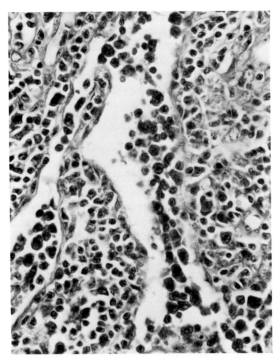

Fig. 18.7 Infectious mononucleosis. A cervical lymph node showing atypical lymphoid 'blast' cells in the lymphoid tissue and sinuses. The Paul–Bunnell test was positive. × 490. (Dr J. F. Boyd: preparation supplied by Dr J. R. S. More.)

of acute virus hepatitis, but aggregates of immunoblasts in the portal areas and sinusoids may be more conspicuous.

During infection, heterophil agglutinins for sheep red cells appear in the blood in some, but not all, cases. Their detection by the Paul–Bunnell test is in wide diagnostic use.

Following a chance observation of the development of antibodies to Epstein–Barr virus (EBV, p. 304) in a technician during an attack of glandular fever, investigations of students at Yale University showed that the appearance of such antibodies was a regular feature of infectious mononucleosis. Similar observations have since been made by other workers, and it is now certain that the EB virus is the causal agent of infectious mononucleosis. However, EBV antibody has been demonstrated in a high proportion of healthy individuals: infection commonly occurs in childhood and confers immunity, usually without causing clinical illness. In higher socio-economic classes (as at Yale), the virus is often first encountered in

adolescence, when it is more prone to cause overt illness before immunity is established.

The virus probably enters and replicates in pharyngeal epithelial cells, and throat washings have been shown to be infective. It is commonly transmitted in the prodromal stage of the disease by kissing. It binds to B lymphocytes by surface receptors and the viral genome becomes integrated into the DNA (p. 305) and transforms the B cells which, like Burkitt lymphoma cells, will proliferate indefinitely in culture. Replication occurs in occasional B cells with release of virions, which colonise more B cells. The transformed B cells possess EBV-determined surface antigens and stimulate an intense T-cell response, and this is reflected in the large numbers of atypical lymphoid cells, most of which are T immunoblasts, in the blood and lymphoid tissues. Only a small proportion of these cells are virus-transformed B cells. The T immunoblasts are cytotoxic for the latter, and destroy them, thus terminating the infection. The initial pharyngitis may be due to destruction of epithelial cells by viral replication and possibly by the cytotoxic T immunoblasts, but it is aggravated by secondary infection.

Infectious mononucleosis can thus be regarded as a virus-induced B-cell lymphoma which is eliminated by a vigorous T-cell response to the transformed cells. Antibodies to EBV persist and prevent binding to and invasion of B cells on subsequent infection, so that immunity is permanent. B cells may continue to harbour the virus in integrated, incompletely expressed form, but there is no evidence of an increased risk of subsequent development of a lymphoma.

Cytomegalovirus infection. In the fetus, the virus (one of the herpesvirus group) can cause fatal infection or a severe encephalomyelitis resulting in mental retardation (p. 757). In postnatal life infection is usually sub-clinical but sometimes causes an illness closely resembling infectious mononucleosis: it is not, however, accompanied by a pharyngitis and the Paul–Bunnell test is negative. Antibodies to EBV do not develop during the illness although they may, of course, already be present in the serum. The virus also causes lesions in immunosuppressed patients, e.g. following renal transplantation.

Measles. In measles, the lymphoid tissues

show formation of multinucleated giant cells, termed Warthin–Finkeldey cells (Fig. 18.8). They are sometimes observed in an appendix or tonsils which happen to have been removed during the incubation period of measles, and it is important not to mistake the changes for anything more sinister. Multinuclear giant cells also develop in the lesions of giant-cell pneumonia which sometimes complicates measles (Fig. 16.28, p. 474): here, they are formed by fusion of epithelial cells.

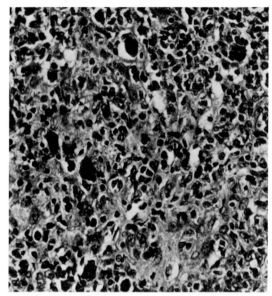

Fig. 18.8 Lymph node in the prodromal stage of measles, showing part of a germinal centre containing Warthin–Finkeldey giant cells. × 320.

Chronic non-neoplastic lymph node enlargement

This occurs in a very large number of conditions and is, of course, a most important clinical sign. The causes may be classified as follows:

(*a*) Reactive hyperplasia, accumulation of lipid and pigments, etc.
(*b*) Chronic infections and sarcoidosis

Many enlargements of lymph nodes are of known cause and readily classified. Others are of unknown aetiology, and some have features which render difficult their classification as either neoplastic or reactive: the term *reticulosis*

was usefully applied to this latter group, but has been used indiscriminately for any systematised cellular proliferation of the lympho-reticular tissue. *Malignant reticulosis* is still used for lympho-reticular neoplastic conditions, but the term *lymphoma* is now preferred.

(a) Reactive hyperplasia, lipid and pigment accumulations

Aggregation of macrophages in the peripheral and especially in the medullary lymph sinuses (formerly termed 'sinus catarrh') occurs in lymph nodes draining sites of chronic or repeated tissue destruction by infection or cancer (Fig. 18.9). It is often seen in the axillary nodes in carcinoma of the breast, and must not be mistaken for secondary cancer. Lymph nodes draining a focus of chronic infection commonly show also the morphological changes of the immune response (p. 137). These combined changes constitute *reactive hyper-*

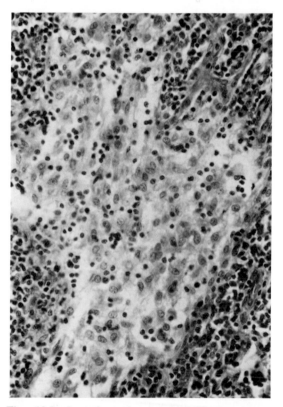

Fig. 18.9 Lymph node showing reactive 'sinus hyperplasia': an enlarged sinus containing increased numbers of macrophages. × 320.

plasia of the lymph nodes. Chronic irritation of long duration leads to a thickening of the stroma; sinuses become obliterated, and ultimately there may be marked fibrosis with atrophy of the lymphoid tissue.

Accumulation of pigments, etc. Pigments of various kinds, carried to the nodes, are taken up by macrophages of the sinuses and medullary cords, where they may persist indefinitely, as is seen in tattooing. The lymph nodes draining the areas affected by certain skin diseases show marked enlargement with accumulation and phagocytosis of melanin and of fat—so-called *lipomelanic reticulosis*. In cases of *anthracosis* carbon particles are dealt with in a similar way and they come to form black masses which replace the lymphoid tissue, with comparatively little fibrous reaction. In *silicosis*, on the contrary, marked fibrosis results from the irritation caused by stone particles, and the nodes become enlarged and indurated. Where there has been local haemorrhage, haemosiderin may be seen in the related lymph nodes, and a remarkable accumulation of haemosiderin occurs in macrophages in lymph nodes etc., in the increased iron storage of *haemosiderosis* (p. 283) and in the lymph nodes draining the liver and pancreas in *idiopathic haemochromatosis* (p. 282). Sometimes the amount is so great that the structure is quite obscured by the masses of pigment, and iron may constitute more than 10 per cent of the dry weight of the nodes. Enlargement of the lymph nodes in lipid storage diseases and in the histiocytoses is mentioned on pp. 566–8.

(b) Chronic infections and sarcoidosis

Tuberculosis. Tuberculous disease of lymph nodes is a very much less common lesion than formerly. It appears first in the group of nodes draining the primary site of entry of the bacilli; thus the cervical, bronchial and mesenteric groups are the commonest to be involved, although where bovine tuberculosis has been eliminated the pulmonary hilar nodes are nearly always the first to be affected.

As elsewhere, tubercles in the lymph nodes may coalesce and then undergo extensive caseation. The process spreads until ultimately the whole node is destroyed. Infection may spread at an early stage to other nodes to form large irregular masses matted together. This is a common feature of primary tuberculosis but is not usually seen with 're-infection' lesions (p. 212). Where infection from milk still occurs, caseous lesions, known as *scrofula*, develop in the cervical nodes. Such lesions, if untreated, may become adherent to the skin, ulcerate and discharge the softened caseous material, and secondary pyogenic infection may occur. Small sinuses thus formed may discharge intermittently for a long time, and disfiguring scarring results: this can be prevented by chemotherapy or surgical treatment. Even without treatment, the lesions usually subside: the caseous material undergoes calcification, while great thickening of the surrounding capsule occurs. In children, primary milk-borne intestinal infection may cause great enlargement and caseation of the mesenteric lymph nodes—*tabes mesenterica*. Healing is usual and calcified mesenteric lymph nodes are still quite commonly encountered.

Sarcoidosis. This is a granulomatous condition of unknown aetiology (p. 216). There is enlargement of lymph nodes and a variable amount of surrounding fibrosis. The pulmonary hilar nodes are usually affected, although other deep and superficial nodes are commonly involved, and also the spleen, lungs and various other organs. The condition is most commonly suspected because of hilar lymph node enlargement, with or without miliary infiltrates in the lung fields, detected on a chest x-ray of a young adult, performed either routinely or because of a febrile illness, cough or other chest symptoms. The affected nodes may be greatly enlarged, greyish or pinkish, and the condition may readily be mistaken clinically for Hodgkin's disease. On microscopic examination the lesion is seen to consist of aggregates of epithelioid cells closely resembling those seen in tuberculous lesions. The epithelioid cells may form tubercle-like follicles without caseation (Fig. 18.10), although there may be a little central fibrinoid necrosis. Multinucleate giant cells may be present, and sometimes they contain curious stellate or conchoid bodies, which may be calcified. The tuberculin test is usually negative in cases of sarcoidosis, and there is evidence that this is due to depression of cell-mediated immunity: delayed hypersensitivity to other antigens, e.g. mumps virus, is also depressed, although the serum contains the usual blood-group and other antibodies, and there may be a raised level of serum IgG.

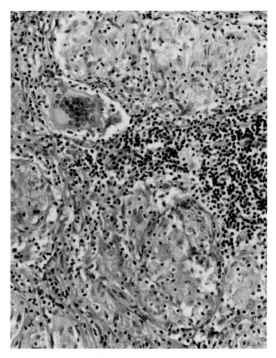

Fig. 18.10 Lymph node in sarcoidosis, showing tubercle-like epithelioid-cell follicles and giant cells but no caseation. × 75.

In some cases, delayed hypersensitivity to tuberculin has been observed to diminish or disappear following the onset of sarcoidosis, and to re-appear following remission. The Kveim test, a granulomatous sarcoid reaction at the site of intradermal injection of a sterilised extract of sarcoidosis lesions, is useful in diagnosis.

Syphilis. Enlargement with induration of the regional nodes draining the primary sore has already been described (p. 218), and also the importance of spread of the spirochaetes by lymphatics and the blood. The skin rashes of the secondary stage are usually accompanied by moderate or slight general enlargement of lymph nodes. In the tertiary stage, gummas are comparatively rare in the lymph nodes.

Histoplasmosis most commonly causes a localised respiratory infection with eventual healing and calcification (p. 224). It may, however, cause a relatively acute generalised infection in which the macrophages in the spleen, lymph nodes, bone marrow, liver and elsewhere are colonised by huge numbers of *Histoplasma capsulatum*. These organs are enlarged and the masses of colonised macrophages may show foci of necrosis similar to tuberculous caseation. A positive skin test, indicating cell-mediated immunity, is of little value in inhabitants of endemic areas where most individuals are positive, and in generalised infection the test may become negative.

Toxoplasmosis. Infection with the protozoon, *Toxoplasma gondii*, may occur at any age and serological tests indicate that approximately 30 per cent of adults in Europe have experienced infection, although very few have had an illness known or suspected to be toxoplasmosis. When, however, infection (usually clinically silent) occurs during pregnancy, the parasite may infect the fetus with serious results. It can colonise almost any type of human cell, including macrophages and the parenchymal cells of most organs. It proliferates within host cells to form pseudocysts containing young forms (bradyzoites) which are released and enter fresh cells. Depending on the stage of pregnancy, the effects range from abortion, stillbirth, a live child with severe abnormalities, or an apparently normal child which may develop relatively mild disease within the first few weeks of life. The most serious effects of fetal infection are encephalomyelitis and choroidoretinitis (p. 762).

Toxoplasmosis acquired after birth may present at any age, but most often in young adults. The commonest feature is lymph node enlargement, either localised or generalised, usually including upper cervical nodes. There may be no other symptoms or a febrile illness, and a wide variety of symptoms may also result from involvement of one or more organs including the lungs, heart and skeletal muscles. There are no typical blood changes. Histologically the main features of the affected lymph nodes are large cells, probably macrophages, scattered singly and in small groups throughout both the cortex and medulla (Fig. 18.11). The sinuses are stuffed with smaller cells of uncertain nature. Plasma cells may also be numerous. Tests for antibodies are exacting: the most satisfactory so far is a dye exclusion test; high or rising titres of antibody are suggestive of infection. Certain diagnosis depends on the inoculation of mice with fresh tissue mash, but this is seldom used.

Human infection usually results from ingestion of oocysts excreted in cat faeces, felines

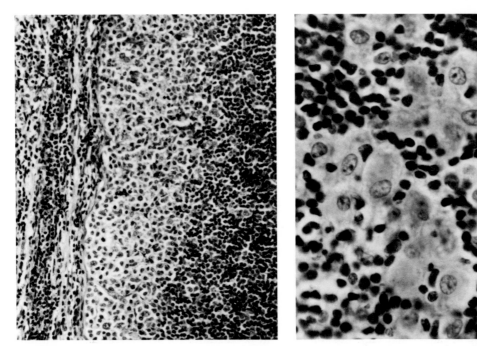

Fig. 18.11   Lymph node in toxoplasmosis. *Left*, a lymphoid sinus filled with pale cells of uncertain origin. × 175. *Right*, showing the large cells, probably macrophages, which are scattered singly and in small groups throughout the node. × 475.

being the only species in which the protozoon is known to complete its life cycle. The oocysts, which are resistant to drying, hatch in the gut, releasing trophozoites and these penetrate the mucosa. Infection may also result from ingestion of undercooked meat from bovines, sheep and pigs which, like man, can be infected by felines.

Resistance seems to depend mainly on cell-mediated immunity, although antibody interferes with the capacity of trophozoites and bradyzoites to colonise fresh cells.

The lymphomas

In view of their cellular variety and proliferative activity, it is not surprising that the lympho-reticular tissues give origin to a group of tumours which vary greatly in their morphology and behaviour.

Although the exact histogenesis of these tumours is often doubtful, there is good evidence that many of them originate from the lymphoid series of cells, while occasional tumours have features suggesting a derivation from the macrophage series. They are grouped together as the lymphomas. Most or all of these tumours will shorten the life-span of the victim, although they vary greatly in malignancy, some types causing death within a few weeks, others only after many years. With most lymphomas, the prognosis lies between these extremes, although surgical excision, x-irradiation and cytotoxic drugs in various combinations without doubt prolong life, and may effect cure in some cases.

Most lymphomas arise in the lymph nodes or other tissues rich in lymphoid cells or macrophages, such as the spleen, bone marrow, liver, skin and gastro-intestinal tract. Lymphocytes and macrophages are, however, almost ubiquitous in the body, and lymphomas can arise from virtually any tissue, including the central nervous system. Although some lymphomas resemble other malignant tumours in forming distinct tumour masses, they include also the lymphoid leukaemias, the cells of which tend to infiltrate the lymph nodes, bone marrow and various other organs diffusely, and also to circulate as single cells in the blood. It is not possible to draw a sharp distinction between the solid and leukaemic types of lymphoma, for the two patterns of growth are commonly associated. Indeed, enlargement of the lymph nodes, and sometimes of the spleen, commonly precedes the development of chronic lymphocytic leukaemia (p. 547).

Classification

As with other tumours, the main purpose in classifying lymphomas is to provide an indication of how a particular example will behave and what form of therapy is likely to be most effective. Unfortunately we have not yet reached the logical stage where classification of all the lymphomas can be based on their cell of origin and morphological features, although rapid progress is now being made.

There is general agreement that *Hodgkin's disease* is a distinct entity, or at least group, different from other forms of lymphoma. The origin of the characteristic cells of Hodgkin's disease is still, however, undecided. The remaining lymphomas are sometimes called *the non-Hodgkin lymphomas*: they form a diverse group, the classification and main features of which are presented on p. 580 *et seq*.

Hodgkin's disease

General features. Although this is the most common form of malignant lymphoma, its exact nature is still uncertain. The distinctive Reed–Sternberg cells and their mononuclear equivalents are widely regarded as the neoplastic elements, but opinion is divided on whether they are derived from lymphoid cells or from cells of the mononuclear phagocyte system.

The disease can develop at almost any age, although there is a peak incidence in early adult life and a second peak in the older age groups. The usual presenting feature is progressive and usually painless enlargement of lymph nodes, most often those of the cervical, inguinal or axillary groups. Early involvement of the abdominal or mediastinal nodes, the pharyngeal lymphoid tissue or the spleen is, however, not uncommon. It is unusual for extranodal sites to be primarily affected, although almost any tissue may be implicated by metastatic spread of the tumour. Constitutional symptoms are sometimes conspicuous, especially in advanced cases; they include an irregular low-grade pyrexia which occasionally assumes a periodic pattern (Pel–Ebstein fever), and an anaemia usually of normochromic normocytic type, sometimes accompanied by neutrophilia. Eosinophilia is less common. An important feature is an early depression of T-lymphocyte function with impairment of cell-mediated immunity. In consequence, patients are unusually prone to various infections, especially tuberculosis and zoster (p. 172), but also fungal and other 'opportunistic' infections by organisms of relatively low pathogenicity. The prognosis varies greatly from death in a few months to survival and good health for many years, even without treatment. The histological pattern and the extent of the disease process at the time of diagnosis have considerable prognostic significance.

Macroscopic changes. Initially the enlarged **lymph nodes** are discrete, soft and rubbery, with a greyish-pink cut surface. In some forms of the disease, however, fibrosis is present from the outset. As they become larger, the nodes tend to become firmer and bound together (Fig. 18.12), and they can produce serious pressure effects, for example on the trachea or mediastinal blood vessels. Foci of non-suppurative necrosis are also commonly observed in the lesions. **The spleen** is frequently involved and enlarged: the lesions develop in the Malpighian bodies, which become expanded and eventually confluent. This process ultimately produces the characteristic German sausage appearance of the cut surface, the pale patches of 'Hodgkin's tissue' resembling flecks of suet (Fig. 18.13). Staging procedures in which splenectomy is carried out (see below) have shown, however, that the spleen may be involved without obvious enlargement, and that splenomegaly may occur in the absence of tumour involvement, presumably due to diffuse hyperplasia of the red pulp. Although the disease is often restricted at first to the lymphoid organs, almost any tissue may be affected at a later

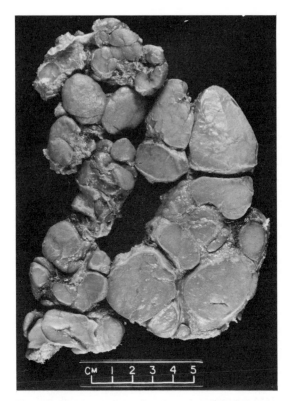

Fig. 18.12 A group of enlarged cervical lymph nodes in Hodgkin's disease. The largest nodes are becoming matted together.

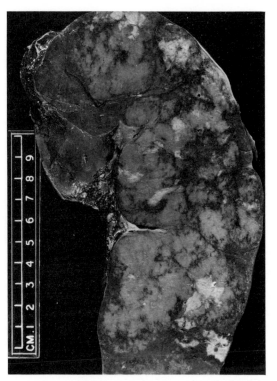

Fig. 18.13 Advanced involvement of the spleen in Hodgkin's disease. The neoplastic tissue is seen as pale, irregular patches on the cut surface. The whitish areas are foci of necrotic neoplastic tissue.

stage, the lesions appearing as infiltration and replacement of the normal tissue by patches of 'Hodgkin's tissue' with the appearances described above. Lesions occur especially in the **liver**, **kidneys** and **bone marrow**: involvement of the vertebrae may lead to pressure on the spinal cord with paraplegia: focal or diffuse lesions in the **lungs** are not uncommon (Fig. 18.14), especially if the mediastinal nodes are affected, and ulcerating tumour masses occur in the **gastro-intestinal tract**.

Microscopic appearances. The diagnosis is usually made readily by biopsy of an enlarged lymph node. The tissue of the node may be partly or completely replaced. The essential feature, without which the diagnosis cannot be made, is the presence of **Reed–Sternberg cells**. In its most characteristic form, this cell measures 40 μm or more in diameter, and has an intricate double or bi-lobed nucleus, each component of which has a vesicular appearance due to condensation of chromatin peripherally, and a large central eosinophilic nucleolus (Fig.

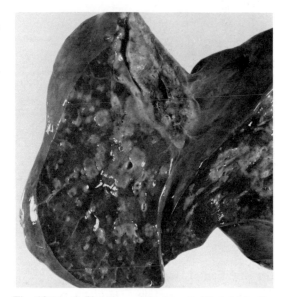

Fig. 18.14 Infiltration of the lung in Hodgkin's disease. In this instance the neoplastic tissue is seen as discrete pale patches: in some cases it is more diffuse. × 0·3.

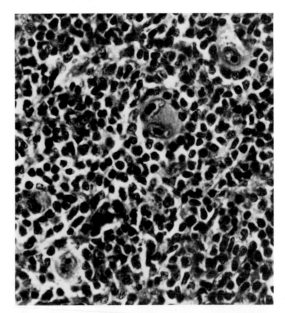

Fig. 18.15 Hodgkin's disease of lymphocyte-predominant type. Field chosen to show Reed–Sternberg cells, one of which shows the characteristic 'mirror-image' nuclei with large nucleoli. × 520.

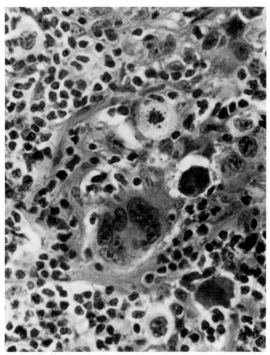

Fig. 18.16 Hodgkin's disease showing numerous neoplastic reticulum cells, including a multinucleated Reed–Sternberg cell. There was a mixed cell infiltrate in this case. × 450.

18.15). The cytoplasm is abundant, usually faintly eosinophilic, and sometimes vacuolated. Reed–Sternberg cells may be much larger with more complex or multiple nuclei (Fig. 18.16). Mononuclear cells with otherwise similar features are also present and appear to represent the main proliferating elements of the tumour: these neoplastic cells (termed here, without commitment on their origin, *neoplastic reticulum cells*) lie in a variable reactive cellular infiltrate which may be predominantly lymphocytic, or may be of *mixed cellular pattern*, including also plasma cells, macrophages, neutrophil and eosinophil leukocytes. Sometimes a sarcoid type of reaction with epithelioid cells and even Langhan's giant cells is seen and is liable to cause diagnostic difficulties. There is invariably some increase in reticulin fibres, particularly in the late stages, and abundant collagen is also formed in some variants of the disease.

Classification of Hodgkin's disease

For prognostic purposes, Hodgkin's disease has been sub-divided, on the internationally agreed Rye classification, into four major types as follows.

(1) Lymphocyte-predominant (15 per cent of cases). Formerly termed *Hodgkin's paragranuloma*, the important feature of this variant is the sparsity of Reed–Sternberg cells, lying among a cellular infiltrate consisting mainly of mature lymphocytes (Fig. 18.15). There may, however, be small aggregates of macrophages and sometimes sarcoid-like follicles. Eosinophils and other reactive cells are scanty or absent and capsular thickening and reticulin deposition are minimal, although sometimes a nodular pattern develops (see below).

(2) Nodular sclerosing type (40 per cent of cases). In this type, the lymph node capsule is thickened and fine or coarse bands of collagen sub-divide the node into nodules of various sizes (Fig. 18.17). Within the nodules the neoplasm may show a mixed cellular reaction (see above) but lymphocytes are usually predominant. The Reed–Sternberg cells show extensive cytoplasmic vacuolation and are called *lacunar cells* (Fig. 18.18): this feature is regarded by some as characteristic of this type of Hodgkin's disease, which typically is confined to the lower

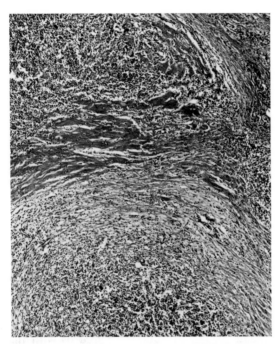

Fig. 18.17 Nodular sclerosing Hodgkin's disease in a lymph node. In this instance, the collagen dividing the 'Hodgkin's tissue' into nodules is abundant and the diagnosis is obvious. × 50.

cervical lymph nodes, mediastinum and sometimes upper abdominal nodes. In some instances the thymus appears to be first involved, and the condition has been misnamed *granulomatous thymoma*.

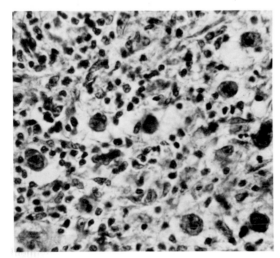

Fig. 18.18 Nodular sclerosing Hodgkin's disease in a lymph node, showing lacunar cells with vacuolated cytoplasm. × 375.

(3) Mixed-cellularity type (30 per cent of cases) corresponds to some of the cases formerly classified as *Hodgkin's granuloma*. Typical Reed–Sternberg cells and their mononuclear equivalents, commonly showing mitotic activity, are numerous, and lie in a mixed cellular infiltrate of neutrophils, eosinophils, macrophages, plasma cells and lymphocytes (Fig. 18.16). Reticulin fibres are sometimes abundant, with early collagen formation but this is diffuse and does not result in nodularity.

(4) Lymphocyte-depleted type (15 per cent of cases) includes cases previously classed as *Hodgkin's sarcoma*. The histological picture in such cases is dominated by Reed–Sternberg cells and their mononuclear equivalents (Fig. 18.19). Lymphocytes are sparse and other reactive cells, including eosinophils, are variable in number. Fibrous tissue varies greatly in amount, but in some cases is very abundant and diffuse.

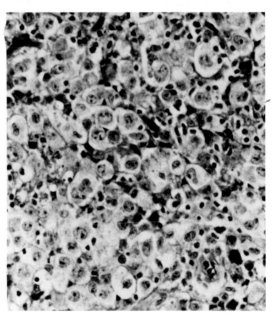

Fig. 18.19 Lymphocyte-depleted Hodgkin's disease. Most of the cells are neoplastic reticulum cells and lymphoctes are few. × 520.

Course of the disease

Hodgkin's disease often appears to start in a single lymph node or group of nodes, and may spread either by lymphatics or by the bloodstream to adjacent or distant tissues, both lymphoid and non-lymphoid. When limited to one area of the body, local ablation, e.g. by radio-therapy, is effective and sometimes apparently curative. Once the lesions are widely disseminated, systemic chemotherapy provides the only hope of controlling its otherwise relentless progress. The extent of the disease is thus critical in determining the prognosis and in planning therapy. To assess this accurately, clinical examination must be supplemented by at least bone marrow biopsy and abdominal lymphangiography, and many now advocate laparotomy with splenectomy and liver biopsy to detect and determine the extent of abdominal involvement. By these methods the disease can be subdivided into four stages (Table 18.1).

Table 18.1   Staging of Hodgkin's disease, based on the Ann Arbor system

STAGE I	Confined to a single lymph node or group of nodes.
STAGE II	Confined to upper or lower part of body, i.e. all lesions *either* above *or* below the diaphragm.
STAGE III	Involving lymph nodes above *and* below the diaphragm, with or without lesions in other tissues.
STAGE IV	Widespread involvement of one or more non-lymphoid tissues, with or without lymph node involvement.

There can be little doubt that the more extensive the disease the worse, in general, is the prognosis, and most patients surviving for ten years or more were initially diagnosed in stage I. The prognosis can also be correlated with the histological type. In general, the outlook is most favourable when lymphocytes are abundant and Reed–Sternberg cells sparse. Thus the lymphocyte-predominant type is associated with a much longer survival than the lymphocyte-depleted type, while the mixed-cellularity type has an intermediate prognosis.

The histological type also correlates quite well with the clinical stage, most cases of lymphocyte-predominant Hodgkin's disease presenting in stage I. The great importance of staging, however, is best illustrated by the nodular sclerosing type. This shows no tendency to undergo transitions to other forms of the disease, and provided it is in stage I the outlook is good: indeed, most of the patients surviving for many years belong to this group. In stages II and III, however, this variant has

a prognosis scarcely better than the mixed-cellularity type. Apart from the nodular sclerosing type, Hodgkin's disease is unfortunately prone to progress to a worse type, i.e. from lymphocyte-predominant to mixed-cellularity and to lymphocyte-depleted.

Non-Hodgkin lymphomas (NHL)

Apart from Hodgkin's disease, in which the nature of the malignant cell is uncertain, nearly all the lymphomas arise from cells of the B and T series of lymphoid cells. Occasional tumours do, however, originate from macrophages and are termed *malignant histiocytomas*, although usually included in the NHL group. Because they are readily identified as neoplasias of the macrophage system, monocytic leukaemia and the rare histiocytic medullary reticulosis (p. 585) are not usually classified as NHL.

While any classification of this diverse group of tumours must at present be provisional, the scheme set out in Table 18.2 accords with the

Table 18.2   Classification of the non-Hodgkin lymphomas

	Cell type
Low-grade malignancy	
Lymphocytic	B or T
Lymphoplasmacytic	B
Follicular	B
Mixed cell type	B
Centrocytic	B
Plasmacytic	B
High-grade malignancy	
Lymphoblastic	'Null', B or T
Large cell type	B or T
Histiocytic	Macrophage

view that these tumours can be broadly divided into two groups, one of **low-grade** and the other of **high-grade malignancy**. It also accepts the reality that cellular morphology in histological sections is likely to remain the mainstay of identification until more sophisticated immunological, ultrastructural and histochemical methods become widely available. It is becoming increasingly apparent that most lymphomas, and virtually all of those within the low-grade group, are derived from B lymphoid cells and that their morphological features are related to the stages in the life cycle of the lymphocyte sub-population to which they belong. Identification of cell type, particularly of the highly malignant lymphomas, is aided by examination of sections of approximately 1 μm thickness. However, this is not yet widespread practice, and accordingly we have prepared illustrations from the traditional paraffin-embedded tissue.

While all lymphomas are to be regarded as malignant they exhibit great variation in natural behaviour. The low-grade types of NHL, which arise almost exclusively in adult life, are often widely disseminated within the lymphoreticular tissues by the time they cause symptoms, and they often become leukaemic. They nevertheless may respond well to chemotherapy and the patient usually survives for years rather than months, although in some instances the tumour evolves into a highly malignant form. By contrast, the high-grade malignancy types of NHL quite often arise in childhood or adolescence and while they may also be widely disseminated at presentation, some are initially localised and only later become disseminated, their behaviour being similar to carcinoma. Staging procedures like those used in Hodgkin's disease are therefore of greater importance in the highly malignant types of NHL: in most instances, however, these tumours are fatal within a short period of time.

Non-Hodgkin lymphomas of low-grade malignancy

(a) Lymphocytic lymphoma. This tumour, which usually progresses slowly, occurs most often in adults over the age of 40 years, and in most cases appears to arise in the bone marrow producing the clinical and haematological features of chronic lymphocytic leukaemia (CLL) (p. 547). There is often generalised lymphadenopathy with hepatosplenomegaly and in some instances this dominates the clinical picture and leukaemia does not develop. Histologically there is a diffuse monotonous infiltration of neoplastic small lymphocytes (Fig. 18.20, *upper*). In lymph nodes this results in loss of the normal architectural features and, in addition, nucleolated pro-lymphocytes and even blast cells may be found lying singly or in groups ('proliferation centres'). When blast cells are numerous the disease tends to be more

aggressive. Most tumours in the group are of B cell type, only a few having T cell characteristics. *'Hairy cell' leukaemia* (B cell), *pro-lymphocytic leukaemia* (B or T) and the *Sézary syndrome* (T cell)—p. 548—are all considered to be variants of lymphocytic lymphoma.

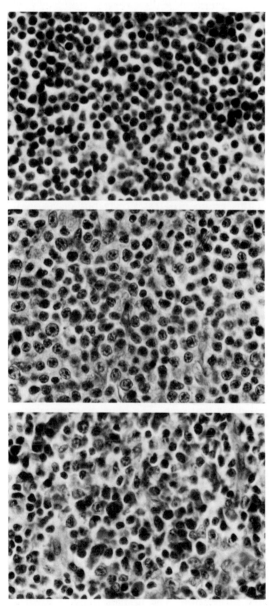

Fig. 18.20   Lymph nodes showing examples of diffuse lymphoma of low-grade malignancy. *Top*, lymphocytic type (from a case of chronic lymphocytic leukaemia). *Middle*, centrocytic type (also from a case of lymphoid leukaemia). *Bottom*, lymphoplasmacytic type (Waldenström's macroglobulinaemia). × 520.

(b) Lymphoplasmacytic lymphoma. These tumours show considerable variation in cellular morphology and clinical expression. Histologically the neoplastic infiltrate, which is diffuse, differs from lymphocytic lymphoma in consisting not only of small lymphocytes but also of plasma cells and cells with intermediate features (plasmacytoid lymphocytes Fig. 18.20, *lower*); immunoblasts and even germinal centre cells may, however, be found in some cases so that a wide spectrum of cells within the B lymphoid range is represented. The clinical features may resemble those of CLL but the condition can present as a localised tumour, sometimes in an extranodal site. A striking feature in some cases is the production of large amounts of immunoglobulin by the tumour cells: usually this is of the IgM class and is associated with the clinical syndrome of *Waldenström's macroglobulinaemia* (p. 551). In general, the tumours in this group progress slowly but occasionally they evolve into highly malignant lymphomas.

(c) Follicular lymphoma. This is one of the most common types of NHL: it is essentially a tumour of late adult life and is rarely encountered in individuals less than 30 years of age. The neoplastic cells have the features of the B cells normally found in germinal centres. Follicular lymphoma usually arises in a lymph node, less often in some extranodal site such as skin or intestinal tract. While it may remain localised for some time, in most cases it is widely disseminated, with generalised lymphadenopathy and splenomegaly, when the patient is first seen. The bone marrow is often involved and CLL develops in about 25 per cent of cases. Follicular lymphoma is perhaps the least malignant of the lymphomas but it has a tendency to change, sooner or later, into a highly malignant phase which is rapidly fatal and is often accompanied by a blood picture resembling acute lymphoblastic leukaemia (ALL) of B cell type.

Histologically the characteristic feature of the tumour is the formation of follicular structures (Fig. 18.21) which mostly consist of an admixture of two types of lymphoid cell in variable proportion. The first of these, known as the **cleaved follicle centre cell** or **centrocyte**, is variable in size but relatively small and has an irregularly-shaped or indented nucleus and indistinct cytoplasm (Fig. 18.22, *upper*); while the other cell, the **non-cleaved follicle centre cell**

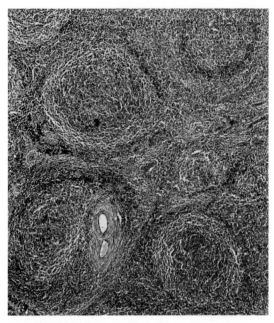

Fig. 18.21   Follicular lymphoma involving a lymph node. There are numerous follicles of roughly equal size. × 35.

or **centroblast**, is generally larger and has a round nucleus with two or more distinct nucleoli often peripherally placed (Fig. 18.22, *lower*). In an affected lymph node the neoplastic follicles resemble reactive germinal centres but usually have a more monotonous appearance due to a predominance of small centrocytes, and macrophages containing nuclear debris (p. 138) are scarce or absent. The neoplastic follicles also tend to have less well defined margins and to compress the interfollicular tissue, and the neoplastic infiltrate invariably extends beyond the sub-capsular sinus. In some cases the follicular structure is lost and there is extensive and profuse proliferation of follicle centre cells: this may be accompanied by the formation of collagen bands which is associated with a relatively good prognosis. Conversely, a predominance of centroblasts and prominent mitotic activity (Fig. 18.22, *lower*) implies a more aggressive course and possibly indicates transformation into a highly malignant phase.

In the bone marrow, neoplastic follicles can often be readily demonstrated (Fig. 18.23) and usually consist of aggregates of centrocytes which may also appear in the peripheral blood.

(d) Lymphoma of mixed type is characterised histologically by an admixture of small and large lymphoid cells which are generally found to be centrocytes and centroblasts; presumably this tumour represents a diffuse variant of follicular lymphoma.

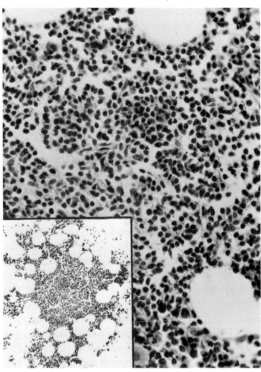

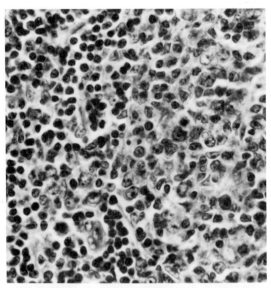

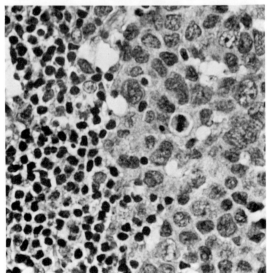

Fig. 18.22 *Above*, follicular lymphoma of predominantly small cleaved cell (or centrocyte) type. *Below*, follicular lymphoma of large-cell (centroblast) type. Each photograph shows the edge of a follicular lesion, the lymphoma cells being on the right, and adjacent lymphoid tissue, containing small lymphocytes, on the left. × 520.

Fig. 18.23 Follicular lymphoma of small-cell type in a needle biopsy of the bone marrow. *Inset*, at low magnification, showing the follicular pattern.

(e) Malignant lymphoma of centrocytic type is also a diffuse neoplasm of germinal centre cell type but consists exclusively of small centrocytes (Fig. 18.20, *middle*). Like follicular lymphoma it often becomes widely disseminated and may be associated with a leukaemic blood picture; it does not, however, appear to transform into a 'blast' cell phase.

(f) Plasmacytic lymphoma. The commonest of these is the bone marrow neoplasm known as multiple myeloma (p. 549): other tumours consisting of plasma cells are uncommon but are being increasingly recognised in the gastro-intestinal tract and may also arise in lymph nodes.

Non-Hodgkin lymphomas of high-grade malignancy

(a) Lymphoblastic lymphoma. By definition, tumours in this group consist of lymphoid 'blast' cells with a high nuclear—cytoplasmic ratio and nuclei mostly smaller than those of normal macrophages. In fact, the nature of cells with this morphology is uncertain, but some at least appear to be lymphocyte precursors. Not surprisingly, it may not always be possible to determine the lymphocyte subpopulation to which they belong. It is also notable that tumours of these cells often arise in the so-called primary lymphoid organs, i.e. bone marrow and thymus, and that many arise during childhood and adolescence. The pathological features of these highly malignant lymphoblastic tumours is variable. Some are leukaemic from the outset, the best example of this being the common type of ALL of childhood which is a marrow-derived lymphoblastic neoplasia of 'non-B non-T' cell type (p. 544). Others become leukaemic after a variable phase of solid growth, often in the mediastinum and possibly originating in the thymus. Tumours of this kind are generally of T cell origin and predominantly affect males in late childhood or adolescence (**Sternberg tumour**). The blast cells may have a distinctive convoluted nuclear morphology. In a third form of lymphoblastic tumour, solid tissue growth is the dominant feature and leukaemia, if it develops at all, is a late event. Some tumours in this category are known to be of B cell origin and some of these may be of germinal centre derivation, Burkitt's tumour (p. 304) being the classic example. Many other solid lymphoblastic tumours arising both in childhood and in adult life are difficult to classify: these may arise in many different sites such as pharyngeal lymphoid tissue, the gut-associated lymphoid tissue, the skin and lymph nodes.

(b) **Large cell lymphoma.** Formerly included within the term *reticulum cell sarcoma*, it is now recognised that these highly malignant tumours constitute a heterogeneous group; most seem to arise from transformed lymphocytes but others are derived from large germinal centre cells or possibly from cells of the mononuclear phagocyte system (see below). A feature of all these tumours is that the nuclei of the neoplastic cells are as large or larger than those of normal macrophages. Exact identification of the cell of origin is often difficult if not impossible, but the effort is worthwhile since the prognosis is better in some types than in others. The stage of the disease at the time of diagnosis is also critically important; only when it is localised is there any hope of controlling the disease, even

for a short time. The most dangerous and probably the most common member of this group is the tumour of *B immunoblasts* which tends to arise in individuals whose immunity system is defective in some way due, for example, to congenital or acquired immunodeficiency disease, prolonged immunosuppression by drugs, or simply old age. The tumours may arise either in lymph nodes or in an extranodal site and characteristically the tumour cells have vesicular nuclei with large central nucleoli and dense, sharply defined pyroninophilic cytoplasm (Fig. 18.24, *upper*). Tumours consisting exclusively of *centroblasts* are essentially similar in terms of behaviour and show only minor morphological

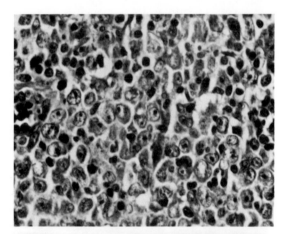

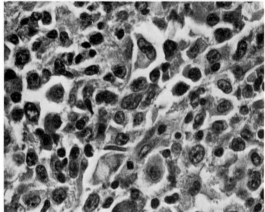

Fig. 18.24 Lymph nodes showing examples of highly malignant lymphomas. Both would formerly have been called 'reticulum-cell sarcoma'. Electron microscopy and immunohistology showed the lymphoma above to be of B immunoblastic type, and the lower to be a 'histiocytic lymphoma'. × 520.

differences. They can be identified with certainty only when they evolve from a pre-existing follicular lymphoma (see above). Tumours of *large centrocytes* appear to be less malignant and are worth distinguishing from other tumours in the group. Tumours of *T immunoblasts* have recently been identified and tend to be less aggressive; the nuclei are more irregular in shape and have less prominent nucleoli and the cytoplasm tends to be more abundant and pale staining.

(c) **Histiocytic lymphoma.** While it is somewhat illogical to include tumours of the mononuclear phagocyte system within the malignant lymphomas, it has become increasingly accepted that some initially localised tumours within the so-called large cell group (Fig. 18.24, *lower*), and arising especially in the gastrointestinal tract, are truly of histiocytic (macrophage) origin as revealed by their ultrastructural features, their possession of certain cytoplasmic enzymes (e.g. muramidase) and their phagocytic activity. These tumours vary in behaviour but may be highly aggressive. The term **histiocytic medullary reticulosis** (p. 568) is applied to a rapidly advancing form of histiocytic neoplasia in which the neoplastic process is widely disseminated within the lymphoreticular tissues from the outset. The condition is characterised by hepatosplenomegaly, lymphadenopathy and pancytopenia caused by phagocytosis of the formed elements of the blood. Most cases have been encountered in East Africa and the Far East but the condition is world-wide. It has also been observed as a complication of coeliac disease.

Conditions resembling lymphomas

Immunoblastic lymphadenopathy (IBL). In this recently described condition, which mainly affects old people, there is widespread lymphadenopathy and hepatosplenomegaly, associated with various disturbances including anorexia, weight loss, cutaneous rashes, haemolytic anaemia and polyclonal hypergammaglobulinaemia. The cause of IBL is uncertain;

it may originate from a hyperimmune state possibly related to hypersensitivity to drugs, etc. The affected lymph nodes show extensive loss of normal architecture and there is a conspicuous proliferation of arborising thick-walled blood vessels. Most of the cells present are immunoblasts and plasma cells. Amorphous eosinophilic intercellular material is also an important feature, and indeed the lymph nodes often appear distinctly hypocellular. The condition is usually rapidly fatal and death may be precipitated by the development of frank immunoblastic lymphoma.

Malignant lymphoepithelioid-cell lymphoma ('Lennert's' lymphoma). Like IBL (see above) this condition has only recently become recognised as a cause of lymph node enlargement, especially in older individuals. Clinically, lymphadenopathy may be associated with fever and weight loss and occasionally the nasopharyngeal lymphoid tissue is primarily attacked. Affected lymph nodes show loss of normal architecture due to infiltration of lymphocytes and immunoblasts, accompanied by conspicuous focal aggregation of epithelioid macrophages. Eosinophils are sometimes numerous. The nature of this condition is uncertain. In some instances it may be a variant of IBL, whereas in other cases it is suspected to be a developing form of malignant lymphoma, possibly of T-cell type. In any event the outlook is poor, median survival being not much more than one year, but in some cases the disease has persisted for many years. Occasionally a frank immunoblastic lymphoma develops.

Lymph node tumour metastases

It must be emphasised that lymphocytic spread and formation of metastatic tumours in the lymph nodes is an extremely important feature of all forms of carcinoma (p. 333) with the exception of basal cell carcinoma of the skin. Usually the draining nodes are enlarged first, but eventually more distant nodal metastases commonly develop. Most types of sarcoma tend to spread especially by the bloodstream, but lymph node involvement is by no means rare, particularly in rhabdomyosarcoma and synovial sarcomas.

The Thymus

The development of the thymus and the advances in our understanding of its major role in the immune response are described in Chapter

5, while the immunological deficiences resulting from defective thymic development are considered on pp. 169–72. The changes in the thymus in myasthenia gravis, and their possible significance, are dealt with on p. 936. It remains to provide a brief account of thymic tumours, all of which are rare.

Tumours of the thymus

Primary thymomas are of several types, all of which are rare.

Epithelial and lymphocytic tumours. Tumours containing both epithelial cells and lymphocytes are least uncommon. They usually consist of nodules, and may be predominantly epithelial, predominantly lymphocytic or may show widely differing ratios of the two cell types in different parts of the tumour and sometimes within single nodules. The epithelial cells may be plump and ovoid, spindle-shaped or rounded, or they may show acinar formation and resemble tumours of the endocrine glands, and two or more types of epithelium may be present in the same tumour. These tumours may be encapsulated, and intersected by dense fibrous stroma, or may extend locally to involve the adjacent tissues, including the major blood vessels, pleura, lung and pericardium. Most tumours are symptomless, and are detected incidentally by x-ray, or cause pressure symptoms, but not uncommonly a thymoma is accompanied by myasthenia gravis, or more rarely by systemic lupus erythematosus. hypogammaglobulinaemia or pure red-cell aplasia. The significance of these associations is not known, but it is noteworthy that the last two may respond to removal of the tumour, while the response of myasthenia gravis is more variable (pp. 936-7).

Very rarely, tumours of mixed epithelial-lymphocytic type, or purely epithelial tumours, are anaplastic and more highly malignant, and squamous carcinoma has been observed.

Teratoma also occurs in the thymus, and may be wholly well-differentiated or have poorly-differentiated areas.

Seminoma of the thymus resembles closely the commoner testicular tumour, and is highly radio-sensitive.

Lymphoid neoplasms may originate in the thymus. The condition sometimes termed *granulomatous thymoma* appears to be the nodular sclerosing form of Hodgkin's disease involving the thymus and often the mediastinal lymph nodes. *Sternberg's tumour* (p. 584) appears to originate, at least in some instances, in the thymus, which may be involved in various other forms of lymphoma.

References and Further Reading

The spleen

Chilcote, R. R., Bachner, R. L. and Hammond, D. (1976). Septicaemia and meningitis in children splenectomised for Hodgkin's disease. *New England Journal of Medicine* **295**, 798–800.

Constantopoulos, A., Najjar, V. A. and Smith, J. W. (1972). Tuftsin deficiency: a new syndrome with defective phagocytosis. *Journal of Pediatrics* **80**, 564–72.

Hodgkin's disease: classification and staging

Lukes, R. J. and Butler, J. J. (1966). The pathology and nomenclature of Hodgkin's disease. *Cancer Research* **26**, 1063–74.

Lukes, R. J. *et al.* (1966). Report of the Nomenclature Committee. *Cancer Research* **26**, 1311.

Rappaport, H. *et al.* (1971). Report of the Committee on Histological Criteria Contributing to the Staging of Hodgkin's Disease. *Cancer Research* **31**, 1864–5.

Non-Hodgkin lymphomas

Burke, J. S. and Butler, J. J. (1976). Malignant lymphoma with a high content of epithelial histiocytes (Lennert's lymphoma). *American Journal of Clinical Pathology* **66**, 1–9.

Carr, I., Hancock, B. W., Henry, L. and Ward, A. Milford (1977). *Lymphoreticular Disease*, pp. 214. Blackwell Scientific, Oxford, London, Edinburgh and Melbourne.

Henry, K., Bennett, M. H. and Farrer-Brown, G. (1978). Classification of the non-Hodgkin's lymphomas. In *Recent Advances in Histopathology*, No. 10, pp. 275–302. Ed. by P. P. Anthony and N. Woolf. Churchill Livingstone, Edinburgh.

Lennert, K. (1978). *Malignant Lymphomas other than Hodgkin's Disease*, pp. 833. Springer-Verlag, New York and Heidelberg.

Lukes, R. J. and Collins, R. D. (1975). New approaches to the classification of the lymphomata. *British Journal of Cancer* **31**, Supplement 11, 1–28.

Lukes, R. J. and Tindle, B. H. (1975). Immunoblastic lymphadenopathy. A hyperimmune entity resembling Hodgkin's disease. *New England Journal of Medicine* **292**, 1–8.

19

Alimentary Tract

I: The Oral Cavity, Salivary Glands and Pharynx

The oral cavity

In general, the tissues of the mouth are subject to the same types of lesion found in other sites but these often show distinctive features peculiar to the mouth. In addition there are a number of specific lesions related to the teeth and their supporting structures.

The most frequent diseases in the mouth are dental caries and non-specific chronic inflammation of the soft tissues immediately related to the teeth. The principal aetiological agents in both of these diseases are the oral bacteria. The bacterial flora of the mouth is complex. Bacteria in the mouth are found in saliva, adherent to the epithelium and also in adherent deposits on tooth surfaces. These deposits are *dental plaque* consisting of bacteria in an organic matrix mainly of bacterial but also of salivary origin. Calcium salts may be deposited in dental plaque to form hard, adherent *dental calculus.*

The teeth

Teeth consist of three specialised calcified tissues (Fig. 19.1): the **dentine** which consists of a thick layer of calcified collagenous tissue surrounding the soft tissues of the pulp, the **enamel**, which forms the hard outer layer of the crown, and is non-cellular, consisting largely of calcium apatite crystals with a delicate organic matrix, and thirdly the **cementum**, which overlies the dentine of the root(s). At the apex of each root is an apical foramen through which vessels and nerves enter the pulp.

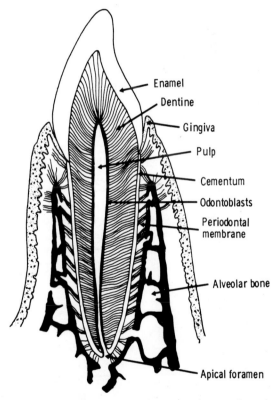

Fig. 19.1 Cross section of an anterior tooth and related tissues.

Developmental abnormalities

Tooth development and eruption of the first dentition and then the second dentition begin at about 3 months of intrauterine life and continue until the early 20s. During this period many developmental abnormalities can occur in the number of teeth, in their form and colour, in the structure of individual tooth elements and the times of eruption and shedding of teeth. These abnormalities result from various factors, both genetic and environmental. An example of iatrogenic disease is the unsightly permanent staining of the calcified dental tissues which results from administration of tetracycline during tooth development.

Dental caries is the progressive destruction, by bacteria and their products, of the calcified tissues of the teeth exposed to the oral environment. Caries itself, and consequent inflammation of the tooth pulp, are the commonest causes of tooth loss up to middle age.

Dental caries usually starts in two principal areas of the tooth, the fissures on the occlusal or biting surfaces of posterior teeth and the areas between teeth (*interproximal caries*). Both of these are areas of relative stagnation (p. 176) in which plaque is likely to accumulate because of lack of friction from normal chewing and from contact with a mucosal surface. The bacteria within the plaque produce various organic acids. The amount of acid produced and resulting pH are dependent on a number of factors, among which the thickness of the plaque and the concentration of dietary sugars appear to be particularly important. The initial attack upon enamel (Fig. 19.2) is by the acid, which produces decalcification and removal of part of the organic matrix. At first this is a painless process, but, as the lesion extends through the enamel, dentine is involved and the pain of

toothache starts. Bacteria do not enter the enamel until decalcification has so weakened the structure that breakdown has occurred to form a cavity. At this stage the acid conditions within the cavity particularly favour the growth of *Lactobacilli*, which appear to be the main organisms involved in dentine caries. The organisms initially penetrate the dentinal tubules, but then cause softening and distortion of the dentine by a combination of decalcification and proteolytic breakdown of the collagen matrix (Fig. 19.3). The carious dentine becomes yellow by absorption of pigment from bacterial metabolic products and from the mouth; the process then extends through the dentine towards the dental pulp.

Dental caries may also start at the neck of the tooth either by involving the cementum and then the dentine, or, if cementum is deficient, by directly attacking the dentine. This form of caries is more common in older patients in whom recession of the gingiva is common.

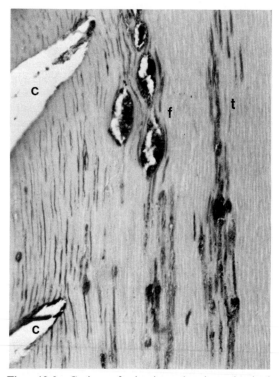

Fig. 19.3 Caries of dentine showing dentinal tubules with bacteria (t) which in places have accumulated in liquefaction foci (f) and in other areas spread along the incremental growth lines giving dentine clefts (c). × 110.

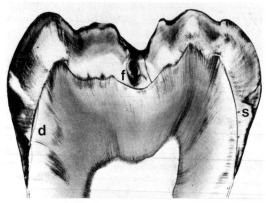

Fig. 19.2 Ground section of a molar tooth crown showing early smooth surface enamel caries (s), fissure caries (f) and early dentine caries deep to enamel caries (d). × 6.

In the very early stages of enamel caries, the damage due to acid attack of enamel is reversible, but thereafter the process of caries of enamel and dentine is progressive except in unusual circumstances where the area becomes self-cleaning and the lesions may be arrested.

Lesions of the dental pulp. The dental pulp is a vascular connective tissue confined within the rigid pulp chamber and root canals in the dentine. The most frequent and clinically significant lesions of the pulp are inflammatory lesions (*pulpitis*) due to the extension of the carious process into dentine and eventually to the pulp. Physical injury, e.g. heat and chemical irritation from filling materials, may also give rise to inflammation in the pulp.

Pulpitis may be acute or chronic. The pathological processes of acute pulpitis are the same as in other acute inflammatory lesions. Because these changes are occurring within the rigid confines of the pulp chamber there is increase in pressure due to inflammatory exudate. Consequently acute pulpitis is very painful and may proceed quickly to necrosis of the pulp.

If the insult to the pulp is less severe, chronic pulpitis may result: it is characterised by infiltration of lymphocytes and plasma cells and there is loss of specialised cells such as odontoblasts. The pulp may eventually undergo necrosis, which is often symptomless. Clinically the non-vital tooth lacks lustre and may be discoloured by the leaching of products of the necrotic pulp into the dentine. In children, a large carious cavity penetrating quickly to the pulp may result in a large opening into the pulp chamber, leading to open pulpitis from which exudate can drain. A mass of granulation tissue forms in the pulp and may extend, as a *pulp polyp*, into the carious cavity.

Periodontal disease

Acute inflammation of the gingiva can arise from various physical, chemical and infective causes. *Acute ulceromembranous gingivitis* (*Vincent's infection*) is a distinctive condition in which there is necrosis of the interdental papillae with variable spread to other parts of the gingiva. It is characterised by a localised overgrowth of two commensal organisms, *Fusibacterium fusiforme* and *Borrelia vincenti* but the exact relationship of these to the disease is not clear.

Chronic inflammation is very common in the periodontal tissues and is the most frequent cause of tooth loss in older individuals. A number of local and systemic factors are involved, but of these the most important is the *bacterial plaque around the neck of the tooth*.

For clinical convenience the lesions are divided into **chronic gingivitis** where the disease is confined to the gingiva and **chronic periodontitis** where the process involves the deeper tissues, causing retraction towards the root apex of the part of the gingiva attached to the tooth. As in most examples of chronic inflammation, there is both tissue destruction and proliferation of new tissue in attempted repair, but there is a net tissue loss. Many mechanisms of tissue destruction have been described involving polymorphonuclear leucocytes, macrophages and both humoral and cell mediated immune mechanisms. It is probable that all of these are operative in different situations. The later stages of the disease involve the alveolar bone supporting the teeth. Osteoclastic resorption occurs and progresses to the formation of areas of deepening of the gingival sulcus, termed *periodontal pockets*: these contain a mixture of necrotic tissue and anaerobic bacterial plaque. Infrequently there is an acute exacerbation of infection in such pockets and a *periodontal abscess* can arise.

Periapical lesions. A variety of lesions can occur in the tissues related to the root apices of teeth. The most frequent of these arise from spread of infection from pulpitis, through the apical foramina of the tooth, to reach the periodontal membrane. This can result in an acute **periapical abscess**, a very painful condition which may be accompanied by cervical lymphadenopathy and generalised fever and malaise. Pus tracks through the adjacent bone and, after the periosteum is breached, a soft tissue abscess—a **gumboil**—develops and later discharges.

More frequently periapical infection follows a low grade pulpitis and a **periapical granuloma** develops. This consists of a mass of granulation tissue heavily infiltrated with chronic inflammatory cells. There is resorption of surrounding bone, seen radiographically as a periapical radiolucency (Fig. 19.4). Acute exacerbation of a periapical granuloma may result in an acute periapical abscess and conversely a periapical granuloma can develop

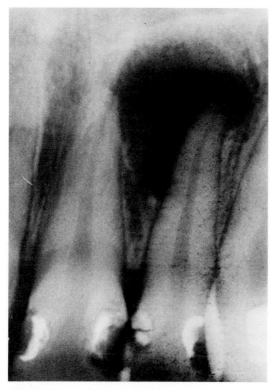

Fig. 19.4 Radiograph of upper anterior teeth with large restorations. The upper lateral incisor is non-vital and a radiolucency is present in the bone around the apex of the tooth.

after an acute periapical abscess has pointed and drained.

Epithelial-lined cysts of the jaws

A number of different types can occur: they can be classified into *odontogenic cysts*, in which the epithelium is derived from the dental epithelial tissues, and *fissural cysts* which arise in areas of fusion of embryonic processes.

Odontogenic cysts may be further subdivided into *inflammatory* and *developmental cysts* and categorised by their position in relation to the teeth. The commonest is the *dental cyst* (synonyms, *radicular* or *periapical cyst*) which is an inflammatory cyst developing from a peri-apical granuloma. Epithelial remnants related to the root are stimulated to grow and cyst formation occurs. If the affected tooth is extracted, the cyst may be left in the bone and remain as a *residual cyst*. The most frequent of the developmental odontogenic cysts is the *dentiger-*

ous cyst which arises in the reduced enamel epithelium around the crown of a tooth which has failed to erupt. Closely related is the *eruption cyst* which presents as a bluish fluctuant swelling overlying the crown of an erupting tooth.

The odontogenic cysts described above are lined by non-keratinised stratified squamous epithelium which occasionally includes a few mucus-secreting cells. These cysts are usually symptomless unless infected and can grow to several centimetres with considerable bone destruction. They must be differentiated from the *odontogenic keratocyst* (synonym—*primordial cyst*) which has a distinctive keratinised stratified squamous epithelial lining (Fig. 19.5). Its

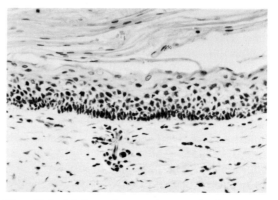

Fig. 19.5 Lining of an odontogenic keratocyst showing a thin regular parakeratinised epithelium with a distinctive columnar basal cell layer. × 140.

relationship to the teeth is variable but frequently it is not directly related to any one tooth. It occurs anywhere in the jaws, the most common site being in the mandibular molar area, often extending up into the vertical ramus of the mandible. The importance of this cyst lies in the frequency with which it recurs after attempted surgical removal, because of the friable nature of the lining and the presence of related small daughter cysts.

Fissural cysts. Two types of intra-osseous developmental fissural cysts are described: the *nasopalatine cyst*, which arises in the nasopalatine canal in the midline of the anterior part of the hard palate, and the *globulo-maxillary cyst*, which arises between the upper second incisor tooth and the canine tooth in the line of fusion of the globulo-maxillary process and the lateral nasal process. A similar type, the *nasolabial cyst*, occurs in the upper lip below the ala of the nose, but this is within the soft tissues. The fissural cysts are usually lined by epithelium with numerous mucus secreting cells, but areas of non-keratinised stratified squamous epithelium may also be present.

Oral mucosa

The oral epithelium is conventionally divided into three structural varieties. (*a*) The loose, mobile mucosa of the cheeks, lips, floor of mouth, ventral surface of tongue and soft palate is known as *lining mucosa* and is non-keratinised: (*b*) The mucosa of the hard palate and gingivae, and the alveolar mucosa which covers the edentulous ridges after tooth loss, is *masticatory mucosa* and is keratinised: (*c*) The specialised lining of the dorsum of the tongue is keratinised *gustatory epithelium*. Although the oral epithelia are grouped into these three types, there is wide variation in histological appearances even within individual types. The supporting connective tissues also show wide variation between the loose corium of lining mucosa and the dense mucoperiosteum of the hard palate.

The oral mucosa is subjected to numerous physical insults and is exposed to vast numbers of micro-organisms, and to food and other material introduced into the mouth. Oral epithelium has a high rate of cell turnover. In almost all lesions of oral mucosa, physical trauma and infection will play a role, and this may be superimposed upon a previously normal or an abnormal mucosa. It is not surprising that these circumstances produce complex changes in disease which are not yet fully documented or understood.

Developmental abnormalities of oral epithelium. Apart from Fordyce's disease—the presence of pale yellowish sebaceous glands in the lining mucosa, especially of the cheeks—developmental abnormalities of oral mucosa are rare.

Infections. Oral mucosa is frequently subject to infection, both as a primary event or superimposed upon some preceding disease.

Fungal infection is usually due to *Candida sp.* which are part of the oral flora of over half the population. *Candida albicans* is the most frequent of these and the lesions have been cate-

gorised into several types. *Thrush* is an acute condition found most often in young children or debilitated adults and is characterised by detachable white fungal plaques on the epithelium. *Chronic atrophic candidiasis* is found under upper dentures. The mucosa is a fiery red due to an inflammatory reaction to fungi which are mainly in the interstices of the fitting surface of the denture. Alternatively candidal hyphae may be found in adherent hyperkeratotic lesions as *chronic hyperplastic candidiasis* (*candidal leukoplakia*).

Angular cheilitis (Fig. 19.6) is a painful cracking at the angles of the mouth often of multifactorial aetiology. With the loss of natural teeth and muscle tone, folds occur which may be moistened by saliva. Infection with *Candida albicans* and *Staphylococcus aureus* is frequent. Underlying nutritional deficiencies, notably of the B group of vitamins and of iron, can predispose to the condition.

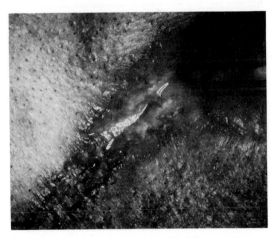

Fig. 19.6 Angular cheilitis showing typical moist skin fissuring.

Virus infections. The most frequent viral infection of oral epithelium is caused by *Herpes simplex*. This occurs in the primary form as *acute herpetic gingivo-stomatitis* characterised by extensive painful ulceration and generalised upset. *Secondary or recurrent herpetic lesions* are more frequent, especially on the lips where the initially vesicular phase is followed by ulceration and crusting. Several other viral diseases also produce vesicular lesions of mucosa which then ulcerate, e.g. the Koplik's spots of measles.

Dermatoses. A number of diseases can involve the skin and mucosae. The skin manifestations of these diseases are discussed in Chapter 26. The oral mucosal features are similar, but frequently not so clearcut, making diagnosis more difficult. Lichen planus (Fig. 19.7) is the most frequent of the dermatoses which affect the mouth. Other examples include pemphigus, benign mucous membrane pemphigoid, erythema multiforme and lupus erythematosus.

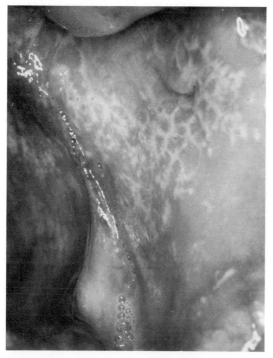

Fig. 19.7 Lichen planus of the cheek mucosa showing a reticular pattern of keratinised striae.

Recurrent oral ulceration (Aphthous ulceration). Recurrent ulcers, either singly or in crops, are a common and troublesome problem. In many cases these are of unknown aetiology, but in some patients they are associated with vitamin B group deficiencies, iron deficiency, or various food allergies.

Leukoplakia. Leukoplakia is a clinical descriptive term for a white patch on the oral mucosa which cannot be attributed to a specific disease, such as lichen planus or lupus erythematosis. It is not a pathological entity. Chronic irritation and smoking are the most commonly implicated aetiologic factors, but in many cases of leukoplakia the causal factors are quite unknown.

Leukoplakia is seen when there is keratosis of a normally unkeratinised site or hyperkeratosis of a site where keratin is normally present. Histologically the viable cell layers of the epithelium may show acanthosis or atrophy and a variable inflammatory infiltrate is present. In most cases there is no epithelial dysplasia, but a small proportion do show dysplasia and can proceed to squamous-cell carcinoma. It is now generally agreed that this is unusual: for example, in a large series of patients followed up carefully, malignancy developed in 4 per cent during a 20-year period. In certain sites, however, leukoplakia has been shown to be more prone to become malignant, particularly in elderly people. These are the floor of the mouth and the ventral surface and lateral margins of the tongue. Leukoplakia arising on an atrophic epithelium or showing as areas of white upon an erythematous background (*speckled leukoplakias*) is also more likely to proceed to carcinoma. Speckled leukoplakias often appear to be associated with superficial infestation by *Candida albicans*.

Pigmentation. Melanin pigmentation, especially of the gingiva, is frequent in coloured races but is very infrequent in whites. Melanin pigmentation of the lips and buccal mucosae occurs in Addison's disease. Perioral melanin pigmentation is a feature of the rare Peutz-Jeghers syndrome (p. 650).

Ingestion of various heavy metals can give rise to dark blue or black pigmented lines around the gum margins, where the pigment is deposited in soft tissues as sulphides following reaction with bacterial products from the dental plaque.

Soft tissue swellings

Fibrous overgrowths of the oral mucosa are a common response to chronic irritation. These may occur on labial or buccal mucosa when they are best designated simply as *fibrous overgrowths*, although the older term *fibroepithelial polyps* may still be used. A frequent site is in relation to the margins of old and ill-fitting dentures where the term denture-induced hyperplasia is used (Fig. 19.8).

An **epulis** is a localised swelling on the

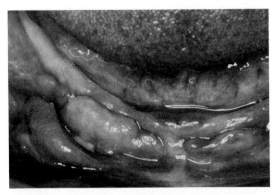

Fig. 19.8 Denture-induced hyperplasia of the lower labial sulcus with folds of fibrous overgrowth provoked by the margin of an old ill-fitting denture.

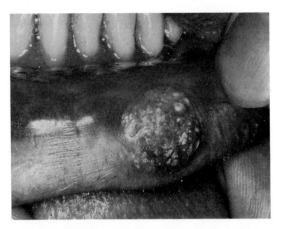

Fig. 19.9 Small exophytic squamous-cell carcinoma of the lower lip.

gingiva. The common type is a reaction to chronic irritation, e.g. from dental calculus or the rough margin of a carious cavity or filling; it consists of a mass of highly cellular fibrous tissue frequently with metaplastic bone formation. Less commonly, such lesions consist of highly vascular granulation tissue and are then described as **pyogenic granulomas**: this may occur during pregnancy—*pregnancy epulis*.

Giant cell epulis is a distinctive lesion consisting of numerous multinucleated giant cells in a vascular stroma. The giant cell epulis is a superfical lesion with minimal bone involvement, but intra-osseous lesions, such as *central giant cell granuloma* or *osteitis fibrosa cystica* may mimic a giant cell epulis if they extend outwith the bone.

Haemangiomas and less frequently **lymphangiomas** can arise in the oral mucosa and submucosa.

Tumours of the oral mucosa

Tumours arise from any of the tissues of the oral mucosa, but the most frequent neoplasms are epithelial. **Squamous cell papilloma** may occur at any site on the oral mucosa. The most frequent malignant tumour is **squamous-cell carcinoma**, which accounts for more than 90 per cent of oral malignancies. Despite the fact that early recognition should be possible, many oral cancers have a bad prognosis because the tumours are not recognised and treated when small. Although squamous-cell carcinoma can occur at any oral site, more than half the lesions involve either the lower lip (Fig. 19.9) or

the lateral border of the tongue (Fig. 19.10). Carcinoma of the lower lip is much more frequent in males and exposure to sunlight appears to be an important causal factor. The lesion is most often seen as an ulcer which fails to heal. Histologically it is usually a well-differentiated squamous carcinoma which shows slow local spread and involves lymph nodes relatively late.

Intra-oral carcinomas as a generalisation have a poorer prognosis the further posteriorly in the mouth they arise. Although some appear to develop from recognised premalignant lesions, over three-quarters of carcinomas develop in clinically normal mucosa. The earliest lesions are red rather than white and are symptomless. As successful treatment is dependent upon

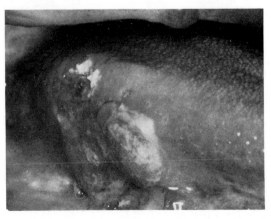

Fig. 19.10 Squamous cell carcinoma of the lateral margin of the tongue and lingual sulcus.

early diagnosis, it is important that lesions of the oral mucosa which do not relate to obvious causes, or which fail to respond to the removal of obvious causes, be examined microscopically.

Other tumours occur rarely in the mouth. They include the usually-benign granular cell myoblastoma, malignant lymphomas of the tonsils and palate, and tumours of the minor salivary glands.

Odontogenic tumours. The lesions designated odontogenic tumours are a group of several rare lesions, of widely differing pathology, derived from the dental soft and hard tissues. Some of these lesions are neoplasms but several are hamartomas. The most important of the odontogenic neoplasms is the *ameloblastoma* which is an epithelial neoplasm of distinctive appearance (Fig. 19.11). Ameloblastomas are

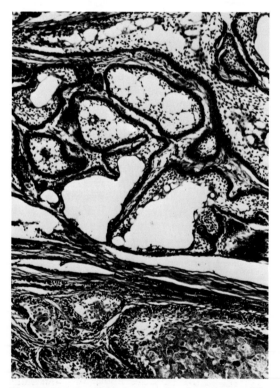

Fig. 19.11 Ameloblastoma, showing the proliferated epithelium in spaces enclosed in a well-defined stroma. In places, the epithelium forms a loose network. The appearances resemble the enamel organ. The lower part of the field shows a histological variant of an ameloblastoma in which granular cells are present.

most frequent in the molar region of the mandible and are locally aggressive, often producing extensive bone destruction. When the tumour mass contains enamel and dentine the term *odontoma* is used. A complex odontoma consists of a disorganised mass of dental tissues, whereas a compound odontoma consists of numerous small teeth.

The salivary glands

Inflammation of the parotid and other salivary glands is most often due to the virus of **mumps**, which gives rise to an early viraemic phase. The chief lesion in mumps is an acute inflammatory swelling, mainly of the parotids, with oedema and interstitial mononuclear cell infiltration. Usually this subsides without permanent damage to the glands. It may be accompanied by orchitis and by pancreatitis, both of which are more prone to result in some degree of atrophy. Mumps virus is also a relatively common cause of aseptic meningitis (p. 755).

Suppurative parotitis occurs as a complication of prolonged febrile illnesses, infection usually reaching the gland by way of Stensen's duct. Infection is prone to occur if the duct is partially obstructed by a calculus.

Salivary calculi occur most often in the submaxillary gland. The calculus is round or elongated and may project from the orifice of the duct which it partially occludes. Salivary calculi are composed chiefly of calcium carbonate and phosphate. The obstruction thus caused is apt to lead to atrophy and fibrosis of the gland (Figs. 19.12).

Sjøgren's syndrome occurs mostly in women of middle age. There is dryness of the mouth due to lack of saliva with consequent extensive dental caries. There may also be *keratoconjunctivitis sicca*. Many cases also suffer from chronic polyarthritis of rheumatoid type. The lacrimal, conjunctival and salivary glands are often swollen: they are extensively infiltrated by lymphocytes and plasma cells, the glandular acini are atrophic and may disappear, and the ducts show epithelial proliferation to form masses of cells, among which lie accumulations of homogeneous eosinophilic material (Fig. 19.13). Various auto-antibodies may appear in the serum, including antinuclear antibodies, precipitins to cellular constituents and rheumatoid factor. The syndrome is sometimes

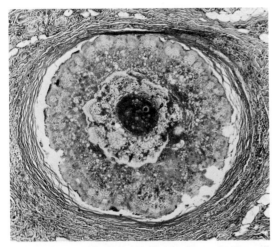

Fig. 19.12a Calculus obstructing duct of submaxillary gland. × 55.

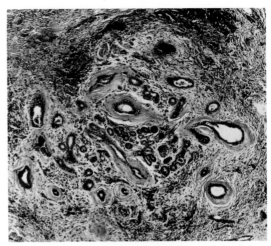

Fig. 19.12b Atrophy and fibrosis of submaxillary gland with chronic inflammatory infiltration, resulting from duct obstruction. × 55.

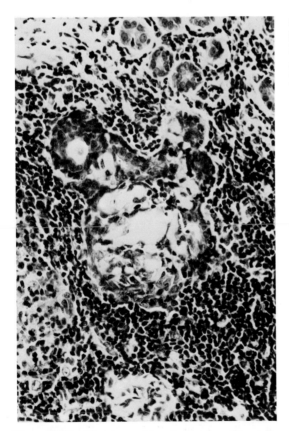

Fig. 19.13 The parotid gland in Sjøgren's syndrome, showing heavy infiltration with lymphocytes, loss of glandular tissue and proliferation of duct epithelium to form a cellular mass containing foci of pale-staining hyaline material. × 320.

associated with chronic thyroiditis and its immunological accompaniments. The condition long known as Mikulicz's disease is now recognised as the same condition, with prominent lacrimal gland enlargement.

Uveo-parotid fever. This is one of the important lesions of sarcoidosis (p. 216) in which iridocyclitis and parotid swelling occur, sometimes involving the facial nerve and causing paralysis. The glands may be considerably enlarged due to the presence of chronic inflammatory infiltrates in which sarcoid follicles are found.

Salivary gland tumours

These tumours are not very common, but notably variable in histology and difficult to treat. About 20 per cent are malignant, and even the benign ones are difficult to resect completely and (except for the adenolymphoma) often recur. Eighty per cent occur in the parotid, ten per cent in the submandibular gland, and ten per cent in the minor glands. More than might be expected occur in the palate, and very few in the sublingual glands. Theories to explain the histological diversity are numerous, and none satisfactory. Similar tumours occur in the lachrymal, nasal and sweat glands.

Pleomorphic salivary adenoma (PSA). Over two-thirds are of this type. They form firm slow-growing nodules, apparently well defined (Fig. 19.14). Most characteristically they consist

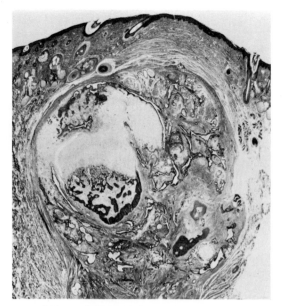

Fig. 19.14 A small pleomorphic salivary adenoma of the lower lip. The tumour is roughly rounded and sharply defined. The pale part of the mushroom-shaped area within it is cartilage, which shows formation of bone trabeculae, seen as dark areas. × 7.

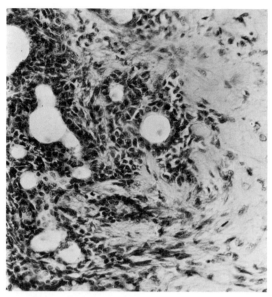

Fig. 19.15 Pleomorphic salivary adenoma, showing gland-like epithelial structures, from which cells appear to be streaming off into the connective tissue stroma. × 200.

of an epithelial element made up of small ducts and cysts surrounded by more or less solid masses of cells which probably correspond to myoepithelium of the normal gland, and which stream off into the stroma (Fig. 19.15). This stroma is usually infiltrated with connective-tissue mucin ('myxoid') and in about one case in seven shows metaplasia to cartilage: it was this combination of epithelial tissue with cartilage that gave rise to the old name of '*mixed parotid tumour*'. These tumours are benign and do not metastasize, but they often recur (sometimes after decades). This is largely due to the fact that small outgrowths of the tumour often protrude through the capsule and are left behind if close excision is done, while wide excision is made difficult by the facial nerve and other important structures. Occasionally a frank carcinoma arises in a pre-existing PSA.

Rarer variants include the **monomorphic adenoma** (strands or tubes of small dark cells), the **mucoepidermoid tumour** (combining squamous and mucoid epithelial elements) and the **acinic cell tumour** (closely resembling parotid acinic cells). The last two are usually malignant though generally at a low level.

Adenolymphoma (Fig. 19.16) the second com-

monest tumour, is basically a papillary cystadenoma, with a characteristic two-layered epithelium of tall pink-staining (mitochondrion-rich) cells, and with abundant lymphoid tissue filling the stroma. In distinction from all other

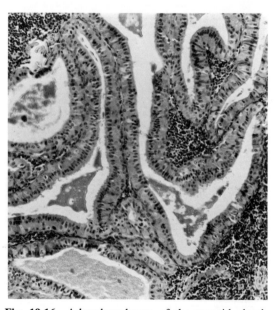

Fig. 19.16 Adenolymphoma of the parotid gland, showing the papillary architecture, with lymphoid stroma. × 130.

tumours of these glands, they occur chiefly in older men, are almost entirely limited to the parotids, may be multiple and bilateral, and are *always benign*. Work in Glasgow by Ian Brown has recently shown that adenolymphomas contain large amounts of IgA, apparently formed in the lymphoid tissue and secreted by the epithelial cells into the lumen: the epithelium only shows its characteristic morphology when in contact with lymphoid tissue and engaged in IgA transfer. It is probable that this finding is related to the presence of IgA in the normal saliva, and suggests that this is derived from the lymphoid foci normally present in the parotid gland.

Adenoid cystic carcinoma is the commonest malignant tumour, and, though slow-growing and slower to metastasize, is rarely if ever cured. It consists of masses of small dark-staining cells which show a characteristic sieve-like or 'cribiform' pattern (Fig. 19.17) and has a particularly striking tendency to infiltrate along nerves.

Besides the varieties already mentioned, occasional ordinary **adenocarcinomas** and even **squamous-cell carcinomas** occur, and **malignant lymphomas** (sometimes apparently arising in Sjögren's lesions of long standing) are also not very rare.

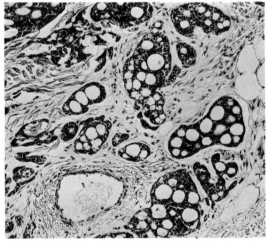

Fig. 19.17 Adenoid cystic carcinoma showing the characteristic architecture. ×90.

Pharynx

Tonsillitis. Acute tonsillitis is a common cause of sore throat. Haemolytic streptococci are the commonest infecting agents and give rise to acute inflammatory swelling with purulent exudate in the tonsillar crypts—*follicular tonsillitis*. The infection occasionally extends more deeply and involves the whole tonsil and adjacent tissues with frank suppuration; this is known as *quinsy*. From such a lesion streptococcal cellulitis may spread widely into the neck—*Ludwig's angina*—or even into the mediastinum or may give rise to a retropharyngeal abscess.

Acute streptococcal tonsillitis occurring alone or in scarlet fever is the usual antecedent infection in rheumatic fever and post-streptococcal glomerulonephritis. Chronic enlargement of the tonsils and adjacent lymphoid tissue commonly results from colonisation by one or other of the many adenoviruses.

Vincent's angina is a painful necrotic ulcerating lesion on the fauces characterised by a patch of yellowish-white false membrane surrounded by an area of acute inflammation, and may be difficult to distinguish from diphtheria (p. 436). It is due to the symbiotic action of fusiform bacilli and the spirochaete *Borrelia vincenti*. Vincent's infection in its most severe form is probably responsible for the lesions on the cheek known as *noma* or *cancrum oris*, and it also gives rise to a severe ulcerative and necrotic gingivitis. A similar lesion is found in established scurvy, due to vitamin C deficiency.

Blood dyscrasias. Swelling, haemorrhage and ulceration of the gingivae occur in the acute leukaemias, particularly in the monocytic form, and necrotic ulceration occurs on the fauces, pharynx and larynx in various conditions characterised by extreme reduction in the number of circulating polymorphonuclear leukocytes, i.e. in *agranulocytosis* (p. 512).

Diphtheria is an acute inflammation which affects most frequently the fauces, soft palate and tonsils, but may also attack the nose, or the larynx and trachea; it occurs chiefly in young children, but may also affect adults. The causal organism, *Corynebacterium diphtheriae*, exists in three main forms, *mitis*, *intermedius* and *gravis*, and infections with the last type tend to be more severely toxic and also to show greater local inflammatory reaction. The organisms remain strictly localised at the site of infection and the systemic effects are due to the formation and absorption of a powerful exotoxin which may cause myocardial damage and toxic fatty change in the organs; the mechanism of cellular injury is outlined on p. 8. The local lesions are characterised by the formation on the affected surfaces of a false membrane composed of fibrin and leukocytes. In the fauces, palate and tonsils the stratified squamous epithelium becomes permeated by exudate which forms a fibrinous coagulum in which the epithelium is incorporated; it then undergoes extensive necrosis under the influence of the diphtheria toxin. The whole false membrane is dull greyish-yellow and it can be detached only with difficulty owing to the attachment of the dead epithelium to the underlying tissues. When it is removed a bleeding connective tissue surface is laid bare. In *gravis* infections, membrane formation may be less obvious but inflammatory congestion and swelling are more marked and the cervical lymph nodes may be much swollen.

Diphtheria of the nasopharynx and of the larynx is described on p. 437.

Immunisation programmes are largely responsible for the present low incidence of diphtheria in many parts of the world.

Tumours of the pharynx are included with those of the oral cavity on pp. 593–4.

II: Oesophagus

General considerations. The oesophagus is a muscular tube, lined by squamous epithelium and adapted to bear without injury the rapid passing of food over its surface. It has marked powers of resistance and is a rare site of primary bacterial invasion, but damage to the mucosa of the lower end from regurgitated gastric juice is fairly common. Oesophageal obstruction can arise from various lesions, the most important being carcinoma of the oesophagus and invasion by bronchial carcinoma.

Circulatory disturbances

Oesophageal varices. The submucosal veins in the lower oesophagus and cardia of the stomach communicate with both the portal and systemic venous systems. In cases of portal hypertension, most frequently due to *hepatic cirrhosis*, these veins become distinctly varicose (Fig. 19.22): they may rupture, causing severe and often fatal haemorrhage.

Other causes of oesophageal haemorrhage. *Peptic reflux oesophagitis* (p. 597), particularly with ulceration, is a cause of bleeding of the lower oesophagus, and haemorrhage can also occur from *laceration of the mucosa at the cardia* during vomiting (p. 600). Rarely severe haemorrhage occurs as a result of impaction of a sharp *foreign body*, e.g. a fish bone, in the oesophagus: suppuration and ulceration develop and may involve the aorta or other large vessel: an *ulcerated oesophageal carcinoma* may similarly cause haemorrhage. Rarely an *aortic aneurysm* ruptures into the oesophagus.

Inflammatory conditions

As already mentioned, primary infections of the oesophagus are rare. Occasionally the lesion of diphtheria extends into, or arises primarily in, the oesophagus. In the rare but distinctive form of disseminated herpes simplex infection encountered in early infancy, the virus sometimes gains entry through the oesophagus. The characteristic lesion associated with South American trypanosomiasis (Chagas' disease) is described below.

'Opportunistic infections' (p. 174) may, however, occur in the oesophagus in states of debility or reduced immunity, and are often caused by organisms normally of low virulence. **Thrush,** caused by the yeast-like fungus *Candida albicans,* is the most common infection of this type and is characterised by the formation of irregularly raised opaque whitish patches consisting of swollen and sodden epithelium infiltrated by the septate mycelial threads and spores of the fungus (Fig. 19.18). The infection may have spread from the mouth or throat and can extend more distally in the gastrointestinal tract or even invade the bloodstream to produce generalised lesions.

Oesophagitis can arise from non-infective causes. The most common example of this is *peptic oesophagitis* caused by regurgitation of gastric juice from the stomach (see below). The

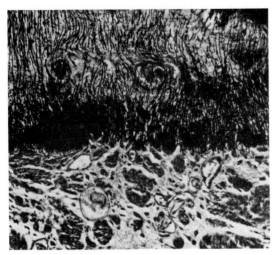

Fig. 19.18 Thrush of oesophagus, showing mycelial threads penetrating the wall. × 115.

accidental or intentional swallowing of corrosive or irritating fluids can cause severe, even fatal, injury to the oesophagus. Concentrated strong acids or alkalis, for example, produce extensive necrosis and sloughing of the oesophageal wall. More dilute solutions lead to superficial destruction followed by inflammatory changes. If the patient survives, scarring may result in fibrous stricture.

Peptic or reflux oesophagitis. This important clinical disturbance is caused by a defect in the mechanism which normally prevents reflux of gastric juice into the lower oesophagus. This mechanism is not completely understood but appears to depend upon three main components: (1) the intrinsic sphincter action at the lower end of the oesophagus which is partially dependent upon gastrin, (2) the attachment of the cardio-oesophageal junction to the diaphragmatic hiatus, and (3) the maintenance of the cardio-oesophageal angle, probably by a muscular sling extending over the body of the stomach. This anti-reflux mechanism tends to become defective if there is an increase in intra-abdominal pressure, due for example to obesity or pregnancy, and particularly if this is associated with acid hypersecretion in the stomach and low levels of serum gastrin. These factors tend to be associated also with the development of **hiatus hernia**, i.e. the herniation of the upper part of the stomach with its peritoneal covering through the diaphragmatic hiatus (Fig. 19.19). Hiatus hernia of the *sliding type*, in which

there is upward displacement of the cardia through the hiatus, aggravates the degree of reflux. The *'rolling' type* of hernia, in which the gastric fundus passes into the thorax alongside the cardia, does not predispose to reflux, although it may be a cause of gastro-oesophageal haemorrhage.

Reflux of gastric juice damages the squamous epithelium of the lower oesophagus. Initially there is elongation of the connective tissue papillae and infiltration of polymorphs: later, superficial ulceration develops which, if it persists, leads to marked fibrosis in the deeper layers of the oesophageal wall. It is notable, however, that peptic ulceration of the squamous epithelium of the lower oesophagus does not penetrate deeply as it does in the stomach (p. 608). The main clinical consequences of these pathological phenomena are oesophageal pain, usually readily recognisable as 'heartburn', but sometimes resembling angina pectoris (p. 400), haemorrhage sometimes leading to iron-deficiency anaemia, and stricture of the lower oesophagus.

Peptic oesophagitis is usually made worse by lying in bed, and symptoms of it are very common in hospital patients.

Diagnosis of peptic oesophagitis at necropsy is not easy, for considerable digestion of the lower oesophagus can occur after death, the wall being discoloured, soft and shreddy, and often perforated. Accordingly, the diagnosis of peptic oesophagitis at necropsy requires histological confirmation of an inflammatory reaction.

Deep **chronic peptic ulceration** of the oesophagus is uncommon. It occurs when the lower oesophagus is lined by columnar epithelium of gastric type (Barrett's syndrome). This may occur as a congenital abnormality but more often arises as a metaplastic change in recurrent reflux oesophagitis and in sliding hiatus hernia (Fig. 19.19).

Spontaneous rupture of the oesophagus

This unusual condition occurs in previously healthy men, usually when a heavy meal has been followed by violent vomiting. The lesion takes the form of a longitudinal slit, most often in the left posterior position, just above the diaphragm. The acid gastric contents are dis-

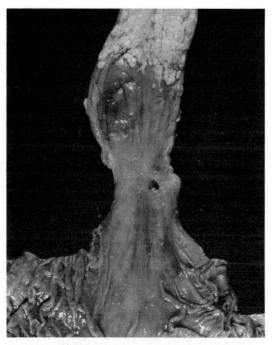

Fig. 19.19 Sliding hiatus hernia with chronic peptic ulceration in Barrett's syndrome.

charged into the pleural cavity directly or after first distending the posterior mediastinum. The appearance of the lesion indicates that it is brought about by sudden overdistension of the lower oesophagus in the act of vomiting, but digestion by the strongly acid gastric juice may also be a factor. Peptic ulceration of stomach or duodenum is often present.

Severe vomiting, usually associated with heavy alcohol intake, may also lead to brisk haematemesis as a result of laceration of the mucosa in the vicinity of the cardia. The damage, however, usually affects the gastric rather than the oesophageal mucosa. (Mallory-Weiss syndrome.)

Oesophageal obstruction

Obstruction of the oesophagus usually has an *organic* basis. In some instance, however, a primary organic lesion cannot be recognised and the obstruction is apparently due to *muscular dysfunction* ('*functional obstruction*').

Organic obstruction

This may arise in a number of different ways. (1) The lumen of the oesophagus may actually be occluded, usually by tumour, either benign or malignant, although occasionally by a foreign body. (2) Disease within the wall of the oesophagus may lead to stenosis of the lumen; again malignant tumours are most often implicated. Fibrous stricture may, however, arise as a complication of hiatus hernia, the swallowing of corrosive or scalding fluids, trauma, or as a congenital defect. (3) The oesophagus may be compressed from outside, e.g. by a mediastinal tumour or cyst, aortic aneurysm, enlargement of the left atrium following mitral stenosis, congenital malformation of the great vessels, or pharyngeal diverticulum. (4) Diseases affecting the neuromuscular co-ordination of the oesophagus may interfere with normal deglutition. Progressive systemic sclerosis and Chagas' disease are suitably included in this group, and also disorders of the central nervous system which interfere with deglutition.

Progressive systemic sclerosis. This is a connective tissue disease (p. 941) which may produce widespread systemic lesions, the skin of the hands and face (acrosclerosis) and the kidneys being especially affected. Dysphagia is not uncommon, and is due to replacement of the oesophageal musculature by fibrous tissue which, if diffuse, leads to pronounced interference with peristaltic activity. Shortening of the oesophagus causing reflux oesophagitis may be an additional complication.

Chagas' disease (South American trypanosomiasis). The protozoon parasite (*Trypanosoma cruzi*) which causes this interesting disease appears to be capable of exerting a toxic effect on the autonomic ganglia of various viscera, especially the heart, oesophagus and colon. In the oesophagus, there may be widespread destruction of the ganglia of the myenteric plexus, leading to disturbance of peristalsis and the development of a clinical picture very similar to that of achalasia (see below).

'Functional' obstruction

The most important 'functional' disturbance is *achalasia of the oesophagus*, although other functional disorders have been described, e.g. diffuse spasm, sometimes associated with organic lesions of the gastro-intestinal tract, especially peptic ulcer, gall-bladder disease and hiatus hernia. Dysphagia may also occur from dysfunction of the upper end of the oesophagus in anaemic women (Kelly–Patterson or Plummer–Vinson syndrome, p. 539): the constriction can be visualised radiologically and by oesophagoscopy, and is sometimes described by the vague term *oesophageal web*: since it is not seen at necropsy, and is usually cured by treating the anaemia, it appears to be due to muscle spasm.

Achalasia of the oesophagus. In this condition there is pronounced narrowing of the terminal part of the oesophagus with dilatation proximally. It usually develops in early adult life and leads to dysphagia and regurgitation of food; later there may be more serious obstruction. Oesophageal narrowing is usually at the diaphragmatic level and marked dilatation of the oesophagus results (Fig. 19.20), with compensatory muscular hypertrophy of the wall. The narrowing was formerly attributed to muscular

spasm, hence the term '*cardiospasm*'; there is probably, however, a primary disturbance of motility with defective transmission of peristaltic waves to the cardia and subsequent failure of relaxation of the cardiac sphincter. The cause of this disturbance remains uncertain. Degenerative changes have been described in the myenteric ganglia, and it is probable that achalasia is an acquired abnormality of autonomic innervation; the close similarity to the oesophageal disturbance in Chagas' disease supports this hypothesis. Incision of the oesophageal wall through to the mucosa at the level of obstruction (Heller's operation) appears to be the most satisfactory form of surgical treatment in severe cases.

Diverticula

Two varieties of local dilatation are observed in the oesophagus, namely the *pulsion diverticulum* and the *traction diverticulum*.

The pulsion diverticulum is caused by forcible distension during the act of swallowing. It is usually not noticeable till early adult life but may be due to a congenital weakness or deficiency in the muscle of the inferior constrictor of the pharynx; it is therefore more correctly termed a *pharyngeal* pouch or diverticulum. Once a diverticulum has formed, as may result from repeated stretching of the deficiency in the wall during swallowing of food, it tends to become distended with food and gradually extends downwards behind the wall of the oesophagus, tilting the tube forwards so that the mouth of the sac comes to lie in line with the upper pharynx. The sac ultimately becomes permanently distended by food and may compress and obstruct the adjacent oesophagus, with consequent severe dysphagia and weight loss.* Such a diverticulum is lined by mucous membrane supported by connective tissue, but its wall usually contains no muscle; it becomes ulcerated. Less commonly, a diverticulum occurs anteriorly and bulges between the trachea and the oesophagus.

The traction diverticulum of the oesophagus is produced by the contraction of connective tissue pulling the wall outwards, usually by the adhesion to the wall of the tube of a mass of

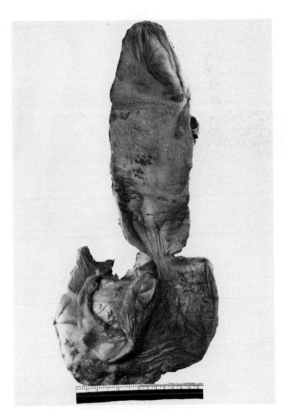

Fig. 19.20 Achalasia of oesophagus. Note the great dilatation with numerous superficial ulcers. ×0·25.

---

* 'Bloody' Judge Jeffries had a pharyngeal pouch, the discomfort of which may have contributed to the severity of his sentences.

calcified tuberculous lymph nodes or occasionally a mass of silicotic nodes. A pouch with a sharp apex is the result, and this is stretched and increased both by further scarring and by the movements of the oesophagus. Ulceration of the diverticulum may occur and may lead to perforation, resulting in gangrenous mediastinitis which may extend to the pleura and other parts.

Rarely a diverticulum occurs opposite the bifurcation of the trachea as a congenital abnormality, arising in the same way as a communication between the oesophagus and trachea (see p. 601). Such diverticula are sometimes lined by columnar epithelium.

Tumours

Benign tumours. These are all rare. Lipoma, fibroma and leiomyoma may all occur, leiomyoma probably being the least rare and occasionally reaching a large size. Benign tumours tend to project into the lumen as polyps.

Malignant tumours

Carcinoma of the oesophagus. Carcinoma is by far the commonest malignant tumour in the oesophagus. It occurs usually after the age of forty-five, and is much commoner in men than in women. The commonest site is at the level of the bifurcation of the trachea, the lower and upper ends being next in order of frequency. There is, however, a distinct sex difference in the sites of incidence. About three-quarters of cases of cancer in the hypopharynx and upper end of the oesophagus occur in women, whereas over 80 per cent of cancers elsewhere in the oesophagus occur in men.

Oesophageal carcinoma shows remarkable geographical variation in incidence. Although not uncommon in this country its incidence is much greater in certain parts of China and the U.S.S.R., and in parts of Africa where contaminated alcoholic drinks are suspected as a causal factor. Fungal contamination of maize grown upon poor soil has also been incriminated. There is a remarkably high incidence in Curaçao, probably attributable to eating food that is too hot. Little is known about the causation of oesophageal cancer in Western Europe and North America apart from a possible

association with heavy alcohol intake. The long-suspected relationship of iron-deficiency anaemia and dysphagia with post-cricoid carcinoma in women has never been firmly established.

Naked-eye appearances. There are two chief types. *Scirrhous carcinoma* grows round the tube and induces a fibrous reaction, causing progressively severe stenosis. The *soft* or *encephaloid* type involves a greater length of the oesophagus, forms irregular projections into the lumen and thus tends to cause occlusion (Fig. 19.21). At the same time, the destruction of the muscular tissue by infiltration interferes with contraction. The tumour may spread upwards and downwards in the submucous tissue, and forms secondary nodules which raise the mucosa, giving a false appearance of multifocal origin.

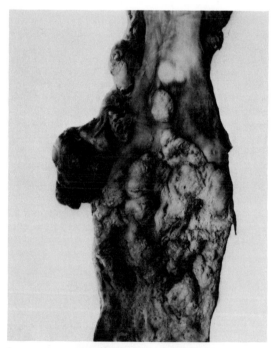

Fig. 19.21 Extensive ulcerating carcinoma in middle part of oesophagus.

In addition to causing obstruction, the tumour may spread to the trachea or a bronchus, and ulcerate through the wall. Infected fluids are then likely to pass down the bronchi and cause *aspiration pneumonia*. Rarely ulceration into the aorta may result in fatal haemorrhage. Metastases also occur in the local lymph nodes, and occasionally also in the internal organs, especially the liver; but death is usually caused by oesophageal obstruction.

Microscopic appearances. In nearly all cases the tumour is a poorly keratinised squamous carcinoma; rarely it resembles oat-cell bronchial carcinoma. Adenocarcinoma has also been described, but many examples are due to extension of a gastric carcinoma. Tumours arising from the oesophageal glands are uncommon; they present the features of muco-epidermoid or adenoid cystic carcinomas found in the salivary glands (p. 595 *et seq.*).

Sarcoma is rare. It resembles the softer varieties of carcinoma, but its growth may be more massive. Rhabdomyosarcoma of the oesophagus is extremely rare.

Congenital abnormalities

In addition to stenosis or dilatation, already mentioned, there may be various degrees of atresia of the oesophagus. The commonest of these is a condition in which the upper part forms a blind sac which is separated from the lower part, while the latter is patent and communicates with the trachea closely above its bifurcation. Sometimes the oesophagus is patent throughout, but there is a small communication with the trachea, through which food may pass into the trachea and cause a suppurative or necrotising pneumonia. A congenital diverticulum is a lesser degree of this malformation.

III: Stomach

General considerations. The two most important pathological conditions in the stomach are peptic ulcer and carcinoma. Bacterial infection as a cause of serious disease in the stomach is comparatively rare. Gastric juice rapidly destroys most vegetative bacteria entering with food, and when digestion has been completed, and the stomach contents pass on to the intestine, the stomach soon returns to a state of virtual sterility. Nevertheless ingested tubercle bacilli, *Salmonellae*, *Brucellae* and dysentery bacilli can all successfully evade the chemical barrier of the gastric secretion and no doubt more easily if there is defective acid secretion or stasis. Acute inflammation of the gastric mucosa may be due to swallowing irritating fluids or food contaminated with bacterial, e.g. staphylococcal, toxins. It is also likely that the stomach can be affected by some of the enteroviruses and perhaps other viruses also.

Chronic gastritis of the acid-secreting mucosa has the features of an organ-specific auto-immune disease. The chronic inflammation which frequently occurs in the antral mucosa appears to be due to agents which damage the surface epithelium, such as bile and alcohol.

Circulatory disturbances

Chronic congestion of the gastric mucosa is seen as part of the general picture of congestive cardiac failure (p. 398) and may account for the anorexia observed in this condition. Mucosal congestion may also result from portal hypertension and may be accompanied by dilatation of submucosal veins, usually in association with oesophageal varices (Fig. 19.22).

Mucosal haemorrhage and haemorrhagic erosions. Petechial haemorrhages of 1–3 mm. diameter, sometimes with mucosal erosion, occur in various conditions including infective fevers, purpuric states (p. 556) and chronic mucosal congestion (Fig. 19.23). More extensive haemorrhage, commonly associated with multiple mucosal erosions * and even acute ulcers is, however, more often due to the ingestion of aspirin and similar anti-inflammatory agents, or is associated with severe states of shock or uraemia. The term **acute haemorrhagic gastritis** is sometimes given to these more extensive changes (see below).

Haematemesis, or vomiting of blood, is due to *severe* haemorrhage from the oesophagus or proximal part of the gastro-intestinal tract.

* *Erosion* is the term used for ulceration of the mucosa which does not extend deep to the lamina muscularis mucosae. An *acute ulcer* is defined as extending into the submucosa.

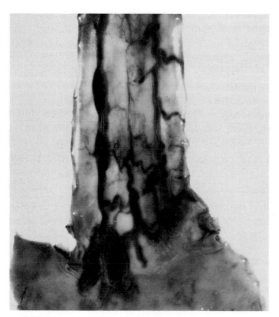

Fig. 19.22 Oesophagus and cardiac end of stomach, showing large dilated varicose veins from a case of cirrhosis of the liver. Death was due to haemorrhage from the large varicosity at the cardia.

When less severe, the blood tends to track distally, and is recognised by black discolouration of the stools (**melaena**).

The commonest causes of *serious haemorrhage* are peptic ulcer, either in the stomach or duodenum, and oesophageal varices (Fig. 19.22) with portal hypertension, usually due to hepatic cirrhosis. Carcinoma of the stomach frequently causes haemorrhage, but this is rarely severe. Haemorrhagic erosions (see above) are a common cause of gastric haemorrhage. Diffuse haemorrhage is seen in haemorrhagic diatheses, in severe septic conditions, in yellow fever where it gives rise to 'black vomit', in acute liver failure, and occasionally without discoverable cause as a terminal event.

Blood shed into the stomach becomes mixed with gastric juice and acquires a brownish or almost black colour, or there may be fragments of brownish coagulum, resembling coffee grounds, mixed with the fluid. Altered blood may also pass into the intestine. In cases of rapidly fatal haemorrhage the stomach may be filled by a large coagulum which forms a cast of the interior and the colour of the blood may be little altered.

Acute gastritis

Acute inflammation of the gastric mucosa is usually due to aspirin-type anti-inflammatory agents, alcohol, or bacterial toxins in contaminated food, especially staphylococcal enterotoxin. In the most severe form, known as **acute haemorrhagic gastritis**, there is extensive oedema and focal erosion of the mucosa (Fig. 19.24), commonly associated with mucosal or submucosal haemorrhage. This has been observed especially following aspirin ingestion and in severely shocked patients; the mechanism is thought to be similar in both instances, namely the back-diffusion of hydrogen ions into the mucosa. In aspirin poisoning, acute ulceration

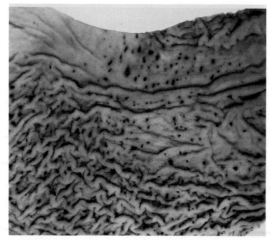

Fig. 19.23 Multiple minute haemorrhagic erosions of the gastric mucosa. × 0·75.

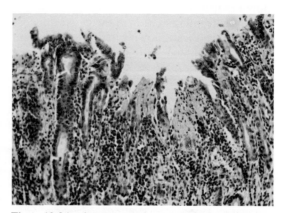

Fig. 19.24 Acute erosive gastritis. There is superficial loss of the surface epithelium with fibrinoid necrosis and polymorph infiltration. × 205.

may lead to haematemesis, and even perforation has been described.

Corrosive gastritis. The ingestion of strong acid or alkali leads to variable destruction of gastric tissue usually associated with haemorrhage and sometimes with perforation. There may be marked gastric scarring should the patient survive. Acid tends to produce coagulative tissue necrosis, whereas alkali more often causes tissue liquefaction. Mild acids, e.g. oxalic or acetic, and arsenic, produce more superficial mucosal ulceration and gastritis. Some chemicals, e.g. phenol or mercuric chloride, actually fix the gastric tissues. For details, special works on toxicology should be consulted.

Acute bacterial gastritis. As mentioned earlier, bacterial infection is an unusual cause of acute gastritis, but *acute infective gastritis*, together with acute enteritis, is seen in 'food poisoning' due to *Salmonellae* and in *Yersinia* infections (p. 638). Rarely, extensive suppuration in the submucosa and muscle layer may develop when pyogenic bacteria, especially streptococci, gain entrance from an ulcerated carcinoma or from injury by a foreign body.

Chronic gastritis

Chronic inflammation of the gastric mucosa is extremely common. The increased use of endoscopic biopsy has helped to distinguish between two main types, a **diffuse** type which affects the acid-secreting mucosa of the stomach and has all the features of an organ-specific auto-immune disease, and a **multifocal** type which usually appears first in the antral mucosa or at the junction between antrum and body, but can involve both types of mucosa. The multifocal type appears to be caused by irritation of the mucosa, e.g. by reflux of bile or excessive alcohol.

Diffuse chronic gastritis

In this form of gastritis, the changes may initially be focal, but in many cases they are progressive, and as the condition becomes more advanced, it extends to involve the whole of the **acid-secreting mucosa**. It may be accompanied by multifocal chronic gastritis of the antrum, but the association is probably coincidental.

Pathological changes. Macroscopic examination of the gastric mucosa *in vivo* is of little value in diagnosing chronic gastritis. Microscopically, three stages can be recognised— *chronic superficial gastritis*, *atrophic gastritis* and *gastric atrophy*.

In **chronic superficial gastritis**, the gastric pits or foveolae are increased in length, and the superficial lamina propria is infiltrated with lymphocytes and plasma cells, together with a few neutrophil and eosinophil polymorphs (Fig. 19.25*b*).

In **atrophic gastritis**, the inflammatory changes are similar to those of chronic superficial gastritis, but extend more deeply into the mucosa and are accompanied by various degrees of loss of the specialised (parietal and chief) cells of the mucosal glands. In its extreme degree, the acid-secreting mucosa is diffusely affected and thinned and there is virtually complete loss of the specialised glandular cells (Fig. 19.25*d*). The glands appear fewer and their specialised cells are replaced by simple mucus-secreting epithelium similar to the surface mucosa (*pseudo-pyloric metaplasia*) or show *intestinal metaplasia* characterised by the presence of goblet cells, absorptive cells with a brush border and Paneth cells (Fig. 19.25*c*). The altered glands may show irregular cystic change. The lamina propria is relatively increased and appears as broad areas of vascular tissue heavily infiltrated with lymphocytes and plasma cells and occasionally containing lymphoid follicles with germinal centres ('*follicular gastritis*'). There is marked atrophy and loss of glands and the mucosa is appreciably thinned and the rugae inconspicuous. In less severe atrophic gastritis the changes are focal, affecting patches of mucosa in a part or the whole of its thickness, while the intervening areas of mucosa may show superficial gastritis, or may be normal.

In **gastric atrophy** the fundal mucosa is diffusely atrophic, with virtually complete replacement of parietal and chief cells by metaplastic mucus-secreting glandular epithelium, and increase of loose vascular connective tissue in the lamina propria. The appearances resemble closely those of severe atrophic gastritis except for the much smaller numbers of lymphocytes and plasma cells in gastric atrophy.

Aetiology. The evidence from biopsy studies suggests strongly that the three stages of chronic gastritis described above are indeed different degrees of the same process. The destructive inflammatory changes begin superficially and as they extend towards the base of the mucosa lead to progressive loss of the specialised glandular cells. When all or virtually all of the

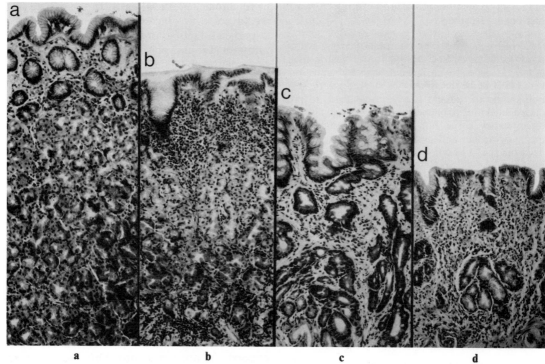

Fig. 19.25 Chronic gastritis of acid-secreting mucosa. All × 100. **a** Normal mucosa. **b** Superficial gastritis and atrophic gastritis affecting the deep part of the mucosa. **c** Complete loss of parietal and chief cells with intestinal metaplasia. **d** Complete atrophic gastritis. The remaining glands are of simple mucus-secreting type. In **b**, **c** and **d**, the full thickness of the mucosa is shown.

specialised cells have been destroyed, the inflammation subsides, leaving the appearances of gastric atrophy.

Diffuse chronic gastritis is widely regarded as one of the organ-specific auto-immune diseases; the evidence for this may be summarised as follows:

(1) *Auto-antibodies* are commonly present in the serum of patients with chronic gastritis, and their incidence increases with the extent of the gastric mucosal changes. Auto-antibody to membrane lipoprotein of gastric parietal cells can be detected by immunofluorescence (Fig. 19.26) or complement-fixation tests in the serum of over 80 per cent of patients in whom severe grades of gastritis have resulted in pernicious anaemia (p. 535). Two auto-antibodies to intrinsic factor, a product of the gastric parietal cells, are also associated with severe chronic gastritis. One of these combines with the part of the intrinsic factor molecule which binds vitamin B_{12}, and the other with a site on the molecule distant from the B_{12}-binding site: they interfere respectively with binding of B_{12} by intrinsic factor, and with absorption of the complex from the ileum (p. 535). These latter antibodies are observed only occasionally apart from pernicious anaemia, in which their combined incidence is more than 50 per cent.

(2) *Associated conditions.* The organ-specific auto-immune diseases tend to occur in association with one another (p. 163), and the common association of various grades of chronic thyroiditis and thyrotoxicosis with chronic gastritis supports the auto-immune nature of the latter. Moreover, the rarer members of the group—primary adrenocortical atrophy, and primary hypoparathyroidism—are frequently accompanied by chronic gastritis.

(3) *Familial tendency.* Like the other auto-immune diseases, chronic gastritis shows a familial tendency, and chronic thyroiditis commonly occurs in members of the same families.

(4) *Age and sex.* Like chronic thyroiditis, chronic gastritis occurs mostly in the middle-aged and elderly, and in women more often

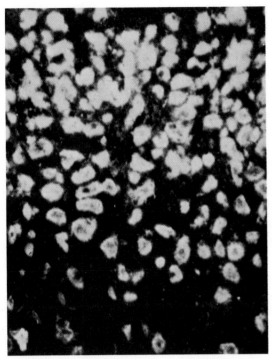

Fig. 19.26 Indirect immunofluorescence test for parietal-cell antibody. The parietal cells fluoresce brightly, indicating the presence of the antibody in the serum being tested.

than men; the female sex preponderance is not, however, nearly so marked as in chronic thyroiditis or thyrotoxicosis.

(5) *Experimental chronic gastritis.* Administration to monkeys of injections of preparations of gastric fundal mucosa incorporated in Freund's adjuvant (p. 114) has been reported to induce *experimental chronic gastritis* accompanied by both antibody and cell-mediated immunity to gastric parietal cells.

The mechanism of the production of the changes in chronic gastritis in man has not been fully established. Auto-antibodies to parietal cells do not appear to play a major pathogenic role, and it is more likely that a delayed hypersensitivity reaction against the specialised gastric glandular cells is largely responsible for the destructive changes. Auto-antibodies to intrinsic factor do, however, contribute to the failure of absorption of B_{12} in pernicious anaemia, especially when they are present in the gastric juice, where they inhibit the function of any intrinsic factor produced by the atrophic mucosa (p. 535).

Physiological disturbances. Chronic diffuse gastritis seldom causes local symptoms, but deficiencies of gastric function occur and correlate with the extent of loss of specialised cells. Thus in superficial gastritis there is little functional upset; with progressing glandular atrophy varying degrees of hypochlorhydria develop, culminating eventually in complete achlorhydria as seen in severe atrophic gastritis. Even at this latter stage, some intrinsic factor is still secreted, and megaloblastic anaemia is not common. In the extreme gastric atrophy of pernicious anaemia, there is, however, absence of hydrochloric acid and pepsin, and near or complete absence of intrinsic factor, from the gastric juice.

Multifocal chronic gastritis

This term has been applied to those common forms of non-specific chronic gastritis which have non-immunological causes and tend initially to attack the antrum or junctional zone between antrum and body of stomach in a patchy fashion, although the lesions may become extensive throughout the gastric mucosa and may be confluent in advanced cases. The aetiology is not entirely clear but there is evidence that chronic alcoholism and bile reflux may be of importance; chronic gastritis of this kind is also common following gastro-enterostomy and in the vicinity of gastric ulcers, and may be found in the antrum in patients with duodenal ulcer.

Histologically the lesions tend to progress like those of the diffuse type of chronic gastritis (see above) but more active lesions of inflammation with neutrophil infiltration are more often seen in the gastric pits, and there is often degradation of the surface epithelium with evidence of increased epithelial cell turnover. This is probably a consequence of direct injury to the surface mucosa by the causal factors with consequent back-diffusion of hydrogen ions. While the functional effects of this are generally less marked than in diffuse chronic gastritis, the lesions are thought to be more often a cause of dyspeptic symptoms, and it is widely held that multifocal chronic gastritis predisposes to the development of peptic ulcer and possibly of gastric carcinoma.

Chronic gastritis and mucosal atrophy are common in cases of pyloric stenosis, but it is doubtful whether the various saprophytic micro-organisms which colonise the stagnating gastric contents in this condition (p. 613) cause the mucosal changes.

Other types of chronic gastritis

Granulomatous gastritis. The presence of a sarcoid reaction in the gastric mucosa or deeper tissues sometimes occurs without apparent reason, but it may be a manifestation of sarcoidosis (p. 216) or of tuberculous origin. Sometimes it complicates peptic ulceration or gastric carcinoma, and there is always the possibility that it represents an unusual expression of Crohn's disease (p. 620). Tuberculous ulcers sometimes develop in the stomach in patients with advanced pulmonary tuberculosis.

Hypertrophic gastritis. This rather ill-defined term is applied to lesions in which there is macroscopic enlargement of gastric rugae. This may be due to the increase in parietal cell mass that results from gastrin-producing tumours (p. 1034) or is found in some patients with duodenal ulcers. The most important cause, however, is *Ménétrier's disease* in which there is marked thickening of the gastric mucosa due chiefly to elongation and tortuosity of the foveolae. The aetiology is not clear. The main clinical effect is loss of protein into the gastric lumen and hypoalbuminaemia.

Peptic ulcer

By far the most important type of ulceration found in the stomach is peptic ulceration, in which the action of gastric juice is primarily concerned. It is often referred to simply as *gastric ulcer*. Peptic ulceration is encountered, however, not only in the stomach but also in other parts of the alimentary tract exposed to gastric juice: it is especially common in the first part of the duodenum and is occasionally found in the lower part of the oesophagus (p. 599). It is also seen in relation to heterotopic gastric mucosa, e.g. in a Meckel's diverticulum (p. 655) or at the umbilicus. Furthermore, in cases where gastrojejunostomy has been performed, peptic ulceration may take place in the part of the jejunal wall exposed to the action of gastric juice, especially when this is of high acidity. Apart from these circumstances, however, peptic ulceration distal to the duodenal bulb is rare.

Incidence. The incidence of the different types of peptic ulcer has changed considerably since the beginning of the century. Before that time the prevalent type was the acute perforating ulcer (Fig. 19.33) which was usually found in the anterior wall of the pylorus or duodenum and predominantly affected anaemic young women. After World War I gastric ulcer became much commoner in men and to a lesser extent in older women. At the present time, gastric ulcer is more common in men than in women at all ages up to 65, but thereafter the sex difference becomes less marked: on the other hand duodenal ulceration, which became more frequent at about the same time, is much commoner in men in all age groups and is between 4 and 10 times as common as gastric ulcer in the general population. Gastric ulcer was formerly considered to be a disease of the lower income groups, but it is doubtful if this is now the case, and duodenal ulcer had never shown any social or economic clustering. Both types of ulceration show a familial incidence.

Naked-eye appearances. Depending on the depth of penetration, peptic ulcers are usually classified (somewhat artificially) into three main types—*acute*, *subacute* and *chronic*.

(*a*) *Acute peptic ulcer* involves only the mucosa and submucosa in the ulcerative process (Fig. 19.27); it is usually small, but may occasionally reach 1–2 cm diameter. The ulcers

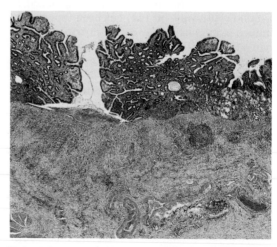

Fig. 19.27 A small acute peptic ulcer which has penetrated superficially into the submucosa. × 12.

may be single or multiple and, unlike chronic ulcers, have a wide distribution in the stomach. In the duodenum, however, they are usually restricted to the first few centimetres. They rarely produce symptoms other than haemorrhage, which may be severe when a mucosal artery in the base of an acute ulcer is eroded (Fig. 19.34, p. 611). This type of ulcer usually heals without a visible scar. Acute ulcers usually develop in states of stress, e.g. in shock, during severe illnesses, in association with burns or following surgical operations and in neurological disturbances.

(*b*) *Subacute peptic ulcers* are usually fewer in number than the acute type, and more often single. They extend down to the muscular coat, the superficial part of which may be involved; like chronic ulcers, they tend to be found on the lesser curvature of the stomach and they may represent a transition from the acute to the chronic type.

(*c*) *Chronic peptic ulcer.* Complete penetration of the muscular coat is regarded as the most important criterion of chronicity in a peptic ulcer (Figs. 19.30, 19.31). In about 90 per cent of cases it is solitary. In most other cases there are two ulcers, and in the duodenum they may face one another on the anterior and posterior wall ('kissing ulcers'). Occasionally a chronic ulcer is found both in the stomach and duodenum, and in most instances the duodenal ulcer appears to develop first.

Chronic gastric ulcers seem to arise mainly in antral mucosa close to the junction between antrum and body. Accordingly, the commonest site in the *stomach* is the lesser curvature between 5 and 10 cm from the pylorus, the pyloric canal being the next most frequent site. In the duodenum over 99 per cent arise in the first 2–3 cm, i.e. in the duodenal bulb. Their occurrence in other parts of the stomach and duodenum is rare, and should make one look for some unusual cause.

Chronic ulcers are usually ovoid and larger than subacute or acute ones (Figs. 19.28, 19.29). The majority, however, are less than 2·5 cm across, and larger ulcers should raise the suspicion of an ulcerated tumour. The base of the ulcer may be formed by the outer part of the gastric or duodenal wall, the floor being usually smooth and fibrous with fibrous induration of the surrounding tissues. More frequently, however, fibrous adhesions have de-

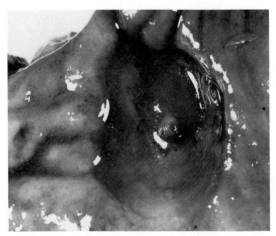

Fig. 19.28 A chronic gastric ulcer, showing an eroded artery from which fatal haemorrhage occurred. × 2.

veloped over the ulcer and the base is firmly fixed to adjacent tissues; large ulcers often penetrate into adjacent tissues, usually the pancreas or liver. When this advanced stage has been reached, the ulcer margin is smooth with overhanging edges, the crater is deep and the floor is firm and nodular, being formed by a fibrosed layer of the eroded organ. Occasionally a gastro-colic fistula develops when the ulcerative process extends into the transverse colon.

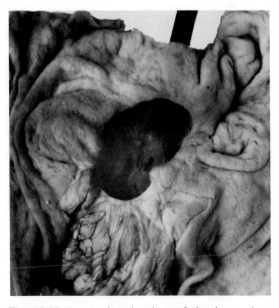

Fig. 19.29 Large chronic ulcer of duodenum just beyond the pylorus. The ulcer had perforated at the margin, as indicated by the pointer. × 0·8.

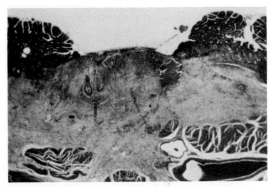

Fig. 19.30 Early chronic gastric ulcer, showing fibrous replacement of muscular coat. × 7.

Microscopic appearances. Peptic ulcers usually have a sharply demarcated outline. The ulcer crater is lined by a thin layer of necrotic debris and neutrophil polymorphs overlying a layer of eosinophilic necrotic tissue ('fibrinoid necrosis'—p. 274), beneath which is a layer of granulation tissue showing some leukocytic infiltration. In chronic ulcers the muscle coat is interrupted and at either side of the ulcer merges into the fibrous tissue which forms the outer layer of ulcer lining and may extend for some distance beyond it. The muscle coat thus ends high up in the lateral walls of the crater (Fig. 19.31). Endarteritis obliterans is often

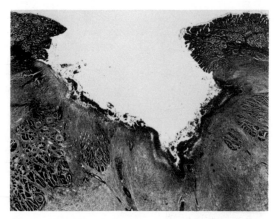

Fig. 19.31 Chronic gastric ulcer at later stage, showing breach of muscular coat. × 7.

conspicuous in the arteries in the ulcer base. At the margin of the ulcer, the mucosal epithelium may show active regenerative changes; fragments of mucosa may also be 'buried' in fibrous tissue during the ulcerative process,

and give a false impression of malignant change (see p. 612).

Chronic gastric ulcers are always surrounded by a zone of active chronic gastritis and more extensive chronic gastritis (p. 607) is common. Similarly, active duodenitis is present around duodenal ulcers. It is not known whether duodenitis of this kind can produce dyspeptic symptoms in the absence of frank ulceration.

Results and complications of peptic ulceration

(1) Healing and scarring. Acute peptic ulcers usually undergo healing and leave no visible scar. Healing is the rule also in the subacute type and is common in chronic ulcers, even when large, as is shown by the common necropsy finding of contracted scars in the ulcer-prone sites. If the ulcer has been superficial, the scar may be merely a small depression with a smooth whitish surface; if, however, it has penetrated more deeply, there is often a radiating indrawing of the surrounding mucous membrane, so that a stellate appearance results (Fig. 19.32). Scarring of an ulcer at or near the

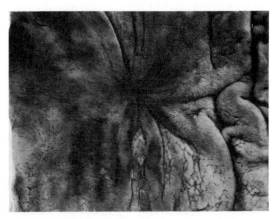

Fig. 19.32 Healed gastric ulcer with stellate scar. × 1.

pylorus commonly results in **pyloric stenosis,** and the stomach may gradually become enlarged due to repeated retention of food and secretion. The muscle of the pylorus is apt to be thickened and oedematous, and the appearance may suggest scirrhous carcinoma; only microscopic examination can rule this out.

Stenosis of the duodenum or pyloric antrum by the scarring of chronic ulcers has a similar effect, and ulcers higher up on the lesser curvature of the stomach may, by scarring and contraction, produce the deformity of '*hour glass*' stomach.

(2) Perforation. When an ulcer perforates rapidly (Fig. 19.33), gastric contents escape either into the general peritoneal cavity or into the lesser sac. The pain, abdominal rigidity and symptoms of collapse which follow are usually dramatic and are caused by the acid gastric contents; these are virtually sterile at first, but without prompt surgical treatment, organisms soon flourish and **acute peritonitis** results. Air from the stomach comes to lie between the liver and diaphragm where it is visible radiologically. After successful surgical treatment of the perforation, there is a risk that infected material lodged between the liver and diaphragm may become sealed off by fibrinous exudate and cause a **sub-phrenic abscess** which may later infect the pleura. In other cases infection of the peritoneum may occur without actual perforation, and the peritoneal surface becomes glued to adjacent parts by fibrinous exudate. This is more likely to happen with ulcers on the posterior aspect of the lesser curvature, where the stomach is less motile than elsewhere. The inflammation may produce localised fibrous adhesions or rarely localised suppuration. Very rarely, bacterial invasion of a portal tributary may produce secondary abscesses in the liver (p. 695). In the duodenum, ulcers situated anteriorly perforate most frequently. Some peptic ulcers penetrate the wall of the gut rapidly, sometimes without preceding symptoms.

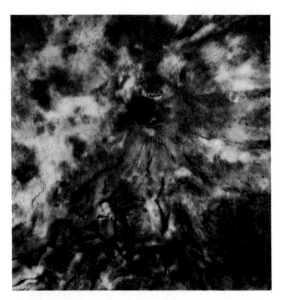

Fig. 19.33 Acute perforating ulcer. × 1.

Such '*acute perforating ulcers*' (Fig. 19.33) have become relatively uncommon.

(3) Haemorrhage. This is common and varies greatly in degree. Minor but continued loss of blood is caused by the erosion of small blood vessels in the base of an ulcer, and may only be detected by chemical examination of the stools or by the development of iron-deficiency anaemia (p. 538). More severe bleeding, giving rise to 'coffee-ground' vomit or 'tarry' stools (melaena) is usually due to involvement of a larger submucosal artery in the base of an acute or chronic ulcer (Fig. 19.34). The most dramatic form of haemorrhage, however, is caused by a deeply penetrating chronic ulcer

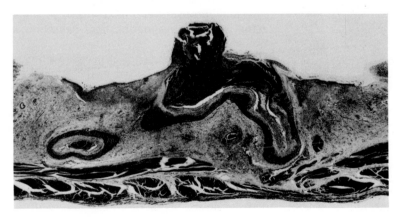

Fig. 19.34 Superficial acute ulcer of stomach which has eroded an artery and caused fatal haemorrhage. × 10.

eroding a major artery lying outside the gastric or duodenal wall (Fig. 19.28). In the case of lesser curve ulcers, the left gastric artery may be affected; whereas posteriorly-situated duodenal ulcers may erode the gastro-duodenal artery. A catastrophic event of this kind usually produces massive haematemesis which may be fatal. Large vessels incorporated in an ulcer base commonly show endarteritis obliterans, but if the ulcer is rapidly progressive this fails to develop satisfactorily, and rupture, sometimes preceded by aneurysm formation, takes place. The vessel, surrounded by fibrous tissue, is unable to contract properly, and only the development of an occlusive thrombus will stop the bleeding. Accordingly, urgent surgical intervention is often essential.

(4) Development of carcinoma: ulcer-cancer. Although it cannot be doubted that carcinoma sometimes develops in a chronic gastric ulcer,

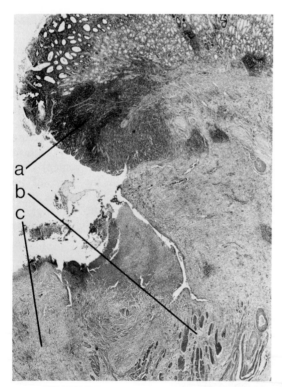

Fig. 19.35 Ulcer-cancer of stomach. A chronic peptic ulcer showing the characteristic complete breach of the muscle coat. A focus of early carcinoma was detected microscopically at **a** in the overhanging margin of the ulcer crater: **b** muscle coat: **c** fibrous base of ulcer.

its frequency has probably been overestimated in the past. One reason for this lies in the difficulty in distinguishing between a chronic peptic ulcer which has undergone malignant change and a carcinoma which has ulcerated. Complete interruption of the muscle coat is good evidence of pre-existing chronic peptic ulceration (Fig. 19.35).

Cancer develops in the continuously regenerating epithelium at the ulcer margin (Figs. 19.35, 19.36) and tends to encircle the ulcer crater, spreading outwards into the submucosa and muscular coat, but not usually invading far into the fibrous ulcer floor. By contrast, a carcinoma developing without peptic ulceration often invades the muscular coat but practically never destroys it entirely and even in advanced cases remains of muscle are to be found between cancer cells. Another important point is that irregular growth and displacement of epithelium at the margin of a peptic ulcer may give a false impression of malignant change.

Taking these factors into consideration, it is unlikely that cancer develops in more than 1 per cent of chronic gastric ulcers, although it is probable that there is an increased tendency for carcinoma to develop in a stomach bearing a chronic peptic ulcer. *Carcinoma does not arise in chronic duodenal ulcers.*

Aetiology of peptic ulcers

Although it is convenient to discuss the causes of peptic ulceration in general, chronic gastric and duodenal ulcers differ in some respects, including age and sex distribution, occupational incidence and familial tendency; their causes may therefore differ. It may also be necessary to distinguish aetiologically between acute and chronic ulcers. In any case, no single factor is clearly responsible and causation is complex.

The possible importance of **genetic factors** in the pathogenesis is reflected in the familial incidence (p. 608), and in the relationship between duodenal ulcer and individuals who do not secrete blood-group substances into the gastric juice and belong to blood group O. **Environmental factors** must be responsible for the changing incidence of peptic ulcer during this century and for 'epidemics' of the disease which may be localised or affect certain age groups in the community. Geographical variations in incidence also emphasise the importance of environment. Peptic ulcer is essentially a disease of developed, industrialised communities. Factors such as dietary habits, drugs (especially aspirin) and occupational or social stresses may be important. Cigarette smoking is also a contributory factor, especially in gastric ulcer, and may account for the association between peptic ulcer and chronic bronchitis.

It seems necessary to explain firstly the development of a mucosal lesion, and secondly why it does not heal like a wound made in a normal stomach. Local ischaemia due to thrombosis, embolus or vascular spasm has been postulated as a cause of the initial injury, but lacks supporting evidence.

The only entirely consistent finding associated with peptic ulceration is the presence of gastric acid, which is undoubtedly responsible for the special features of this disease. *Peptic ulcer does not develop in patients with histamine-fast achlorhydria and is caused by interference with the capacity of the gastro-intestinal mucosa to resist digestion by gastric acid*, due either to impaired mucosal resistance or to hypersecretion of gastric juice, or possibly both. The nature of the mucosal defence mechanism is complex and depends among other things upon the secretion of mucus and the presence of inhibitors of gastric secretion. Interference with these protective factors appears to be of particular importance in the pathogenesis of **gastric ulcer**. In this disease, gastric secretion may be normal but is often reduced due to the presence of chronic gastritis. Indeed gastric ulcers tend to develop during certain phases in the evolution of chronic gastritis, which impairs the defensive capacity of the mucosa. There is also evidence that dietary factors may be of particular importance in the pathogenesis of gastric ulcer.

By contrast, gastric hypersecretion appears to be of major significance in the pathogenesis of **duodenal ulcer**, and a substantial minority of affected individuals have an increased parietal-cell mass. In others, the acid secretory capacity is normal but the acid response to meals is exaggerated, possibly as a result of a defect in the feedback mechanism which controls gastric secretion (Sircus, 1974).

Although the role of humoral stimulants of gastric secretion in the pathogenesis of peptic ulcer in general is uncertain, there is no doubt that excess of such substances is capable of causing a fulminating ulcer diathesis. This is observed in the Zollinger–Ellison syndrome (p. 1034) in which a single or multiple pancreatic islet-cell tumours secrete large amounts of gastrin. These pancreatic tumours may be associated with tumours of other endocrine glands such as the parathyroids, adenohypophysis, adrenal medulla, etc., and with medullary carcinoma of C cell origin of the thyroid, etc.—the multiple endocrine adenoma syndrome (p. 1034). In these cases, peptic ulceration takes place not only in the common sites but also in unusual areas, e.g. the greater curvature of the stomach and distal duodenum. There is evidence that a raised level of blood calcium promotes an increase in gastric secretion, and this may account for the high incidence of peptic ulceration in patients with hyperparathyroidism.

Dilatation of the stomach

This may arise as a result of obstruction caused for example by the scarring associated with gastric or duodenal ulceration (p. 610), carcinoma, congenital pyloric hypertrophy (p. 617) and occasionally from the presence of fibrous peritoneal adhesions in the pyloric region. In such instances there may be varying degrees of hypertrophy of the gastric muscle coat: repeated vomiting may lead to serious metabolic effects, e.g. hypokalaemic alkalosis (p. 644). Chronic gastritis and mucosal atrophy are common in the chronically dilated stomach, and acid secretion is often greatly reduced. In such cases, various saprophytic bacteria and fungi grow in the retained gastric contents, with production of gas, etc. from fermentation. It is, however, doubtful if this is responsible for mucosal changes.

Occasionally, acute dilatation takes place in the absence of obstruction. This is usually a complication of surgery, similar to paralytic ileus (p. 645), but has been observed as a consequence of diabetic coma.

Tumours

Benign tumours

Benign epithelial tumours or *neoplastic polyps* are rare, but if larger than 1 cm in diameter should be regarded as potentially malignant. Most mucosal polyps are hyperplastic or regenerative, possibly arising as a consequence of mucosal damage, and some are hamartomatous: neither of these has malignant potential. The commonest benign tumour is the *leiomyoma*, which is sometimes multiple: it arises from the muscular layer and projects into the lumen. Although usually small, it may show a characteristic type of clean punched-out ulceration and can produce very brisk bleeding. The histological appearances of well-differentiated smooth muscle tumours is, however, misleading, for some of them invade locally and even metastasise: completeness of excision is therefore important. Lipoma, fibroma, neurofibroma, (associated with generalised neurofibromatosis) and glomangioma (p. 348) may also occur.

Gastric carcinoma

Carcinoma is by far the most important tumour in the stomach, both numerically and clinically, and is also one of the commonest internal malignant tumours in man. There is considerable geographical variation in its incidence, which has shown a slight fall in this country in recent years. It still, however, remains the commonest internal carcinoma in many countries, with a particularly high incidence in Iceland, Finland and Japan. Men are affected twice as often as women, and the disease is commoner in the poorer economic groups. The maximum incidence is over 50 years of age. The five-year survival rate is of the order of 10 per cent.

Aetiology. No specific cause of gastric carcinoma has been identified but certain predisposing factors are recognised. Some families have an unusually high incidence, and **genetic influences** may be involved in a proportion of cases, perhaps indirectly, as in the association with pernicious anaemia. It has been established that, in caucasians, blood group A is associated with a significantly higher incidence of gastric cancer than other blood groups, in contrast to the high incidence of peptic ulcer in those of group O. It is also likely, from the variations in the incidence of gastric cancer between communities, that **environmental factors**, such as the diet and methods of cooking, are important. Specific dietary factors have not been identified, but the consumption of salted or pickled food may be associated with an increased risk. The composition of the soil and the extent of background radiation have been investigated to explain geographical variations in incidence but further epidemiological studies are clearly required.

Precancerous lesions. Of *local gastric factors*, the importance of *gastric ulcer* has already been discussed (p. 612). There remains the possible relationship of *chronic gastritis* to carcinoma. Certainly the two lesions co-exist in a high percentage of cases and there is a notable degradation of cell type and replacement of the superficial mucosa by cells of intestinal type, especially in the pyloric antrum. The aetiological relationship remains unsettled, but the incidence of gastric carcinoma in patients with pernicious anaemia, adequately maintained on vitamin B_{12}, is about three times that in the general population in a comparable age group.

Macroscopic appearances. Almost half of all gastric carcinomas arise in the pylorus or pyloric antrum, most of the remainder being found either in the body of the stomach or in the cardia. In a small percentage of cases the tumour exhibits a diffuse infiltrative pattern and the primary site cannot readily be recognised. The distribution of carcinoma thus differs from that of peptic ulcer, which in the great majority of cases is confined to the lesser curvature (p. 609).

Gastric carcinoma presents various naked-eye appearances. In many cases, the tumour projects into the gastric lumen, producing an irregular *nodular* pattern, and sometimes large *fungating* masses are formed. Another common appearance is produced by the *scirrhous* tumour, which occurs mainly in the pyloric region, and infiltrates deeply into the gastric wall producing a marked scirrhous reaction (Fig. 19.36); in this type, *ulceration* is almost always present but, in contrast to chronic peptic ulceration, tends to be shallow without complete penetration of the muscle layer, and the edge is either nodular or shows loss of the normal rugose mucosal pattern. In the less common *mucoid* type, which also arises most often in the pylorus, the gastric wall is markedly thickened and is obviously gelatinous (Fig. 19.37). *Diffuse carcinoma* (Fig. 19.38) is also uncommon but is distinctive in that the deeper layers of the gastric wall are extensively infiltrated and thickened without obvious mucosal involvement (*leather-bottle stomach* or

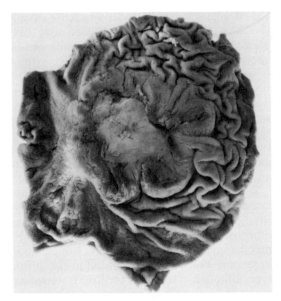

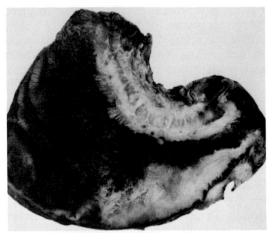

Fig. 19.37 Mucoid carcinoma at pylorus, showing great infiltration and thickening of the wall (anterior part of stomach viewed from behind). ×0·5.

Fig. 19.36 Ulcerating scirrhous carcinoma of stomach, with thickened, raised margin and ulcerated base.

linitis plastica). Sometimes the infiltrate extends into the lower oesophagus and duodenum. In contrast, some rare forms of gastric cancer spread extensively in the mucosa or submucosa without deeper involvement—the so-called *superficial spreading cancer*.

The appearance of *early gastric cancer* is becoming more widely recognised by the widespread use of endoscopic techniques, especially in Japan which has an exceptionally high incidence of gastric carcinoma. Cytological techniques in expert hands may also be of value in the early detection of gastric carcinoma.

Spread of gastric carcinoma. *Local spread* is usually prominent. The muscularis is infiltrated most extensively in the *ulcerative scirrhous* and *diffuse* types and involvement of the oesophageal and duodenal muscle coat is not unusual. The duodenal mucosa is rarely invaded,

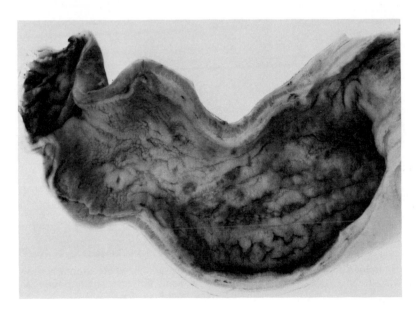

Fig. 19.38 Diffuse carcinoma of stomach. Note the general thickening of the wall without a localised tumour mass and with little ulceration. ×0·7.

but the oesophageal mucosa is often involved by tumours of the fundus or cardia. The gastric serosa is penetrated early, with direct extension to surrounding structures such as the greater and lesser omentum, liver, pancreas, spleen, diaphragm and abdominal wall. Invasion of the peritoneum may lead to *transcoelomic spread.* Numerous minute nodules may be scattered throughout the peritoneal cavity and the greater omentum may come to form a hard, palpable contracted mass in the epigastrium. The ovaries are not infrequently involved via the peritoneum. If the tumour is of the 'signet-ring' cell type with a prominent fibrous tissue reaction, bilateral ovarian metastases are referred to as 'Krukenberg tumours' (p. 966).

Lymphatic spread is early and frequent and is probably the most important factor in determining the feasibility of surgical removal. From the primary focus in the mucosa, the tumour spreads to the wide network of submucosal lymphatics (Fig. 19.39) and through the muscularis to the serosal lymphatics and thence to the para-gastric lymph nodes which are usually the first to be involved. Extension may take place into the mucosa from the submucosal lymphatics to form numerous nodules, giving a false impression of multifocal origin. Lymphatic spread is often extensive, especially in *diffuse carcinoma*, involving lymphatics in the omentum, mesentery and wall of the intestine; it may take the form of diffuse permeation without formation of tumour nodules. Lymph node metastases are usual in the upper abdomen, and more distant nodes may also be involved.

Blood spread occurs by the portal venous system, usually resulting in early metastasis to the liver, and eventually to the lungs. Various other organs, including the brain and bones, may be involved. Blood spread is less common in mucoid cancer, and is unusual in the diffuse type, although in the latter the liver is sometimes involved by lymphatic permeation.

Microscopic appearances. In most cases the tumour is an **adenocarcinoma**, often rather poorly differentiated (Fig. 19.40). In areas of

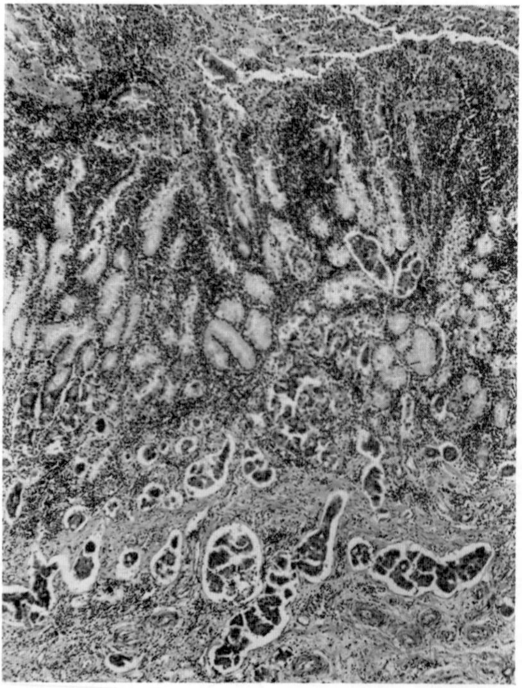

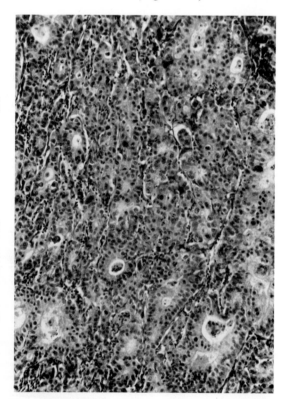

Fig. 19.39 Stomach wall, showing infiltration of lymphatics by carcinoma cells, which, in places, are growing upwards through the muscularis mucosae into the mucosa. Note the severe chronic gastritis. × 30.

Fig. 19.40 Adenocarcinoma of the stomach showing formation of acini but also solid, poorly differentiated areas. × 130.

high incidence it is thought to arise usually from the metaplastic 'intestinal' epithelium of the gastric mucosa in chronic gastritis (p. 605). Some, however, are composed of solid masses of anaplastic cells. Mixed patterns are observed in both ulcerative and fungating tumours. In the diffuse type the cells often occur singly or in small groups throughout the thickness of the gastric wall: they may be small and difficult to recognise, but some of them have the characteristic '*signet-ring*' *cell* appearance (Fig. 19.41) in which the globule of mucin confirms their identification as cancer cells. In the mucoid type, the cells are bathed in extracellular mucin. (Fig. 12.17, p. 331).

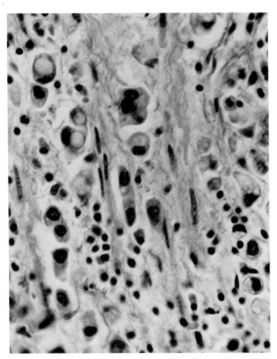

Fig. 19.41 Diffuse type of carcinoma in muscular coat of stomach. The cells are irregularly scattered, some containing mucous globules and others showing atrophic change. × 600.

Associated conditions. Achlorhydria or hypochlorhydria is usual in gastric carcinoma, and in many cases is due to the chronic gastritis which precedes or accompanies the tumour.

The absence of hydrochloric acid, aided by stasis due to pyloric obstruction and infection of necrotic tumour tissue, leads to the growth of micro-organisms of various kinds and secondary bacterial infection of the ulcerating tumour may account, in part, for the *cachexia* with '*secondary*' *anaemia* (p. 540) observed clinically in gastric cancer. *Iron-deficiency anaemia* may also occur from chronic blood loss: *macrocytic anaemia* is rare and due to atrophic gastritis, i.e. pernicious anaemia. It is also well recognised that when gastric carcinoma becomes widespread it may be associated with a low-grade *microangiopathic haemolytic anaemia*, possibly caused by the seeping of tumour mucin into vessel walls and widespread microvascular thrombosis. This type of anaemia is often accompanied by a leukoerythroblastic blood picture due to bone-marrow metastases.

Cancer of the stomach is one of the tumours sometimes accompanied, or even preceded, by the appearance in the skin of multiple warty hyperkeratotic patches, especially about the folds or flexures—so-called *acanthosis nigricans*.

Other malignant tumours of the stomach

Various types of sarcoma may arise in the stomach, but these constitute less than 5 per cent of malignant neoplasms of the stomach.

Leiomyosarcoma (p. 346) is perhaps the commonest of these. It tends to be more localised than carcinoma and usually takes the form of a large fungating mass projecting into the lumen. Ulceration and necrosis are common.

Malignant lymphoma, often of plasma cell type (p. 583), may form a localised mass or a more diffuse infiltrative growth causing enormous thickening of the whole gastric wall. When localised to the stomach, the prognosis after surgery is better than for carcinoma.

Carcinoid tumours may also arise occasionally in the stomach, but differ from the commoner carcinoids in the intestine both in morphology and in their secretory effects (p. 648).

Congenital abnormalities

The most important of these is **stenosis of the pylorus**. It is not uncommon, symptoms appearing usually about two to three weeks after birth, and by obstruction and persistent vomiting may lead to death. Obstruction is due to muscular hypertrophy of the wall at the pylorus, and this may extend back over a considerable distance, gradually fading off, or may be more localised and in the form of a discrete band (Fig. 19.42). The circular muscle fibres are especially increased, and narrowing of the lumen is sometimes severe. It is usually regarded as a hypertrophy produced by spasmodic

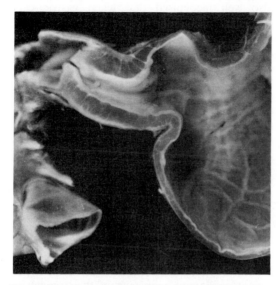

Fig. 19.42 Congenital stenosis of pylorus. The anterior wall at the pylorus has been cut away to show the greatly hypertrophied muscle at the pyloric antrum. × 1·2.

contraction at the pylorus, but the nature of the exciting agent or neuromuscular abnormality is not known. Its increased incidence in siblings, and especially in twins, of affected infants suggests a genetic predisposition, and it has been claimed to be due to a Mendelian recessive gene. Against this, however, the incidence in affected families is less than the expected 1 in 4 and the condition is six times commoner in male than in female infants. Relief of the obstruction by incision of the hypertrophied muscle is usually necessary and effective. Occasionally some degree of congenital pyloric stenosis may persist into adult life, and if symptoms are produced the condition is then liable to be mistaken for carcinoma.

Diverticula occur in the pyloric and fundal regions of the stomach, but they are rare. Occasionally the stomach is congenitally narrowed about the middle, producing the so-called 'hour-glass' contraction, but this occurs more frequently as the result of scarring around a chronic gastric ulcer (p. 611). Persistent vomiting and failure of a neonate to thrive may also be due to congenital deficiency in the enzymes necessary for the metabolism of the sugars— galactose, lactose or sucrose—and these rare conditions may be mistaken for congenital pyloric stenosis.

IV: The Intestines

Introduction

The pathology of the intestine is influenced considerably by the normal presence of bacteria in its lumen: lesions of the intestinal wall, whether due to ischaemia, neoplasia or of unknown cause, e.g. Crohn's disease and ulcerative colitis, are prone to undergo secondary bacterial infection, with the usual forms of inflammatory response. In addition, various pathogenic bacteria and parasites find a suitable environment in the intestine, and **infection** is much more important than in

the stomach. Extensive mucosal lesions, particularly in the small intestine, can result in **malabsorption syndromes**, and a large number of conditions can cause **intestinal obstruction**. Finally, **carcinoma** is very common in the colon and rectum, but rare in the small intestine.

Although the small and large intestines each have their own specific diseases, these are relatively few, and most pathological processes affect them both similarly. For that reason the intestine is considered as a whole in most of the account which follows.

Ischaemic bowel disease

In most instances, ischaemic damage is due to partial or complete occlusion of the major mesenteric arteries. Complete occlusion usually leads to haemorrhagic infarction and gangrene of variable extent limited to the areas supplied by the artery involved (Fig. 19.72, p. 645). Narrowing of the mesenteric arteries, usually resulting from degenerative vascular disease in elderly individuals, does not, as a rule, produce pathological change unless there are also hypotensive episodes, e.g. in cardiac failure, which aggravate the intestinal ischaemia. The effects depend upon the duration of the ischaemic episode and vary from full thickness necrosis with subsequent gangrene to slight mucosal damage which heals completely. Occasionally more extensive mucosal and sub-mucosal necrosis takes place and subsequent healing leads to fibrous thickening of the bowel wall, sometimes with stricture formation. In addition, bacterial infection of the damaged mucosa produces inflammatory change so that the ischaemic lesion resembles inflammatory bowel disease, although its true origin may be revealed by the presence in the bowel wall of haemosiderin-laden macrophages indicating previous haemorrhage. The term 'ischaemic colitis' has been applied to such lesions which occur especially in the watershed zone between the areas supplied by the superior and inferior mesenteric arteries, i.e. in the vicinity of the splenic flexure of the colon.

There is also a group of ischaemic intestinal lesions in which major vascular obstruction does not appear to be implicated since the pathological changes tend to be patchy and can involve both the small and large intestine in apparently random fashion. Such lesions, which are sometimes extensive, develop in various clinical circumstances, including intestinal obstruction, states of shock following surgical operations or myocardial infarction, uraemia and cardiac failure. The clinical picture is that of severe circulatory collapse associated with abdominal pain, diarrhoea and blood loss per rectum: the condition is usually fatal. The generic term **ischaemic enterocolitis** has been given

to this group. In its most severe form, the intestinal mucosa shows extensive haemorrhage and necrosis which may involve the entire thickness of the bowel wall. In some cases there may be extensive pseudomembrane formation on the mucosal surface (Fig. 19.43). Fibrin thrombi have been demonstrated in the mucosal blood vessels in the various forms of ischaemic disease. The cause of ischaemic lesions of this kind is not clear: inadequate perfusion of the intestine during episodes of hypotension may be significant, but disseminated intravascular coagulation (p. 556) and local factors such as raised intraluminal pressure might be contributory factors.

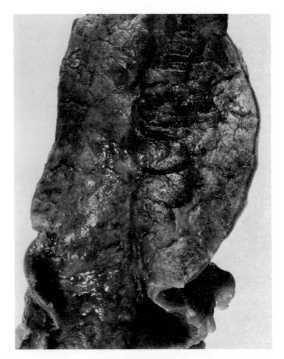

Fig. 19.43 Ischaemic colitis in an elderly woman. The lesion was multifocal in the transverse and descending colon. The area illustrated shows pseudomembranous inflammation, but there were older lesions with submucosal fibrosis and narrowing. Although ischaemic, the exact causation of such lesions is not clear (*see text*).

Conditions of uncertain aetiology

Gastro-enteritis of infancy

This infection, which can become epidemic in nurseries, carries a high mortality, usually attributable to fluid and electrolyte depletion resulting from diarrhoea and vomiting, in infants under two years of age. Despite this, the pathological changes are seldom impressive, although intestinal mucosal biopsies have shown epithelial damage associated with some increased leukocytic infiltration in the lamina propria and moderate degrees of villous atrophy (p. 640). Indeed, villous atrophy may persist for some weeks after the acute episode and produce transient malabsorption. In fatal cases the liver often shows marked fatty change. The pathogenesis is sometimes uncertain but some serological types of *Esch-*

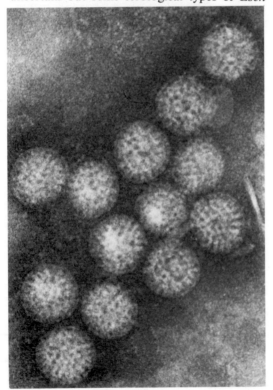

Fig. 19.44 Human rotavirus in a direct electron micrograph of centrifuged faecal extract. The complete virus particles, with the outer surface layer, are illustrated. × 200 000. (Professor C. R. Madeley, Department of Virology, University of Newcastle upon Tyne.)

erichia coli (for example 0111, 055 and 0119) are commonly blamed. Recently, virus particles have been demonstrated by electron microscopy, both in duodenal biopsies and in the faeces, in a substantial proportion of cases in which pathogenic bacteria have not been isolated. Of the various types which have been described, the best recognised are the *rotaviruses*, so-called because of their cart-wheel morphology (Fig. 19.44).

Crohn's disease (regional enteritis)

Although this is a relatively uncommon condition it is becoming increasingly recognised as a cause of lesions throughout the alimentary tract, from mouth to anus. Most commonly, however, the terminal part of the ileum is initially and often mainly involved.

Clinical features. Young adults of both sexes are most frequently affected, and there is some evidence of familial incidence, although this is not striking. The symptoms are ill-defined at first, mild diarrhoea and vague abdominal pain being the usual complaints. Later, subacute or chronic intestinal obstruction develop and may require excision of the narrowed segment of bowel. The disease runs a prolonged course, with long remissions, and recurrence after operation occurs in about 50 per cent of cases. Malabsorption and protein-losing enteropathy can result from repeated and extensive involvement of the small intestine.

Naked-eye appearances. The changes are most often observed in the distal ileum. 'Skip lesions' separated from the main lesion by apparently healthy bowel are sometimes found, and distal extension into the caecum and ascending colon is common. The colon may also be involved primarily, especially in the older age groups, and many cases of segmental or right-sided forms of colitis, previously classified as cases of ulcerative colitis (p. 622), are, in fact, examples of Crohn's disease. The lesion is characterised by intense oedematous thickening of the bowel wall, the submucosa being especially involved, and there is marked narrowing of the lumen (Fig. 19.45). Ulceration of the oedematous mucosa is invariable and often assumes a linear form to produce the typical 'cobblestone' appearance (Fig. 19.46). Fissures penetrating

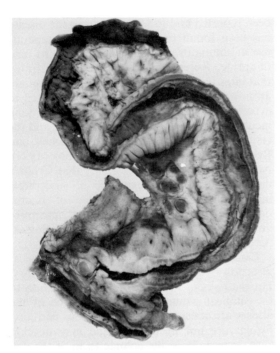

Fig. 19.45 Crohn's disease, showing diffuse thickening of the wall of the lower part of the ileum, with narrowing of its lumen.

the entire thickness of the bowel wall, and sometimes developing into fistulas opening into adjacent loops of intestine or the urinary bladder, are characteristic. The mesentery is usually thickened and oedematous and the regional lymph nodes conspicuously enlarged.

Microscopic appearances. It is characteristic of Crohn's disease that the *inflammatory changes extend throughout the entire thickness of the bowel wall* (c.f. *ulcerative colitis, below*). The most constant change is focal lymphocytic infiltration, usually most prominent in the submucosa. Of greater diagnostic value, however, is the presence, in about 60 per cent of cases, of *epithelioid-cell granulomas* which resemble closely those of sarcoidosis: they may occur in all the layers of the bowel wall and even in the mesentery and mesenteric lymph nodes. Sometimes they arise in relation to lymphoid aggregates, but more often they are found in and around lymphatic channels (Fig. 19.47). It is notable, however, that lymphatic obstruction and dilatation are almost invariably found in early cases, and lymphatic obstruction is thought to be of primary importance in the pathogenesis of the disease. Certainly this accounts for the *marked oedema* which is always

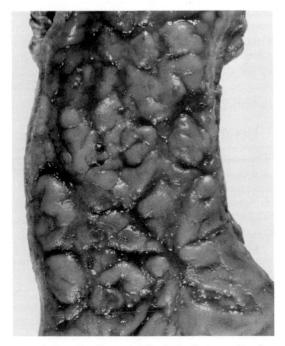

Fig. 19.46 The ileum in Crohn's disease, showing the 'cobblestone' appearance of the fissured, oedematous mucosa.

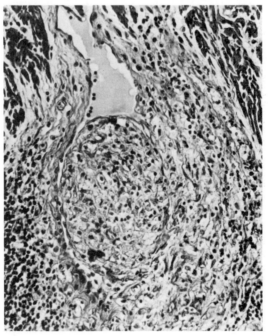

Fig. 19.47 Crohn's disease, showing a granulomatous lesion occluding a lymphatic in the muscle coat of the ileum. × 200.

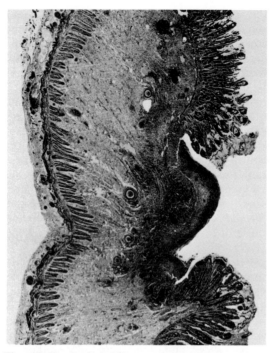

Fig. 19.48 Crohn's disease showing oedematous thickening, especially of the submucosa, with focal inflammatory infiltration and ulceration. × 12.

most conspicuous in the submucosa (Fig. 19.48) and is mainly responsible for the thickening of the bowel wall and mesentery in the early stages of the disease. *Fibrosis*, however, becomes increasingly prominent in more chronic cases. The mucosal changes, such as *ulceration* and subsequent *metaplasia* to pyloric type glands, are mainly due to *secondary infection* of the lesions, (although the epithelioid-cell follicles are occasionally found in the lamina propria, particularly in the colon). A further change of diagnostic value is the presence of *fissures* which arise from ulcer bases and may penetrate the whole thickness of the bowel wall. Microscopically, they are lined by granulation tissue with foci of suppuration due to secondary bacterial infection. Although the destructive inflammatory lesions of Crohn's disease are usually of patchy distribution, it has been demonstrated recently that, at least in the colon, mucosal inflammation may be diffuse.

Aetiology. There is no convincing evidence that Crohn's disease is related to sarcoidosis (p. 216), which rarely affects the intestinal tract. It is of interest, however, that as in sarcoidosis, abnormalities of cell-mediated immunity have

been reported and in some instances the disease has been found to respond to the therapeutic use of immunosuppressive drugs such as azathioprine. Recently it has been demonstrated that intestinal lesions in Crohn's disease contain an infective agent which can be transmitted to experimental animals, although there is a long incubation period before lesions appear and the results are as yet unconfirmed (Mitchell and Rees, 1970; Cave, Mitchell and Brook, 1973). Nevertheless there is a possibility that Crohn's disease is caused by exposure of susceptible individuals to a particular type of microorganism, possibly a virus, and that susceptibility is determined by some immunological peculiarity.

Complications. As mentioned above, surgical resection of narrowed bowel may be necessary, but the risks of fistula formation in relation to the surgical wound and of recurrence of the disease are considerable. Spontaneous peri-anal fistulas are not uncommon and may develop early, especially in the colonic form of the disease: the detection of epithelioid-cell granulomas in the wall of such fistulas is of diagnostic help. Iron-deficiency anaemia is common, and occasionally a macrocytic anaemia results from interference with vitamin B_{12} absorption, which takes place exclusively in the ileum. Other features of malabsorption syndrome may develop, especially in diffuse jejuno-ileal forms of the disease (p. 639). As in ulcerative colitis, systemic complications may occur. These include arthritis, uveitis and skin lesions.

Ulcerative colitis

The cause of this moderately common condition is not known. It behaves as a distinct clinical and pathological entity, although it may be difficult to distinguish, particularly in the early stages, from other inflammatory diseases of the colon, notably Crohn's disease.

Clinical features. The disease mainly affects young adults of both sexes and is characterised by episodes of diarrhoea with the passage of blood per rectum. Malaise, anorexia and weight loss vary greatly in degree. Most cases follow a chronic relapsing course with exacerbations and remissions. Some are mild and possibly self-limiting, but a few run a more severe, continuous course and fulminating rapidly fatal forms are by no means rare.

Naked-eye appearances. Ulcerative colitis typically involves the sigmoid colon and rectum (proctitis) either alone or in continuity with the remainder of the colon. The entire colon is affected in about half of the cases, and in such instances the terminal ileum may also be inflamed. In some cases, the proximal colon, with or without the terminal ileum, is principally affected. It is now recognised, however, that many such 'segmental' or 'right-sided' forms of colitis are examples of Crohn's disease (p. 620) and others may have an ischaemic origin.

In its early phases, sigmoidoscopy shows the colonic mucosa to be deeply congested, velvety in appearance and to bleed easily (Fig. 19.49). Punctate erosions herald the onset of ulceration, which usually begins in the rectum or sigmoid and is found initially at the tips of the mucosal folds overlying the longitudinal muscle bands. Later the ulcers coalesce, giving rise to large irregular areas of mucosal denudation associated with extensive muco-purulent discharge and haemorrhage. Between the ulcers, especially in chronic cases, the surviving mucosa becomes swollen and hyperplastic (Fig. 19.50) and in some instances numerous polypoid excrescences are seen, a condition known as *pseudo-polyposis*. Attempts at healing take place during remissions, but fibrous thickening and stenosis of the lumen are relatively uncommon. During relapses, the colon is spastic and the early loss of the normal sacculation produces a characteristic radiological appearance.

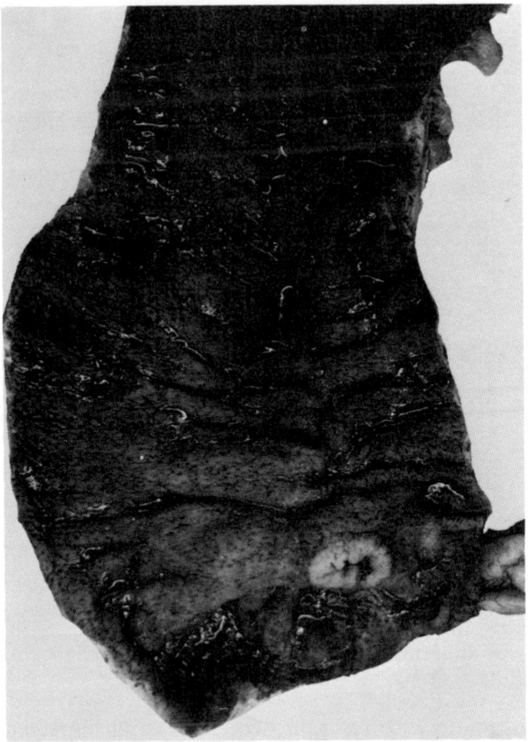

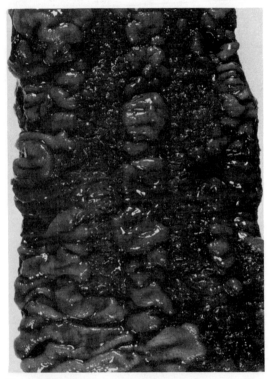

Fig. 19.50 The colon in chronic ulcerative colitis. The mucosa is extensively ulcerated and the surviving portions are swollen and hyperplastic with many undermined bridges of mucosa. × 0·8.

In severe cases or during exacerbations the colon may become greatly dilated—'*toxic dilatation*' (see below) and the stretched wall may perforate.

Microscopic appearances. Unlike Crohn's disease, it is the mucosa which is primarily involved in ulcerative colitis. During active phases it is congested and densely infiltrated with leukocytes, especially plasma cells. The formation of *crypt abscesses* (Fig. 19.51*a*),

Fig. 19.49 The caecum in early ulcerative colitis. Intense congestion, haemorrhage and multiple pinpoint ulcers of mucosa. The appendicular orifice is shown, and in this case is not affected. × 0·7.

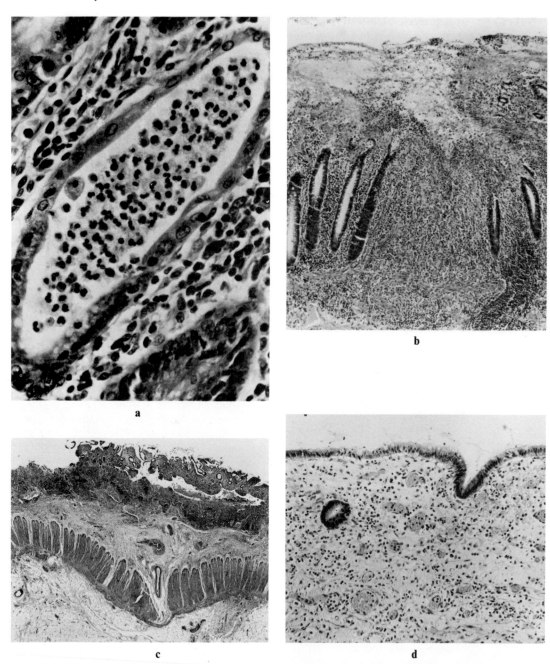

Fig. 19.51   Ulcerative colitis. **a** Crypt abscess. × 425. **b** Early mucosal ulceration with purulent exudate. × 70. **c** Chronic stage: complete loss of mucosa on the left, with undermining of surviving mucosa on the right. × 13. **d** Healing stage showing granulation tissue covered by a simple mucosa. × 115.

characterised by accumulation of neutrophils, eosinophils, red cells and mucus within crypt lumina, is a conspicuous feature, although by no means specific for ulcerative colitis. The epithelial lining of the crypts degenerates and ultimately breaks down, releasing infected material into the lamina propria mucosae. This lesion is a prelude to the appearance of frank ulceration (Fig. 19.51b), which is produced by the coalescence of ruptured crypt abscesses in the deeper parts of the mucosa. *Ulceration seldom extends more deeply than the submucosa* and the base is formed by vascular granulation tissue (Fig. 19.51c) containing large numbers of plasma cells and lymphocytes, the latter becoming increasingly conspicuous in chronic cases. The pseudo-polyps observed in chronic cases consist of islands of surviving hyperplastic mucosa and tags of granulation tissue; true polypoid adenomas (p. 650) are rare, although carcinoma is a common complication in long-standing cases. Surface re-epithelialisation of ulcerated areas may take place but the healed mucosa contains few glands (Fig. 19.51d). An increase in Paneth cells in the crypts of Lieberkühn is noted especially in the proximal colon; the significance of this is uncertain.

Complications. The most urgent of **local complications** is *perforation of the colon*, which is usually associated with pronounced dilatation of the colon ('*toxic dilatation*'). This complication may be due to superimposed infection, or precipitated by the use of antispasmodic drugs. *Peri-anal fistulae* may be troublesome in some cases. Although simple fibrous strictures are uncommon, it is now recognised that the development of *carcinoma* of the colon is a considerable risk. It occurs most commonly in cases in which the entire colon is involved, the onset is early in life and the disease has been present for 10 years or more; the risk is such as to provide an indication for total colectomy in some instances.

By repeated biopsy, it is possible to detect the development of premalignant change, which usually starts in a flat (as opposed to polypoid) mucosa: the changes include nuclear pleomorphism, hyperchromatism, loss of polarity and increased mitotic activity in the epithelial cells (Morson, 1978).

The various **systemic complications** include fever and leukocytosis, and debilitating diarrhoea with haemorrhage and exudation leads to protein depletion and anaemia. Arthritis, iridocyclitis and skin lesions, such as erythema nodosum and pyoderma gangrenosum, are seen in a proportion of cases. There appears to be an association between joint disease, especially ankylosing spondylitis, and chronic inflammatory disease of the intestine. Liver disease, of which chronic pericholangitis is the most characteristic and frank cirrhosis the most severe, is not infrequent in ulcerative colitis.

Aetiology. The cause of ulcerative colitis remains an unsolved problem. The disease is commonest in affluent societies and shows a familial incidence. No specific micro-organism has been isolated, although it is notable that certain types of colonic infection, especially amoebiasis (p. 635) may closely resemble ulcerative colitis pathologically. *A search for Entamoeba histolytica and other known pathogens should always be undertaken in suspected cases.* The possibility that ulcerative colitis has an immunological basis is tenuous. Antibodies which react with colonic epithelium (and also with *Esch. coli* 0119 B14) are present in the serum in some cases, and there is evidence also of cell-mediated immunity to colonic epithelium, but these findings have not been shown to be specific for ulcerative colitis, and may be secondary phenomena.

Other non-specific intestinal lesions

Eosinophilic gastro-enteritis. In this disease segments of the stomach or small intestine are extensively infiltrated by eosinophils and often markedly oedematous. When the submucosa is mainly affected, obstructive symptoms predominate; if the mucosa in involved there may be malabsorption or protein-losing enteropathy. It is probably an allergic reaction to dietary constituents or metazoan parasites and is often accompanied by eosinophil leukocytosis.

Inflammatory fibroid polyp is a term applied to certain localised lesions of stomach or small bowel, in which exuberant granulation tissue accompanied by eosinophilic infiltration produces a mass which protrudes into the lumen of the gut and may cause intussusception. The cause is not known.

Non-specific ulcers of the intestine. Solitary ulcers of a non-specific nature are occasionally encountered both in the small bowel and colon. In most instances the causation is unknown. Recently, however, it has been suggested that administration of enteric-coated tablets of potassium chloride in association with the diuretic chlorothiazide is responsible in some instances.

Solitary ulcer of the rectum. This term is used to describe a recurrent ulcerative condition, which usually affects young adults and presents a distinctive appearance in rectal biopsies. The mucosa shows variable inflammatory change with irregular superficial ulceration, and fibro-muscular thickening of the lamina propria. There may also be displacement of crypt epithelium into the submucosa with subsequent cyst formation. These changes are thought to be related to muscular spasm possibly related to chronic straining at stool, and have also been observed in association with rectal prolapse.

Colitis cystica profunda. This rare condition is to be regarded more as a pathological phenomenon than as a distinct disease entity. It is caused by the displacement of epithelium into the colonic submucosa with subsequent cyst formation. It is commonly a consequence of mucosal inflammation and may be observed in the vicinity of solitary ulcers (see above). Cyst formation in the mucosa (*colitis cystica superficialis*) has been described in pellagra and in malabsorption states.

Functional disorders of the colon. In clinical practice it is by no means uncommon to encounter patients who have symptoms associated with constipation and excessive mucus secretion, although organic lesions cannot be demonstrated.

'Mucous colitis', in which membranous structures composed of inspissated mucus are passed by the bowel, is probably a variant of this syndrome.

Although a variety of names has been attached to such states, the term 'irritable colon syndrome' is most commonly employed, and finds justification in the fact that the colon may be found to exhibit unusual irritability or hypermotility. The causation is obscure—indeed this syndrome may possibly include more than one disease entity—although previous organic disease, for example dysentery, psychological disturbance and dietary indiscretion might be involved.

Appendicitis

Acute appendicitis

This lesion is of the highest importance because of its frequency and serious complications. Individuals of either sex and of virtually any age may be affected but the disease is commonest in children and young adults.

Naked-eye appearances. The condition occurs in three forms: *simple acute*, *suppurative* and *gangrenous* appendicitis. The first two of these types are different degrees of severity of the same condition; the third has special features of its own. Perforation may occur in both suppurative and gangrenous types.

In all cases, the whole thickness of the wall is involved. In the earlier stages of simple or suppurative appendicitis, the appendix is swollen, tense and markedly congested, and there may be a little fibrin on the surface (Fig. 19.52). When the appendix is cut across, the mucosa bulges owing to the swelling, and turbid exudate may escape from the lumen.

In other cases the changes are of greater severity. The primary inflammatory lesion may

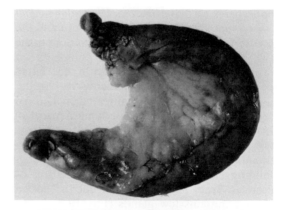

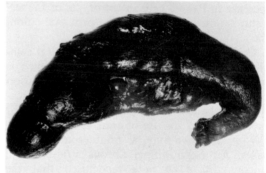

Fig. 19.52 Acute appendicitis. *Above,* showing swelling and congestion and dulling of the serosal surface by fibrin. *Below,* gangrenous appendicitis, showing swelling, haemorrhage and fibrin deposition.

progress to a small abscess in the wall, and this may perforate. There may occur also more general suppuration and necrosis with multiple abscesses and perforations. The presence of a concretion (faecolith) in the lumen may predispose to perforation because, in acute appendicitis, the swollen wall becomes stretched over the concretion with consequent ischaemia and gangrene.

Gangrenous appendicitis (Fig. 19.52) is due to acute appendicitis complicated by thrombosis of the veins in the meso-appendix, with consequent haemorrhage and arrest of the circulation. In some cases, however, gangrene develops early and rapidly and affects the whole appendix apart from any vascular lesion: in such cases, gangrene is due to obstruction at the outlet of the appendix and distension with faecal material, or to the presence of a faecolith (see above). Experimentally a closed portion of small intestine filled with faecal material becomes gangrenous within a short time, and many cases of so-called fulminating, i.e. gangrenous, appendicitis are of this nature. The great danger of gangrenous appendicitis is the early development of general peritonitis due to mixed bacterial infection, including anaerobes.

Microscopic appearances. In most cases of acute appendicitis, there is an acute inflammatory reaction involving the entire thickness of the appendicular wall, with a fibrinopurulent exudate on the peritoneal surface. This inflammatory reaction probably originates from a focus of mucosal ulceration, possibly in the deeper parts of the epithelial crypts with subsequent extension into the lamina propria (Fig. 19.53). Several foci of inflammation are some-

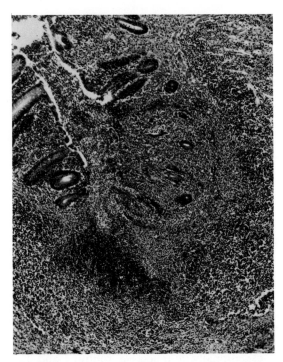

Fig. 19.53 Acute appendicitis, showing a local ulcerative lesion in mucosa with commencing abscess formation beneath. × 60.

times observed, but the changes are usually most marked in the distal part (i.e. the blind end) of the appendix. Sometimes the inflammation is localised and can easily be missed on cursory examination. In some patients with an appendicitis-like syndrome the only changes seen are pus cells in the appendicular lumen, associated with either foci of polymorph infiltration in the superficial parts of the mucosa, or occasional crypt abscesses. The clinical significance of such limited forms of appendicitis is debatable since similar changes are sometimes seen in appendices removed prophylactically during the course of some other operation, e.g. hysterectomy.

Clinical features. Acute appendicitis presents typically as colicky abdominal pain in the umbilical region, due to spasmodic contractions of the inflamed appendix. This is followed by a continuous 'burning' pain, tenderness and rigidity of the abdominal muscles, in the vicinity of the appendix. These latter features are due to irritation of the parietal peritoneum by the inflamed appendiceal serosa, and they may be inconspicuous or absent when the appendix is retrocaecal. Vomiting, pyrexia, increased pulse rate and neutrophil leukocytosis are inconstant features.

The diagnosis of acute appendicitis is often difficult and gangrenous appendicitis may be accompanied by remarkably slight clinical upset. The results of delay in removing an acutely inflamed appendix (see below) are so serious that exploratory laparotomy is often necessary in cases where the diagnosis is far from certain.

Results. Acute appendicitis gives rise to important complications. In some cases there is merely a slight amount of fibrinous exudate on the surface, which does not spread and may afterwards become organised, resulting in local adhesions. In others, a localised collection of pus may form around the appendix—**appendix abscess.** Sometimes an escaped concretion is present in the pus. The pus may track upwards alongside the caecum and ascending colon and between the surface of the liver and the diaphragm. Alternatively, an abscess may develop in, or extend into, the pelvic cavity. Such abscesses may be persistent, with increasing surrounding fibrosis, or they may discharge, e.g. from the pelvis into the rectum. In other cases, **generalised peritonitis** may develop, and this can happen very rapidly in gangrenous appendicitis. Other complications of appendicitis are due to infection of the veins. There may be a local septic phlebitis, and from this emboli may be carried to the liver, where they set up secondary abscesses. Rarely, a spreading thrombosis with secondary suppuration may extend up the portal vein—*portal pylephlebitis* (p. 695).

Aetiology. Although the lesions of acute appendicitis are due to *bacterial infection*, the factors which trigger it off are still largely unknown. There is even uncertainty about which organisms primarily invade the wall, although there is no doubt that the important effects are caused by coliform bacilli, streptococci and anaerobic bacteria, all of which are normally present in the lumen. It seems certain, however, that *obstruction* of the appendicular lumen is involved in many cases and, as already mentioned, gangrenous appendicitis is often produced in this way. Less easy to explain is the cause of the obstruction; foreign bodies and intestinal parasites, e.g. *Oxyuris vermicularis*, have been blamed from time to time, but in many cases are absent. A more promising suggestion is that obstruction is caused, particularly in childhood, by swelling of the appendicular lymphoid tissue, due possibly to viral infection, or, as has recently been demonstrated, by infection with *Yersinia enterocolitica*, an organism also known to produce acute mesenteric lymphadenitis (which incidentally can mimic acute appendicitis clinically). The part played by faecal concretions, or faecoliths, which are hard masses of faeces mixed with mucus and occasionally calcium salts, is difficult to assess, since these are commonly found even in normal appendices. As explained above, a *concretion* is likely to cause ischaemia and gangrene in an acutely inflamed appendix. It is notable that appendicitis, like diverticular disease (see below), is essentially a disease of developed societies, and it might well be that, as Burkitt has claimed, refined diets lacking in roughage are of importance in its pathogenesis.

Recurrent and chronic appendicitis and mucocele of the appendix

Recurrent acute appendicitis is not unusual in cases where the initial attack has been relatively mild and has been treated conservatively. If there is no history of an acute attack, recurrent abdominal pain without localising symptoms is unlikely to be due to appendicitis.

Fibrous thickening of the wall of the appendix, especially in young people, may be a consequence of acute inflammation. Occasionally, fibrosis may be the result of persistent chronic infection—the so-called *chronic appendicitis*—and there may be no history of an acute attack. It is conceivable that mild attacks of abdominal pain in the region of the appendix are due to this ('appendicular dyspepsia').

It should be emphasised, however, that in older individuals asymptomatic appendicular fibrosis is extremely common and can almost be regarded as a normal ageing process.

A common result of a localised lesion of the appendix is obliteration of the lumen at that point, whilst elsewhere the mucosa may be comparatively well preserved. This may be readily explained by the commonly focal nature of acute appendicitis. When localised obliteration is present, dilatation of the distal portion of the lumen may follow (Fig. 19.54). This may be slight, or there may be a cyst-like enlargement filled with mucus—**mucocele**.

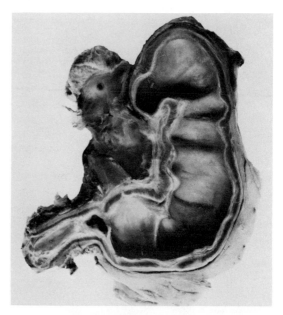

Fig. 19.54 Chronic appendicitis with obliteration at proximal end and mucocele of the distal portion.

Occasionally a mucocele ruptures and the mucus leaks into the pertoneum, where it becomes organised, resulting in peritoneal adhesions. The condition known as *pseudomyxoma peritonei* may be produced in this way; it is more likely, however, that serious forms of this condition, in which mucous-secreting cells seed throughout the peritoneum, are due to mucous-secreting neoplasms of the appendix. Another quite common lesion is a *diverticulum*, which may project on the surface of the appendix, and is due to distension of part of the wall in which the muscle coat has been weakened, possibly by previous inflammation.

Diverticular disease

A diverticulum consists of protrusion of the mucous and submucous coats through the muscle of the wall: the projecting pouch has no muscle coat, and is properly called a 'false diverticulum', in contrast to a true diverticulum, e.g. Meckel's (p. 655), which has a complete layer of muscle like the bowel.

(a) Small intestine. Diverticula are uncommon in the small bowel. The duodenum is most often involved, followed by the jejunum and ileum in that order. The diverticula may be single or multiple and are invariably found along the mesenteric border of the bowel in close relationship to the entry-sites of the blood vessels. They may enlarge to over 3 cm in diameter.

Pathological effects. Small-bowel diverticula are seldom encountered before adult life; they probably cause abdominal symptoms more often than is generally realised. Frank inflammatory change, haemorrhage and obstruction are, however, rare complications. More often malabsorption similar to that in the 'blind-loop syndrome' (p. 642) is the principal feature: it is caused mainly by abnormal and excessive bacterial proliferation in the diverticula. Bacterial uptake of vitamin B_{12} before it can reach its main absorptive site in the distal ileum leads to vitamin B_{12} deficiency and megaloblastic anaemia, and it is probable that bacteria are also responsible for the steatorrhoea which is sometimes observed. Oral broad-spectrum antibiotics lead to improvement in both vitamin B_{12} and fat absorption.

(b) Colon. Multiple diverticula of the colon are very common in later adult life: in this country about one person in ten is affected, although in only 20 per cent of cases does the condition produce symptoms. The sigmoid colon is most often involved, although diverticula may occur at a higher level, including the caecum. Characteristically they lie in two rows between the mesenteric and the anti-mesenteric taeniae and are related to the entry of blood vessels into the colonic wall. They commonly extend into the appendices epiploicae. Small depressions at first, they enlarge and become spherical or flask-shaped (Fig. 19.55), usually less than 1 cm in diameter. Diverticula frequently contain inspissated faeces and it is notable that muscle hypertrophy and thickening of

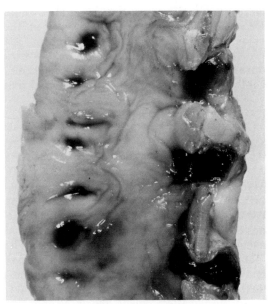

Fig. 19.55 Part of the sigmoid colon cut open to show the mucosal surface in diverticulosis. There are two longitudinal rows of diverticula: those on the right have been opened and can be seen to herniate through the muscle coat of the bowel.

the peri-colic fat are commonly observed in the adjacent bowel.

Pathological effects. Inflammatory change in the diverticula (*diverticulitis*) is the common cause of clinical symptoms, which are usually encountered in the older age groups. Acute inflammation leads to a syndrome resembling appendicitis with localisation of pain to the left side of the abdomen. This condition may progress to peri-colic abscess formation and even to free perforation into the peritoneal cavity and acute peritonitis. The development of fistulae between the colon and adjacent organs, especially the bladder, is not uncommon. More chronic diverticulitis leads to fibrous thickening of the colonic wall with some degree of intestinal obstruction, and the lesion may be mistaken macroscopically for carcinoma. There is no evidence that diverticular disease is a precancerous condition. Rarely severe rectal haemorrhage occurs, probably due to erosion of blood vessels in the diverticular wall.

Aetiology. It is generally accepted that diverticula are caused by high pressure within the bowel lumen leading to protrusion of the mucosa through points of weakness in the bowel wall. The latter are usually related to the entry of blood vessels from the mesocolon. Recent studies suggest that, at least in the colon, diverticula are associated with the generation of localised areas of unusually high intraluminal pressure by abnormal segmental contraction of the bowel musculature, and that the muscle hypertrophy related to diverticula is a morphological expression of this effect. It is notable that diverticular disease is mainly restricted to developed societies and the consumption of refined foods lacking in roughage may be the most important aetiological factor.

Specific bacterial infections

Many inflammatory conditions of the intestines, both acute and chronic, are produced by bacilli of the typhoid-coli group the most serious lesions being produced by *Salmonella typhi* and organisms of the *paratyphoid group*. The food-poisoning bacilli (*Salmonella typhimurium* and others) cause acute diffuse mucosal inflammation of the small or large intestine. The *dysentery bacilli* affect chiefly the large intestine and cause both acute and chronic lesions. In all these cases, and also in *cholera*, infection is acquired by ingesting the specific microorganisms in food or water contaminated by the excreta of cases of the disease or of carriers of the infection. Contamination by handling of food, or by the activities of flies, gives rise to sporadic cases or small outbreaks, but major epidemics are virtually always due to seepage of sewage into water supplies. An additional source of infection in food poisoning by *Salmonellae* is the soiling of food by the faeces of infected mice or rats. Bacteria of the genus *Campylobacter* have recently been implicated in outbreaks of infective diarrhoea, as have *rotaviruses* in infantile gastro-enteritis (p. 620). Chronic infections of the intestines are caused by *Myco. tuberculosis* and *Actinomyces israelii*. Many *viruses* that produce no apparent lesion of the gut are nevertheless excreted in the faeces and are invasive when ingested, e.g. poliomyelitis virus, Coxsackie virus.

The enteric fevers

This term is used to describe the illnesses caused by acute infections with *S. typhi* (typhoid fever) or *S. paratyphi* (paratyphoid fever).

Typhoid fever

This disease is caused by the Gram-ve bacillus *Salmonella typhi*. Corresponding with the clinical illness there are inflammatory changes and necrosis in the lymphoid tissue of the bowel, followed by healing.

Course. After an incubation period of about two weeks, the ingested organisms, which have already invaded the lymphoid tissues of the small intestine, enter the bloodstream, probably via the lymphatics. Bacteraemia is accompanied by progressive fever of insidious onset, sometimes with a 'staircase' rise: after a further week the characteristic rose spots appear in the skin. In the first week of the fever blood cultures are usually positive, thus confirming the diagnosis. About the end of ten days, immunity begins to develop and the organisms disappear from the blood stream. Thereafter they persist in the liver and biliary passages and re-enter the small intestine in large numbers from the bile so that they are then readily detected in the faeces. During the bacteraemic phase, the lymphoid tissues of the gut and draining lymph nodes become acutely inflamed and progress through the stages described below. It is significant that the gallbladder bile is invariably infected during the bacteraemic phase, and the wall of the viscus may become inflamed, producing a typhoid cholecystitis. These phases in the distribution of the organisms are of decisive importance in the bacteriological diagnosis of the disease. The course may be modified considerably by previous immunisation, and diagnosis may then be difficult both clinically and bacteriologically.

Naked-eye appearances. Re-infection of the lymphoid tissue of the gut by organisms in the bile leads to the development of lesions which are usually most marked in the Peyer's patches of the distal ileum, although solitary lymphoid follicles more proximally and distally are also affected. The lymphoid patches initially show an inflammatory swelling which is followed,

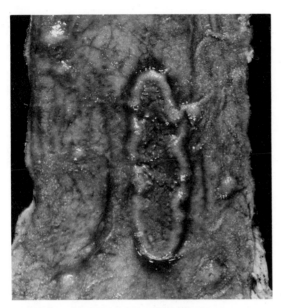

Fig. 19.56 The lower ileum in typhoid fever, showing necrosis and ulceration of the Peyer's patches and solitary lymphoid follicles.

usually about the tenth day of the illness, by necrosis and subsequent ulceration (Figs. 19.56, 19.57). Healing usually begins about the end of the third week and is complete by the fifth week in uncomplicated cases. The ulcers have a

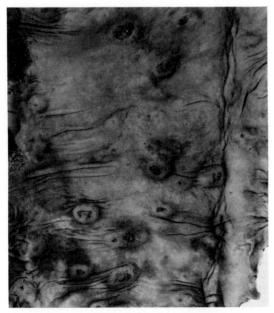

Fig. 19.57 Colon in typhoid fever showing swelling and ulceration of the lymphoid follicles.

yellowish-brown or black colour, correspond in shape and extent to the lymphoid patches, and tend to have soft, shreddy, undermined margins. Healing of these ulcerated lesions leaves a smooth silky scar which never shows any tendency towards stricture formation. *Severe haemorrhage* sometimes occurs from these necrotic ulcerated lesions, although a more serious complication resulting from extensive necrosis is *perforation of the small bowel* with usually fatal generalised peritonitis. Clinically this latter event is seldom accompanied by the dramatic symptoms associated with gastroduodenal perforation, possibly because the alkaline intestinal contents have less irritant effect on the peritoneal cavity.

Microscopic appearances. The early changes are those of acute inflammation, but neutrophil polymorphs are absent. The enlargement of the Peyer's patches (Fig. 19.58) is thus due to

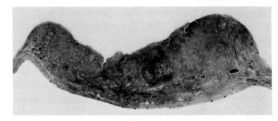

Fig. 19.58 Peyer's patch in the early stage of typhoid fever, showing the marked inflammatory swelling and commencing necrosis. × 5.

congestion, oedema and the infiltration of inflammatory cells, predominantly lymphocytes, plasma cells and macrophages. Haemorrhage and fibrinous exudation often contribute to the inflammatory swelling. These inflammatory changes may extend deeply to involve the muscularis propria (Fig. 7.4, p. 185) and even the serosal coat. As the inflammatory lesion progresses, patchy necrosis develops with extensive nuclear karyorrhexis and the surrounding macrophages, sometimes called typhoid histiocytes, typically ingest the nuclear debris as well as extravasated red cells. The development of necrosis may well represent a delayed hypersensitivity reaction to bacterial antigens. Polymorphs are only seen in relation to ulceration and secondary infection. The **mesenteric lymph nodes** are commonly enlarged and show changes closely similar to those in the Peyer's patches (Figs. 18.5, p. 570 and 2.4, p. 10). The development of focal necrosis can lead to softening and rupture of the lymph node with subsequent peritonitis.

Associated lesions. The most characteristic change in the blood is a low leukocyte count— usually below 4×10^9/litre (4000/μl)—due to a decrease of neutrophil polymorphs: this is associated with diminished granulopoiesis in the bone marrow. Similarly the *spleen* (p. 563), although commonly enlarged, contains few neutrophils, contrary to what might be expected in a severe bacterial infection. Typhoid fever is associated with a great variety of lesions which are widely distributed and may arise during the course of the disease or later: they are due to endotoxaemia (p. 178) and bacteraemia. **Endotoxaemia** may be responsible for the fever and produces degenerative changes in several organs, e.g. myocardial damage, which may precipitate heart failure, and focal necrosis of the abdominal muscles (Zenker's degeneration), which is characteristic. The liver and kidneys also show toxic injury. Typhoid endotoxaemia probably also impairs resistance to invasion by other bacteria and the well recognised development of *laryngitis*, *bronchitis* (sometimes an early symptom) and *pneumonia* may well be due to this. **Bacteraemia** brings about acute enlargement of the spleen and probably accounts for the characteristic rose-coloured spots in the skin. In some patients, infection persists in the gallbladder, with or without cholecystitis, and less commonly in the urinary tract. This is the pathological basis of the **carrier state**, since *patients thus affected excrete bacilli in the faeces or in the urine for varying periods and are commonly the source of outbreaks of typhoid fever.* Other lesions produced by circulating bacilli include endocarditis, meningitis and arthritis. Periostitis and osteomyelitis may develop after the acute illness, even years later. Perichondritis involving the costal and laryngeal cartilages are also well recognised complications.

Paratyphoid infections

Infections caused by the paratyphoid organism are not uncommon, paratyphoid B being the most frequent of the enteric fevers in West Europe. In some cases the disease has the general features of typhoid, though usually less severe. There is a similar involvement of the lymphoid tissue, especially the Peyer's patches and solitary follicles of the small intestine, with swelling of mesenteric nodes and spleen; but the necrotic and ulcerative processes are less marked and usually limited to the lower part of the ileum. In other cases a generalised mucosal inflammatory reaction is found, and there is little implication of the lymphoid tissue; sometimes enteritis is associated with marked gastritis. The 'carrier' condition may result also from paratyphoid infections, as has been described above in typhoid fever.

Other Salmonella infections

Many species of *Salmonellae* have been implicated in local outbreaks of bacillary food infection throughout the world. The most important of these are *S. enteritidis* and *S. typhimurium*. Such organisms produce an acute gastro-enteritis with fever, vomiting and diarrhoea developing 12–14 hours after eating the contaminated food. In most cases recovery is complete, but death from water and electrolyte depletion may occur in severe cases. It is also becoming increasingly recognised that *acute colitis* may be due to salmonellae (Day *et al.*, 1978).

Cholera

This disease is caused by *Vibrio cholerae* or its subtypes and is a classical example of a waterborne infection capable of causing explosive epidemics. Profuse watery diarrhoea is the outstanding clinical feature and the stools are often described as having a colourless 'rice-water' appearance. Diarrhoea leads to the loss of about 30 litres of fluid during an illness lasting 3–6 days, and the depletion of water and electrolytes, especially sodium and potassium, is extremely severe and often fatal.

Until recently it was considered that the pathological basis for the severe diarrhoea was an acute inflammation of the small intestine, especially its distal part, and occasionally of the large bowel in addition. Intestinal biopsies have failed, however, to demonstrate loss of the integrity of the surface epithelium, and *Vibrio cholerae*, which is present in large numbers in the intestinal lumen, is now known to cause diarrhoea by producing an exotoxin which increases the net flow of fluid and electrolytes from the plasma into the lumen of the gut, particularly in the jejunum. The mechanism differs from that of inflammatory exudation, and the fluid has a low protein content. It is probable that cholera toxin exerts its effect by stimulating adenyl cyclase activity, thus increasing adenosine monophosphate which affects the equilibrium of fluid and electrolytes between the mucosal cell and gut lumen. Oral administration of glucose and electrolyte solutions has been shown to be of great therapeutic value. Although the organisms are largely confined to the intestinal tract, they can become established in the gallbladder and lead to a carrier state which, although usually of short duration, may last as long as four years. It has also become apparent that the number of cases of cholera is far exceeded by the number of individuals who become infected and excrete the vibrio without developing the disease.

The **El Tor vibrio**, first isolated in Sinai, is closely related to *V. cholerae* and has been responsible for recent outbreaks of a cholera-like illness in various parts of the world.

Tuberculosis

Intestinal tuberculosis was formerly common, but in many countries the incidence is now low, partly because infection of milk by bovine tubercle bacilli has been eliminated, and partly as a consequence of the falling incidence of pulmonary tuberculosis. Three main forms of intestinal tuberculosis are recognised.

(a) Primary infection. The small bowel was formerly a common site for the primary tuberculous complex in children who had ingested cow's milk containing bovine tubercle bacilli. As elsewhere, the site of entrance of the organisms is inconspicuous, although this probably means that the lesion has been minute and has not spread, rather than that the bacilli have invaded without producing any lesion. The prominent change is produced in the mesenteric lymph nodes, which become greatly enlarged and caseous (tabes mesenterica). In favourable circumstances, the condition remains localised, and the calcified mesenteric nodes still quite often observed in the elderly represent the result of intestinal infection in early life. Occasionally, however, the disease spreads from the nodes to the peritoneal cavity leading to tuberculous peritonitis (p. 657).

(b) Secondary infection. Intestinal lesions used to be a common complication of open pulmonary tuberculosis, especially in children. This secondary form of intestinal tuberculosis, caused by swallowing sputum containing tubercle bacilli, causes ulcers of the intestine, but with only slight involvement of the mesenteric lymph nodes.

The small intestine is the common site of the lesions, which usually occur in the Peyer's patches or solitary lymphoid follicles. Initially, caseating tubercles develop in the mucosa and the submucosa, and subsequent mucosal breakdown leads to the formation of small ulcers, which become progressively enlarged by direct spread of the organisms to adjacent parts of the mucosa. Ultimately large ulcers are produced and these tend to extend by spread of infection along the lymphatics, transversely to the longitudinal axis of the bowel; sometimes indeed they encircle the gut (Fig. 19.59). The larger ulcers have an irregular outline, undermined edges and raised nodular margins (Fig. 19.60). The floor is uneven or granular and may be coated by caseous material, but tubercles are

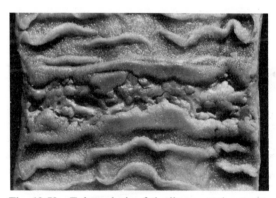

Fig. 19.59 Tuberculosis of the ileum causing transverse ulceration.

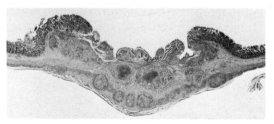

Fig. 19.60 Small tuberculous ulcer of small intestine with thickened and irregular margins and floor. Note the tubercles beneath the serosal surface: these are often visible at laporotomy. ×6.

rarely visible. The serous coat overlying the ulcer is often thickened and opaque and the presence of visible tubercles along the lines of serosal lymphatics may be of diagnostic value. Histologically, the tuberculous lesions are similar to those observed elsewhere: the ulceration extends through the mucosa into the submucous layer and there may be varying degrees of fibrous replacement of the muscular coat. Tubercles are usually found throughout the entire thickness of the bowel and in the related mesenteric lymph nodes, although the nodes are seldom as grossly affected as in the primary form.

Tuberculous ulceration rarely causes gross haemorrhage, and perforation into the peritoneal cavity is uncommon. The formation of fistulae between adjacent loops of bowel, initiated by the development of adhesions, may, however, lead to short-circuiting of bowel contents and malabsorption: the effects thus contrast with those of typhoid ulceration. The peritoneum may show frank tuberculous lesions (p. 657) or simply multiple fibrous adhesions which may cause mechanical obstruction of the bowel.

(c) 'Hyperplastic caecal tuberculosis'. This is usually secondary to pulmonary tuberculosis and is now rare in Europe and North America. It consists of gross fibrous thickening of the wall of a length of the caecum or ascending colon with ulceration of the surface and caseating tubercle follicles. Because it causes obstruction and is sometimes palpable, the lesion may be clinically suggestive of carcinoma. Pathologically, it may be confused with Crohn's disease affecting the caecum, and demonstration of tubercle bacilli by microscopy, culture or animal inoculation is important in order to make the differential diagnosis between the two conditions.

The **appendix** is occasionally affected in cases of intestinal tuberculosis. The changes are similar to those in the intestine and in some cases a faecal fistula develops following appendicectomy. More often, however, this sequence is attributable to Crohn's disease.

The dysenteries

The term dysentery was originally used to denote conditions of severe inflammation and ulceration of the colon, with diarrhoea, tenesmus and the passage of blood and mucus in the stools. Two main types of dysentery are distinguished, namely, *bacillary* and *amoebic*.

Bacillary dysentery

Bacillary dysentery is produced by bacilli of the *Shigella* species, of which there are several varieties, distinguishable by their serological and fermentative reactions. The mildest type is usually caused by *Shigella sonnei*, and in children is often called ileocolitis; more severe infections are caused by *Sh. flexneri*, and the most severe tropical form by *Sh. dysenteriae* (*Sh. shigae*), which produces a powerful exotoxin. The lesion is essentially inflammation of variable intensity in the colon, though the lower end of the ileum is sometimes also affected.

In mild cases the main features are intense mucosal inflammation with oedema, haemorrhage and excess mucus secretion. There may be some fibrinous exudation on the mucosal surface, but this is much more marked in severe cases in which there is extensive pseudomembrane formation with mucosal necrosis, and subsequent ulceration. The ulcers extend in an irregular manner and tend to have shredded margins. It is usual for healing to take place after the acute phase and the re-epithelialised ulcers assume a smooth and even appearance in contrast to the surrounding mucosa. The disease may, however, be prolonged and relapses are quite frequent. Such subacute or chronic cases are characterised by repeated ulceration and healing and can lead to polypoid mucosal irregularity with fibrous scarring and subsequent stenosis of the bowel. Bacillary dysentery may also be complicated by pyogenic bacterial infection of the portal venous system and focal suppuration in the liver.

Microscopically, the colonic mucosa shows intense inflammatory reaction in the lamina propria and polymorphs can be seen surrounding the mucosal crypts and invading the epithelial surfaces. The appearances resemble early ulcerative colitis (p. 622). The presence of numerous polymorphs admixed with red cells and mucus in the faeces is of presumptive diagnostic value.

Amoebic dysentery

This is caused by *Entamoeba histolytica*. The disease is only rarely acquired in temperate climates, but is common in tropical and sub-tropical countries, a fact not easily explained since entamoeba cysts are found in the faeces of a small proportion of people in this country who have not been abroad.

Naked-eye appearance. The organisms, swallowed in the cystic stage in food or water, are freed in the gut by digestion of the cyst wall, and enter the wall of the large intestine through the mucosa to settle in the submucous tissue where they produce tissue necrosis. Accordingly, the first lesion visible to the naked eye is the formation of swollen congested patches in the mucosa, the central parts of which become soft and somewhat yellowish as necrosis occurs (Fig. 19.61). The mucosa then gives way and an

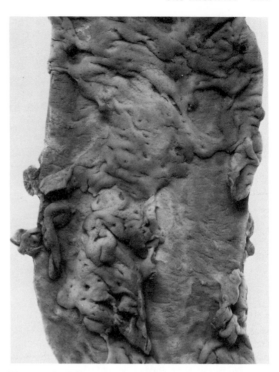

Fig. 19.62 The colon in chronic amoebic dysentery, showing irregular smooth areas where the mucosa has been destroyed.

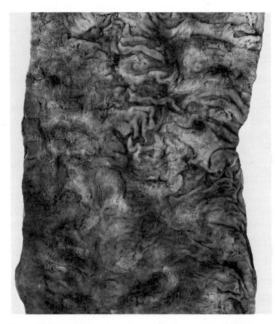

Fig. 19.61 The colon in early amoebic dysentery, showing irregular swelling of the mucosa, but, as yet, no obvious ulceration.

ulcer is formed with shreddy and undermined margins. Such ulcers, as they spread, become confluent first in their deeper parts, so that a probe may be passed under the mucosa from one to the other; the bridges then give way and the ulcerated areas are greatly increased. Accordingly a considerable part of the bowel may have lost its mucosa, while in the intervening parts fragments of mucosa in process of disintegration and separation are present (Fig. 19.62).

Microscopically the most prominent changes are found in the submucosa which shows intense inflammatory oedema but with remarkably little leukocytic infiltration. Subsequent necrosis takes place in the tissues around the entamoebae and may become extensive. The mucosa overlying the submucosal lesions initially shows non-specific inflammation. Later, however, ulceration develops and amoebae can be readily detected in ulcer bases (Fig. 19.63) and in mucosal exudate. Occasionally in chronic cases tumour-like masses of granulation tissue may form in relationship to mucosal ulceration ('amoeboma'). The mucosa overlying submucous lesions commonly becomes secondarily infected and shows changes similar to those of ulcerative colitis (p. 622). In suspected cases of the latter disease, it is thus most important to examine the stools for the presence of amoebae (see below).

Results and complications. When the acute stage of amoebic dysentery has passed off, attempts at healing may occur. The necrotic

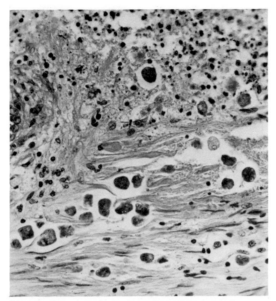

Fig. 19.63 Section through the base of an amoebic ulcer of the colon. The upper part of the field (nearest to the lumen) consists of necrotic tissue and exudate; below this, amoebae are seen in the submucosa where they have digested the surrounding tissue but have induced remarkably little cellular reaction. × 200.

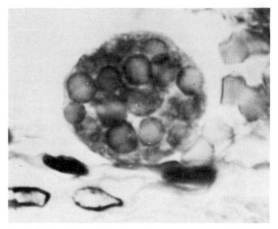

Fig. 19.64 Amoebic dysentery: an entamoeba containing red cells is seen in a venule in the base of an ulcer of the colon. × 1100.

tissue is thrown off and the epithelium grows over the denuded areas. But the process is often interrupted, and just as in bacillary dysentery, the disease may become protracted and pass into a chronic condition. Overgrowth of fibrous tissue is apt to occur in the deeper coats with resulting strictures. Enterostomy or faecal fistula in the presence of active amoebic infection may be followed by spread of amoebae into the skin, where they produce a severe necrotising ulceration. The passage of entamoebae to the liver in the portal blood (Fig. 19.64) gives rise to amoebic hepatitis and in some cases a tropical abscess develops in the liver (p. 696) or occasionally in the brain where it is often fatal.

Diagnosis. *In the acute phase* the stools contain blood and mucus but, in contrast with bacillary dysentery, pus is absent. The mucus is thus clear and in it vegetative amoebae showing active movements are readily found on microscopic examination of a fresh preparation, examined without delay on a warm stage; the ingestion of red cells by the amoebae is diagnostic. *In the chronic phase*, vegetative forms are absent from the faeces, and the diagnosis depends on the detection of cysts.

Antibiotic-associated pseudomembranous colitis

It is becoming increasingly recognised that various antibiotics, especially those of the clindamycin–lincomycin group and ampicillin, may be complicated by diarrhoea, and in many cases pathological changes can be found in the colon and occasionally also the distal ileum. In severe cases, which may be complicated by circulatory collapse and may be fatal, this takes the form of *pseudomembranous colitis*, characterised macroscopically by the appearance of raised yellowish-white plaques on the colonic mucosa (Fig. 19.65), which otherwise appears normal or at most slightly congested.

Histologically this disease process is initiated by focal damage to the intestinal epithelium with underlying acute inflammation. Subsequently a prominent adherent exudate or 'pseudomembrane', consisting of strands of fibrin and mucus with enmeshed neutrophils, arises from these foci of damage (Fig. 19.66). In severe cases the underlying mucosa shows progressive necrosis and crypt dilatation.

Recent studies have shown that pseudomembranous colitis of this kind is due to the action of exotoxin produced by *Clostridium difficile* under the promoting influence of antibiotics (p. 176). It now seems unlikely that similar pathological changes are caused by staphylococcal superinfection, although staphylococci can pro-

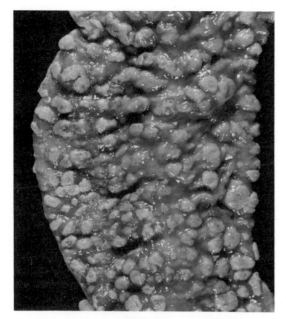

Fig. 19.65 Pseudomembranous colitis, showing the typical discrete raised patches of pseudomembrane and normal intervening mucosa. × 0·7.

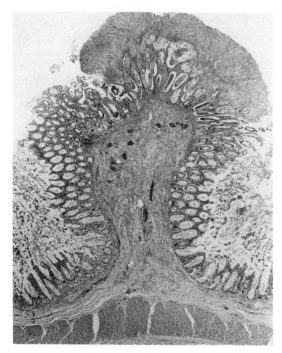

Fig. 19.66 Pseudomembranous colitis, showing one of the lesions. The mucosal glands are dilated and undergoing necrosis beneath the pseudomembrane. The thrombosis of submucosal blood vessels is a late event. × 12.

duce more widespread severe inflammatory changes in the intestinal mucosa.

Pseudomembrane formation may also be seen in association with other intestinal disturbances such as ischaemic disease (p. 619) and bacillary dysentery (p. 634).

Actinomycosis

As a path of entry for the branching, colony-forming Gram + ve bacterium *Actinomyces israelii*, the intestine comes next to the mouth in order of frequency. The lesions consist of suppuration and ulceration (p. 221) of the wall of the gut, with a tendency to spread to involve the peritoneum or adjacent loops of gut, abdominal wall, etc. with formation of sinuses and fistulas. The wall of the appendix seems to be the most common portal of entry; acute appendicitis may result and appendicectomy is liable to be followed by local recurrence and formation of fistulas. In some cases, the infection spreads beyond the appendix, usually to the wall of the caecum, before causing localising symptoms. In the peritoneum, loculated abscesses between the coils of intestine may discharge into the bowel. Diagnosis can usually be made by finding colonies of *Actinomyces* on microscopic examination. Secondary actinomycotic abscesses may occur in the liver.

Intestinal schistosomiasis

This disease, which is common in various tropical and subtropical parts of Africa and other countries, is produced by the dioecious trematode, *Schistosoma mansoni*. The adult parasites lodge in the tributaries of the portal vein (Fig. 19.67), especially those in the colonic wall, and the females lay eggs in the surrounding tissues: many of these pass through the mucosa into the lumen of the gut with little reaction and are excreted, but some become arrested in the tissues and induce a granulomatous reaction (Fig. 19.68) with formation of lesions, particularly in the rectum, similar to those caused in the bladder by *Schistosoma haematobium* (p. 867). The eggs are oval, measuring about 140 μm in length, and have a small lateral spine near one end. The reaction is chronic inflammation, with macrophage granulomas around the ova and granulation tissue formation progressing to fibrosis in the mucous and submucous coats, resulting in nodular and polypoid projections of the mucosal surface (Fig. 19.69). Ulceration with haemorrhage occurs, and sometimes there is gross fibrous thickening of the wall.

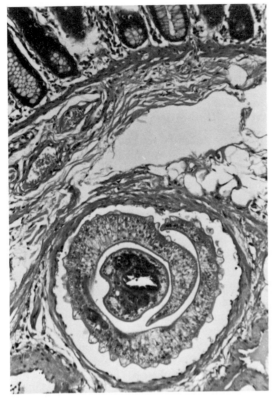

Fig. 19.67 Schistosomiasis. Wall of colon, showing *S. mansoni* adults in cross section. The female lies in connubial bliss in the gynaecophoric canal of the male. × 200.

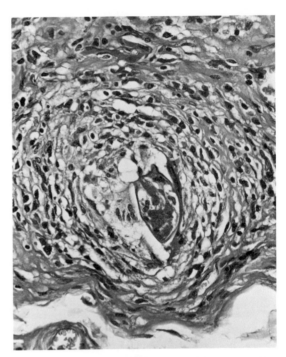

Fig. 19.68 Ovum of *S. mansoni* with surrounding granulomatous reaction in the wall of the colon. × 300.

Granulomatous lesions may be observed in other tissues, particularly the liver and lungs. In the liver, they develop in relation to the portal tracts and lead to a condition sometimes referred to as 'pipe-stem cirrhosis' (Fig. 20.47, p. 698); portal hypertension with splenomegaly arises from obstruction of the portal radicles. Unlike the urinary type, intestinal schistosomiasis does not appear to predispose to the development of carcinoma; even so, it is an all too frequent cause of chronic ill-health in the tropics. The adult parasites may live and continue to produce ova for over 20 years.

The life-cycle of the parasite is similar to that of *S. haematobium* (p. 867).

Schistosoma japonicum causes similar lesions in both the small and large intestines, and the liver is often extensively affected owing to the large number of ova produced by this species.

Other specific intestinal infections

(a) Yersinial disease. Bacteria of the genus *Yersinia*, especially *Y. enterocolitica* and *Y. pseudotuberculosis*,

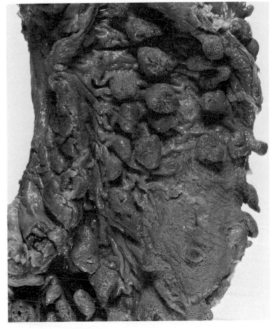

Fig. 19.69 Schistosomiasis of large intestine, showing multiple polypoid nodules projecting from mucosal surface.

are capable of producing a variety of acute inflammatory lesions in the alimentary tract. These organisms have a predilection for the gut-associated lymphoid tissue, and are responsible for some cases of acute ileitis, acute appendicitis (p. 628) and acute mesenteric adenitis, any of which may be associated with acute pharyngitis. Histologically the characteristic feature of these infections is the development of foci of suppuration within lymphoid aggregates and in the case of *Y. pseudotuberculosis* those lesions may be surrounded by a mantle of macrophages, resembling closely the lesion of lymphogranuloma inguinale (p. 569).

(b) Clostridial disease. It is well recognised that some self-limiting cases of *food poisoning* are due to the ingestion of food contaminated by *Cl. welchii*. In malnourished individuals, however, the ingestion of heavily contaminated food may produce a severe and often fatal form of *necrotising enteritis*. This has been observed, especially in children, in E. Africa and New Guinea, where it is known as 'pig-bel' since it follows the consumption of infected porcine offal at wedding feasts. The most dramatic form of clostridial disease is *botulism*, which is caused by the ingestion of improperly cooked food in which *Cl. botulinum* has been permitted to grow and produce a powerful exotoxin capable of producing muscular weakness and paralysis. Death commonly results from respiratory paralysis and aspiration pneumonia.

(c) Staphylococcal disease. Some of the most dramatic forms of *food poisoning* are due to the ingestion of food contaminated with staphylococcal enterotoxin, which is capable of producing acute gastroenteritis. Fortunately it is self-limiting. Staphylococcal *infection* may be implicated in some cases of antibiotic associated diarrhoea.

(d) Campylobacter infections. It has recently been shown that infections with the vibrio-like organisms of the Campylobacter genus are often responsible for infective diarrhoea. The inflammatory lesions are sometimes found in the small intestine but an acute colitis is a commoner finding.

(e) Lymphogranuloma inguinale. This is the least rare cause of an inflammatory stricture of the rectum, particularly in women, in whom the infection tends to spread by the lymphatics from the genitalia to the rectum and peri-rectal tissues (p. 569).

As elsewhere, the rectal lesion is a chronic inflammation with necrosis and suppuration. Ulceration may extend round the whole circumference and scarring then results in stricture. The lesion may also result in recto-vaginal fistula, or discharge on to the perineum.

Mucosal inflammation and ulceration may also occur in the rectum in syphilitic and gonococcal infections.

The malabsorption syndrome

The products of digestion of food are absorbed almost exclusively from the small intestine, and accordingly most extensive pathological processes in the small intestine interfere with this important function to some degree. The absorption of some nutrients may be restricted to certain relatively well-defined parts of the small bowel; iron, for example, is absorbed mainly from the duodenum and vitamin B_{12} from the distal ileum. Depending thus upon the extent, site and nature of the disease process, the absorption of some constituents of the diet may be affected more than others. In severe cases, all nutrients including protein, fat, carbohydrates, vitamins, minerals and even water may fail to be adequately absorbed. Failure to absorb fat is the most prominent feature in most cases and on it depend some of the other deficiencies.

Clinical features. The clinical manifestations of malabsorption vary accordingly. The most common symptom is chronic diarrhoea; the stools are pale, bulky and foul-smelling and contain an excess of fat (**steatorrhoea**) and of nitrogenous material. In severe cases, loss of weight, muscle wasting, dehydration and hypotension are prominent features. Hypoglycaemia with a low glucose tolerance curve (p. 1031) indicates failure of carbohydrate uptake. Hypoproteinaemia, associated with oedema, may be the result not only of impaired amino-acid absorption, but also of protein leakage into the bowel lumen (**protein-losing enteropathy**)—a feature of many gastro-intestinal diseases. Vitamin deficiences are common, and symptoms of beri-beri, pellagra, scurvy and rickets in children, may be presenting features of the syndrome. Anaemia frequently dominates the clinical picture; usually it is microcytic and attributed to iron deficiency but macrocytic anaemia following failure to absorb vitamin B_{12} or folic acid is by no means unusual. It is rare for all of those features to be noted together, and any one deficiency may predominate; biochemical tests, however, usually reveal more extensive malabsorption than is clinically evident.

Peroral intestinal biopsy. This technique, now widely used, is of great help in the diagnosis and investigation of malabsorptive disturbances. Biopsy makes it possible to assess not only the morphological state of the mucosa but also the enzyme content of the absorptive epithelium and the bacterial content of the intestinal lumen.

Under the dissecting microscope, the normal jejunal mucosa has tall, slender finger-shaped villi interspersed with occasional broader leaf-shaped villi, which are more conspicuous in the duodenum. The villi measure about 400 μm in height and usually account for about 70 per cent of the total mucosal thickness. In tropical residents, however, the villi are more often leaf-shaped and may even fuse to form short ridges. Histologically, moreover, they appear shorter and broader than their temperate counterparts. The cause of this geographical variation in jejunal morphology is not known.

The absorptive epithelial cells lining the villi are formed in the crypts of Lieberkühn and gradually ascend the villi before being extruded into the lumen after a life-span of about 3 days. These cells are the principal source of the digestive enzymes of the succus entericus, and the final stage in the digestion of many nutrients takes place in the vicinity of the innumerable microvilli which form the epithelial surface. Malabsorptive disturbance may be caused by deficiency of intestinal enzymes, especially the disaccharidases.

Villous atrophy (Fig. 19.70) is the commonest pathological change in mucosal pattern. In the *partial* form (PVA) the villi show extensive fusion with the formation of long ridges or convolutions; histologically they appear shorter and broader than normal, although the crypts are enlarged and hyperplastic. The villous epithelium often shows degenerative change, and there is little doubt that the fundamental disturbance is a shortening of the life-span of these cells with compensatory hyperplasia of the generative crypt cells. There is often increased cellular infiltration in the lamina propria mucosae, plasma cells being most conspicuous. In the more severe *subtotal* form (SVA) villous

fusion is more advanced and the mucosa appears completely flat both under the dissecting microscope and histologically. Epithelial degenerative changes are also more prominent.

Villous atrophy is not a specific change. It is however, characteristic of the two major primary malabsorption disorders, namely *tropical sprue* and *coeliac disease*, the latter being by far the commonest cause of severe villous atrophy in this country. Less often it is found following gastro-enteritis in childhood. Some degree of villous atrophy is also commonly associated with some forms of hypogamma-globulinaemia, although this has been attributed to complicating giardiasis. In the tropics, kwashiorkor is a recognised cause of villous atrophy. Minor villous changes have also been described in many other diseases, although the association is inconstant and of dubious significance.

In malabsorptive states, intestinal biopsy may reveal other important pathological changes. The lesions of Whipple's disease (see below) and amyloidosis (p. 272) are unmistakable and congenital agammaglobulinaemia can be recognised by absence of plasma cells in the lamina propria. In the rare intestinal lymphangiectasia, there is diffuse dilatation of mucosal lymphatics which is associated with malabsorption of fat, lymphopenia and protein-losing enteropathy (p. 639). Congenital absence of β-lipoprotein produces a complex syndrome in which there is a curious spiny abnormality of red cells (acanthocytosis), cerebellar dysfunction, retinal abnormality and fat malabsorption. Distension of villous epithelial cells by neutral fat, in an otherwise normal intestinal biopsy, is the diagnostic feature. It is unusual for Crohn's disease or tumour to be detected by biopsy techniques, although the rare, so-called Mediterranean type of intestinal lymphoma produces a typical appearance (p. 552). Intestinal parasites capable of causing malabsorption, e.g. *Giardia lamblia*, can be detected by intestinal biopsy and also in the stools.

Primary malabsorptive disorders

This group includes *coeliac disease* (idiopathic steatorrhoea or gluten enteropathy), *tropical sprue* and the rare *Whipple's disease*.

Coeliac disease. This term is used to describe one of the most important causes of intestinal malabsorption in this country and includes both the childhood form of the disease and the adult condition formerly called idiopathic steatorrhoea. In this disease, malabsorption is characteristically associated with severe diffuse abnormalities of the intestinal mucosa, and *withdrawal of the wheat protein gluten from the*

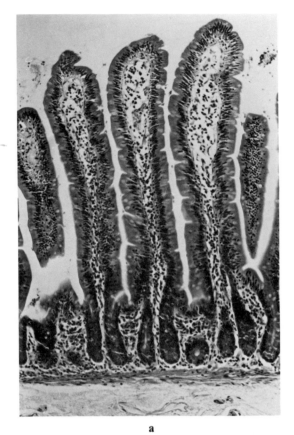

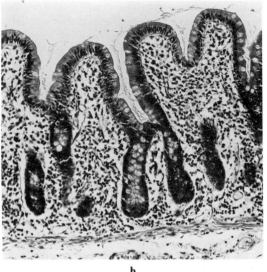

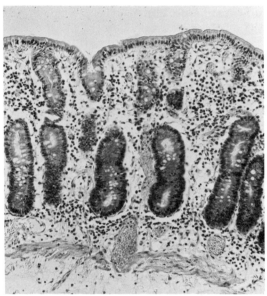

Fig. 19.70 Villous atrophy of jejunum: **a** normal jejunal mucosa; **b** partial villous atrophy; **c** subtotal villous atrophy. × 150. (Material obtained by peroral biopsy.)

diet brings about both clinical and morphological remission. The mucosal abnormality takes the form of villous atrophy (see above) which is most marked and usually subtotal in the proximal jejunum, and becomes progressively less severe, i.e. partial, more distally. There is an associated heavy infiltration of the lamina propria with plasma cells and a marked increase in the number of lymphocytes between the surface epithelial cells. In some cases, especially those

with a poor response to therapy, there is collagen deposition beneath the epithelial surface, but American workers regard this as a disease entity ('collagenous sprue') distinct from coeliac disease. Withdrawal of dietary gluten leads to a reversal of the mucosal changes, initially in the distal small bowel and later in the upper jejunum which, particularly in adults, may never revert entirely to normal. It seems clear that gluten is in some way responsible for the mucosal damage, but the mechanism involved is not known. Coeliac disease has a strong familial tendency and patients have a strikingly high incidence of histocompatibility antigens HLA-B8 and DW3. While an inherited enzyme defect cannot be discounted as a causative factor, it seems more likely that coeliac disease is caused by a genetically-determined abnormal immune response to gluten. Certainly the nature of the mucosal inflammatory reaction is consistent with this and antibodies and cell-mediated immunity to α-gliadin, a constituent of gluten, and antibody to reticulin fibres, are commonly detectable. There is also evidence of impaired immune responsiveness to various exogenous antigens and splenic atrophy is commonly observed in adult patients (p. 562).

In some cases there is an association with *dermatitis herpetiformis* (p. 1061). There is an increased incidence of neoplasia of the alimentary tract, especially malignant lymphoma of the small bowel, usually of macrophage (histiocytic) type. This may be preceded by episodes of ulceration ('ulcerative jejunitis').

Tropical sprue is a disease encountered in certain areas in the tropics and sub-tropics, Africa being an exception. There is malabsorption resulting in severe emaciation and chronic diarrhoea, and macrocytic anaemia from deficiency of B_{12}, folate or both. Villous atrophy, usually partial and less often subtotal, is the characteristic change found at jejunal biopsy. This lesion, and the malabsorptive disturbance, are relieved by removal of the patient from the tropical environment and by oral broad-spectrum antibiotics, but a gluten-free diet has little or no beneficial effect. Folic acid may also cause some improvement. The cause of the disease remains uncertain, but abnormal bacterial colonisation of the upper small bowel is probably involved.

Whipple's disease. This rare and interesting disease affects mostly adult males in middle age. Malabsorption is usually the presenting feature, although other signs and symptoms such as generalised lymphadenopathy, arthropathy, skin pigmentation and chronic cough may be encountered. Jejunal biopsy is diagnostic: the mucosal lamina propria is stuffed with large granular macrophages containing glycoprotein which stains strongly with the periodic acid-Schiff technique for mucopolysaccharides (Fig. 19.71). The regional lymph nodes, and occasionally other tissues, e.g. brain and heart valves, contain

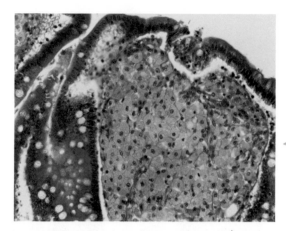

Fig. 19.71 Whipple's disease of small intestine, showing infiltration of the mucosa with granular macrophages. × 230.

similar cells. Neutral fat accumulates in lymphatic channels. Electron microscopy has demonstrated that the abnormal glycoprotein within macrophages consists of unidentified bacteria and bacterial debris. Moreover, the disease responds to oral antibiotics. It would, however, be premature to assert that Whipple's disease is a form of specific infection, especially in view of the age and sex incidence.

Secondary malabsorption

Many disease processes can interfere with absorption. Most of these are discussed elsewhere, and only a brief account will be given here. Classification is most rationally based upon the mechanism thought to be mainly involved in causing malabsorption, although it should be appreciated that more than one mechanism may be operating in any individual disease.

(a) **Chronic intestinal disease** may cause malabsorption if extensive areas of the mucosa are affected. Examples include Crohn's disease, tuberculosis, tumours (especially malignant lymphoma), amyloidosis, radiation injury and connective tissue disorders such as systemic sclerosis.

(b) **Abnormal bacterial proliferation** in the small bowel interferes not only with the absorption of vitamin B_{12} but also to some extent with fat absorption. It results from stasis in the intestinal lumen, especially that produced by short-circuit operations which leave stagnant loops of bowel (**the blind-loop syndrome**). Stasis occurs also in jejunal diverticulosis (p.

629), in chronic intestinal obstruction, and in the blind loop resulting from some techniques of partial gastrectomy; malabsorption may complicate these conditions.

(c) Other mechanisms which may cause malabsorption include *biochemical defects* such as disaccharidase deficiency, agammaglobulinaemia and abetalipoproteinaemia; *endocrine disturbances*, including the carcinoid syndrome (p. 649) and the Zollinger–Ellison syndrome (p. 1034); *lymphatic obstruction*, congenital or acquired, e.g. as a result of tuberculosis or tumour; *circulatory disturbances*, especially mesenteric

vascular insufficiency; and *drug therapy*, e.g. phenindione, neomycin.

(d) Inadequate digestion must always be considered as a cause of malabsorption and may be due to disease of the liver and biliary tract or to exocrine pancreatic insufficiency. Malabsorption following gastro-jejunostomy, alone or with partial gastrectomy, is largely a consequence of disordered digestion. There is inadequate mixing of food with pancreatic enzymes and bile as a result of interference with the normal anatomical relationships.

Intestinal Obstruction (Ileus)

Passage of intestinal contents is dependent on the patency, viability and normal contractions of the gut. Accordingly, 'obstruction' may result from *mechanical compression or occlusion* of the intestine, from *ischaemia*, and from *neurological disturbances* interfering with contractility. The effects of obstruction depend on whether it is sudden or gradual, complete or partial, and on its level in the gut.

The following are the chief **mechanical causes** of intestinal obstruction:

(*a*) *Constriction from outside*—for example, by a hernial sac, by special conditions such as volvulus or intussusception, or by fibrous peritoneal adhesions. This is the commonest cause of acute mechanical obstruction.

(*b*) *Stenosis caused by thickening and contraction of the wall* is produced by diverticular disease, ischaemic stricture, Crohn's disease, tuberculosis and, of course, primary or secondary malignant tumours, most commonly carcinoma of the colon. The obstruction from these causes is usually incomplete and chronic, but complete obstruction may supervene by impaction of inspissated faecal masses in the narrowed portion of bowel.

(*c*) *Actual obstruction of the lumen.* This may result from impaction of a large gallstone or other foreign body or by the growth of a tumour into the lumen, usually malignant but sometimes a benign polyp.

(*d*) *Pressure from outside*, for example by a large tumour in the pelvis; obstruction is not often complete from such a cause.

The nervous type of obstruction is called *paralytic or adynamic ileus* and may occur after handling of the intestines at operation, or it may result from peritonitis. The principal **vascular lesion producing obstruction** is occlusion of the mesenteric vessels by embolism or thrombosis. In the type of mechanical obstruction seen in group (*a*) above, vascular obstruction is commonly superadded and the subsequent course is then modified. When the blood supply is intact the obstruction is said to be **simple**, when it is seriously impaired the term **strangulation** is applied.

A length of strangulated gut rapidly becomes haemorrhagic and necrotic. Bacteria proliferate in its bloodstained contents and invade the necrotic wall, producing **gangrene**. Toxaemia is very severe and may be fatal before the distended gangrenous loop ruptures.

The results of intestinal obstruction

The site of the obstruction is important in determining both the effects and the prognosis. High intestinal obstruction is in general more acute in onset, more rapid in its progress and more likely to be complete than low intestinal obstruction which is usually of slow onset, is often incomplete and is less rapidly fatal.

Acute obstruction. When a portion of the small intestine is suddenly obstructed, e.g. by passing under a fibrous peritoneal band, the part above contracts actively for a time and then passes into a condition of paralytic distension. There are probably both increased secretion from the wall and diminished absorption, and thus the bowel becomes distended with fluid in which there is abundant growth of bacteria. The fluid is passed back to the stomach by antiperistalsis and is vomited. Its exact composition depends on the site of the obstruction, but since nearly 8 litres of fluid are secreted into the gut daily, of which all but 100 ml are normally reabsorbed, the volume of fluid available for loss by vomiting or by pooling in the gut is obviously considerable.

If the obstruction is at the **pylorus** or **duodenum** the fluid lost is predominantly acid in reaction with a high Cl⁻ content. This results in a depletion of plasma chloride, and the urinary excretion of chlorides is then diminished or absent. Since sodium, the ion which normally balances the Cl⁻ ion, is not lost, carbonic acid is retained to take the place of the lost chloride and the plasma bicarbonate content therefore rises. This state of *alkalosis* is shown clinically by drowsiness and slow shallow respiration and can be demonstrated on analysis by a rise in the CO_2 combining power. A further complication is the development of *tetany* due to a fall in the ionised serum calcium, as a result of the alkalosis. Extracellular potassium deficiency may be superadded—*hypokalaemic alkalosis*. If the fluid loss is great enough, oliguria and *extrarenal uraemia* may follow, the blood urea being markedly raised terminally.

Obstruction in the *jejunum* results in the loss by vomiting of a fluid which contains saliva, gastric juice, bile, pancreatic juice and succus entericus. This leads to depletion of Na⁺, K⁺, and Cl⁻. The CO_2 combining power remains normal, without marked disturbance of the acid-base balance. Although in high obstruction there is a tendency towards acidosis, it is the loss of fluid and electrolytes that leads rapidly to a fall in blood volume, dehydration, haemoconcentration and finally death. Fluid and electrolyte replacement is therefore essential to prolong life until surgical intervention can be undertaken.

Chronic obstruction. In low intestinal obstruction the absorptive area of the gut proximally is extensive, and depletion of water and electrolytes is often delayed. Ultimately, however, dehydration due to vomiting does take place and the vomitus becomes brown and foul-smelling—the so-called faecal or stercoral

vomit. The dominant and dangerous factor in this form of obstruction is distension of the gut with fluid and with gas mainly derived from swallowed air. Prolonged increase of intraluminal pressure impairs the viability of the bowel wall, with subsequent diffusion of toxic bacterial products into the peritoneal cavity where they are absorbed and produce toxaemia and death. Relief of distension by intubation is thus critically important and sustains life until surgical intervention can be undertaken. The fluid lost by intubation is predominantly alkaline and this leads to acidosis and a low CO_2 combining power. Parenteral infusion of normal saline should thus be supplemented by lactate or carbonate. A further complicating factor is potassium depletion which leads to weakness and muscular paresis and may superimpose a state of adynamic ileus on the existing obstructive lesion (see below). In this context it must be appreciated that potassium is an intracellular ion and the plasma level does not reflect accurately the state of the cells. Caution must therefore be exercised in interpreting the biochemical analysis of the plasma as a basis for potassium replacement. In partial chronic obstruction, prolonged intermittent gut distension leads to hypertrophy of the bowel muscle proximal to the obstructive lesion. Also the pressure of faecal accumulation impairs mucosal viability and predisposes to bacterial invasion which leads to the formation of a mucosal exudate and ultimately to mucosal breakdown and ulceration. This so-called *stercoral ulceration* can take place some distance proximal to the obstruction and sometimes leads to perforation and faecal peritonitis. The effects of chronic stricture, especially in the colon, are aggravated if the regurgitation of faecal material proximally is prevented, for example by an all too competent ileo-caecal valve (closed loop obstruction). In this situation stercoral ulceration is likely to occur in the caecum even when the stricture is in the distal colon, and the caecum may rupture.

Vascular causes of obstruction

Apart from strangulation these are chiefly embolism of thrombosis of the superior mesenteric artery, but thrombosis of the mesenteric veins will produce the same result. This is sometimes seen when a thrombus occluding the portal vein extends backwards to obstruct the mouths of the splenic and superior mesenteric veins.

Haemorrhagic infarction with gangrene of a segment of bowel quickly supervenes (Fig. 19.72), and death follows from toxic absorption and peritonitis.

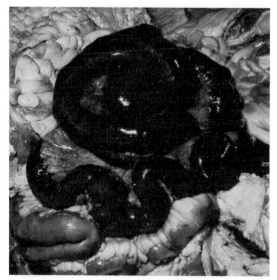

Fig. 19.72 Haemorrhagic infarction of the small intestine due to thrombosis of the superior mesenteric artery. The infarcted bowel is black and would soon have become gangrenous.

Neural causes of obstruction

Paralytic ileus. In this condition the motor activity of the bowel is impaired without the presence of a physical obstruction. Sometimes it is due to over-activity of the sympathetic nervous system, and may then be relieved by antagonistic drugs, but in other cases toxic damage to the bowel muscle causes the paralysis. Lowering of the potassium level of the plasma greatly aggravates the condition. It is seen most often in association with peritonitis or it may follow operations on the abdomen, frequently of a minor nature. It may result also from intestinal infections or severe toxaemia. The whole intestine may be affected and may become greatly distended. The condition is serious and if untreated will result in death in much the same way as in acute mechanical obstruction. Following intubation and drainage of the distended bowel, its contractility may return, particularly if electrolyte and fluid balance can be restored.

Hirschsprung's disease. This is a rare congenital condition characterised by an enormous accumulation of faeces in the greatly enlarged colon which comes to occupy much of the swollen abdomen. There may be periods of weeks or months without defaecation, and repeated attacks of obstruction. The distension may extend as far as the caecum, but at first affects mainly the lower colon. The grossly hypertrophied and dilated colon tapers rather abruptly into a narrow rectal segment joining sigmoid to anus. There is congenital absence of the para-sympathetic ganglion cells of both Auerbach's and Meissner's plexuses for a distance of 5–20 cm below the dilated sigmoid, i.e. corresponding to the narrow segment of rectum. In consequence there is overaction of the sympathetic, which normally inhibits the propulsive contraction of the intestinal wall and stimulates contraction of the internal anal sphincter. The disease is thus one of neuromuscular incoordination. While lumbar sympathectomy has proved helpful in some cases, the results have not always been permanent and excision of the defective narrow segment and anastomosis of the sigmoid to the anus has proved more effective.

Hernia

This term is applied to any protrusion of a portion of viscus outside its natural cavity. Protrusion of the bowel usually occurs in a pouch of the peritoneum, which projects on the surface of the body, forming an **external hernia**. The term **internal hernia** is applied when the swelling does not present to an external surface. Two major factors are involved in the formation of a hernia—local weakness and increased pressure. *Local weakness* is usually congenital, notably at the umbilicus or the inguinal canal; occasionally it results from the stretching of the scar of an operation wound— **incisional hernia**. *Increased intra-abdominal pressure* is usually caused by muscular exertion, coughing and straining at stool.

External hernias. The commonest are the *inguinal, femoral* and *umbilical hernias*. Those arising at other sites in the abdominal wall are termed *ventral hernias. Inguinal hernias* are of two types, *indirect*, where the hernia follows the inguinal canal lateral to the inferior epigastric artery, and *direct*, which passes medial to the artery and projects through the external abdominal ring. The femoral hernia passes under Poupart's ligament medial to the femoral vessels. Examples of **internal hernia** are seen when the protrusion occurs through an aperture in the diaphragm, through the foramen of Winslow, or into a pouch in the jejuno-duodenal fossa, the pouch then passing behind the peritoneum. The common external hernias usually contain a loop of small intestine, though in the larger ones omentum or other structures may also be present. So long as it is possible to return the contents into the abdominal cavity, the hernia is termed **reducible**. When this is impossible owing either to the bulk of the contents or to adhesions which have formed within the hernial sac, the hernia is termed **impacted**.

The most serious result of hernia is strangulation, i.e. obstruction of the blood flow through the herniated gut. This may occur by the addition of a fresh loop of bowel to the sac or by accumulation of faeces and gas. Strangulation may develop when the hernia is first formed, a portion of bowel being forced into a tight aperture; this is not uncommon in a femoral hernia. The changes following strangulation have already been described (p. 643).

Intussusception

In this condition a length of intestine is invaginated into the portion below. This usually has serious consequences and presents clinically as an acute surgical emergency. An exception to this is the multiple form observed quite often at necropsy, particularly in children dying from various causes, and presumably due to irregular bowel contraction around the time of death (agonal intussusception). The clinically important forms are also most often observed in infancy and early childhood. This is probably because the intestinal lymphoid tissue, especially in the distal ileum, is prone to undergo swelling in childhood, and because it protrudes into the intestinal lumen, is propelled distally by peristaltic activity, drawing the adjacent bowel with it. Viruses of the echo or adenovirus groups may be responsible for the lymphoid swelling and have been isolated from the intestinal contents and mesenteric lymph nodes in children with intussusception. An inverted Meckel's diverticulum projecting into the intestinal lumen also predisposes to intussusception, and in adults polypoid intestinal tumours are the usual cause.

Naked-eye appearances. In intussusception of the ordinary type three layers of bowel are seen on section, two layers formed by the doubling of the invaginated length of bowel, and one layer consisting of the wall of the bowel into which the invagination has occurred. Thus it consists of an entering tube, a returning tube and an ensheathing tube (Fig. 19.73). The commonest site is at the ileocaecal valve, and usually the valve forms the apex of the intussusception and is passed along the large intestine. The apex may ultimately reach the rectum, and the whole lesion forms a fairly firm sausage-shaped mass, which is palpable during life. This type of intussusception is called **ileocaecal**. More rarely the small intestine is passed through the ileocaecal valve into the colon—**ileocolic** type—and there may also be combinations of those two types with more complicated invaginations. For example, the ileocaecal valve may be passed along for only a short distance, so that the tip of the appendix may be

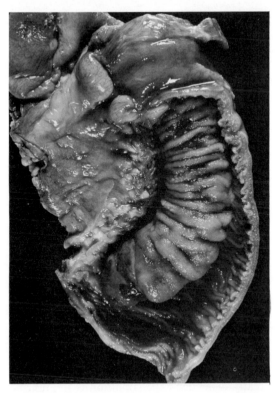

Fig. 19.73 Intussusception of the small intestine. The ensheathing section of gut has been cut open to show the invaginated loop, which is passing downward. The invaginated loop shows early haemorrhagic necrosis at the apex (near lower margin of excision) and near the entrance (at the top of the photograph).

still visible, and then coils of the small intestine may be passed down through the valve and firmly impacted. Intussusception also occurs in the small intestine or the transverse colon, but it is comparatively rare. Intussusception of the appendix has been recorded, but it is very rare; it occurs chiefly in children.

Results. The important effects of intussusception are interference with the blood supply and mechanical obstruction of the bowel. The vessels of the invaginated part are stretched and also compressed; venous obstruction, oedema and extensive haemorrhage result. Accordingly the passage per anum of a mixture of blood and mucus is a common sign of intussusception, but pure blood may be passed. Unless the intussusception can be reduced (i.e. reversed), the haemorrhagic, ischaemic bowel becomes infarcted and gangrenous, and in most cases death results from obstruction or general peritonitis unless early excision is performed. In some cases, however, the serosa of the invaginated bowel becomes glued by fibrinous exudate at its point of entry, to the serosa of the ensheathing bowel: general peritonitis is thus prevented and the gangrenous invaginated bowel may then slough off and be passed in fragments along the lower bowel. The fibrinous serosal adhesions organise. In this way, natural amputation and union may restore the continuity of the gut and effect cure.

Volvulus

In this condition a loop of bowel is twisted or rotated through 180° or more, so that the lumen is effectively obstructed at the point of twisting and the venous drainage is prejudiced. It occurs particularly in the sigmoid colon (Fig. 19.74), especially when this is heavily loaded with faeces and the mesocolon is unusually long. The twisted loop becomes increasingly distended with gas and fluid and blood flow is further impaired. The wall of the gut becomes congested, haemorrhagic and ultimately gangrenous. In some cases a portion of bowel is found to be enormously distended, filling a large part of the abdominal cavity. Volvulus of the small intestine may occur also, but it is less common; the favouring conditions are the same, and sometimes the approximation of the

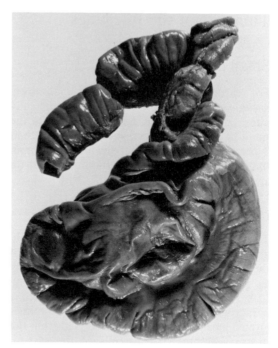

Fig. 19.74 Volvulus of sigmoid colon.

ends of the loop is due to local adhesions around calcified mesenteric lymph nodes. In children, however, volvulus of the small bowel is much commoner than in adults. More rarely two loops of intestine become intertwined and then the symptoms are very severe.

Intestinal obstruction by foreign bodies

The most common cause of this type of obstruction is a large composite gallstone, which has entered the duodenum through a fistulous track developing between gallbladder and bowel; commonly there is little or no history of symptoms to indicate choleithiasis. The calculus passes along the intestine but may become impacted, usually about a metre proximal to the ileocaecal valve. Even the largest stone is smaller than the diameter of the fully relaxed bowel, so muscle spasm must contribute to the impaction. Unmasticated food may act similarly, for example obstruction of the ileum by a mass of dried fruit. Gastro-enterostomy predisposes to the passage of large masses of undigested food into the intestine, and thus to obstruction.

Tumours of the Intestines

Small intestine

For reasons which are obscure, the small bowel has a surprisingly low incidence of clinically important tumours. Epithelial neoplasms of the small bowel, for example, account for less than 2 per cent of all intestinal (including colonic) tumours. Nevertheless the tumours that do arise form an interesting group.

Carcinoid tumour (argentaffinoma)

This arises from certain specialised cells, which, although located within the epithelial surface of the gastro-intestinal tract, are thought by many to be of neural crest origin. These cells belong to a widely distributed family of cells with a paracrine (local endocrine) function sometimes termed **apud cells**, an acronym derived from the property common to all cells of the system, namely, **a**mine-**p**recursor **u**ptake and **d**ecarboxylation (p. 1034). While tumours arising from these endocrine cells have been given the generic name **apudoma**, those occurring in the gut are more commonly called **carcinoid tumours**, since in the appendix (their commonest site of origin) they are clinically benign despite an appearance of infiltration resembling carcinoma. Both in the appendix and in the ileum, which is also a common primary site, carcinoid tumours arise from the most distinctive intestinal representative of the apud system, namely the *argentaffin cell*, so named because of its capacity to form cytoplasmic deposits of metallic silver from silver salts. This histologically demonstrable property is related to its secretion of 5-hydroxytryptamine (5HT). Carcinoids only rarely occur in the stomach and large intestine, and in these sites they may arise from a different member of the apud system, since the cells often fail to show the argentaffin reaction unless a reducing agent is added (argyrophilia). Carcinoid tumours are usually found by chance in or near the tip of appendixes removed surgically, often for acute appendicitis. Although sometimes only a few millimetres in diameter, they can occlude the distal lumen of the appendix and have a distinctive yellowish-brown colour.

In the small intestine, especially in the lower ileum, carcinoids are commonly multiple. They form small button-like swellings in the mucosa, one or more of which shows deep penetration of the muscular wall which may be locally hypertrophied (Fig. 19.75). Lymphatic invasion is often widespread in the affected segment. Ileal carcinoids are not benign like those in the appendix, and as a consequence both intestinal obstruction (Fig. 19.76) and metastases to the mesenteric lymph nodes and liver occur; characteristically these secondary deposits grow exceedingly slowly.

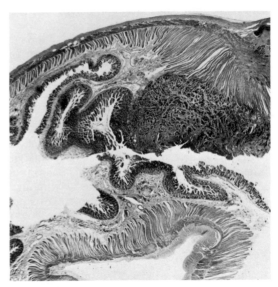

Fig. 19.75 Carcinoid tumour of ileum, seen as the darkly-stained tissue invading the circular muscle coat, which is greatly hypertrophied, and causing stenosis. There were hepatic metastases and the carcinoid syndrome developed. × 2·5.

Microscopically, carcinoid tumours consist of small clear cells, closely packed in alveolar formation (Fig. 19.77), throughout the whole thickness of the appendicular or ileal wall. The yellowish colour is due to lipids, some of which are doubly refracting. As stated above, the tumour cells contain granules which reduce silver salts—hence called argentaffin cells. In the appendix, carcinoid tumours are commonly related to old inflammatory lesions and the cells are often associated with proliferated nerve fibres.

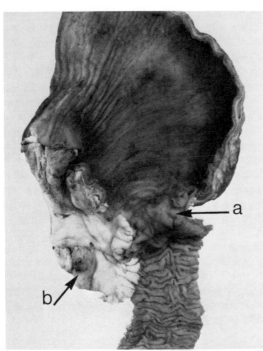

Fig. 19.76 Carcinoid tumour of ileum causing obstruction. Note the dilatation and hypertrophy of the bowel above the tumour **a** and secondary deposit in the mesenteric lymph node **b**.

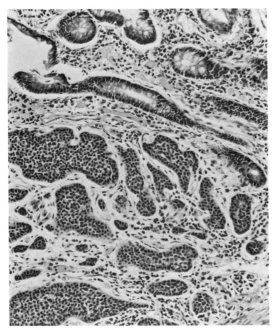

Fig. 19.77 Carcinoid tumour of ileum, showing clumps of small polygonal epithelial cells infiltrating the mucosa. × 125.

The carcinoid syndrome. Large hepatic secondary growths of carcinoid tumours are sometimes, but not invariably, accompanied by attacks of flushing of the face, diarrhoea and bronchospasm. There may also be pulmonary stenosis. These effects are due to the secretion of large amounts of 5HT and other compounds by metastatic tumour cells in the liver. 5HT is inactivated by amine oxidase in the liver cells, and so long as the tumour is confined to the drainage area of the portal circulation systemic effects are not produced. Hepatic metastases, however, set free 5HT into the systemic circulation. 5HT is a potent vasodilator, and smooth-muscle stimulant; it may also stimulate fibroblastic proliferation and so cause the subendocardial fibrosis in the right atrium and ventricle and the pulmonary stenosis which is a late feature of the syndrome. The left side of the heart is less often involved, since 5HT is inactivated also in the lungs. Excessive diversion of tryptophane to the metabolism of massive secondary deposits may induce symptoms of pellagra. 5HT is converted by the enzyme amine-oxidase to 5-hydroxyindoleacetic acid (5HIAA), which is excreted in the urine where its quantitative estimation affords a valuable clinical test for the presence of large argentaffin tumours. The flushing attacks are often precipitated by alcohol or sympathetic stimulation: they are not due to 5HT, but probably to kallikrein, which is also secreted by the tumour cells, and activates the kinin system (p. 55).

Carcinoids ('adenomas') of the bronchi (p. 500) secrete 5-hydroxytryptophane, possibly because they lack the enzyme decarboxylase required to convert this substance to 5HT. Carcinoids of the stomach may also secrete histamine in addition to 5HT and kallikrein. Colonic carcinoid tumours rarely give rise to the syndrome.

Other tumours of the small intestine

Connective tissue tumours. Members of this group, such as leiomyoma, lymphangioma and lipoma, are quite common but seldom cause symptoms unless they protrude into the intestinal lumen and produce intussusception. Occasionally a leiomyoma ulcerates and leads to intestinal blood loss and iron-deficiency anaemia. *Leiomyosarcoma*, the only malignant tumour of this group that is at all common, presents clinically like its benign variant but tends to recur after operation and sometimes metastasises to the liver. The behaviour of smooth muscle tumours of the gut often belies their histological appearances, and it is very difficult to classify them as benign or malignant.

The Peutz–Jeghers syndrome. This interesting hereditary disorder is transmitted as a Mendelian dominant of high penetrance. Multiple epithelial-lined highly differentiated polyps are found in the small intestine, especially the jejunum, and are associated with melanotic pigmented spots on the lips and oral mucosa, and sometimes on the fingers and toes. The polyps cause recurring attacks of intussusception and sometimes iron deficiency anaemia due to blood loss, but rarely undergo malignant transformation. Grossly, they may be sessile or pedunculated and resemble the neoplastic polyps of the large intestine, but the epithelium consists of a mixture of the several normal cell types found in the small intestine, and they have a branching muscular stroma derived from the muscularis mucosae. Because of these features they are regarded as hamartomas (p. 358) rather than true neoplasms. Single polyps of this type, without other features of the syndrome, also occur in the stomach and intestines (Morson, 1978).

Carcinoma. This is surprisingly uncommon in the small bowel, being rather less frequently encountered than lymphoid tumours. Length for length, the proximal parts of the small bowel are more often affected than the distal. In appearance and behaviour carcinomas of the small intestine are very similar to those of the colon (p. 652). Intestinal obstruction and the effects of haemorrhage are the most common modes of presentation, but diagnosis is not often made early enough to allow curative excision. The causal factors are unknown, although occasionally carcinoma arises as a complication of coeliac disease.

Lymphoid neoplasms. Although generalised forms of lymphoma may metastasise to the intestinal tract, it is important to realise that lymphomas may arise primarily in the small intestine, where they are at least as common as carcinomas. These primary intestinal lymphomas, which may be multiple, ulcerate deeply (Fig. 19.84) and may cause perforation. Less often they cause obstruction. Most of these tumours are of B–lymphocyte type: some

show plasma-cell differentiation, while others show signs of germinal centre derivation and may consist mainly of centrocytes (see p. 582). The tumours which complicate coeliac disease (p. 640) seem, however, to be of histiocytic (macrophage) origin (p. 585). When lymphoma is associated with malabsorption or villous atrophy, it is probable that there is underlying coeliac disease, but this is not always the case: in some instances, malabsorption arises as a complication of the lymphoma, as in the peculiar form of intestinal lymphoma described in young adults mainly of East Mediterranean origin. The entire mucosa of the small bowel is swollen by a diffuse pleomorphic infiltrate of plasma cells, lymphocytes, eosinophils and undifferentiated lymphoid cells. The neoplastic condition called α-*chain disease* is probably a variant of this 'Mediterranean lymphoma', the distinctive feature being that the tumour cells, which tend to be more differentiated, produce the heavy chain of IgA immunoglobulin (p. 552).

Large intestine

Although connective tissue tumours and lymphomas are rare in the large intestine, both benign and malignant epithelial tumours are all too common and constitute a major problem in terms of management and prevention.

Benign neoplastic polyps (adenomas)

These tumours are the commonest types of polyp of the colon and rectum. They present a spectrum of macroscopic and microscopic appearances, and are classified as *tubular*, *tubulovillous* and *villous adenomas*. In spite of these names, the cells of all these tumours show various degrees of aberration (atypia) and *they all have a tendency to undergo malignant change to adenocarcinoma*.

Tubular adenoma is usually a small (less than 1 cm diameter) pedunculated nodule with a smoothly lobulated surface (Fig. 19.80). Microscopically (Figs. 12.10, 12.11, p. 327) it is seen to consist of closely-packed neoplastic epithelial tubules resembling the tubular glands of colonic mucosa but less regular in size and shape and lined by closely-packed epithelial cells.

Villous adenoma is really a papilloma but is now included with the adenomas (World

Health Organization Classification) because of the occurrence of all gradations between villous and tubular tumours. The villous adenoma is usually over 1 cm in diameter when detected and is typically a sessile papillary tumour composed of numerous fronds which project into the gut lumen (Fig. 19.78). Each frond consists of a fine vascular stromal core lined by a single layer of epithelium.

Tubulo-villous adenoma presents features of both the above adenomas, having a mixed tubular and villous structure in various proportions. In most instances the tubules lie deep to blunt, short villi.

The adenomas can occur anywhere in the colon and rectum. They may be single or multiple, and one or more is found incidentally in approximately 10% of necropsies. In general, the distribution of adenomas throughout the large intestine is similar to that of carcinomas, and one or more adenomas are found in about 25% of colons excised for carcinoma. Villous adenomas have a predilection for the rectum and sometimes secrete sufficient albuminous or potassium-rich fluid to cause hypoalbuminaemia or hypokalaemia. Otherwise, colorectal adenomas are usually symptomless, but sometimes give rise to melaena and very rarely to intussussception. Their predisposition to undergo carcinomatous change is reflected in the various degrees of cellular aberration of their epithelium, including pleomorphism, nuclear hyperchromasia, loss of polarity, crowding of cells and an increase in mitoses. Tumour size also correlates with malignant transformation, and villous adenomas, regardless of size, have a greater tendency to become malignant.

Confirmation that excision of a colorectal adenoma is complete requires careful histological examination of the excision margin, which should include the adjacent normal colonic mucosa around the base of the tumour.

Adenomatosis (polyposis) coli. This hereditary disorder is usually transmitted as a Mendelian dominant but in some families either with very poor penetrance or as a recessive character. It is characterised by the development of literally hundreds of adenomatous polyps in the large intestine (Fig. 19.79). The condition does not usually appear until late childhood or early adult life. Since each of the many polyps appears to share the predisposition to become malignant, the onset of carcinoma of the colon

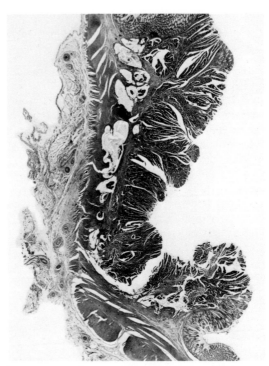

Fig. 19.78 Villous adenoma of rectum. There is malignant infiltration of the wall by mucoid carcinoma. × 3.

is almost inevitable, usually about 15 years after the development of adenomatosis. The adenomas themselves may be symptomless for many years and frequently the presenting features are caused by the development of one or more carcinomas.

Other polypoid lesions

Non-neoplastic polyps occur in the large bowel, and are not to be confused with the true tumours already described. The **metaplastic polyp** is a small, raised, pale, sessile lesion not infrequently encountered in middle or later adult life. Histologically there is localised papilliform hyperplasia of the epithelium lining the surface and upper parts of the crypts. This lesion lacks the hyperchromatism of the polypoid adenoma and does not appear to be premalignant. **Hamartomatous polyps** of the Peutz-Jeghers type (p. 650) are found occasionally in the colon. In childhood, globular polypoid lesions, sometimes quite large, are encountered in the rectum: histologically they consist of intensely inflamed mucosa in which

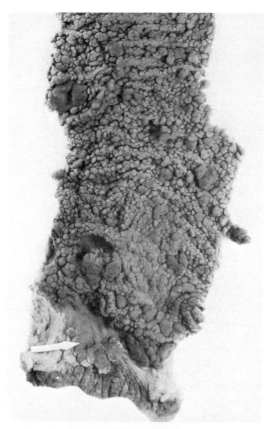

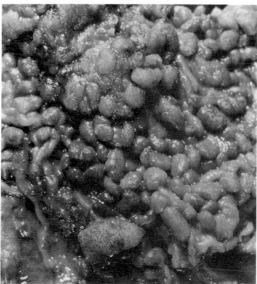

Fig. 19.79 Polyposis coli. *Above*, innumerable small polyps and several larger ones are present. Two small cancers have developed just above the anal margin. × 0·5. *Below*, showing the appearance of the individual polyps. × 2·5.

the crypts are markedly dilated and cystic, and are frequently ulcerated. These so-called **juvenile polyps** do not show epithelial dedifferentiation and may be hamartomatous in nature. Apart from adenomatosis coli, true colonic adenomas are seldom observed in children. Finally, mention must be made of the condition known as **benign lymphoid polyposis of the rectum**, in which multiple polypi, consisting of masses of lymphoid tissue, showing numerous germinal centres and covered by normal rectal epithelium, develop in the rectum, especially in young women. The condition is of unknown causation but, as the name implies, does not have malignant potential.

Carcinoma of the large intestine

This is one of the commoner malignant tumours. It occurs mainly among older people. The rectum is the commonest site, especially in males; next follows the sigmoid colon, the caecum and ileo-caecal valve and the flexures. The overall incidence is about the same for males and females.

Aetiology is largely unknown, although carcinoma of the large bowel is principally a disease of urban communities, low-fibre diet being a possible aetiological factor. As already explained, benign neoplastic polyps (especially adenomatosis coli) and ulcerative colitis are predisposing conditions. In ulcerative colitis, and in adenomatosis coli, carcinoma tends to develop 10–15 years after the onset and thus may affect relatively young people.

Naked-eye appearances. When carcinoma begins in an adenomatous polyp, infiltration of the stalk and base occurs so that the tumour appears like a button fixed to the bowel wall; subsequently the centre breaks down leaving a necrotic ulcer with raised everted ('rolled') edges (Fig. 19.80). The base is then fixed to the muscular coat, which is ultimately breached by progressive ulceration. Spread in the submucous and subserous lymphatics also occurs so that the tumour gradually encircles the bowel wall. The majority of cancers of the colon are scirrhous, and cause contraction and stricture; some, however, are soft and fungating, and others are mucoid and gelatinous. The more slowly growing types especially tend to encircle the bowel, forming a ring-shaped growth and thus producing narrowing or complete obstruc-

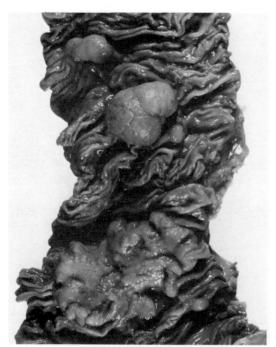

Fig. 19.80 Part of the caecum and ascending colon showing two tubular adenomas (*above*), the larger of which has the typical smoothly lobulated surface. The ulcerated carcinoma (*below*) has originated in a third adenoma.

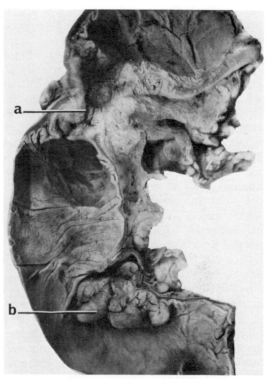

Fig. 19.81 Carcinomatous stricture (**a**) of the colon: note proximal hypertrophy of the colon wall. There is also a polypoid adenoma (**b**) distal to the carcinoma.

tion. The bowel above the obstruction undergoes great, sometimes enormous dilatation, while its wall becomes hypertrophied (Fig. 19.81). The raised intraluminal pressure may interfere with mucosal blood flow and an ischaemic enterocolitis, sometimes with pseudomembrane formation, may develop proximal to the tumour. In other cases, frank ulceration occurs, especially in the caecum (so-called *stercoral ulceration*): perforation and peritonitis may result. Fungating cancers form a large projecting mass which ulcerates and eventually causes obstruction (Fig. 19.82) The mucoid type may, as in the stomach, lead to widespread infiltration and thickening of the wall, and may spread to the peritoneum.

Microscopic appearances. Practically all intestinal cancers are adenocarcinomas, some being highly differentiated, while others are anaplastic and the arrangement of the cells is irregular (Fig. 12.15, p. 330). This is the usual variety that complicates ulcerative colitis.

Spread and prognosis. These tumours tend to spread circumferentially in the wall of the large intestine and also directly through the wall to

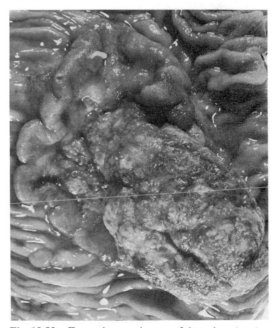

Fig. 19.82 Fungating carcinoma of the colon showing ulceration. Note the raised margin of the ulcer.

the serosa. Occasionally extensive spread occurs in the peritoneal cavity. Lymphatic spread, with metastases in the mesocolic lymph nodes, often occurs quite early, while blood spread to the liver or elsewhere is usually relatively late. Using *Duke's staging*, patients in which the tumour is confined to the intestine (stage A) have a cure rate approaching 100 per cent, unless the tumour has penetrated the whole thickness of the wall (stage B), when the cure rate falls to 70 per cent. Lymph-node metastases (stage C) reduce the cure rate to approximately 30 per cent.

Colonic carcinomas are among the tumours which secrete a glycoprotein (**carcino–embryonic antigen** or **CEA**) which is produced also by normal fetal endodermal tissues (p. 317). Detection of CEA in the serum has not provided a reliable diagnostic test, for it is present in trace amounts in the serum of normal subjects and in increased amounts in various types of cancer, in inflammatory bowel disease and in some other non-neoplastic conditions. Nevertheless, assay of CEA may be helpful in the management of patients with carcinoma, for the level falls after removal of the tumour and a subsequent increase suggests recurrence or metastases.

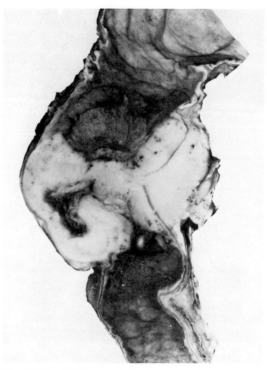

Fig. 19.83 Malignant lymphoma of the ileo-caecal region.

Other malignant tumours

Malignant lymphomas occur, particularly in the caecum and rectum, but are less common than in the small intestine. They may form a large mass and cause obstruction (Fig. 19.83) or ulcerate and sometimes perforate. Leiomyosarcoma is rare.

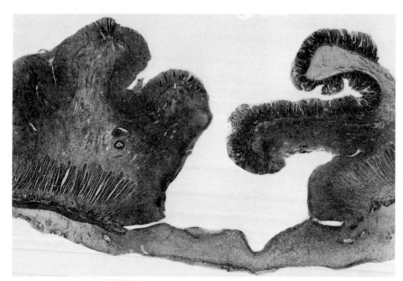

Fig. 19.84 Malignant lymphoma of small intestine, showing deep but sharply localised ulcerative penetration of the wall. ×6.5.

Tumours of the anal canal

Malignant tumours are uncommon. Most are *squamous carcinomas*, often with a 'basaloid' pattern, i.e. resembling rodent ulcer of the skin: some show a mixture of squamous and mucin-secreting elements (*muco-epidermoid carcinoma*). These tumours all tend to metastasise to both pelvic and inguinal nodes, and the prognosis is then poor. *Malignant melanoma* also occurs in the anal canal, where it is almost always fatal.

Secondary tumours of the intestines

Apart from invasion by peritoneal and lymphatic spread, intestinal metastases are extremely uncommon, though metastatic melanoma is seen occasionally, and also the lymphoid neoplasm *struma reticulosa* of the thyroid (p. 1029) has a notable tendency to metastasise to the gut. The peritoneum is a common site for secondary carcinoma (p. 659) and the bowel may become invaded from the serous surface and its lumen considerably contracted.

Congenital Abnormalities

The commonest of these is the **Meckel's diverticulum**, which represents the proximal end of the omphalomesenteric duct. The diverticulum usually measures about 2–3 cm in length, and is narrower than the small intestine (Fig. 19.85). Occasionally it is adherent at the umbilicus and in some cases a fistula is present; or again, there may be obstruction at the proximal end, sometimes merely by a fold, and accumulation of mucus occurs so that an *enterocyst* results. A Meckel's diverticulum rarely leads to any serious results, but when it is adherent it may cause volvulus of the small intestine or, even more serious, strangulation. Acute inflammation of a Meckel's diverticulum presents features similar to those of acute appendicitis, and requires similar surgical treatment. Sometimes heterotopic acid-secreting gastric mucosa is present and may lead to peptic ulceration of the diverticulum with perforation or haemorrhage. In the adult the diverticulum occurs usually about a metre above the ileo-caecal valve, and at about half that distance in young children. Carcinoma has very rarely been observed to develop in the apex of a Meckel's diverticulum.

   Stenosis or actual **atresia** may occasionally occur in the intestines. In the small intestine, the commonest site is at the orifice of the common bile duct or at the ileo-caecal valve. Part of the intestine may be absent, usually along with other malformations. The commonest site of atresia, however, is at the lower end of the rectum. Sometimes a dimple in the

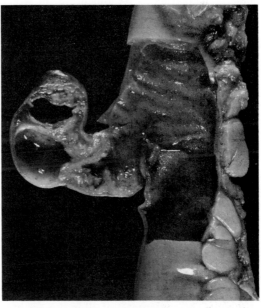

Fig. 19.85 Meckel's diverticulum. In this instance there was pancreatic tissue in the wall and a cystic space. (Dr. John S. Currie.)

skin, representing the anus, is separated from the lower end of the rectum by a thin layer of tissue—the condition being known as **imperforate anus.** In other cases of atresia of the lower end of the rectum, however, the lower end of the bowel communicates with the bladder or urethra in the male and with the vagina in the female.

V: The Peritoneum

Acute peritonitis

Because it contains the gastro-intestinal tract, with its heavy bacterial flora, the peritoneal cavity is liable to bacterial infection, and because of its potential volume and large surface area, acute bacterial infection of the whole peritoneal cavity is a severe, often fatal condition. It is therefore not surprising that the cavity is guarded by potent defence mechanisms. Like other serosal membranes, there are a large number of readily available macrophages in or on the mesothelial lining. These cells are particularly numerous in the omentum, in which they are aggregated in visible 'milk spots'. Even the mild irritation of perfusion by 'physiological' solutions, as in peritoneal dialysis, releases huge numbers of macrophages into the cavity. This phenomenon does not, of course, exclude the usual emigration of polymorphs and subsequently monocytes from the venules in the inflamed peritoneal surfaces. A second important defence mechanism is localisation of an infected focus by the omentum and adjacent viscera. These tissues become glued together by fibrin deposition on their surfaces and so tend to wall off the site of infection from the rest of the cavity.

Causes. Acute bacterial peritonitis is nearly always due to infection from one of the abdominal viscera, in most instances the gastro-intestinal tract. Any breach in the integrity or viability of the wall of the tract is likely to cause local or general peritonitis. The list of causes is thus long. The commonest of all in this country is acute appendicitis, but perforation of a peptic ulcer and acute diverticulitis of the colon are also frequent causes. Others include perforation of typhoid ulcers, usually in the ileum; rupture of the large intestine proximal to an obstruction or in severe ulcerative colitis; penetrating abdominal woulds; perforation of an ulcerated tumour of the intestine, particularly a lymphoma; devitalisation of the gut due to mesenteric vascular thrombosis; or strangulation of part of the gut by herniation, volvulus, etc.

Acute peritonitis can also arise from an acutely infected gallbladder, either by rupture of the wall or spread of the bacteria through it. Acute haemorrhagic pancreatitis, acute salpingitis and acute cystitis may also result in peritonitis. Haematogenous peritonitis is relatively uncommon.

Appearances. The features of acute peritonitis depend on the types of bacteria responsible and the nature of the causal lesion. When the infection is due to escape of bacteria from the gut, the infection is likely to be a mixed one, although one or other species of bacteria may predominate. *Escherichia coli* infection is extremely common, either alone or associated with the other species. Various streptococci, including anaerobes, and *Clostridium welchii*, *Bacteroides*, and various Gram −ve bacilli are all encountered. Pneumococcal peritonitis used to be encountered as an apparently primary phenomenon in young girls, but is not often seen now in this country.

When virulent bacteria enter the peritoneum, or when heavy infection occurs, as in perforation of an ulcer or gangrenous appendicitis, general peritonitis is likely to result. With less virulent bacteria or more gradual infection, the spread may be limited, either by rapid elimination of the bacteria or by formation of fibrinous adhesions around the infected site.

In **generalised peritonitis**, the surfaces are inflamed and the exudate varies in amount and appearance. In haemolytic streptococcal peritonitis, formerly a common puerperal infection, there may be only a little serous or haemorrhagic exudate. With coliform bacilli and the other bacteria mentioned above, exudate is usually more abundant and turbid or frankly purulent, and there is usually a deposit of fibrin on the serosal surfaces. When peritonitis has resulted from perforation of a peptic ulcer, there may be accumulation of air beneath the diaphragm, detectable by radiography: the leakage of acid gastric juice results in a haemorrhagic exudate, and this is seen also when there has been leakage of bile. In acute haemorrhagic pancreatitis the affected surfaces show fat necrosis and the exudate is haemorrhagic: the changes may be generalised or limited to the lesser sac.

The appearances of **localised peritonitis**

depend on the causal organisms and the site affected. If infection is mild, it may resolve without suppuration, although there may be residual adhesions; this is seen when gonococcal salpingitis progresses to pelvic peritonitis. Frequently, however, local acute peritonitis results in suppuration as, for example, when an acutely inflamed appendix becomes surrounded by omentum, loops of gut, etc., and a periappendicular abscess results: this may occur also in relation to an acutely inflamed diverticulum, or when perforation of a peptic ulcer occurs in the lesser sac.

General peritonitis may be overcome, and yet leave residual foci of infection, e.g. a collection of pus in the pelvis or between the liver and diaphragam (subphrenic abscess) walled off by adhesions between adjacent structures.

Effects. Acute generalised peritonitis is an extremely serious, often fatal condition, firstly because the cavity is so large and has such a great surface area from which toxins are absorbed, and secondly because the intestines bathed in bacterial toxins are very likely to develop *paralytic ileus* (p. 645). These factors result in *severe toxaemia* and also *gross dehydration* and disturbance of electrolyte and acid–base balances from loss of fluid into the peritoneal exudate, the paralysed gut, and by vomiting. The result is a combination of *endotoxic and hypovolaemic shock* which is very likely to be fatal unless effectively treated. In many instance, bacteraemia or septicaemia develops.

Recovery may be complicated by residual abscesses, as mentioned above, or by organisation of deposited fibrin to form fibrous adhesions between loops of gut (Fig. 19.86) and the parietal peritoneum, etc.: such adhesions carry a risk of subsequent intestinal obstruction by kinking of the gut or internal hernia.

Chronic peritonitis

As stated above, abscess formation may result from localised or generalised peritonitis, and may persist for weeks or months unless drained. As elsewhere, the persistent abscess becomes enclosed in dense fibrous tissue, which may intefere with the function of the loops of intestine usually forming the wall.

Tuberculous peritonitis is much less common than formerly: it may be general or localised. The origin of the generalised type may be a cas-

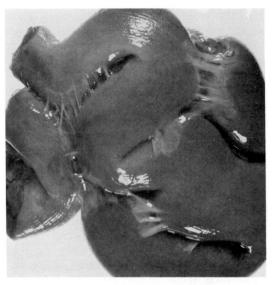

Fig. 19.86 Fibrous adhesions between loops of small intestine, resulting from organisation of fibrin deposited during acute peritonitis.

eous mesenteric lymph node, or the bacilli may reach the peritoneum from a tuberculous Fallopian tube, either directly through its covering or by way of its abdominal opening. In other cases where no gross lesion can be found, the infection is probably by the bloodstream, a small focus forming from which dissemination afterwards occurs. The appearances vary widely in different cases. There may be an eruption of minute grey tubercles all over the peritoneum, with or without a sero-fibrinous effusion. The omentum is often extensively involved and forms a large mass across the upper part of the abdomen. In other cases, there may be caseation, either in scattered foci or diffusely. Lastly, cases are encountered in which the tubercles are comparatively scanty and where the chief result is formation of adhesions, sometimes with serous effusion between them. When chronic tuberculous peritonitis is associated with ulcers of the intestine, ulceration between adjacent loops of the bowel may lead to the formation of multiple fistulae, and may result in the malabsorption syndrome.

Non-bacterial peritonitis

As already mentioned, acute peritonitis results from the irritant effect of gastric juice or bile when these escape into the peritoneal cavity, and also from leaking pancreatic enzymes in acute pancreatitis. All these conditions are likely to be complicated by the supervention of bacterial peritonitis.

There are a number of miscellaneous conditions in which chronic peritonitis or fibrous thickening of the peritoneum occurs in the absence of bacterial infection.

The former use of *talc*, and more recently *starch*, to lubricate surgical gloves led, in some instances, to the development of a granulomatous peritoneal reaction with consequent fibrous adhesions. Peritoneal involvement by *carcinoma*, e.g. from the stomach, colon or ovary, often results in an inflammatory exudate and adhesions (see below). The term *chronic hyperplastic peritonitis* is sometimes used to describe hyaline fibrous thickening of the visceral peritoneum, often over the liver and spleen, but sometimes also the omentum and mesentery. It is usually accompanied by ascites. The term 'sugar-iced liver' (Zuckergussleber) has been applied: in appearance, it resembles the hyaline pleural plaques attributable to inhalation of asbestos, and indeed this may be the cause in some cases. Hyaline thickening involving all the serous sacs is sometimes called *Concato's disease*, while involvement of the pericardium and hepatic peritoneum is termed *Pick's disease*. Very striking thickening of the posterior peritoneum may also occur in the carcinoid syndrome, possibly due to a desmoplastic effect of 5HT (p. 649).

Retroperitoneal fibrosis

In this condition, there is extensive formation of fibrous tissue retroperitoneally. It tends to cause trouble by constricting the ureters. While the aetiology is not known, the condition has been associated with Riedel's thyroiditis, and also with taking the drug methysergide.

Ascites

Serous effusion into the peritoneum occurs in cases of general oedema of both the cardiac and renal types, and is sometimes abundant; some fluid may accumulate also in severe anaemias and wasting diseases. The most severe ascites, however, results from portal obstruction, and the accumulation of fluid often leads

to enormous distension of the abdomen: the commonest cause is cirrhosis of the liver, and in cases which develop primary liver cancer, thrombosis of the portal vein often occurs, the ascitic fluid then accumulating very rapidly and becoming bloodstained. Thus endophlebitis of the hepatic veins (Budd-Chiari syndrome) is accompanied by gross ascites. In the above conditions the fluid is a transudate and there is no formation of fibrin in the peritoneum, but in cases of portal cirrhosis it is not uncommon for a mild infection to become superadded, and occasionally tuberculous peritonitis. Accumulation of inflammatory exudate is, of course, a prominent feature of acute peritonitis, and occurs in some cases of tuberculous peritonitis. Peritoneal carcinomatosis also commonly induces an inflammatory, sometimes haemorrhagic, exudate.

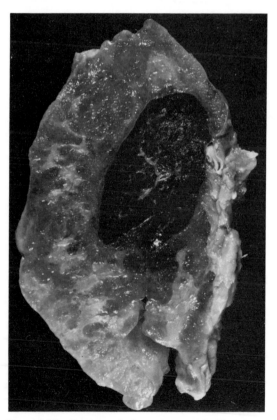

Fig. 19.87 Section of the spleen embedded in a large mass of mucoid carcinoma.

Tumours

Primary tumours of the peritoneum are rare, and in most cases they take origin not from the serous layer but from some adjacent structure. For example, *lipoma* may arise from the appendices epiploicae; *fibroma* takes origin from the connective tissue and sometimes from the sheaths of the nerves in *neurofibromatosis*; and *lymphangioma* occasionally arises from the lymphatics of the mesentery. *Mesothelioma* of the peritoneum presents features like those of mesothelioma of the pleura but is less frequent, and the same caution in the interpretation of the appearances is required. In both situations there is an association with inhalation of asbestos (p. 501).

Secondary tumours of the peritoneum are comparatively common, especially in cases of gastric and ovarian carcinoma. They may be extremely numerous and very minute and may be mistaken macroscopically for tubercles. As mentioned above, they may induce a haemorrhagic inflammatory exudate; or there may be larger nodules and diffuse infiltration. The omentum is very frequently involved and becomes contracted into a hard irregular mass. In some cases of cancer the chief lesion is a very diffuse infiltration with thickening of the serous layers, but with little nodular formation; by such a process the mesentery may become greatly thickened and shrunken. This often results from *linitis plastica* of the stomach, and is accompanied by marked ascites. In mucoid carcinoma the peritoneum is sometimes overgrown by enormous soft translucent tumour masses (Fig. 19.87). Metastases of melanoma are not infrequent and the peritoneum may be studded with enormous numbers of small black nodules; these tend to be specially numerous in the omentum and mesentery.

As in the other serous cavities, the lining cells may desquamate and multiply in ascitic fluid, sometimes developing bizarre morphological features which make them very difficult to distinguish from cancer cells.

Extensive lymphatic permeation by carcinoma is often readily seen in the peritoneum (Fig. 19.88).

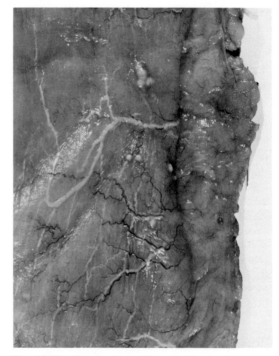

Fig. 19.88 Permeation of lymphatics in the serosa of the small intestine by gastric carcinoma cells. × 2·5.

References and Further Reading

Cove, D. R., Mitchell, D. N. and Brooke, B. N. (1975). Experimental animal studies of the aetiology and pathogenesis of Crohn's disease. *Gastroenterology* **69**, 618–24.

Day, D. W., Mandal, B. K. and Morson, B. C. (1978). The rectal biopsy appearances in Salmonella colitis. *Histopathology* **2**, 117–31.

Mitchell, D. N. and Rees, R. J. W. (1970). Agent transmissible from Crohn's disease tissue. *Lancet* **ii**, 168–71.

Morson, B. C. (1978). *The Pathogenesis of Colorectal Cancer*, pp. 164. Saunders, Philadelphia, London and Toronto.

Morson, B. C. and Dawson, I. P. M. (1979). *Gastro-intestinal Pathology*, 2nd edn., pp. 805. Blackwell Scientific, Oxford, London, Edinburgh and Melbourne.

Sircus, W. (1979). The enigma of peptic ulcer. *Scottish Medical Journal* **24**, 31–7. (An excellent review on aetiology.)

Sobin, L. H., Thomas, L. B., Percy, Constance and Henson, D. E. (Eds.) (1978). *A Coded Compendium of the International Histological Classification of Tumours*, pp. 116. World Health Organization, Geneva.

Whitehead, R. (1979). *Mucosal Biopsy of the Gastro-intestinal Tract*, 2nd edn., pp. 202. Saunders, London.

20

Liver, Biliary Tract and Exocrine Pancreas

The Liver

The anatomical unit: acinus or lobule? The structural unit of the liver has long been considered to be the lobule, arranged around a central hepatic venule and with portal tracts at its periphery (Fig. 20.1a). In fact, the lobule only forms a unit in so far as blood from it drains into one central venule. It receives portal venous and hepatic arterial blood from several portal tracts, and its bile drains into several small bile ducts. On the basis of elegant microcirculatory studies, Rappaport and his colleagues (1954) have defined the basic structural unit as the **simple acinus** (Fig. 20.1b); this is the parenchyma receiving blood from a single terminal portal venule and hepatic arteriole (termed together the *axial vessels* of the acinus) and passing its bile into a single small duct in the same portal tract. The simple acinus lies between two hepatic ('centrilobular') venules into which its blood drains.

The simple acinus is subdivided into three zones (Fig. 20.1b). The hepatocytes in zone 1 (**periportal zone**) are those nearest to the axial vessels: they receive blood rich in nutrients and oxygen and are metabolically more active than cells in the other zones. Zones 2 (**mid-zone**) and 3 (**perivenular zone**) are more peripheral to the axial blood supply; the cells of zone 3 are metabolically least active, are most susceptible to hypoxic damage and are at the microcirculatory periphery of the acinus. The three or more simple acini relating to the preterminal branches of a portal venule and hepatic arteriole together form a **complex acinus** (Fig. 20.2a), the central part or core of which is made up of zones 1 of the simple acini, the intermediate part of zones 2, while zones 3 are peripheral and continuous with zones 3 of adjacent complex acini (Fig. 20.2b). Finally, aggregates of three or four complex acini, deriving their blood supply

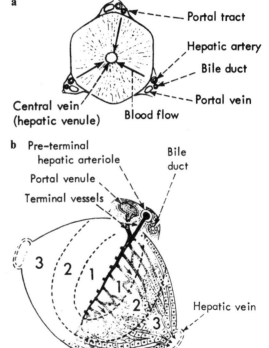

Fig. 20.1 **a** Diagrammatic illustration of the hepatic lobule arranged around a single central (hepatic) vein into which its blood flows. **b** Diagrammatic illustration of the simple acinus arranged around the terminal branches of the hepatic artery, showing its blood draining into two hepatic vein branches.

from a single portal vein branch and hepatic arterial branch, are termed **acinar agglomerates**.

Although the three zones of the simple acinus correspond loosely to the peripheral, mid-zonal and centrilobular zones of the traditional lobule, study of Fig. 20.1 will make it clear that the correspondence is inexact. Lesions of hepatocytes which are influenced by

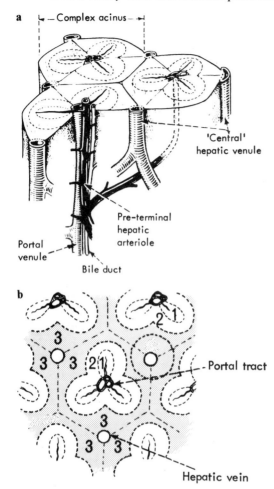

Fig. 20.2 **a** Diagrammatic illustration of the complex acinus comprising three simple acini but deriving its blood from a single pre-terminal branch of the hepatic artery. **b** Diagrammatic illustration showing the relationship between adjacent complex acini, and how there is continuity between zones 3, i.e. the microcirculatory periphery of the acini.

their relationship to axial vessels and differences in their metabolic activities are more readily understood and described on the basis of the acinar concept. In practice this applies to most lesions of hepatocytes, and although in previous chapters we have adhered to the traditional concept of the lobule, which is still widely used, we shall refer in this chapter mainly to the acinus as the anatomical and functional hepatic unit.

Patho-physiology

The liver has a very large number of important physiological functions. It is involved in the intermediary metabolism of proteins, carbohydrates and fats, in the synthesis of a number of plasma proteins such as albumin and fibrinogen, the production of various enzymes and the formation and secretion of bile. It is also responsible for the detoxication of endogenously produced waste products or exogenously derived toxins and drugs, and in the storage of proteins, glycogen, various vitamins and metals. Accordingly, the liver is liable to injury from a variety of causes, and injury to it may have profound metabolic effects.

The major causes of liver disease

Injury from metabolic disturbances. In experimental animals specific dietary deficiencies can produce fatty liver and liver cell necrosis. Similarly in man, protein malnutrition, e.g. in kwashiorkor, can produce marked fatty change and there is evidence that malnutrition may considerably exacerbate other forms of injury. Specific enzyme deficiencies may cause various hepatic storage diseases (p. 668) or failure of biliary secretion (p. 715).

Injury from toxins and poisons. The liver cell is especially liable to injury because of its function of taking up and dealing with many metabolites, toxic substances, drugs and poisons. The vast number of chemicals used industrially and pharmacologically provide an ever-increasing hazard to the liver, particularly as it has been shown that certain chemicals are harmless to most individuals, but can cause extensive liver damage in individuals with a special susceptibility, as yet unpredictable. A wide spectrum of hepatotoxic effects may be produced by the numerous drugs now in clinical use (p. 705). The liver also receives blood draining the gastro-intestinal tract, and is exposed to poisons and toxins absorbed from the gut.

Lesions of the biliary tract affect the liver in two ways. Biliary obstruction, if sufficiently prolonged, results in biliary cirrhosis, and the bile ducts are also the most common route of bacterial infection of the liver.

Certain virus infections damage the liver severely, causing acute hepatitis with extensive necrosis of liver cells. They include Type A (infectious hepatitis), Type B (serum hepatitis) and Type 'non-A : non-B'. Progression to chronic hepatitis is a complication of Type B and Type non-A : non-B.

Hypoxia. Owing to their active and complex metabolism, liver cells are readily injured by hypoxia, as in shock, venous congestion or anaemia.

Tumours. Primary tumours of the liver are relatively uncommon in this country though of great frequency in parts of Africa and the Far East; they are commonly associated with cirrhosis. The liver is a very common site of metastatic carcinoma, particularly from primary tumours of the gastro-intestinal tract.

Pathological effects of disturbed hepatic function

Disturbances of function resulting from lesions of the liver and biliary tract are varied and complex in their effects. They may be considered under three major headings: hepatocellular failure, portal hypertension and biliary obstruction. These are described more fully later in this chapter, but brief summaries of their main features are helpful at this point.

Hepatocellular failure arises when total liver cell function falls below the minimum required to maintain a physiological state. It results from loss of a large number of liver cells from various causes, and/or from impaired function of liver cells, usually attributable to chronic interference with hepatic blood flow; both factors may be involved, especially in hepatic cirrhosis. The more important effects include: **(a) changes in nitrogen metabolism** with a rise in the blood level of toxic nitrogenous compounds produced by bacteria in the gut and normally metabolised by the liver cells; these compounds affect especially the central nervous system, causing hepatic encephalopathy which consists of neuropsychiatric and locomotor disturbances, delirium, convulsions and sometimes 'hepatic coma'; **(b) failure to remove bilirubin** from the blood, to conjugate it and excrete it in the bile; **(c) failure to produce plasma proteins** in normal amounts, particularly albumin, but also fibrinogen, prothrombin and various other clotting factors; **(d) hormonal disturbances** attributable to interference with hepatic metabolism of various steroid and other hormones; **(e) circulatory disturbances** of obscure nature, with cyanosis and a hypervolaemic hyperkinetic circulation.

Portal hypertension. This is caused by obstruction to the blood flow through the liver. As a result, veins which provide an anastomosis between the portal and systemic systems enlarge and some of the portal blood is shunted directly into the systemic circulation instead of passing through the liver. Some of these dilated anastomotic channels, notably in the submucosa of the oesophagus, may rupture and bleed; furthermore the bypassing of the liver increases the blood level of toxic compounds absorbed from the gut, thus aggravating the effect of hepatocellular failure on the central nervous system.

Biliary obstruction. This results from obstruction of the common hepatic or common bile duct or from stagnation of bile in the biliary canaliculi without major duct obstruction. The effects include: (*a*) re-absorption of conjugated bilirubin into the blood, producing **obstructive jaundice**; (*b*) re-absorption of other constituents of bile, such as bile acids and cholesterol; (*c*) malabsorption of fats and fat-soluble vitamins because of the lack of bile salts in the intestine, producing **steatorrhoea** and effects arising from the **deficiency of vitamins A, D, E and K**; (*d*) prolonged cholestasis resulting in **liver cell necrosis** and eventually in **cirrhosis**. Secondary bacterial infection of the biliary tract—*ascending cholangitis*—is an important complication of major duct obstruction.

Circulatory Disturbances

The total hepatic blood flow is approximately 1·5 litres per minute, three-quarters of the blood being supplied by the portal vein and one-quarter by the hepatic artery. Thus, although hepatic arterial blood has a higher oxygen saturation (95 per cent) than portal vein blood (85 per cent), the latter normally provides approximately 70 per cent of the hepatic oxygen requirement. Mixing of the two blood supplies takes place in the liver sinusoids, blood flow through which is controlled by sphincters at their portal and venular ends: flow of arterial blood into the sinusoids may be intermittent, with consequent variations in the proportion of arterial and portal venous blood.

Hepatic arterial obstruction

The hepatic artery is rarely severely obstructed by disease. Fatal infarction has followed accidental ligation of the main trunk or its branch to the right lobe, but in other instances adequate collateral circulation has prevented this. Obstruction of smaller intrahepatic branches is usually without effect because of adequate collateral circulation. However, local infarction may occur in polyarteritis nodosa and has also been described in acute bacterial endocarditis.

Portal venous obstruction

The normal portal venous pressure is 7 mm of mercury, and the *most important effect of portal venous obstruction, whatever the site or cause, is portal hypertension* (p. 692). Impairment of the portal venous blood flow can arise from obstruction of the hepatic veins, hepatic sinusoids, intrahepatic portal vein branches, or of the portal vein itself. *The commonest and most important cause of obstruction is hepatic cirrhosis.* Other intrahepatic causes include congenital hepatic fibrosis (p. 704), schistosomiasis (p. 697) and metastatic or primary carcinoma of the liver.

Obstruction of the portal vein itself is uncommon. It can result from thrombosis, which may occur apparently spontaneously or may complicate (a) umbilical sepsis in the neonatal period, (b) intra-abdominal sepsis, (c) direct invasion by tumour, (d) myeloproliferative disorders, (e) splenectomy, especially in a patient with a normal pre-operative platelet count, and (f) portal hypertension. Obstruction of the portal vein without thrombosis may result from pressure by tumours in or around the porta hepatis.

The effects of *complete portal vein obstruction* depend on the site. If it is in the portal vein alone, nothing dramatic happens, but when it extends to occlude the ostium of the splenic vein, then the blood cannot drain via the splenic and gastro-oesophageal anastomoses and venous infarction of the bowel follows. In patients surviving portal venous thrombosis, new vascular channels develop in the portal fissure,

so that a cavernous type of tissue is formed. *Occlusion of a branch of the portal vein* may sometimes be followed by 'red infarction' (Fig. 20.3), especially when venous congestion is also present. Such lesions, however, are not complete infarcts but are due to sinusoidal engorgement and atrophy of liver cells (p. 248).

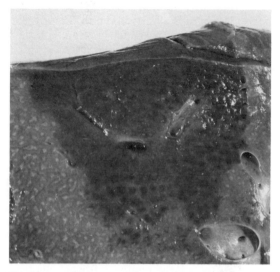

Fig. 20.3   Subcapsular 'red infarct' of the liver.

Hepatic venous obstruction

Obstruction of the major hepatic veins, clinically producing the Budd–Chiari syndrome, is rare. In many instances it is due to endophlebitis with superadded thrombosis, the aetiology being unknown. Compression by tumour masses or direct spread of tumour in the hepatic vein or the terminal inferior vena cava predisposes to thrombotic venous occlusion, and spontaneous thrombosis of these vessels may occur in myeloproliferative disorders or in thrombophlebitis migrans. Intense engorgement of the liver results, with sinusoidal dilatation, perivenular (centrilobular) congestion and haemorrhage, and atrophy and necrosis of liver cells (Fig. 20.4). Ascites is usually severe, and death results from hepatocellular failure.

Veno-occlusive disease of the liver occurs in Jamaica and certain other tropical countries, probably as a result of drinking various plant or herbal medicines—'bush teas'. The active agents are alkaloids of the pyrrolizidine group present in plants of the genera *Senecio* (rag-

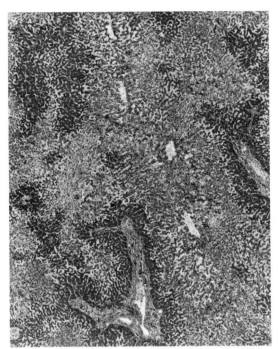

Fig. 20.4 Liver in Budd–Chiari syndrome due, in this instance, to carcinomatous obstruction of the inferior vena cava; there is extensive perivenular hepatocyte necrosis and haemorrhage, and prominent sinusoidal dilatation. × 28.

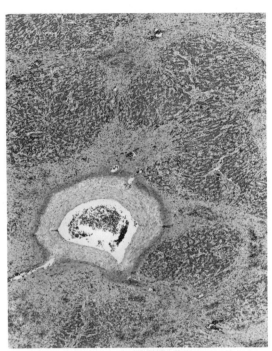

Fig. 20.5 Liver in veno-occlusive disease. There is extensive perivenular hepatocyte loss with replacement fibrosis and marked intimal fibrosis of the hepatic vein branch. × 28.

wort), *Crotalaria* and *Heliotropium*. Liver damage also occurs in animals that eat these plants, and has been produced experimentally. Changes are seen first around the hepatic venules with obliteration of sinusoids and hepatocellular injury. Later the hepatic vein radicles show sub-intimal oedema and progressive fibrosis, which may proceed to complete occlusion (Fig. 20.5). Death may result from liver failure in acute cases, but a chronic stage may develop with perivenular fibrosis and nodular hyperplasia progressing to cirrhosis. A similar condition may result from irradiation of the liver, and has also been associated with certain drugs, e.g. urethane.

Circulatory disturbances due to systemic disease

Acute circulatory failure and shock. In cardiac, hypovolaemic and bacteraemic shock the circulation through the liver is impaired. This results from a fall in both hepatic arterial and portal venous blood flow as part of the general circulatory failure. Initially the microcirculatory periphery (zone 3) of the acinus is injured, but involvement of zones 2 and 1 may occur in prolonged shock. Ischaemic hepatocyte necrosis (Fig. 20.6) of varying distribution patterns results, surrounding which there is usually an acute inflammatory reaction with infiltration of polymorphs. Biochemically these changes are reflected by elevations of serum aminotransferases, which are sometimes as high as in acute viral hepatitis, and by variable increases in serum bilirubin levels.

Venous congestion. In the systemic venous congestion of *acute cardiac failure* the liver is enlarged, often tender, and microscopy shows sinusoidal dilatation and congestion in the perivenular areas. *In chronic cardiac failure* the changes are more marked (p. 228), with liver cell loss resulting from the continued effects of hypoxia and compression by the dilated sinusoids. Clinically there may be mild jaundice, moderate or sometimes marked elevation of the serum aminotransferase levels and also a reduced rate of hepatic inactivation of various

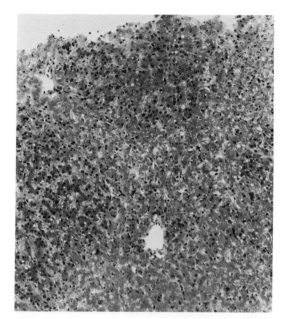

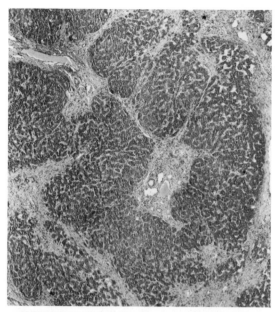

Fig. 20.6   Liver in acute circulatory failure: note the perivenular necrosis of hepatocytes extending in a radiate pattern and producing bridging necrosis between adjacent branches of hepatic veins. × 80.

Fig. 20.7   Liver in chronic venous congestion: perivenular fibrosis has occurred with septate linkage between hepatic vein branches. Note the large portal tract (*central*) surrounded by surviving hepatic parenchyma. This corresponds to so-called cardiac cirrhosis. × 40.

drugs. In very prolonged venous congestion, perivenular (centrilobular) hepatocyte loss may be fairly extensive and replacement fibrosis takes place; sometimes fibrous septa link adjacent hepatic venous branches, resulting in architectural disorganisation (Fig. 20.7): although still called 'cardiac cirrhosis' this seldom, if ever, progresses to a true cirrhosis. The prognosis in hepatic venous congestion is that of the cardiac disease causing it.

Degenerations and Metabolic Disorders

Atrophy

The chief cause of general atrophy of the liver is starvation, in which it becomes shrunken and brown. This is seen also in senility. The cells, especially in the perivenular zones, are shrunken, and often contain granules of lipofuscin (p. 285).

Pressure atrophy occurs around tumours and cysts in the liver, in amyloidosis, and focal atrophy is widespread in cirrhosis. The so-called cough furrows occurring in chronic bronchitis consist of grooves on the anterior and upper surfaces of the liver. They are due to localised atrophy caused by the pressure of diaphragmatic contraction during coughing and are of little importance.

Hyperplasia and hypertrophy

These occur commonly as a compensatory process, the liver cells both multiplying and enlarging, and often becoming multinucleate. These processes are prominent where there has been extensive liver cell necrosis, e.g. in viral or drug-induced hepatitis (Fig. 20.8), and in cirrhosis. The changes are often focal and the surrounding liver tissue may be compressed and atrophic. Hyperplasia and hypertrophy occur in the residual liver following experimental partial hepatectomy. Even when as much as two-thirds of the liver are removed, the weight of the organ may be restored within a few weeks. In fact, restoration occurs so rapidly that

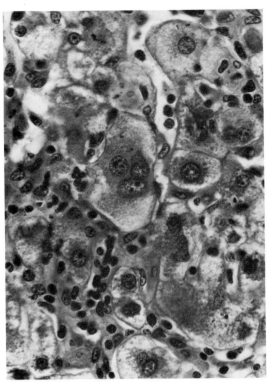

Fig. 20.8 Multinucleated liver cells, in the stage of recovery after acute hepatitis. × 450.

attempts to study diminished hepatic function by this method have usually failed.

Fatty change

A general account of fat metabolism has been given on pp. 24–8. Because of their central role in fat metabolism, the liver cells are particularly prone to undergo fatty change, i.e. to accumulate in their cytoplasm droplets consisting mainly of neutral fat, and in adults a minor degree of fatty change is probably within physiological limits. In *pathological obesity* (p. 27) severe fatty change occurs in the liver, the accumulation of fat beginning and being greatest in periportal hepatocytes (Fig. 2.18, p. 26). The liver cells, in addition to taking up a high proportion of dietary fat absorbed from the intestine and fatty acids released from the depots, are also active in the synthesis of fat from glucose and amino acids. The relative importance of these processes depends on the amounts of carbohydrate, fat and protein in the diet.

In addition to the causes of general fatty change (p. 25)—hypoxia, starvation and wasting disease, and numerous chemical and bacterial toxins—fatty change in the liver may also result from chronic malnutrition, alcohol abuse (p. 681) and in the rare conditions of acute fatty liver of pregnancy (p. 705) and Reye's syndrome (p. 703).

Fatty change in chronic malnutrition is a controversial topic of some importance because of the prevalence of malnutrition in many parts of the world. Severe malnutrition gives rise to a syndrome termed *kwashiorkor*, which affects infants and young children in many parts of southern and central Africa, in tropical America, and extensively in the Far East. The syndrome is a complex one, attributable to a diet severely deficient in high-grade protein, less deficient in total calories, and with additional features due to vitamin deficiencies. Growth is impaired, the liver is severely fatty (Fig. 20.9), the pancreas is atrophic, the plasma albumin is low and there is nutritional oedema. It seems likely that the fatty liver is the result of impaired lipoprotein synthesis due to the protein deficiency, perhaps aggravated by inadequate

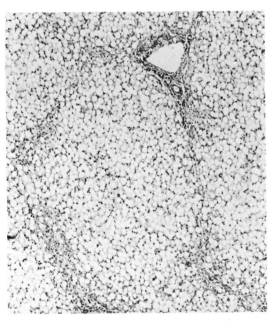

Fig. 20.9 Fatty liver in kwashiorkor. In addition to vacuolation of each liver cell by a large globule of fat, there is an increase in connective tissue in the form of fine strands running through the parenchyma. × 40. (Preparation kindly lent by Professor R. S. Patrick.)

carbohydrate intake. There is no evidence that the fatty liver in malnutrition progresses to cirrhosis.

Haemosiderosis

Haemosiderin pigment gives a blue staining reaction with prussian blue stain (Perls' reaction). The normal adult liver contains approximately 0·3 g of iron, but more than half of this is in the form of ferritin, and the amount of haemosiderin is not sufficient to give a prussian blue reaction (p. 281). In infancy the liver normally gives an iron reaction and this becomes more marked in wasting conditions of children.

Excess iron deposition occurs (*a*) in primary haemochromatosis (p. 282); (*b*) in conditions of excessive blood destruction, e.g. haemolytic anaemias of all types; (*c*) following multiple blood transfusions in some chronic blood disorders; (*d*) in alcoholic liver disease and (*e*) from ingestion of excessive amounts of iron, either in medicines or in the diet. This is common in the South African Bantu whose staple diet of porridge is prepared in iron pots. Excessive iron deposits in the liver may involve only the parenchymal cells in the early stages of primary haemochromatosis, whereas in the other conditions of iron overload both parenchymal cell and Kupffer cell siderosis occur. The haemosiderin appears as brownish-yellow granules in the liver cells. Deposits initially tend to be more marked in the periportal hepatocytes. Subsequently there may be diffuse hepatocellular deposition.

Amyloid disease

In this condition (pp. 269–74) the liver becomes larger, firmer and elastic and is often palpable during life. Amyloid disease does not usually produce jaundice or ascites, but the latter may occur as part of the general oedema in the nephrotic syndrome due to amyloid disease of the kidneys. The amyloid is irregularly deposited in the perisinusoidal space and compresses neighbouring hepatocytes (Fig. 10.4, p. 271).

Glycogen storage diseases

Glycogen storage diseases (p. 30) result from a number of enzyme defects, and the ultimate diagnosis depends on the demonstration of the specific defect. The liver cells are involved in Types I, II, III, IV, VI and VIII, and the intracellular site of glycogen storage varies in the different types: light and electron microscopy thus reveal diagnostically useful changes. Hepatocellular adenomas may develop in Type I and cirrhosis in Type IV.

Excessive accumulation of glycogen occurs also in other forms of metabolic disturbance, e.g. in diabetes mellitus. The histochemical recognition of glycogen is described on p. 31.

Lipid storage diseases

In these conditions abnormal amounts of *lipids* (other than triglyceride fats) accumulate, mainly in cells of the mononuclear-phagocyte system, the Kupffer cells being consistently involved in Gaucher's disease (cerebroside accumulation) and Niemann–Pick disease (sphingomyelin). Hypercholesterolaemic lipid storage diseases rarely affect the liver.

Other metabolic disorders

Many other inherited metabolic disorders affect the liver, and involvement is severe in some, e.g. galactosaemia, alpha-1-antitrypsin deficiency, Wilson's disease and erythropoietic protoporphyria. Although these conditions are rare, preventive measures or treatment may be helpful and so clinical awareness and early recognition are important.

Liver Cell Necrosis

Necrosis of liver cells, of greater or lesser extent, occurs in many diseases of the liver, and also in many other conditions, such as severe infections, wasting diseases and cardiac failure, in which liver cell injury is neither the most important nor the most characteristic feature. Infarction (p. 248) needs no further description here.

Necrosis may affect: **(a) single scattered liver cells** which die one by one (*necrobiosis* or *apop-*

tosis), and are recognised as shrunken, deeply eosinophilic granular cells with a pyknotic nucleus which is eventually extruded leaving the *acidophilic* or *'Councilman' body*; **(b) small groups of hepatocytes**, irregularly distributed (*focal necrosis*) in relation to which macrophages and lymphocytes may accumulate. Such foci may result from many types of liver injury, but are common in severe toxaemia, particularly when due to infections within the portal drainage area. Focal necrosis also occurs in acute viral and drug-induced hepatitis; **(c) large groups of hepatocytes** (*confluent necrosis*) as in severe viral hepatitis, drug-induced and acute ischaemic liver injury. In severe viral hepatitis, confluent necrosis may extend between contiguous hepatic venules or between hepatic venules and portal tracts ('central-central' and 'central-portal' bridging necrosis); **(d) extensive areas of the liver** (*massive hepatic necrosis*),

which represents a more severe degree of confluent necrosis and may be a sequel to viral hepatitis or drug injury. Clinically, it results in fulminant acute hepatocellular failure with a mortality approaching 80 per cent.

The factors which determine the topographical distribution of hepatic necrosis are not known but presumably include the zonal differences in enzyme distribution, cell metabolism and quality of blood supply. Ischaemic injury affects the perivenular zones of the acini (Fig. 20.6) as do many drugs and toxins, e.g. alcohol and paracetamol. Other agents produce periportal injury, e.g., phosphorus, while yellow fever characteristically affects zone 2 of the acinus, producing a 'mid-zonal' pattern of necrosis.

Massive liver cell necrosis is described later as a complication of viral hepatitis, and 'piecemeal necrosis' is defined as a characteristic feature in many forms of chronic hepatitis.

Hepatitis

Hepatitis literally means any inflammatory lesion of the liver. In practice the term is not used for focal lesions, such as an abscess, but only when there is diffuse involvement of the liver. This may be either acute or chronic, and in some instances acute and chronic hepatitis may be present simultaneously.

Hepatitis may be further classified on an aetiological basis, and some types are best dealt with under separate headings, e.g. alcoholic hepatitis, drug-induced hepatitis, and chronic hepatitis in Wilson's disease, haemochromatosis and biliary disease. Cirrhosis represents a late, irreversible and progressive stage of chronic hepatitis, and it also will be discussed separately (p. 687).

In this section we deal with (i) *acute viral hepatitis* due to the well-recognised Type A and Type B viruses, the more recently described non-A: non-B Type, and other acute virus and virus-like infections; and with (ii) *chronic hepatitis*, often of unknown cause, and sub-classified into chronic persistent and chronic active types.

Acute viral hepatitis

This is an acute infection characterised by diffuse hepatitis with widespread liver cell necro-

sis. There are two well-characterised types, A and B, and a recently recognised 'non-A:non-B type' which may, however, include a number of different virus infections.

Type A (infectious hepatitis) is a naturally acquired infection, has an incubation period of 15–40 days, and occurs endemically and as epidemics. The infective agent is a picornavirus and associated 27 nm particles occur in the blood and faeces during early infection and have been demonstrated in the liver-cell cytoplasm in experimental animals. In contrast to Type B hepatitis, only one serotype of Type A hepatitis has been identified in world-wide studies. The highest natural incidence occurs in children under 15, boys and girls being equally affected, with a higher frequency in the lower socio-economic classes. It is estimated that 50–75 per cent of the community may be infected during epidemics, but in most of them the infection is anicteric and often subclinical. Faeces and blood become infected 3–4 weeks after exposure to the virus, and remain infective for about 3 weeks. Specific immunity is established after recovery from Type A hepatitis and protective antibody is demonstrable in the serum. Active immunisation is still not possible, but passive immunisation with pooled human IgG has been shown to prevent clinical disease.

Type B (serum hepatitis) has an incubation period of 50–180 days; it is most frequently transmitted by blood and blood products, but may also be transmitted naturally from an infected person, e.g. sexually, and also from mother to child. It is a particular hazard in renal transplantation and dialysis units and among intravenous drug addicts. The disease occurs in any age group; it is more severe than Type A, with a higher mortality, and infection may result also in the development of a carrier state or in progression to chronic liver disease.

In 1964, Blumberg and his colleagues described a lipoprotein complex in the blood of an Australian aborigine, using as antibody the serum of a much-transfused haemophiliac. This complex they called **Australia (Au) antigen**; subsequently it was shown by them (1967) and others to be particularly associated with cases of serum hepatitis. Accordingly, it is now generally known as hepatitis B antigen (**HB Ag**), and

is demonstrable by various serological techniques of differing sensitivities—agar diffusion precipitation, complement fixation, immuno-electrophoresis, haemagglutination inhibition, immuno-electron microscopy, solid phase radio-immunoassay and others (Burrell, 1980).

Electron microscopy (Fig. 20.10) shows two morphologically distinct viral components which are also known to represent two serologically distinct antigens. The 42 nm Dane particle is regarded as the complete infective virion of hepatitis B. The central core of the Dane particle, hepatitis B core antigen (*HBcAg*), contains DNA polymerase, circular twin-stranded DNA, and protein antigens; the core antigen is equivalent to the nucleocapsid antigen of other viruses. Viral replication occurs in the liver cell nuclei, and core particles may appear free within the liver cell cytoplasm, but are demonstrable in the serum only within complete Dane particles. The outer envelope of the Dane particle is antigenically distinct from HBcAg, and is referred to as hepatitis B sur-

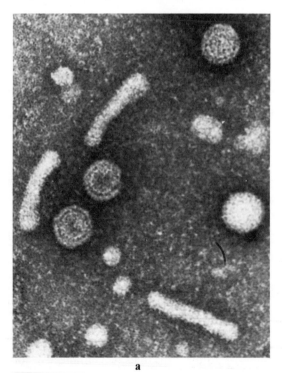 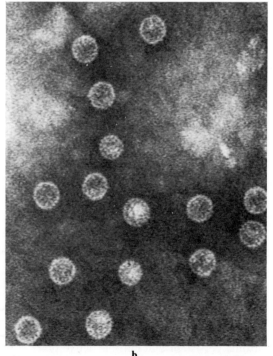

| a | b |

Fig. 20.10   Electron micrographs showing the morphological forms of the HB Ag. **a** This shows the small spheres and tubular structures (20 nm diameter) together with the larger double-shelled Dane particles (42 nm diameter). The small spheres, tubules and outer coat of the Dane particle comprise HBsAg. The inner part of the Dane particle is HBcAg. × 300 000. **b** A preparation of purified core particles—HBcAg. × 300 000. (Dr. June Almeida.)

face antigen (*HBsAg*). It is produced in excess in the liver cell cytoplasm and appears in the serum, both as the coating material of Dane particles and also as 20 nm spherical particles and tubular structures (Fig. 20.10).

HbsAg is not serologically homogeneous, and various antigenic markers have been described. All **subtypes** contain three such antigens, 'a', 'd' or 'y', 'w' or 'r'. These subtypes—adw, adr, ayw, and ayr—do not appear to differ in their clinical effects, but are of considerable value in epidemiological studies. A number of other antigen/antibody systems have been described in hepatitis B, and of these the 'e' antigen (*HBeAg*) appears to be clinically important. Its presence is closely related to Dane particle formation; its persistence in the serum is thus associated with infectivity and active chronic liver disease.

The distribution of the HB antigens within the liver cells has been demonstrated by immunofluorescence techniques, direct electron microscopy and immuno-electron microscopy. HBcAg is found mostly in the nuclei (Fig. 20.11) and to a lesser extent in the cytoplasm; it always acquires a surface antigen coating before entry into the serum. Excess of HBcAg in the nucleus may occasionally be recognisable by light microscopy as 'sanded nuclei', containing a granular eosinophilic inclusion (Fig. 20.11). HBsAg is found exclusively in the liver cell cytoplasm; it is present in the smooth endoplasmic reticulum, and the cytoplasmic deposits produce characteristic 'ground-glass' hepatocytes (Fig. 20.12) which are readily recognisable on routine haematoxylin and eosin or trichrome stains, but are rendered more conspicuous by orcein or by aldehyde thionine. It should be emphasised that the liver-cell distribution of these antigens has been demonstrated mainly in chronic carriers of hepatitis B or patients with chronic hepatitis as a sequel to the acute infection. 'Sanded' nuclei and 'ground-glass' hepatocytes are not seen in the acute clinical attack.

The patterns of antigen and antibody response in the acute classical attack, with elimination of the virus and full clinical recovery, is shown in Fig. 20.13. The development of antibody to HBsAg (HBsAb) appears to be delayed, but it is regarded as the protective antibody. HBcAb titres fall gradually after the acute illness and it may eventually become undetectable. While recovery with elimination of the virus is the outcome in most patients, some become chronic carriers and others develop chronic hepatitis and progress to cirrhosis. The incidence of carriers in the community shows marked geographic variation, being of the order of 0·1 per cent in this country, whereas in parts of Africa and South-East Asia it is as high as 20 per cent. In some carriers there is no previous history of hepatitis; they are asymptomatic and are detected when being tested for suitability as blood donors. Vertical transmission from the mother to child during delivery is considered to be an important mode of infection in countries with high carrier rates. The host factors which determine these sequelae are not fully understood, but it is thought that they result from inadequate humoral and cell-mediated immune responses. There is evi-

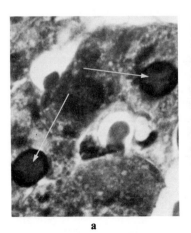 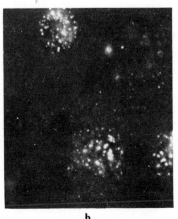 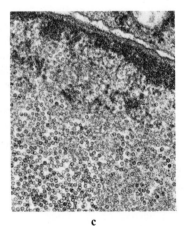

a   b   c

Fig. 20.11 Hepatitis B core antigen. (**a**) Nuclear excess of antigen producing 'sanded nuclei' (*arrows*). × 150. (**b**) Specific immunofluorescence for core antigen: note the granular nature of the intranuclear deposits. (**c**) Intranuclear core particles demonstrated by electron microscopy: the nuclear membrane runs transversely across the upper part of the illustration. × 43 000. (Professor L. Bianchi, University of Basel, Switzerland.)

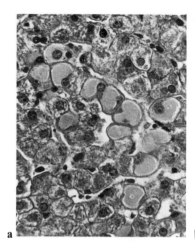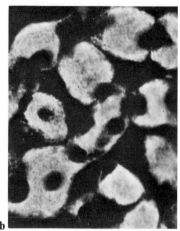

Fig. 20.12 Hepatitis B surface antigen. (**a**) Cytoplasmic excess of antigen producing 'ground-glass hepatocytes' with an intracytoplasmic homogeneous inclusion. Masson's trichrome. × 250. (**b**) Specific immunofluorescence for surface antigen showing uniform cytoplasmic staining; the nuclei are negative. (Fig. 20.12b, Professor L. Bianchi, University of Basel, Switzerland.)

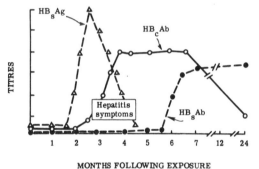

MONTHS FOLLOWING EXPOSURE

Fig. 20.13 Humoral immune response in hepatitis B infection and with clinical recovery (see text).

dence that **the chronic carrier state** may be of two types: (a) *HBsAg predominant,* in which HBsAg is present in the serum, ground-glass hepatocytes are numerous in liver biopsy, and there is minimal expression of HBcAg and so possibly low infectivity; (b) *HBcAg predominant,* in which there is continued viral replication in hepatocyte nuclei, with abundant circulating Dane particles and high infectivity.

The main significance of the discovery of the hepatitis B virus and its complicated antigen/antibody systems has been as follows: (a) it allows screening of potential blood donors and may thus reduce the incidence of direct transmission of Type B hepatitis; (b) it has resulted in specific diagnostic and retrospective tests for infection and this has greatly increased our knowledge of the epidemiology of the disease and of its clinical behaviour; (c) it has provided information on the possible relationships of Type B hepatitis to chronic liver disease and hepatocellular carcinoma; (d) it has raised the

possibility of active and passive immunisation, and perhaps eradication of the disease.

Type Non-A:Non-B hepatitis was first described following blood transfusion after serological exclusion of other known hepatitis viruses and with the demonstration of a transmissible agent which induces hepatitis in chimpanzees. Prospective studies have indicated that it is now responsible for more than 70 per cent of post-transfusion hepatitis. At least two types of non-A:non-B have been postulated. However the infective agent(s) have not been identified nor have antigenic markers been detected. Carrier states occur, and there is evidence of an increased risk of progression to chronic hepatitis following the acute disease.

Clinical and biochemical features

The clinical and biochemical features of the three types are very similar, but Type B is regarded as being most severe and is more often fatal. These types are compared in Table 20.1.

The early clinical features are severe nausea, anorexia, intolerance of fat, often retching, vomiting and fever. A 'serum-sickness-like' syndrome may be seen, with arthralgia and occasionally skin rashes. There is often epigastric pain and the liver is enlarged, tender and the site of a dull ache. Jaundice develops 3 to 9 days after this prodromal illness and reaches a peak in 10 days, during which period the stools are pale and the urine dark. The spleen is palpably enlarged in a third of patients. These features subside in 2–6 weeks but full clinical recovery may take several more weeks. An initial leukopenia is seen in the pre-icteric stage, succeeded

Table 20.1 Comparative aspects of Types A, B and non-A:non-B hepatitis

	Type A	Type B	Non-A:non-B
Mode of spread	Oro-faecal (parenteral)	Parenteral (oro-faecal and sexual)	Parenteral ? others
Incubation period (days)	15–40	50–180	10–90
Age affected	Younger age groups	Any age	Any age
Clinical episode	Mild: mortality rate 1% or less	Severe: mortality rate variable up to 15%	Moderate but tendency for clinical fluctuation
Markers identified	HA Ag-27 nm particles HA Ab	HB-associated antigens and particles*	Not yet identified
Carrier states and chronic hepatitis	No	Yes**	Yes***
Transmissible experimentally to:	Marmoset Chimpanzee	Chimpanzee	Chimpanzee

*See text for discussion of antigen/antibody systems.   ***Chronic sequelae prominent.
**Association also with hepatocellular carcinoma (p. 701).

by a lymphocytosis with, in a small proportion of cases, atypical lymphocytes resembling those found in infectious mononucleosis. The serum bilirubin level is between 80 and 250 μmol/litre (4–12 mg/100 ml) and this is mainly in the conjugated form. Serum alkaline phosphatase levels do not usually exceed 30 King-Armstrong units/dl. Serum aspartate aminotransferase (SGOT) and alanine aminotransferase (SGPT) levels may reach levels greatly in excess of 1000 iu/litre early in the disease and then fall rapidly with the onset of jaundice. The one-stage prothrombin time is usually prolonged, and this measurement provides the best single indication of the severity of the hepatitis.

Most patients recover completely from an attack. Mortality rates are lower in Type A than in Type B, but vary in different communities and outbreaks from 1 to 20 per cent. In very severe cases, death results acutely from fulminant liver failure due to massive hepatic necrosis. The hepatitis may progress, sometimes with fluctuations in severity, and cause death from liver failure in 3–8 weeks: this occurs more frequently in females. In some cases jaundice is deeper and persists for weeks or even months—*cholestatic hepatitis*—but eventually with complete recovery. The development of chronic carrier states and of chronic active hepatitis and cirrhosis are discussed later. The so-called *post-hepatitis syndrome* with vague features—undue fatigue, dyspepsia and

hepatic pain—occurs in a small number of patients.

Pathological changes

There is diffuse hepatic involvement, with acute degenerative changes in scattered hepatocytes accompanied by a predominantly mononuclear cell infiltrate of the portal tracts and parenchyma, Kupffer cell reactive hyperplasia and varying degrees of hepatocyte regenerative activity (Fig. 20.14).

There is great variation in the degree of injury of individual liver cells: many cells appear normal, but there may be single or focal hepatocellular necrosis. The cells may be enlarged, with granular cytoplasm tending to be condensed round the nucleus—ballooning degeneration (Fig. 20.15); others show acidophilic degeneration, with shrinkage of the cells, increased cytoplasmic eosinophilia, pyknosis and eventually extrusion of the nucleus, leaving the acidophilic or Councilman body (Fig. 20.16). With necrosis and eventual lysis of single cells or groups of cells, there is disruption of liver cell plates, but the reticulin framework remains intact. An inflammatory infiltrate, mainly of lymphocytes, very occasional plasma cells and a few polymorphs, is intimately related to the liver cell necrosis and is also a regular finding in the portal tracts. Kupffer cells show reactive hyperplasia; many contain phagocytosed

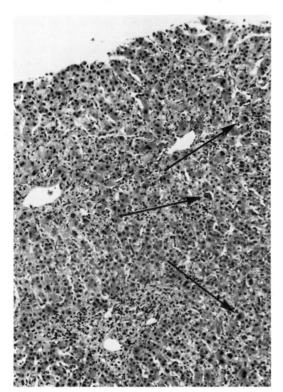

Fig. 20.14 Liver in viral hepatitis. There is a moderately intense mononuclear cell infiltrate of the portal tract (*lower centre*), and a more intense diffuse parenchymal cell infiltrate with liver cell degeneration and a number of acidophilic bodies (*arrowed*). × 120.

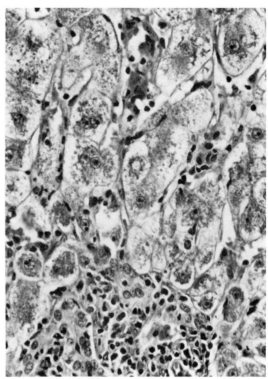

Fig. 20.15 Liver in viral hepatitis showing ballooning degeneration of liver cells and foci of liver cell necrosis. Note also the portal tract inflammation (*lower centre*). (Professor R. S. Patrick). × 465.

cellular debris, bile pigment and lipofuscin granules, and they contribute to the striking increase in cellularity so characteristic of the histological appearance. Biliary stasis is usually not severe but intracytoplasmic bile pigment granules and occasional bile thrombi are seen. Electron microscopy shows irregular swelling of the endoplasmic reticulum of hepatocytes to form vesicles, detachment of the membrane-associated ribosomes and enlarged phagosomes containing altered mitochondria and organelle debris. None of these electron-microscopic changes is specific. The mechanisms of the liver cell injury are not understood.

The acute liver cell injury is brief, and before the attack has subsided clinically, hypertrophy and hyperplasia are seen among surviving hepatocytes with the formation of binucleate and multinucleate cells (Fig. 20.8).

In unusually severe cases there may be more extensive loss of liver cells. Confluent necrosis

occurs and lysis of the groups of injured hepatocytes produces an empty reticulin framework which later collapses. These more extensive areas of confluent necrosis peculiarly affect certain zones and extend between adjacent hepatic veins and between hepatic veins and portal tracts ('central-central' and 'central-portal' bridging hepatic necrosis: Fig. 20.17). Such extensive lesions may result in fulminant hepatic failure. Survival depends on the regenerative power of the spared parenchyma, and with survival there is usually a restoration of normal architecture.

Acute viral hepatitis with massive necrosis

This consists of confluent necrosis of all or nearly all the parenchymal cells in large areas of the liver, often more extensive in the left lobe. When almost the whole of the parenchyma is destroyed, death results from fulminant hepatic failure.

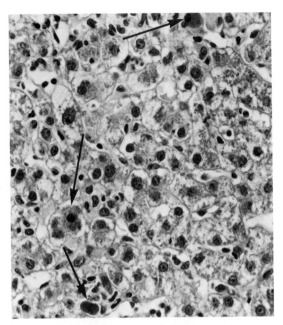

Fig. 20.16 Liver in viral hepatitis: perivenular area showing a number of ballooned hepatocytes, a diffuse mononuclear infiltrate, and a number of acidophilic (Councilman) bodies (*arrowed*) one of which lies free in a sinusoid. × 360.

Massive liver cell necrosis may occur as an unusual complication in acute viral hepatitis and is commoner in Type B. Certain chemicals used therapeutically and in industry produce massive liver cell necrosis in a small proportion of individuals at risk. When death occurs within a few days, i.e. before autolysis of the dead liver cells, the liver is approximately normal in size and is strikingly yellow owing to bile-staining. Subsequently the dead cells disappear, the affected parts of the liver become shrunken, soft and red due to sinusoidal congestion and local haemorrhage (Fig. 20.18). If the patient survives for weeks or months, proliferation of the surviving parenchyma produces pale nodules varying in size to over a centimetre, and scarring occurs in the area of liver cell loss. These changes result in a shrunken nodular liver—*postnecrotic scarring* or *multiple nodular hyperplasia*. The variation in size of nodules and the breadth of intervening fibrous tissue bands are much greater than in cirrhosis (Fig. 20.19). The prognosis is still poor, and death may result from a recurrence of massive necrosis, from chronic hepatocellular failure, or from portal hypertension.

The patterns of massive necrosis due to viral

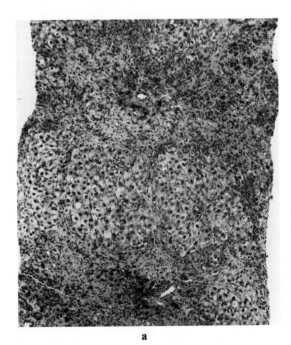

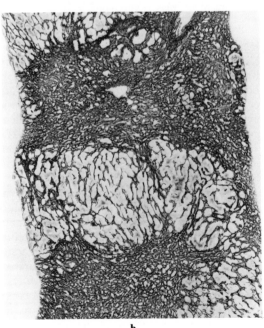

a   b

Fig. 20.17 Liver in viral hepatitis: acute Type B infection with bridging confluent necrosis. Note the extensive confluent necrosis of liver cells, producing collapse of the reticulin framework and central–central and central–portal bridging. Full uneventful recovery occurred in this patient. **a** H & E. × 60. **b** Gordon and Sweet's reticulin. × 60.

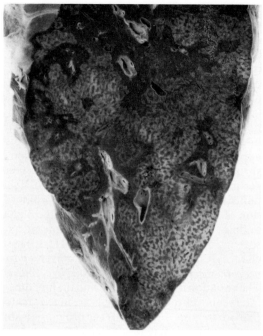

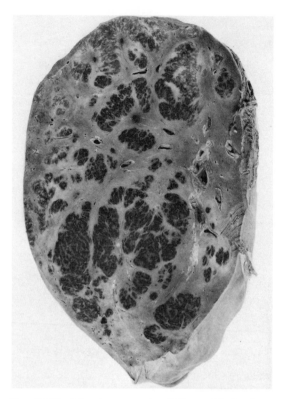

Fig. 20.18 Massive necrosis of liver, three weeks after the onset of jaundice. Note the irregular dark areas from which the dead liver cells have been absorbed, and the portions showing persisting liver structure which were deeply jaundiced. These latter areas had undergone necrosis shortly before death.

Fig. 20.19 Massive necrosis of liver with fatal recurrence. The pale areas consist of fibrous tissue, the liver cells having undergone necrosis in the initial attack and subsequent autolysis. The dark areas consist of tissue in which the liver cells survived the initial attack, but were destroyed in a rapidly-fatal recurrence. × 0·9.

hepatitis, drugs or chemicals are microscopically similar. Initially there is extensive liver cell death, with only a few surviving periportal hepatocytes, and with little inflammatory cell reaction (Fig. 20.20). Subsequently there is extensive autolysis of dead cells with consequent collapse of the reticulin framework (Fig. 20.21). There is a moderately intense mononuclear cell infiltrate, and after a few days early fibrosis and hepatocyte regeneration may be noted.

It is not clear why massive hepatic necrosis occurs in some cases of viral hepatitis, usually a fairly benign condition, or following therapeutic doses of various drugs in certain susceptible individuals. While there are reports that acute viral hepatitis may run a more severe course in malnourished people, there is little evidence that this is a factor in massive hepatic necrosis in this country.

Hepatitis due to other viruses

Acute hepatitis may occur as an unusual complication of *rubella* or of *herpes simplex* in in-

fancy and childhood, but rarely in adults. In *infectious mononucleosis* due to the Epstein–Barr virus, abnormal lymphoid cells may accumulate in the portal tracts and sinusoids, and a mild form of clinical hepatitis may occur with focal liver cell necrosis and slight cholestasis. *Cytomegalovirus* hepatitis is a feature of the generalised form of infection with this virus, which occurs in neonates infected *in utero*. In older children and adults, this virus can cause hepatitis closely resembling acute viral hepatitis (Type A or B) and may sometimes occur as part of an illness resembling infectious mononucleosis particularly in immunosuppressed patients.

Yellow fever, caused by a Group B arbovirus, occurs sporadically and in epidemics in certain parts of Africa and tropical America. The disease occurs in monkeys and is transmitted to

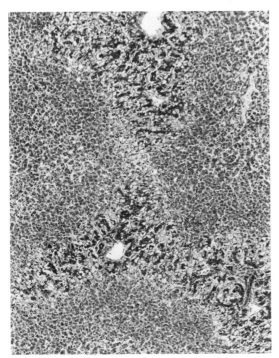

Fig. 20.20 Massive liver cell necrosis in paracetamol overdosage: the hepatocytes in the periportal zones have survived and appear darkly stained. × 60.

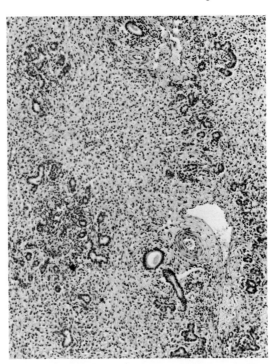

Fig. 20.21 Massive liver cell necrosis: there are virtually no surviving hepatocytes and the parenchyma comprises dilated capillary-like structures. Early duct proliferation is seen around portal tracts. × 75.

man by the bite of *Aedes aegyptii* and certain other mosquitoes. It varies in severity from a mild unsuspected febrile illness to a fatal combination of fulminant massive hepatic necrosis, acute renal failure and marrow depression with leukopenia and thrombocytopenia. The hepatic lesion consists of mid-zonal necrosis and fatty infiltration in mild cases. Acidophilic or hyaline liver cell necrosis is prominent, producing the classical Councilman body. The kidneys show proximal tubular necrosis.

Chronic hepatitis

Chronic hepatitis may be conveniently defined as inflammation of the liver continuing without improvement for at least six months. It is a primary disease of liver and can be viral, drug-induced or of unknown aetiology.

Chronic inflammation is also a feature of alcohol-induced liver injury, long-standing biliary obstruction, Wilson's disease and other metabolic disorders; while these conditions may also be associated with morphological features similar to those about to be described, and also

run a chronic course, they are not usually included in the definition of chronic hepatitis.

Chronic hepatitis has been subdivided into a relatively benign form, **chronic persistent hepatitis**, in which the inflammation is confined to the portal areas, and a more aggressive form, **chronic active hepatitis**, in which there is portal and parenchymal involvement with progressive fibrosis ending in cirrhosis. These definitions are based on morphological criteria, and have replaced former terms such as subacute hepatitis, lupoid hepatitis, juvenile cirrhosis, etc. The clinical and pathological features of chronic hepatitis will first be outlined, and aetiological mechanisms will then be discussed.

Chronic persistent hepatitis

This is a mild disease, with a benign course, and characterised clinically by symptoms of fatigue, malaise, vague upper abdominal pain and sometimes intolerance of dietary fat. The liver may be tender and slightly enlarged. Biochemical tests show a moderate elevation of aminotransferase levels, but levels of IgG are within the normal range.

Liver biopsy shows a moderately intense mononuclear cell infiltrate of the portal tracts, with a normal architecture, intact limiting plates, little or no significant increase in portal fibrous tissue and only minimal parenchymal cell necrosis (Fig. 20.22).

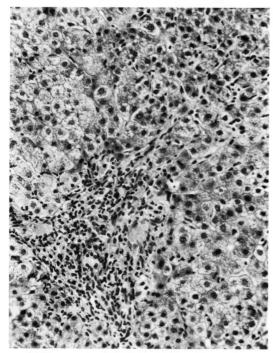

Fig. 20.22 Chronic persistent hepatitis. There is a mononuclear cell infiltrate confined to the portal tract in the lower left quadrant with little or no involvement of the hepatic parenchyma. × 205.

This entity is thought to be a sequel to a subclinical or clinical attack of acute viral hepatitis. Although progression to cirrhosis has not been reported, development of the picture of chronic active hepatitis has been described in a few cases, and cases of chronic active hepatitis have changed to a pattern of chronic persistent hepatitis following treatment.

Chronic active hepatitis

Clinical features. Without treatment, this condition usually progresses to cirrhosis, although some cases may subside spontaneously. In our experience there is a female to male preponderance of 3 to 1, but it is well recognised that HB-associated chronic active hepatitis (see below) is more common in males. The condition occurs mainly between 20 and 50 years of age, but is seen also in older people. The onset may be acute in about a third of patients and indistinguishable from an acute viral hepatitis, or it may be insidious with non-specific symptoms of anorexia, tiredness, vague upper abdominal pain and often amenorrhoea. There may be evidence of hepatocellular failure, but the disease tends to fluctuate in severity. There is hepatomegaly, and often splenomegaly which precedes the development of any portal hypertension.

Additional features include arthralgia, skin rashes, pleural effusions, thrombocytopenia, leukopenia and proteinuria attributable to glomerular lesions; they occur in various degrees and combinations. Some patients also may have chronic inflammatory bowel disease, chronic thyroiditis, Sjøgren's syndrome, and other diseases of possible auto-immune aetiology.

Biochemical tests show elevations of aminotransferase levels, usually over 100 iu/litre. The occurrence and degree of jaundice varies; when present it is usually associated with a moderate rise of the serum alkaline phosphatase level. Hyperglobulinaemia, predominantly of IgG, is a frequent finding. In the later stages, more advanced changes of hepatocellular dysfunction and cirrhosis are manifest, e.g. hypoalbuminaemia and prolongation of the prothrombin time.

Morphologically, chronic active hepatitis is a continuing progressive inflammation with liver-cell degeneration and necrosis accompanied by fibrosis of variable extent and distribution, progressing to cirrhosis in a proportion of cases. The liver may be of normal size or enlarged. For a long time the surface is smooth but eventually it becomes nodular. The most significant histological lesion is **piecemeal necrosis** (Fig. 20.23), which is defined as 'the destruction of liver cells at an interface between parenchyma and connective tissue, together with a predominantly lymphocytic or plasma cell infiltrate' (Bianchi *et al.*, 1977). The inflammatory cells infiltrate between liver cells, which show *feathery degeneration* (swelling and irregular cytoplasmic vacuolation) and eventual necrosis. Fibrosis occurs early, and when regenerative activity occurs groups of hepatocytes surroun-

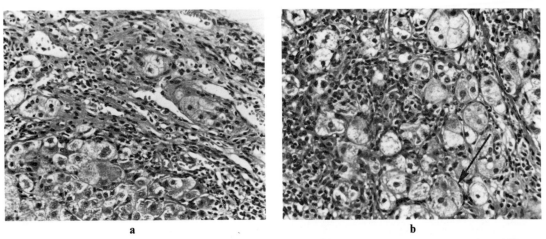

a   b

Fig. 20.23 Chronic active hepatitis with piecemeal necrosis. Note in **a**, the irregular margin between fibrous septum and parenchyma, with trapping of liver cells within the fibrous tissue, and a lymphocytic and plasma cell infiltrate extending among liver cells. In **b**, the extension of inflammatory cells between liver cells is also evident: note the feathery degeneration of the liver cells and the formation of liver-cell rosettes (*arrowed*), an indication of regenerative activity. **a** and **b** × 225.

ded by fibrous tissue produce pseudoglandular rosettes (Fig. 20.23b).

Histologically, two broad categories of chronic active hepatitis are recognised: (a) chronic active hepatitis with predominantly portal and periportal inflammation and piecemeal necrosis affecting the periportal hepatocytes. Extension of this necrosis and accompanying fibrosis results in fibrous septa linking portal tracts, and there is also extension into the parenchyma producing progressive distortion of the normal architecture (Fig. 20.24); (b) chronic active hepatitis with bridging hepatic necrosis; in this form hepatic necrosis and fibrosis extend between adjacent hepatic veins and between hepatic veins and portal tracts: there is also piecemeal necrosis of hepatocytes at the margins of the septa (Fig. 20.25). Both forms usually progress to a macronodular cirrhosis, but this tends to develop more rapidly in (b) than in (a).

In both groups the features of acute hepatitis may be superimposed, particularly during clinical relapse, and this produces a more generalised parenchymal involvement. When chronic active hepatitis is a sequel to hepatitis B infection then 'ground-glass' hepatocytes (p. 671) may be identified. Remission may occur spontaneously, with greatly reduced intensity of the inflammatory and destructive processes, and may also be produced by treatment with corticosteroids and azathioprine. The prognosis,

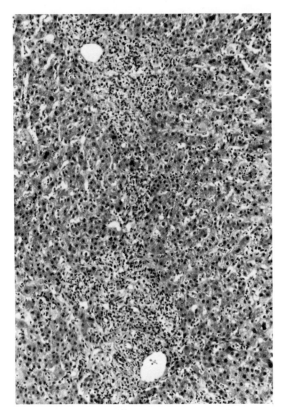

Fig. 20.24 Chronic active hepatitis: the inflammation here is predominantly portal and periportal with early portal–portal bridging: there is also diffuse inflammation within the parenchyma. × 120.

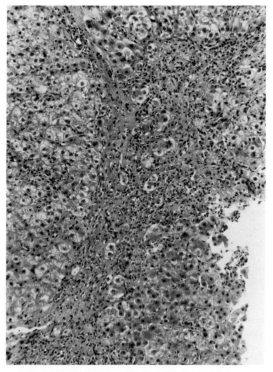

Fig. 20.25 Chronic active hepatitis with central–central and central–portal bridging septa causing architectural distortion and there is well-marked piecemeal necrosis at the fibrous/parenchymal interface. × 120.

however, is variable. About 50 per cent of patients survive longer than 5 years, but recent reports suggest that this figure is increased by better therapeutic management.

Recently a *chronic lobular hepatitis* has been described, in which the histological features are indistinguishable from those of acute viral hepatitis, but these persist for years. The diagnosis is dependent on serial biopsy in patients with biochemical evidence of hepatitis. It is not known whether progressive fibrosis occurs. Some are HB-associated, but in others a non-A:non-B aetiology is suspected.

The aetiology of chronic active hepatitis is controversial. HB antigen studies have shown that about 6 per cent of patients with Type B hepatitis fail to eliminate the virus and progress to chronic active hepatitis with persistence of HBsAg in the serum and of both surface and core antigens in the liver. This occurs also in some cases of non-A:non-B, but not in Type A hepatitis. *There is thus a virus-associated type of chronic active hepatitis.* In a proportion of patients (60 per cent of ours) *auto-antibodies* are found in the serum. These include antinuclear factor and smooth muscle antibodies: a positive LE cell test, rheumatoid factor and microsomal antibody are less frequent. None of these antibodies is specific for chronic active hepatitis, and there is no evidence that these are of aetiological significance. Currently the auto-antibody-associated disease is termed 'lupoid hepatitis'. There is usually no evidence of hepatitis B infection in such cases, and lupoid hepatitis is included by many in the group of auto-immune diseases although future studies may show Type non A: non B to be causal in some patients.

The elevation of serum immunoglobulin levels, the lymphocyte and plasma cell infiltrate in the liver, and the clinical response to immunosuppressive therapy all suggest that immune mechanisms are important in the pathogenesis of this disease. The differences in incidence relating to sex, the development of the disease in only a small percentage of Type B hepatitis patients, its rare occurrence in association with certain drugs (methyldopa and isoniazid) and the increased incidence of the HLA antigens A1 and B8 in patients with 'lupoid' hepatitis, also indicate that individual host factors are important. The cause of the persistence of viral infection in some cases is not known. The possible mechanisms of auto-immunisation are discussed elsewhere (p. 164). It seems that in both groups (viral and lupoid) the liver cells are the target of an aberrant and aggressive immune reaction, but the interplay between host factor and possible viral, drug or other aetiological agents remains obscure.

Alcoholic Liver Disease

The changes in the liver brought about by high alcohol consumption include *fatty liver, alcoholic hepatitis, hepatic fibrosis* and *cirrhosis*. Fatty change alone is considered to be a reversible disorder although when it is very severe, cholestasis and hepatocellular failure may develop; alcoholic hepatitis is considered to be the precursor of cirrhosis. *Excess alcohol consumption alone has now been shown to produce these hepatic lesions in man without any other obvious nutritional abnormality, and their degree and severity are related to the amount and duration of alcohol abuse.* This is supported by the experimental production of the entire spectrum of alcoholic liver injury in baboons on a nutritionally adequate diet.

Alcoholic fatty liver

Under controlled conditions, alcohol administration has been shown to produce hepatic fatty change regularly in man. After a single dose of alcohol, the fatty acids which accumulate in the liver are derived from fat depots, whereas with chronic alcohol intake they are predominantly of dietary origin, mobilisation of fat from adipose tissues being inhibited in this state, probably by acetate circulating as an end product of alcohol metabolism.

The relationships between alcohol metabolism and accumulation of fat in the hepatocyte are outlined in Fig. 20.26. Alcohol is broken down mainly by oxidation by alcohol dehydrogenase (ADH) in the cell sap. This results in the generation of hydrogen ions, and is reflected by an increase in the reduced nicotinamide adenine dinucleotide:nicotinamide adenine dinucleotide ratio (NADH:NAD), with a resultant change in reduction–oxidation (redox) potential. Some alcohol is also metabolised by microsomal enzymes in the smooth endo-

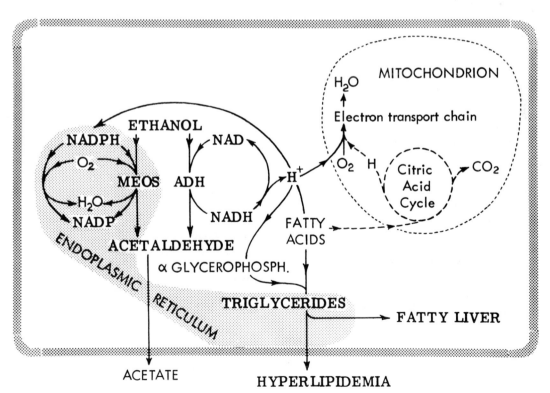

Fig. 20.26 Alcohol metabolism and fatty change in the liver cell, schematic representation. ADH = alcohol dehydrogenase; MEOS = microsomal ethanol oxidising system. Pathways that are decreased by alcohol are represented by interrupted lines. (Modified after and printed with permission from Professor C. S. Lieber.)

plasmic reticulum (SER), this pathway being known as the microsomal ethanol oxidising system (MEOS): it is dependent on the reduced form of NAD phosphate (NADPH), or an NADPH generating system. Normally it is thought that the ADH:MEOS ratio for alcohol metabolism is approximately 3:1, but in chronic alcohol abuse with an increase in SER a greater amount may be metabolised via the MEOS.

This increase in the SER is a well recognised feature of alcoholic liver damage, and it seems likely that induction of a number of microsomal enzyme systems may accompany this increase in SER and contribute to some of the other effects of alcohol on hepatocyte fat metabolism. In addition, the mitochondria are damaged by alcohol: they become swollen, sometimes markedly so, producing giant forms with disorganisation of the cristae, associated with increased fragility and permeability of the mitochondrial membrane.

The cumulative effects of these changes on hepatocyte fat metabolism are as follows: (*a*) increased lipogenesis *per se*; (*b*) accumulation of fatty acids, mainly because the NADH: NAD redox changes inhibit their oxidation via the citric acid cycle; this is aggravated by the direct damage to mitochondria. In addition there is an increase in the concentration of α-glycerophosphate and this results in trapping of fatty acids in the hepatocytes. These fatty acids are then esterified in the endoplasmic reticulum to triglycerides, some of which accumulate in the hepatocytes. In addition, however, increased lipoprotein synthesis occurs in the SER and some of these triglycerides are thus transported into the circulation, producing hyperlipidaemia; (*c*) cholesterol esters also accumulate, and there is evidence that this is partly due to increased cholesterol production in the SER and partly to a reduced cholesterol catabolic rate.

The mechanisms thus combine to produce hepatic fatty change, which can be detected after only two days of excess alcohol. Similarly, stopping alcohol results in a rapid mobilisation of the stored fat.

Alcoholic hepatitis and cirrhosis

In contrast to our understanding of alcohol-induced fatty liver, the metabolic events that lead to the development of alcoholic hepatitis and cirrhosis are still not understood. Both the volume of alcohol and the duration of alcohol abuse relate to the development of these lesions. Estimates suggest that a daily consumption of 80–160 g alcohol per day ($\frac{1}{3}$ to $\frac{2}{3}$ of a bottle of spirits, 1–2 bottles of wine or 4–8 cans of beer) for at least 5 years represents a hepatotoxic level of alcohol abuse. However, there are undefined host factors which determine susceptibility, and clinical evidence suggests that alcoholic hepatitis develops in only about 35 per cent of chronic alcoholics and only one third of these (i.e. 12 per cent of alcoholics) progress to cirrhosis.

In alcoholic hepatitis there is ballooning degeneration and necrosis of hepatocytes, associated with a neutrophil polymorph reaction (Fig. 20.27). Fatty change is usually also present. Characteristically the hepatitis develops around the hepatic vein branches (Fig. 20.28). Amorphous irregular eosinophilic aggregates of **Mallory's hyalin** (Mallory bodies—Fig. 20.29a) are seen within the cytoplasm of some hepatocytes; it has a fibrillar pattern on electron microscopy and represents an accumulation of microfilaments within the damaged cells. Giant mitochondria may also be noted (Fig. 20.29b). Fibrosis is an early feature, showing a striking pericellular distribution, and, with continued liver cell loss, producing fibrous septa with replacement of the parenchyma and obliteration

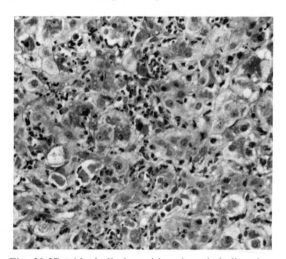

Fig. 20.27 Alcoholic hepatitis—there is ballooning degeneration of liver cells, and liver cell necrosis with a related neutrophil polymorphonuclear cell infiltrate. Mallory's hyalin is also identifiable. × 230.

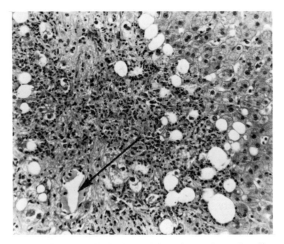

Fig. 20.28 Alcoholic hepatitis—the perivenular distribution of the lesion is evident (*hepatic vein arrowed*). There is well marked liver cell necrosis, neutrophil polymorphs are present in large numbers, and there is ballooning degeneration of liver cells, some fatty change and early fibrosis. × 150.

of sinusoids. In some instances the changes progress rapidly with diffuse parenchymal involvement, an intense polymorph infiltration, peripheral leucocytosis, and portal hypertension with progressive ascites and hepatocellular failure develop.

With continuing alcoholic hepatitis there is progressive fibrosis and scarring; fibrous septa extend and form links between contiguous perivenular areas and between perivenular areas and portal tracts. The liver architecture is increasingly distorted, fibrous contraction occurs and eventually a regular micronodular cirrhosis is established (see Fig. 20.30). If there is still further parenchymal cell loss and fibrosis, with accompanying nodular regeneration, the end-stage liver may show a mixed or macronodular cirrhosis.

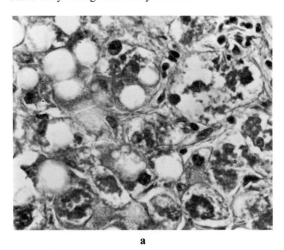

a

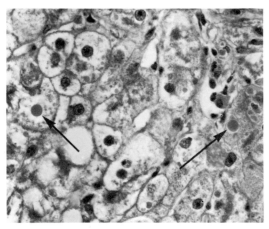

Fig. 20.29 Alcoholic hepatitis. **a** Mallory's hyalin is seen as irregular dark intracytoplasmic inclusions within swollen hepatocytes. × 310. **b** giant mitochondrion (*arrowed*) within a liver cell. × 350.

Cirrhosis

Definition. Cirrhosis is a condition involving the entire liver in which the parenchyma is changed into a large number of nodules separated from one another by irregular branching and anastomosing sheets of fibrous tissue. It results from long-continued loss of liver cells, with a persistent inflammatory reaction accompanied by fibrosis and compensatory hyperplasia. The progressive loss and regeneration of liver cells occurs focally and leads to disruption of the normal architecture, so that the portal tracts and hepatic veins are spaced irregularly in the nodules of surviving parenchyma, as well as being embedded in the fibrous septa. The condition is irreversible and the fibrosis and architectural distortion interfere with the flow of blood through the liver, with the result that, in most cases, loss of liver cells continues, even in the absence of the original cytotoxic agent (e.g. alcohol) and death usually results from hepatocellular failure, portal hypertension or a combination of both.

It is important to emphasise that the changes of cirrhosis affect the whole liver. Localised scarring caused, for example, by syphilitic gummas, is not included within the term cirrhosis; nor are mild degrees of more generalised hepatic fibrosis unaccompanied by loss of lobular architecture.

Pathological features

The liver may be of normal size or enlarged if there is fatty change of the liver cells or excessive development of hyperplastic regenerating nodules. Usually, however, it shrinks as the disease progresses, due to loss of liver cells exceeding regeneration, and terminally may weigh less than 1 kg. The surface is diffusely nodular and on section the parenchyma is seen to be divided up everywhere into rounded nodules, separated by bands of fibrous tissue (Figs. 20.30, 20.31). The colour varies considerably, depending on whether or not there is severe fatty change, on the presence or absence of cholestasis, and on the degree of congestion. Recently-divided liver cells are deficient in lipochrome, and the nodules are thus often paler than normal liver parenchyma.

Microscopy of the nodules shows loss of normal architecture, the portal tracts and central veins having lost their regular spacing. This is associated with foci of liver cell atrophy and loss, and foci of hypertrophy and hyperplasia, so that in some parts of a nodule the cells are small, and in others they are enlarged and include binucleate forms (Fig. 20.32).

The fibrous tissue runs in septa between parenchymal nodules: it may contain fine or dense collagen fibres, and varies in its vascularity depending on the duration of the cirrhotic process. It tends to involve the portal tracts, but also envelops hepatic veins. Some nodules are partially divided by incomplete septa extending into them. Collagen develops in relation to damaged liver cells, which presumably stimulate its production by fibroblasts or the perisinusoidal cells of Ito. Fibroblasts are not, however, conspicuous in early experimentally-induced cirrhosis. Commonly, single and small groups of liver cells are entrapped within the fibrous septa. Increased numbers of small bile duct elements are also present in the fibrous tissue—so-called 'ductular proliferation' (Fig. 20.33). Cholestasis is not usually marked (except in biliary cirrhosis, p. 687), but is seen focally in some cases and may develop terminally in hepatocellular failure.

Lymphocytes, and less commonly plasma cells, infiltrate the connective tissue and less frequently the parenchymal nodules. The infiltrates vary considerably in degree from case to case, and may be focal. Feathery degeneration of liver cells (p. 678) may be observed especially at the margins of the nodules, and this, particularly if associated with heavy lymphocytic infiltration, is an indication that the cirrhotic process is progressing actively. In necropsy material there is often extensive recent liver cell necrosis, attributable to terminal failure of the circulation.

Classification of cirrhosis

The differentiation of cirrhosis into various types has some clinical significance, and elucidation of the causes of cirrhosis, and thus eventually its prevention, are dependent on distinguishing between various types. Cirrhosis may be classified on an aetiological basis or on the morphological appearances of the liver.

The morphological divisions are into a **micronodular** or regular cirrhosis in which the nodules are of approximately the same size, i.e. up to 3 mm in diameter; a **macronodular** or irregular cirrhosis in which the nodules are of variable size and may range up to 1 cm in diameter; and a **mixed** type in which both small and large nodules are present (Figs. 20.30, 20.31). The value of this classification is doubtful. In our experience the correlation between aetiological factors and post-mortem hepatic morphology is poor. In the end-stage liver the distinctive morphological features of most aetiological types have largely disappeared. Furthermore the same aetiological factor may produce different morphological patterns. However, it is becoming increasingly apparent that examination of liver biopsy material reveals features which correlate with aetiological factors, and it now

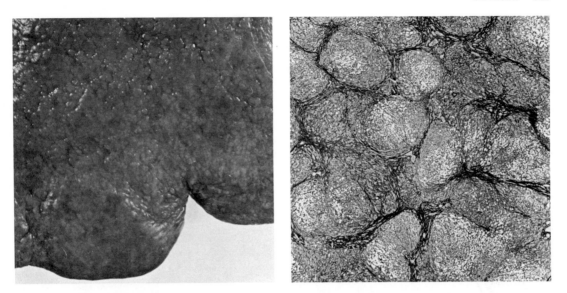

Fig. 20.30 Micronodular cirrhosis. *Left*, showing the fine uniform nodularity of the liver surface. × 0·75. *Right*, microscopy shows regular nodular regeneration: the hepatocytes in many of the nodules show marked fatty change. (Gordon and Sweet's reticulin.) × 20.

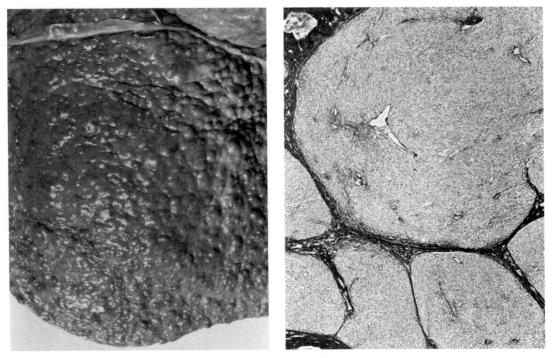

Fig. 20.31 Macronodular cirrhosis. *Left*, surface view, showing the coarse irregularity, with considerable variation of nodular size. × 0·75. *Right*, microscopy shows the variation in nodular size. (Gordon and Sweet's reticulin.) × 20.

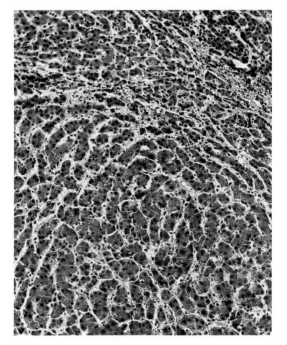

Fig. 20.32   Early cirrhosis of liver, showing hypertrophy of the liver cells in part of a nodule, and stretching and atrophy of the adjacent cells in upper part of field. × 90.

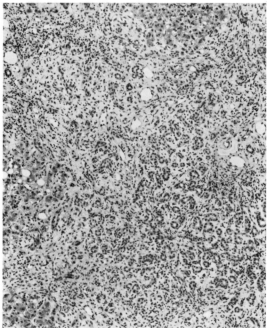

Fig. 20.33   Hepatic cirrhosis. Ductular proliferation in fibrous septa. × 83.

seems appropriate to give an aetiological classification and describe the pathological features most commonly found in each type. Such a classification is given in Table 20.2.

In our experience in this country, alcoholic cirrhosis comprises 30–35 per cent of all cases of cirrhosis, post-viral 15–20 per cent, 40–45 per cent are cryptogenic and the remainder form a miscellaneous group.

The features of some of these will now be briefly outlined.

Alcoholic cirrhosis

The pathological features have already been described. Alcoholic cirrhosis is commoner in men than in women, and develops mainly between 40 and 70 years of age, although recently younger cases have occurred, reflecting alterations in social drinking habits.

The degree of fatty change in the liver tends to diminish as the disease progresses. Reduction in size of the liver, if present, is usually slight, the weight being 1·2 kg or more. The early pattern of the cirrhosis is micronodular with loss of acinar architecture (Fig. 20.30), but

Table 20.2   Classification of Cirrhosis

Acquired

Alcoholic

Post-hepatitic or post-viral

Of unknown aetiology

> Cryptogenic
> Indian childhood cirrhosis

Biliary cirrhosis

> Primary (of unknown aetiology)
> Secondary (due to bile duct obstruction)

Congenital

Inborn errors of metabolism

> Haemochromatosis
> Thalassaemia
> Wilson's disease
> Alpha 1—antitrypsin deficiency
> Galactosaemia
> Type IV glycogen storage disease
> Tyrosinosis
> Fructose intolerance.

with further liver-cell loss and nodular hyperplasia the liver may show a mixed or a predominantly macronodular appearance.

The margins between nodules and fibrous septa are in most places fairly regular, the septa are narrow and composed of mature connective tissue, bile duct proliferation is slight, and lymphocytic infiltration is usually not heavy. The presence of Mallory's hyalin (Fig. 20.29a) is a useful diagnostic marker; it is, however, seen also in Wilson's disease, Indian childhood cirrhosis and in primary biliary cirrhosis.

Hepatic encephalopathy is less common than in post-viral cirrhosis. Additional but inconstant features include muscle wasting, anaemia, vitamin B and C deficiency, polyneuritis, alcoholic gastritis and peptic ulceration, chronic pancreatitis, Dupuytren's contracture and the mental changes of chronic alcoholism.

It is important to recognise this type of cirrhosis because it progresses more slowly than most other types, and improvement may result from abstinence from alcohol.

Post-viral (post-hepatitic) cirrhosis

The liver is usually smaller than in alcoholic cirrhosis, and fatty infiltration is slight or absent. It may be reduced to about 1 kg and the pattern of cirrhosis is usually macronodular (Fig. 20.31). The normal architecture is not completely lost, and can be detected in parts of some of the nodules. The liver cells vary considerably in size, multiple and large nuclei being common, and in places the margin between nodules and fibrous septa is irregular. The septa are thicker than in alcoholic cirrhosis, are often composed of younger, more cellular connective tissue, and are often, but not always, heavily infiltrated with lymphocytes. Bile duct proliferation is usually marked.

Post-hepatitic cirrhosis is commoner in women than in men, and occurs usually at a younger age than alcoholic cirrhosis, although the range is wide. In those cases which result from chronic active hepatitis, many of the additional features of this condition may persist. For example, the spleen is often palpable at an early stage, there may be skin rashes, arthropathy, leukopenia, etc., the serum IgG level may be high and there may be various autoantibodies. The disease has a poor prognosis, progressive portal hypertension and hepatocellular failure usually being more rapid than in alcoholic cirrhosis. There is also a higher incidence of liver cell carcinoma, especially where there is associated persistent HB antigenaemia.

Cryptogenic cirrhosis

Morphologically this group is a heterogeneous one. Most cases show a macronodular pattern, but micronodular and mixed patterns are also observed.

Biliary cirrhosis

Long-continued cholestasis, whether of extra- or intrahepatic origin, can lead to cirrhosis. Two varieties are recognised.

(*a*) *Primary biliary cirrhosis* in which a non-suppurative destructive process of unknown aetiology affects intrahepatic bile ducts.

(*b*) *Secondary biliary cirrhosis* resulting from prolonged mechanical obstruction of the larger biliary passages.

Primary biliary cirrhosis. This is an uncommon condition, occurring predominantly in middle-aged women, the female preponderance being 8 or 9 to 1. Clinically, the onset is insidious, frequently with pruritus and sometimes with a period of vague ill-health before jaundice appears. There is frequently a marked degree of hepatomegaly. The level of jaundice may fluctuate, and is initially usually mild. The serum alkaline phosphatase level is disproportionately high when compared with the increase in conjugated bilirubin. Serum aminotransferase levels are mildly raised and cholesterol levels may be markedly elevated. After a duration varying from months to many years, death results from liver failure or complications of portal hypertension. In longstanding cases malabsorption develops, and there may be osteomalacia and osteoporosis. There may also be features of secondary hypersplenism with varying degrees of leukopenia, thrombocytopenia and anaemia.

Although the clinical and biochemical features are those of obstructive jaundice, the large intrahepatic and extrahepatic bile ducts are patent. The most conspicuous change is an infiltration of lymphocytes and plasma cells in and around the epithelium of the smaller (50 μm or less) intrahepatic bile ducts. The epithelium shows degenerative changes in some areas and becomes heaped up in others (Fig. 20.34), and there is gradual destruction and loss of these smaller bile ducts. Macrophage granulomas resembling sarcoid follicles are found in about one-third of the cases and may be intimately related to bile ducts (Fig. 20.35). Later there is extension of the chronic inflammatory cell infiltrate to lie among the periportal parenchymal cells, and this is accompanied by portal fibrosis and cholestasis, usually most marked in the periportal areas. Accumulation of protein-bound copper in the periportal liver cells is a late feature and of unknown significance. Eventually irregular loss and nodular regeneration of liver cells complete the picture of cirrhosis, which is usually of a micronodular pattern. Mallory's hyalin is seen in 25 per cent of cases.

Aetiology. In this disease the initial lesion is an inflammatory destructive process involving septal and interlobular bile ducts. Later, parenchymal cell necrosis is superadded, probably due to cholestasis, and progresses to cirrhosis. In nearly all cases the serum contains, in

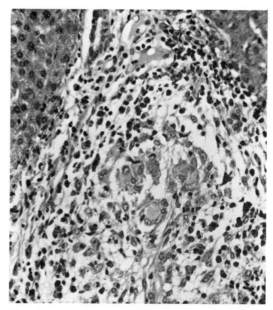

Fig. 20.35 Primary biliary cirrhosis, showing a miliary granuloma with formation of giant cells, lying in a portal area which is heavily infiltrated with lymphoid cells. × 350.

high titre, an antibody which reacts with a non-organ specific mitochondrial antigen. Demonstration of this antibody by indirect immunofluorescence provides a valuable confirmatory diagnostic test. The lymphocytic and plasma-cell infiltration of the portal tracts and bile duct epithelium, the occurrence of the mitochondrial antibody and the commonly elevated serum IgM levels, raise the probability that immune reactions are involved in this disease. Catabolism of some of the complement components is increased and there is evidence of circulating immune complexes in most cases. Sensitisation to an antigen present in bile has been demonstrated in some patients, but its significance is not yet known.

Secondary (obstructive) biliary cirrhosis. Unrelieved obstruction to the outflow of bile from the liver from any cause results, in time, in secondary biliary cirrhosis. The rate of development of cirrhosis is extremely variable, and depends partly on the degree of obstruction. In some cases, and particularly when obstruction is due to gallstones, an ascending bacterial cholangitis is superadded and, if severe, leads to necrosis and abscess formation (Fig. 20.36). In obstruction due to neoplasms, e.g. cancer of the head of the pancreas, the period of survival is

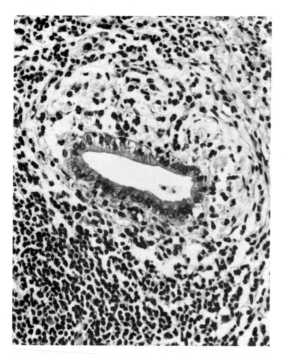

Fig. 20.34 Primary biliary cirrhosis, showing an intrahepatic bile duct with surrounding inflammatory reaction. The duct epithelium is unduly basophilic with vacuolation of the cells lining the upper margin. × 350.

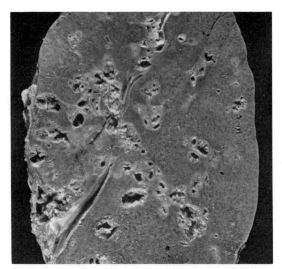

Fig. 20.36 Liver slice from a case of large duct obstruction and ascending cholangitis: numerous abscesses, some of which show central breakdown, are present in the parenchyma. × 0·6.

limited and death often results before cirrhosis has developed.

The early changes following biliary obstruction consist of cholestasis, bile accumulation developing in the hepatocytes, bile canaliculi and Kupffer cells, particularly in the perivenular zones (Fig. 20.37), and in the small bile ducts. Subsequently the larger bile ducts become dilated and filled with concentrated bile. After weeks or months a progressive inflammatory reaction develops in the portal

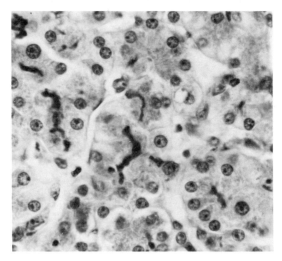

Fig. 20.37 Perivenular cholestasis in early extrahepatic obstruction. × 390.

tracts, which become oedematous and infiltrated with lymphocytes, plasma cells and significant numbers of polymorphs (Fig. 20.38). Bile duct proliferation develops, and there is fibroblast proliferation and development of fibrous septa extending irregularly into the parenchyma and linking up with adjacent portal tracts. Periductal fibrosis is often also a feature.

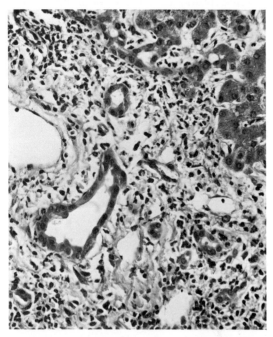

Fig. 20.38 Extra-hepatic obstruction with oedema of the portal area, a prominent neutrophil infiltrate, some of which is closely related to the bile ducts, and early duct proliferation. × 250.

Single or small groups of liver cells become pigmented, swollen and show feathery degeneration. Aggregates of such necrotic cells may form distinct '**bile infarcts**'. Rupture of canals of Hering adjacent to the portal tracts may occur with escape of bile to form **bile lakes**. Biliary granulomas may also be a feature. Loss of liver cells and fibrosis result eventually in disturbance of architecture and, together with the development of regenerating nodules, progress to a micronodular cirrhosis. Possibly because the cholestasis interferes with their function, the hepatocytes show marked hyperplasia, and consequently the liver is enlarged: it is also firm from the increase in fibrous tissue, deeply jaundiced and the surface is usually finely nodular. Portal hypertension may eventually supervene, but death results more often from liver failure or intercurrent infection.

The cirrhosis appears to be due to the harmful effect of retained bile upon liver parenchymal cells; in some cases this is aggravated by the occurrence of ascending bacterial cholangitis. In man, the best example of pure obstructive biliary cirrhosis without infection is seen in congenital biliary atresia (Fig. 20.39) which may involve either the extrahepatic or intrahepatic biliary tree. In the extrahepatic variety there is marked jaundice and death

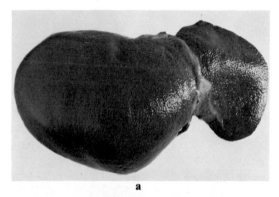

a

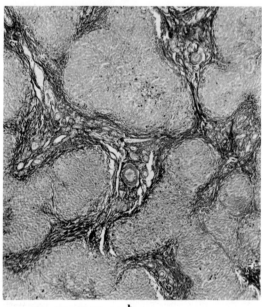

b

Fig. 20.39 Secondary biliary cirrhosis. The liver of a child with congenital atresia of the biliary tract. (**a**) uniform fine nodularity of the surface. × 0·7. (**b**) micronodular cirrhosis with cholestasis. × 25. (Dr. A. M. MacDonald.)

occurs within a few months of birth. Patchy atresia of smaller intrahepatic bile ducts sometimes has a more prolonged course with survival into early adult life: secondary biliary cirrhosis develops, as described above, but is of a fine pattern with portal–portal linkages predominant.

Congenital cirrhosis

Many of the metabolic abnormalities listed in Table 20.2 can cause cirrhosis in childhood. In addition, there are other causes of cirrhosis in childhood, e.g. *Indian childhood cirrhosis* which is common in 1–3-year-olds in that country. It is of unknown aetiology, but gross accumulation of copper in the liver cells has been demonstrated recently. Biliary cirrhosis may result from congenital intra- or extrahepatic biliary atresia, and from fibrocystic disease (p. 721).

Wilson's disease (Hepatolenticular degeneration) is an inherited disorder of copper metabolism determined by a pair of autosomal recessive genes, and with a prevalence of 1 per 200 000 of the population. Increasing amounts of copper accumulate in and damage the liver, the lenticular nuclei, the kidneys and the eyes. The aetiological biochemical abnormality in Wilson's disease is found in the liver: there is an increase in the hepatic lysosomal copper concentration presumed to be due to defective excretion of copper via the bile. This defect is associated in most patients with reduced hepatic synthesis of the serum copper glycoprotein, caeruloplasmin. The accumulation of copper in the liver begins in infancy, and in time excess amounts diffuse from liver to blood and accumulate in and damage other target organs.

In the liver, fatty change, hepatocellular necrosis and fibrosis, sometimes morphologically resembling chronic active hepatitis, and with Mallory's hyalin in a proportion of cases, progress at variable rates to produce a macronodular cirrhosis. The changes in the nervous system are described on page 770. There is excess urinary copper excretion, and defective tubular absorption leads to amino-aciduria. In the eyes, deposits of copper in Descemet's membrane of the cornea produce the diagnostic Kayser-Fleischer rings. Treatment with D-penicillamine by increasing urinary copper excretion is of clinical value.

Haemochromatosis. A general account of this disease, and of other conditions causing gross iron overload, is given on pp. 282–3. The liver is the major organ affected, but iron deposition and fibrosis of the pancreas and other viscera is also present. There is a characteristic pattern of hepatic fibrosis, and in the later stages a micro-nodular cirrhosis is established. Excess iron deposits are present in hepatocytes, Kupffer cells, fibrous septal macrophages and in bile duct epithelium. Increased amounts of lipo-fuscin are also present in hepatocytes.

The development of cirrhosis and the intensity of iron deposition are not closely correlated. However, the iron deposition is considered to be fibrogenic, and removal of iron by repeated venesection results in some reduction of the fibrosis. Primary carcinoma of the liver may develop in both treated and untreated patients.

Pathogenesis of cirrhosis

Cirrhosis results from long-continued loss of liver cells, accompanied by compensatory liver cell hyperplasia and nodule formation, and by a chronic inflammation and progressive repla-cement fibrosis, i.e. chronic hepatitis. It is, in fact, the outcome of prolonged hepatocellular necrosis, the cause of which is, more often than not, unknown. *Eventually the irregular liver-cell hyperplasia and fibrosis interfere with blood flow to such an extent that, whatever the initial cause of the injury, hepatocyte loss continues as a result of ischaemia and the changes become pro-gressive, leading to death from hepatocellular failure and/or portal hypertension* (Fig. 20.40). In experimental animals liver cell injury, e.g. by CCl_4, is followed by replacement of any liver cells destroyed and a return to normality. This also occurs after repeated liver injury unless the CCl_4 is administered at intervals of less than 10 days, when complete regeneration does not occur and the lesion progresses to cirrhosis (Fig. 20.41).

The possible aetiological factors in human cirrhosis have already been enumerated, but in over 40 per cent of cases in this country none of these factors can be incriminated and the aetiology remains unknown. Whereas in secon-dary biliary cirrhosis the progression to cirrho-sis is predictable, in alcohol abuse only 10 per cent of patients develop cirrhosis. Similarly, in acute Type B viral hepatitis only a small per-

LIVER CELL INJURY
by

alcohol
hepatitis B virus
chronic cholestasis
etc.   } + HOST FACTORS

→ Progressive hepatocyte necrosis

Chronic inflammation → Fibrosis → Ischaemia

Liver cell regeneration → Hyperplastic nodules

CIRRHOSIS

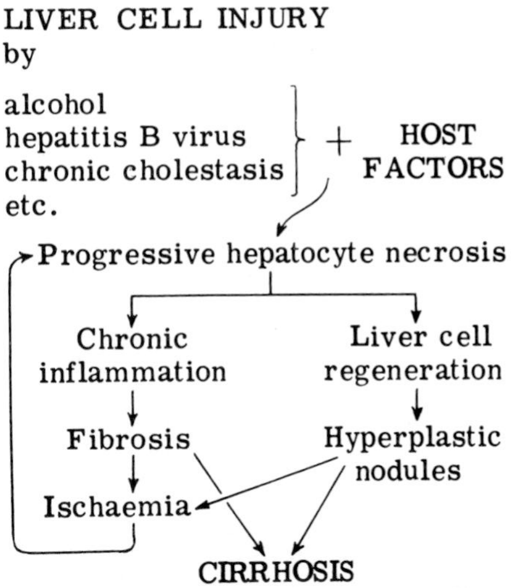

Fig. 20.40 The pathogenesis of cirrhosis.

centage progress to chronic active hepatitis and cirrhosis (p. 671). In others the chronic hepatitis is sub-clinical and after some years of apparent well-being the patients present with manifesta-tions of cirrhosis.

In cryptogenic cirrhosis there is, by defini-tion, no history of any previous acute liver dis-ease and the stage of morphological progressive

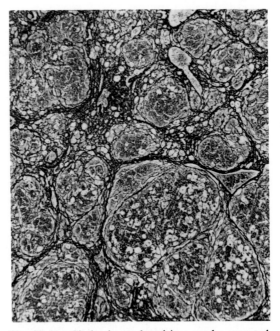

Fig. 20.41 Cirrhosis produced in a rat by repeated inhalation of carbon tetrachloride (see p. 20). (Gordon and Sweet's reticulin.) × 40.

chronic hepatitis has been clinically silent. While some such cases are probably the result of an episode of viral hepatitis, more sensitive tests for evidence of previous virus infection must be developed before this relationship can be elucidated.

It is now generally accepted that, in spite of apparently contrary experimental evidence in rats, malnutrition *per se* is not a cause of cirrhosis in man, although it may be a contributory factor and may aggravate the effects of alcohol abuse and of viral hepatitis.

The sequence of events in the development of cirrhosis is summarised diagrammatically in Fig. 20.40. Predisposing factors, such as known metabolic defects, may explain occasional cases, but usually the nature of such factors is not clear. The progression from an acute to a chronic hepatitis may be due to persistence of the aetiological agent, as has been shown in some cases of Type B virus hepatitis, or may be the result of auto-immunisation or some other cytotoxic immunological reaction, as has been postulated in some cases of chronic active hepatitis and in primary biliary cirrhosis. Similarly the factors responsible for initiating hepatic fibrosis also remain obscure, but the importance of the fibrosis in the progression of the cirrhosis and in the development of the secondary effects of cirrhosis is not in doubt. Fibrosis is a feature of chronic inflammation of any sort and so is to be expected in chronic hepatitis.

Effects of cirrhosis

Cirrhosis has two important effects, **portal hypertension** and **hepatocellular failure** which are described below. It is the major cause of these two conditions, particularly when they occur together. **Liver-cell carcinoma** arises in 10–15 per cent of all cirrhotic patients in this country, the incidence varying with sex and with different types of cirrhosis.

Portal Hypertension and Hepatocellular Failure

Portal hypertension

The normal portal venous pressure is 7 mm of mercury. Portal hypertension occurs when there is interference with the blood flow within the liver or obstruction of the portal vein (p. 664). The obstruction may be **post-sinusoidal** as in cirrhosis, veno-occlusive disease, hepatic vein obstruction, alcoholic hepatitis and congestive cardiac failure, or **pre-sinusoidal** as in schistosomiasis, congenital hepatic fibrosis and portal vein obstruction. Massive splenomegaly with increased splenic blood flow can also cause portal hypertension in the absence of obstruction. Effects of portal hypertension result from some of the portal blood by-passing the liver and entering the systemic veins at sites of portal-systemic anastomosis. In cirrhosis, in addition, some of the blood which does enter the liver does not perfuse the liver cells adequately and is shunted into the hepatic veins.

Portal-systemic anastomoses at the following sites become enlarged, with varicosity of the veins.

(i) in the lower oesophagus and upper gastric fundus, between the left gastric vein (portal) and the azygos minor vein (systemic).

(ii) in the lower rectum and anus, between the superior haemorrhoidal (portal) and the middle and inferior haemorrhoidal veins (systemic).

(iii) in the falciform ligament between the left branch of the portal vein and the superficial veins of the anterior abdominal wall, via the para-umbilical veins.

(iv) at points of contact between abdominal viscera and the posterior abdominal wall.

The most important anastomoses are those at the gastro-oesophageal junction, where **spontaneous rupture of the large submucosal varices** (Fig. 19.22, p. 604) results in bleeding which may be fatal and also contributes to the development of hepatocellular failure (see below).

Portal hypertension results in **splenomegaly**, due primarily to passive congestion, but often with lymphoid hyperplasia. *Hypersplenism* (p. 565) may result in anaemia, thrombocytopenia and granulocytopenia. Focal haemorrhages may occur in the spleen and produce siderotic fibrotic nodules (Gamna Gandy bodies).

Portal hypertension is a major factor in the production of **ascites** (p. 658). Portocaval, lieno-renal or other surgical shunt procedures may be carried out to reduce the hypertension and thus the risk of bleeding from oesophageal varices. These procedures, however, are of limited value in patients with portal hypertension and cirrhosis, for they increase the danger of hepatic encephalopathy (see below).

Hepatocellular failure (liver failure)

Although the liver has a large functional reserve and a high regenerative capacity when injured, liver insufficiency, manifested by failure of the liver cells to perform adequately their various functions, occurs both in patients with severe acute liver injury and in advanced cases of chronic liver disease. **Acute liver failure** occurs in severe viral hepatitis, as an adverse reaction to certain drugs, as a result of drug overdose or poisoning by certain hepatotoxic chemicals, in massive liver cell necrosis of unknown cause, and occasionally in severe fatty infiltration of the liver. Hepatic failure results directly from the parenchymal cell injury and is a manifestation of the degree of hepatocellular damage. **Chronic liver failure** is most often due to cirrhosis. It may occur even in patients with a relatively large amount of surviving liver tissue, and is attributable in part to the interference with hepatic blood flow which results from the disturbed architecture and fibrosis of the liver. Acute or chronic hepatic failure may be precipitated by factors such as gastro-intestinal bleeding, the use of diuretic or narcotic drugs, bacterial infection, paracentesis, portacaval shunt and other surgical operations.

Because of the multiple functions of the liver, acute or chronic hepatic insufficiency gives rise to a complex syndrome, which includes neurological disturbances, jaundice, defects of blood coagulation and renal failure. Additional features include ascites and oedema, endocrine and circulatory disturbances, but these occur mainly in chronic failure. The mechanisms involved in these manifestations of liver failure are discussed below.

Neurological disturbances comprise mental confusion with apathy, disorientation or excitement, a coarse flapping tremor and muscular rigidity, and finally coma. These are accompanied by characteristic changes in the electro-encephalogram and by a number of biochemical abnormalities. All these features are reversible, and morphological changes have been observed only in the astrocytes, the nuclei of which are enlarged, sometimes to 25 μm in diameter; the chromatin is condensed around the nuclear membrane, and the nucleolus is unduly conspicuous. In occasional cases, however, progressive brain damage may occur. In acute liver failure, cerebral oedema is often a significant contributory cause of death.

The neurological disorder is probably due to a metabolic disturbance, for it is potentially fully reversible: it is of multifactorial aetiology and in individual cases the following factors are probably involved in various combinations.

(i) Failure of the liver to remove potentially toxic agents: in particular, nitrogenous bacterial metabolites absorbed from the gut may avoid detoxication in the liver, due to liver cell loss and/or portasystemic by-pass of the liver. An increased nitrogen load from a high protein intake or haemorrhage from oesophageal varices often precipitates hepatic encephalopathy. In most cases there is an increased level of ammonia in the blood, and this probably contributes significantly to the hepatic coma, although the correlation is imperfect and other metabolic products of intestinal bacteria have also been implicated. Increase in serum aromatic amino acids, and/or a decrease in branched-chain amino acids, increase in serum short-chain fatty acids and mercaptans, may also be important.

(ii) Increased cerebral sensitivity to a variety of agents, possibly due to interference with oxidative metabolism via the citric acid cycle and consequent ATP depletion.

(iii) Changes in vascular permeability, particularly affecting the blood brain barrier.

(iv) The hypotension, anoxia and electrolyte disturbances which accompany hepatic failure.

(v) Loss of (unidentified) factors normally produced by liver cells and regarded as essential for normal neuronal function.

The nature of the functional neuronal changes in hepatic encephalopathy is even less certain.

Jaundice is usual in acute hepatocellular failure, its severity reflecting the degree of hepatocellular damage. In very severe cases, however, death may result before jaundice has become conspicuous. In chronic failure the degree and type of jaundice depends upon the nature of the liver disease. In secondary biliary cirrhosis, obstructive jaundice precedes and accompanies the development of hepatic dysfunction. In other cirrhoses, jaundice is a late but bad prognostic sign, and is usually only of mild or moderate degree. The precise mechanisms of the hyperbilirubinaemia are uncertain, but are considered to be most likely due to failure of hepatocytes to excrete bilirubin.

Coagulation defects result primarily from defective synthesis of a number of coagulation factors by the liver, notably prothrombin, fibrinogen and factors V, VII, IX and X. There may also be thrombocytopenia (accompanied sometimes by anaemia and leukopenia) due to hypersplenism, and, particularly in acute failure, disseminated intravascular coagulation with consumption of clotting factors.

Renal failure may develop in both acute and chronic hepatic failure. Acute renal failure may result from hypotension due to bleeding from oesophageal varices. Impairment of renal function without morphological damage may also occur terminally in hepatic failure: this is characterised by reduced glomerular filtration rate and progressive oliguria, but without a fall in urine osmolarity. The mechanisms remain uncertain but the renal failure is reversible with improvement in hepatic function.

Ascites and oedema. Ascites does not result from hepatocellular failure unless there is also portal hypertension, as in cirrhosis. In chronic liver failure there is diminished production of plasma albumin, with a consequent fall in plasma osmotic pressure. The portal hypertension increases the intravascular hydrostatic pressure in the microvasculature of the gut, and in addition there is leakage of hepatic lymph because of obstruction to its outflow from the liver. Secondary hyperaldosteronism (p. 258) occurs in some cases, and may, by inducing sodium retention, aggravate the oedema and ascites. The causation of secondary hyperaldosteronism, and why it occurs in some cases and not others, is not clear. Peripheral oedema is due mainly to the fall in plasma osmotic pressure.

Endocrine disturbances. In chronic liver failure there is, in both sexes, a tendency to depression of libido, sterility and loss of body hair. In men, the testes are frequently atrophic, and occasionally one or both breasts are enlarged (*gynaecomastia*). These effects result from failure of hepatic inactivation of oestrogens, which have a stimulating effect upon the breast and may also suppress the production of pituitary gonadotrophin, thus explaining the testicular atrophy. The exact mechanisms of the menstrual irregularities, secondary amenorrhoea and breast atrophy which occur in women are not clear. Two well-known vascular changes in liver failure are exaggerated mottling, due to patchy congestion, of the skin of the palms—the so-called '*liver palms*'—and the development in the superior vena caval drainage area of small leashes of dilated vessels in the superficial dermis, radiating out from a central arteriole—the '*spider naevus*'. Both these features may occur in normal pregnancy and probably have a hormonal basis.

Circulatory disturbances. A hyperkinetic circulation characterised by peripheral vasodilatation and an increase in circulation rate, cardiac output and blood volume may occur in hepatic failure. This may possibly result from circulating vaso-active substances or may be due to impaired sympathetic responsiveness. Cyanosis with arterial hypoxia is not uncommon and finger clubbing develops in a small percentage of patients.

Other features. In hepatocellular failure, particularly when acute, the breath has a peculiar sweetish smell termed '*foetor hepaticus*', possibly due to failure of the liver to detoxify substances absorbed from the gut. *Fever* is also common in acute failure, but profound *hypothermia* has been described in chronic failure. *Bacteraemia*, particularly with coliform organisms, is also a complication. General ill-health with anorexia, wasting and vomiting is common.

Non-Viral Infections of the Liver

The common virus infections of the liver have been dealt with on p. 669 *et seq.* Accordingly this account deals with infections by bacteria and protozoa, and infestation by metazoan parasites.

Pyogenic infections. Because of improvements in diagnostic facilities and the earlier use of antibiotics, pyogenic infection of the liver is less common than it used to be, and when it does occur it is usually due to extension of bacteria within the biliary duct system—**ascending cholangitis.** *Escherichia coli,* either alone or with other bacteria, is the commonest causal organism. Bile duct obstruction is the most important predisposing cause, and because bacterial infection commonly accompanies stones, obstruction by a stone is especially liable to be complicated by suppurating cholangitis. The process extends into the liver tissue, giving rise to multiple abscesses in which the pus is characteristically bile-stained.

Multiple abscess formation in the liver also results from suppurative phlebitis affecting the veins around a septic focus in the abdomen or pelvis, e.g. acute appendicitis, diverticulitis of the colon, or infected haemorrhoids: the infection may reach the liver by **septic emboli** or by **portal pylephlebitis.** Umbilical sepsis in the neonate sometimes spreads to the intrahepatic portal vein radicles via the umbilical vein.

Abscesses may also develop in the liver in septicaemia or pyaemia, but these are less frequent and less important than in various other organs.

Actinomycosis. Actinomycosis occurs in and around the appendix, from where it may extend to the liver by the portal venous system or by direct spread. Multiple abscesses form in the liver separated by granulation and fibrous tissue, and produce a honeycomb appearance. The abscesses contain thick greenish-yellow pus, and the characteristic yellowish or greyish sulphur granules, which comprise aggregates of the branching filament of the causal organism—*Actinomyces israelii* (p. 221).

Leptospirosis. The spirochaete *Leptospira icterohaemorrhagiae* causes endemic chronic renal infection in rats, and can survive in water or damp conditions for some time after excretion in rat urine. It can penetrate the intact human skin or may gain entry via the respiratory or oral routes, and after an incubation period of 10–15 days causes an intense febrile illness (**Weil's disease**) with conjunctivitis, renal tubular damage, a haemorrhagic tendency, jaundice, focal myocardial and skeletal muscle necrosis and often a mild lymphocytic meningitis. The disease occurs chiefly in sewer workers, agricultural workers and fish handlers. Various other leptospira, including *L. canicola* from dogs, can cause a similar but usually milder disease in man.

Liver biopsy may show liver cell degeneration, prominent mitotic activity of the hepatocytes and sometimes focal necrosis, cholestasis and haemorrhages. In some cases, however, the changes are slight. After death, the liver cells are often rounded and separated from one another (Fig. 20.42). This may be a post mortem change but it is certainly seen when necropsy has been performed within a few

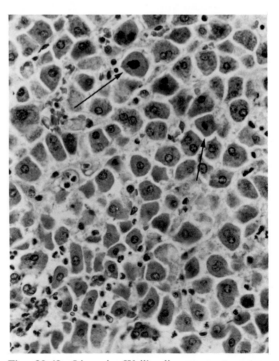

Fig. 20.42 Liver in Weil's disease: post-mortem liver showing separation and rounding of hepatocytes, proliferative activity (*arrows*) and focal liver cell necrosis with a related inflammatory cell exudate (*lower left*). × 400.

hours of death, and is sometimes helpful in suggesting the diagnosis.

The mortality rate is about 15 per cent. Death may occur in the first week, when haemorrhagic consolidation of the lungs may be the most conspicuous lesion. Later, death is usually due to renal failure, which in these patients is almost always accompanied by evident hepatic involvement.

Syphilis. The liver is frequently affected in both congenital and acquired syphilis. In **congenital syphilis**, the commonest lesion is a diffuse interstitial pericellular fibrosis, proliferating fibroblasts extending between the sinusoidal endothelium and the liver cells producing compression or ischaemic atrophy of the hepatocytes. A dense interstitial mononuclear cell infiltrate is also present. Miliary gummas (p. 220) are not uncommon. In fatal cases, spirochaetes are usually abundant throughout the liver. In **acquired syphilis**, a diffuse hepatitis, sometimes with miliary granulomas, may occur in the secondary stage. Hepatic gummas were a common feature of tertiary syphilis before effective treatment became available. They were typically rounded, might be multiple and became very large (>10 cm). They presented the usual features of central necrosis and peripheral fibrosis which might extend as dense radiating bands into the surrounding parenchyma. Healing usually occurred even without treatment, and scarring was extensive, producing gross distortion of the liver—*hepar lobatum*. The adjacent tissues usually became adherent to the liver. Amyloid disease, sometimes irregular in distribution, was also a common complication.

Relapsing fever. This is a spirochaetal disease, caused by various species of *Borrelia*. It may be louse- or tick-borne. Large epidemics have occurred in the past and sporadic outbreaks are encountered in various parts of the world. Jaundice occurs in severe infections, accompanied by biochemical evidence of liver cell injury. In fatal cases there is perivenular necrosis and a moderate generalised inflammation of the liver.

Tuberculosis. Tuberculous lesions are less common in the liver than in most other organs. In generalised tuberculosis miliary tubercles occur, and are distributed irregularly in the parenchyma: sometimes they are large enough to be visible to the naked eye and may have a caseous bile-stained centre. Rarely, a few large caseous lesions result from blood spread, and may be identifiable only by the finding of tubercle

bacilli. Tuberculous cholangitis is extremely rare, and probably results from ulceration of a tuberculous nodule of the liver into a bile duct.

Other causes of tubercle-like granulomas in the liver. Lesions resembling tubercle follicles occur in the liver in several non-tuberculous conditions. They consist of aggregates of epithelioid cells, often with one or more multinucleated giant cells which may contain various cytoplasmic inclusions, and show little or no central necrosis. Such lesions occur in most cases of sarcoidosis and brucellosis, and are seen frequently in tuberculoid leprosy and histoplasmosis; they occur sometimes in secondary syphilis and in chronic berylliosis due to inhalation of beryllium compounds. Tubercle-like follicles are seen also in rather less than 40 per cent of liver biopsies from patients with early primary biliary cirrhosis and around impacted ova in schistosomiasis. Occasionally granulomas are found incidentally in the liver in individuals not obviously suffering from tuberculosis or any of the above conditions; their significance is unknown.

Protozoal parasites

Hepatic amoebiasis. This is a complication of amoebic dysentery (p. 634), brought about by amoebae entering colonic venules and passing by the portal vein to the liver, which they then colonise. Liver lesions may be the presenting clinical feature, or may occur only many years after the colonic lesions have apparently subsided.

In the liver they multiply in the sinusoids, releasing a proteolytic enzyme which digests the liver tissue producing a cavity—the so-called 'tropical abscess'. For reasons unknown, there is usually a single 'abscess', most often in the upper part of the right lobe and measuring up to 15 cm in diameter. It may ulcerate through the diaphragm into the lung and discharge via the bronchus, or less commonly may rupture into the pericardial or peritoneal cavities.

Macroscopically, the lesion has a compressed fibrous capsule, with an irregular shaggy necrotic inner wall and the cavity contains thick glairy fluid, often chocolate-coloured or showing admixture of blood (Fig. 20.43). On microscopic examination the contents include necrotic liver cells, granular debris and a varying number of red cells. Only a few neutrophils are

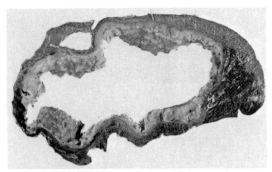

Fig. 20.43 Sagittal section of right lobe of liver, extensively replaced by a large amoebic 'abscess': some surviving liver parenchyma on the right.

present and the lesion is thus not really an abscess. *Entamoeba histolytica* may be demonstrable in the inner aspects of this necrotic wall (Fig. 20.44), but are rarely present in the fluid.

Malaria. In the incubation period, malarial parasites develop within hepatocytes but they do not bring about permanent hepatic damage. In the stage of blood infection, colonised erythrocytes are phagocytosed by Kupffer cells, which show marked hypertrophy and hyperplasia and contain abundant dark brown granules or 'malarial pigment'.

Kala-azar (visceral leishmaniasis). The liver is usually enlarged, and there is hyperplasia of the Kupffer cells which are distended by large

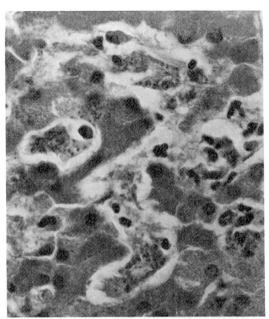

Fig. 20.45 Liver in Kala-azar: distended Kupffer cells laden with Leishman–Donovan bodies are easily seen. × 650.

numbers of Leishmann–Donovan bodies (Fig. 20.45). There may be some fibrosis, but cirrhosis does not result.

Metazoal parasites

Schistosomiasis. Infestation with *Schistosoma mansoni*, in which the adult worms colonise the veins of the colon, is prevalent in Egypt and various other parts of Africa, in the West Indies and parts of South America. *S. japonicum* infestation occurs in Japan, China and the Philippines, and the worms are present in the veins of the small intestine. Both species produce large numbers of ova, some of which enter the portal venous circulation and impact in the liver. Adult worms may also colonise the larger portal vein branches, and deposit their eggs in the adjacent liver tissue. The life cycles of the parasites are similar to that of *S. haematobium* (p. 867), which only rarely involves the liver.

The worms evoke both an antibody response and cell-mediated immunity in the host. In experimental animal infections there is evidence that the adult worms are protected by a coating of mucopolysaccharide which may be of host origin, and which acts as an immunological barrier and prevents hypersensitivity reactions.

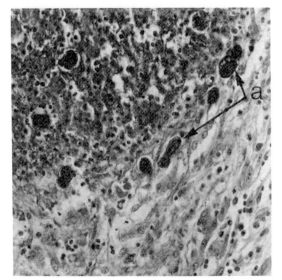

Fig. 20.44 Amoebic abscess of liver showing numerous amoebae (**a**) in the necrotic margin of a small recent lesion. × 200.

When ova are inappropriately laid in the tissues, however, they lack this coating and stimulate a delayed hypersensitivity reaction characterised by accumulation of epithelioid macrophages and lymphocytes and eventually dense fibrosis.

The morphological features of the human disease (Fig. 20.46) are, in general, consistent with similar immunological phenomena, but these have not been proven. Where there is extensive fibrosis of portal areas, the picture is that of 'pipe-stem' fibrosis, with irregular attenuated fibrous septa extending into the parenchyma (Fig. 20.47) but cirrhosis does not result. Portal hypertension may develop with marked enlargement of the spleen and there may be haemorrhage from oesophageal varices. Hepatocellular function is well maintained, and relief of portal hypertension by portacaval anastomosis may be of more clinical benefit than in cirrhosis.

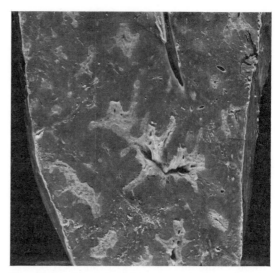

Fig. 20.47 Liver in schistosomiasis, showing the pale areas of fibrous tissue around the portal veins.

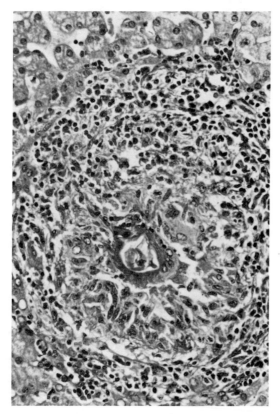

Fig. 20.46 *Schistosoma mansoni* infestation of liver, with a granulomatous reaction surrounding an ovum impacted in a portal vein branch. × 250. (Preparation kindly lent by Mr. C. Campbell.)

Hydatid disease. Hydatid is the cystic stage of *Echinococcus granulosus*, a small (3–6 mm long) tapeworm, and occurs most commonly in sheep, but also in cattle, pigs and men. Infection results from swallowing the ova shed in the faeces of dogs, which harbour the adult worm in the small intestine. Dogs become infected by eating the offal of infected sheep, cattle or pigs, thus enabling the life cycle to be completed. The disease in man results from close contact with infected dogs and possibly from eating contaminated vegetables. It is commonest in sheep-farming communities, notably in Australia, New Zealand and South America: in the United Kingdom it is uncommon except in parts of Wales.

The ingested ova have a chitinous coat which is digested by gastric juice, liberating the embryos. They invade the veins of the gastrointestinal tract and reach the liver via the portal vein, where most of them lodge. A few may pass into the pulmonary or systemic circulation, producing cysts in the lungs and other organs, e.g. muscles, kidneys, spleen and brain.

The commonest type of hydatid is a cyst of up to 20 cm diameter, usually multilocular due to the presence of daughter cysts, and with a thick wall comprising the inner germinal layer and an outer non-nucleated hyaline laminated layer, which in turn is surrounded by a layer of host granulation tissue; sometimes the liver is

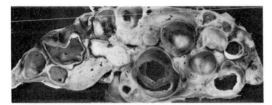

Fig. 20.48 Liver in hydatid disease, with multiple sharply circumscribed cysts replacing much of the organ. (Professors R. A. Joske and M. N.-I. Walters.)

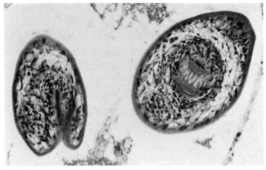

Fig. 20.49 Scolices of *Echinococcus granulosus* showing their rows of hooklets by which they become attached to the brood capsule. (Professor R. A. Joske and Dr. L. R. Matz.)

the site of a mass of small cysts, each approximately 6 mm in diameter (Fig. 20.48). Brood capsules bud from the germinal layer, and scolices are formed within the brood capsule from buds which develop on its inner surface (Fig. 20.49). The cysts contain straw-coloured fluid and rupture of brood capsules into this releases their scolices which form 'hydatid sand'.

The cysts occur most commonly in the right lobe of the liver. The symptoms are those of a slowly expanding lesion. The parasites may die in the cystic stage, which then undergoes calcification. The diagnosis is made radiologically or on scintiscanning of the liver, and by the demonstration of hypersensitivity to an intra-

dermal injection of hydatid antigen (the *Casoni test*).

Clonorchiasis and fascioliasis result from invasion of the biliary tree by the larvae of the Chinese liver fluke (*Clonorchis sinensis*) and the sheep fluke (*Fasciola hepatica*) respectively. Clonorchiasis results from eating inadequately cooked or raw fish. It can produce biliary obstruction and ascending cholangitis, and is characterised by marked proliferation of bile-duct-like elements (Fig. 20.50). Portal hypertension may develop, and there is a high incidence of

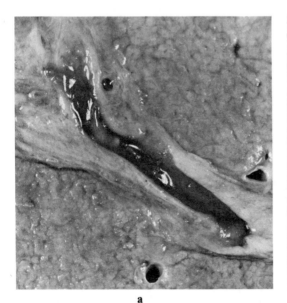

a

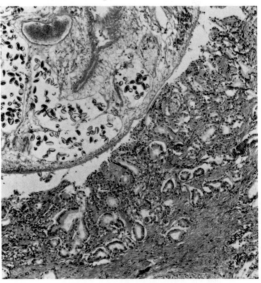

b

Fig. 20.50 Liver infestation by *Clonorchis sinensis*. **a**, fluke lodged in a bile duct, which shows thickening of its wall and surrounding fibrosis. **b**, microscopic appearances with a fluke in the lumen, and proliferation of duct-like elements in the wall of the bile duct. × 177.

cholangiocarcinoma. Fascioliasis is characterised by a cholangitis.

Ascariasis, i.e. infestation of the intestine by the round worm *Ascaris lumbricoides* is widely distributed throughout the world, but is particularly prevalent in Africa and the Far East. It commonly affects children, and in over a third of cases is associated with direct invasion of the common bile duct, producing obstruction and cholangitis.

Tumours of the Liver

Benign tumours

Benign tumours of the liver are rare, comprising approximately 5 per cent of all hepatic neoplasms. They include: (*a*) **liver cell adenomas**, which bear a close microscopic resemblance to normal liver tissue, the cells forming regular trabeculae two or three cells thick. Bile canaliculi are present and appear normal but bile ducts are absent. These tumours are usually very vascular and are not always encapsulated. An increased incidence due to the use of oral contraceptive pills and sex hormone therapy has recently been reported; (*b*) **bile duct adenomas** are very rare and are usually an incidental finding. These are less than 1 cm in diameter, and are composed of small bile duct elements in a fibrous stroma. Intrahepatic bile duct *cystadenomas* are also rare, but sometimes large, tumours; (*c*) **haemangiomas**, usually cavernous, dark purple owing to the contained blood, and sharply demarcated from the surrounding hepatic tissue, are not uncommon. Most are less than 2 cm in diameter, but some are larger. They are usually superficial and may be mistaken for infarcts by the casual observer.

Malignant tumours

Liver cell carcinomas account for approximately 85 per cent of primary malignant tumours of the liver, bile duct carcinomas for approximately 5–10 per cent, and the remainder consist of relatively rare tumours including haemangiosarcomas, hepatoblastomas, and mesenchymal tumours.

Liver cell (hepatocellular) carcinoma

This tumour shows marked geographic variation in incidence. In this country it is present in less than 1 per cent of all necropsies, whereas in parts of Africa and Far East Asia it is 5–6 times more common. In both low- and high-incidence areas 80–90 per cent of cases occur in males, and the tumour supervenes on cirrhosis (predominantly of macronodular type) in 70–80 per cent of cases. In cases without pre-existing cirrhosis, the male:female ratio is 2:1. *In low-incidence areas* the tumour arises usually after the age of 50, and while the incidence of cirrhosis is often high the proportion of cases in which malignancy supervenes is low, estimates varying from 5 to 15 per cent: the tumour develops as a late complication of long-established cirrhosis. By contrast, *in high-incidence areas* the tumour arises in a much younger age group. The incidence of cirrhosis in these areas is uncertain; it appears to be high, but not high enough to explain the high frequency of liver cell carcinoma; in such areas there is a much greater risk of tumours supervening in cirrhosis, some estimates being as high as 50 per cent, and clinical features of the tumour and of cirrhosis often present virtually simultaneously.

Aetiological factors. The precise relationship between cirrhosis and liver cell carcinoma is uncertain. Whereas we have previously subscribed to the view that the cirrhosis was a premalignant lesion, neoplasia supervening on the longstanding and continued hyperplasia of the cirrhotic liver, we feel that, on the basis of the epidemiological facts just presented, two other possibilities must be considered. These are (i) that both the cirrhosis and the tumour are caused by one agent, and (ii) that the cirrhotic liver is peculiarly predisposed to the carcinogenic effects of a variety of chemical and/or microbiological agents.

Experimentally, liver cell carcinoma has been produced in rats by feeding with mouldy peanuts, and this has been attributed to *aflatoxins* which are products of the mould *Aspergillus flavus*. These and other *mycotoxins* and *plant toxins* may contaminate stored foods and cereals, and this may explain in part the geographical variation in incidence in man. *Chemical carcinogens*, notably *o*-aminoazotoluene and *p*-dimethylaminoazobenzene (butter yellow) produce liver tumours in experimental animals without an intervening cirrhosis (p. 300), the incidence being increased by a diet low in protein or deficient in cystine and methionine. Accordingly *protein deficiency* may be synergistic in promoting the development of liver cell cancer in man, and may help to explain geographic variations in incidence. Recent attention has been focussed on the possible role of *nitrosamines*, compounds which can be synthesised from nitrites and secondary amines in the gastro-intestinal tract, and which produce experimental liver tumours. Nitrites (and nitrates) are common food additives, and the possibility that some nitrosamines are carcinogenic for man has been raised.

The tumour cells produce α-fetoprotein which exceeds 10 ng/ml in the serum in 85 per cent of cases.

There is growing epidemiological evidence of an association between *hepatitis B virus* infection and liver cell carcinoma. Firstly, markers of hepatitis B infection (e.g., HBsAg), have been detected in 80–90 per cent of patients with liver cell cancer, even in some areas with a low overall incidence of HB infection: secondly, liver cell dysplasia (Fig. 20.51), regarded as a premalignant change, is a common feature of cirrhosis in places with a high incidence of carcinoma, and shows a significant association with HBs antigenaemia: thirdly, liver cell

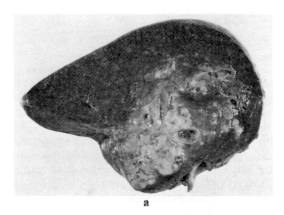

a

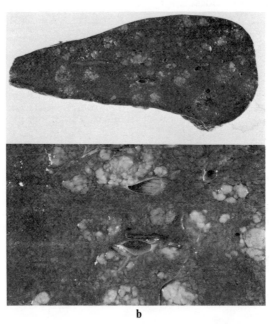

b

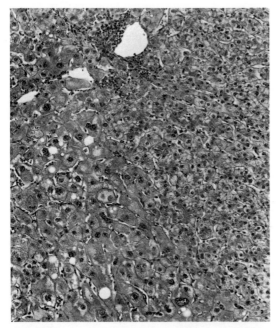

Fig. 20.51 Liver cell dysplasia: there is a focal increase in liver cell size, with nuclear pleomorphism and some binucleate and multinucleate cells. This section was from the right lobe of liver in a patient with a liver cell carcinoma in the left lobe. × 80.

Fig. 20.52 Liver cell carcinoma. **a**, arising as a single large mass and with evident permeation of surrounding portal vein branches. **b**, arising as multicentric foci throughout the liver (shown also at higher magnification).

carcinoma appears to occur more frequently in HB-associated cirrhosis; fourthly, hepatitis B infections and chronic carrier states are common in those parts of the world where there is a high incidence of liver cell carcinoma; transmission of HB infection from mother to child has been demonstrated, and such early infection in high-incidence areas could be a factor in the observed early development of liver cell cancer. However, while the evidence for an association between virus and tumour is indeed strong, evidence for a direct oncogenic role for HB is lacking, and the virus might be a 'passenger' rather than the 'driver' in tumour development.

Macroscopically the tumour may form a single large mass (Fig. 20.52a), often sharply defined, with central necrosis, haemorrhage and irregular bile-staining. In other cases the tumour is apparently multicentric (Fig. 20.52b), and there is also a type in which extensive nodular infiltration involves a considerable part of the liver. Extensive permeation of intrahepatic portal vein branches is a common feature; extrahepatic metastases occur in less than half the cases, mostly in the lungs and lymph nodes.

Microscopically the tumour cells closely resemble hepatocytes, their arrangement being more or less trabecular, and with intervening sinusoids (Fig. 20.53). Canaliculi, sometimes containing bile, may be seen.

Bile duct carcinoma (cholangiocarcinoma)

Primary tumours composed of cells resembling biliary epithelium (Fig. 20.54) are much less common than liver cell tumours. They are not usually associated with cirrhosis, and there is no difference in sex incidence. In the Far East, where these are relatively frequent, about 65 per cent of cases are associated with infestation by the liver flukes *Clonorchis sinensis* or *Opisthorchis viverrini*.

Hepatoblastoma and haemangiosarcoma

These are both very rare. Hepatoblastomas are congenital tumours of childhood and are composed of mixtures of epithelial and mesenchymal elements. Haemangiosarcomas are angioformative tumours: there is current interest and concern over their postulated association with exposure to vinyl chloride monomer (p. 312).

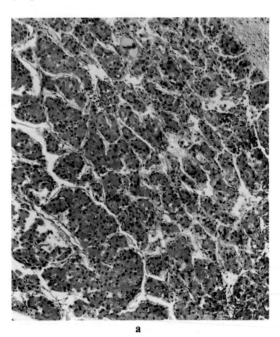
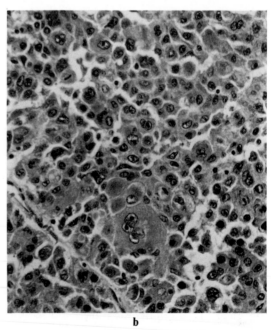

a   b

Fig. 20.53   Liver cell carcinoma. **a**, trabecular arrangement with endothelial lined sinusoids separating the aggregates of tumour cells. × 77. **b**, individual tumour cells resembling hepatocytes and with some binucleate and giant cell forms. × 250.

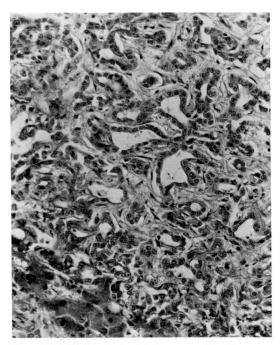

Fig. 20.54 Bile duct carcinoma—an adenocarcinomatous pattern resembling bile ducts, with a related fibrous reaction. × 200.

Secondary tumours

The liver is a very common site of secondary carcinomas of all kinds, notably from the

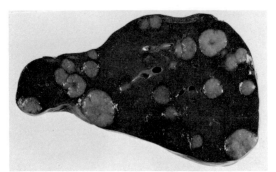

Fig. 20.55 Multiple secondary deposits in liver from a primary carcinoma of oesophagus.

gastro-intestinal tract, lung and breast. Secondary carcinoma may develop as one or two main masses, but often the whole organ is permeated by tumour nodules (Fig. 20.55). The liver becomes enlarged and its surface is beset with nodular elevations, some of which may show umbilication owing to central necrosis. The organ may come to weigh 5 kg or more. Intrahepatic cholestasis and jaundice may develop from pressure on bile duct radicles.

Sarcomas also frequently metastasise to the liver, and may produce marked hepatomegaly: Leukaemic infiltration and metastatic spread by malignant lymphoid neoplasms are common.

Other Disorders of the Liver

Liver diseases in childhood: congenital malformations

Many of the forms of liver disease which can occur in childhood are dealt with elsewhere. They include the congenital forms of cirrhosis, Indian childhood cirrhosis, biliary cirrhosis due to bile duct atresia or as a complication of fibrocystic disease of the pancreas, congenital syphilis, and the various metabolic storage diseases in which there may be hepatic involvement. There remain a few miscellaneous conditions which merit a brief description.

Neonatal hepatitis. This is a presumed virus infection of the liver and is sometimes familial. Cytomegalovirus, hepatitis B, herpes simplex and rubella viruses are all possible causes, while

some metabolic disorders, e.g. galactosaemia and alpha-1-antitrypsin deficiency, and also biliary atresia, may also produce a histological picture of hepatitis. Diffuse giant cell transformation of liver cells, often with 30–40 nuclei, is a striking feature of neonatal hepatitis (Fig. 20.56).

Reye's syndrome affects children up to 10 years old. A mild upper respiratory infection is followed by convulsions, vomiting, fever, coma and sometimes death. There may be hypoglycaemia and raised serum ammonia levels. The aetiology is uncertain, and while viral infection is suspected, the profound metabolic disturbances are unexplained. The liver is usually enlarged and shows very severe microvesicular fatty change (Fig. 20.57), which is seen also in other viscera.

Cystic disease of the liver. Congenital cysts in the liver are rare and are usually associated with cystic

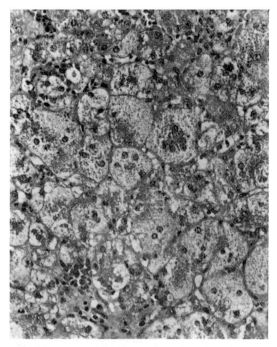

Fig. 20.56 Neonatal hepatitis: many of the liver cells are enlarged and multinucleate forms are evident: there is also intrasinusoidal extra-medullary haemopoiesis. × 190.

disease of the kidneys; the latter condition, however, occurs much more commonly alone. The cysts vary greatly in size and number; the liver may be studded with them, there may be only a few, or they may comprise microscopic hamartomatous lesions—*von Meyenburg complexes*. They usually contain a clear

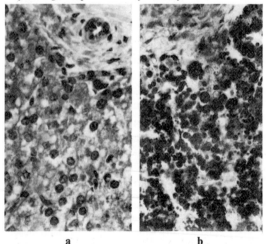

a   **b**

Fig. 20.57 Liver in Reye's syndrome: there is a severe degree of microvesicular fatty change. **a** H & E. × 250. **b** Oil Red O × 250.

fluid, have a cuboidal epithelial lining, and probably originate from the bile ducts.

Congenital hepatic fibrosis. This is regarded by some workers as a form of cystic disease of the liver. It may be familial and is sometimes accompanied by cystic disease of the kidneys. Bands of dense fibrous tissue extend irregularly throughout the liver, but the normal architecture is preserved between these. Within the fibrous bands there are numerous mature bile duct elements lined by cuboidal epithelium (Fig. 20.58). Affected individuals present in childhood or early adult life with portal hypertension, and when this is relieved surgically the prognosis is usually good because hepatocellular function is normal (c.f. cirrhosis). However, there appears to be an increased susceptibility to cholangitis.

Focal nodular hyperplasia. This is a benign hamartomatous lesion in which there is a focal aggregation of hyperplastic liver cell nodules separated by fibrous septa, and which may be mistaken for tumour. The lesion is usually func-

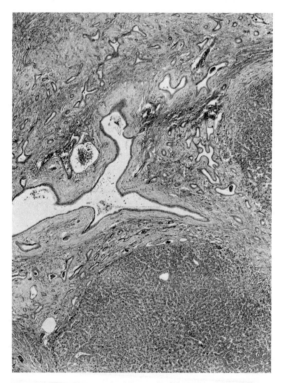

Fig. 20.58 Congenital hepatic fibrosis: wide fibrous septum within which are numerous mature bile duct elements, some of which contain inspissated bile. × 31.

tionally and histologically benign, although a few instances of portal hypertension have been reported where the lesion has arisen in the region of the porta hepatis.

Liver disease in pregnancy

Pregnancy may modify the clinical course of certain hepatic diseases. *Massive hepatic necrosis*, possibly viral, may be more severe in pregnancy, occurring particularly in the last trimester.

A benign form of **intrahepatic cholestasis** may recur with each pregnancy and is probably due to increased levels of steroid hormones.

Acute fatty liver of pregnancy occurs usually in the last trimester, and is commonly fatal. There is widespread fatty accumulation in hepatocytes, but of an unusual appearance (Fig. 20.59). A similar morphologic appearance may occur with tetracycline toxicity, and the lesion appears to result from depressed hepatocyte protein synthesis with resultant accumulation of fat.

Liver in eclampsia. The liver is not usually injured in eclampsia, but in fatal cases there are often foci of periportal necrosis and haemorrhage with fibrin thrombi within related portal capillaries and sinusoids and plasmatic vasculo-

sis (p. 808) of hepatic artery branches (Fig. 20.60). Perivenular necrosis and haemorrhage, if present, are manifestations of shock. These lesions are probably ischaemic and due to hepatic involvement in the disseminated intravascular coagulation now regarded as of pathogenic significance in pre-eclampsia and eclampsia.

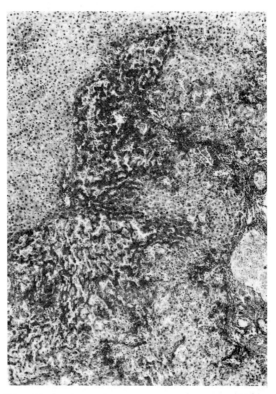

Fig. 20.60 Liver in eclampsia, showing necrotic liver cells separated by fibrin (darkly stained) and haemorrhage. × 75.

Drug and toxic liver injury

The liver plays a central role in the metabolism of many drugs and chemicals, and drug-induced hepatic injury is now one of the commonest forms of iatrogenic disease. Indeed, *in any patient presenting with liver disease or with unexplained jaundice, the possibility of a drug-induced lesion should always be considered.* Many of the pathological features already described in this chapter can be reproduced by drugs—hepatocellular injury and necrosis (sometimes massive), both acute and chronic hepatitis, hepatic fibrosis and cirrhosis,

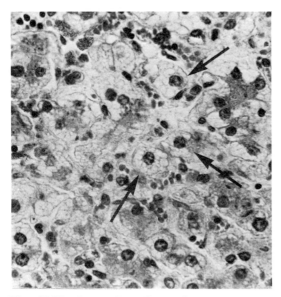

Fig. 20.59 Acute fatty liver of pregnancy: the hepatocytes are enlarged and contain multilocular droplets of fat arranged circumferentially round the nucleus (arrows). × 400.

vascular injury, hepatic neoplasia, and cholestasis by various mechanisms. It is not proposed to list the drugs which have hepatotoxic side-effects but merely to outline the hepatic disease patterns which may occur and to give examples of those drugs or agents which may produce them.

As with drug reactions in general, those affecting the liver may be divided into two main classes: (a) those which are *predictable*, i.e. they occur in most individuals taking the drugs in sufficient amount, the severity being related to the dose of the drug; they usually have similar effects in experimental animals and may either cause direct structural injury to liver cell components (membranes, etc.), or interfere with liver cell metabolism and result in secondary structural damage; (b) those which are *unpredictable* or *idiosyncratic*, i.e. they occur in only a proportion of individuals taking the drug, and are usually not dose-related; similar lesions are not produced regularly in experimental animals, and injury may be the result of host hypersensitivity or due to some individual metabolic aberration which renders a particular drug toxic.

Hepatocellular injury and necrosis. Fatty change may occur with tetracycline and in phosphorus poisoning; many drugs can produce focal necrosis, and massive necrosis can be caused by various industrial agents, including chlorinated hydrocarbons such as carbon tetrachloride and, seen increasingly in this country, by paracetamol overdosage. The poisonous mushroom *Amanita phalloides* also causes massive hepatic necrosis.

Hepatitis. Acute drug-induced hepatitis closely resembles classical viral hepatitis, and may be virtually indistinguishable in liver biopsy. Isoniazid, halothane and methyldopa are examples and in severe cases fulminant hepatic failure results from massive liver cell necrosis. With methyldopa and isoniazid progression to a condition resembling chronic active hepatitis has been described.

Cirrhosis has resulted from the prolonged use of methotrexate, e.g. for the treatment of leukaemia or psoriasis.

Vascular injury. Veno-occlusive disease due to pyrrollizidine alkaloids has been described earlier: urethane and radiotherapy may each cause a similar lesion, while hepatic vein thrombosis has been associated with the use of contraceptive steroids. Anabolic and contraceptive steroids may also produce periportal sinusoidal dilatation, and a rare condition *peliosis hepatis* (seen also in patients with advanced tuberculosis) in which blood-containing cysts up to 1 cm in diameter form, usually in the perivenular zones.

Hepatic neoplasia. An increased incidence of adenoma of the liver has resulted from the use of contraceptive steroids: regression of this lesion after withdrawal of the drug suggests, however, that it is not a true tumour. Long-term use of anabolic and contraceptive steroids is currently suspected of increasing the risk of liver cell carcinoma. Thorotrast, once used extensively in vascular angiography, carries a serious risk of liver cell and bile duct carcinomas and also haemangiosarcoma of the liver, which has recently been associated also with exposure to vinyl chloride monomer.

Jaundice occurs in most drug-induced liver injuries, and may be a prominent feature, for example in *intrahepatic cholestasis* which results regularly from *high dosage* of C17-alkylated anabolic and contraceptive steroids and as an idiosyncratic reaction to chlorpromazine and other drugs of the phenothiazine group. *Unconjugated hyperbilirubinaemia* may result from drug-induced haemolysis or from interference with conjugation of bilirubin in the liver, e.g. by novobiocin.

It is clear that many drugs are potential hepatotoxins and, in addition, many chemicals used in industrial processes may have hepatotoxic and possibly carcinogenic effects. The need for continued surveillance for such effects cannot be over-emphasised, and a careful occupational and drug history should be taken in patients with liver disease.

The Gallbladder and Bile Ducts

Function of the gallbladder

The relatively watery bile from the liver is stored in the gallbladder and concentrated by the absorption of water and electrolytes. Accordingly, with the addition of mucin from the mucosa, gallbladder bile becomes thick and mucoid. The normal structure of the mucosa is well suited to this absorptive function (Fig. 20.61). This concentrating ability of the gallbladder facilitates its radiological examination, in that certain iodine-containing compounds taken orally or administered intravenously are excreted and concentrated in the bile and, being radio-opaque, allow the gallbladder and the extrahepatic biliary system to be visualised.

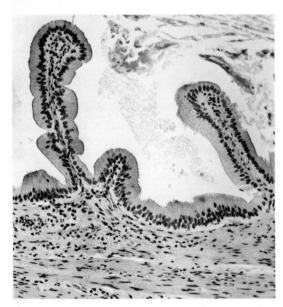

Fig. 20.61 Normal human gallbladder, showing delicate villous folds of mucosa covered by tall columnar epithelium. × 180.

The gallbladder bile is discharged into the duodenum in response to the entry into the duodenum of food, particularly fatty foods. When the food enters the duodenum the gallbladder discharges a proportion of its contents, and thereafter only small quantities are passed at intervals: there is always a relatively large amount of bile retained in the gallbladder. Between these periods of discharge there is probably a steady flow of hepatic bile into the gallbladder where it is concentrated.

The release of bile into the duodenum is due to contraction of the gallbladder accompanied by relaxation of the sphincter of Oddi. This is mediated humorally by cholecystokinin which is secreted by the duodenum in response to the presence there of fatty food.

Gallstones (Cholelithiasis)

Gallstones are formed from constituents of the bile—cholesterol, bile pigments and calcium salts—in various proportions, along with other organic material. They form usually in the gallbladder, but may also develop in the extrahepatic biliary tree and occasionally within intrahepatic ducts.

There is marked geographic variation in incidence, cholesterol stones being uncommon in developing countries. There is a very high incidence in North American Indians. Gallstones are commonest in late adult life, in women, especially multiparous, and in association with diabetes and obesity. In patients who have undergone ileal resection there is an increased tendency for stone formation due to a decrease in the bile-acid pool.

Pathogenesis

The exact mechanisms of stone formation remain debatable, and it seems likely that changes in the composition of the bile, local factors in the gallbladder and biliary tract infection are predisposing causes.

Composition of the bile. Cholesterol is the main constituent of most gallstones. It is synthesised in the liver and excreted in the bile, where it is kept in solution by the formation of micelles comprising cholesterol, phospholipids and bile salts. The phospholipids, also insoluble in water, are mainly (96 per cent) lecithins and small amounts of lysolecithin and phosphatidyl ethanolamine. The primary bile acids are synthesised in the liver from cholesterol, the most important ones being cholic acid and chenodeoxycholic acid: they are secreted in the bile as conjugates of the amino acids glycine and taurine, the glycine/taurine conjugate ratio being 3 to 1. In the colon the primary bile acids are dehydroxylated to form the secondary bile acids, deoxycholic and lithocholic acid. These major bile acids, together with other minor ones, constitute the bile acid pool, approximately 2–4 g in man, and more than 85 per cent of this is reabsorbed daily from the distal small intestine and colon and re-cycled.

The primary bile acids act as detergents in the bile and thus help to keep the cholesterol and phospholipids in true solution as mixed micelles. The ratio of cholesterol to bile acids and phospholipids determines cholesterol solubility.

Gallstones tend to form when there is a relative excess of cholesterol to bile acids and phospholipids—so-called '*lithogenic bile*'. This may result either from an increase in bile cholesterol or a decrease in the bile-acid pool: these changes are commonly found in patients with gallstones, but are unexplained.

Local factors in the gallbladder. These must have some part to play in the actual precipitation of stones. Not all patients with cholesterol stones secrete lithogenic bile. The parts played in stone formation by the gallbladder mucosa, the mucus and glycoprotein which it secretes, and the effects of local stasis are not known. There may also be a feedback effect on bile composition from the gallbladder and lithogenic bile shows a return to more normal composition following cholecystectomy.

Infections. It is doubtful whether infection is involved in the formation of cholesterol or pigment stones. The bile is sterile in most patients with such stones. Infection may, however, enhance the effects of local factors already mentioned and thus contribute to increase in size of stones and the formation of additional and mixed ones.

Types of stone

Stones containing predominantly cholesterol are by far the commonest, whereas bile pigment stones and calcium carbonate stones are comparatively rare. **Cholesterol stones** can be classified as *mixed* or *laminated*, *pure*, and *combination* or *compound cholesterol* stones (Fig. 20.62).

Mixed or *laminated gallstones.* These, the commonest type, are always multiple and often very numerous (Fig. 20.62c). They are some-

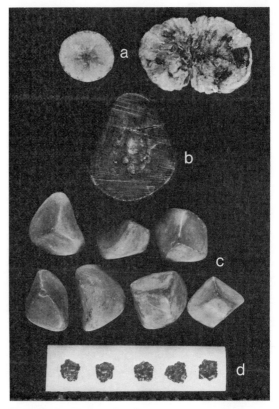

Fig. 20.62 Types of gallstones. **a** Two cholesterol stones; **b** Combination stone: a cholesterol core coated by laminated surface deposits of mixed composition; **c** multiple faceted mixed stones; **d** bile-pigment stones.

times associated with and secondary to a solitary cholesterol stone. They vary greatly in size—from 1 cm or more in diameter to the size of sand grains, are irregular in shape and often faceted. On section they have a distinctly laminated structure, dark brown and paler layers alternating. These layers consist chiefly of cholesterol and bile pigment respectively, both containing also an admixture of calcium salts and organic material. The layers are thicker at the angles. The faceting is due to growth of the stones in contact with one another. Their colour varies greatly from white, grey, brownish-yellow, pinkish, brown or almost black according to the nature of the covering layer and the stage of oxidation of the bile pigment. Mixed gallstones occur in very variable numbers; occasionally there may be hundreds of small stones. They may lie free in the bile, which may be mixed with inflammatory exu-

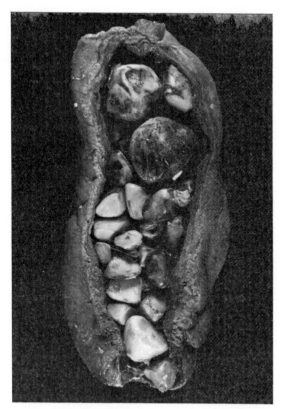

Fig. 20.63 Gallbladder filled with numerous gall-stones of mixed type. The wall is thickened and fibrosed due to chronic cholecystitis.

date or pus, or they may be tightly packed together within a contracted gallbladder with thickened wall (Fig. 20.63).

The *pure cholesterol stone*. This is usually solitary, oval, and may reach over 3 cm in length. It is pale yellow or almost white, soapy to the touch and of low specific gravity, often floating in water. Some are almost transparent with a frankly crystalline surface (Fig. 20.62a). When broken across, the stone shows a crystalline structure composed of sheaves of cholesterol crystals which radiate outwards from the centre. The core is sometimes dark owing to the incorporation of bile pigment between the crystals, but there is no break in the continuity of their formation, and no trace of lamination. Some specimens of solitary cholesterol stones, however, have a laminated cortex (i.e. concentric deposits) composed of bile pigment and calcium salts, the pigment causing the darker markings (Fig. 20.62b). This is due to a secondary deposit, which occurs when the gallbladder wall becomes inflamed by super-added bacterial infection. Stones of this class may be called *combination* or *compound cholesterol stones*. They constitute the largest gallstones. Occasionally a contracted gall-bladder contains two or three barrel-shaped combination cholesterol stones placed end to end.

Bile pigment stones. Such stones are usually multiple, black, irregular in form or occasionally somewhat stellate (Fig. 20.62d). They are composed chiefly of bile pigment, and may be friable or hard. They are often present in chronic haemolytic anaemias and are due to excess of bile pigment in the bile, but are encountered also occasionally in the absence of increased red cell destruction. The gallbladder usually appears normal.

Calcium carbonate stones. These also are rare. They are multiple, small, pale yellowish and fairly hard.

Cholesterosis of the gallbladder

This unimportant condition results from the patchy deposition of doubly refractile choles-terol esters within mucosal macrophages. This produces distinct yellowish flecking of the mucosa giving the appearance of so-called 'strawberry gallbladder' (Fig. 20.64). The lipid deposits may increase in size to form poly-poidal nodules. It is associated with cholesterol stones, solitary or mulberry, in one-third of cases.

Cholecystitis

Inflammation of the gallbladder is one of the commonest causes of abdominal pain, and frequently necessitates cholecystectomy.

Acute cholecystitis

Acute cholecystitis is nearly always associated with the presence of stones. It has been shown repeatedly that in the early stages of acute cholecystitis, bacteria cannot usually be cultured from the gallbladder. It is therefore thought that the initial inflammation is chemically induced. Obstruction to the outflow

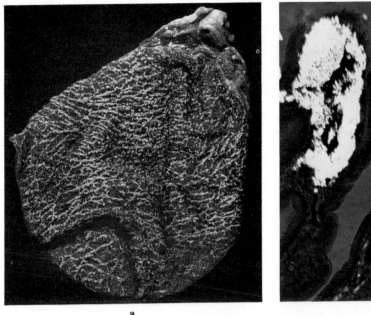
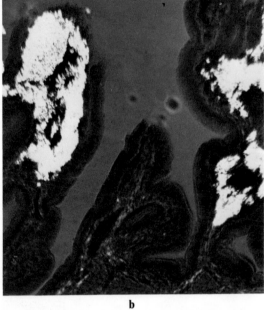

a   b

Fig. 20.64   Cholesterosis of gallbladder. **a**, the characteristic macroscopic pattern of 'strawberry gallbladder'. **b**, deposits of cholesterol esters in papillae, viewed by polarised light. × 90. (Professor W. A. Mackey.)

of bile due to a stone results in the bile becoming hyperconcentrated and this produces an irritant effect with consequent inflammation. Secondary bacterial infection may then occur, aggravating the inflammatory reaction. The organisms are thought to reach the gallbladder via the lymphatics, and are most commonly *Esch. coli.* or *Strep. faecalis.* Acute cholecystitis rarely occurs in the absence of stones, and is then usually associated with a source of infection elsewhere.

Pathologically, acute cholecystitis may be merely a mild catarrhal inflammation, or more severe—fibrinous, pseudo-membranous, haemorrhagic or suppurative. These more severe types occur especially when there is continued obstruction of the cystic duct either by stone or by superadded inflammatory oedema and exudate. The lumen may then become filled with pus—*empyema of the gallbladder.* Abscesses may also form in the wall, or there may even be necrosis or gangrene of the wall with rupture into the peritoneal cavity. In acute cholecystitis, fibrin deposition on the serosal surface may be organised, resulting in fibrosis and adhesions. The condition is often recurrent and may become chronic.

Chronic cholecystitis

This may result from repeated attacks of acute cholecystitis. In many patients, however, the disease is one of insidious onset, accompanied by dyspeptic symptoms or biliary colic. Gallstones are almost always present. The gallbladder wall is shrunken and shows marked fibrous thickening (Fig. 20.65). The lining is irregular, and there may be distinct pouches, especially when numerous stones are present. The contents may be clear, turbid or frankly purulent. The lining epithelium sometimes extends normally as downgrowths between the muscle bundles to form gland-like structures known as *Rokitansky–Aschoff sinuses.* This becomes much more marked in some cases of chronic cholecystitis, and there may be multiple complex epithelial overgrowths within the wall, which have occasionally been mistaken for adenocarcinoma (Fig. 20.66). Previously referred to as 'cholecystitis glandularis proliferans', the condition is now known as *adenomyomatosis of the gallbladder* and is benign. It may rarely occur in the absence of stones, and produce inflammation and symptoms resembling biliary colic.

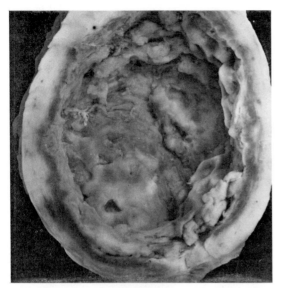

Fig. 20.65 Chronic cholecystitis, showing great thickening of wall. The gallbladder was packed with small rounded stones.

Complications of cholelithiasis and cholecystitis

Gallstones and infections of the gallbladder are so intimately related that the complications associated with them are best considered together. Some of these have been referred to already.

Gallstones, single or multiple, may lead to no noticeable symptoms—so-called silent stones. When a stone becomes impacted in Hartmann's pouch or in the cystic duct, great distension of the gallbladder results: the bile pigments are absorbed and the contents become clear and mucoid—mucocele of the gallbladder (Fig. 20.67). In the presence of infection, however, the contents become turbid or purulent—empyema of the gallbladder. Inflammation of the wall may progress to necrosis, with escape of the contents into the peritoneal cavity producing localised or generalised peritonitis.

Stones may also obstruct the common bile duct, producing biliary colic, extrahepatic obstruction and jaundice (p. 715). If the stone

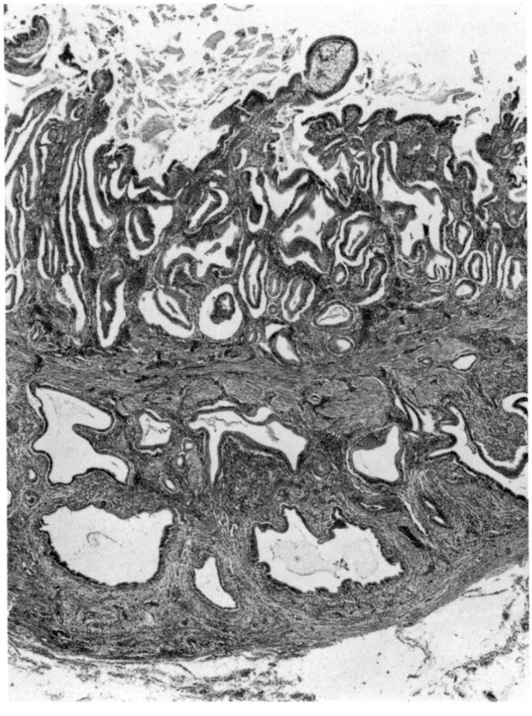

Fig. 20.66 Chronic cholecystitis showing extensive penetration of fundus of gallbladder by epithelial-lined spaces lying between muscle and serosa. (Rokitansky–Aschoff sinuses.) × 20.

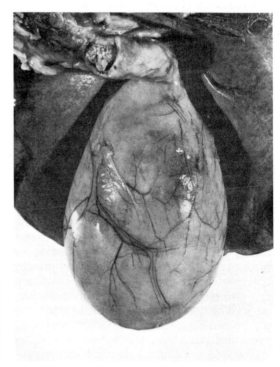

Fig. 20.67 Mucocele of the gallbladder. A stone is impacted in the cystic duct producing distension of the gallbladder, the contents of which have become clear and mucoid. Note how this accentuates the vascular markings on the serosa.

remains loose in the duct, the jaundice may be intermittent. Secondary bacterial infection is common, resulting in ascending cholangitis. In only a small proportion of cases does obstruction of the bile duct by stones lead to secondary biliary cirrhosis.

In chronic cholecystitis the wall becomes thickened and may be contracted over a mass of closely packed stones: there are often adhesions around the gallbladder and a stone or stones may ulcerate in one of several directions. A large stone of the compound cholesterol type may, for example, ulcerate through into the duodenum or less frequently into the colon. It may pass along the bowel, or may become arrested at some part of the small intestine, chiefly by contraction of the muscular coat, and may produce acute intestinal obstruction, which is then termed *gallstone ileus*. Ulceration into the portal vein with the setting up of portal pyaemia has been recorded.

Lastly, the irritation produced by gallstones may lead to carcinoma of the gallbladder, or, more rarely, of the large ducts.

Tumours of the biliary tract

Benign tumours, such as fibroma, lipoma and papilloma, are all very rare. Rarely, a large papilloma may obstruct the outflow with much distension of the gallbladder.

Carcinoma of the gallbladder is uncommon, and gallstones are an important factor in its causation, being present in fully 80 per cent of cases of cancer. The commonest site is the fundus and next is the neck of the gallbladder. It is usually of the slowly-growing, infiltrating type, but sometimes it is a soft growth with a tendency to necrosis. Occasionally the gallbladder may be practically destroyed and its cavity represented by a small irregular space in which gallstones may be present. It may invade the liver (Fig. 20.68) and may also give rise to numerous metastases. In most cases it is an adenocarcinoma, sometimes a cancer of spheroidal cell or mucoid type. Squamous cell carcinoma, arising secondarily to metaplasia of the lining epithelium, also occurs.

Carcinoma occurs also in the *large bile ducts* and is usually a small and slowly growing tumour. The two commonest sites are the lower end of the common bile duct (Fig. 20.69) and

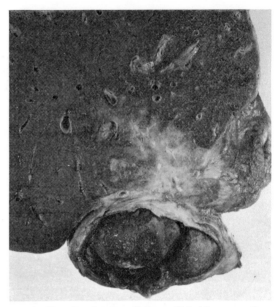

Fig. 20.68 Carcinoma of the gallbladder spreading directly into the overlying liver.

the junction of the cystic and hepatic ducts, the latter being more frequent; this site is also commonly involved by secondary lymphatic spread from carcinoma of the gallbladder.

Of the very many individuals who develop gallstones, less than 2 per cent develop carcinoma of the gallbladder; the incidence of bile-duct carcinoma is also low, although it is often not possible to determine whether a tumour around the ampulla has originated from bile duct or pancreas.

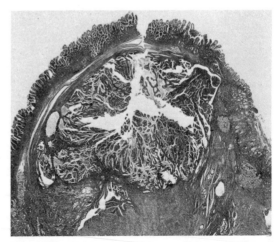

Fig. 20.69 Primary carcinoma of the ampulla of Vater causing obstructive jaundice. × 6.

Congenital anomalies of the gallbladder and bile ducts

A large number of abnormalities of the gallbladder have been described and may affect its size, shape, position, relation to the liver, etc. Gallstones may occur more frequently at a younger age in association with these anomalies.

Varying degrees of extrahepatic *biliary atresia* may occur and may result in secondary biliary cirrhosis. The rare *choledochal cyst* comprises a sac-like dilatation of a part or all of the biliary tract, and is associated with jaundice and cholangitis.

Jaundice

Staining of the tissues with bilirubin or bilirubin complexes is known as **jaundice** or **icterus**. When the serum level of these pigments exceeds about 34 μmol/litre (2 mg/100 ml), generalised jaundice develops. According to the severity and duration of the condition the skin and conjunctiva present various degrees of yellow staining up to deep orange colour and in very chronic cases it becomes olive-green owing to formation of biliverdin. The internal organs also are pigmented except the brain and spinal cord, which are not usually affected. In *icterus gravis neonatorum*, however, there may be bile staining of areas in the central nervous system, usually localised to the grey matter of the basal nuclei—the so-called *kernicterus*—but sometimes affecting the cortex (p. 746). The presence of the pigment in the blood in a case of marked jaundice is readily shown by the colour of the serum. Bile pigment may also be excreted in the urine and in the sweat; the tears, however, are not coloured, nor are the saliva, gastric juice or bile-duct epithelial secretion.

When the cause of the jaundice has been removed the skin may remain stained for some time after the serum bilirubin level has returned to normal, owing to the strong affinity of the elastic tissue for bilirubin. A rise of serum bilirubin from the normal level of 3–14 μmol/litre (0·2–0·8 mg/100 ml) up to 34 μmol/litre (2 mg/100 ml) is not usually accompanied by visible jaundice, but is sometimes called 'latent jaundice'. The term 'localised jaundice' is seldom used but it is seen around a bruise, the escaped haemoglobin being broken down to bilirubin.

Before considering further the features and types of jaundice, it is necessary to give an outline of the normal bile pigment metabolism.

Bile pigment metabolism

More than 80 per cent of the bile pigment is derived from the breakdown of effete mature red cells. Approximately 6 g of haemoglobin are broken down daily, mainly in macrophages, in man chiefly in the spleen, bone-marrow and liver, and the steps have already been described (p. 278). The remaining 20 per cent is derived in part from non-haemoglobin haem-containing pigments, e.g. myoglobin, catalase and cytochromes, and in part from ineffective erythropoiesis during red cell maturation (p. 531). Excessive production of this latter erythropoietic component may occur in thalassaemia, congenital porphyria and in dyserythropoietic or shunt hyperbilirubinaemia. Approximately 300 mg of bilirubin are produced daily.

Following release from macrophages, bilirubin (sometimes called **unconjugated bilirubin** to distinguish it from bilirubin glucuronides—see below) circulates in the plasma and is preferentially taken up by the hepatocytes. Within these cells it is transported by bilirubin-binding 'z' and 'y' proteins to the endoplasmic reticulum where it is conjugated with glucuronic acid, a reaction catalysed by the enzyme uridine diphosphate glucuronyl transferase. Both mono- and diglucuronide conjugates are formed, and possibly also sulphate and carbohydrate conjugates whose importance is uncertain. These conjugates are water soluble, and are referred to as **conjugated bilirubin**; they are rapidly excreted directly into the bile canaliculi and hence pass into the bile. Conjugated bilirubin is converted in the intestine into **stercobilinogen**, the normal brown faecal pigment. A small fraction of the stercobilinogen is reabsorbed from the gut, and most of this passes back to the liver where it is re-excreted into the bile—the entero-hepatic circulation of bile pigment. A minute amount (1–3 mg daily) of the re-absorbed stercobilinogen is excreted in the urine as **urobilinogen**.

To understand the clinical, biochemical and morbid anatomical features of the different types of jaundice, it is necessary to appreciate that *unconjugated bilirubin is water-insoluble and remains in solution in the plasma only as a rather firm complex with albumin. Consequently, it does not readily pass through capillary walls, and its increase in the plasma is not accompanied by bilirubinuria.* Nevertheless, unconjugated bilirubin is capable of staining the tissues, although the form in which it escapes from the plasma remains unknown. *Another feature of unconjugated bilirubin is its solubility in lipids, which may explain the bilirubin-staining of the brain in neonates with high plasma levels of unconjugated bilirubin.* The brain damage which may result is due to the toxic effects of bilirubin on nerve cells. By contrast, *conjugated bilirubin is water-soluble, and increased levels in the plasma are always accompanied by its appearance in the urine: it is relatively insoluble in lipids and causes neither staining of, nor damage to, the central nervous system.*

The biochemical estimation of serum bilirubin employs the **van den Bergh reaction**. When Ehrlich's diazo reagent, a mixture of sulphanilic acid and sodium nitrite, is added to a solution of bilirubin, the pigment becomes diazotised to give a blue-violet compound which can be assayed colorimetrically. Conjugated bilirubin gives an *immediate* or *direct* reaction, and the *total* bilirubin is then measured after treatment with alcohol which splits the unconjugated or indirect-reacting bilirubin from its bilirubin–albumin complex.

Classification of jaundice

Jaundice may result from:

(1) Increased bilirubin production.
(2) Interference with hepatic uptake of bilirubin.
(3) Interference with hepatic conjugation of bilirubin.
(4) Interference with hepatic excretion of bilirubin.
(5) Combinations of 2–4 resulting from reduction in functional hepatic cell mass.

While it is of diagnostic and therapeutic importance to determine which of the above five factors is responsible for the development of jaundice, in practice it is found that more than one factor is often concerned. For example, the anaemia resulting from increased red cell destruction may cause liver cell injury, as also does prolonged obstruction of the biliary tract, whether or not accompanied by infection. Thus *jaundice is frequently attributable to more than one factor, and diagnosis of the underlying condition is sometimes very difficult.*

(1) Increased bilirubin production

(a) Haemolytic (acholuric) jaundice. This is not uncommon and is due to increased red cell destruction, either acute or chronic (see p. 518), with consequent production in the macrophage system of increased amounts of bilirubin, up to 1·5 g daily. Normally, the liver is capable of extracting, conjugating and excreting such large amounts of bilirubin, and jaundice is thus latent or mild. The agent causing the haemolysis may, however, also damage the liver, or the anaemia resulting from haemolysis may depress liver function, and in these circumstances jaundice is more pronounced. In infants, the rate of red cell destruction is relatively high, and the liver is deficient in the enzymes necessary for conjugation of bilirubin, particularly when birth is premature. Accordingly, *icterus neonatorum* is a common condition, and is likely to be especially severe in infants with haemolytic anaemia due to maternal iso-antibodies (p. 527). Exchange blood transfusions may be necessary to keep the plasma bilirubin below 250 μmol/litre (15 mg/100 ml), the level at which there is a real danger of brain damage from kernicterus (p. 746).

In haemolytic jaundice, most of the bilirubin in the plasma is unconjugated, and thus bile pigment is absent from the urine (*acholuric jaundice*). The amount of urobilinogen in the urine is, however, usually much increased.The faeces are dark from the excessive amounts of bile pigment excreted.

(b) Dyserythropoietic (shunt) hyperbilirubinaemia. This is associated with ineffective or abnormal red cell maturation resulting in the premature destruction of erythrocyte precursors in the marrow: there is an unconjugated bilirubinaemia but with a normal peripheral blood red cell survival time. The disease is rare, familial and the mode of inheritance is not defined.

(2) Interference with hepatic uptake of bilirubin

Gilbert's disease. Although rare, this is the commonest form of familial non-haemolytic acholuric jaundice. It is apparently due to a 'dominant' defect of a single autosomal gene which impairs either transport of bilirubin to the liver, or uptake of bilirubin by the liver. Mild intermittent acholuric jaundice results. The condition is, however, rather poorly defined.

(3) Interference with hepatic conjugation of bilirubin

(a) Physiologial or neonatal jaundice. This is a common condition, particularly in premature babies. It is due to relative deficiency of glucuronyl transferase in the neonatal liver. The jaundice usually improves 2–3 weeks post-partum as the enzyme attains normal levels.

(b) Inherited defective bilirubin conjugation. In the very rare *Crigler-Najjar syndrome*, deficiency of glucuronyl transferase results in very high levels of unconjugated bilirubin. In Type I, in which the enzyme is absent, kernicterus within the first two years of life is the usual cause of death, whereas in Type II, with a variably reduced enzyme activity, normal survival may occur.

(4) Interference with hepatic excretion of bilirubin

(a) Intrahepatic inherited. In the rare *Dubin–Johnson syndrome*, there is a partial failure of the liver cells to secrete conjugated bilirubin into the bile canaliculi, and as a consequence conjugated bilirubin is regurgitated into the blood and intermittent jaundice results. The other constituents of the bile are secreted normally, and the serum alkaline phosphatase level is not raised. A curious feature is accumulation of granules of brown pigment in hepatocyte lysosomes, as yet of uncertain nature but possibly melanin-like. Little or no disability results from this syndrome, which is believed to be due to a single gene defect with 'dominant' transmission. A second, and genetically related condition, is the *Rotor syndrome* in which there is failure to secrete conjugated bilirubin but no accumulation of brown pigment in the liver cells.

In a further rare condition—*benign idiopathic recurrent intrahepatic cholestasis*—multiple recurrent attacks of cholestasis occur in the absence of large duct obstruction, the jaundice persisting for some months, but without producing any evidence of progressive or permanent liver damage.

(b) Intrahepatic acquired. This occurs in primary biliary cirrhosis, and also as a complication of therapy with certain drugs (p. 706).

Drug-induced cholestasis occurs as an idiosyncrasy in a small proportion of patients taking phenothiazine derivatives, notably chlorpromazine, and appears unrelated to dosage. It is reversible, at least in most cases, on discontinuing the drug. Cholestasis results also from administration of methyl testosterone and certain other C17-alkyl-substituted testosterones, and does not depend upon idiosyncrasy, being produced regularly by a sufficient dosage of such compounds.

(c) Extrahepatic biliary obstruction is the commonest cause of jaundice in middle and old age: it is termed **obstructive jaundice**. Major duct obstruction is caused chiefly by gallstones lodging in the common bile duct, and by carcinoma of the head of the pancreas or of the lower end of the common bile duct. Less commonly, it arises from scarring of bile ducts due to previous inflammation and ulceration by gallstones, and from accidental injury or ligation of the common bile duct during operations in this area. Other causes include congenital malformations of the major duct system, and involvement of the ducts in tumours or tuberculosis affecting the lymph nodes and surrounding tissues in the portal fissure.

When due to gallstones, the obstruction may be sudden and complete, or intermittent if the stone or stones move along the common bile duct; it is often accompanied by biliary colic. In carcinomatous involvement or scarring of the ducts, obstruction, and hence jaundice, are usually of more gradual onset, progressive and often painless. As in all forms of obstructive jaundice the serum alkaline phosphatase is greatly raised.

Apart from jaundice and its effects, major duct obstruction, particularly if caused by gallstones, is likely to be complicated by superadded suppurative cholangitis, and in unrelieved obstruction the patient does not usually survive long enough to develop secondary biliary cirrhosis (p. 688).

(5) Reduction in functional hepatic cell mass (hepatocellular or toxic jaundice)

This type of jaundice is also common. It results from damage to liver cells, e.g. by viruses, bacterial or hepatocellular toxins. It is a feature of the various forms of viral hepatitis and leptospirosis (Weil's disease), where the organisms are actually present in the liver, and it occurs occasionally in typhus, pneumonia, septicaemia, relapsing fever, smallpox, etc. It is seen also in some forms of snake bite, in poisoning with various chemicals and toxins—trinitrotoluene, phosphorus, amanitine and amanita toxin from various fungi, etc. Except in biliary cirrhosis, jaundice is usually a late complication of hepatic cirrhosis, and is then likely to be attributable to liver cell necrosis and hepatocellular failure.

Two factors are concerned in the production of hepatocellular jaundice: (*a*) damage to the liver cells may interfere with the passage of bile along the bile canaliculi: in other words, a degree of intrahepatic cholestasis arises. Focal necrosis or swelling of the liver cells, and disorganisation of the liver cell plates and fibrosis (as in cirrhosis), may thus cause focal cholestasis; (*b*) removal of unconjugated bilirubin from the blood, its conjugation and discharge into the bile canaliculi, may all be impaired as a result of liver cell injury. The relative importance of these two factors varies in different cases, and may also change, as liver cell injury progresses, in the individual case.

The Exocrine Pancreas

The pancreas is composed of two kinds of tissue with distinct functions. Firstly, the **acinous or exocrine glandular tissue**, which produces the digestive secretion of the gland, of pH 7·5–8·0 and containing bicarbonate, amylase and lipase which are secreted in their active form, and trypsinogen and chymotrypsinogen which are converted to the active enzymes trypsin and chymotrypsin in the duodenum. Secondly, the **islets of Langerhans or endocrine glandular tissue**, which secrete several hormones—insulin and glucagon, which are of importance in carbohydrate metabolism, and somatostatin and pancreatic polypeptide whose precise function is uncertain. The pathology of the islets is dealt with in Chapter 26.

Exocrine pancreatic function can be assessed by measuring the volume and enzyme content of pancreatic juice obtained by duodenal aspiration following a standard small meal of gruel—the Lundh test. Evidence of structural pancreatic abnormalities may be seen on plain x-ray films of the abdomen or by a barium meal; special radiological procedures include hypotonic duodenography, angiography, radioisotope scanning, and more recently ultrasonography, C–T scanning and endoscopic cannulation of the pancreatic duct. In acute pancreatitis some enzymes are released into the circulation and may be measured in serum and urine.

Degenerative changes

Focal necrosis occurs in infections, fatty change in various poisonings, and sometimes amyloid change from the usual causes. Fatty replacement occurs in obesity, and is often a marked feature when the glandular tissue becomes atrophied, e.g. after obstruction of the duct. Atrophy of the gland, with consequent functional deficiency, accompanies fibrotic lesions and obstructions of the duct, described below; symptomless atrophy occurs also in wasting diseases, and to a lesser degree as a senile change. Abnormal smallness of the pancreas without any other change occurs in some cases of diabetes in young subjects, but its nature and significance are doubtful. Pigmentation from deposition of granular haemosiderin, sometimes considerable, is common in haemochromatosis (p. 282) and may be accompanied by diabetes. When the pancreatic tissue is injured in various ways, it is attacked by its own enzymes, and necrosis results. Thus small circumscribed areas of dull yellowish necrotic tissue are a common necropsy finding. They are seen especially after operations on the pancreas, in acute and chronic pancreatitis, and in obstruction of the ducts; they are often accompanied by patches of necrosis in the fat around the pancreas (Fig. 20.70b). Fine fibrosis and dilatation of the pancreatic ducts and acini may occur in uraemia ('*uraemic pancreatitis*').

Experimentally the administration of ethionine to rats has resulted in pancreatic degeneration and necrosis, apparently by antagonising methionine and interfering with protein synthesis.

Pancreatitis is classified into acute and chronic forms, which are now believed to be two distinct entities. Acute pancreatitis rarely proceeds to the chronic form, even when it is of the recurrent variety. Chronic relapsing pancreatitis is a further variant.

Acute pancreatitis (acute haemorrhagic necrosis of the pancreas)

In most cases this condition is essentially an acute necrosis with haemorrhage in greater or lesser degree; in the later stages secondary infection leading to *suppuration* and even to *gangrene* may occur. These changes characterise stages in the condition rather than distinct varieties. In cases dying very rapidly after the onset of symptoms there may be patchy necrosis of the pancreas with only a light haemorrhagic speckling, indicating that necrosis precedes haemorrhage, but in others of longer duration the whole organ may be deep purple-black owing to diffuse interstitial haemorrhage.

Clinical features. This is a not uncommon clinical emergency. It occurs most frequently after the age of 40 and is commoner in women. Predisposing factors are summarised in Table 20.3. Primary acute pancreatitis (i.e. not preceded by a surgical operation, trauma or duct cannulation) accounts for 90 per cent of cases.

Clinical onset is sudden with abdominal pain, vomiting and collapse, and may simulate gastro-duodenal perforation. Shock may be marked, with hypotension, and sometimes may lead to acute renal failure. Hypocalcaemic tetany and hyperglycaemic coma may complicate the picture. There is a marked degree of hypoxia with arterial Po$_2$ levels of less than 60 mm of mercury, and thus the patients are bad operative risks. Amylase and lipase are released into the circulation and their measurement in the serum, and of amylase in the urine, are of diagnostic value. **Recurrent acute pancreatitis**

Table 20.3 Predisposing factors in acute pancreatitis

Common factors		Minimal factors
Primary acute pancreatitis		
Biliary disease (gallstones and cholecystitis)	50%	Ampullary/pancreatic cancer
		Drugs
Alcoholism	20–40%	Hyperlipoproteinaemia (Friedrichson's types I and V)
		Hypothermia
		Virus infection
		Hyperparathyroidism
		Previous 'blind-loop' operation
		Pregnancy
		Scorpion bites (Trinidad)
		Worms/flukes in common bile duct (S.E. Asia)
Secondary acute pancreatitis		
Post operative	65%	
A blow or penetrating injury	25%	
Duct cannulation	10%	

Primary cases exceed secondary cases in a ratio of 9:1.

should lead to careful investigation for possible causal factors, such as gallstones or alcohol abuse, for correction of these will usually prevent further episodes.

The peritoneal cavity generally contains bloodstained serous fluid, and numerous patches of *fat necrosis* result from the liberation of pancreatic lipase from the damaged parenchyma; fat is hydrolysed, the glycerol being absorbed, while the firm yellowish-white patches represent fatty acids. These patches are specially numerous in the region of the pancreas and in the greater omentum (Fig. 20.70b), but occur elsewhere. The haemorrhage into the pancreas and tissues around may be so extensive that at operation a dark mass is seen through the peritoneum of the lesser peritoneal sac. The cut surface of the pancreas varies; in some cases it is almost uniformly haemorrhagic, in others there is a mixture of dull yellowish areas of necrosis with haemorrhage between and around (Fig. 20.70a), and sometimes necrosis predominates.

On **microscopic examination**, necrosis, haemorrhage and inflammation are associated in varing proportions. Haemorrhage may be the outstanding feature, the whole tissue of the

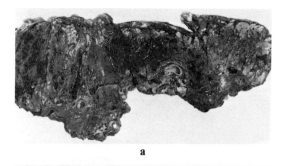

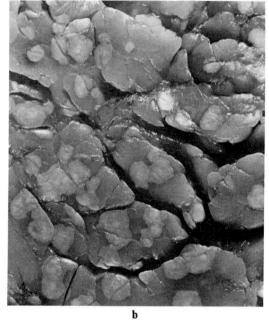

Fig. 20.70 **(a)** Acute haemorrhagic pancreatitis. × 0·6. **(b)** Part of the greater omentum from the same case, showing pale patches of fat necrosis. × 1·7.

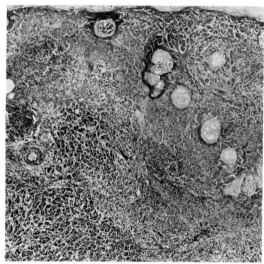

Fig. 20.71 Acute pancreatitis. The pale-staining necrotic area with fat necrosis is seen top right, with surviving pancreas below. × 38.

gland being infiltrated with blood, while diffuse necrosis of the acini is seen at places. Venular thrombi are commonly seen, usually associated with a vasculitis which may be caused by trypsin release. Fibrinoid necrosis of blood vessels is common in severe cases and this leads to subsequent haemorrhage. In early lesions, large numbers of polymorphs are seen in areas of parenchymal and fat necrosis (Fig. 20.71). Later, when large areas of pancreas are necrotic, polymorphs are usually absent from the necrotic areas and the appearances resemble those of coagulative necrosis secondary to infarction. These cases in particular are associated with venular thrombi, and this, together

with the finding of markedly reduced pancreatic blood flow late in the disease process in experimental animals, suggests a final ischaemic mechanism. All the appearances may be interpreted as the result of some toxic agent, which kills the parenchyma and also acts on the vessels, leading to thrombosis and haemorrhage. Superadded bacterial infection is common and may be severe, progressing to suppuration with abscess formation or gangrenous pancreatitis, often with generalised peritonitis.

The aetiology of acute pancreatitis is not clear and probably several mechanisms are involved which can ultimately lead to the same clinico-pathological state. In pancreatitis associated with gallstones it has been shown that in up to 90 per cent of cases the attack of pancreatitis has been secondary to the passage of gallstone(s) from the gallbladder into the common bile duct and thence to the duodenum, possibly with temporary arrest at the ampulla of Vater. Much has been written about the anatomy of the ducts at the ampulla, following the observation by Opie of a case of fatal pancreatitis where a gallstone was found impacted in the ampulla. In about 80 per cent of individuals in general (and of patients with fatal acute pancreatitis) the pancreatic and common bile ducts open into a common channel in the ampulla, thus allowing the possibility of reflux of bile into the pancreatic duct. The initiating mechanism of pancreatitis associated with alcohol abuse is unknown and largely uninvestigated.

Undoubtedly there is activation of lipolytic and proteolytic enzymes within the parenchyma and this contributes to the subsequent necrosis in the gland. Pancreatic enzymes can be activated by duodenal juice, bile and possibly certain bacteria. However, instillation of active enzymes into the pancreatic duct at normal physiological pressure does not result in pancreatitis in experimental animals, and it is not known how the enzymes penetrate the pancreatic duct mucosal barrier in acute pancreatitis.

Suppurative pancreatitis may occur apart from secondary infection in acute pancreatitis, and is then usually caused by passage of bacteria along the ducts, or by direct spread from a local focus of infection, e.g. from an infected pancreatic tumour, or inflammatory diseases of the duodenum. Pancreatitis may occur as a rare complication of mumps and is thought to be due to viral infection of the organ.

Chronic pancreatitis

It is important to distinguish between **chronic relapsing pancreatitis**, which may follow repeated attacks of acute pancreatitis, and **true chronic pancreatitis**, which presents with no previous history of acute attacks. Both forms can lead to malabsorption and/or diabetes mellitus.

Chronic relapsing pancreatitis is most frequently associated with alcohol abuse or previous blunt abdominal trauma, but acute pancreatitis of any origin occasionally progresses to this disorder. Clinical separation from recurrent acute pancreatitis is dependent on the patient being entirely asymptomatic between attacks of recurrent acute, whereas with chronic relapsing there is continuous abdominal pain and discomfort. The two are, however, different stages of the same disease process: it is frequently associated with scarring and distortion of the main pancreatic duct.

True chronic pancreatitis is relatively uncommon in this country, but is encountered more in France, and is related to heavy wine drinking. It is curious that, whereas no particular type of alcohol beverage is associated with acute pancreatitis, chronic pancreatitis is more frequent where wine is the main form of alcohol intake. *Duct obstruction* from whatever cause may be an important factor in its development, and proteinaceous deposition on the inner lining of both small and large pancreatic ducts is the most widely held explanation for the diffuse changes present in the pancreas. Chronic pancreatitis, often with diabetes, is also a regular feature of haemochromatosis (p. 282), in which excessive parenchymal iron deposits appear to play a causal role. Areas of fibrosis in the pancreas may be produced, as in other organs, by arteriosclerosis. A form of diffuse interstitial pancreatitis has also been described in congenital syphilis.

In chronic pancreatitis the gland becomes firmer, sometimes enlarged, but more often shrunken. Microscopy shows fibrosis and atrophy of the glandular elements (Fig. 20.72). The fibrosis may be chiefly between the lobules—*interlobular*—or there may be a more diffuse fibrosis between the acini—*intralobular*. In the connective tissue, the small ducts may be unduly prominent. The islets of Langerhans suffer less than the glandular acini, but they also may be implicated in the fibrosis when it is intralobular in distribution, and thus diabetes may result. *The histological distinction between chronic pancreatitis and carcinoma of the pancreas may be very difficult* (cf. Figs. 20.72b and 20.74).

Obstruction of pancreatic ducts

Obstruction of the main duct may be caused by a pancreatic calculus, occasionally by a gallstone impacted in the ampulla of Vater, by scarring, or by pressure of a tumour, most frequently cancer of the head of the pancreas. Obstruction leads to irregular dilatation of the large ducts. The smaller ducts may be similarly affected and may occasionally show cyst-like distension. The result, as in other organs, no doubt depends on whether the obstruction is constant or intermittent, but two changes are prominent: atrophy of the exocrine cells and overgrowth of the connective tissue. In long-standing cases only shrunken remains of the parenchyma are found in the connective tissue. Sometimes the atrophy is accompanied by extensive replacement of the gland by adipose tissue without loss of shape (lipomatosis). The islets of Langerhans are not affected by the atrophic process, and on the contrary they

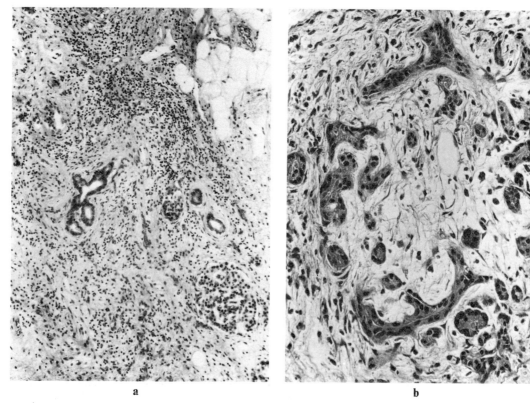

Fig. 20.72 **a** Chronic pancreatitis with diffuse fibrous replacement of exocrine pancreas: a surviving islet is present (*lower right*) and there is a chronic inflammatory cell infiltrate of the interstitium. × 100. **b** Chronic pancreatitis: surviving acinar elements in fibrous tissue showing compression and distortion. × 250.

appear more numerous than usual, owing to the loss of acinar tissue. Even when the exocrine tissue has almost gone, groups of virtually unchanged islets remain. Similar results follow experimental ligation of the pancreatic duct in animals; here also the persistence of the islets is striking. This explains why diabetes does not, as a rule, follow ligation of the main duct.

In view of the effects of pancreatic duct obstruction, it is curious that pancreatic tissue of normal microscopic appearance is sometimes seen in teratomas: it seems most unlikely that such tissue could have a patent duct system.

Pancreatic calculi

Rarely small concretions, composed of calcium carbonate and a little phosphate, form in the pancreatic ducts. They seldom exceed 5 mm, and may be numerous and minute. They are irregularly rounded or elongated, whitish and usually hard. In addition to

causing obstruction in varying degree, they may lead to secondary bacterial infection, with acute or chronic inflammatory change as the result.

Cysts

The most important variety is the single 'pancreatic cyst' which forms a large rounded swelling, sometimes of over 10 cm diameter. The cyst usually contains a colourless fluid, clear or slightly turbid, though sometimes there may be an admixture of altered blood. The pancreatic enzymes are present in the fluid for a time, and may be detected by the usual tests; later, however, they disappear. The formation of such a cyst has been observed after injury, and this is regarded as the usual cause. The layer of peritoneum over the pancreas is torn and there then occurs an escape of blood and pancreatic secretion into the lesser peritoneal sac, the fluid becoming localised by adhesions. The condition is thus really a *pseudo-cyst* which is situated outside the pancreas. A similar condition may follow an attack of acute pancreatitis, but the cause is often obscure. A cystic form of adenoma sometimes occurs in the pancreas. In *Lindau's disease* (p. 791), cysts may occur in the pancreas along with haemangiomas in the cerebellum. Hydatid cysts also occur in and around the pancreas.

Cystic fibrosis (Fibrocystic disease of the pancreas)

This disease is due to a generalised abnormality of exocrine gland secretion involving pancreas, bowel, lungs, biliary tree and sweat glands. In the newborn it may give rise to intestinal obstruction by inspissated meconium (*meconium ileus*), sometimes resulting in perforation and *meconium peritonitis*. In older children respiratory infections, and eventually bronchiectasis, are common and in about 25 per cent of cases the liver shows focal portal and periportal fibrosis in relation to bile concretions in cholangioles: the fibrosis is usually mainly subcapsular, but an irregular type of biliary cirrhosis may develop. Failure of pancreatic exocrine secretion produces a malabsorption syndrome (p. 643). There is an increased sodium chloride content of the sweat both in affected individuals and in presumed heterozygotes, and this provides a useful diagnostic test and a test for studies of the genetic inheritance of the disease.

The inheritance is autosomal recessive, but apparently with some genetic heterogeneity. It is not uncommon, occurring in approximately one per 2000 live births in caucasians. The precise aetiology is unknown, postulated mechanisms including defective function of cholinergic autonomic nervous control, absence of an enzyme, or some other type of inherited metabolic disorder. The pancreas is small, firm and gritty, the cysts rarely being visible to the naked eye. On section the acini and ducts are dilated and filled with tough yellowish eosinophilic secretion which contains abundant mucin (Fig. 20.73). Subsequent fibrosis, both inter-and intra-lobular, may lead to loss of the normal lobulation.

Tumours

Apart from carcinoma, tumours are rare in the pancreas. Fibroma, lipoma, lymphangioma,

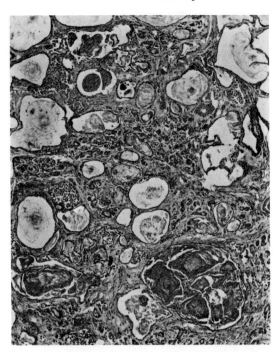

Fig. 20.73 Fibrocystic disease of the pancreas. The ducts are filled with eosinophilic laminated secretion; the acini are either markedly atrophied or much dilated. × 50. (Professor G. L. Montgomery.)

adenoma and cystadenoma have been described; the last mentioned may reach a considerable size.

Carcinoma of the pancreas nearly always occurs in the head, less frequently in the body, rarely in the tail; it is usually a scirrhous adenocarcinoma, which may mimic the pancreatic acinar structure (Fig. 20.74), but sometimes the cells are quite irregularly arranged. Cancer of the head of the pancreas nearly always leads to obstruction of the main ducts, with exclusion of the pancreatic secretion from the intestine. The common bile duct also is usually obstructed, causing jaundice. Cancer of the tail or body of the pancreas may be clinically silent until effects arise from metastases. Pancreatic cancer also causes bizarre clinical effects due to unexplained venous thrombosis, peripheral neuropathy and myopathy.

It usually appears in the sixth decade and is twice as common in men as in women. The incidence has increased greatly and in some American surveys of alimentary tract cancers, it ranks second in frequency only to cancer of

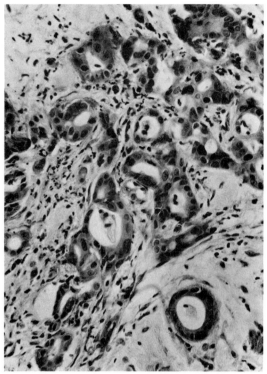

Fig. 20.74 Adenocarcinoma of pancreas, showing a regular acinar pattern and with a related scirrhous reaction. × 250.

the large intestine. It is sometimes accompanied by anomalies of carbohydrate metabolism, and is twice as common in diabetics as in the general population. The possibility of pancreatic cancer should therefore be considered in late-onset unstable diabetes, or development of instability in a previously stable diabetic.

Tumours of the islet cells are described on p. 1034, in the account of disorders of the endocrine part of the pancreas.

Congenital abnormalities

Developmental abnormalities of the pancreas and variations in the arrangement of its ducts are not uncommon. Occasionally the tissue of the head surrounds the adjacent part of the duodenum as a circular band, and stenosis may be produced. This is known as 'annular pancreas'. Foci of ectopic pancreatic tissue also occur, and may be single or multiple. The commonest site is in the submucosa of the jejunum, though occasionally they occur in the duodenum and even in the stomach. Ectopic pancreas is sometimes found in the apex of a Meckel's diverticulum and also in an ordinary 'false diverticulum' of the small intestine.

References

Bianchi, L., De Groote, J., Desmet, V. J., Gedigk, P., Korb, G., Popper, H., Poulsen, H., Scheuer, P. J., Schmid, M., Thaler, H. and Wepler, W. (1977). Acute and chronic hepatitis revisited. *Lancet* **ii**, 914–19.

Blumberg, B. S. (1964). Polymorphism of serum proteins and the development of iso-precipitins in transfused patients. *Bulletin of the New York Academy of Medicine* **40**, 377–86.

Blumberg, B. S., Gerstley, B. J. S., Hungerford, D. A., London, W. I. and Sutnick, A. I. (1967). A serum antigen (Australia antigen) in Down's Syndrome, leukaemia and hepatitis. *Annals of Internal Medicine* **66**, 924–31.

Burrell, C. J. (1980). Serological markers of hepatitis B infection. In *Clinics in Gastroenterology*, Vol. 9, No. 1, pp. 47–63. Ed. by Sheila Sherlock. Saunders, London, Philadelphia and Toronto.

Rappaport, A. M., Borowy, Z. J., Lougheed, W. M. and Lotto, W. N. (1954). Subdivision of hexagonal liver lobules into a structural and functional unit; role in hepatic physiology and pathology. *Anatomical Record* **119**, 11–34.

Further Reading

Anthony, P. P. and Woolf, N. (Eds.) (1978). *Recent Advances in Histopathology*, No. 10, pp. 356. Churchill-Livingstone, Edinburgh and London.
Chapter 8: Causation of liver disease: recent developments. P. J. Scheuer.
Chapter 9: Alcoholic liver disease. R. N. M. MacSween.
Chapter 10: Tumours of the liver. P. P. Anthony.

Bouchier, I. A. D. (Ed.) (1973). Diseases of the Biliary Tract. In *Clinics in Gastroenterology*, Vol. 2, No. 1, pp. 215. Holt-Saunders, Eastbourne.

Howat, H. T. and Sarles, H. (Eds.) (1979). *The Exocrine Pancreas*, pp. 540. Holt-Saunders, Eastbourne.

MacSween, R. N. M., Anthony, P. P. and Scheuer, P. J. (Eds.) (1979). *Pathology of the Liver*, pp. 458. Churchill-Livingstone, Edinburgh and London.

Popper, H. (Ed.) (1975). Cirrhosis. In *Clinics in Gastroenterology*, Vol. 4, No. 2, pp. 463. Holt-Saunders, Eastbourne.

Sherlock, Sheila (1975). *Diseases of the Liver and Biliary System*, 5th edn., pp. 821. Blackwell Scientific, Oxford and London.

Sherlock, Sheila (Ed.) (1980). Virus Hepatitis. In *Clinics in Gastroenterology*, Vol. 9, No. 1, pp. 228. Holt-Saunders, Eastbourne.

Wright, R., Alberti, K. G. M. M., Koran, S. and Millward Sadler, G. H. (Eds.) (1979). *Liver and Biliary Diseases*, pp. 1345. Saunders, London, Philadelphia and Toronto.

21

The Nervous System

I: The Brain

Introduction

The nervous system is composed of two types of tissue both of which are involved in varying degree in disease processes. The first consists of the highly specialised nerve cells and their processes and also the neuroglial cells, all of which, except microglia, are of neuro-ectodermal origin: the second comprises the meninges, the blood vessels and their supporting connective tissue, all derived from mesoderm, and phagocytic cells, similar in many respects to corresponding tissue found in other systems of the body. Some diseases of the nervous system are similar to those observed in other organs—for example, inflammation, diseases of the blood vessels and tumours. Others are primary diseases of the neuron involving its cell body, its axon or its myelin sheath and in this group the aetiology is often obscure although certain virus infections, metabolic disturbances and nutritional deficiencies, particularly of the vitamin B group, may cause direct damage to nerve cells. Even in those diseases where the primary damage is to the neuron, the most conspicuous pathological abnormalities are often reactive changes in the neuroglia, the microglia (p. 728) or the blood vessels. Indeed quite severe derangement of neuronal function may occur in the absence of obvious structural abnormalities in neurons.

Applied anatomy

The arrangement of the meninges and the distribution of the cerebrospinal fluid (CSF) are intimately concerned with the spread of pathological processes. The dura mater acts as the periosteum to the cranial bones but it can be stripped from the skull by haemorrhage or exudation into the potential **extradural space**, the former secondary to tearing of a meningeal blood vessel by a fracture and the latter from spread of infection, e.g. mastoiditis, in the adjacent bone. The dura and the outer surface of the arachnoid are normally in contact but the **subdural space** can more readily be distended by blood or pus than the extradural space. The arachnoid forms a continuous sheet in contact with the dura, while the pia follows the convolutions of the brain. The space between the pia and arachnoid, known as the **subarachnoid space**, is traversed by delicate trabeculae of connective tissue into a series of intercommunicating spaces filled with CSF. Apart from the cisterna magna and the cisterns at the base of the brain, the subarachnoid space is broadest in the sulci. **The major cerebral arteries and veins** run in the subarachnoid space, and from the arteries small **nutrient vessels** pass into the cortex. The nutrient arteries to the basal ganglia and other deep structures enter the base of the brain at the **perforated areas**.

As an artery penetrates the brain it carries a sheath of pia with it, the resulting potential perivascular space (often known as the **Virchow–Robin space**) between the vessel wall and the invaginated pia being continuous with the subarachnoid space (Fig. 21.1). As the vessels become smaller the two layers fuse to form a reticular perivascular sheath which can be followed as far as precapillary vessels but not to the capillaries themselves. **The foot processes of astrocytes** form a cuff in apposition to and completely surrounding the Virchow–Robin space and the capillaries of the brain.

Micro-organisms and their toxins readily spread throughout the subarachnoid space,

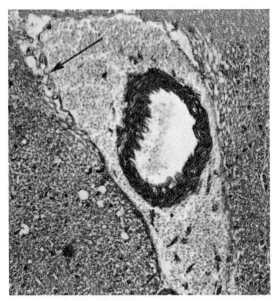

Fig. 21.1 Haemorrhage into Virchow–Robin space. The blood shows the relation of the small artery to the brain tissue. Note the pia (*arrow*). (Professor A. C. Lendrum.) × 100.

which may become filled with inflammatory exudate. The inflammatory process may then spread into the brain around the nutrient blood vessels which become surrounded by collections of leukocytes. The ventricular system com-municates with the subarachnoid space by means of the exit foramina in the roof (Magendie) and lateral recesses (Luschka) of the fourth ventricle. Cerebrospinal fluid passes freely through these foramina and, in certain disease processes, so also do blood, pus, micro-organisms or, more rarely, tumour cells. The circulation of the CSF is dealt with in greater detail in relation to hydrocephalus (p. 732).

Examination of the CSF often provides valu-able information about diseases of the nervous system. Specimens are ordinarily obtained by lumbar puncture but ventricular or occas-ionally cisternal puncture may sometimes be indicated. The pressure of the CSF should always be measured, as either an increase or a decrease may be of diagnostic value. Micro-biological, serological, cytological and bio-chemical investigations on the CSF are routine procedures.

Normal CSF is clear and colourless, does not coagulate and has a specific gravity of 1·006. It contains about 0·15–0·45 g/litre protein, about 2·8–4·4 mmol/litre (50–80 mg/100 ml) glucose, and approximately 128 mmol/litre sodium, and 128 mmol/litre chloride. A few mononuclear cells may be found in normal fluid but rarely more than 4 per μl. (See Table 21.1, pp. 768–9.)

The Reactions of the Nervous System to Disease

Neurons

The neuron (Fig. 21.2) is one of the most com-plex and specialised cells in the body, and its high, aerobic, glycolytic metabolic activity ren-ders it particularly susceptible to many disease processes. Since neurons are incapable of divid-ing after the first few weeks of extra-uterine life, any brain damage associated with loss of neurons is structurally irreversible. The neuron can be thought of as a conducting unit, and may be afferent or efferent, neurotransmitter or neuroendocrine. It consists of three main parts, the **perikaryon** or cell body, from which extend the **dendrites** and the **axon** (Fig. 21.2a). Their perikarya, which vary greatly in size, are the principal constituents of grey matter where they tend to be arranged in layers, as in the cerebral cortex, or in aggregates as in the basal ganglia. A particularly conspicuous feature in the perikarya, especially in large neurons, is the presence of the **Nissl granules** which are com-posed of rough endoplasmic reticulum and interspersed free ribosomes. Silver stains de-monstrate **neurofibrils** in the cytoplasm while **microtubules** and collections of finer tubular filaments known as **neurofilaments** can be iden-tified with the electron microscope. **Mito-chondria** are particularly numerous in dendrites and in the pre-synaptic region. **Lysosomes** are also found; and a particularly characteristic fea-ture in larger nerve cells is a progressive in-crease in their **lipofuscin** content with age. Some neurons however—particularly those in the ventral horns of the spinal cord (Fig. 21.2a) and in the inferior olivary nuclei—contain a con-

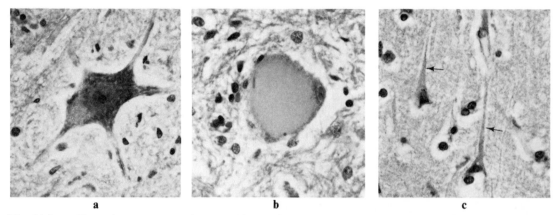

a   b   c

Fig. 21.2 a. Normal motor neuron in ventral horn of spinal cord. The dark granules within the cytoplasm are the Nissl granules. The pale area is the region occupied by lipofuscin. **b.** Similar neuron showing the features of central chromatolysis. Note the pale homogeneous cytoplasm and the eccentric nucleus. **c.** Neurons showing the features of ischaemic cell change. They are shrunken and contain dark hyperchromatic nuclei. All × 400.

siderable amount of lipofuscin even in early adult life. Certain neurons, e.g. those in the substantia nigra and the pigmented nucleus of the pons, contain **neuromelanin.**

Reactions of the neuron to disease take several forms. **Central chromatolysis** occurs in the perikaryon when the axon has been severed, and is seen in its most characteristic form in the related nerve cell bodies when the main trunk of a cranial or spinal motor nerve is transected. It can also occur as a response to certain viral infections and in certain deficiency states, particularly of the vitamin B group. At first the Nissl granules may be hyperchromatic but they rapidly lose their configuration and break down into dust-like particles before they disappear. A few granules may persist in the periphery of the cell but most of the cytoplasm becomes pale, swollen and homogeneous, and the nucleus eccentric (Fig. 21.2b). This response to injury is accompanied by increased metabolic activity and the cell may recover, particularly when the central chromatolysis has occurred as the result of damage to a cranial or spinal nerve root. By contrast, if the axon damaged is in the central nervous system, the perikaryon is more likely to degenerate and disappear. This is known as **retrograde degeneration.**

Another common abnormality is **ischaemic cell change** and is usually attributable to an inadequate supply of oxygen, but an essentially similar sequence of changes occurs in hypoglycaemia (see p. 745). The perikaryon shrinks and often takes the form of a slim triangle, Nissl granules disappear and the cytoplasm becomes intensely eosinophilic. The nucleus becomes pyknotic, and then fragments (Fig. 21.2c). A particularly characteristic feature of recent necrosis of neurons is the presence of small, dark granules known as encrustations on the surface of the perikaryon and its dendrites. Some neurons, particularly the Purkinje cells of the cerebellum, become swollen rather than shrunken; the Nissl substance disappears, the cytoplasm becomes pale and expanded and the nucleus pyknotic. This is known as **homogenising cell change.** Sometimes the dead nerve cells are removed by phagocytes (neuronophagia—see below) but more commonly, particularly in infarcts, they undergo progressive autolysis and disappear. Moderate neuronal loss is very difficult to recognise histologically unless there are also some reactive changes in the neuroglia.

Another common degenerative change in neurons is **simple atrophy**. This occurs in many of the slowly progressive degenerative diseases of the nervous system, such as motor neuron disease (p. 776). The nerve cells appear smaller than normal and lipofuscin accumulates in the cytoplasm.

There are many other but less common intrinsic degenerative changes in neurons, e.g. the appearance of inclusion bodies in certain viral infections and in Parkinsonism, neurofibrillary degeneration in some types of dementia, and distension of the cytoplasm with lipid-laden lysosomes in certain inborn errors of metabolism, but these will be dealt with later in the chapter. Abnormalities are readily brought about in neurons if the functioning of their intracellular oxidation–reduction enzyme systems is impaired as a result of some deficiency state, particularly in association with vitamin B deficiency (pp. 780–1).

When the perikaryon of a neuron is destroyed, its axon degenerates; axons separated from their cell bodies by trauma, infarction, etc., degenerate in the same way. The process is known as **Wallerian degeneration** and is well seen when peripheral nerves are transected. The axon distal to the point of transection shrinks, becomes irregular and then breaks up into fragments which are later absorbed. The myelin sheath reacts at the same time and the complex lipids are broken down into simpler lipids and, ultimately, neutral fat. Globules of lipid may be seen three or four days after damage to the axon and thereafter the fatty globules are gradually absorbed by phagocytes. The Schwann cells proliferate to form cords of cells within endoneural tubes. Degeneration of the central part of the axon usually extends for one or two segments proximal to the level of transection. The perikaryon undergoes central chromatolysis (see above). An essentially similar degeneration occurs in axons within the central nervous system when they are transected. The lipids produced by the degeneration of myelin are absorbed by macrophages and when large tracts are affected, lipid-laden macrophages may be present for many months.

Wallerian degeneration of the long tracts in the spinal cord will be dealt with in more detail later (p. 773) but it should be observed here that two principal staining techniques are used to demonstrate loss of myelin. The first of these—the Marchi technique—is used as a positive technique to demonstrate recent or active breakdown of myelin: the unsaturated fatty acids formed during this process are stained black, while normal myelin remains unstained. In the later stages, however, when most of the breakdown products have been removed, the demyelinated areas remain pale with conventional stains for myelin, e.g. the Weigert–Pal method and its modifications. Negative techniques of this type are used also to demonstrate loss of myelin in conditions other than Wallerian degeneration, e.g. multiple sclerosis (see p. 765).

Repair of neural tissue is described on p. 94. It should, however, be emphasised that, while the axons of peripheral nerves can regenerate, particularly if the endoneural tubes remain, there is no structurally significant regeneration of axons in the central nervous system.

Another form of secondary degeneration is **trans-neuronal** or **trans-synaptic atrophy**. This occurs in neurons whose principal afferent connections have been destroyed: examples are atrophy of the neurons in the external geniculate body after lesions in the retina or optic nerves, or in the nucleus gracilis and nucleus cuneatus when the posterior columns of the spinal cord have degenerated. Trans-synaptic degeneration is sometimes 'retrograde', i.e. it can occur in cells whose axons make synaptic connections with cells which have been destroyed.

Cerebral atrophy

Diffuse atrophy of the brain is due to a progressive loss of neurons, particularly within the cerebral cortex. When the process is advanced, the convolutions become more rounded and firmer than normal and the sulci widened, so that there is an excess of CSF in the subarachnoid space. The pia-arachnoid, especially over the vertex, may become thickened and opalescent while the surface of the hemispheres often appears gelatinous because of the increase in the CSF in the subarachnoid space.

The full extent of the atrophy is often not obvious until the meninges have been stripped from the surface of the brain. As the neuronal loss is accompanied by the disappearance of their axons and myelin sheaths, the white matter also shrinks and this is accompanied by enlargement of the ventricles. The histological changes underlying atrophy vary with the many different causes, e.g. senile and pre-senile dementia, ischaemia, subacute encephalitis and, to a more limited degree, as part of the changes in old age, but the two constant abnormalities are **loss of neurons and reactive gliosis**.

Neuroglia

The neuroglia includes astrocytes, oligodendrocytes and ependymal cells, all of which are of neuro-ectodermal origin.

Astrocytes. The astrocytes, which form the

astroglia, constitute the principal supporting tissue of the central nervous system. They are stellate cells with numerous fine branching processes, which lie in a mucopolysaccharide ground substance. *Protoplasmic* astrocytes and *fibrillary* astrocytes may be distinguished; the latter have fibres in their cytoplasm, which join cell to cell, and their processes are longer and straighter. Normally protoplasmic astrocytes are found mainly in the grey matter, and fibrillary astrocytes in the white matter and subpial glial layer. Both forms are attached to the walls of capillaries and other small vessels by one or more processes with swellings at their ends, the so-called foot processes. Similar expansions unite with the fibres of the pia.

In general, the reactions of astrocytes resemble those of fibroblasts. They are less susceptible to injury than neurons but where the injury is severe, as in an infarct or an acute inflammatory lesion, they undergo necrosis and disintegration. In less severe injury, astrocytes enlarge, proliferate and produce glial fibrils in increased amount. *This process is known as* **gliosis** *and it occurs in almost all conditions where damage is inflicted on any part of the central nervous system.* Where gliosis is recent and active, many enlarged cell bodies are seen, but in the late stages the cell bodies shrink and all that can be seen is a dense network of glial fibrils—*fibrillary gliosis.* The brain tissue is then firmer than normal and may have a grey translucent appearance.

Oligodendrocytes. The oligodendrocytes are small cells so named because of their few short protoplasmic processes. They are very numerous and occur as *perineuronal satellites* in the grey matter, and as rows of closely apposed nuclei in relation to myelinated nerve fibres— the *interfascicular oligodendroglia.*

Developing axons invaginate into oligodendrocytes which then form the characteristic laminated myelin sheath. Oligodendrocytes play an important role in the maintenance of myelin, and in some of the leukodystrophies (p. 767), loss of interfascicular oligodendrocytes appears to precede obvious degeneration of myelin. Very little is known about the causes or significance of reactive changes in the oligodendrocytes apart from the *acute swelling* which occurs in many acute toxic processes and the proliferation of perineuronal satellites around degenerating neurons. The latter process is

known as *satellitosis* and has to be distinguished from neuronophagia (see below).

Ependymal cells. These form a single layer of cells lining the ventricular system and the central canal of the spinal cord. They are columnar and have a ciliated, free (i.e. luminal) surface, immediately deep to which there is a line of small oval bodies known as blepharoplasts. Processes from the deep surface of the cells merge with the underlying neural tissue.

Ependymal cells show few reactive changes. Thus when the ventricles distend as in hydrocephalus, the ependyma is stretched and then broken, but the ependymal cells do not proliferate to fill the defects. A common but non-specific reaction to chronic irritation is the appearance of numerous small excrescences on the ventricular surface—**granular ependymitis.** This is, in fact, due to focal proliferation of groups of subependymal astrocytes (Fig. 21.3).

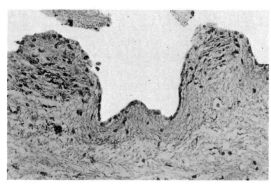

Fig. 21.3 Granular ependymitis in the floor of the fourth ventricle. × 112.

Microglia

Microglial cells are small, with an elongated hyperchromatic nucleus, scanty cytoplasm and delicate cytoplasmic processes. They belong to the mononuclear-phagocyte system (p. 72).

Microglia do not appear in the central nervous system until the vessels are formed, and are few in number until shortly before birth: they are derived from monocytes which emigrate from the small blood vessels and invade the neural tissue from the pia. They often lie close to blood vessels.

Although normally inconspicuous, microglial cells are capable of enlarging and becoming active macrophages, although it is not known how many of the macrophages seen in various lesions of the CNS are derived from microglia and how many consist of monocytes that have emigrated from the venules.

As in other tissues, macrophages are seen in the CNS in inflammatory lesions and where there is tissue destruction, in which they become laden with lipids from broken-down nervous tissue: such '*lipid macrophages*' may be present for some months following necrosis of brain tissue, e.g. in infarcts (Fig. 21.4). When neurons are selectively killed, e.g. by hypoxia or by viruses, they become surrounded by micro-

glia, and sometimes polymorphs, and undergo phagocytosis. This is known as *neuronophagia* (Fig. 21.45, p. 759), a feature which must be distinguished from non-specific satellitosis by oligodendroglia.

In some conditions, e.g. subacute encephalitis, microglia increase in length and become slightly thicker than normal: these are referred to as '*rod cells*'.

The meninges and blood vessels

While gliosis readily occurs when there is any damage to the brain, *production of fibrous tissue is seen only when the process is severe enough to damage blood vessels*. For instance, when suppuration occurs within the brain, fibroblastic proliferation along with the formation of new blood vessels leads to the production of a distinct capsule around the abscess cavity. Gliosis occurs within and around the fibrous capsule, and this combined glial and fibroblastic reaction is often referred to as a *gliomesodermal reaction*. Proliferation of capillary blood vessels is the rule in infarcts and other hypoxic lesions and in relation to rapidly growing cerebral tumours.

The reactions of the meninges will be considered in the section on meningitis (p. 746).

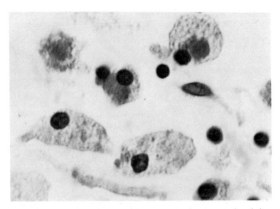

Fig. 21.4 Lipid-laden phagocytes in a cerebral infarct. × 750. (Professor A. C. Lendrum.)

The Pathology of Intracranial Expanding Lesions

Various pathological processes, such as tumour, haematoma, or a massive recent cerebral infarct, have in common the feature of increasing the bulk of the brain. *As the brain is enclosed within the rigid cranium, there is very little free space to accommodate these various expanding lesions with the result that they ultimately produce an* **increase in intracranial pressure**. An essentially similar state is produced by an extracerebral intracranial expanding lesion such as an extradural or subdural haematoma or a meningioma. There is, however, **a stage of spatial compensation** during which the intracranial pressure remains within normal limits. This compensation is brought about principally by a reduction in the volume of CSF both within the ventricles and within the subarachnoid space, by a reduction in the volume of

blood within the intracranial veins, and less commonly by actual loss of brain tissue. When all the available space has been utilised *there is a critical point at which a further slight increase in the volume of the intracranial contents causes an abrupt increase of intracranial pressure and deterioration, often rapid, in the patient's condition*. Near this critical point, arteriolar vasodilatation due to a short period of increased arterial P_{CO_2} may be sufficient to produce this effect. Clearly the compensatory mechanisms will fail more rapidly when the lesion is expanding rapidly, e.g. an intracerebral haematoma, than one of similar size that has developed slowly, e.g. a meningioma. Indeed in the latter instance there is often also local pressure atrophy and loss of brain tissue. Expanding lesions also cause distortion of the brain and it must be emphasised that *distortion and displacement of the brain and any associated increase in intracranial pressure are often of greater significance with regard to the immediate survival of the patient than the nature of the lesion or the amount of cerebral tissue destroyed by it.*

The sequence of changes in the brain caused by a **supratentorial intracerebral expanding lesion** follows a fairly standard pattern. As the lesion expands so also does the hemisphere. The CSF in the subarachnoid space is displaced and the convolutions become flattened against the dura, the sulci are progressively narrowed and the surface of the brain, when exposed *post mortem*, looks dryer than normal. Cerebrospinal fluid is also displaced from the ventricular system with the result that the lateral ventricle on the same side as the lesion becomes smaller while the contralateral ventricle may become larger. Further expansion of the affected hemisphere leads to distortion of the brain and a shift to the opposite side of the midline structures, viz. the interventricular septum, the anterior cerebral arteries and the third ventricle (Fig. 21.5). Such displacement is readily seen radiologically by ventriculography, carotid arteriography or CAT scanning. Then, depending to some extent on the site of the expanding lesion, internal herniae develop. Thus the cingulate gyrus frequently herniates under the free margin of the falx cerebri above the corpus callosum—the so-called **supracallosal** or **subfalcine hernia** (Fig. 21.5). However, the most import-

ant hernia associated with a supratentorial expanding lesion is a **tentorial hernia**, viz. protrusion of the medial part of the ipsilateral temporal lobe through the tentorial opening (Fig. 21.6). The herniated brain tissue compresses and displaces the midbrain which is pushed against the contralateral rigid edge of the tentorium. The pressure may be sufficient to produce a distinct groove (*Kernohan's notch*) on the surface of the midbrain at this point. *Compression of the aqueduct* may then block the free flow of CSF from the lateral ventricles and this further increases the intracranial pressure.

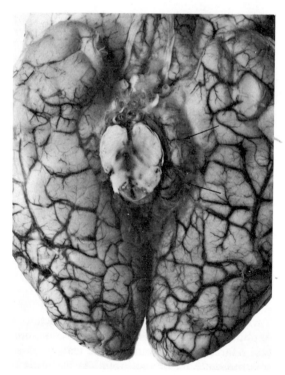

Fig. 21.6 Increased intracranial pressure due to a supratentorial tumour. Note displacement of brain stem and medial and downward displacement of the medial part of the temporal lobe—a tentorial hernia. The deep groove (*arrows*) indicates the position of the edge of the tentorium.

Other features associated with a tentorial hernia are caudal displacement of the brain stem, compression of the third and sixth cranial nerves with resultant disturbances of eye movement and pupillary reflexes and, less commonly, infarction of the ipsilateral medial occipital cortex due to selective compression of the

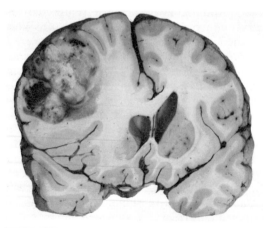

Fig. 21.5 Increased intracranial pressure due to frontal lobe tumour. Note displacement of the lateral ventricles, midline shift and supracallosal hernia.

posterior cerebral artery over the tentorium. A common terminal event in raised intracranial pressure is *haemorrhage into the midbrain and pons* (Fig. 21.7), usually involving the tegmentum adjacent to the midline. The precise pathogenesis of this haemorrhage is obscure but it is presumably a combination of caudal displacement of the brain stem, obstruction to venous drainage and stretching of arteries.

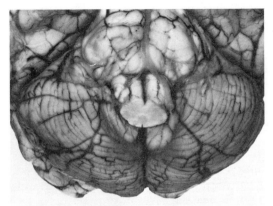

Fig. 21.8 Increased intracranial pressure. Tonsillar hernia resulting from a diffuse astrocytoma of the pons.

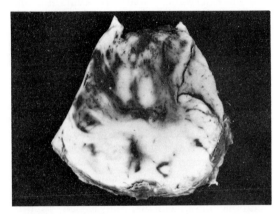

Fig. 21.7 Secondary haemorrhage into the pons caused by increased intracranial pressure.

Similar abnormalities are brought about by extracerebral intracranial expanding lesions, although flattening of the ipsilateral convolutions is often not so pronounced. If the increase in volume of the brain is more diffuse, as in generalised cerebral oedema, both lateral ventricles and the third ventricle are reduced in size. There may also be bilateral tentorial herniae. A frequent clinical sign of raised intracranial pressure is **papilloedema** due to compression of the retinal vein where it traverses the subarachnoid space in the optic nerve sheath.

A supratentorial expanding lesion may also cause a **tonsillar hernia (cerebellar cone)**, viz. impaction of the cerebellar tonsils in the foramen magnum (Fig. 21.8) but this type of hernia is more constant when the lesion lies below the tentorium. The tonsils compress the medulla and interfere with the function of the vital centres within it, particularly the respiratory centre. The hernia, by obstructing the flow of CSF through the fourth ventricle and the exit foramina, may in turn further increase the intracranial pressure so that a vicious circle is set up.

In a patient with an intracranial expanding lesion, lumbar puncture can precipitate cerebellar coning or tentorial herniation, with serious consequences. Even if only a small amount of CSF is withdrawn, more may leak into the spinal extradural space via the puncture wound in the meninges. *Lumbar puncture is therefore contra-indicated in all cases where an intracranial expanding lesion is suspected.* An exception to the rule is a suspected case of bacterial meningitis, when lumbar puncture is an essential step in establishing the diagnosis (pp. 747–8).

Prolonged increase in intracranial pressure may result in erosion of certain parts of the skull and these changes can often be seen on radiological examination. The most common examples are erosion of the posterior clinoid processes and, in children, thinning of the inner table of the skull over the convolutions, the so-called convolutional markings or beaten-brass appearance (Fig. 21.9).

The clinical features of raised intracranial pressure include headache, vomiting, a raised systolic blood pressure with a slow pulse and high pulse pressure, and diminished consciousness passing into coma. Ophthalmoscopy reveals papilloedema.

Cerebral oedema

An increase in the volume of brain tissue is a potent factor contributing to an increase in intracranial pressure. In some situations the term 'brain swelling' is preferable to 'cerebral oedema' since the increase in the volume of the brain tissue may be due simply to vasodilatation:

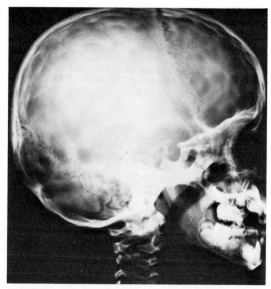

Fig. 21.9 Prolonged increase of intracranial pressure in a child. Note thinning of the skull.

ent to cerebral contusions, brain abscess and certain tumours. It is often particularly severe around metastatic tumours or meningiomas when a relatively small lesion may produce severe oedema in the adjacent brain. Indeed the oedema may constitute the major part of the 'expanding lesion'. In vasogenic oedema, there is increased permeability of the small vessels, resulting in escape of proteins and electrolytes into the extracellular space. It occurs not only in obviously inflammatory lesions but also in areas of physically traumatised brain tissue and around brain tumours: the oedema fluid diffuses into the adjacent white matter. On microscopic examination of stained sections, the abnormal tissue is pale and the tissue constituents appear to be separated by accumulated fluid. Astrocytes enlarge and if the oedema has been present for some time there is some tissue breakdown and the appearance of lipid-laden macrophages.

Cytotoxic oedema is less common in clinical situations although it may be present in some metabolic derangements, but it can be produced experimentally by various noxious agents such as triethyltin. In cytotoxic oedema there is basically a disturbance of cellular osmoregulation, the blood-brain barrier to proteins remains relatively intact and the oedema is intracellular.

this may occur in association with hypoxia or hypercapnia or be due to loss of vasomotor tone, as may occur in association with any acute brain damage. Thus vasodilatation can be a major factor contributing to brain swelling in acute head injuries (p. 738).

True cerebral oedema may be *vasogenic* or *cytotoxic*. Vasogenic oedema is common adjac-

Hydrocephalus

Definition. Hydrocephalus denotes an increase in the amount of CSF within the skull, and by far the commonest cause of **primary hydrocephalus** is obstruction to the flow of CSF. **Secondary hydrocephalus** is an increase in CSF which is compensatory for loss of neural tissue, e.g. from cerebral atrophy, when the hydrocephalus is less important since there is no increase in the total volume of the intracranial contents and so no rise in intracranial pressure. The increase of CSF may be in the ventricles, in the subarachnoid space or in both.

The source and circulation of cerebrospinal fluid

The main source of CSF is the choroid plexuses of the ventricles but some may be formed on the surface of the brain and spinal cord, for it is known that ionic exchange between blood and CSF can occur widely and is not restricted to the choroid plexuses. The total volume of the CSF is about 120–150 ml and it is renewed several times per day. The fluid formed in the lateral ventricles passes by the foramina of Monro to the third ventricle and then by the aqueduct of Sylvius to the fourth ventricle. It then passes through the foramina of Magendie and Luschka in the roof and lateral recesses respectively of the fourth ventricle to reach the subarachnoid space of the cisterna magna and basal cisterns. Thereafter it spreads through the subarachnoid space over the surface of the brain and spinal cord and is absorbed into the blood through the arachnoid granulations (arachnoid villi) which project into the dural venous sinuses (Fig. 21.10).

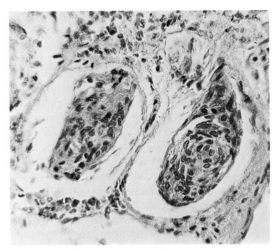

Fig. 21.10 Two arachnoid granulations lying in small dural veins.

Primary hydrocephalus

This is most often caused by obstruction to the free flow of CSF. Obstruction is most likely to occur where the channel is narrow, e.g. in the aqueduct or at the exit foramina of the fourth ventricle, but obstruction may also occur in the subarachnoid space itself.

Obstruction to the flow of CSF results in expansion of that part of the ventricular system which lies proximal to the obstruction. Thus, if the obstruction is in the third ventricle, both lateral ventricles enlarge symmetrically; if at the exit foramina in the roof of the fourth ventricle, the entire ventricular system enlarges. Obstruction at any of the above sites results in **non-communicating hydrocephalus**, i.e. the CSF cannot pass from the ventricular system to the subarachnoid space. By contrast, in obstruction of the subarachnoid space at the base of the brain, the entire ventricular system again enlarges but hydrocephalus is of **communicating type**. The site of obstruction in primary hydrocephalus can be detected by withdrawing CSF, injecting air into the lumbar subarachnoid space or into the ventricles and following its distribution by x-rays on moving the patient into various positions. Alternatively, CSF may be withdrawn from the ventricles and radio-opaque fluid injected.

It is convenient to divide obstructive hydrocephalus into **congenital** and **acquired** types but the distinction is not always clear-cut. Other possible causes of primary hydrocephalus are increased production or impaired absorption of CSF. Increased production is rare but may contribute to the hydrocephalus associated with a secreting papillary tumour of the choroid plexus (Fig. 21.75, p. 786). Decreased absorption of CSF is theoretically possible, but its occurrence in man has been questioned.

(1) Congenital hydrocephalus

This condition may be present at birth in such degree as to interfere with parturition. More often it is only slight at birth and afterwards increases. The head may become enormously enlarged and tends to become quadrangular, the vertex becomes flattened and the frontal bone projects over the orbits. The sutures are greatly widened and the fontanelles much enlarged, their closure being long delayed. There is a corresponding enlargement of the brain, the convolutions being broadened and flattened and the sulci shallow. Distension of the lateral ventricles may be so great that the brain around them is sometimes less than a centimetre wide (Fig. 21.11). If the third ventricle

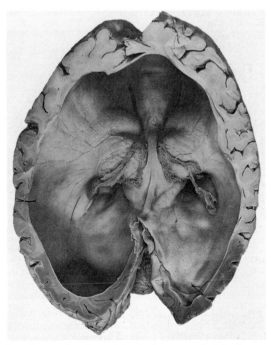

Fig. 21.11 Section of brain in congenital hydrocephalus, showing enormous dilatation of the lateral ventricles.

is involved its floor becomes greatly ballooned and extremely thin. It is remarkable how the brain can adapt itself to its altered shape and although considerable interference with mental function is usual, in a very few cases the child may be surprisingly intelligent.

One of the commoner causes of congenital hydrocephalus is the **Arnold–Chiari malformation** (Fig. 21.12): this consists of a tongue-like

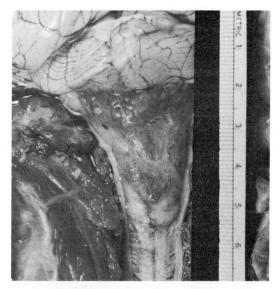

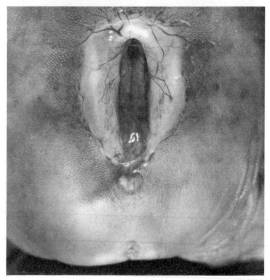

Fig. 21.12 The Arnold–Chiari malformation (*above*). The inferior part of the cerebellum protrudes as a tongue-like mass through the foramen magnum. Meningomyelocele (*below*) is almost always present. (Dr. A. A. M. Gibson.)

prolongation of the inferior cerebellar vermis through the foramen magnum and lying dorsal to the greatly elongated medulla. The lower part of the fourth ventricle thus lies in the upper part of the vertebral canal and the foramen magnum is blocked by the displaced tissue from the posterior fossa. Cerebrospinal fluid can flow out of the main exit foramina in the fourth ventricle—the hydrocephalus is, therefore, of communicating type (see above), but as the CSF is unable to re-enter the cranial cavity it cannot reach the main sites of reabsorption. The entire ventricular system thus becomes grossly enlarged. A meningomyelocele (p. 772) is an almost invariable accompaniment of the Arnold–Chiari malformation, and other features include a small posterior fossa, a poorly developed tentorium cerebelli and fusion and 'beaking' of the colliculi.

Other relatively common congenital abnormalities which give rise to hydrocephalus are faulty development of the aqueduct, and atresia of the foramina of Luschka and Magendie: in the former, hydrocephalus is confined to the third and lateral ventricles; in the latter there is in addition enlargement of the aqueduct and of the fourth ventricle. The ballooning of the roof of the fourth ventricle in these latter cases is usually so severe as to cause distortion of the inferior surface of the cerebellum.

Congenital hydrocephalus occurs also in the absence of any apparent developmental malformation. One cause of this is intra-uterine meningitis or ventriculitis, e.g. due to toxoplasmosis in which the inflammatory process produces obliterative changes in the subarachnoid space or in the ventricular system, particularly in the aqueduct. It seems likely, too, that some cases of hydrocephalus which are apparently congenital in type are a consequence of neonatal meningitis or subarachnoid haemorrhage resulting from cerebral birth injury, either of which may evoke a fibroblastic reaction leading to obliteration of the subarachnoid space and obstruction to the flow of CSF.

(2) Acquired hydrocephalus

Any expanding lesion within the skull, e.g. a tumour, an abscess or a haematoma can obstruct the flow of CSF, but the effects of the lesion depend less on its nature than on its location. Even a small lesion in a vital site, e.g.

adjacent to a foramen of Monro or close to the aqueduct, will cause hydrocephalus, whereas larger lesions elsewhere in the cerebral hemispheres may not interfere with the circulation of CSF. In general, *expanding lesions in the posterior fossa are particularly prone to cause hydrocephalus because they readily compress the aqueduct and the fourth ventricle.* Common examples are a tumour of the acoustic nerve, a meningioma or a tumour in the fourth ventricle. Acquired obstruction of the exit foramina or of the subarachnoid space is almost always due to meningitis; this may be acute, as in acute purulent meningitis, or subacute, as in tuberculous meningitis; in both, the subarachnoid space is at least partly occluded by exudate. If the inflammation does not resolve, fibroblastic proliferation leads to obliteration of the subarachnoid space particularly in the basal cisterns (Fig. 21.13) and around the midbrain which is closely embraced by the rigid tentorium cerebelli. Such an occurrence is common in the later stages of tuberculous meningitis and sometimes is a late result of acute purulent meningitis particularly if effective treatment is delayed.

A relatively uncommon cause of hydrocephalus occurring after early childhood is progressive gliosis around the aqueduct. The aetiology of this is obscure but it is probably a hamartomatous proliferation (p. 358) of astrocytes.

Secondary hydrocephalus

Symmetrical enlargement of the ventricles may be secondary to a generalised reduction in the amount of brain tissue, as in senile dementia or general paralysis of the insane. If there is only local loss of cerebral tissue, the adjacent ventricle enlarges; a common example of this is enlargement of one lateral ventricle when there is an old infarct in the territory supplied by the ipsilateral middle cerebral artery (Fig. 21.26, p. 744).

In recent years, there has been increasing recognition of a syndrome characterised by dementia, a disturbance of gait and hydrocephalus, apparently without increased intracranial

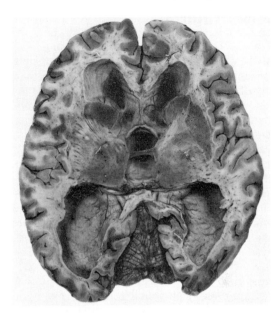

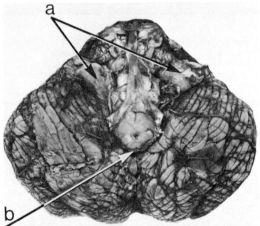

Fig. 21.13 Hydrocephalus due to occlusion of the foramina of Luschka (**a**) and Magendie (**b**) by fibrous adhesions.

pressure. The syndrome is usually referred to as '**normal pressure hydrocephalus**' but a better term would be intermittent hydrocephalus, for monitoring of the ventricular fluid pressure has shown that there may be significant rises during sleep. Some patients with this syndrome improve if a ventricular shunt operation is undertaken.

Head Injuries

In the United Kingdom trauma is responsible for more deaths in all age groups under 45 than any other single cause, and *brain damage resulting from a head injury is the most important factor contributing to death or serious incapacity due to trauma.* In civilian practice the great majority of head injuries are of the *non-missile (blunt)* type where the head suddenly accelerates or decelerates. This is associated with transient deformation of the skull, which may fracture, and linear or rotational movements of the brain within the skull which produce **immediate impact damage** to the brain, such as focal contusions and diffuse damage to nerve fibres. The clinical manifestations range from mild concussion to coma persisting until death. Other damage directly attributable to impact may be **delayed**, i.e. the process is initiated at the moment of impact but the clinical manifestations may not become apparent for some hours or even days: the commonest of these are intracranial haemorrhage and brain swelling which are sometimes referred to as **primary complications** of the head injury. **Secondary complications** include brain damage attributable to raised intracranial pressure and distortion of the brain, ischaemic or hypoxic brain damage, or infection.

(1) Immediate impact injury

Fracture of the skull

There is a tendency to exaggerate the importance of a fracture of the skull, for many patients with simple fractures may have suffered no significant brain damage, while about 20 per cent of fatal head injuries do not have a fracture. A fracture, however, does indicate that the blow has probably been of considerable force and that there is a greater likelihood of brain damage. There are some specific features associated with fractures which are important. Thus a fracture may be depressed, causing local pressure on the brain, and if there is also a laceration of the scalp the fracture is a potential source of subsequent intracranial sepsis. Any fracture of the base of the skull provides a potential source of infection from the nasal passages, the paranasal sinuses

or the middle ear. The presence of such a fracture may be shown by a CSF rhinorrhoea or otorrhoea. Other complications of a fracture are laceration of a meningeal artery leading to the formation of an extradural haematoma (see below), or injury to the carotid artery within the cavernous sinus giving rise to a carotico-cavernous fistula.

Contusions and lacerations

These are the classical features of focal brain damage directly attributable to impact. They may occur at the site of impact, particularly if there is a depressed fracture, but in any non-missile head injury they tend to involve the frontal poles, the orbital gyri, the temporal poles and the inferior and lateral surfaces of the anterior halves of the temporal lobes (Fig. 21.14). These regions are vulnerable because movement of the brain within the skull brings them into forcible contact with bony protuberances in the base of the skull. Contusions are usually asymmetrical and they may be more extensive on the side opposite the one that has suffered the impact ('*contre coup*' injury): thus severe frontal contusions may occur in association with an occipital impact. Contusions may be superficial, when they tend to be restricted to the crests of gyri, but they may extend through the full thickness of the cortex into the adjacent white matter and be associated with some intracerebral haemorrhage and oedema.

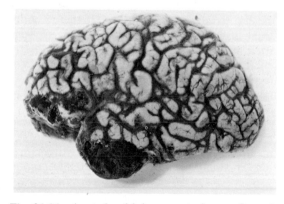

Fig. 21.14 Acute head injury: contusions at frontal and temporal poles.

Old healed contusions are represented by golden-brown shrunken scars which have such a characteristic distribution and appearance that it is often possible to state with certainty at necropsy that a patient has experienced a head injury in the past.

Diffuse damage to white matter

There is now considerable evidence to suggest that nerve fibres can be torn at the moment of impact as a result of shear strains produced by movement, particularly rotational, of the brain within the skull. This type of brain damage may occur in the absence of conventional contusions, and if the patient dies soon after the injury the only macroscopic abnormalities in the brain may be small haemorrhagic lesions in the corpus callosum and in the dorso-lateral quadrant of the rostral brain stem (Fig. 21.15) adjacent to one or both superior cerebellar peduncles. Some patients with this type of brain damage who experience no further complications of their injury may survive in a vegetative state for up to a year or so. At necropsy the brain may appear remarkably normal on inspection apart from small healed contusions. Dissection shows ventricular enlargement due to a reduction in the white matter, and small shrunken cystic lesions in the corpus callosum

and in the dorso-lateral quadrant of the rostral brain stem, i.e. in the situations where haemorrhagic lesions are seen in patients who die shortly after their injury. The principal histological abnormality in these patients is Wallerian-type degeneration in the cerebral and cerebellar hemispheres, the brain stem and the spinal cord. The clinical features of diffuse brain damage are often referred to as primary brain stem injury, but in such cases the damage is not restricted to the brain stem.

(2) Primary complications

Intracranial haemorrhage

Extradural haematoma results from haemorrhage from a meningeal vessel, usually the middle meningeal artery. As the haematoma develops, it gradually strips the dura from the skull to form a large ovoid mass (Fig. 21.16) that progressively compresses the adjacent brain. Although the tear in the meningeal artery is usually directly attributable to a frac-

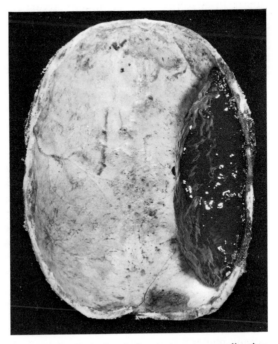

Fig. 21.16 Extradural haematoma complicating fracture of the skull. The specimen shows the undersurface of the vault of the cranium from which the dura has been removed.

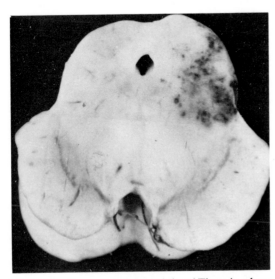

Fig. 21.15 Immediate impact injury. There is a haemorrhagic lesion in the dorso-lateral quadrant of the midbrain.

ture of the skull, it sometimes occurs without a fracture, particularly in children. The initial injury is often apparently mild. Thus many patients, whether or not they lose consciousness immediately after the injury, experience a lucid interval of some hours before developing headache and becoming drowsy. As the haematoma enlarges the patient lapses into coma and may die from the effects of raised intracranial pressure unless the haematoma is evacuated. Extradural haematomas occasionally occur in the frontal or the parietal regions, or within the posterior fossa.

Subdural haematoma results from laceration of small 'bridging' veins or of larger veins running into the main venous sinuses. In contrast to extradural haematoma, which usually remains localised, the blood tends to spread diffusely over one or both hemispheres.

Acute subdural haematoma is a common necropsy finding if death has occurred soon after a head injury. The haematoma is often thin and may not have contributed significantly to the patient's death since such patients often have extensive contusions and lacerations of the brain. In some cases, however, an acute subdural haematoma may be much larger and unless surgically evacuated can produce coma and death from raised intracranial pressure. Some patients with acute subdural haematoma experience a lucid interval similar to that classically associated with extradural haematoma.

Chronic subdural haematoma presents weeks or months after what may have seemed at the time to have been a trivial head injury. Indeed many patients deny any history of head injury. The precise aetiology is not clear but the clot becomes encapsulated in a fibrous membrane and slowly increases in size, probably as a result of repeated small haemorrhages. Because chronic subdural haematoma is particularly common in old people who already have some cerebral atrophy and because the haematoma expands very slowly, it may become very large—often 2–3 cm thick—before symptoms appear. In untreated cases, however, death is usually due to brain damage secondary to increased intracranial pressure (Fig. 21.17). Chronic subdural haematoma is not uncommonly bilateral.

Intracerebral haemorrhage usually occurs in association with contusions of the brain and so traumatic haematomas are most often seen in

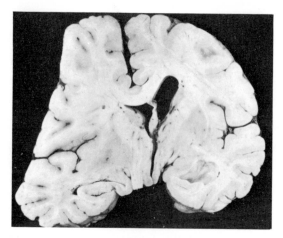

Fig.21.17 Severe distortion of the brain caused by a chronic subdural haematoma.

the frontal and in the temporal lobes. They are often multiple and vary greatly in size. They may also occur deep within the hemispheres where they are presumably due to shear strains affecting small vessels at the moment of impact.

(3) Secondary complications

Not all of the brain damage found in fatal head injury is directly attributable to impact. If an intracranial haematoma develops, much of the brain damage, particularly in cases of extradural haematoma, is due to **raised intracranial pressure** and distortion of the brain (p. 729).

Brain swelling (p. 732) is a further factor that may contribute to a high intracranial pressure in a head-injured patient. Thus there is almost always some swelling around contusions and lacerations. In patients with an acute subdural haematoma, there is often diffuse swelling throughout the ipsilateral cerebral hemisphere. Diffuse swelling may also affect both cerebral hemispheres, particularly in children.

Hypoxic brain damage is frequently observed in patients dying from non-missile head injury. Some of the causes of this are well recognised, e.g. cardiorespiratory arrest or status epilepticus, the latter being particularly frequent in children. Other hypoxic brain damage may be a direct consequence of raised intracranial pressure, but there remains a fairly large group of cases who develop focal infarction in the cerebral cortex or in the basal nuclei, the pathogenesis of which is not clearly understood. A further fairly common complication of a head injury is **infection** due to the spread of micro-organisms through a compound fracture or a fracture of the base of the skull. The infection usually presents as *meningitis* and its onset is not restricted to the early post-traumatic period, because a small traumatic fistula from the subarachnoid space to one of the major air sinuses in the base of the skull may persist. *Intracranial abscess* is a rarer complication and is usually secondary to a penetrating injury.

Clinical implications of head injury

Since the pathogenesis of brain damage due to a head injury is complex, the clinical spectrum is wide. Immediate impact damage is the beginning of an evolving process which may range from progressive improvement without complications, as in most patients with so-called concussion, to death. The period of disturbed consciousness and the interval between the injury and the return of continuous memory—**post-traumatic amnesia**—are probably closely related to the degree of diffuse brain damage: if this is mild, the patient may only be transiently dazed; if it is severe the patient will remain in a vegetative state until death. By contrast, immediate impact damage of focal type, i.e. contusions, may have relatively mild clinical effects and even severe cerebral contusions may cause little or no permanent cerebral dysfunction. But even if the initial injury appears only trivial, there is the possibility of primary or secondary complications such as intracranial haematoma, raised intracranial pressure, hypoxic brain damage or infection. Thus in a personally studied series of 151 patients with fatal non-missile head injuries, who had been referred to a neurosurgical unit because their neurological state had been causing concern, 58 were found to have talked at some time after their injury, i.e. they had ap-

parently recovered in some measure after their injury, only to deteriorate and die later. *The management of head-injured patients has therefore to be based on the knowledge that complications occur only too frequently, and that at least some of these are avoidable.*

Head injury is an important cause of **symptomatic epilepsy**. About 10 per cent of patients admitted to hospital with a non-missile head injury develop fits. These tend to occur in the first week after injury (*early epilepsy*) or are delayed until 2–3 months or more after the injury (*late epilepsy*). Early epilepsy occurs more commonly after severe or complicated head injuries, although children under 5 may develop it after apparently trivial injuries. Factors predisposing to late epilepsy include a depressed fracture and an acute intracranial haematoma. Fits are less liable to recur in patients with early epilepsy than in those who develop late epilepsy. With missile (i.e. penetrating) head injuries, the incidence of epilepsy is about 45 per cent.

Trauma to the spinal cord

Injuries of the spinal cord, like those of the brain, are of all degrees of severity. In cases of fracture-dislocation, bullet wounds, etc., the cord may be directly lacerated, or even torn across. Apart from such extreme cases, the cord may be damaged by acute flexion or extension of the neck, when haemorrhage may occur outside or inside the dura or within the spinal cord itself. There may also be infarction of the cord. Haemorrhage occurs especially immediately dorsal to the grey commissure, and tends to extend upwards and downwards through several segments. In cases of haemorrhage into the cord, or *haematomyelia*, the blood is broken down and ultimately an elongated pigmented encapsulated cavity may result, which may simulate syringomyelia (p. 778).

Circulatory Disturbances

Cerebrovascular disease falls into two principal categories—spontaneous intracranial haemorrhage and ischaemic brain damage. Both are often referred to as 'strokes'.

Spontaneous intracranial haemorrhage

The two common causes of spontaneous intracranial haemorrhage are primary intracerebral haemorrhage and rupture of an aneurysm on a major cerebral artery.

Intracerebral haemorrhage

Primary intracerebral haematomas occur mostly in patients with hypertension. About a century ago Charcot came to the conclusion that the haemorrhage occurred from miliary aneurysms on small perforating cerebral arteries but this has only become generally accepted in recent years as a result of postmortem micro-angiographic studies which have clearly demonstrated the existence of micro-aneurysms on these arteries. They are usually multiple, tend to occur on arteries less than 250 μm in diameter and may attain a diameter of 2 mm. They occur mainly in hypertensive subjects over the age of 50. In contrast, micro-aneurysms are rare in normotensive individuals although a few can be demonstrated in some people over the age of 65.

The commonest site for hypertensive intracerebral haemorrhage is in the region of the basal ganglia and the internal capsule (Fig. 21.18). Other fairly common sites are the pons (Fig. 21.19) and the cerebellum. Subcortical haemorrhage also occurs but is rare. The haematoma usually increases in size rapidly, causes severe local destruction of tissue, and produces a sudden rise in intracranial pressure and rapid distortion and herniation of the brain (p. 730).

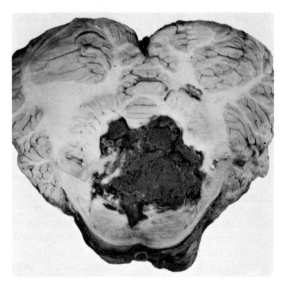

Fig. 21.19 Hypertensive haemorrhage into the pons.

The blood may rupture into the ventricles or through the surface of the brain directly into the subarachnoid space. The clinical onset is usually sudden and patients with large intracerebral haematomas rarely survive for more than a few days, death often being precipitated by secondary haemorrhage into the brain stem as a result of raised intracranial pressure.

The appearance of the haematoma at necropsy varies with its duration. A recent haematoma is composed of ordinary dark coloured clot. If the haematoma is not large enough to be rapidly fatal, its periphery has a brownish colour after about a week and there are early reactive changes in capillaries and astrocytes in the adjacent brain. This brownish colour then spreads throughout the entire haematoma while gliosis leads to the formation of a poorly-defined capsule. If the patient survives, the clot is ultimately completely absorbed and replaced by yellow fluid to form a so-called **apoplectic cyst** (Fig. 21.20).

Ruptured intracranial aneurysm

Aneurysms develop on the major arteries at the base of the brain in about 1–2 per cent of the adult population, and they are quite common incidental findings at necropsy. They are often referred to as **congenital** or **berry aneurysms**, but the developmental abnormality is a defect

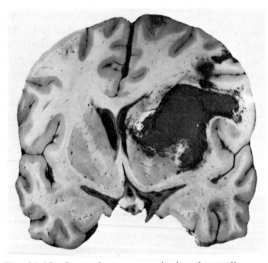

Fig. 21.18 Large haematoma in basal ganglia, resulting from chronic hypertension.

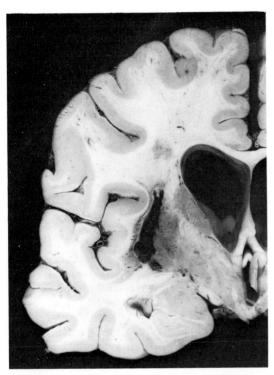

Fig. 21.20 Old apoplectic cyst on left side of brain. The cyst is centred on the external capsule and the outer part of the lentiform nucleus.

in the medial coat of the artery at the bifurcations of the larger cerebral arteries within the subarachnoid space. Subsequent degeneration of the internal elastic lamina, probably due to early atheroma, may predispose to the development of the aneurysm. The arterial wall at the bifurcation then commences to bulge and an aneurysm forms which may vary in size from a small projection 2–3 mm in diameter to a sac measuring 2–3 cm across.

The commonest sites for these aneurysms are the bifurcation of a middle cerebral artery within the Sylvian fissure, the junction of the anterior communicating artery with an anterior cerebral artery, and the junction between an internal carotid and posterior communicating artery. Aneurysms may also occur on the basilar artery and its branches. About 10–15 per cent of patients who present with symptoms due to an aneurysm are found to have multiple aneurysms, usually two or three but sometimes five or more.

Aneurysms usually rupture at their fundus and produce **subarachnoid haemorrhage**. This may be limited to the immediate vicinity of the aneurysm but frequently there is severe and extensive haemorrhage into the subarachnoid space. Blood may also track into the brain to produce an **intracerebral haematoma** (Fig. 21.21), and if its fundus is embedded in brain

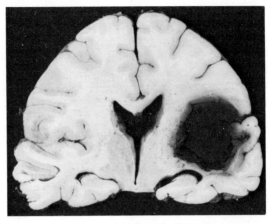

Fig. 21.21 Ruptured aneurysm. Haemorrhage from an aneurysm on the middle cerebral artery has produced a haematoma in the Sylvian fissure and in the adjacent brain.

tissue—a not uncommon occurrence—intracerebral haemorrhage may occur without any subarachnoid haemorrhage. Anterior communicating aneurysms tend to burst into the frontal lobe while posterior communicating aneurysms and middle cerebral aneurysms commonly rupture into the temporal lobe. Thus patients with ruptured intracranial aneurysms may have the clinical and pathological features of an acute expanding lesion in addition to subarachnoid haemorrhage. Such intracerebral haematomas often in turn rupture into the ventricles.

Another complication of a ruptured aneurysm is **infarction**, most commonly in the region of the brain supplied by the affected artery. This is probably partly attributable to arterial spasm, and the swelling which occurs in a recent infarct (pp. 743–4) may cause further displacement and distortion of the brain.

In many fatal cases of ruptured intracranial aneurysm there is a history of a previous small subarachnoid haemorrhage and in such cases examination of the brain may reveal the presence of altered blood pigment in the meninges adjacent to the aneurysm.

Rarer causes of intracranial aneurysm are

infected emboli (mycotic aneurysms, p. 388) and atheroma.

It should be emphasised that subarachnoid haemorrhage and ruptured intracranial aneurysm are not synonymous terms; the former may be the result of an acute head injury or haemorrhage from a vascular malformation (see below) or it may be secondary to a primary intracerebral haemorrhage tracking into the ventricles or through the surface of the brain; moreover, a ruptured aneurysm may cause an intracerebral haematoma or a cerebral infarct without any significant subarachnoid haemorrhage.

Other causes of spontaneous intracranial haemorrhage

Probably the commonest of these is haemorrhage from a **vascular malformation**, which may range in size from small capillary angiomas to massive lesions composed of a plexus of large, often thick-walled vascular channels (Fig. 21.22). They usually occur on the surface of the brain or the spinal cord but sometimes lie deep in the brain. When a vascular malformation ruptures it may produce a massive intracerebral haematoma which is rapidly fatal but a more frequent result is mild subarachnoid haemorrhage. Many of these lesions are compatible with long survival, perhaps punctuated by episodes of subarachnoid haemorrhage.

Other causes of spontaneous intracranial

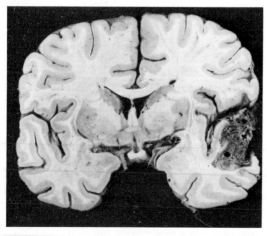

Fig. 21.22 Vascular malformation. There is a plexiform mass of vessels in the superficial part of the temporal lobe.

haemorrhage include haemorrhage into tumours and haemorrhagic diseases. Thus cerebral haemorrhage is a common fatal complication in acute leukaemia.

Spontaneous intracerebral haemorrhage sometimes occurs in normotensive subjects: the pathogenesis is not clear but it may be related to the occasional micro-aneurysms found in normotensive subjects, to degenerative vascular disease or to rupture of a small vascular malformation within the brain.

Ischaemic brain damage

The brain receives its blood supply from the internal carotid and vertebral arteries, sometimes called the *extracranial cerebral arteries*, from which the major *intracranial cerebral arteries* arise. *A* **cerebral infarct** *occurs when the blood flow to any part of the brain falls below the critical level necessary to maintain the viability of brain tissue.* In contrast to the *diffuse* selective neuronal loss that may occur in various hypoxic states, not necessarily due to reduction of cerebral blood flow (p. 745), an infarct is essentially a *focal* lesion and may be restricted to a small discrete lesion in the grey or white matter or may affect a large part of the brain. The reduction in blood flow may result in the death of only the most susceptible cells, viz. the neurons, but usually it is more severe, producing necrosis also of the neuroglial cells and, slightly less commonly, of microglia and blood vessels also. Occlusion of a cerebral artery is not essential for infarction: indeed an episode of severe hypotension or transient cardiac arrest may cause cerebral infarction in the absence of arterial disease, but more usually there is stenosis and/or occlusion of a major extracranial or intracranial cerebral artery. *The critical reduction in the blood flow to a particular region of the brain needs to last for only several minutes to produce an infarct.* If the reduction is transient, blood flow through the infarct may return to normal. When the cerebral circulation is already compromised by pre-existing arterial stenosis, infarction is particularly liable to occur in any hypotensive state, e.g. following myocardial infarction.

The principal local cause of an *inadequate cerebral blood flow* is **atheroma**: this may result only in stenosis, but the artery may become occluded by the formation of thrombus on an atheromatous plaque. Other vascular diseases leading to a reduced arterial lumen with or without thrombosis are *arteritis* (e.g. in polyarteritis nodosa, giant cell arteritis, tuberculous meningitis and syphilitic endarteritis). A cerebral artery may also be blocked by an **embolus** which usually comes from vegetations on the mitral or aortic valve cusps in cases of infective endocarditis or from mural thrombus in patients with auricular fibrillation or a myocardial infarct. Transient neurological symptoms, the so-called 'transient ischaemic attacks' are often due to emboli of platelet aggregates (p. 234) or lipid from ulcerated atheromatous plaques in the carotid or vertebral arteries.

An infarct may occur in any part of the brain although the middle cerebral arterial territory is most frequently involved. The size of the infarct depends to a considerable extent on the degree of occlusive arterial disease and the available collateral circulation. Collateral channels exist between the major cerebral arteries on the surface of the brain and in the circle of Willis, but anastomoses do not exist within the brain. Depending on the site of vascular occlusion, an infarct may therefore affect an entire arterial territory or only part of it, while if the blood flow through two adjacent arterial territories is affected, infarction may be restricted to the **boundary zone** between them.

Arterial obstruction

Cerebral infarction may result from occlusion of arteries within the cranium or in the neck. The commonest intracranial site of occlusion is the middle cerebral artery. The commonest extracranial site is at the origin of an internal carotid artery and, if the collateral circulation is or becomes inadequate, the usual site of infarction is in the distribution of the middle cerebral artery on the same side. In some cases thrombosis extends along the internal carotid artery into the middle and anterior cerebral arteries to produce infarction of a large part of the cerebral hemisphere. When the vertebral arteries are the more severely involved, ischaemic changes occur characteristically in the brain stem, the cerebellum and the part of the cerebral hemispheres supplied by the posterior cerebral arteries, i.e. the occipital lobes. Cerebral infarction is often the result of a combination of systemic circulatory insufficiency and stenosis of the extracranial or intracranial cerebral arteries, or of both. Occlusion of an internal carotid artery in the neck is usually secondary to atheroma, but it may also occur after closed injuries to the neck.

Structural changes in a cerebral infarct

A cerebral infarct may be pale or haemorrhagic: this depends (*a*) on whether or not some blood flow has been restored through the infarct and (*b*) on whether or not necrosis of vessel walls has occurred, thus allowing the extravasation of blood into the necrotic tissue. An intensely haemorrhagic infarct may superficially resemble a haematoma but the distinctive feature of a haemorrhagic infarct is the preservation of the intrinsic architecture of the affected tissue (Fig. 21.23). A pale infarct less

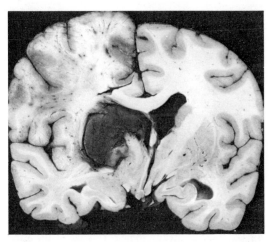

Fig. 21.23 Recent infarct in left cerebral hemisphere. The basal ganglia show the features of haemorrhagic infarction; the posterior part of the frontal lobe above the Sylvian fissure shows those of pale infarction. Note that the affected hemisphere is swollen and that there is displacement of the midline structures to the right.

than 24 hours old may be difficult to identify macroscopically, but thereafter the dead tissue becomes slightly soft and swollen and there is a loss of the normal sharp definition between grey and white matter. At this stage histological examination will show ischaemic necrosis of neurons, pallor of myelin staining and sometimes polymorphonuclear leukocytes in relation, to necrotic vessel walls. If the infarct is large it may swell to the extent of producing the typical features of an acutely expanding intracranial lesion and raised intracranial pressure (see p. 729). Within a few days, the infarct becomes distinctly soft and the dead tissue disintegrates: hence a cerebral infarct is often referred to as a '**softening**' (Fig. 21.24). Microscopic examina-

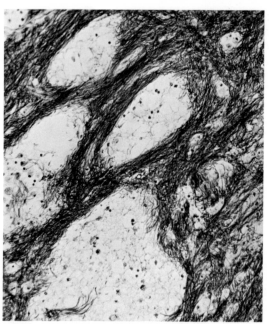

Fig. 21.25 Glial fibrils and spaces containing fluid in an old infarct. × 140. (Professor A. C. Lendrum.)

(Fig.21.26). The meninges overlying an old cortical infarct are thickened and opaque and underneath there is usually an adherent layer of brownish-yellow cortical tissue composed of

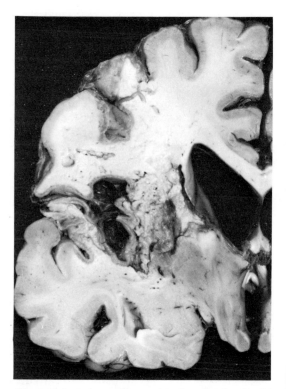

Fig. 21.24 Infarct of a week's duration in the left cerebral hemisphere. The dead tissue is disintegrating and there is already some shrinkage of the affected cortex.

tion at this stage will show phagocytes filled with globules of lipid produced by the breakdown of myelin (Fig. 21.4), and, around the dead tissue, enlarged astrocytes, and early capillary proliferation. Eventually the dead tissue is removed, lipid phagocytes become scanty, a fibrillary gliosis occurs and the lesion ultimately becomes shrunken and cystic. The cysts are often traversed by small vessels and glial fibrils (Fig. 21.25). If the infarct has been haemorrhagic, a proportion of the phagocytes will contain haemosiderin. Shrinkage of the affected region is usually accompanied by enlargement of the adjacent lateral ventricle

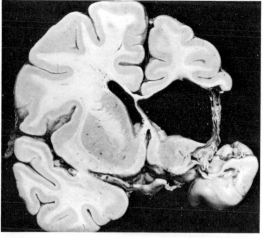

Fig. 21.26 Infarct of several years' duration in the right cerebral hemisphere. The dead tissue has been completely removed. The lateral ventricle is separated from the surface of the brain by a narrow web of tissue composed of leptomeninges, ependyma and a few glial fibrils.

enlarged astrocytes and occasional lipid phagocytes. Beneath this the cortex is usually
cystic and traversed by strands of thick astrocytic fibres. A consequence of infarction is
Wallerian degeneration in the nerve fibres that
have been interrupted. Thus if the infarct involves the internal capsule, there is progressive
degeneration and shrinkage of the corresponding pyramidal tract in the brain stem and in the
spinal cord.

Other aspects of ischaemic brain damage

A diminished blood supply to the brain may
lead to loss of nerve cells without frank infarction. The neuroglia remains alive, with the
result that focal neuronal loss is accompanied
by a fibrillary gliosis. This process is analagous
to the ischaemic atrophy with fibrosis which
occurs as the result of arterial narrowing in the
kidneys and other organs. Areas of sclerosis
produced in this way are a prominent feature in
dementia of arteriopathic type, and they are
common also in general arterial disease, especially in old people.

Venous obstruction

The most important form of this results from
thrombosis in one of the sinuses. Two types of
thrombosis are usually distinguished, *marantic*
and *septic*: in the latter there is often suppuration within the sinus. *Marantic thrombosis* is
most frequent in poorly nourished children
during the course of acute infections, e.g.
gastro-enteritis; but it may occur in adults in
wasting diseases, e.g. malignant tumours, or as
a complication of infective fevers. Impaired circulation and possibly bacterial infection of low
virulence may be causal factors. The commonest site is the superior sagittal sinus, and,
when obstruction is complete, intense engorgement of the superficial veins occurs. There may
also be irregular zones of intensely haemorrhagic infarction in the parasagittal parts of the
cerebral hemispheres. In thrombosis of the
straight sinus, similar haemorrhagic areas are
present in the walls of the third ventricle. *Septic
thrombosis* is the result of direct spread of organisms from an adjacent septic lesion (p. 749).

Cerebral hypoxia

Neurons are particularly susceptible to hypoxia, and consciousness is lost within a few
seconds of complete oxygen deprivation. Their
supply of oxygen depends on the cerebral
blood flow which in turn depends on the cerebral perfusion pressure, i.e. the difference between the systemic arterial pressure and the
cerebral venous pressure. Since the most important factor maintaining an adequate oxygen
supply to the brain is the cerebral blood flow,
there are inbuilt protective mechanisms to pre-
serve it. This mechanism is known as *autoregulation* which can be defined as the maintenance
of a relatively constant blood flow in spite of
changes in perfusion pressure. Autoregulation
is brought about mainly by changes in the cerebrovascular resistance—when arterial pressure
falls, cerebral arterioles dilate; when arterial
pressure increases, cerebral arterioles constrict.
In consequence, blood flow is maintained
within normal limits even when the systemic
arterial pressure falls to as low as 50 mmHg,
provided the subject is in the prone position.
At arterial pressures lower than this, cerebral
blood flow falls rapidly. Autoregulation may
be impaired in chronic hypertension, in hypoxic
or hypercapnic states, and in a wide range of
acute conditions producing brain damage, e.g.
head injuries and strokes.

Because of the susceptibility of neurons to
hypoxia, the vital factor with regard to the ultimate clinical outcome in many medical emergencies, e.g. cardiorespiratory arrest, a severe
episode of hypotension, carbon monoxide or
barbiturate intoxication or status epilepticus, is
whether or not satisfactory resuscitation can be
achieved before the occurrence of irreversible
hypoxic brain damage. Hypoglycaemia has an
essentially similar effect because neurons require glucose as well as oxygen for their metabolism. The neuronal damage varies in its
distribution; thus it tends to be *focal* and
accentuated in the boundary zones between
major arterial territories when there is a severe
but transient episode of hypotension, whereas it
is *diffuse* in more generalised disturbances of the
supply of oxygen or glucose to the brain as in
cardiac arrest, status epilepticus, carbon monoxide poisoning and severe hypoglycaemia.

Many patients who suffer severe diffuse
hypoxic brain damage die very soon after the

episode, and the brain may appear entirely normal macroscopically. Indeed it may still appear normal macroscopically even if the patient has survived deeply comatose for a few days. Provided the patient has survived for more than about 12 hours, however, microscopic examination will disclose widespread and severe neuronal necrosis. There are minor variations in the distribution of the neuronal necrosis but the neurons in the brain that are selectively susceptible to oxygen deprivation are those in the Ammon's horns (hippocampus), in the third, fifth and sixth layers of the cerebral cortex (particularly within the sulci), and in certain of the basal nuclei, and the Purkinje cells in the cerebellum.

With the passage of a few days, the dead neurons disappear and reactive changes in astrocytes, microglia and capillaries become intense. If the patient survives for more than a few weeks, the affected regions become shrunken and cystic as in a conventional infarct.

Kernicterus. When severe jaundice occurs in infancy it carries the risk of brain injury: necrosis of

neurons and bile staining are seen particularly in the hippocampus and basal nuclei (hence *kernicterus* or *nuclear jaundice*) and sometimes in the cerebral cortex, and are followed by gliosis. If not fatal, the brain injury is likely to cause choreo-athetosis, spasticity and often mental deficiency.

Pathogenesis. The condition is particularly likely to occur when the plasma level of *unconjugated* bilirubin exceeds 250 μmol/litre (15 mg/100 ml), and by far the commonest cause of this in full-term infants is haemolytic anaemia due to fetal-maternal Rh incompatibility (p. 527). Other causal factors include functional immaturity of the liver in premature infants, liver injury of various kinds and genetically determined defects of bilirubin conjugation (p. 715). Hypoxia during labour or at birth, or due to severe anaemia, may be contributory factors and the administration of excess vitamin K analogues (for haemorrhagic disease of the newborn) tends to aggravate haemolysis and so may increase the jaundice.

In the fetus, bilirubin is excreted by the placenta, and so jaundice only becomes severe after birth. This can be prevented by exchange blood transfusion which, by removing antibody and replacing the sensitised fetal red cells by compatible cells, is especially effective in preventing kernicterus in Rh incompatibility.

Bacterial Infections of the Nervous System

Since the brain and spinal cord are relatively well protected from bacteria, infections of the nervous system are not particularly common. But once micro-organisms have gained access to the nervous system, the infection may spread rapidly by way of the CSF pathways. The severity of the clinical illness depends on the virulence of the infecting agent and the susceptibility of the host, but many micro-organisms which are relatively non-pathogenic elsewhere in the body may cause serious and often fatal infection of the nervous system.

Inflammation of the meninges—**meningitis** —and inflammation of the brain—**encephalitis** —will be considered separately since, although both are usually present in any severe inflammatory process one is almost always much more severe than the other.

Meningitis

Meningitis may involve the dura—**pachymeningitis**—or the pia and the arachnoid—**leptomen-**

ingitis. The latter is by far the commoner, and is usually referred to simply as meningitis.

Pachymeningitis

Acute inflammation of the dura is practically always due to extension of inflammation from the bones of the skull. The underlying infection may be chronic suppurative otitis media or mastoiditis, or the infection may be a sequel to a depressed fracture of the skull. When pyogenic organisms spread from the bone, suppuration occurs between bone and dura and an **extradural abscess** may form. The dura becomes swollen and softened, and the infection may penetrate through it and spread widely over the hemisphere to form a **subdural abscess**. The organisms may also spread to the subarachnoid space, setting up either localised or general **leptomeningitis**. Further effects of spread, such as the production of cerebral abscess, are described below. The dura is occasionally the site of gummatous lesions in syphilis (p. 752).

Leptomeningitis

This is produced by the spread of micro-organisms throughout the subarachnoid space. They provoke an inflammatory reaction and exudate is added to the CSF, which is a good culture medium for many bacteria.

Causal organisms are many and varied. Acute purulent meningitis is caused most often by *Neisseria meningitidis* (meningococcus), *Streptococcus pneumoniae* (pneumococcus) and the haemophilus group. *Escherichia coli* is fairly common in infants. Some viral diseases of the nervous system, and also subarachnoid haemorrhage, can produce symtoms suggestive of acute bacterial meningitis. Less frequent causes of meningitis are *Mycobacterium tuberculosis*, the ordinary pyogenic cocci, the bacilli of the coli-typhoid group, the anthrax bacillus, *Treponema pallidum*, leptospirae and various fungi.

Routes of infection. (*a*) *Infection by the bloodstream*. Most cases of meningitis are of haematogenous origin. In meningococcal meningitis (*cerebrospinal fever*), for example, infection is spread by droplet infection from carriers who harbour the micro-organism in the nasopharynx. Spread is favoured by poor hygienic conditions, especially overcrowding, and thus the disease tends to occur in epidemic form among recruits in overcrowded barracks, refugees in camps, etc. In susceptible persons the meningococci pass from the nasopharynx to the meninges by the bloodstream and during epidemics cases of fatal meningococcal septicaemia can occur without meningitis, death sometimes occurring within a few hours of infection. A characteristic feature of meningococcal septicaemia is the occurrence of a haemorrhagic rash from which the old name 'spotted fever' is derived (Fig. 21.27).

(*b*) *Infection from an adjacent lesion*. Leptomeningitis may result from spread of infections in the middle ear or in any of the air sinuses in the base of the skull, or through an open depressed fracture. It should be emphasised that acute leptomeningitis is a fairly common complication of a fracture of the base of the skull as a result of direct spread of organisms from air sinuses or the nasopharynx.

(*c*) *Iatrogenic infection* can occur from the introduction of micro-organisms at operation or by lumbar puncture with non-sterile instruments. This is rare, but as the infecting agents

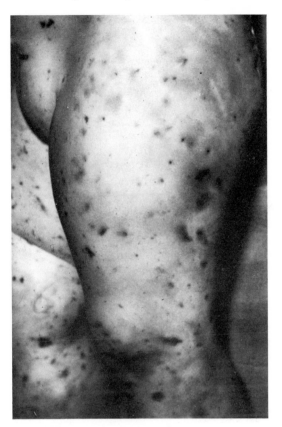

Fig. 21.27 Acute meningococcal septicaemia, showing the haemorrhagic rash.

are introduced directly into the subarachnoid space, a generalised meningitis rapidly ensues.

Structural changes. Exudate accumulates in the subarachnoid space and is most easily seen where the space is wide, i.e. within sulci (Fig. 21.28) and at the base of the brain, where it accumulates around the optic chiasma and in the adjacent cisterns. It varies markedly in appearance, even in the same type of infection. There may merely be excess of turbid fluid in the sulci, or the exudate may be abundant, yellowish and fibrinous or purulent. Some degree of hydrocephalus is common since the exudate interferes with the flow of CSF.

The inflammation frequently extends into the ventricles: they contain turbid CSF and a coating of fibrin is seen on their walls and on the choroid plexuses. Exudate is also abundant in the spinal subarachnoid space, particularly on the dorsal surface of the cord.

Diagnosis. *The CSF must be examined as*

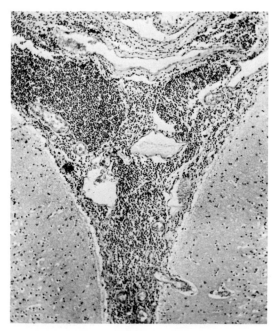

Fig. 21.28 Acute pneumococcal meningitis: section of cerebral cortex showing distension of the subarachnoid space with purulent exudate. × 55.

soon as possible whenever meningitis is suspected, even if there is some clinical evidence of increased intracranial pressure (p. 731), for this is the only means by which the diagnosis can be established and the causal agent identified. The CSF is usually turbid and may be distinctly purulent. Microscopic examination shows it to contain numerous polymorphonuclear leukocytes. The protein content is raised and the sugar reduced or absent (Table 21.1, pp. 768–9). The causal organisms are often apparent, although in some cases they can be obtained only by culture. In early acute meningitis, particularly in children, the first specimen of CSF may be normal in every respect. This is difficult to explain, but a subsequent lumbar puncture only 24 hours later may show all the features of a florid acute meningitis.

Treatment. Vigorous early treatment with the appropriate antibiotic usually results in resolution of the infection with little or no residual damage. If treatment has been inadequate or started too late for resolution of the inflammatory exudate to occur, the disease may pass into a subacute or chronic phase. Formerly this was not uncommon in young children, particularly with meningococcal meningitis, and the

disease was then referred to as *posterior basal meningitis*. The meninges become thickened and oedematous and the exudate organised leading to obliteration of the foramina in the roof of the fourth ventricle and/or some degree of obstruction in the subarachnoid space, and consequent hydrocephalus (p. 735). Various cranial nerves may be involved with resulting paralyses. Similar chronic changes can occur in the spinal meninges with widespread involvement of nerve roots. Bacteria are usually scanty in such chronic cases. Closely similar structural changes may be brought about by the tubercle bacillus (see p. 750) and by *Haemophilus influenzae*.

'*Aseptic' or viral meningitis* is described on p. 755.

Bacterial encephalitis

Bacterial encephalitis is usually suppurative (i.e. a *brain abscess*) but non-suppurative encephalitis may result from extension of inflammation from an active meningitis. The degree to which this occurs varies greatly. In some cases it is striking how little leukocytic infiltration there is along the blood vessels; in others the perivascular spaces are crowded with leukocytes and there may occasionally be superficial infarction and suppuration in the cortex. In tuberculous meningitis there is usually marked involvement of the cortex due to obliterative arteritis and thrombosis in many of the arteries in the subarachnoid space.

Brain abscess

The causative organisms are many, anaerobic streptococci, diphtheroids and coliforms, etc. being encountered in addition to the common pyogenic cocci. They reach the brain, as in meningitis, by direct spread or by the blood stream.

Direct spread of bacteria. This is usually a consequence of pyogenic infection in the bones or sinuses of the skull or of a compound fracture. The most important cause is chronic suppurative otitis media or mastoiditis. The bone is eroded by a chronic osteitis and infection reaches the dura to produce an *extradural* or a *subdural abscess* (p. 746). The inflammation extends to the leptomeninges and a generalised meningitis may ensue but more frequently the inflammation is limited by local adhesions. The bacteria may then cause suppuration in the cortex before extending more deeply into the brain, but more often the subsequent abscess is separated from the surface of the brain by an intact layer of cortex; in fact, in some cases of middle ear disease, the caries may not even have reached the surface of the bone. The precise route of infection in these cases may be via small blood vessels. The emergent veins from the bone drain into a venous sinus, into which the veins of the brain also discharge, providing a possible route of infection.

If the middle ear infection spreads upwards through the tegmen tympani, the abscess occurs in the temporal lobe (Fig. 21.29). If infection spreads from the mastoid antrum, or from the middle ear, to the posterior aspect of the petrous bone, the abscess occurs in the cerebellum; in such cases the sigmoid sinus may be involved and thrombosed. In some cases with chronic middle ear disease, abscesses may be found both in the temporal lobe and in the cerebellum.

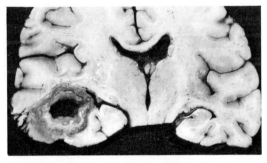

Fig. 21.29 Cerebral abscess. There is an encapsulated abscess in the left temporal lobe, secondary to chronic suppurative otitis media.

As elsewhere, an abscess in the brain becomes limited by a pyogenic membrane which, unless the infection extends very rapidly to involve the meninges or ventricles, soon becomes a well-defined capsule composed of young connective tissue, new capillaries, enlarged astrocytes and lipid phagocytes. In the adjacent cerebral tissue there are varying degrees of oedema, reactive gliosis and infiltration by lymphocytes and plasma cells, particularly in the perivascular spaces. The symptoms of an abscess are often vague and by the time the diagnosis is made it may contain thick greenish-yellow pus commonly with a foul odour because of the mixed bacterial flora. An abscess

may remain latent for some months, but it commonly enlarges and becomes multilocular, and finally may rupture into a ventricle or the subarachnoid space.

Otitis media and mastoiditis. Disease of the middle ear, mastoid antrum and air cells, resulting from spread of infection along the Eustachian tube from the pharynx, is commoner in children than in adults. It often starts as a complication of streptococcal tonsillitis, but in infants pneumococci are often responsible. Mixed infections are also common. Acute suppurative inflammation of the lining of the tympanic cavity develops and, if this progresses, the mucous membrane is destroyed and replaced by a layer of granulation tissue; the tympanic membrane is often perforated allowing access to a very mixed bacterial flora. The bone becomes eroded by osteitis and infection may reach the dura, giving rise to local pachymeningitis, acute leptomeningitis, cerebral abscess, sinus thrombosis, etc. A similar sequence may follow acute suppuration in the frontal sinus, the resulting abscess being in the frontal lobe, but this is more rare.

Septic sinus thrombosis. This results from spread of pyogenic infection to the wall of a sinus, most frequently to the sigmoid sinus from the mastoid or middle ear. The process is similar to septic venous thrombosis (p. 201) with infection and sometimes suppuration of the thrombus. Extension of thrombosis into the jugular vein often prevents the dissemination of septic emboli from the sinus, so that pyaemia is unusual.

Haematogenous abscesses occur most frequently in the parietal lobes but may appear in any part of the brain and are often multiple. When solitary they may become large and develop a thick gliomesodermal capsule before being diagnosed. The source of the septic embolus may be anywhere in the body but the primary site is often in the lung. In the past, there was a particularly close association between suppurative bronchiectasis and brain abscess, but fortunately infection in bronchiectasis can now usually be adequately controlled by antibiotics. Individuals with congenital cyanotic heart disease are, however, still prone to develop a brain abscess. Multiple small acute abscesses occur in pyaemia, while in a patient dying with subacute infective endocarditis numerous small perivascular inflammatory foci are almost always found in the brain. Such lesions may be seen as minute haemorrhagic foci but frequently they are identifiable only on microscopic examination.

Yeasts and fungi are rarer causes of haematogenous brain abscess (p. 763).

Tuberculosis

Involvement of the nervous system is a not uncommon feature of tuberculosis. It is always secondary to tuberculosis elsewhere in the body and usually presents as a *subacute meningitis*. Less commonly it takes the form of a *tuberculoma*.

Tuberculous meningitis

The bacilli reach the brain by way of the bloodstream: this may be simply one manifestation of miliary tuberculosis, usually in association with a primary complex, but sometimes it is a complication of chronic pulmonary or renal tuberculosis in adults. Less commonly the infection may spread to the meninges by direct spread from tuberculosis of a vertebral body. Another mode of infection is by way of a small haematogenous caseous lesion in the cortex of the brain.

On reaching the meninges the bacilli proliferate and spread throughout the subarachnoid space where their presence induces a diffuse leptomeningitis characterised by both exudation and formation of tubercles. At first the CSF is clear or faintly turbid, but later the exudate in the subarachnoid space becomes thick and gelatinous or caseous (Fig. 21.30). As is usual in meningitis, the exudate is most abundant in the basal cisterns (Fig. 21.31) and in the sulci: the exudate itself, and deposited fibrin, obscure the surface features of the base of the brain, brain stem and cord. Tubercles are seen

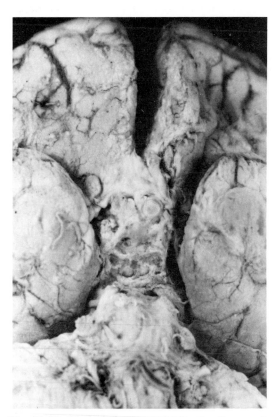

Fig. 21.30 Tuberculous meningitis, showing exudate which obscures structures at base of brain. A few tubercules can be seen on the frontal lobes.

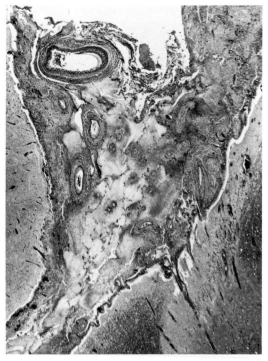

Fig. 21.31 Tuberculous meningitis. Chiasmal cistern, showing soft fibrinous exudate filling the subarachnoid space, with cellular exudate in the walls of vessels. × 8.

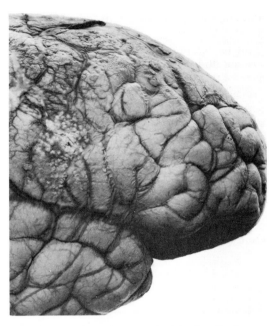

Fig. 21.32 Tuberculous meningitis: localised eruption of tubercles on the surface of the hemisphere in the region of the Sylvian fissure.

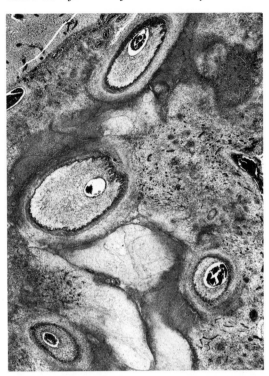

Fig. 21.33 Cerebral arteries in chronic tuberculous meningitis, showing obliterative endarteritis. × 15.

most readily when the exudate is thin: they appear as grey nodules, 1–2 mm in diameter, adjacent to the blood vessels in the subarachnoid space (Fig. 21.32). Microscopically, the subarachnoid space may at first contain many polymorphonuclear leukocytes but these are soon replaced by macrophages, lymphocytes and desquamated pia-arachnoid cells. Fibrin from the exudate is deposited in the subarachnoid space and may later undergo organisation. The tubercles are seen to be poorly formed, rounded cellular aggregates with central caseation: the cells are mainly macrophages which show incomplete transformation to epithelioid cells while giant cells are relatively small or absent.

Vascular involvement is a prominent feature. In the early stages this may take the form of an acute necrotising arteritis in which the vessel walls are infiltrated with polymorphs and fibrin. Later, and particularly in prolonged cases where effective treatment has been started relatively late, there is an intense reactive endarteritis which leads to considerable thickening of the intima (Fig. 21.33). In consequence, there is quite often focal infarction of the adjacent superficial brain tissue and of

cranial and spinal nerves, these infarcts accounting for some of the focal neurological signs which occur in patients with tuberculous meningitis.

Some degree of hydrocephalus is an almost invariable accompaniment of tuberculous meningitis since the tough exudate readily obstructs the free flow of CSF.

The CSF in tuberculous meningitis is under increased pressure. It is often clear but more frequently has an opalescent appearance. A fine fibrin web may appear on standing. The number of cells is raised, often to over 200 per μl: usually they are mostly lymphocytes and plasma cells with a few macrophages, but polymorphs may be present and may occasionally exceed the lymphocytes, especially in the earliest stages of the disease. The protein is increased and the glucose and chlorides are diminished. Tubercle bacilli can usually be found on microscopic examination of the centrifuged deposit or of the fibrin web which forms in the fluid on standing. It is essential to administer the appropriate antibiotics to all suspected cases, even when tubercle bacilli cannot be found in the CSF. Delay in starting treatment may allow the pathological changes to progress to a point from which return to normal is impossible.

Tuberculomas

These are frequently encountered in regions such as East Africa, India and South America where tuberculosis is common, and in some localities they account for a considerable proportion of all intracranial expanding lesions. They occur particularly in children and young adults and may be multiple. The commonest sites are the cerebellum (Fig. 21.34) and brain stem. They are usually firm, dull yellow, with a grey fibrous, or more highly vascular, red capsule.

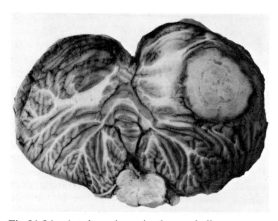

Fig.21.34   A tuberculoma in the cerebellum.

Syphilis

Syphilitic lesions of the central nervous system used to be common and serious. They fall into two groups. Firstly, lesions occurring in the late secondary and tertiary stages, which involve connective tissues and the blood vessels; these comprise meningitis, gummas and endarteritis, either singly or combined. Secondly, *neurosyphilis*, which includes tabes dorsalis and general paralysis of the insane; these occur much later than the tertiary stage, and involve the nervous tissue directly.

Syphilitic meningitis may involve the dura, the leptomeninges, or both. Syphilitic *leptomeningitis* most commonly affects the base of the

brain, where it causes a diffuse thickening of the meninges, usually with superficial involvement of the brain. The affected meninges are swollen and gelatinous, and there may be patches of gummatous necrosis. Various cranial nerves, especially the optic and oculomotor nerves, become involved. The process may obstruct the foramina of the fourth ventricle and cause hydrocephalus.

Microscopy shows a fibroblastic reaction and a heavy infiltrate of lymphocytes and plasma cells (Fig. 21.35) and commonly reactive endarteritis (Fig. 21.36) with consequent focal infarction in the adjacent cortex. Cellular infiltration occurs round the small penetrating vessels and there is gliosis in the outer layers of the cortex.

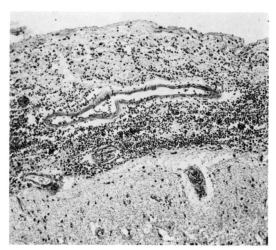

Fig. 21.35   Syphilitic leptomeningitis, showing thickening and lymphocytic infiltration of the meninges. × 50.

Similar lesions occur in the spinal meninges, in which endarteritis and infarction of the cord are prominent. The rare *hypertrophic cervical pachymeningitis* is produced mainly by syphilis: the dura and arachnoid are thickened and adherent, gliosis occurs in the spinal cord, and the nerve roots may be compressed and undergo atrophy.

Meningeal *gummas* may be multiple in syphilitic meningitis. When they arise in the leptomeninges, they extend inwards and are irregular. Gummas of the dura are usually flattened and may cover a large part of a hemisphere (Fig. 21.37): they may erode the skull and/or compress the adjacent brain tissue.

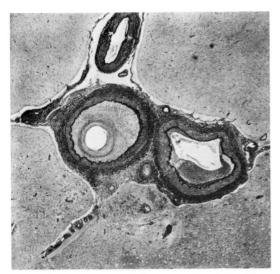

Fig. 21.36 Syphilitic endarteritis of the anterior cerebral arteries. There is also a well-marked syphilitic meningitis. Multiple small infarcts were present in both hemispheres. × 28.

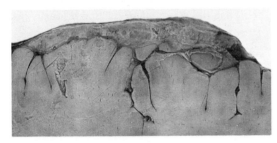

Fig. 21.37 Section of hemisphere showing a large gummatous mass arising in the dura. × ½.

Neurosyphilis

This includes two conditions, *general paralysis of the insane* and *tabes dorsalis*, which occur in a small proportion of patients some years after the tertiary lesions and usually 5–20 years after contracting syphilis. They affect men much more often than women and may occur together. They may also occur in congenital syphilis, usually from 10 years of age onwards. The changes in the nervous tissue in these conditions are not due to vascular disease.

General paralysis of the insane (GPI) is a subacute encephalitis with widespread lesions in the nervous system; the resulting symptoms are motor, sensory and psychiatric. *Treponema pallidum* has been demonstrated in the brain. The Wassermann reaction is usually positive in both blood and CSF.

Structural changes are most marked in the frontal lobes, where the gyri are atrophic and the sulci widened, with a corresponding increase in CSF. The pia and the arachnoid are thickened and opaque and are unduly adherent to the brain. There may be chronic subdural haematomas. The ventricles are enlarged as a result of cerebral atrophy (secondary hydrocephalus) and there is a granular ependymitis (Fig. 21.3, p. 728).

Microscopically, the cortical grey matter is much more cellular than normal, although the number of neurons in it is greatly reduced. The cells include lymphocytes and plasma cells, which are most numerous in the space around the small nutrient vessels, and rod cells (p. 729), many of which contain granules of haemosiderin, and which are sometimes conspicuous also in the deep tissues. There is a general increase in glial fibres, while enlarged and branched astrocytes ('spider cells') are conspicuous, particularly in the superficial cortex and around small blood vessels. Gliosis may extend to the white matter. With effective treatment, active inflammation subsides, leaving residual gliosis, both general and cortical, and loss of nerve cells.

Cerebrospinal fluid. The cells are usually increased to over 50 per μl—mostly lymphocytes but with some macrophages and plasma cells. Protein, particularly IgG, is usually much increased. On immuno-electrophoresis, much of the IgG in the CSF separates into a number of discrete bands, indicating its production in the CNS by plasma cells derived from a small number of B-cell clones. The Lange test gives a paretic pattern (Table 21.1, p. 768) and the CSF almost invariably gives a positive Wassermann reaction.

Tabes dorsalis (locomotor ataxia). The lesion in this late syphilitic disorder is a slowly progressive degeneration of the posterior roots of the spinal nerves and their upward extensions in the posterior columns of the spinal cord. The posterior roots entering the lumbar enlargement of the cord are mainly or solely affected in most cases, but in some the cervical enlargement is affected (*cervical tabes*).

In sections stained by the Weigert–Pal method (Fig. 21.38) the posterior roots, posterior horns and posterior columns all appear pale from loss of myelinated fibres. At higher levels

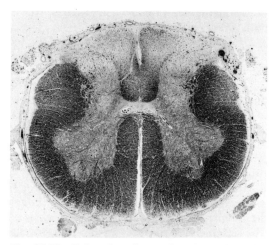

Fig. 21.38 Tabes dorsalis: section through lumbar enlargement of cord, showing the degeneration in the posterior roots and posterior columns. × 8. (Weigert–Pal method.)

in the cord the posterior roots appear relatively or completely normal, and the posterior column degeneration is confined to the medial (gracile) tract as in ascending degenerations in general (p. 773). Degenerative changes may involve the sensory cranial nerves, and involvement of the optic nerves with visual loss is common.

Clinically, there is early loss of proprioceptive sense in muscles and joints in the lower limbs, with loss of co-ordination and ataxia.

The posterior root lesion also interrupts the spinal reflex arc, with absence of the knee-jerk, etc. and loss of muscle tone with a characteristic stamping gait. There is also loss of pain sense, and consequent trophic changes are common, e.g. deep ulceration of the soles of the feet, and neuropathic arthropathy (*Charcot's disease*—p. 923). Some common clinical features are not satisfactorily explained, for example, the *Argyll-Robertson phenomenon* in which the pupils contract normally during accommodation but not in response to light, abdominal crises which simulate acute surgical emergencies and attacks of 'stabbing pain' in the lower limbs.

In *cervical tabes* the pathological changes are similar and result mainly in disturbances of function in the upper limbs.

The CSF in tabes shows an increase of cells, usually to over 50 per *μ*l.; they are mainly lymphocytes but with some macrophages. The protein is normal or slightly raised and, as in GPI, IgG is usually raised and of oligoclonal origin. The Lange test usually gives a luetic reaction (Table 20.1, pp. 768–9) and the Wassermann reaction is usually positive.

The mechanism of nervous tissue injury in GPI and tabes dorsalis is obscure: spirochaetes have been detected with some difficulty in the CSF and affected nervous tissue. Even without treatment, only a small proportion of patients develop neurosyphilis.

Virus Infections of the Nervous System

Most patients with a viral infection of the CNS present as cases of either '*aseptic' leptomeningitis* or *encephalitis*, although some degree of both (meningo-encephalitis) is usually present. In some types of encephalitis due, for example, to the polioviruses (i.e. viruses which colonise neurons), the most severe lesions occur in the spinal cord, where there is selective involvement of motor neurons: in such cases the term *paralytic disease* is often appropriate clinically. Aseptic meningitis is the commonest clinical illness but relatively little is known about its pathology since it is rarely fatal. Encephalitis, on the other hand, usually causes severe and frequently fatal brain damage.

Acute virus diseases of the nervous system have long been recognised but only relatively recently has the nature of **persistent virus infections**, e.g. subacute sclerosing panencephalitis (p. 760), and **slow virus infections**, e.g. kuru (p. 761), been appreciated.

Pathogenesis

Most viruses reach the nervous system by way of the bloodstream, i.e. there is a viraemia, often after primary viral multiplication in lymphoid tissue. They may enter the body by various routes, e.g. infection of the skin or mucous membranes (herpes simplex virus), by way of the alimentary tract (enteroviruses), through injured skin (B virus of monkeys), or introduction through the skin by the bite of an arthropod (arboviruses). A few viruses may reach the nervous system by travelling along peripheral nerves (rabies virus). Polioviruses travel readily along nerves in experimental animals, but the natural route of infection in man is by the bloodstream.

The clinical features of virus infections of the nervous system frequently occur late in the course of the infection when viraemia is subsiding and circulating antibody has appeared. This has led to the concept that at least a proportion of the brain damage is brought about by immunological reactions to viral antigens in the nervous system. Only a small proportion of individuals infected by potentially *neurotropic viruses* (i.e. viruses with a predilection for the nervous system) develop clinical evidence of neurological disease.

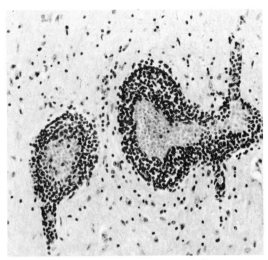

Fig. 21.39 Section of posterior part of medulla in encephalitis lethargica, showing the extensive perivascular infiltration by lymphocytes and plasma cells. × 170.

General features of virus encephalitis

The reactions of the brain and spinal cord to virus infections tend to be similar in all types of virus encephalitis but they vary both in their intensity and distribution throughout the nervous system.

In fatal acute viral encephalitis, there may be no macroscopic abnormalities in the nervous system, but in some varieties there is congestion, swelling, softening, or focal haemorrhage in the more severely affected regions. Microscopically, the most prominent and widespread abnormality is the presence of lymphocytes, macrophages and plasma cells in the meninges and around small vessels (often referred to as **perivascular cuffing**) throughout the brain and spinal cord (Fig. 21.39). The next most characteristic feature is **necrosis of nerve cells** and **neuronophagia** (Fig. 21.45), when the dead neurons become engulfed by macrophages, or less commonly by polymorphs.

In the more florid types of encephalitis, necrosis may not remain restricted to nerve cells but may spread to involve grey and white matter, e.g. in herpes simplex encephalitis. In certain forms of encephalitis, e.g. herpes simplex encephalitis and subacute sclerosing panencephalitis, **intranuclear inclusions** may be found in neurons or astrocytes (Fig. 21.41). If the patient lives for some time after the acute illness, the areas that have borne the brunt of the damage may be shrunken and cystic (Fig. 21.42).

In aseptic meningitis, abnormalities are virtually restricted to infiltration of the subarachnoid space by mononuclear cells and perivascular cuffing in the superficial layers of the cortex.

Essentially similar abnormalities are found in the CSF in all acute virus infections of the nervous system. It is often under increased pressure and there is characteristically an increase of leukocytes (50–500/μl, usually lymphocytes, plasma cells and large mononuclear cells) and of protein (0·5–2 g/litre, 50–200 mg/100 ml) whereas the sugar content is normal.

Aseptic meningitis

Although usually not a severe illness, viral leptomeningitis, commonly termed aseptic meningitis, is a *very common* acute infection of the nervous system, particularly in children. It is caused by many viruses but those most frequently implicated in Britain are the *enteroviruses* and *mumps virus*. Enterovirus meningitis is a summer disease and is often seen as an epidemic in which one or perhaps two enteroviruses predominate. The virus is spread by the faecal–oral route. In mumps meningitis, which does not show the striking seasonal incidence of enterovirus meningitis, there is no accompanying parotitis in about 50 per cent of cases.

Viruses of the herpes group

The nervous system may be affected by at least four viruses in the herpes group—herpes simplex, varicella-zoster, B virus of monkeys and cytomegalovirus. All are DNA viruses of similar morphology.

Herpes simplex virus

This causes three types of disease in the CNS. The most severe is *acute necrotising encephalitis* which at present is the commonest type of acute encephalitis in Western Europe. The others consist of *foci of necrosis* throughout the brain associated with similar lesions in other organs and tissues in disseminated herpes simplex virus infection in infants, and *aseptic meningitis* (see above).

Acute necrotising encephalitis. This is fulminating and often rapidly fatal. Its most characteristic feature is selective, bilateral but asymmetrical involvement of the temporal lobes with gross, irregular patches of necrosis. In a fatal case there is usually flattening of the convolutions and raised intracranial pressure, while the more severely affected temporal lobe is soft, swollen and often focally haemorrhagic (Fig. 21.40). There is often also an ipsilateral tentorial hernia (see p. 730). Necrosis usually

occurs also in the insulae and in the cingulate gyri. *Microscopic examination* shows diffuse infiltration of the meninges and perivascular spaces by lymphocytes and plasma cells, and where necrosis has occurred, there are numerous plasma cells and hypertrophied microglia in the affected brain tissue. In the cortex adjacent to the zones of necrosis, intranuclear inclusion bodies may be found

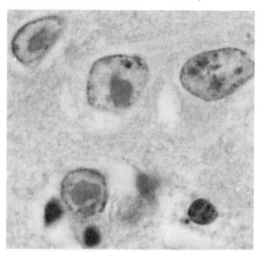

Fig. 21.41 Acute necrotising encephalitis. Note the presence of intranuclear inclusion bodies. × 1200.

within neurons and astrocytes in some cases (Fig. 21.41). Neuronophagia is seen widely throughout the brain and spinal cord. The diagnosis of herpes simplex encephalitis during life rests on the isolation of virus from a brain biopsy taken through a burr hole in the skull. Virus cannot usually be isolated from the CSF. If the patient survives the acute phase, the necrotic tissue becomes shrunken and cystic (Fig. 21.42).

Zoster

This is a disease of adults, caused by the same virus that causes varicella (chickenpox). During the illness there is often a rise in the antibody titre against the virus to levels above those commonly seen in varicella. Adults with zoster sometimes infect susceptible children, typical varicella resulting. The reverse, however, is very rare, and it appears that zoster is the result of recrudescence of a latent infection with varicella virus in a partially immune subject. Zoster results from acute inflammation of

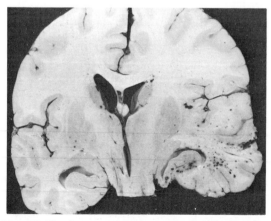

Fig. 21.40 Acute necrotising encephalitis due to Herpes simplex virus. Within the swollen right temporal lobe there are many small haemorrhagic foci.

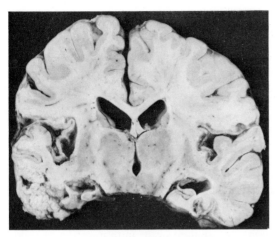

Fig. 21.42 Acute necrotising encephalitis. This patient survived for several weeks. The affected regions are now shrunken and focally cystic. The left temporal lobe is more severely affected than the right one.

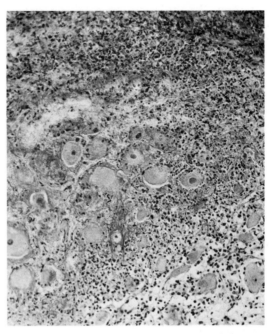

Fig. 21.43 Section of posterior root ganglion in zoster, showing inflammatory infiltration and destruction of nerve cells. × 160.

a posterior root ganglion, most commonly one of the lower cervical or dorsal ganglia. In one type of zoster the Gasserian ganglion is affected. Along the course of the nerve related to the affected ganglion, pain and hyperalgesia occur, followed by erythema and the formation of vesicles which contain a serous or haemorrhagic exudate. The acutely inflamed ganglion is swollen by haemorrhagic exudate and heavily infiltrated with lymphocytes, while the nerve cells show various degrees of acute injury (Fig. 21.43): many of them undergo necrosis while in other areas they appear almost normal. The inflammatory process may extend into the dorso-lateral quadrant of the spinal cord at the level of the affected ganglion. Central chromatolysis is commonly seen in the neurons of the anterior horn and there may be paresis.

As a result of the nerve cell injury, secondary degeneration (shown by Marchi's method) can be traced along the nerve fibres to their peripheral distribution, and also proximally through the posterior nerve roots and for a distance upwards in the posterior columns of the cord. Later, secondary fibrosis occurs in the root ganglia which have been damaged.

What produces reactivation of the latent virus is not clear, but physical trauma to the affected part seems to be a fairly frequent precipitating factor. Immunological disturbances may also be involved, for zoster is common in patients with a malignant lymphoma, in whom the lesions may become disseminated with a generalised varicelliform rash, particularly in patients treated with cytotoxic drugs and corticosteroids. In such cases there may also be a multifocal necrotising encephalomyelitis.

B-virus encephalomyelitis

B virus is a natural parasite of monkeys in which it causes stomatitis and viraemia, and is very similar to herpes simplex in man. Transmission to man is by a monkey bite or by contamination of a skin wound by saliva or tissues from an infected monkey. The human disease is an acute encephalomyelitis with paralysis of cranial nerves and the respiratory muscles, usually progressing to coma and death within two weeks. Histological examination shows a **multifocal necrotising encephalitis** affecting grey and white matter, sometimes with a particular predilection for the spinal cord.

Cytomegalovirus

Involvement of the nervous system by cytomegalovirus is mainly due to infection acquired *in utero*. In the neonate, it causes an acute, often severe, disseminated necrotising encephalomyelitis with selective involvement of periventricular tissue. Cytomegalic inclusions may be found in various types of cell. Survivors are often mentally retarded; the principal abnormalities in the brain are hydrocephalus and periventricular calcification. Infection early in pregnancy may lead to developmental malformations such as microgyria (p. 772).

Enteroviruses

The most important enteroviruses are the polioviruses, Coxsackie and ECHO viruses. All are small RNA viruses. They are a frequent cause of *aseptic meningitis* but they may also cause *paralytic disease*, e.g. acute anterior poliomyelitis, which is classically associated with the polioviruses, but is caused occasionally by other enteroviruses, particularly Coxsackie A7. Indeed in countries where a vigorous poliovirus vaccination programme has been undertaken Coxsackie virus may now be a commoner cause of paralytic disease than the polioviruses. Overt paralysis probably occurs in no more than about 1 per cent of individuals infected with the most pathogenic poliovirus—type I.

Acute anterior poliomyelitis

This is an acute encephalomyelitis affecting especially severely the anterior horns of the spinal cord, and leading to destruction of the motor neurons, with corresponding paralysis and subsequent atrophy of the related muscles.

Epidemiology and virology. Before the introduction of poliovaccine, this was the commonest acute encephalomyelitis caused by a neurotropic virus. It may occur sporadically but also in both major and minor epidemics. Three types of poliovirus have been distinguished and immunity to one type does not protect against the others. Most cases of paralytic poliomyelitis are caused by type I virus.

In man the natural route of infection is by the mouth and the virus multiplies in the alimentary tract. It is often present in the nasopharyngeal secretions of a person suffering from the disease but is most readily isolated from the faeces, where it may persist for long after the acute illness. There is an early viraemia and the infection reaches the central nervous system by crossing the blood–brain barrier.

In the past, endemic poliomyelitis was a disease affecting young children almost ex-

clusively. In the large epidemics of paralytic disease which swept through countries with a high standard of living (and hygiene) in the years before and just after World War II, there were however proportionately more cases in adults. The infectivity rate of poliovirus is high but most of those infected develop either no symptoms or only a mild febrile illness. Only a few develop severe neurological lesions, which may appear after a brief temporary remission of fever. There is good evidence that the development of paralytic disease may be determined by factors such as muscular fatigue during the initial stage of the illness or by local tissue damage, e.g. by intramuscular injections, such as those used in the immunisation of children by combined prophylactics, especially those containing alum. Adults are also more likely than children to develop paralysis when infected with poliovirus. The occurrence of epidemics of paralytic disease in countries with high standards of hygiene was attributable to the relatively low incidence of infection in childhood, and adults encountering the virus for the first time were at greater risk of developing severe, paralytic disease. By contrast, in countries with poor standards of hygiene, most people encounter the infection in childhood, and so the risk of paralytic disease is less.

Structural changes. The virus selectively attacks the neurons in the ventral horns of the spinal cord, particularly in the lumbar and cervical enlargements, which are affected asymmetrically. Macroscopic examination in an acute case reveals little beyond congestion of the meninges over the affected part of the cord and of the ventral horns which, in severe cases, may be necrotic and haemorrhagic.

Microscopic examination reveals extensive inflammatory infiltration of the leptomeninges, with lymphocytes, plasma cells, and some polymorphonuclear leukocytes, but no fibrin. The infiltrate extends along the perforating vessels, especially branches of the anterior spinal arteries (Fig. 21.44).

In the anterior horns, where inflammation is usually most marked in the medially placed cell groups, there is intense congestion and oedema along with the cellular infiltration; some of the smallest vessels may be thrombosed and there may be capillary haemorrhages. The nerve cells are affected in varying degree. Some undergo acute necrosis, and are removed by phago-

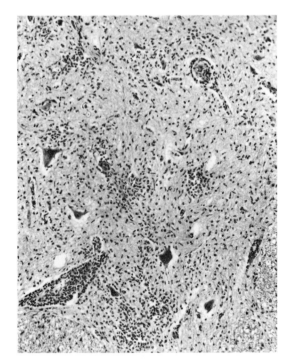

Fig. 21.44 Ventral horn of lumbar cord in poliomyelitis fatal on the 5th day. Note the perivascular cuffing, the general inflammatory infiltration and neuronophagia of dead nerve cells.

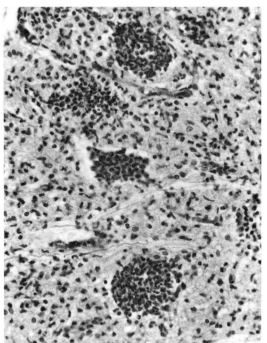

Fig. 21.45 Ventral horn of lumbar cord in acute poliomyelitis (5th day). Each of the dense cellular aggregates is a dead neuron which is obscured by polymorphs and macrophages (neuronophagia).

cytes—neuronophagia (Fig. 21.45). If the nerve cell dies, disintegration of its axon and myelin sheath follows. Other nerve cells show varying degrees of central chromatolysis, though it is remarkable how little altered some of them are, even when surrounded by inflammatory change. There may be little change in the adjacent white matter beyond perivascular cuffing by mononuclear cells.

Sometimes the virus affects the motor nuclei in the medulla, causing acute bulbar paralysis. There are also lesions in the cerebral cortex, characteristically localised to the motor and pre-motor areas, but there tends to be no generalised involvement of the cortex.

Effects. The more acute changes usually pass off in a few days, but the infiltrate of lymphocytes and plasma cells may persist for some months. In the acute illness, there is paralysis of the muscles supplied by damaged neurons. Since many of the less severely injured neurons recover, the paralysis may improve considerably. The destructive lesions in the cord are followed by removal of the degenerated tissue by macrophages, with subsequent gliosis. Gradually the affected parts shrink, and if the lesion has been severe, the ventral horns become very small, and the anterior nerve roots thin. The permanently affected muscle fibres undergo typical neurogenic atrophy (Fig. 23.68, p. 935). Owing to the unopposed action of the unaffected muscles, deformities of the limbs, including various forms of club-foot etc., develop. The bones in the affected limbs may show atrophy, being reduced both in thickness and in density (Fig. 2.33, p. 39).

Rabies

Rabies is still a major problem in Central and Eastern Europe, in India and in some parts of North and South America. Its incidence in animals is increasing in Europe. The virus enters the body in the saliva of biting animals and reaches the CNS by travelling along peripheral nerves. The major reservoirs of the virus are the fox, the skunk and the jackal, although most human cases result from the bite of a rabid dog. Vampire bats seem to be an important source of infection in some regions. The incubation period of the disease in man is usually between one and two months: rabies may be of the restless type, corresponding to the 'furious' rabies of dogs, or, much less commonly, of the paralytic type. Spasm of the muscles of deglutition on attempting to drink water is a prominent and early symptom, and accounts for the old name, *hydrophobia*.

Microscopically, rabies encephalitis is predominantly a polio-encephalitis since perivascular cuffing by lymphocytes and plasma cells and microglial hyperplasia occur principally in the grey matter. Neuronophagia is common, as are larger aggregates of macrophages. The pathognomonic histological feature of rabies, however, is the **Negri body**, which is a large sharply defined, rounded or oval acidophilic cytoplasmic inclusion body. They may lie anywhere within the cytoplasm of a neuron, including its dendrites, and two or more may be seen in the one cell. The largest bodies are usually seen in the pyramidal cells of the hippocampus and in Purkinje cells in the cerebellum. Virus particles have not been identified in Negri bodies, and it has been suggested that they store nucleoproteins until a proper template for virus assembly is formed. Negri bodies are found only after infection with 'street' virus and do not occur after the virus has become 'fixed' by laboratory passage.

In classical rabies the dorsal root ganglia, lower brain stem and hypothalamus are principally affected. In the paralytic form, abnormalities are more severe in the lower parts of the spinal cord and in the medulla.

When someone is bitten by a dog suspected of having rabies, the animal should not be killed, for its survival for a week excludes the diagnosis. Rabies can be diagnosed in animals by the histological identification of Negri bodies in the brain.

Arboviruses

The only shared attributes of arboviruses are that they are transmitted from host to host by blood-sucking insects (**ar**thropod–**bo**rne **viruses**), and that they are all RNA viruses. They multiply in both vertebrate and invertebrate hosts. An arthropod vector is infected by sucking blood from a vertebrate and, after an incubation period, the virus reaches the salivary gland of the arthropod whose bite infects a new host: after an interval during which viral replication occurs, there is a period of viraemia during which other arthropods may become infected. Man is not the natural host for any arbovirus but, during periods of epizootic spread among the natural hosts (usually wild birds and small mammals), he may become infected.

Several arboviruses can cause severe encephalitis in man, e.g. *St. Louis encephalitis, Eastern and Western equine encephalomyelitis* and *Japanese B encephalitis*, all of which are mosquito-borne. The structural changes are in general those of a disseminated encephalitis (p. 755), sometimes with focal necrosis in vessel walls. Tick-borne arboviruses are responsible for *Russian spring–summer encephalitis* and *louping ill*.

Encephalitis lethargica

This was the first pandemic encephalitis in modern times, and its sudden appearance, rapid pandemic spread and subsequent disappearance are not the least of its mysterious features since its cause was never established. It is however generally accepted that the disease was a virus encephalitis. A small epidemic with a mortality rate of about 50 per cent occurred in Vienna in the winter of 1916–17. The disease than spread through Western Europe, and reached North America towards the end of 1918. The epidemic reached its peak in Britain in 1924. It had virtually disappeared from there by 1926.

The symptoms were those of an acute generalised encephalitis, often with disturbed sleep rhythm and extreme lethargy by day. The mortality averaged about 25 per cent. A high proportion of patients who survived developed permanent Parkinsonism (see p. 771).

If the patient died in the acute stages of the disease, there was characteristically intense congestion of the meninges, the cerebral cortex, the basal ganglia and the brain stem. Microscopical examination showed infiltration of the meninges and perivascular cuffing by lymphocytes and plasma cells (Fig. 21.39) and sometimes haemorrhages into perivascular sheaths and adjacent tissue. Thrombosis of small vessels was sometimes present. Although many nerve cells showed evidence of chromatolysis, neuronophagia was slight.

Subacute sclerosing panencephalitis (SSPE)

First described in children as subacute inclusion body encephalitis, and later as subacute sclerosing leukoencephalitis, subacute sclerosing panencephalitis is a **persistent virus infection** of the nervous system caused by the measles virus. It is a rare form of prolonged encephalitis, occurring mainly between the ages of 4 and 20 years, and usually fatal in 6 weeks to 6 months. In the early stages there are personality changes and intellectual deterioration, followed by a stage of periodic involuntary movements, and finally profound dementia and decerebrate rigidity.

SSPE occurs some years after an apparently uncomplicated attack of measles. Its pathogenesis is not understood, but it appears to be due to reactivation of measles virus which has remained latent in the brain since the time of primary infection. There are high levels of both IgM and IgG classes of antibodies to measles virus in the blood and CSF. The CSF antibody levels are not only higher than the serum levels, but on immune-electrophoresis of the CSF they separate into distinct bands, indicating that antibody-producing plasma cells in the CNS are derived from a small number of B lymphocyte clones. Measles virus antigen has been detected in brain tissue obtained by biopsy in cases of SSPE, and complete virus has been isolated from such biopsies.

In measles and some other virus infections, cell-mediated immunity to various antigens is reduced. It is not known what role this plays in SSPE.

At necropsy, the brain may appear almost normal, but the white matter is often abnormally firm. Microscopic examination shows the features of a subacute meningo-encephalitis with widespread cuffing of vessels throughout the brain with lymphocytes and plasma cells. Neuronophagia is common, and varying numbers of residual neurons contain intranuclear and/or cytoplasmic inclusion bodies. There is also considerable gliosis in the white matter.

Subacute spongiform encephalopathy

The discovery and investigation of **kuru** has been one of the most dramatic occurrences in the entire field of diseases of the nervous system in the past two decades. It is a subacute disease of the brain characterised by microcystic degeneration in the grey matter, referred to as *status spongiosus*, associated with loss of neurons and a great excess of hypertrophied astrocytes. These changes are particularly severe in the cerebellar system. Kuru is restricted to the Fore tribe and their tribal neighbours in the Eastern Highlands of New Guinea. Its peculiar importance is that it was the first progressive degenerative disease of the nervous system of man to be transmitted to another

animal, first the chimpanzee but later to other primates, by injecting extracts of brain tissue from patients with the disease. It is therefore now classified as a **slow virus infection** although the agent, which is filterable and capable of replicating, has not been identified. Cannibalism was the primary mode of transmission, and the incidence of the disease has subsided since this practice ceased.

A second progressive degenerative disease of the nervous system, **Creutzfeldt–Jakob disease**, has been shown to be transmissible to other primates (and accidentally to man). It is a progressive dementia of world-wide distribution, again characterised by status spongiosus and astrocytosis. Kuru and Creutzfeldt–Jakob disease along with two transmissible diseases of the nervous system in animals—*scrapie* of sheep and *mink encephalopathy*—are now classified as *subacute spongiform encephalopathies*. All appear to be due to slow viruses, have an exceptionally long incubation period, and have an unremitting and always fatal progressive course. The transmissible agents have so far not been shown to be antigenic in that antibody has not yet been demonstrated.

Progressive multifocal leukoencephalopathy (PML)

This condition is caused by a papovavirus morphologically similar to polyoma virus. As its name implies, PML is characterised by multiple foci of degeneration in the brain, particularly in the white matter. The most characteristic macroscopic feature is the presence of multiple small grey foci distributed widely but usually asymmetrically in the white matter. These foci can coalesce to form large grey areas which may become frankly cystic. Histological examination shows multiple foci of demyelination associated with which there are lipid phagocytes, abnormal oligodendrocytes containing large hyperchromatic nuclei within which ill-defined inclusion bodies occur, and usually large and bizarre astrocytes. Most patients who develop the disease already have a disseminated malignant lymphoid neoplasm or leukaemia and it has been suggested that the virus may remain latent following a symptomless primary infection. Antibody to the virus is common in the community. It may attack the brain when immunological deficiency develops, due to the lymphoma or to immunosuppressive therapy, e.g. cytotoxic drugs.

Other Infections of the Nervous System

Protozoal infections

The commoner protozoa which cause infections of the nervous system are *Toxoplasma gondii* and some amoebae. Various trypanosomes produce a meningo-encephalitis, sleeping sickness, well known in Central Africa, being an example.

Toxoplasmosis. Congenital toxoplasmosis results from a primary maternal infection during pregnancy. Infection in early pregnancy may lead to abortion, a little later to a stillborn infant, and still later to a live-born child with clinical manifestations of the disease, which, however, may not appear until the early weeks of life. In babies who survive the congenital or neonatal infection, there is often residual mental retardation, epilepsy and chorioretinitis. In fatal cases there is extensive granulomatous destruction of the brain (Fig. 21.46) and often hydrocephalus. Parasites may be found in the granulomas, both free and within cells (including macrophages) in which they form pseudocysts (Fig. 21.47).

Amoebiasis. *Primary amoebic meningo-encephalitis* is a relatively recently recognised disease of man, caused by free-living amoebae traditionally regarded as being non-pathogenic in man. Numerous cases have now been reported from all parts of the world, the amoebae usually belonging to the Naegleri

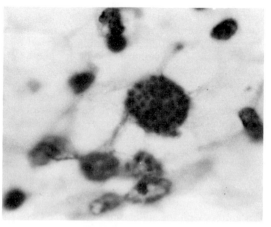

Fig. 21.47   Congenital toxoplasmosis. A pseudocyst containing many parasites: a few are also seen in the cell below (from same case as 21.46). × 900.

group. The amoebae reach the nasal sinuses when exposed to contaminated water, and spread through the olfactory plate into the skull. The disease is an acute meningo-encephalitis, most patients dying within about a week. At necropsy there is a fibrino-purulent exudate in the subarachnoid space, necrotising vasculitis and necrosis in the superficial parts of the cortex. Amoebae are found in the exudate, and the diagnosis may be made during life by identifying amoebae in the CSF.

Amoebic abscess. Although uncommon, amoebic abscess in the brain is one of the most frequently encountered fatal complications of amoebic dysentery (p. 634). The abscess may not appear until many years after the first attack of amoebic dysentery: it is usually single and contains reddish-brown or pinkish creamy fluid. It usually presents clinically as a rapidly expanding intracranial lesion (p. 729).

Cerebral malaria is almost always due to *Plasmodium falciparum*. In fatal cases there are numerous petechial haemorrhages throughout the brain.

Metazoal parasites

Cysticercosis may involve the brain. The larvae of the pork tapeworm, *Taenia solium*, may reach the brain, where they usually produce multiple small cysts measuring up to about 1 cm in diameter. They are a cause of epilepsy where cysticercosis is prevalent. The larva exists as a mural nodule in the cyst, which usually becomes surrounded by a collagenous capsule. When the larva dies, the cyst may become calcified. **Hydatid cysts** may also occur in the brain

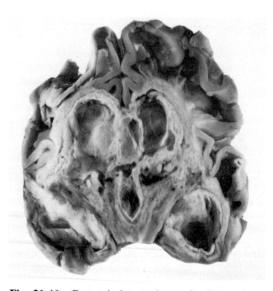

Fig. 21.46   Congenital toxoplasmosis. Coronal section of brain of a 2 months' old infant. Note the enlarged ventricles with necrotic lining, and extensive cystic and gelatinous degeneration of the hemispheres.

(p. 698). **Schistosomiasis** may be a cause of granulomas in all parts of the central nervous system including the spinal cord.

Fungal infections

Fungal infections of the nervous system are invariably secondary to infection elsewhere in the body but lesions at the portal of entry may be small and readily overlooked. The brain, therefore, may appear to be the only organ involved. In other cases, infection of the nervous system may simply be one of the manifestations of a generalised infection. Some fungi, e.g. *Cryptococcus neoformans* and *Coccidioides immitis*, may produce disease in man in the absence of predisposing factors other than increased exposure to the particular fungus. Apart from cryptococcosis (torulosis), these infections are extremely rare in Britain. Both meningitis and brain abscesses caused by fungi are, however, encountered with increasing frequency as opportunistic infections in patients with depressed immunity (p. 169 *et seq.*).

Cryptococcosis. The commonest clinical presentation of infection with *Cryptococcus neoformans* (p. 224) is as a subacute meningitis. The exudate in the subarachnoid space is rather gelatinous and usually contains masses of encapsulated cryptococci. Flask-shaped cysts filled with cryptococci in the superficial layers of the cortex are frequently found. Inflammatory changes in the brain and subarachnoid space are often remarkably mild but occasionally there is a granulomatous reaction very similar to that seen in tuberculous meningitis.

Opportunistic fungal infections. These are caused mainly by *Candida albicans*, *Aspergillus fumigatus* and *Nocardia asteroides*. They generally produce multiple brain abscesses of various sizes (Fig. 21.48). In the acute stages the abscesses may resemble haemorrhagic infarcts but later they usually become encapsulated. Candida may also cause a florid meningitis. Histological examination usually discloses abundant fungus, particularly at the edges of the abscesses. Accurate identification, however, depends on culture. *Mucormycosis* is a rarer opportunistic infection. It has a particular predilection for uncontrolled diabetic patients. Infection usually commences in the paranasal sinuses and spreads directly into the anterior fossa of the skull to produce selective involvement of the frontal lobes.

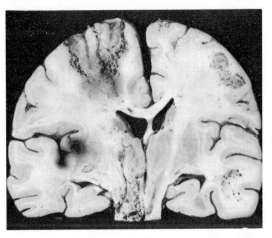

Fig. 21.48 Opportunistic fungal infection. There are several acute haemorrhagic lesions. The causal fungus was *Candida albicans*.

Demyelinating Diseases

This is a convenient term to bring together a number of disorders characterised by loss of myelin unrelated to specific fibre systems or particular arterial territories. The group includes **acute** conditions associated with considerable cellular exudation, and **chronic** disorders, in which there is conspicuous fibrillary gliosis in the demyelinated areas, but forms intermediate in both clinical and pathological features are not very rare. Examples of the chronic type are **multiple** or **disseminated sclerosis** in which the lesions are focal and not specially perivascular, and **diffuse cerebral sclerosis** in which the process is more generalised but may affect certain areas of the brain more severely than others. In the acute disorders the demyelination is usually strikingly perivascular and may develop very rapidly as in **acute disseminated encephalomyelitis**, which usually occurs as a complication of an acute virus infection, or in **acute haemorrhagic leukoencephalitis**, a condition in which the aetiology is still unknown.

An acute demyelinating encephalomyelitis (**experimental allergic encephalomyelitis**, or **EAE**) can be produced in various species of animals by injection of homogenised neural tissue, of the same or a different species, emulsified in Freund's adjuvant. The disease develops after a latent period of 10 days or more, and is believed to be due to the development of an immune response to neural tissue antigen in the inoculum and a subsequent immunological reaction with the animal's own neural tissue. The antigen is a basic protein present in myelin and an encephalitogenic fragment has been isolated and synthesised but differs for different species. The presence of antibody in the serum does not correlate well with the occurrence of the disease, and there is strong evidence that the lesions result from a delayed autohypersensitivity reaction in which sensitised lymphocytes and possibly macrophages react directly with the encephalitogenic component(s) of myelin.

The changes of EAE vary depending on the experimental detail and the animal species: in some species however they are similar to those of acute disseminated encephalomyelitis in man, which develops 10 days or so after the predisposing virus infection: a similar immunological reaction may be involved. Although EAE can be induced by one injection of antigen in Freund's adjuvant, its production in monkeys without the use of Freund's adjuvant requires many injections. An acute demyelinating encephalitis of similar nature sometimes results in man from multiple injections of anti-rabies vaccine prepared from infected rabbit spinal cord. Vaccine prepared from duck embryo appears to be safer.

Acute disseminated encephalomyelitis

This disease is known also as **post-infectious encephalitis** or **acute perivascular myelinoclasis** because of the rapid occurrence of perivascular demyelination. It develops as a sequel to various acute virus diseases such as measles, rubella or varicella, to respiratory infections presumed to be viral, and as a complication of primary vaccination against smallpox (**post-vaccinial encephalitis**) and anti-rabies inoculation (see above). Post-vaccinial encephalitis occurs mainly in older children and adults, about 10 days after primary vaccination.

The focal lesions in the nervous system are mainly around small venules throughout the brain and spinal cord, but often affect the ventral half of the pons, the deeper layers of the cerebral cortex, the thalamus and the white matter of the cerebral hemispheres with particular severity. The characteristic histological features are perivenular demyelination (Fig. 21.49) associated with inflammatory oedema and perivenular infiltration, mainly by lymphocytes and macrophages. Demyelination occurs very rapidly, being sometimes almost complete within 4 days. Axons show only slight damage, nerve cells adjacent to the perivascular demyelination may show mild degenerative changes and there may be a slight increase of mononuclear cells in the leptomeninges. The lesions are therefore quite different, both in character and distribution, from those of acute viral encephalitis due to the presence of any known virus in the central nervous system.

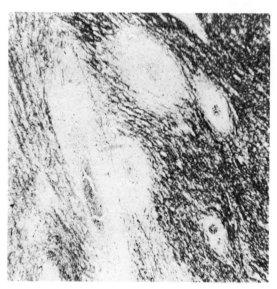

Fig. 21.49 Acute demyelinating encephalomyelitis following measles. A section showing perivascular demyelination in the white matter of the brain. (Loyez stain: myelin stained block.) × 60.

Aetiology. It is widely accepted that acute disseminated encephalomyelitis represents an immunological reaction in the CNS: from its similarity to experimental allergic encephalomyelitis, it seems likely that the predisposing virus infection leads to the development of an immune response against neural tissue antigen(s), and that a delayed hypersensitivity reaction is responsible for the lesions. The possibility of an immune reaction against the virus, or virus-infected cells cannot, however, be completely excluded as the cause.

Acute haemorrhagic leukoencephalitis

This relatively uncommon disease may also occur as a sequel to any one of several possible viral infections but it may develop during apparently normal health. It occurs also as a complication of septic shock. The course is rapid and fulminating, death occurring within a few days. At necropsy the brain is swollen and congested and there are numerous petechial haemorrhages particularly in the white matter, the naked-eye appearances being very similar to those observed in cerebral fat embolism.

Microscopic examination shows focal necrosis of the walls of venules and arterioles, perivascular haemorrhage and loss of myelin, often with emigration first of polymorphonuclear and later of mononuclear cells, cerebral oedema and an inflammatory exudate in the leptomeninges. The grey matter is relatively spared. Some consider that acute haemorrhagic leukoencephalitis is simply a particularly severe form of acute disseminated encephalomyelitis, but the different distribution of the focal lesions suggests that the pathogenesis may not always be the same.

Multiple or disseminated sclerosis (MS)

This fairly common disease is characterised by patchy demyelination and gliosis of the CNS. It usually starts before 50 years of age and most often in adolescents and young adults. Typically, the course is episodic, acute attacks of demyelination occurring at irregular intervals, and resulting in increasing motor disability and sensory loss. In some cases, however, the intervening periods of remission extend over years, and the rate of progress and severity vary considerably. In many cases, the disease becomes relentlessly progressive in the later stages, and occasionally is steadily progressive from the start. A common early symptom is an acute unilateral optic neuritis which progresses to some degree of optic atrophy.

Structural changes. The clinical episodes of MS are caused by patchy demyelination of irregular distribution in the brain and spinal cord, the area of demyelination being referred to as a *plaque*. Acute lesions are yellowish and soft; they are rounded or irregularly shaped and

measure up to 10 mm or so across. Microscopically, the changes are those of acute demyelination (p. 727) with infiltration by lipid-containing macrophages and perivascular cuffing by lymphocytes and plasma cells. As the plaque ages, the cellular infiltration subsides and vascular thickening and gliosis occur, but without much contraction or distortion. The partial clinical recovery from the disabling effects of the acute lesions is probably due to subsidence of inflammatory oedema in and around the acute lesions since the demyelinated axons may persist and function for a long time. Many eventually undergo Wallerian degeneration. Nerve cells included in a plaque usually show little or no abnormality. Old plaques are firm, grey and slightly translucent. They are readily visible in the unstained brain or cord (Fig. 21.50) and are seen as conspicuous pale

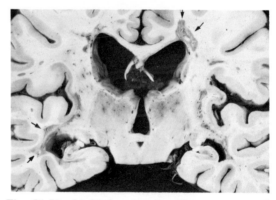

Fig. 21.50 Multiple sclerosis. There are several well-defined round or oval grey plaques of demyelination in each cerebral hemisphere and a group of coalescent plaques (*arrows*).

areas in sections stained by the Weigert–Pal method, which demonstrates complete loss of myelin and a fairly sharp line of demarcation from the adjacent normal tissue (Fig. 21.51). Smaller plaques, up to a few millimetres across, are usually round or oval; larger ones are irregular, and may result from the confluence of smaller plaques. In the typical case with a prolonged episodic course, most of the lesions seen at necropsy are old ones: they vary greatly in number, size and distribution, but are usually most easily seen in the white matter of the cerebrum, particularly at the angles of the lateral ventricles and at the junction of the cortex with the white matter. Plaques do, however, occur also in the cortex and central grey matter. They are common in the brain stem (Fig. 21.51), particularly around the aqueduct and 4th ventricle and in the spinal cord. If there is a history of retrobulbar neuritis, a plaque can usually be found in the optic nerve.

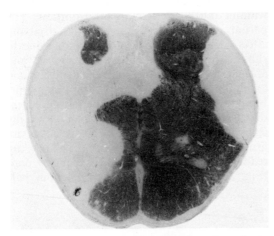

Fig. 21.51 Multiple sclerosis. Section through the lower part of the medulla. The demyelinated plaques appear pale. (Weigert–Pal method.)

The CSF in MS may contain more than 5 lymphocytes per μl, particularly during acute episodes, when lipid-containing macrophages and plasma cells may also be present. Protein levels may be normal or slightly increased; IgG is often moderately increased and, as stated below, may be oligoclonal: the demonstration of a 'paretic' reaction in the Lange colloidal gold test is a less sensitive indication of changes in protein content.

Aetiology. Genetic and environmental factors both appear to be of importance in MS. Genetic factors are suggested by a very high incidence (70 per cent) of the HLA antigen DW2 in patients as compared with the normal population (16 per cent) and slightly increased incidences of HLA-A3 and B7. Epidemiological studies point to an environmental factor of importance in childhood, for there is a relatively high incidence of MS in the higher latitudes of both Northern and Southern Hemispheres and yet people who migrate from one area to another after about the age of 14 retain the incidence of their childhood locality. There is an increased incidence of MS among siblings and parents of patients with the disease, but it is not known whether this is attributable to genetic or environmental factors or to a combination of both.

There is evidence of an immune reaction in the CNS in MS, notably an increase of lymphocytes in the CSF, and of lymphocytes and plasma cells in the acute lesions. As in subacute sclerosing panencephalitis, neurosyphilis and the Guillain–Barré syndrome, immuno-electrophoresis of concentrated CSF produces discrete bands of IgG, indicating IgG production by plasma cells derived from a small number of B lymphocyte clones in the CNS (p. 125). These immunological factors could be interpreted as indicating either a response to a neurotropic virus or an auto-immune response to a nervous tissue component, as in experimental allergic encephalomyelitis (p. 763). In support of a viral infection, the titres of antibody to measles virus are relatively high in both the serum and CSF, but antibodies to some other viruses are also raised. Recently the presence of small virus-like particles has been reported in the serum, nervous and other tissues in MS, and these have been claimed to induce prolonged neutropenia in mice, and neutralising antibodies to this agent have been reported in the serum of MS patients (Henle *et al.*, 1975). There is, however, considerable doubt as to the significance of this agent. However, the disease does not resemble known persistent or slow virus infections of the CNS (subacute sclerosing panencephalitis, Creutzfeldt–Jakob disease and kuru) and the evidence for detection of a virus is conflicting. As regards an auto-immune aetiology, antibodies which, together with complement, cause demyelination of nerve tissue cultures have been detected in the serum of MS patients, but occur also in other, non-demyelinating diseases. Also, acute demyelination complicating rabies prophylaxis in man (p. 764) and in experimental allergic encephalomyelitis (both of which appear to have an auto-immune pathogenesis) occurs as a single acute episode and is perivenular, in contrast to the recurrent acute episodes of MS, in which the plaques are much larger and show no obvious relationship to small vessels.

In conclusion, the lesions of MS present features suggestive of an immunological reaction, but there is no strong evidence pointing to either a virus or a component of nervous tissue as the antigen. Claims that the lesions result from a biochemical disturbance have also been made, but lack strong supporting evidence.

Neuromyelitis optica is a disease of adults characterised by rapid loss of vision and the occurrence of extensive demyelinating lesions, particularly in the optic nerves and spinal cord but also in the cerebral hemispheres. The disease is commonly preceded by fever; it runs a more acute course and the lesions are more severely destructive than in multiple sclerosis, but the two diseases cannot be sharply distinguished.

Diffuse cerebral sclerosis

This is rather a complex group of rare diseases which have in common *diffuse demyelination* and *gliosis* in the white matter of the cerebral hemispheres and sometimes also in the cerebellum, the brain stem and the spinal cord. Most forms are genetically determined and occur in childhood: these are termed the **leukodystrophies**, and have also been referred to as *dysmyelinating diseases* in the belief that the myelin is biochemically abnormal before it degenerates. Other cases, however, are apparently non-familial, start in adult life, and show inflammatory changes in addition to demyelination.

Sudanophilic cerebral sclerosis

In this type of diffuse sclerosis the breakdown of myelin follows the conventional pattern (p. 727).

Sudanophilic cerebral sclerosis is commoner than the other types of diffuse sclerosis and it occurs both in childhood, when it may be familial (i.e. a leukodystrophy), and in adult life as a sporadic disease. It is a progressive disease, characterised by mental deterioration, blindness and spastic paralysis. In subacute cases, death occurs within a few months, but more frequently the patient survives for one or two years. There is widespread degeneration of the cerebral white matter notably in the occipital lobes (hence the common occurrence of early visual impairment), but any part of the cerebral hemispheres, cerebellum or brain stem may be affected. Typically, the subcortical arcuate fibres are spared and stand out as a conspicuous white band in the affected areas. In Weigert–Pal preparations, the demyelination is seen to be less sharply demarcated than in multiple sclerosis and shades off marginally into normally stained white matter. In the affected areas microglial cells stuffed with sudanophilic lipid are abundant while the degree of fibrillary gliosis varies with the duration of the disease. Axon cylinders are usually lost in the lesions but, apart from occasional neurons showing central chromatolysis, the grey matter is normal.

Some cases of this type of diffuse sclerosis in males are associated with adrenal insufficiency which may precede the onset of the neurological illness, may coincide with it, or may remain subclinical. The disease is known as **adrenoleukodystrophy** and the single most reliable test to establish the diagnosis is adrenal biopsy. The characteristic feature is the presence of ballooned vacuolated cortical cells which contain linear lamellar bodies with distinctive fine structural features. Similar cytoplasmic inclusions occur in the brain. It has been suggested that the overwhelming majority of males with sudanophilic cerebral sclerosis are in fact instances of adrenoleukodystrophy, and that cases occurring in males without adrenal atrophy and in females may represent a variant of multiple sclerosis. The term *Schilder's disease* has been used in the past for diffuse sclerosis of sudanophilic type. If the term has to be retained, it should probably now be restricted to cases of adrenoleukodystrophy.

Metachromatic leukodystrophy

This is a rare familial disease occurring mainly in children between 2 and 5 years old but not confined to this age group. It is progressive and tends to run a course of 1 or 2 years. The basic defect is a genetically-determined deficiency of arylsulphatase, a useful diagnostic test for which can be performed on the blood leukocytes. In contrast to myelin destruction in other diseases, in this condition myelin is not broken down into neutral fat and cholesterol esters but into metachromatic material containing sulphatides which is PAS positive and is stained brown by cresyl violet or thionine in an acid solution.

At necropsy the brain feels unusually firm and the white matter may be somewhat greyer and more translucent than normal. The subcortical arcuate fibres are usually not spared. Microscopic examination demonstrates widespread loss of myelin in the white matter, the fibre systems which mature last being the most severely affected. The demyelinated areas contain large quantities of intracellular and extracellular metachromatic material which can only be demonstrated satisfactorily in frozen sections since much of it dissolves during the usual histological processing. Sudanophilic lipid is present only in small amounts in perivascular phagocytes. Metachromatic material is not restricted to white matter since it can also be demonstrated in neurons and peripheral nerves. It may also be present in the urine and in many other tissues, e.g. liver, pancreas, adrenal and kidney.

A rarer type of leukodystrophy is **Krabbe's disease**. There is a deficiency of the enzyme galactocerebroside β-galactosidase. The striking histological feature is the presence of large fused multinucleated macrophages, known as globoid cells (p. 29).

Table 21.1 The Cerebrospinal Fluid in health and

	Normal	Acute pyogenic meningitis	Tuberculous meningitis	Acute virus infection with meningo-encephalitis
Pressure (horizontal posture)	60–150 mmH$_2$O	Increased—probably to 200 mm or more	Increased to as much as 300 mm or more	Increased sometimes to 250 mm
Appearance	Clear and colourless	Turbid or frankly purulent	Clear or slightly opalescent. A fine fibrin coagulum may form on standing	Clear or slightly opalescent
Cell content per μl	0–4 leukocytes (all lymphocytes)	Markedly raised 500–5000 polymorphs at first, mononuclears later	Increased up to 500 lymphocytes; some polymorphs at first	Increased 50–500 lymphocytes, some polymorphs at first
Protein g/litre	0·15–0·45	0·5–2·0 average; up to 10 g	0·5–3·0 usually; if spinal block present, may rise to over 10 g	0·5–2·0; 0·5–1·0 in paralytic polio
Glucose mg/100 ml (mmol/litre)	50–80 (2·8–4·4)	Absent or greatly reduced	Decreased to 20–30 (1–1·5)	Normal
Bacteriology	Sterile	Causative organisms present; type confirmed by culture	Tubercle bacilli in fibrin coagulum or in deposit. Positive cultures usually obtained	Sterile
Lange's colloidal gold test	Normal, i.e. 0000000000	May be normal or meningitic, e.g. 0012344320	Normal or meningitic	Normal or meningitic. Weak paretic or luetic in poliomyelitis
Wassermann Reaction	Negative	Negative	Negative	Negative

Other Disorders of the Central Nervous System

Neuronal storage diseases

In this group of diseases there is abnormal accumulation of certain metabolites within neurons. As in storage disorders mainly affecting other tissues (pp. 28–32), the neuronal storage diseases are genetically determined, usually become apparent in childhood and often in infancy, they are due to a deficiency in one or more lysosomal enzymes necessary for catabolism, and the metabolite which cannot be further degradated accumulates in the neuronal cytoplasm. Thus the affected neurons have a ballooned appearance, the storage material can be demonstrated histochemically, and electron microscopy demonstrates phagosomes containing non-metabolisable residues. Some of these phagosomes have highly distinctive morphological features diagnostic of a specific storage disorder.

There is some similarity in the clinical and pathological features of all neuronal storage disorders, although there are features specific to individual diseases. In the early stages, the storage leads to neuronal dysfunction. Ultimately the cell dies and disappears and there is atrophy of the brain and gliosis in grey and white matter. Thus there is retardation or progressive deterioration of mental and motor functions, apathy, lassitude, spastic or flaccid paralysis, fits, often visual disturbances and ultimately coma and death.

Based on the observed enzyme defects, there are more than 20 known storage diseases which involve neurons: in many the neuronal disorder is the most prominent feature of the disease but in others there is also involvement of other tissues.

One of the commonest is **Tay–Sachs disease**, the classical infantile type of amaurotic family idiocy. A particularly characteristic sign of this disease, but not restricted to it, is the cherry red spot at the macula due to retinal involvement. Since the abnormal metabolite is ganglioside GM$_2$, this condition is now best referred to as GM$_2$ gangliosidosis. The missing enzyme is hexosaminidase A and the abnormal phagosomes with highly distinctive fine structural features are known as membranous cytoplasmic bodies. There are also other types of gangliosidosis.

in certain diseases as obtained by lumbar puncture

General paralysis of the insane	Tabes dorsalis	Multiple sclerosis	Subarachnoid haemorrhage	Complete spinal block (Froin's syndrome)
Normal	Normal	Normal	Raised often to 300 mm or more	Low: CSF may have to be actively withdrawn
Normal	Normal	Normal	Frankly bloodstained: on centrifugation, supernatant is yellow	Yellow, opalescent and tends to clot
Up to 100 (lymphocytes)	Up to 50–100 (lymphocytes)	Slight increase to 20–100 (lymphocytes)	Many red cells and some leukocytes	Slight increase of lymphocytes
0·5–1·0 Oligoclonal IgG	0·3–0·6 Oligoclonal IgG	0·3–0·6 Oligoclonal IgG	Normal in the early stages. Slight rise later	More than 30 g
Normal	Normal	Normal	Normal	Normal
Sterile	Sterile	Sterile	Sterile	Sterile
Paretic, e.g. 5544321000	Luetic, e.g. 123321000	Paretic, rarely luetic or may be normal	Normal	Meningitic
Positive	Positive in 80% of cases	Negative	Negative	Negative

Other lysosomal storage disorders involving the nervous system include infantile Gaucher's disease (deficiency of β-glucocerebrosidase), Niemann–Pick's disease (deficiency of sphingomyelinase), type II glycogenosis (Pompe's disease, deficiency of acid α-glucosidase), the mucopolysaccharidoses and certain syndromes previously classified as types of amaurotic family idiocy (e.g. Batten's disease).

Other inborn errors of metabolism involving the nervous system

Phenylketonuria and galactosaemia are the most important of these because they can be detected by screening tests on the urine of infants, and brain damage can be prevented or reduced by exclusion of the precursor substances from the diet.

In **phenylketonuria**, inherited as an autosomal recessive, absence of the active enzyme phenylalanine hydroxylase, which converts phenylalanine to tyrosine, leads to accumulation of phenylalanine in the blood and tissues and excretion of phenylpyruvic acid in the urine. Epileptiform seizures, severe mental deficiency and some failure of myelination are the principal findings.

In **galactosaemia** there is hepato-splenomegaly, cataract and mental retardation associated with inability to metabolise galactose owing to absence of the enzyme galactose-1-phosphate uridyl transferase; consequently galactose-1-phosphate rises to toxic levels and is excreted in the urine.

Despite the severe mental derangement no specific pathological abnormality has been recognised in the brain in these serious disorders. As in most enzyme disorders, the defective enzyme may be absent or produced in an abnormal form.

The dementias

Dementia is brought about by more or less extensive destruction or disorganisation of the brain, particularly the cerebral cortex, by one or more pathological processes. The personality coarsens, intellect and memory become impaired and the individual ultimately becomes demented. In many patients dementia is secondary to some other primary abnormality in the brain, such as a deeply seated tumour or diffuse processes such as general paralysis of the insane, leukodystrophy or subacute sclerosing panencephalitis. By far the commonest type of secondary dementia however is that produced by **ischaemic brain damage**, this being referred to as *multi-infarct* or *arteriopathic* dementia.

Multi-infarct dementia often has a rapid onset and a fluctuating course. Most patients are over 60 and are hypertensive. Examination of the brain will usually disclose widespread atheroma of the major cerebral arteries. In slices of the brain the characteristic abnormality is the presence of old infarcts: their distribution appears to have little correlation with the development of dementia, and it seems more likely that dementia occurs after a certain volume of the brain—perhaps about 100 ml—has been destroyed. The ventricles are usually enlarged: the enlargement may be symmetrical if there are multiple small infarcts in each hemisphere, or asymmetrical if the infarcts involve mainly one hemisphere.

There remains a group of **primary organic dementias**, usually relentlessly if slowly progressive, in which there are fairly specific pathological changes in the brain. Common to all is cortical atrophy, the gyri becoming rounder and firmer than normal and the sulci widened, and secondary hydrocephalus.

Alzheimer's disease and senile dementia. These two types of dementia show the same pathological features but Alzheimer's disease is the term used when the onset is pre-senile, i.e. before the age of 60. The pathological findings in both types resemble a gross exaggeration of those of the normal ageing processes in the brain. Death usually occurs a few years after the onset of the disease. Cortical atrophy is widespread but more conspicuous at the frontal and temporal poles. Histological examination reveals a generalised loss of neurons, reactive gliosis and vast numbers of senile (Alzheimer) plaques in the cortical grey matter (Fig. 21.52). The plaques are composed of masses of small argyrophilic granules and filaments often with a core of amyloid material. In addition, there are tangles of coarse neurofibrils (Alzheimer's neurofibrillary change) in many of the larger nerve cells of the cerebral cortex. It has been established recently that the levels of many biochemical markers are reduced in the brain in Alzheimer's disease. There is however, a relatively severe loss of choline acetyl transferase, suggesting a selective loss or dysfunction of cholinergic neurons.

Pick's disease is classed as a pre-senile dementia. Cortical atrophy from loss of neurons is particularly intense in the frontal and temporal lobes, giving the brain a distinctive naked-eye appearance. The consequent degeneration of axis cylinders probably accounts for the loss of myelin, reactive gliosis and

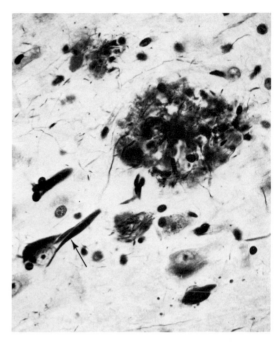

Fig. 21.52 Alzheimer's disease. Note the presence of a typical senile plaque composed of filamentous and granular material. A neurofibrillary tangle is seen in a neuron (*arrow*). King's amyloid stain. × 250.

considerable shrinkage of the underlying white matter. Some of the surviving neurons are greatly swollen by a globular mass of intracellular argyrophilic material.

Huntington's chorea. This disease of middle adult life is characterised by coarse choreiform movements, progressive mental deterioration and, in some cases, striatal rigidity. It is believed to be inherited by an autosomal dominant gene. In addition to widespread cortical atrophy, there is selective atrophy and loss of nerve cells in the caudate nucleus and the putamen.

Hepatolenticular degeneration (Wilson's disease). This is a rare condition which occurs mainly in adolescents and young adults, shows a familial tendency, and is probably due to an autosomal recessive character which determines an inborn error of copper metabolism (see p. 690). The main changes in the brain are in the putamen and caudate nucleus, which become soft, shrunken, and ultimately cystic. Neuronal loss is accompanied by a fibrillary gliosis and the occurrence of large astrocytes with strikingly vesicular swollen nuclei. These are termed *Alzheimer astrocytes*: they are found in cases of chronic liver failure of any cause and may be widely distributed throughout the grey matter. The lesions in the nervous system in hepatolenticular degeneration are due to metabolic disturbances dependent partly on the deposition of copper. The greenish-brown discoloration of the cornea near the limbus, known as the *Kayser–Fleischer ring*, is due to deposition of copper. The resulting symptoms are mainly muscular tremors and spasticity. The condition is associated with cirrhosis of the liver, which is also due to the defect in copper metabolism mentioned above.

Acquired hepatocerebral degeneration is also recognised. The acute forms are associated with massive liver-cell necrosis when the principal abnormality in the brain is the occurrence of Alzheimer astrocytes. A chronic form is seen in individuals with a large porto-systemic venous shunt as occurs in cirrhosis (p. 692). Alzheimer astrocytes again appear in the brain but there may also be microcystic degeneration in the caudate nucleus, the putamen, and the deeper layers of the cortex.

Creutzfeld–Jakob disease is described on p. 761 and **normal-pressure hydrocephalus** on p. 735.

The psychoses. In many quite common psychiatric disturbances, including schizophrenia and the involutional psychoses, there are no identifiable structural abnormalities in the brain. They are therefore still classified as functional disorders.

Parkinsonism (paralysis agitans)

This is a common disease of the elderly which affects men more often than women. It develops gradually and, if untreated, is permanent and tends to get worse. The predominant clinical features are involuntary tremor and muscular rigidity: the fixed facial expression, dribbling of saliva and tottering gait are characteristic and are brought about by a selective and progressive destruction of the pigmented dopaminergic neurons in the substantia nigra and locus coeruleus in the brain stem. Associated with the destruction of neurons (the cause of which is unknown), granules of pigment may be seen lying free in the parenchyma and within microglia. There is also some fibrillary gliosis. Frequently some of the residual pigmented neurons contain large intracytoplasmic inclusion bodies known as Lewy bodies. In advanced cases, depigmentation of the substantia nigra is readily apparent macroscopically. A similar clinical syndrome may sometimes occur in association with small infarcts in the rostral brain stem, and typical Parkinsonism, with the pathological changes noted above, was a common sequel to encephalitis lethargica (p. 760)—*post-encephalitic Parkinsonism*.

Disorders of the nervous system in cancer

The nervous system may be implicated by malignant tumours arising elsewhere by direct or metastatic invasion of the brain, spinal cord and peripheral nerves, or by compression of the cord by extradural deposits. Indirect effects also occur in the nervous system, the commonest being a *peripheral neuropathy* which may be predominantly motor or sensory, or of mixed type. The most conspicuous histological abnormalities in the cases with sensory symptoms are loss of neurons in the dorsal root ganglia and degeneration of the dorsal roots, posterior columns of the spinal cord and peripheral nerves. In predominantly motor neuropathies, histological changes are usually slight although there may be various degrees of neurogenic atrophy of muscle. Other conditions in this group are a *myasthenic syndrome*, a *diffuse encephalomyelitis* characterised by intense perivascular cuffing by lymphocytes and affecting particularly the medial parts of the temporal lobes ('limbic encephalitis'), and *subacute cerebellar atrophy* characterised by an extensive loss of Purkinje cells and degeneration of the long tracts—motor and sensory—in the spinal cord. These changes are found most often in, but are not confined to, cases of *bronchial carcinoma*. The neurological symptoms not infrequently precede local ones caused by the tumour itself. In long-standing malignant lymphomas, and in widespread involvement of the lympho-reticular tissues by other conditions, e.g. carcinomatosis and sarcoidosis, the brain may show many irregularly disposed areas of demyelination and an unusually severe degree of astrocyte hyperplasia. The term *progressive multifocal leukoencephalopathy* is applied to this condition (p. 761).

Congenital abnormalities of the nervous system

Defects of the brain are many and the anatomical changes are often complex; we can only summarise the main ones. **Anencephaly** is a condition in which there is a deficiency of the cranial vault with absence of the brain, although there is often a small sac with the remains of cerebral tissue on the exposed base of the cranial cavity, the base also being small. The condition, which is incompatible with life, is sometimes associated with non-closure of the spinal canal or *rachischisis*.

Occasionally there is a deficiency in the cranial bones and a sac-like protrusion is present. This occurs in the line of a suture, is often median in position and usually occipital; or it may be lateral, e.g. at the side of an orbit or the nose. The sac is lined in some instances by the meninges and contains only CSF—**meningocele**. In other cases the sac is lined by neural tissue and sometimes, when the defect is posterior, may contain a considerable part of the cerebrum—**encephalocele**. The term **micrencephaly** means a congenitally small brain. There is deficiency in the convolutions, and the sulci are imperfectly formed; it is associated with various grades of idiocy. The whole brain may be abnormal, but usually the cerebellum and brain stem are less affected than the cerebrum. In other cases, there is a local defect in growth, often associated with a small size of the convolutions or *microgyria*. The cause of micrencephaly is not known: it is not due to early closure of the sutures, as was once supposed. The term **porencephaly** is applied when part of the brain is replaced by a collection of fluid, covered by meninges and sometimes in communication with the ventricles. In the *primary type*, which results from failure of growth of the brain, the edges of the defect are usually smooth. The condition is occasionally bilateral and sometimes accompanied by other defects. In the *secondary form*, the lesion is supposed to be the result of encephalitis, e.g. toxoplasmosis, or of interference with the blood supply during intrauterine life, and a somewhat similar condition may result from injury at the time of birth.

Spinal cord defects. A fairly common abnormality is non-closure of the spinal canal, or **rachischisis**, in which there is a local deficiency in the arches of the vertebrae, the gap being covered posteriorly by soft tissues. The term **spina bifida** is applied to such a condition; a distinct rounded projection is usually present over the site of the defect, which is then known as *spina bifida cystica*. When there is no such projection the term *spina bifida occulta* is applied.

The commonest position of spina bifida is in the lumbo-sacral region, and in all cases the spinal cord extends to a lower level than the normal; in other words, it remains in the position it normally occupies only in the earlier stages of development. In the commonest form, the spinal cord is adherent to the posterior wall of the sac and the term **meningomyelocele** is applied. The dura mater is absent in the sac, over which there is often an area where the skin is deficient (Fig. 21.12, p. 734). At this point there is a smooth membrane in which the spinal cord is incorporated, the cord being open posteriorly, with the openings of the central canal sometimes visible as one or two small depressions. The spinal nerves are spread out on the inner lining of the sac. In another rarer form, the space containing the fluid is a distension of the central canal and is lined by ependyma. In this form, termed **myelocystocele** or **syringomyelocele**, the spinal cord has closed posteriorly, the abnormality having arisen later in development than the previous form. In a third and least common variety, the sac is lined by a hernial protrusion of the arachnoid, and the spinal cord lies normally in relation to the vertebrae. This is called **meningocele**. In all three varieties the dura mater is absent locally. In spina bifida the sac contains CSF. In the first variety, the fluid is in the subarachnoid space in front of the spinal cord; in the second, it is in the dilated canal of the cord, and in the third, it is in the subarachnoid space behind the cord.

Severe forms of meningomyelocele are almost invariably associated with hydrocephalus and the **Arnold–Chiari malformation** (p. 734).

Assays of α-fetoprotein in maternal blood and amniotic fluid are useful in antenatal screening for the above defects.

In **spina bifida occulta**, where there is no swelling to indicate the defect, the skin over the part usually shows abnormalities in appearance and there is sometimes excessive growth of hair on it. Here, also, the cord extends to a lower level in the spinal canal than normally.

Diastematomyelia is the term applied when the cord is split into two by a fibrous or bony spur projecting into the vertebral canal.

Tuberous sclerosis. In this disorder there are multiple foci of hyperplasia of neuroglia and nerve cells in the cortex of the brain and in the subependymal tissue, in association with rhabdomyoma of the heart muscle (p. 430), adenoma sebaceum and other congenital abnormalities. In a few cases one or more of the glial foci give rise to a distinctive subependymal giant-celled type of astrocytoma.

II: The Spinal Cord

The tissue of the spinal cord is similar to that of the brain but the relative frequencies of various lesions are very different. Specific diseases of the spinal cord are described later but so-called *transverse lesions* and the consequent ascending and descending Wallerian degeneration within the cord will be dealt with first.

Transverse Lesions

These occur when partial or complete interruption of the cord is produced by local intrinsic or extrinsic lesions. **Slowly progressive effects** may be produced by *pressure on the cord by extrinsic tumours* in the extradural space, e.g. metastatic carcinoma (Fig. 21.53) or lymphoid neoplasm, or in the subdural space, e.g. meningioma (Fig. 21.84, p. 790) or Schwannoma. *Intrinsic tumours*, e.g. astrocytoma and ependy-

moma, are rarer causes. *Tuberculosis* is still a common cause in various parts of the world. It leads to angular curvature of the spine and tuberculous granuloma, both of which can cause pressure on the cord; this may be so severe that infarction of the cord may occur at this level. **Acute transverse lesions** may be due to *trauma*, usually a fracture-dislocation of the vertebrae, *infarction* when the circulation through the anterior spinal artery is impeded, *haemorrhage*, usually from a vascular malformation, *acute myelitis* (see below) or acute *demyelination* as in neuromyelitis optica (p. 767).

An inevitable consequence of a total or partial transverse lesion of the cord, besides the local damage, is the development of **ascending and descending Wallerian degeneration** in the respective tracts of the spinal cord. Degeneration occurs in those fibres that are separated from their cell bodies by the lesion and, when recent, is best demonstrated by the Marchi technique (p. 727). The degenerating fibres appear black from about a week after onset (Fig. 21.54). The method is applicable until the degenerated myelin has disappeared—that is, for several months. In older lesions, the Weigert–Pal method, which stains the normal myelin black, should be used since, when the degenerate myelin has become absorbed, the affected tract appears as a pale area (Fig. 21.56).

Ascending degeneration

If we take as an example a comparatively recent lesion in the lower dorsal region, the following ascending degenerations are found in a section taken a few segments above the lesion (Fig. 21.54). There is degeneration in the pos-

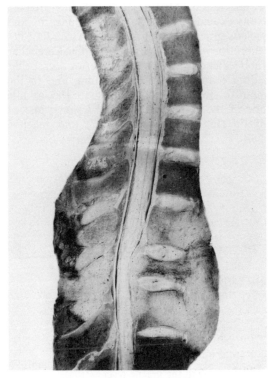

Fig. 21.53 Sagittal section of the vertebral column in lower cervical–upper dorsal region, showing metastatic tumour pressing on the cord.

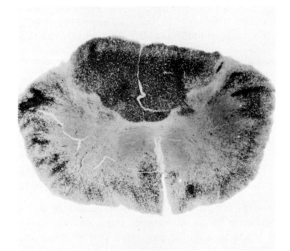

Fig. 21.54   Immediately above the lesion. The whole of the posterior columns and antero-lateral ascending tracts are degenerating.

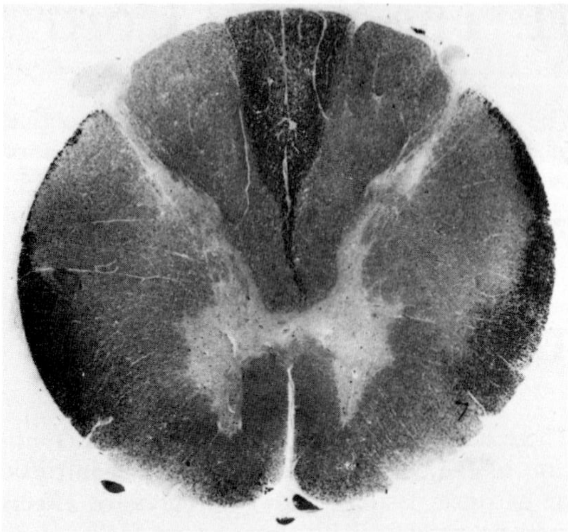

Fig. 21.55   Cervical region. There are fewer degenerating fibres because of the inflow of fibres above the level of the lesion.

Figures 21.54 and 21.55   Ascending degeneration above a recent transverse lesion in the lower dorsal region, stained by Marchi's method: the degenerating fibres appear black.

terior columns (with the exception of a small area dorsal to the grey commissure where there are chiefly commissural fibres) and in the spino-thalamic and spino-cerebellar tracts. In the cervical region, however, the degeneration in the posterior columns is practically confined to the gracile tracts (Fig. 21.55) because the cuneate tract is composed mainly of ascending fibres that have joined the cord above the level of the lesion. Degeneration of the affected axons extends up to the nucleus cuneatus and nucleus gracilis in the medulla. Ascending degeneration in the posterior spino-cerebellar tract extends up to the inferior cerebellar peduncle and into the cerebellum, and in the anterior spino-cerebellar tract to the middle lobe of the cerebellum. In old lesions, loss of myelin (Figs. 21.56 and 21.57) and reactive

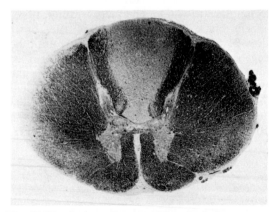

Fig. 21.56   A short distance above the lesion.

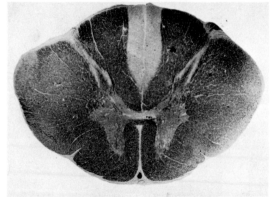

Fig. 21.57   Cervical region. Degeneration appears to be confined to the gracile tract.

Figures 21.56 and 21.57   Ascending degeneration above an old transverse lesion in the dorsal region, stained by the Weigert–Pal method. The degenerated fibres appear pale.

gliosis are more conspicuous in the posterior columns since the inflow of normal myelinated fibres at higher levels masks the relatively slight loss of myelinated fibres in the spino-cerebellar and spino-thalamic tracts.

Descending degeneration

This is most often encountered (*a*) when there is a transverse lesion in the cord, and (*b*) when the lesion is at a higher level. In a section taken from below a *transverse lesion* of the cord the most marked degeneration is in the crossed (lateral) and uncrossed (anterior) pyramidal tracts unless the lesion is low in the cord where the uncrossed tract is no longer present.

The commonest example due to a *lesion at a higher level* is destruction of the motor fibres in the internal capsule by infarction. There is degeneration of the crossed pyramidal tract on the opposite side (Fig. 21.58) and of the uncrossed pyramidal tract on the same side. As the uncrossed pyramidal tract does not usually extend below the upper thoracic segments, its degeneration will not appear in sections of the lower thoracic cord (Fig. 21.59).

Where there is compression of the spinal cord by a gross lesion which also blocks the subarachnoid space, the CSF below the block becomes altered. There is a great increase in protein concentration and the fluid coagulates rapidly after withdrawal; it is often yellow (xanthochromia). There may also be a slight increase in lymphocytes. These changes are grouped under the term 'Froin's syndrome' (see Table 21.1, pp. 768–9).

Prolapsed intervertebral disc

This is a common cause of compression of the nerve roots and more rarely it causes compression of the cord. The intervertebral disc consists of a central nodule of semifluid matrix, the nucleus pulposus, surrounded by a circle of fibrous tissue and fibrocartilage, the annulus fibrosus. The posterior segment of the annulus is thinner and less firmly attached to bone and, following unusual stress, part of the matrix of the nucleus pulposus may herniate through it (Fig. 21.60). The lesion, often termed *'slipped disc'*, may occur after slight injury and symptoms depend on the direction taken by the material extruded from the nucleus pulposus. The herniated material usually tracks postero-laterally around the expansion of the posterior longitudinal ligament, appearing at one side and compressing the spinal nerve root in the intervertebral foramen. Disc protrusions almost always occur in the lumbar spine and L5–S1, L4–L5 and L3–L4 discs are affected in that order of frequency: they also occur occasionally in the cervical spine, principally in C5–6 and C6–7 discs. If the protrus-

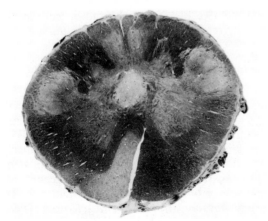

Fig. 21.58 Medulla. The pyramid on one side is degenerated.

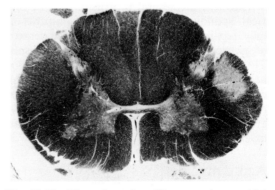

Fig. 21.59 Thoracic region. The crossed pyramidal tract on one side is degenerated.

Figures 21.58 and 21.59 Descending degeneration. Transverse sections through medulla and spinal cord showing descending degeneration from an old lesion of one internal capsule. Stained by Weigert–Pal method: degenerated fibres appear pale.

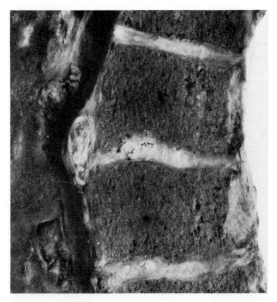

Fig. 21.60 Sagittal section of vertebral column, showing ruptured disc protruding beneath the posterior longitudinal ligament.

ion is small, localised pain is produced by irritation of the posterior longitudinal ligament; if larger, there may be root pain due to pressure on nerves leaving the spinal canal giving rise to the clinical signs and symptoms of sciatica. A single mid-line posterior disc protrusion may cause compression of the cord or obstruction of the anterior spinal artery, and is a rare but important cause of permanent damage to the spinal cord if surgical treatment is delayed. When there are several protrusions, as in cervical spondylosis, the resulting compression may impair the circulation and variable degrees of ischaemia of the spinal cord may result. There may be cavitation of the cord and loss of nerve cells in the severely affected areas, the condition being known as *spondylotic myelopathy*. Even in cervical spondylosis, however, nerve root compression is commoner than myelopathy.

Acute myelitis

This uncommon condition, by definition an acute inflammation of the cord, is more a clinical syndrome than a precise pathological entity. It is usually of acute or subacute onset and is characterised by flaccid paralysis and sensory loss, either of which may be total or partial, below the level of the lesion.

A considerable length of the cord may be affected—*diffuse myelitis*; or the lesion may be confined to one or two segments—*transverse myelitis*. These terms, however, tend to be used for any pathological process, other than external pressure or tumour, which causes intrinsic damage to the grey and white matter of the cord.

Causes. Acute demyelination (p. 763), and infarction of the cord due to impaired circulation through the anterior spinal artery, are probably the commonest causes. In some cases of infarction of the lumbo-sacral cord in adults, there are numerous hyalinised vessels within the cord: this condition is known as *subacute necrotic myelitis*. Other causes of transverse myelitis are acute disseminated encephalomyelitis (p. 764), spontaneous haematomyelia (probably from a vascular malformation) and, more rarely, bacterial infections.

Structural changes. The appearances of the cord vary with the underlying pathological process. In general, however, the affected part of the cord is swollen and soft, the normal architectural markings are blurred and there may be foci of haemorrhage.

If the patient survives the acute stage, there may be some restoration of function. More often the affected part of the cord becomes shrunken, cystic and gliosed, there is ascending and descending degeneration, and the patient is permanently paraplegic.

Lesions of the motor neuron

The main acute disease of lower motor neurons, *acute anterior poliomyelitis*, has already been described (p. 758). Chronic progressive degenerative disease of the motor neurons is usually referred to as *motor neuron disease*.

Motor neuron disease

In motor neuron disease there is a relentless and progressive degeneration of motor neurons of unknown aetiology. The brunt of the damage may fall on the lower motor neurons in the spinal cord (*progressive muscular atrophy*) or on the cranial nerve nuclei in the brain stem (*progressive bulbar palsy*). Some degeneration of upper motor neurons is usual and may be prominent (*amyotrophic lateral sclerosis*). These three variants of *motor neuron disease* occur in middle and late adult life, and are much more frequent in men than in women.

Progressive muscular atrophy. In this variant there is a progressive degeneration of the neurons in the anterior horns of the spinal cord. It usually starts in the cervical enlargement in the neurons related to the small muscles of the hand. The affected muscles show fibrillary twitchings and, gradually, atrophy with corresponding weakness follows. The thenar and hypothenar eminences become markedly wasted, the interossei also become affected, and the hand assumes a characteristic claw-like form. Involvement then extends to the muscles of the arm and shoulder girdle; terminally the symptoms of bulbar paralysis may appear. In the anterior horns there is gradual atrophy and loss of neurons. Gliosis may occur but is usually not marked. The anterior spinal nerve roots become wasted, particularly in the cervical region and in the cauda equina, and appear grey and thin to the naked eye, while in the related muscles there is neurogenic atrophy (Fig. 23.68, p. 935).

Progressive bulbar palsy. This variant of motor neuron disease may appear first, or may follow spinal involvement. There is progressive paralysis and wasting of the muscles of the tongue, lips, jaws, larynx and pharynx; death often occurs by involvement of the respiratory centre, or by foreign matter entering the lungs through the paralysed larynx. The lesions are in the medulla and are of the same nature as those in the cord. They are usually most marked in the hypoglossal and spinal accessory nuclei, but occur also in the nuclei of the vagus and facial nerves, and in the nucleus of the motor part of the trigeminal. Along with the changes in the brain stem there is varying involvement of the nerve cells in the anterior horns and of the pyramidal fibres.

Amyotrophic lateral sclerosis. In cases where there is considerable degeneration of upper motor neurons, there is loss of nerve fibres in the cortico-spinal tracts and consequently various degrees of spasticity. When this is marked, the clinical syndrome is usually called amyotrophic lateral sclerosis. In addition to the atrophic changes in the anterior horns, there is widespread sclerosis and loss of myelin in the lateral and anterior white columns, especially the pyramidal tracts (Fig. 21.61). The changes in the pyramidal fibres usually start first and are most marked at their lower extremities, the process then extending upwards. Atrophic changes, corresponding to those in the anterior horns, occur in the motor cells of the cerebral cortex and here also many disappear.

No sharply dividing line can be drawn between these variants of motor neuron disease. Their names merely emphasise that in any one case, the early stages of the disease may have a particular distribution. In the terminal stages there is often widespread involvement of motor neurons in the brain stem and in the spinal cord, and involvement of the lateral and ventral white columns in the spinal cord.

Friedreich's ataxia

In this disease there is atrophy in both motor and sensory tracts. It often affects more than one member of a family, and so is sometimes called **familial ataxia**; rarely it occurs in successive generations. Isolated cases also occur. It usually begins in childhood and the chief symptoms are ataxia with muscular weakness. Lateral curvature of the spine and talipes equinus often develop, and nystagmus and disturbances of speech are also common. In such cases, the spinal cord is found to be relatively thin and there is degeneration in the posterior and lateral columns (Fig. 21.62). The posterior roots also show degeneration, especially the fibres within the cord, and involvement of the roots and posterior columns may be present in the cervical region as well as lower down; the cells in the posterior root ganglia, however, are little altered. In the lateral columns the pyramidal fibres are degenerate, most markedly at lower levels. The posterior spino-cerebellar tracts are similarly affected, and the cells of the thoracic nucleus show degenerative changes. There may be some degeneration also in the anterior spino-cerebellar and spino-thalamic tracts. The nature of the disease is

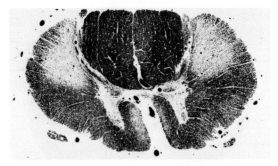

Fig. 21.61 Amyotrophic lateral sclerosis. Section of the spinal cord, showing degeneration in the lateral and anterior columns and preservation of the posterior columns. There is selectively severe involvement of the crossed pyramidal tracts. (Weigert–Pal method.)

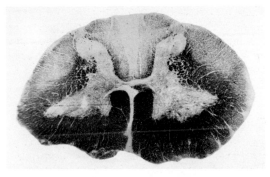

Fig. 21.62 Section of cord in Friedreich's ataxia, showing degeneration in posterior and lateral columns. (Weigert–Pal method.)

obscure. Friedreich's ataxia and *Marie's hereditary cerebellar ataxia* are probably related: the two conditions sometimes overlap and intermediate forms occur, but each affected family presents its own variant. Friedreich's ataxia is frequently associated with a chronic progressive myocarditis, in which focal coagulative necrosis of the muscle fibres is followed by replacement fibrosis.

Other lesions of the spinal cord

Subacute combined degeneration

This type of degeneration formerly occurred in a high proportion of cases of inadequately treated pernicious anaemia, but since highly effective purified preparations of vitamin B_{12} have been available this complication is now much less common. Similar lesions have been found much more rarely in some other chronic diseases, e.g. malabsorption syndromes, leukaemia, diabetes and carcinoma. *Subacute combined degeneration may develop in the 'pre-anaemic stage' of pernicious anaemia.* The administration of vitamin B_{12} in adequate doses is completely effective in preventing the development of neural lesions.

The anatomical changes consist of degeneration in the dorsal and lateral columns of the spinal cord (Fig. 21.63). The process appears to start, and to be most severe and extensive, in the lower thoracic region and then extends upwards and downwards. In the involved segments the degenerate myelin is removed by phagocytes which migrate to the perivascular sheaths. In untreated cases there is practically no glial proliferation and the degenerated areas present an open spongy appearance. With long survival on B_{12} treatment, however, some glio-

sis eventually occurs. The degeneration in the motor tracts may ascend through the internal capsule and degenerative changes may be seen in the Betz cells of the cortex. The symptoms depend on the degree and extent of tract involvement, and consist mainly of ataxia and spasticity. *In view of its progressive, disabling nature, and the arresting effects of B_{12} therapy, early diagnosis is of the utmost importance.*

Syringomyelia

This term is applied to a rare condition in which a cyst-like space or spaces develop within the cord, containing fluid and enclosed by neuroglia. There is considerable controversy over the nature and pathogenesis of syringomyelia. In the past, it was distinguished from hydromyelia (dilatation of the central canal of the spinal cord) on the basis that syringomyelic cavities first appear dorsal to the central canal. There is, however, increasing evidence that, in most cases, syringomyelia is caused by CSF being propelled through a valve-like opening between the caudal extremity of the fourth ventricle and the central canal, i.e. that the cavity is a greatly distended central canal. Individuals with this type of syringomyelia also tend to have a mild developmental abnormality at the cranio-cervical junction, the cerebellar tonsils protruding further through the foramen magnum than usual. Whatever its pathogenesis, however, the structural abnormalities in the cord are fairly stereotyped. The cavity usually extends through several segments of the cervical cord (Fig. 21.64) and, as it enlarges, the cord becomes swollen and feels somewhat soft. On microscopic examination the tissue lining the cavity is composed of enlarged astrocytes and coarse astrocytic fibrils in the rarified tissue around the central

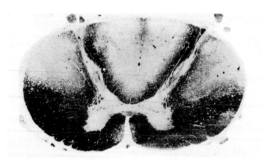

Fig. 21.63 Subacute combined degeneration, showing conspicuous degeneration in both lateral and posterior columns. (Weigert–Pal method.)

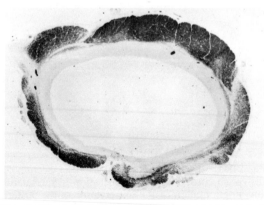

Fig. 21.64 Syringomyelia: junction between cervical and thoracic portion. (Weigert–Pal method.)

cavity. Occasionally syringomyelia occurs in association with tumours affecting the spinal cord.

Effects. These are due principally to destruction of the cord by the enlarging cavity. The first fibres to be affected are the decussating sensory fibres conveying the sensations of heat and pain: the resulting defect, known as *dissociated anaesthesia*, is a selective insensibility to heat and pain in the region corresponding to the involved segments of the spinal cord. Trophic disturbances affect the joints, bone and skin. A neuropathic arthritis occurs, closely similar to that in tabes (p. 753), but, as syringomyelia is usually in the cervical region, the joints of the upper limbs are chiefly involved. The trophic lesions of the skin are various and include vesicles, ulceration and painless whitlows. As the cavity enlarges it ultimately affects the lateral white columns leading to spastic paraplegia, the ventral grey horns leading to neurogenic atrophy of muscles, and the posterior white columns leading to even greater disturbances of sensation.

Acute decompression sickness (caisson disease)

This occurs as a result of barotrauma, due to a rapid reduction in environmental pressure. It is thus a hazard for deep water divers who are brought back to atmospheric pressure without sufficiently gradual decompression, to workers in compressed air, and occasionally to aviators and others subjected to sub-atmospheric pressures.

Symptoms may come on during return to atmospheric pressure or up to more than a day afterwards. In its mildest form the disorder consists of pain in one or more large joints ('bends' or 'diver's cramps'), but bone necrosis may subsequently become apparent (p. 875). In more severe cases, there are complex disturbances, including haemoconcentration and hypovolaemia, sludging of red cells, thrombocytopenia and activation of clotting and fibrinolytic mechanisms. Profound circulatory disturbance occurs and may cause death. Some of the features of decompression sickness are explicable on the basis that nitrogen, which dissolves slowly in the tissues and blood, comes out of solution and forms bubbles on reduction of the environmental pressure, and therefore of the pressure within the body. Other features are not well explained, but may be due to the surface effects of blood or cell/gas interfaces on proteins, platelets, plasma membranes, etc., i.e. an indirect effect of bubbles in the blood and tissues.

This condition is included here because in more serious cases the central nervous system, and particularly the **spinal cord**, is commonly affected. It has been suggested that, because of its high solubility in lipid (including myelin), large amounts of nitrogen under pressure dissolve in the nervous tissue, particularly the white matter, during compression and come out of solution to form bubbles there on too rapid decompression. However, the formation of bubbles in the white matter of the cord has not been demonstrated, and another theory is that, because of its venous drainage, the cord is highly susceptible to pressure fluctuations in the thorax and systemic veins. Such fluctuations occur in acute decompression sickness due to plugging of the alveolar capillaries with bubbles (and sometimes fat emboli).

Spinal cord involvement results in paraplegia, which usually passes off, although permanent disability may result. The cord lesions resemble multiple microscopic foci of infarction.

The likelihood of developing decompression sickness depends on many factors, including individual variations, and although the condition can be prevented by ensuring that decompression is gradual, calculated rates of decompression must include wide safety margins.

III: The Peripheral Nerves

Peripheral neuropathies

Although the terms *neuritis* and *polyneuritis* have often been used in the past to describe virtually all non-traumatic disorders of the peripheral nerves, an inflammatory process within the nerve is rare. Thus the terms *neuropathy* or *polyneuropathy* are often more appropriate. The neuropathies fall into three major categories: (*a*) primary degeneration of the nerve cell (parenchymatous neuropathy), (*b*) dysfunction of the Schwann cell, and (*c*) alterations in the blood supply to the nerve. A true, i.e. inflammatory, neuritis also occurs and is considered after the neuropathies.

Parenchymatous neuropathies

Parenchymatous neuropathies usually affect several nerves more or less symmetrically, i.e. they are polyneuropathies. The first manifestation of the primary abnormality in the nerve cell is degenerative change in the most distal part of the fibre as shown by dissolution of the axon and destruction of the myelin sheath. The myelin is broken up into globules, which undergo phagocytosis: these globules stain with Sudan dyes and are positive with the Marchi reaction (Fig. 21.65). This Wallerian-type de-

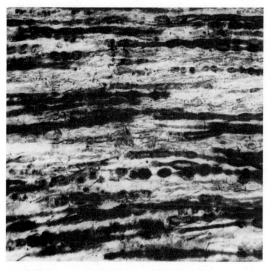

Fig. 21.65 Longitudinal section of peripheral nerve in alcoholic neuropathy showing degeneration of myelin sheaths. (Marchi method.) × about 400.

generation then extends proximally—the so-called 'dying-back' process. In general the longest and largest fibres are affected first and so the earliest neurological disturbance appears in the distal parts of the limbs: the most characteristic are paraesthesiae, muscle weakness, loss of vibration sense and diminished two-point discrimination. Microscopic examination of the proximal part of an affected nerve may show very few abnormal fibres although they may be very numerous in its distal part. In some cases where muscle weakness is considerable, abnormalities in the nerves may be re-

stricted to the small distal radicles actually within the muscle. As the motor fibres degenerate the muscle end-plates lose their innervation and the muscle fibres undergo neurogenic atrophy (see p. 935). If some healthy nerve fibres remain, ineffective regenerative phenomena to re-innervate motor end plates are shown by the presence of collateral and ultra-terminal axonal sprouting. As the degeneration extends proximally, central chromatolysis becomes apparent in the motor neurons in the ventral horns of the spinal cord and in the neurons in the dorsal root ganglia.

The causes of parenchymatous peripheral neuropathy are many and varied. Probably the commonest is **nutritional deficiency**, beri-beri being the most important disease in this group.

Beri-beri is essentially a polyneuropathy which results from the absence or deficiency of vitamin B_1 (thiamine), and is usually caused by a diet consisting exclusively of over-milled cereals, especially rice. The disease, which is encountered principally among rice-eating populations, occurs in two forms. In one—**the 'dry' form**— the peripheral nerves are chiefly affected. Chromatolysis is often prominent in the ventral horns of the spinal cord and in the dorsal root ganglia. The levels of pyruvate in the blood and CSF are raised. In the other, or **'wet' form**, the disturbances are mainly cardiac; the heart becomes dilated, especially the right ventricle, there is general venous congestion, and oedema usually becomes a marked feature. Degenerative changes have been found in the vagi, the phrenic nerves, and the sympathetic system. It may be that the cardiac dilatation is secondary to the lesions in the nerves, but the possibility of a primary change in the cardiac muscle cannot be excluded.

Polyneuropathy can readily be produced in fowls and pigeons by feeding them with milled or polished rice. In the experimentally produced disease rapid recovery takes place when the birds are fed on diets containing the necessary vitamin. The biochemical abnormality is a failure of neural tissue to complete the oxidation of carbohydrate in the absence of co-carboxylase which normally is produced by phosphorylation of thiamine. Consequently carbohydrate metabolism ceases at the pyruvate level and there is an increased concentration of pyruvate in the blood and tissues.

Since the body's requirements of thiamine

are proportional to the amount of carbohydrate metabolised, the deficiency of thiamine is exaggerated by a predominantly carbohydrate diet, and the severity of the effects on neural tissue are attributable to its dependence on carbohydrate oxidation. *In vitro* the metabolic defect of homogenised affected tissue is rectified very speedily by the addition of co-carboxylase, and *in vivo* by the administration of the precursor, vitamin B_1. Substitution of undermilled for milled rice has caused beri-beri to disappear in many places but it has not been established that beri-beri in man is due *solely* to the lack of thiamine, and deficiencies in other members of the vitamin B group may well contribute. Protein deficiency is thought to be partly responsible for the 'wet' form of the disease (p. 257).

Wernicke's encephalopathy. This syndrome is also attributed to thiamine deficiency, but patients with it are likely to be deficient also in other components of the vitamin B complex. The deficiency may be of long duration as in chronic alcoholism or prolonged malnutrition, or it may be acute and occur as a complication of persistent vomiting. Wernicke's encephalopathy caused by acute vitamin deficiency is probably considerably commoner than is generally recognised, but chronic alcoholism remains the commonest underlying cause in well-nourished communities. The disorder was common among prisoners of war in the Far East during the Second World War and was attributed to dietary deficiencies.

Clinically, the onset is acute or subacute: clinical features include disturbances of consciousness, ophthalmoplegia and ataxia with, if untreated, terminal coma. The blood pyruvate level is raised and, if the deficiency state is chronic, there is usually also a peripheral neuropathy. Pathologically there are, in acutely fatal cases, numerous petechial haemorrhages in the mamillary bodies, in the floor and walls of the third ventricle, around the aqueduct, and in the floor of the fourth ventricle. The anterior nuclei of the thalamus may also be involved. In subacute cases, macroscopic abnormalities may be restricted to slight granularity and loss of definition in the affected areas. Histologically there is dilatation and proliferation of capillaries and small haemorrhages: the parenchyma stains palely and there are various degrees of reactive change in astrocytes and microglia. Neurons are relatively spared.

Quite dramatic improvement may follow the administration of the vitamin B group, but good clinical recovery is unlikely if the mamillary bodies are already structurally damaged before treatment is initiated. The mamillary bodies become small and shrunken and often have a brownish discoloration

on section. Such patients usually have a persistent psychosis of Korsakoff type.

Other metabolic disturbances. *Deficiency of nicotinic acid or vitamin B_{12} are other causes of peripheral neuropathy, while a deficiency of various members of the vitamin B group is probably the principal cause of the peripheral neuropathy associated with *chronic alcoholism*. This is brought about partly by the restricted diet and partly by deficient absorption from the alimentary canal because of associated gastrointestinal disturbances.

Various chemicals may produce a parenchymatous polyneuropathy. Examples are triorthocresyl phosphate, dinitrobenzene and carbon disulphide, and certain drugs, e.g. isoniazid. Some metabolic or toxic derangement is probably the cause of *carcinomatous neuropathy* (see p. 771) while an endogenous metabolic defect is the cause of the neuropathy in *acute porphyria*.

In **acute porphyria**, there is usually a history of attacks of colicky abdominal pain followed by the onset of weakness in the legs and arms and sometimes mental disturbances, an association of symptoms suggestive of lead poisoning. The essential lesion is a polyneuropathy, but in spite of paraesthesiae, there is little true sensory loss. In severe cases, paresis may progress rapidly to complete quadriplegia and death. Some run a relapsing course, and others recover completely, though the metabolic abnormality may persist. The condition may be precipitated by drugs, especially allyl-barbiturates, but there is often a hereditary predisposition and the metabolic pigment abnormality may be present in healthy siblings; in some families, the disorder is transmitted as a Mendelian dominant. The diagnosis depends on the recognition of the abnormal chromogen, porphobilinogen, and other pigments in the urine, which darkens on exposure to light, uroporphyrin III being the usual pigment in idiopathic cases. Since these pigments are pharmacologically inert, the actual cause of the symptoms is still obscure. In **chronic congenital porphyria**, on the other hand, the pigment excreted is uroporphyrin I and photosensitisation is a prominent symptom. Cases of the idiopathic disease with neurological symptoms have also been observed in which uroporphyrin I was excreted.

Schwann cell dysfunction

In neuropathies due to dysfunction of the Schwann cell, the characteristic abnormality is *segmental demyelination*, i.e. demyelination of an axon between two nodes of Ranvier. Many segments in a single fibre may be randomly affected. Segmental demyelination affects nerve conduction but a particularly interesting feature is that remyelination may occur. The regenerated myelin, however, usually forms a thinner sheath than normal, while the formation of extra nodes means that the internodal distance becomes reduced. This type of nerve damage in addition to diabetic micro-angiopathy of the vasa nervorum (p. 1033) contributes to the neuropathy in individuals with *diabetes mellitus*, and occurs particularly in *post-diphtheritic paralysis* and in *lead poisoning*.

Continuing hyperplasia of Schwann cells may occur in response to long-standing segmental demyelination. 'Onion bulbs' composed of Schwann cells and collagen fibrils surround individual axons and in the resultant **hypertrophic interstitial neuropathy** subcutaneous nerves may be readily palpable.

Vascular and ischaemic changes

These account for the third major group of neuropathies. In contrast to the types already described, the cause is usually local with the result that the distribution is not symmetrical although sometimes several nerves are affected. Probably the commonest cause is *pressure* such as in 'crutch palsy' or 'Saturday night paralysis'. The duration of the disability depends on the degree of ischaemia produced by the pressure. Abnormalities in the vasa nervorum account for the peripheral neuropathy commonly seen in *polyarteritis nodosa* (Fig. 21.66): the term **mononeuritis multiplex** is often used because of the presence of multiple individual lesions in various nerves. The ischaemia may be sufficient only to produce transient dysfunction but there may be frank infarction with subsequent Wallerian degeneration of the affected fibres. In *peripheral vascular disease of the lower limbs*, caused usually by atheroma, there may be a pronounced reduction in the number of nerve fibres and a progressive increase of fibrous tissue in peripheral nerves.

True peripheral neuritis

The peripheral nerves may also be affected by an inflammatory process—**true peripheral neuritis**—and as the interstitial tissue in the nerve is more severely affected than the nerve fibres themselves, the term *interstitial neuritis* is often appropriate. This type of neuritis may result from the *extension of any type of local tissue inflammation*, e.g. wounds, abscesses, bed-

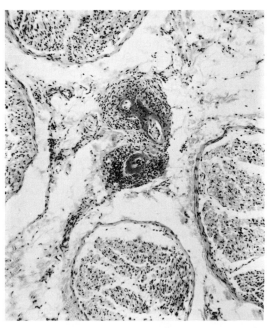

Fig. 21.66 Transverse section of the sciatic nerve in polyarteritis nodosa, showing an acute arterial lesion. × 170.

sores, arthritis, etc., into the nerve. The latter becomes swollen and congested and there is an interstitial inflammatory exudate. A similar though ill-understood process may be responsible for the neuritis of the facial nerve that follows exposure to cold and wet (*Bell's palsy*).

Interstitial neuritis may also be *chronic* from the outset. A striking example of this is seen in *leprosy* (p. 215), where the bacilli enter the supporting sheaths of the nerves, and induce interstitial proliferation of connective tissue followed by atrophy of nerve fibres, leading to paralytic and trophic disturbances. Interstitial neuritis may be produced also by *syphilis*, notably in the cranial nerves at the base of the brain. In any form of *meningitis*, the inflammatory change may spread to and affect the emerging nerves or roots.

Acute infective polyneuritis, often known as the **Guillain–Barré syndrome**, is the most important type of true neuritis. Its incidence is greatest in young adults and in about half the cases it follows a mild 'non-specific' febrile illness, usually a virus infection of the respiratory tract. There is increasing evidence of an association between cytomegalovirus infection and acute infective polyneuritis. In severe cases, there is symmetrical progressive ascending paralysis usually commencing in the lower limbs and then spreading to the arms, the trunk, and the cranial nerves. Sensory disturbance is absent or only mild. Provided the patient can be tided over the acute phase, if necessary with the aid of artificial ventilation, a progressive slow recovery over a period of weeks or months is to be expected. Sudden death, often attributable to a true myocarditis, occurs in a proportion of cases. In a fatal case the main *structural alterations* are seen throughout the length of the peripheral nerves: they consist of oedema, infiltration by lymphocytes and plasma cells, and phagocytosis and destruction of myelin. The CSF shows a highly characteristic, but not invariable, increase of protein to as much as 8g/litre, while the cell count remains normal. The protein includes oligoclonal IgG

(p. 766). This disease closely resembles experimental allergic neuritis produced in animals by injecting homogenates or extracts of nerve tissue incorporated in Freund's adjuvant. The experimental disease appears to be due to a delayed hypersensitivity reaction to a basic protein of peripheral-nerve myelin and has much in common with experimental allergic encephalomyelitis (p. 763). In the Guillain–Barré syndrome, there is evidence of cell-mediated immunity to a constituent of nerve myelin, and a similar condition has been observed following inoculation of rabbit-derived vaccine, containing nerve root material, in the prevention of rabies. The syndrome may thus be an autoimmune polyneuritis. Although antibody to myelin has been reported in the serum, it appears to have little or no pathogenicity *in vivo*.

Tumours of the Nervous System

Many tumours of the nervous system arise intrinsically in neural tissue, i.e. they are neuro-ectodermal tumours. Others arise from the meninges (meningioma) or from cranial and spinal nerve roots (Schwannoma). The brain is also a common site of metastatic carcinoma, and finally there are many relatively rare tumours of the nervous system.

The observed incidence of these various tumour types depends on whether this is based on necropsy reports from a general hospital, or on biopsies and autopsies in a neurological institute. Of a total of about 1500 consecutive primary tumours of the nervous system encountered over a 10-year period in the Institute of Neurological Sciences, Glasgow, approximately 1000 were neuro-ectodermal, 250 were meningiomas, and 65 were Schwannomas. During the same period some 400 cases of metastatic carcinoma in the brain were encountered, but this figure is artificially low because not all patients with suspected cerebral metastases are referred to neurosurgical or neurological wards.

Biopsy through a burr-hole in the skull and examination of smear preparations is invaluable in the immediate identification of brain tumours.

Tumours of neuro-ectodermal origin

These include all the tumours which arise from the primitive medullary epithelium. In the central nervous system these cells consist of the neuroglia (astrocytes, oligodendrocytes and ependymal cells) and the nerve cells. Most neuro-ectodermal tumours are of neuroglial origin and are known collectively as the **gliomas**.

The gliomas

Some gliomas are mature tumours composed of cells that resemble closely astrocytes, oligodendrocytes or ependymal cells, the respective tumours being called **astrocytoma**, **oligodendroglioma** and **ependymoma**. Secondly, there are tumours in which only a proportion of the cells are of this type, the others being pleomorphic and less well differentiated: these are referred to as the **anaplastic variants** of these tumours.

As in other tissues, the general rule usually applies that the more primitive or undifferentiated the cells are, the more rapid is their growth, but in contrast to tumours in other tissues, gliomas cannot be divided into benign and malignant types, for *all gliomas*, whether composed of highly or poorly differentiated cells, *infiltrate the adjacent brain tissue* and are never truly sharply demarcated or encapsulated. Paradoxically the rapidly growing anaplastic forms often appear to be the better demarcated, because they also compress and push aside surrounding tissues. Furthermore, except on very rare occasions and usually after craniotomy, *neuro-ectodermal tumours do not metastasise to other organs*. They may however be disseminated by the CSF to other parts of the nervous system. The individual gliomas thus differ mainly in their degree of cellular differentiation and rate of growth.

Astrocytoma. This is by far the commonest type of glioma. A well-differentiated astrocytoma is a slowly growing whitish tumour, usually poorly defined at its margin where it merges with the surrounding tissue. Some contain abundant glial fibres and are tough, almost rubbery: others have scanty glial fibres and are soft. Cystic change is common (Fig. 21.67) particularly in the cerebellar astrocytoma of childhood.

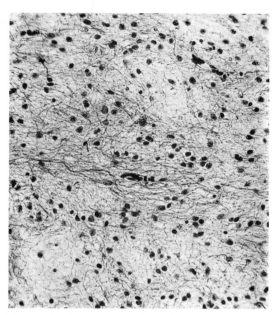

Fig. 21.68 Astrocytoma of relatively low cellularity showing well formed glial fibrils (PTAH). × 260.

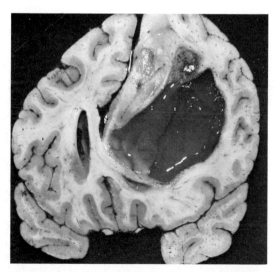

Fig. 21.67 Cystic astrocytoma in right frontal lobe. Tumour tissue is identifiable adjacent to the upper pole of the cyst.

In a *fibrillary astrocytoma*, microscopic examination shows unevenly distributed and often loosely arranged elongated cells separated by glial fibrils (Fig. 21.68). Even in the absence of gross cystic change there are often numerous microcysts. Sometimes the brain tissue is diffusely permeated by tumour astrocytes, often

with remarkable preservation of nerve cells and fibres. The edge of this type of tumour often defies recognition with the naked eye. It is known as *diffuse astrocytoma* or *gliomatosis cerebri* and is particularly common in the brain stem and spinal cord. Other rarer forms of astrocytoma are composed of protoplasmic astrocytes or swollen, so-called gemistocytic astrocytes.

All astrocytomas display a marked tendency

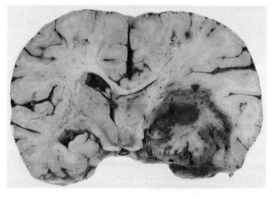

Fig. 21.69 Glioblastoma multiforme of temporal lobe. Note the well-defined margin and haemorrhagic areas within the tumour. There is a pronounced midline shift, virtual obliteration of the lateral ventricle and a supracallosal hernia (see p. 730).

to become *anaplastic:* this may be restricted to one part of the tumour or it may be multifocal. To the naked eye the anaplastic areas are haemorrhagic and necrotic and often appear to have a relatively well-defined edge. The microscopic features of these areas are similar to those of glioblastoma multiforme.

The term **glioblastoma multiforme** may be used for astrocytomas that are highly anaplastic throughout. Such tumours occur in adults, most frequently in the cerebral hemispheres, forming a rapidly growing, apparently relatively well-defined mass with extensive necrosis and haemorrhage. It produces considerable distortion of the brain and often a rapid increase in intracranial pressure (Figs. 21.5, p. 730 and 21.69).

Microscopically a glioblastoma multiforme is richly cellular in the areas that are not necrotic and there are great variations in cell type ranging from closely packed masses of small anaplastic cells to pleomorphic giant cells (Fig. 21.70). Mitoses are often frequent and glial fibrils extremely scanty. Small vessels in and around the tumour may show curious bud-like or 'glomeruloid' endothelial proliferations (Fig. 21.71). Necrosis is usually extensive and frequently elongated tumour cells form a palisade around necrotic foci (Fig. 21.72).

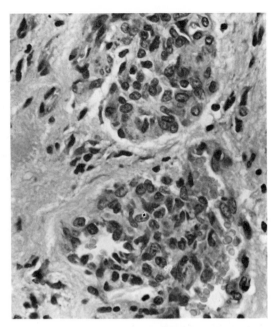

Fig. 21.71 Glomeruloid endothelial proliferation in glioblastoma. × 390.

Ependymoma. This not uncommon tumour is most frequently encountered in children, usually in the fourth ventricle but it occurs

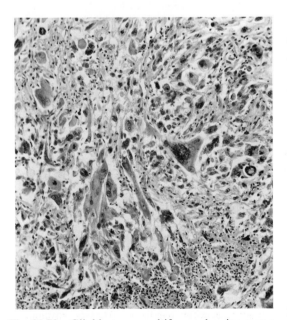

Fig. 21.70 Glioblastoma multiforme showing many aberrant giant cells. × 110.

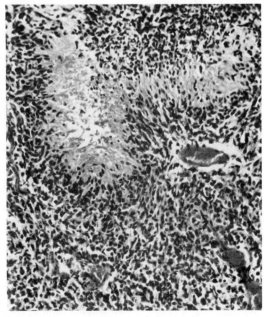

Fig. 21.72 Glioblastoma multiforme, showing a common pattern of central necrosis with peripheral palisading of spindle-shaped cells. × 130.

also in the other ventricles. The tumour cells often have a distinctly epithelial appearance and they are characteristically orientated around small blood vessels but are separated from them by an eosinophilic fibrillary band (Fig. 21.73). Less frequently columnar cells form small canaliculi (Fig. 21.74), and near the free edge of these cells there may be small rod-shaped blepharoplasts. Ependymomas may also become anaplastic as shown by the occurrence of cellular pleomorphism and poor differentiation, haemorrhage and necrosis. Closely related to the ependymoma is the *papillary tumour of the choroid plexus*. This is also most often seen in children, forming a rounded bulky tumour usually in one lateral ventricle. The papillae have a vascular connective tissue core covered by columnar epithelium very similar in appearance to normal choroid plexus epithelium (Fig. 21.75). It frequently causes hydrocephalus.

A curious tumour, the *myxopapillary ependymoma*, arises from the filum terminale in adults. It is slowly growing, markedly gelatinous,

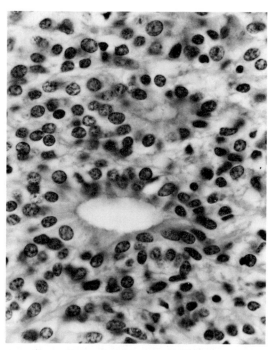

Fig. 21.74 Ependymoma showing a canaliculus lined by columnar cells. × 480.

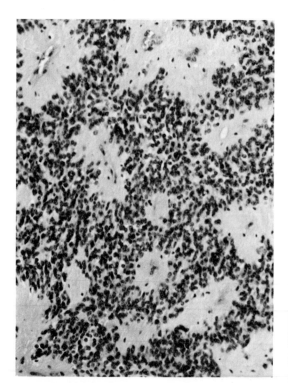

Fig. 21.73 Ependymoma. Note the characteristic perivascular fibrillary haloes. × 125.

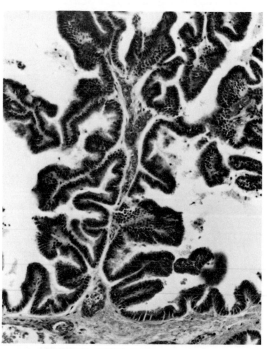

Fig. 21.75 Papillary tumour of the choroid plexus, showing delicate papillary processes covered by cuboidal epithelium. × 200.

and gradually ensheathes the nerve roots of the cauda equina and the caudal part of the spinal cord. The stroma consists of a central vascular core surrounded by mucoid connective tissue and covered in places by cuboidal epithelium (Fig. 21.76); elsewhere the covering cells may form a network between the papillae. This tumour may cause pressure atrophy of the adjacent bones and may even invade them; it is then liable to be mistaken for a chordoma (p. 912).

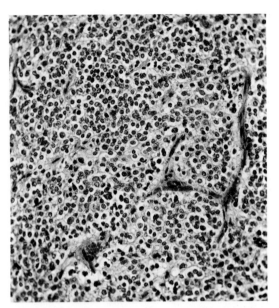

Fig. 21.77 Oligodendroglioma. The tumour is very cellular, the cells being round or oval with distinct cell boundaries. × 125.

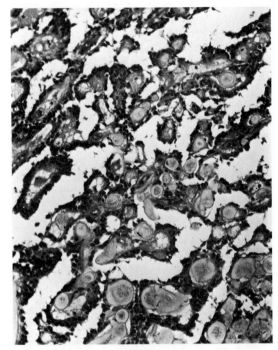

Fig. 21.76 Myxopapillary ependymoma, a papillary structure with very gelatinous stroma, covered by a mainly cuboidal epithelium. × 125.

Oligodendroglioma. In our experience this glioma is rarer than ependymoma. It occurs in the cerebral hemispheres, is slowly growing, rather gelatinous and commonly exhibits numerous small foci of calcification which may be seen radiologically. The cells are uniform, small and rounded, like normal oligodendroglial cells, with somewhat clear cytoplasm and distinct cell-membranes (Fig. 21.77). Cell processes are small and difficult to demonstrate. As with other gliomas, anaplastic change may occur in these tumours.

The above tumours are the commonest types of glioma: other clearly defined variants have not been mentioned because they are rare. Not all gliomas can be placed in a specific category.

Indeed a comprehensive microscopic examination of any glioma may result in the identification of various types of tumour within it and the name applied comes to depend on the most prominent element. In some gliomas both astrocytomatous and oligodendrogliomatous elements are conspicuous. Furthermore each main division exists as a spectrum; at one end there is a mature well-differentiated tumour composed of cells resembling normal glial cells, while at the other there is a highly anaplastic and poorly differentiated tumour. *As all gliomas infiltrate into the adjacent brain, particularly the better differentiated types, total surgical excision is rarely feasible:* radiotherapy is also at best palliative and the ultimate prognosis for a patient with a glioma is usually poor.

Tumours of the neuron series

These include tumours composed of primitive cells, namely *medulloblastoma*, *neuroblastoma* and *retinoblastoma* (p. 803), and tumours containing large ganglion cells, namely *ganglioneuroma* and *ganglioglioma*. The latter types, however, occur very rarely within the central nervous system.

Medulloblastoma. This is the commonest nerve cell tumour of the CNS: it occurs most often in childhood, is a poorly differentiated and rapidly growing cellular tumour and originates in the cerebellum. It forms a soft greyish-white mass protruding into the fourth ventricle and commonly spreads over the surface of the cerebellum as a thin sheet that obscures the normal surface architecture. Seeding of tumour cells by the CSF is usual, and may result in diffuse meningeal tumour or be restricted to small secondary nodules on the nerve roots of the cauda equina. Retrograde spread to the third and lateral ventricles is also common.

Microscopically, its cells are either spherical with little cytoplasm and no fibrils, or somewhat triangular, like short carrots, and arranged around blood vessels and also as rosettes without a central cavity (Fig. 21.78).

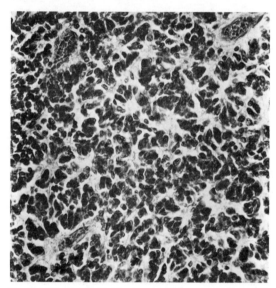

Fig. 21.78 Medulloblastoma. The cells are small and closely packed, but form poorly defined rosettes. × 285.

Neuroblastoma and ganglioneuroma. These, in general, are tumours derived from ganglion cells or their precursors in sites outwith the central nervous system. The majority arise in the adrenal medulla or in sympathetic ganglia but they may also arise in the more distal ganglia of the parasympathetic system. *Neuroblastoma* (sometimes known as sympathicoblastoma) is a primitive, highly malignant tumour whereas *ganglioneuroma* is a mature benign tumour: tumours of an intermediate or mixed character are also encountered.

Neuroblastoma is mainly a tumour of childhood, usually of children under 4 years of age. The commonest sites are the adrenal medulla and the retroperitoneal tissues. A neuroblastoma of the adrenal gland forms a bulky soft cellular and haemorrhagic tumour with extensive necrosis, which destroys the adrenal, spreads rapidly to the upper abdominal lymph nodes, to the liver and notably to the skeleton, secondary tumours in the skull being especially frequent.

Microscopically, the cells are small, round or oval, with little cytoplasm. In many parts they are irregularly arranged, while in places they may form small ball-like masses of cells which sometimes show further differentiation into rings or rosettes, consisting of radially-arranged cells with central cytoplasmic fibrillary projections (Fig. 21.79) which are stained by

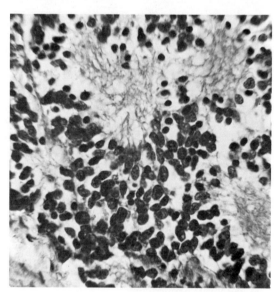

Fig. 21.79 Neuroblastoma. Many of the cells are carrot-shaped and are arranged in well-defined rosettes, the centres of which contain the fine fibrils prolonged from the tapering cells. × 425.

silver impregnation methods, although not so strongly as nerve fibrils. These structures are closely similar to the clumps of neuroblasts which grow out to form the sympathetic system: they are readily seen in the fetal adrenal when it is becoming invaded by neuroblasts which form the medulla of the gland. Rests of undifferentiated neuroblasts are occasionally

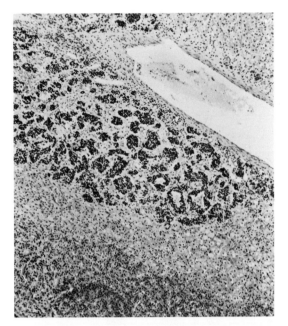

Fig. 21.80 Adrenal medulla of an infant of 9 months, showing masses of undifferentiated neuroblasts. × 60.

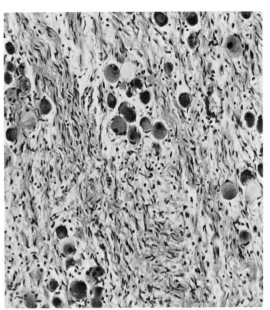

Fig. 21.81 Ganglioneuroma of adrenal, showing abundant mature ganglion cells and non-myelinated nerve fibres.

found in the adrenal medulla in infancy (Fig. 21.80). Some neuroblastomas show partial differentiation, the cells resembling immature neurons.

Ganglioneuroma. This tumour affects older age groups than neuroblastoma and occurs more often in the posterior mediastinum than in the abdomen. It is usually firm, encapsulated like a benign tumour and of rounded or irregular outline. It contains well-formed ganglionic nerve cells, irregularly arranged in a finely fibrillar stroma, and also smaller cells of various forms (Fig. 21.81). There are usually also a large number of nerve fibres, both myelinated and non-myelinated. The tumour is usually benign, but occasionally it is associated with a cellular malignant neuroblastoma.

Neuroblastomas and tumours containing well-differentiated neurons are rare in the CNS: the latter contain also neoplastic neuroglial elements and so are more accurately termed *gangliogliomas* than ganglioneuromas.

The common origin of some of these various tumours is emphasised by the fact that neuroblastic and ganglionic tumours unconnected with the adrenals, e.g. in the thorax, may secrete pressor substances, notably dopamine and noradrenaline, causing severe hypertension.

Tumours of the meninges

The common tumour in this group is the *meningioma*. It is a tumour of the arachnoid and most probably originates from the arachnoid granulations (Fig. 21.10, p. 733).

Meningiomas are solid lobulated tumours, well demarcated from the brain tissue into which they project, forming a depression: they are usually firmly attached by a broad base to the dura. They tend to arise adjacent to the major venous sinuses, commonly parasagittally (Fig. 21.82), or from the base of the skull, often in the region of the olfactory groove when the meningioma projects into the fissure between the frontal lobes (Fig. 21.83). Another common site is the sphenoidal ridge. Rarely a meningioma may arise from the tela choroidea and appear as an intraventricular tumour. Meningiomas may be soft or hard and gritty (see below). Most are benign and can be removed successfully. Some, however, infiltrate the overlying bone, which may be greatly thickened. Very occasional meningiomas metastasise (mostly to the lungs): this may occur following spread into the soft tissues of the scalp after craniotomy, but occasionally from invasion of a venous sinus.

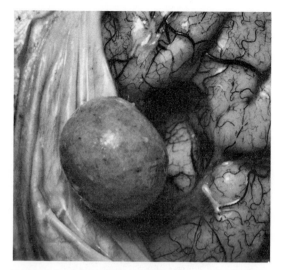

Fig. 21.82 Meningioma attached to dura mater, showing the typical depression of the cerebral cortex from which the tumour is readily withdrawn. × 1·4.

Spinal meningiomas have similar general features, but, owing to their situation, are smaller (Fig. 21.84). They are intradural tumours which arise most frequently on the posterolateral aspect of the cord, and the disturbances at first are chiefly sensory—pain, paraesthesia, etc. Later, various effects up to complete paraplegia may result from pressure on the cord.

Microscopically meningiomas show considerable variation. The most common variety is composed of fibro-cellular tissue with a somewhat whorled appearance owing to the concentric arrangement of the cells (Fig. 21.85). The centres of some of the whorls contain small

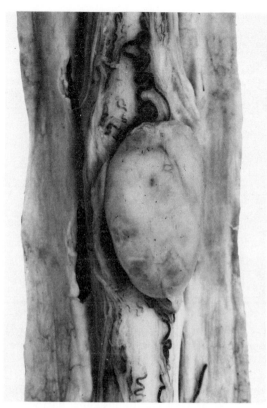

Fig. 21.84 Spinal meningioma compressing the cord. × 1·5.

blood vessels, but others undergo hyaline change and become calcified, resulting in a hard gritty tumour containing numerous spherical calcified particles—*psammoma bodies* (Fig. 21.86). In the more cellular varieties the whorls are composed of rather plump spindle-shaped cells resembling endothelium, but all degrees of transition to the fibrous types are encountered.

Sarcoma very occasionally arises from the meninges and extends widely over its surface. Occasionally a primary *malignant melanoma* occurs as a diffusely spreading tumour in the meninges.

Tumours of vascular origin

Tumours of vascular origin are uncommon, forming about 2 per cent of cerebral tumours. They are divided into *angiomatous malformations*, and the *haemangioblastomas*. The former are not true tumours but are similar to vascular hamartomas elsewhere. They may be chiefly

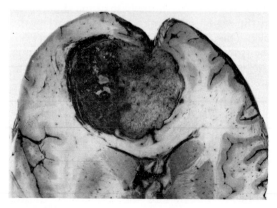

Fig. 21.83 Large meningioma between the frontal lobes.

capillary, venous, or arterio-venous, and their principal importance is as a cause of intracranial haemorrhage (p. 742).

Haemangioblastomas are true tumours arising from vascular elements. They occur most frequently in the cerebellum and are composed of vascular channels or spaces (Fig. 21.87),

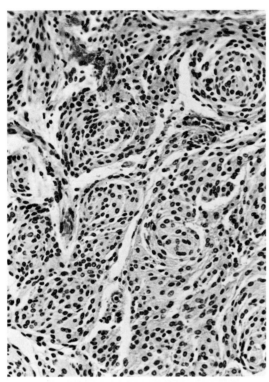

Fig. 21.85 Section of meningioma of common cellular type showing the arrangement of cells and fibres in whorls. × 220.

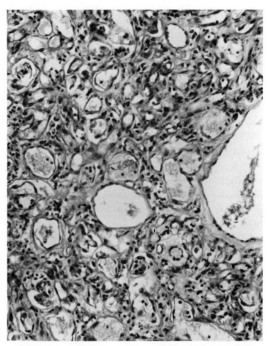

Fig. 21.87 Haemangioblastoma of the cerebellum in a case of Lindau's disease. × 130.

among which there is a large accumulation of lipid-laden cells with an abundant network of reticulin fibres among them. There is a marked tendency to cyst formation: fluid leaking from the vessels comes to form one or more large spaces surrounded by compressed, gliosed brain tissue; the tumour is seen as a nodule in the cyst wall. In **Lindau's disease** a haemangioblastoma of the brain is accompanied by non-vascular cysts in the pancreas (p. 721) or kidneys, and adenomas in the kidneys or adrenals.

Tumours arising in developmental defects

Dermoid and epidermoid cysts, which present clinically as tumours, occasionally affect the nervous system and occur especially at the base

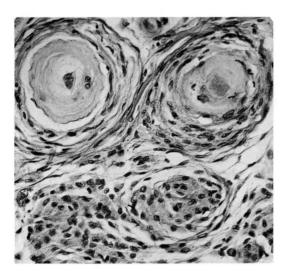

Fig. 21.86 Meningioma, showing fibrocellular masses with concentric arrangement and formation of psammoma bodies. × 350.

of the brain, in the vertebral canal, and in the bones of the skull. An *epidermoid cyst* is well encapsulated, and has a whitish and rather shining appearance (pearly tumour) and rather dry, crumbling contents. The wall is thin and is composed of cells of squamous epithelial type from which keratinised squames are shed into the interior where they accumulate, together with crystals of cholesterol, and thus distend the cyst. In *dermoid cysts*, hairs and sebaceous glands are present. Midline dermoid and epidermoid cysts in the posterior fossa and in the vertebral canal are sometimes connected to the skin surface by a sinus. The opening on the skin may be very small but the sinus provides a route by which the cyst may become infected. *Inclusion epidermoid cysts* in the region of the cauda equina can result from repeated lumbar puncture during childhood.

A somewhat similar partly cystic tumour, is found in children and adults in the region of the pituitary stalk, compressing the gland in the sella turcica and pressing upwards into the third ventricle. These suprasellar tumours probably arise from nests of epidermoid cells derived from the pars tuberalis and they are known as **suprasellar cysts** or **craniopharyngiomas**. Their lining epithelium is in part squam-

ous, but there is also a partial differentiation towards stellate reticulum resembling enamel organ (Fig. 21.88), and the name **adamantinoma** is sometimes applied. The wall is usually partially calcified. The chief clinical features are disturbances of vision and of hypophyseal function (p. 1014). True *Rathke pouch cysts* are intrasellar.

Teratomas are rare intracranial tumours, their chief site being the pineal, where, in boys, their occurrence may be associated with precocious sexual development. They may be well differentiated but more often are of the germinoma type, the histological features being very similar to those of seminoma (p. 997).

Metastatic tumours

Metastatic tumours are very common in the brain and may produce symptoms suggestive of a primary brain tumour before the real origin, e.g. a bronchial carcinoma, is suspected. Metastatic deposits are typically multiple and sharply circumscribed (Fig. 21.89). The tumour

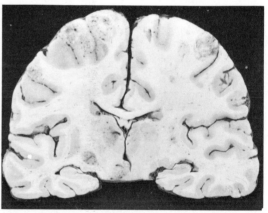

Fig. 21.89 Metastatic carcinoma. Numerous deposits of tumour are present in each cerebral hemisphere.

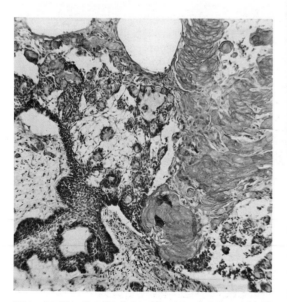

Fig. 21.88 Craniopharyngioma, showing partly squamous, partly 'adamantinomatous' structure. Note the stellate reticulum within the epithelial bands. × 130.

cells tend to spread along the perivascular spaces, ensheathing the blood vessels. Sometimes metastatic carcinoma spreads diffusely throughout the subarachnoid space (*meningeal carcinomatosis*) and the clinical features may be those of a subacute meningitis, but it is usually possible to identify tumour cells in the CSF. The brain may also be infiltrated directly or compressed by tumours arising in the nasopharynx, or by a chordoma growing from the basisphenoid. Secondary tumours within the dura of the spinal cord are rare, but extradural spinal metastases are common.

Effects of tumours

Intracranial tumours may produce **local effects** which will depend on their site, e.g. focal (Jacksonian) epilepsy, paralysis, defects of the visual fields, and also behave as **expanding intracranial lesions** with the effects described on pp. 729–32. An important feature is oedema of the surrounding brain tissue, which usually responds dramatically to steroid therapy.

Tumours of nerve roots and peripheral nerves

These may be solitary or multiple, the latter being especially associated with neurofibromatosis, a disorder inherited as an autosomal dominant. Tumours of nerves are believed to originate from Schwann cells, but some contain a large amount of collagen; hence the sub-division into **Schwannoma** and **neurofibroma**. They do, however, exist as a spectrum, ranging from a discrete paraneural Schwannoma at one end to a poorly delineated plexiform neurofibroma at the other.

Schwannoma. This is typically a rounded or lobulated, often partly cystic, well circumscribed and encapsulated tumour arising from a nerve. These tumours may be intracranial, intraspinal or peripheral. Within the cranium the commonest site of origin is the vestibular portion of the acoustic nerve, but they also occur in association with the trigeminal nerve. An acoustic Schwannoma ('**acoustic neuroma**') takes origin just within the internal auditory meatus, which it invariably expands; and the enlargement may be visible radiologically. The tumour fills the cerebello-pontine angle (Fig. 21.90) and eventually produces severe distortion and displacement of the adjacent brain and some degree of hydrocephalus from compression of the fourth ventricle. When bilateral, they are usually associated with von Recklinghausen's neurofibromatosis (see below). In the spinal canal, Schwannomas occur as intradural tumours on the dorsal nerve roots, mostly in the thoracic region. Their main effect is to compress the spinal cord, but they may extend

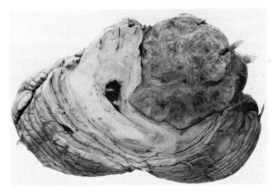

Fig. 21.90 Large Schwannoma of the auditory nerve in the cerebello-pontine angle, which has caused great displacement of the adjacent structures.

through the intervertebral foramen to produce a much larger intrathoracic portion. On peripheral nerves they may occur as isolated single nodules or they may be multiple. The nerve fibres tend to be spread over the surface, especially at one side, and are not incorporated in the tumour.

Microscopic examination shows the tumour

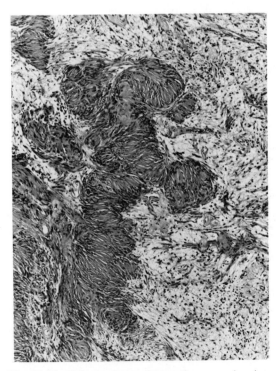

Fig. 21.91 Schwannoma of acoustic nerve, showing whorling and palisading of cells. × 65.

to consist of fibro-cellular bundles in a whorled pattern; within the fasciculi, the cells are closely arranged in parallel fashion with their rod-shaped nuclei forming a characteristic 'palisade' (Fig. 21.91). In other areas the tumour may be of looser texture or even cystic and contain large numbers of fat-laden foamy cells between the fasciculi. The softer and more cellular tumours are prone to repeated local recurrence, and occasionally become frankly sarcomatous.

Neurofibroma may present as a fusiform swelling on a single nerve, but more often a group of nerves are extensively affected by numerous oval and irregular swellings—**plexiform neurofibroma** (Fig. 21.92). If subcutaneous nerves are affected, as not uncommonly occurs in the scalp and neck, the overlying skin becomes firm and nodular and may appear convoluted.

Histological examination shows the nerve to be expanded by large elongated and spindle-shaped cells often separated by mucoid matrix (Fig. 21.93). Residual nerve fibres can be identified in neurofibromas. There is a tendency for local recurrence after excision, and sarcomatous change is not unusual.

In **neurofibromatosis ('von Recklinghausen's disease')**, nodules of various sizes, sometimes numbering hundreds, occur along small nerve branches, especially of the skin, but also in some cases along the visceral branches of the sympathetic. Tumours sometimes arise also from the spinal nerves and their roots within the spinal canal, leading to compression of the spinal cord. The connective tissue of the nodules varies, but is often dense and hyaline; nerve fibres can be traced running through it. Neurofibromatosis is usually associated with multiple pigmented patches in the skin, and lastly, there is occasionally a localised general thickening of the tissues, with nodulation and folding of the skin—a sort of local elephantiasis, to which the name *elephantiasis neuromatosa* has been applied.

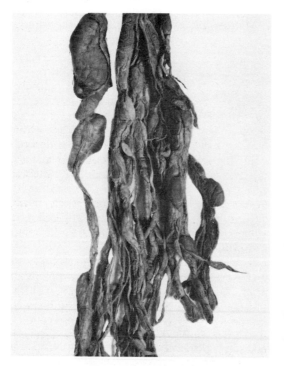

Fig. 21.92   Plexiform neuroma of the sciatic nerve and its branches. Note the numerous nodules of various sizes and forms.

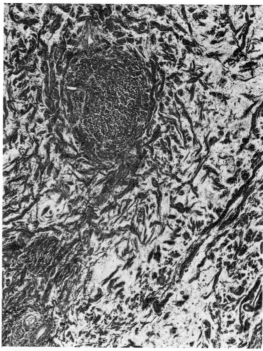

Fig. 21.93   Plexiform neurofibroma showing nerve fibres and loosely arranged interlacing connective tissue bundles. × 120.

IV: The Eye

Introduction

The pathological changes which occur in the eye and the orbital structures are in many respects similar to those described in other systems of the body. However, owing to the particular anatomical and functional properties of the eye, there are some common ocular disease processes which merit separate consideration. Emphasis is therefore placed on inflammatory, neoplastic and degenerative disorders, corneal scarring, glaucoma and degenerative retinopathies, in order to provide suitable examples of pathogenic mechanisms which lead to blindness. The progress of many ocular diseases is followed *in vivo* by a variety of clinical techniques, e.g. slit-lamp microscopy, ophthalmoscopy, angiography and electrophysiological analysis, so that a unique facility exists for clinico-pathological correlation.

Applied anatomy

The structure of the eye is shown diagrammatically in Figs. 21.94 and 21.95. Visual acuity depends upon a transparent focusing system (the cornea and lens), transparent media (the aqueous and vitreous) and a normal photoreceptor and neural conducting mechanism. The metabolism of the cornea and lens is maintained by the circulation of the aqueous fluid, which is produced in the ciliary processes and leaves the anterior chamber via the outflow

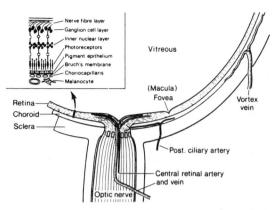

Fig. 21.95 Schematic diagram of the structures of the posterior segment of the eye to show the vascular supply to the choroid, retina and optic disc.

apparatus situated in the inner peripheral cornea adjacent to the root of the iris—the iridocorneal angle. The outflow system is a filter which consists of a series of fenestrated collagenous plates (trabeculae) which are covered by endothelial cells with phagocytic potential—this tissue is limited externally by an endothelial monolayer which lines the circumferential outflow canal of Schlemm (drained by episcleral collector channels). The pressure within the eye is normally 15–20 mmHg and depends upon the rate of aqueous production and the resistance of the outflow system. Any marked variation in pressure—*ocular hypotension* or *hypertension*—whether acute or chronic causes an imbalance in vascular perfusion leading to ischaemic damage to the sensitive neural tissues within the eye.

The retina and the pigment epithelium are maintained by blood flow from two separate arterial systems. The inner two-thirds of the thickness of the retinal tissue are supplied by the branches of the central retinal artery while the outer third (the photoreceptor layer) is maintained by the choriocapillaris, which is supplied by the posterior ciliary arteries. Although the optic nerve is supplied by the central retinal artery and the meningeal arteries, the optic disc or papilla is nourished by blood vessels which are derived from the adjacent (peripapillary) choroid. Because of this vascular

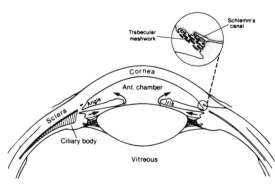

Fig. 21.94 Schematic diagram of the structures of the anterior segment of the eye to show the principal route of aqueous outflow.

arrangement, distinctive patterns of ischaemic damage can occur in the visual sensory system according to the anatomical site of the vascular occlusion or impairment (Fig. 21.96).

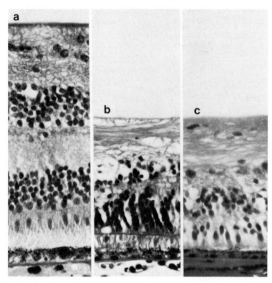

Fig. 21.96 **a** Normal retina: **b** ischaemic atrophy of the inner retina due to occlusion of the central retinal artery: **c** ischaemic atrophy of the outer retina due to posterior ciliary artery occlusion. × 240.

Infections

Pathogenic micro-organisms can invade the eye from the external surface, the adjacent orbital tissues or via the bloodstream. The cellular response is, in general, similar to that observed in other tissues, but the eye is particularly vulnerable because the lens and vitreous are avascular protein-rich structures ideal for the proliferation of many pathogenic bacteria. An ulcer of the cornea due to pyogenic bacterial infection may measure only a few millimetres in diameter, but it will seriously impair vision, and may necessitate removal of the eye by progressing to perforation, ocular hypotonia and endophthalmitis. While numerous types of micro-organisms can cause eye disease, the following are of particular significance.

Viral infections most commonly involve the external surface of the eye, the adenoviruses and herpes simplex being the most important. The **adenoviruses** (types 3 and 8) cause a conjunctivitis in which there is hyperplasia of lymphoid tissue in the oedematous and hyperaemic conjunctival stroma (*follicular conjunctivitis*); this disease often occurs in epidemic form, and can involve the cornea. In **herpes simplex** virus infection, *damage to the cornea* is more important than the associated conjunctivitis: the virus infects the epithelium of the cornea, which it destroys in a particular finger-like or *dendritic* pattern. Herpes keratitis tends to recur and spread to the corneal stroma, inducing neovascularisation and infiltration by lymphocytes, plasma cells and monocytes from the corneal periphery. The corneal lamellae are disorganised and replaced by fibrovascular tissue which causes corneal opacification. Destruction of the stroma of the cornea is aggravated by the release of collagenases from the damaged corneal epithelial cells and the stromal keratocytes. When scarring impairs vision or when ulceration and secondary bacterial infection threaten an endophthalmitis, it is often necessary to replace the involved cornea by a homotransplant (see p. 168).

Trachoma-inclusion conjunctivitis or TRIC infection is caused by chlamydiae (p. 223). Infection with *Chlamydia trachomatosis* is common in the tropical zones and causes 'trachoma', which is responsible for blindness on a massive scale. The organism initially infects the conjunctival epithelium and it can be identified in smears of these cells by the presence of characteristic intracytoplasmic inclusion bodies formed by proliferation of elementary bodies. The superior tarsal conjunctiva is thickened by a dense chronic inflammatory infiltrate containing lymphoid follicles which commonly extends on to and destroys the superficial cornea. The healing stage is associated with extensive corneal and conjunctival scarring and eyelid distortion.

Chlamydia oculogenitalis causes a milder inclusion conjunctivitis in the temperate zones. The lesion is confined to the lower tarsal conjunctiva where there is a low-grade chronic inflammatory infiltration in the stroma. The inclusion bodies observed in the epithelium in this type of TRIC infection can only be distinguished from those of *Chl. trachomatosis* by an immunofluorescent technique.

Bacteria. Primary infections of the conjunctiva and cornea by pyogenic organisms (e.g. gonococcus, Gram +ve cocci, haemophilus, moraxella and pseudomonas) were previously common and serious causes of corneal ulceration, but are now of minor significance in communities in which topical broad-spectrum antibiotics are readily available. Suppurative corneal ulceration, however, is still important as a secondary complication of pre-existing corneal abnormality, advanced glaucoma, mechanical trauma and viral and chlamydial infection. Application of topical steroids may render the cornea more susceptible to infection.

Histological examination of pyogenic ulceration of the cornea (Fig. 21.97) reveals a massive

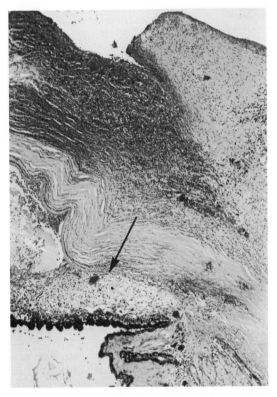

Fig. 21.97 A pyogenic ulcer of the cornea with inflammatory exudation into the anterior chamber and adhesion between the iris and the cornea (*arrow*). × 40.

leukocytic infiltration in the disintegrating corneal stroma. Initially the dense membrane which lines the posterior corneal surface (*Descemet's membrane*), provides resistance to bacterial spread, but toxin diffusion induces migration of polymorphs into the iris and lower part of the anterior chamber (*hypopyon*) and iridocorneal adhesion results. Ultimately Descemet's

membrane prolapses into the corneal deficit (to form a *Descemetocoele*) and, when this ruptures, bacterial penetration is unhindered and abscess formation occurs in the anterior chamber, lens and vitreous.

The eye may be affected in systemic microbial infection, e.g. tuberculosis, syphilis and brucellosis, and usually the uveal tract (the iris, ciliary body and choroid) is involved primarily (*uveitis*). A chronic inflammatory process in the choroid (*choroiditis*) can lead to focal destruction and reactionary proliferation of the pigment epithelium and degeneration in the adjacent retina, which either fuses with the choroid or may be detached by exudation of protein from damaged blood vessels in the choroid and retina. In the iris (*iritis*) and ciliary body (*cyclitis*) the inflammatory process leads to exudation of protein and inflammatory cells into the anterior and posterior chambers and clumps of inflammatory cells adhering to the posterior corneal surface (keratic precipitates) are a classical clinical sign of *iridocyclitis*.

In syphilis and tuberculosis there is widespread destruction of the choroid, ciliary body and iris and the adjacent structures. A similar pattern of tissue destruction is observed in sarcoidosis, fungal infection, protozoal (toxoplasmosis, p. 574) and metazoal (toxocara) infestation, although in the last two examples, the retina is the tissue more severely affected.

It should be noted that many cases of chronic uveitis are of unknown aetiology, although evidence is accumulating to incriminate a hypersensitivity reaction. The inflammatory infiltration in the uveal tract is predominantly lymphocytic, but the end-result is similar to that described above in the chronic bacterial infections, and ophthalmoscopy reveals punched out areas of depigmentation of the fundus. Involvement of the ciliary body leads to ocular hypotension, reactionary fibrosis in the vitreous body, choroidal and retinal oedema and lens degeneration. Contraction of the fibrotic vitreous and exudation into the subretinal space detaches the retina and the end-stage is a striking shrinkage of the eye with massive subretinal fibrosis and secondary ossification (*phthisis bulbi*) (Fig. 21.98). Conversely, ocular hypertension or secondary glaucoma (p. 800) can result from occlusion of the iridocorneal angle by post-inflammatory adhesions between the iris and the cornea (*anterior*

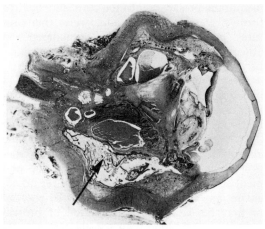

Fig. 21.98   Shrinkage and disorganisation of the eye following inflammation (phthisis bulbi). The retina is detached and the choroid is thickened by oedema and ossification (*arrow*). ×4.

synechiae) or by infiltration of the outflow system by inflammatory cells.

Auto-immune disease

Auto-immune reactions occur in the eye in two established disease entities, *lens-induced uveitis* and *sympathetic ophthalmitis*.

   (1) Lens-induced uveitis. Traumatic breakdown of lens tissue releases lens protein into the anterior chamber or the vitreous and in some circumstances this gives rise to a granulomatous reaction with giant cells due to a complex hypersensitivity reaction involving both auto-antibodies and also delayed hypersensitivity. The inflammatory reaction destroys the lens and the adjacent uveal tissue.

   (2) Sympathetic ophthalmitis. Trauma to one eye which involves damage to or incarceration of either the iris or the ciliary body in the overlying sclera may be followed by a giant-cell granulomatous uveitis in the opposite eye (Fig. 21.99). This secondary inflammatory process may arise months or years after the original injury and results in extensive damage to the second or 'sympathising' eye.

   It is widely believed that release of uveal antigens from the injured eye stimulates a cell-mediated auto-immune response and that the second eye is the target organ of a delayed hypersensitivity reaction. If the first eye is preserved, it too is damaged by a giant-cell granu-

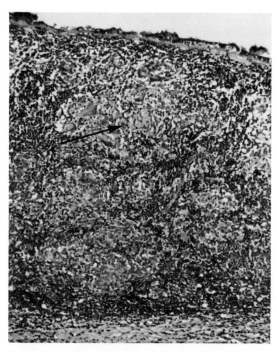

Fig. 21.99   The choroid in sympathetic ophthalmitis; the tissue is infiltrated by a giant-cell granulomatous reaction (*arrow*). ×370.

lomatous reaction in the remaining uveal tissue. Although rare, the threat of occurrence of this complication makes it difficult to decide between surgical repair and immediate removal of the injured eye; the latter abolishes the risk of sympathetic ophthalmitis.

Vascular disease

   Retinal ischaemia and haemorrhage. The pattern of ischaemic disease in the ocular tissues can often be related to the anatomy of the blood supply (p. 795). Complete occlusion of the central retinal artery by atheroma, thrombus or embolism, results in ischaemic atrophy of the inner two-thirds of the retina, while occlusion of the posterior ciliary arteries causes atrophy of the photoreceptor layer (Fig. 21.96). The outer plexiform layer is a zone in which there is inadequate resorption of exudates from damaged capillaries. Exudates which consist predominantly of plasma protein are seen by ophthalmoscopy as discrete pale yellow areas in the retina and are described as *hard exudates*; resorption by lipid-laden glial macro-

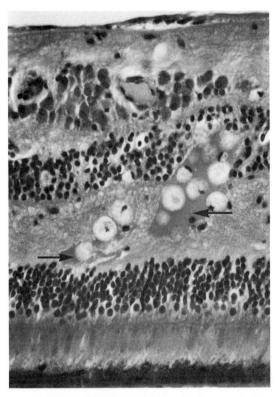

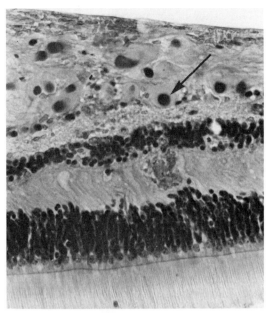

21.101 A micro-infarct in the nerve fibre layer of the retina in which the swollen ends of axons (*arrow*) are seen as large darkly-staining round masses surrounded by paler areas. × 300.

Fig. 21.100 A proteinaceous exudate (*arrow*) in the inner nuclear and the outer plexiform layers; lipid-laden macrophages are prominent. × 300.

phages may take several months (Fig. 21.100). The hard exudate is therefore a clinical manifestation of retinal ischaemia. Another feature is the so-called *soft exudate* which is an ill-defined small white area resembling cotton wool in the inner retina. On histological examination, the cotton wool spot is seen as micro-infarction of the nerve fibre and ganglion-cell layers of the retina. The damaged segment becomes oedematous and contains the swollen ends of disrupted axons (*cytoid bodies*) (Fig. 21.101). Acute focal ischaemia in the retina is most commonly caused by angiospastic arteriolar disease and is a feature of malignant hypertension. When arteriolar disease is so severe that it leads to haemorrhage, the blood tracks within the nerve fibre layer to produce the flame-shaped haemorrhages seen on opthalmoscopy. Accumulation of blood in the outer plexiform layer is due to rupture of capillaries and so-called blot haemorrhages are observed.

Haemorrhages are most prominent when venous outflow is impaired by thrombotic occlusion of the central retinal vein. The visual consequences of venous occlusion are less serious than those of arterial occlusion, because dilatation of collateral venous channels relieves the pressure in the retinal venous system. Retinal oedema often persists and cystic degeneration, particularly in the region of the macula, leads to loss of central vision (Fig. 21.102).

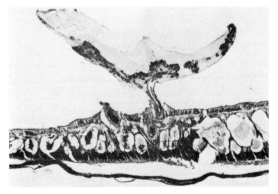

Fig. 21.102 The retina in ischaemic vascular disease due to central retinal vein occlusion. A tree-like growth of blood vessels extends into the vitreous and there is advanced cystic degeneration in the macula. × 40.

One of the important responses to retinal is-chaemia is vasoproliferation from the blood vessels around the ischaemic area. Although this process is potentially beneficial within the retina, the delicate newly-formed vessels penetrate into the vitreous where they are a common source of haemorrhage: contraction of fibrovascular scar tissue ensues and may lead to retinal detachment. It has been suggested that the ischaemic retina produces a *'vaso-proliferative factor'* which is responsible for the fibrovascular proliferation on the anterior surface of the iris with consequent occlusion of the iridocorneal angle and obstruction of aqueous outflow (*secondary closed angle glaucoma* or *neovascular glaucoma*).

The pathological processes described above are exemplified in **diabetic retinopathy** which is an important cause of blindness in diabetes. It is an insidious focal ischaemic arteriolar disease complicated by basement membrane thickening and pericyte degeneration in the capillary walls.

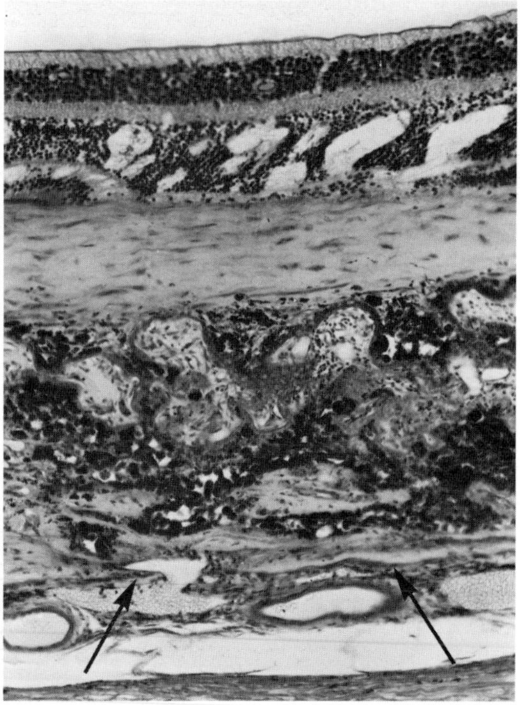

Fig. 21.103 Senile macular degeneration, in which there is a sub-macular mass formed by fibrovascular tissue and proliferating pigment epithelium. Bruch's membrane (*arrows*) is penetrated by a vessel from the choroid. × 100.

The formation of micro-aneurysms in the weakened capillaries is an important feature of diabetes although the same process also occurs in other forms of vascular insufficiency.

Senile macular degeneration. In elderly patients, degeneration of Bruch's membrane in the macular area can result in sub-retinal neo-vascularisation and haemorrhage. The pigment epithelium proliferates and contributes to the submacular fibrous mass (Fig. 21.103). The overlying photoreceptors degenerate and loss of central vision is a serious consequence of this disease.

Retinal detachment. Vascular insufficiency is considered to be an important factor in atrophic degenerative disease in the peripheral retina where microcyst formation and ischaemic chorioretinal scars are often observed. Vitreous traction causes tears in the weakened retina; fluid passes from the vitreous into the subretinal space and this leads to progressive retinal detachment and loss of the visual field.

Glaucoma

Glaucoma is a generic name for a group of diseases in which the intra-ocular pressure increases to a level which impairs the vascular perfusion of the neural tissue and causes blindness. The rise in pressure is usually due to obstruction to the outflow of aqueous, which occurs either as the result of angle closure or as an abnormality in the outflow system.

Closed-angle glaucoma. This may be *primary* or *secondary*. The *primary form* occurs in middle-aged and old people who have a narrow iridocorneal angle and a shallow anterior chamber. In such individuals the iris and lens may come into contact and this interferes with the flow of aqueous through the pupil: pressure builds up behind the iris, which becomes bowed anteriorly and causes further occlusion of the angle. This form of glaucoma is of acute onset, with ocular congestion, corneal oedema and pain.

Narrowness of the iridocorneal angle is attributed to normal variation, and to ageing, which leads to shrinkage of the eye and enlargement of the lens (Fig. 21.104).

Secondary closed-angle glaucoma has many causes, but in enucleated eyes the most common is neovascularisation which 'zips up' crease in intra-ocular pressure leads to an isch-aemic sectorial destruction of the nerve fibres in the optic disc (Fig. 21.105) and this is manifest as a central-field defect which has a characteristic arcuate shape. By light micro-scopy the outflow system in the early stages appears normal, but examination by electron microscopy has shown an accumulation of abnormal collagen in the trabeculae (which narrows the intertrabecular spaces) and in the extracellular spaces of the outer part of the tra-becular meshwork, this increases resistance in the outflow system.

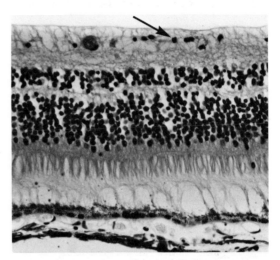

Fig. 21.105 The retina in glaucoma. The nerve fibre layer is atrophic and the ganglion cells are replaced by microglial cells (*arrow*).· (Compare with normal retina, Fig. 21.96.) × 240.

In *secondary open-angle glaucoma*, the out-flow system is obstructed mechanically by exo-genous material, either particulate ·or cellular. In acute or chronic inflammatory disease, in-flammatory cells accumulate within the inter-trabecular spaces, while obstruction by macro-phages occurs after haemorrhage or traumatic release of lens substance into the anterior chamber. The outflow system can also be ob-structed by tumour cell infiltration, e.g. by a primary malignant melanoma of the iris or ciliary body.

The effects of increased intra-ocular pressure

The most serious effects on visual function are due to ischaemic atrophy of the axons in the

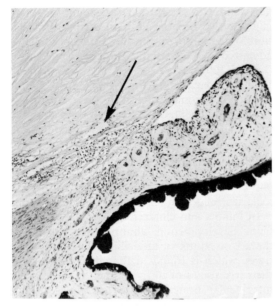

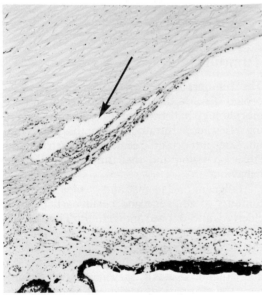

Fig. 21.104 The chamber angle in closed-angle glaucoma (*above*) and open-angle glaucoma (*below*). Note the secondary hyalinisation in closed-angle glaucoma and the preservation of the intertrabecu-lar spaces in open-angle glaucoma. The canal of Schlemm is indicated by arrows. × 75.

the chamber angle (Fig. 21.96): this often com-plicates trauma and inflammatory disease (Fig. 21.104).

Open-angle glaucoma is an insidious disease of the elderly in which a slowly progressive in-

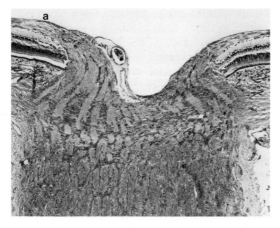

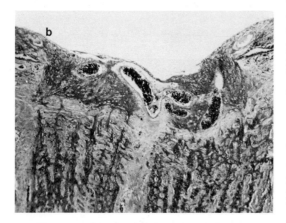

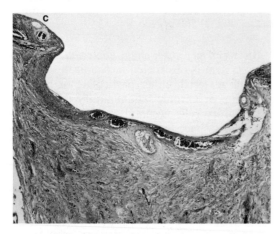

Fig. 21.106   a The normal optic disc: **b** the disc in early glaucoma, showing atrophy of the neural tissue: **c** the disc in advanced glaucoma in which the neural tissue is absent and the lamina cribrosa is bowed posteriorly. × 30.

nerve fibres of the disc and secondary atrophy in the nerve fibre layer of the retina. Excavation or cupping of the disc may become so advanced that it extends into the optic nerve (Fig. 21.106).

The corneal endothelium maintains dehydration of the stroma which is necessary for transparency of the tissue. At high pressure, the cornea becomes oedematous and the epithelium separates (*bullous keratopathy*). At an advanced stage, the uveal tissues become atrophic and fibrosis occurs in ischaemic areas of the iris and choroid; the scleral tissues may stretch to form localised bulges or *staphylomas*.

In infants and children, glaucoma can result from developmental abnormalities in which there is a failure in modelling of the primitive tissue which is found in the chamber angle in the early stages of intra-uterine life. Increasing intra-ocular pressure causes the malleable infantile eye to expand uniformly, and it may become so large that it resembles an ox-eye (*'buphthalmos'*).

Tumours

The tumours of the eyelid, conjunctiva and orbital tissues do not differ significantly in morphology and behaviour from those occurring elsewhere. Intra-ocular tumours are rare, but are important because of their serious effect on vision and their unusual patterns of behaviour.

Malignant melanoma and **benign naevi** are tumours of adult life and occur particularly in elderly white-skinned individuals. They are derived from the spindle-shaped melanocytes of the uveal tract. **Benign naevi** are common and clinically unimportant, but there is some evidence that occasionally they may undergo malignant transformation. **Malignant melanomas** are unilateral and solitary and are most commonly situated in the posterior choroid. The tumour expands the choroid, penetrates Bruch's membrane and initially adopts a characteristic collar-stud shape: alternatively it becomes ovoid (Fig. 21.107). Plasma leaks from the tumour, and from the choroid, into the subretinal space and causes secondary retinal detachment which is often so extensive that visual loss is out of proportion to the size of the tumour. Microscopically the tumour cells are either spindle-shaped (Fig. 21.107) or round

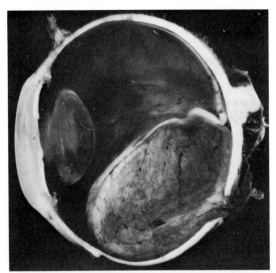

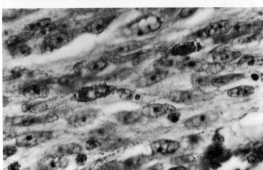

Fig. 21.107 Malignant melanoma of the choroid. *Above*, the gross appearances: the tumour has extended through the sclera. × 2·5. *Below*, microscopy shows this to be an example of the spindle-cell type of tumour. × 525.

(epithelioid). Epithelioid tumours have a much worse prognosis than mainly spindle-cell tumours, which carry a 60 per cent 15-year-survival rate. Growth within the eye leads to disorganisation and often to secondary glaucoma, while extension usually takes place through the intrascleral nerve channels. The choroidal and vortex veins are commonly invaded with consequent blood spread and distant metastasis, especially in the liver. This tumour is notorious for producing multiple rapidly-enlarging liver metastases as long as 20 (symptom-free) years after enucleation of the affected eye (the big liver and glass-eye syndrome). What happens to the tumour cells in the latent interval is a matter for speculation, but current theories invoke an immunological suppression of viable metastases.

Retinoblastoma. This is a tumour of infancy, the incidence of which is gradually rising and is now 1 in 20 000 live births in this country. Six per cent of the cases are familial and the genetic transmission is considered to be an autosomal dominant with poor penetration, although there is also an association with the D chromosome deletion syndrome in a few cases. In approximately half of the patients, the tumour is bilateral and multifocal within the retina.

On gross examination, the retinoblastoma forms a solid pale-grey, partially calcified and partially necrotic mass within the retina. When the tumour fills the vitreous or detaches the retina, a white mass is seen behind the lens, so that reflected light produces a reflex similar to that in the cat's eye. Blindness in the affected eye causes the child to squint. The tumour is

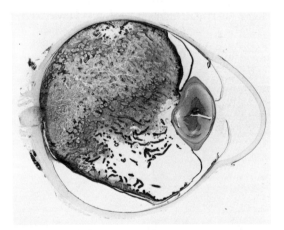

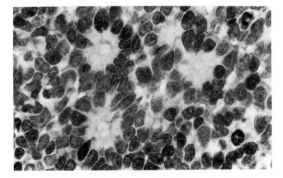

Fig. 21.108 Extensive growth of retinoblastoma within the posterior part of the eye (*above*). × 2·5. The microscopic features include the typical rosettes (*below*). × 525.

composed of small round or oval cells with scanty cytoplasm and a high rate of mitosis. A tendency to differentiation is seen in the formation of 'rosettes', which are circular arrangements of the tumour cells (Fig. 21.108). Extraocular extension occurs either by spread along the optic nerve into the brain or through the sclera into the orbit. Metastases to visceral organs are a late and unusual event. With early enucleation of the eye or radiotherapy, the survival rate is of the order of 90 per cent.

Glioma of the optic nerve occurs in children and adults. In children, proliferation of glial cells within the optic nerve causes proptosis and papilloedema when the nerve becomes thickened and vascular perfusion in the disc is disturbed. Nevertheless nerve conduction survives and tumour growth declines, so that some authorities consider childhood gliomas to be hamartomatous lesions. By contrast, the adult glioma resembles the glioblastoma multiforme (p. 785) in its morphology and behaviour.

References and Further Reading

Blackwood, W. and Corsellis, J. A. N. (Eds.) (1976). *Greenfield's Neuropathology*, 3rd edn., pp. 946. Edward Arnold, London.

Henle, G. *et al.* (1975). Multiple sclerosis-associated agent: neutralization of the agent by human sera. *Infection and Immunity* **12**, 1367–74.

Hume Adams, J., Graham, D. I. and Doyle, David (1981). *Brain Biopsy. The Smear Technique for Neurosurgical Biopsies*. In the Biopsy Pathology Series. Chapman and Hall, London.

Russell, D. S. and Rubinstein, L. J. (Eds.) (1977). *Pathology of Tumours of the Nervous system*, 4th edn., pp. 456. Edward Arnold, London.

Stuart, A. E., Smith, A. N. and Samuel, E. (Eds.) (1975). *Applied Surgical Pathology*, Chapter 18. Blackwell Scientific, Oxford and London.

22

Urinary System

The Kidneys

Fine structure and function

The kidneys are each composed of about one million nephrons, the major functions of which are to remove from the plasma various waste products of metabolism, and to maintain fluid and acid–base balances and normal levels of electrolytes. This is achieved by production of a very large volume of glomerular filtrate, which is subject to selective reabsorption as it passes down the tubules, urine representing what must be discarded for homoeostasis. Compared with most other organs, the blood flow of the kidneys is enormous; nearly all of this passes through the glomeruli, where 22 per cent of the plasma volume (550 ml/min; 800 litres/day) is filtered off, giving a glomerular filtration rate (GFR) of 180 litres per day (120 ml/min). The process of filtration is aided by the unusually high pressure in the **glomerular capillaries** which is due to their unique position between two arterioles. The capillary walls (Fig. 22.1) consist of the vascular endothelium, which is unusual in having cytoplasmic *fenestrations* where the capillary basement membrane is lined only by an extremely thin endothelial membrane. Outside the basement membrane is a layer of visceral *epithelial cells* or *podocytes*, which make contact with the basement membrane by means of cytoplasmic processes—*foot processes* or *pedicels*. In the spaces (*slit pores*) between the foot processes the epithelial lining (*slit membrane*) is also extremely thin. Each glomerulus is composed of several lobules, the structure of which is depicted in Fig. 22.2. The capillary loops lie at the periphery of the lobules, while the core is made up of mesangial cells and basement membrane-like material. *The mesangial cells* have a number of functions:

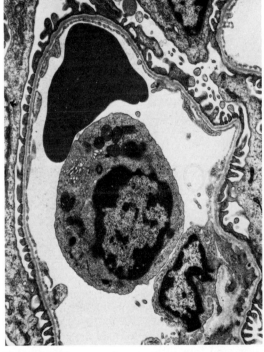

Fig. 22.1 Electron micrograph of glomerular capillary containing a lymphocyte and red cell. Note, from within outwards, the endothelial cytoplasm with fenestrations, the continuous basement membrane, and the foot processes of the epithelium. × 12 000.

they have a structural supportive role, contain smooth muscle fibrils and are contractile and phagocytic. They may also remove from the subendothelial space any macromolecular material which passes through the endothelial fenestrae and transport it to the glomerular hilus and hence to the proximal tubule.

In its passage along the tubules, all but ap-

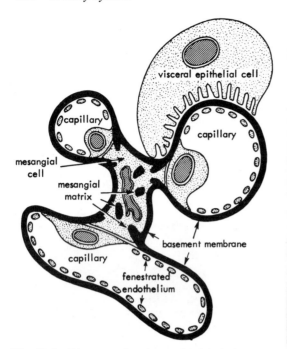

Fig. 22.2 Diagram of a glomerular lobule in cross section.

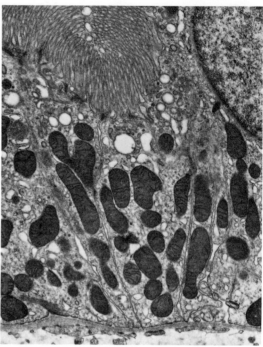

Fig. 22.3 Electron micrograph of parts of two epithelial cells of the proximal convoluted tubule, showing the microvilli (*upper left*) and numerous mitochondria. The basal part of the epithelium rests on a thin basement membrane. × 11 000.

proximately 1·5 litres of the daily 180 litres of glomerular filtrate, and most of its contained solutes, are reabsorbed. This is a process in which the tubule cells exhibit a high degree of selectivity, and some of the fine structural features of the epithelial cells can be related to their special functions. The epithelial cells of the **proximal convoluted tubule** have a prominent brush border, which is seen by electron microscopy to consist of numerous fine, relatively long microvilli (Fig. 22.3): this feature provides a very large surface area for absorption, and four fifths of the fluid in the glomerular filtrate, together with most of its contained glucose, amino acids, and much of its sodium, potassium and phosphate are reabsorbed here. Reabsorption of these solutes is an active process, requiring energy and this may account for the large number of mitochondria in the epithelial cells. A third feature of these cells is the presence of pinocytotic vesicles, which form on the luminal surface of the cells between the bases of the microvilli: there is normally some leakage of plasma proteins into the glomerular filtrate, and this is apparently taken up into these by pinocytosis and presumably metabolised by lysosomal enzymes. When, owing

to various glomerular lesions, there is increased leakage of protein into the glomerular filtrate, the cells of the proximal tubules come to contain protein-rich droplets—*hyaline droplets* (Fig. 22.25, p. 824)—due to excessive protein absorption. Finally, the plasma membrane of the basal surface of the cells of the proximal convoluted tubule shows complicated infoldings which have the effect of increasing the surface area, and are probably important in the passage of reabsorbed fluid into the interstitial tissue, whence it enters the peritubular capillaries.

The cells of the **descending limb of Henle's loop**, and of the thin part of the ascending limb, are relatively simple, and their role in reabsorption is probably largely passive, and dependent on the constitutions of the tubular and interstitial fluids. By contrast, the cells of the **thick part of the ascending limb** have abundant large mitochondria (Fig. 22.4), and it is probable that these cells actively remove sodium chloride from the tubular fluid and pass it into the interstitial fluid. This has two effects; firstly, it

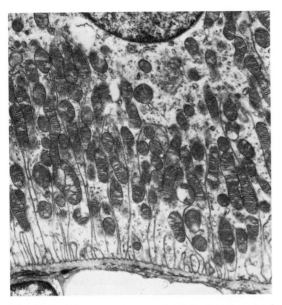

Fig. 22.4 Electron micrograph of the basal part of an epithelial cell of the thick part of Henle's loop. Note large enlongated mitochondria situated between the complex infoldings of the basal cytoplasmic membrane. Portion of cell nucleus at top of picture. × 10 000.

provides a hypertonic interstitial fluid in the renal medulla, and this allows passive reabsorption of water from the descending and thin ascending parts of Henle's limb; secondly, it renders the tubular fluid hypotonic and facilitates further concentration in the distal convoluted tubule. It is probable that *aldosterone* exerts its sodium-retaining effect by stimulating reabsorption of Na^+ by the cells of the thick part of the ascending limb of Henle's loop. There is evidence that, like sodium chloride, urea undergoes partial recirculation in this counter-current system, thus aiding in passive reabsorption of water. This ingenious concentrating mechanism was suggested by Wirz (see Black, 1967) and has since received increasing support. The cells of the thick part of Henle's loop, and of the **distal convoluted tubule**, contain numerous microvesicles, and these may be related to their important functions of deaminating amino acids to produce ammonia, and of providing free hydrogen ion: secretion of NH_4^+ into the lumen by these cells plays an important role in maintaining acid–base balance, and results in an acid urine. Fluid entering the distal convoluted tubule is hypotonic, and isotonicity is restored here by passive

reabsorption of water. As the fluid passes through the medulla in the collecting tubules, passive reabsorption of more water is again possible because the concentrations of sodium chloride and urea in the medullary interstitial fluid are high (see above). It is probable that these final adjustments in concentration are mediated largely by *antidiuretic hormone*, which presumably renders the cells of the distal convoluted and collecting tubules more permeable to water.

In addition to these complex tubular functions, there is evidence that some substances are removed from the blood and actively secreted by the tubular epithelium. For example, creatinine and K^+ are reabsorbed in the proximal convoluted tubule, and the amounts appearing in the urine are dependent largely on their secretion, probably by the cells of the thick part of the ascending limb of Henle's loop and of the distal convoluted tubule. Excretion of administered diodone by the kidneys is dependent mainly on tubular secretion, and it may be used to assess tubular function.

In addition to their homoeostatic and excretory roles, the kidneys secrete renin, an enzyme which acts on a substrate in the plasma to produce angiotensin. The site of renin secretion is located in the granular cells of the afferent glomerular arterioles, which, together with the macula densa and lacis cells, constitute the **juxtaglomerular apparatus** (Fig. 9.34, p. 258). Angiotensin has a direct effect on peripheral vascular resistance, and hence on blood pressure, and also stimulates the secretion of aldosterone by the adrenal cortex. These phenomena, and the fine structure of the juxtaglomerular apparatus, are described on pp. 258–9.

Another function of the kidneys is the production of **erythropoietin**, a factor stimulating the production of red cells.

Renal clearances. The renal clearance of a substance is an estimation of the volume of plasma completely cleared of that substance by the kidneys in one minute. It is calculated by measuring its concentration in the plasma (P,). in the urine (U), and the volume of the urine (V) in ml per minute, and applying the formula

$$Clearance = \frac{U \times V}{P} ml$$

In the case of a substance which passes freely into the glomerular filtrate, and which is neither reabsorbed nor secreted by the tubules, renal clearance is a measure of glomerular filtration rate. This is approximately the case for inulin, which may be administered for the purpose of measuring the renal clearance. Of endogenous substances, clearance of urea is commonly measured, but 30–50 per cent of the urea in the glomerular filtrate is normally reabsorbed, and accordingly the renal urea clearance (approx. 70 ml) is appreciably below that of inulin (approx. 120 ml). The clearance of creatinine is similar to that of inulin, but this results from a combination of reabsorption by the proximal tubule and secretion by the distal tubule, and is therefore not always a true indication of glomerular filtration rate in pathological states of the kidney.

Heterogeneity of nephrons. It has long been known that individual nephrons show morphological and circulatory differences—for example, in the length of Henle's loop. Thurau and his colleagues (see Horster and Thurau, 1968) have shown important functional differences between the majority of nephrons and the one-fifth of nephrons originating in glomeruli close to the cortico-medullary junction. By micropuncture of individual tubules, they showed differences in glomerular filtration rates, and differences in responses to low and high sodium loading. These findings, based on work on rat kidneys, are likely to apply to the kidneys of other mammals, including man, in which case they will necessitate a reconsideration of various aspects of renal function, both normal and in pathological states, since our present views are based largely on the assumption of a functionally homogeneous population of nephrons.

Pathophysiology of renal disease

Many of the diseases described in this chapter result in disturbances of renal function, and these are considered in more detail later. The four major disturbances which are responsible for most of the clinical features of renal diseases are as follows.

(1) Impairment of blood flow through the kidneys can result in **arterial hypertension** (**secondary** or **renal hypertension**): this is encountered commonly in glomerular disease, but can result from extensive renal scarring from various causes, and also from an extra-renal lesion, e.g. narrowing of the main renal artery by an atheromatous patch in the aorta.

(2) **Renal failure ('uraemia')** with accumulation in the body of urea and other nitrogenous waste products and disturbances of water and acid–base balances and of electrolyte levels, can result from *a reduced glomerular filtration rate*, from tubular injury, or from a combination of both. *Since lesions which impair renal blood flow reduce the glomerular filtration rate, it is not surprising that renal failure and hypertension are commonly associated.*

(3) There are a number of diseases which injure the glomerular capillaries and render them abnormally permeable to plasma proteins; heavy and prolonged albuminuria results in fall of the level of plasma albumin, and this can set in motion a train of events leading to generalised oedema. *The combination of proteinuria, hypoalbuminaemia and oedema is known as the* **nephrotic syndrome**.

(4) Glomerular injury can result in the escape of red cells which appear in the urine either in small numbers or sufficient to discolour it. *When there is widespread glomerular inflammation, as in some forms of glomerulonephritis, such haematuria is accompanied by hypertension and oliguria, a combination known as the* **nephritic syndrome**.

Urinary casts. Increased leakage of plasma proteins into the glomerular filtrate results in proteinuria, most of the escaping protein being albumin. This is accompanied by the formation in the distal tubules of solid, cylindrical-shaped bodies, termed casts (Fig. 22.5), *the presence of which in the urine indicates that the proteinuria is attributable to a renal lesion.* When the proteinuria is unaccompanied by escape of cells in the urine, the casts are transparent and are termed *hyaline, colloid* or *protein* casts. Their solid component consists largely of a protein—*Tamm–Horsfall protein*—which is probably secreted normally by the epithelium of the distal convoluted tubule and is precipitated to form casts by the presence of plasma albumin in the tubular fluid. When proteinuria is accompanied by escape of inflammatory cells into the tubular fluid, or desquamation of tubular epithelial cells, these become incorporated into the casts, giving *cellular casts* when the cells are largely intact and *granular casts* when the cells are disrupted. Similarly *blood casts* result from incorporation of red cells escaping into the glo-

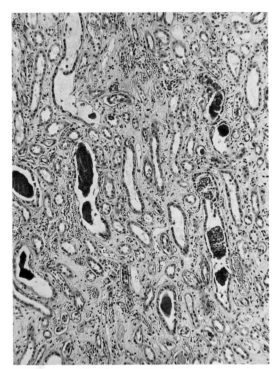

Fig. 22.5 Casts in the distal and collecting tubules. × 90.

merular filtrate or tubule, and *pigmented casts* from incorporation of bilirubin when protein-uria accompanies obstructive jaundice, or haemoglobin or myoglobin in conditions giving rise to haemolysis or breakdown of skeletal muscle respectively.

Renal changes in hypertension

The general features of hypertension and the associated vascular changes, namely arterio-sclerosis and arteriolosclerosis, have already been described (pp. 371–4). The latter are usu-ally more pronounced in the blood vessels of the kidneys than in other organs, and result in various grades of renal injury. In chronic ('benign') essential hypertension, the renal injury is generally slight, and renal failure does not usually occur, but quite commonly there is some scarring of the kidneys. By contrast, the renal vascular lesions in malignant (accele-rated) essential hypertension are severe, and renal failure is a common termination unless the blood pressure can be reduced.

Chronic glomerulonephritis and certain other chronic diseases of the kidneys can result in persistent secondary hypertension (see above) and when this occurs further renal injury ensues, indistinguishable from that seen in benign or malignant essential (i.e. primary) hypertension. A complex picture results, and it is advantageous to consider first the pure lesions of essential hypertension before pro-ceeding to the pathology of the various renal diseases which are complicated by secondary hypertension.

Chronic ('benign') essential hypertension

Pathological changes. The renal changes in this disease are attributable to ischaemia result-ing from arteriosclerosis and arteriolosclerosis (pp. 371–4).

The larger arteries in the kidneys, as else-where, become rigid and thickened, but their lumina are not seriously reduced, and may be enlarged. Similar changes occur in the arcuate arteries, but owing to their smaller calibre, thick-ening of the wall may result in reduction of the lumen: this is not uniform, and since the arcuates are, in effect, end arteries, ischaemia of patches of cortical tissue, seen as coarse depressed scars, may result. More commonly, ischaemia results from changes in the smaller vessels: the interlobular arteries become elon-gated and tortuous, with medial fibrosis and fibro-elastic thickening of the intima resulting in significant narrowing of the lumen. The af-ferent glomerular arterioles are also tortuous and show patchy hyaline thickening, the wall being acellular, homogeneous, eosinophilic, rather refractile and with various degrees of luminal narrowing (Figs. 22.6 and 14.17, p. 373). Regarding the nature of hyaline arteriolar thickening, Lendrum (1969) has shown that at an early stage the hyaline material has the staining reactions of fibrin, and that as it ages the staining reactions come to resemble those of collagen. He has suggested that increased permeability of the vascular endothelium allows exudation of plasma constituents and that these form the hyaline material. He has termed the process *plasmatic vasculosis* and the older hyaline material *pseudocollagen*. This interpretation is now supported by histo-chemical, immunofluorescence, and electron microscopic studies, and provides a satisfactory explanation of the observed changes. These

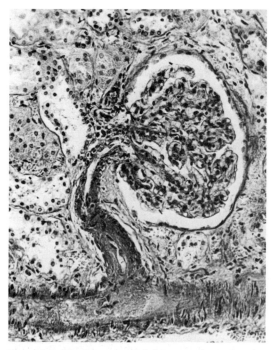

Fig. 22.6 Benign essential hypertension, showing great hyaline thickening of an afferent arteriole. × 180.

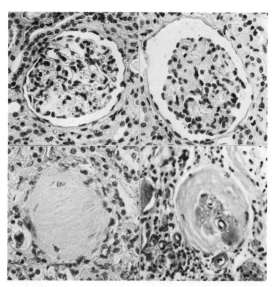

Fig. 22.7 Ischaemic changes in the glomeruli in chronic essential hypertension. The two glomeruli above show partial hyalinisation. The lower left is completely hyalinised and the lower right is collapsed, extensively hyalinised, and encased in fibrous tissue which has formed inside Bowman's capsule. Note its hyalinised afferent arteriole (seen below, containing a leukocyte). × 160.

changes result in glomerular ischaemia, the glomerular tuft becoming shrunken and the capillaries gradually replaced by pale-staining homogeneous material, also believed to result from plasmatic vasculosis: eventually the whole tuft is converted to an acellular hyaline sphere (Fig. 22.7). This change is often accompanied by obliteration of the capsular space. The related tubules become atrophic and inconspicuous, and fibrous tissue, often infiltrated by lymphocytes, develops between the affected tubules and glomeruli. These changes in the small vessels, and consequent loss of nephrons and scarring, are distributed randomly throughout the cortex of both kidneys. It is probable that the arteriolar changes are more important than those in the interlobular arteries, for the ischaemic changes do not follow a lobular pattern, but affect single scattered nephrons, while those around may appear healthy.

The destruction of nephrons described above proceeds very slowly, and at necropsy the kidneys may appear macroscopically normal apart from thickening of the arteries on the cut surface. However, enough nephrons are commonly lost to cause a slight or moderate reduc-tion in size and diffuse thinning of the cortex: the capsule may be somewhat adherent, and the subcapsular surface diffusely and finely irregular (*granular*), contraction of scarred areas resulting in fine depressions (Fig. 22.8). In some long-standing cases, a sufficient number of nephrons may be lost to stimulate hypertrophy in those remaining, and the enlarged, hypertrophied tubules then contribute to the surface granularity (Fig. 22.9), but *the kidneys are seldom very small, and renal function is not significantly impaired*. In those patients who develop heart failure, the blood urea often rises, but this is attributable to inadequate renal blood flow, and is reversible if cardiac output again improves.

Malignant (accelerated) essential hypertension

This may arise *de novo*, usually at 35–45 years of age, or may supervene on benign essential hypertension. In the former case, the kidneys are of normal size, and the subcapsular surface is smooth and spotted with dark red areas due to patches of congestion and haemorrhage. The main renal, segmental and arcuate arteries

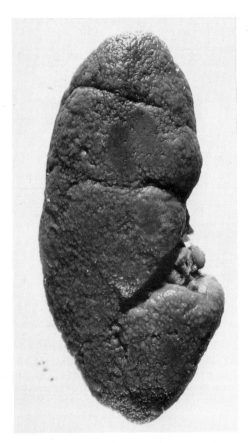

Fig. 22.8 Kidney in longstanding benign essential hypertension, showing slight reduction in size and granularity of the subcapsular surface. × 1.

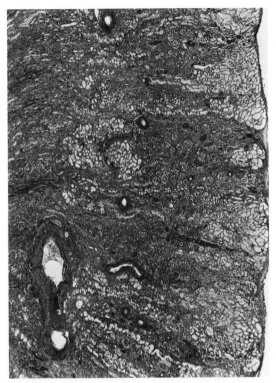

Fig. 22.9 Kidney in benign essential hypertension, showing foci of fine cortical scarring, with enlargement of the tubules in the unaffected cortical areas. Note also the arterial thickening. × 12·5.

show the usual arteriosclerotic changes of hypertension. The interlobular arteries display great intimal thickening, due to formation of fine concentric layers of connective tissue and smooth muscle cells, with very severe reduction of the lumen (Fig. 22.10). They may also show fibrinoid necrosis of the wall, especially at their distal end. The afferent arterioles show fibrinoid necrosis, the wall being thickened, brightly eosinophilic, granular or homogeneous, and containing few or no living cells, but often pyknotic nuclei and red cells (Fig. 22.11): the necrotic material gives the staining reactions of fibrin, and the lumen is often completely obliterated, or occupied by thrombus which merges with the necrotic wall. The conspicuous fibrinoid necrosis may extend into the glomerulus, where it may involve parts or all of the tuft. Other glomeruli are less severely damaged, and

show intense capillary dilatation and congestion. There is often blood or exudate in the capsular space, and occasionally proliferation of the capsular epithelium to form a crescent (p. 822). The glomerular changes are the direct result of acute ischaemia resulting from fibrinoid necrosis of the afferent arterioles: this affects one arteriole after another, and *in untreated patients progresses to renal failure unless death results from cerebral haemorrhage or heart failure.* Even when death has resulted from renal failure, some afferent arterioles are still unaffected and their corresponding glomeruli show little or no change. Some tubules show atrophy, particularly of the proximal convoluted regions; others are of normal size or enlarged and hyaline droplets (p. 806) are conspicuous in the epithelial lining. Eosinophilic casts and sometimes red cells are seen throughout the length of some of the tubules.

Where malignant hypertension has supervened on benign essential hypertension, the

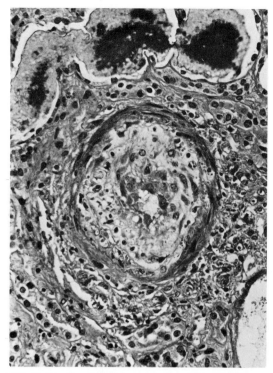

Fig. 22.10 Interlobular artery in malignant hypertension, showing gross intimal fibro-cellular thickening. × 100.

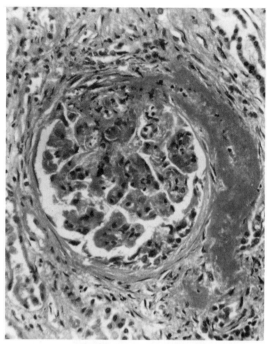

Fig. 22.11 Malignant hypertension. Fibrinoid necrosis of an afferent arteriole and of most of the glomerular tuft. Note also the aggregation of cells in the capsular space (*lower right*) to form a small crescent. × 180.

changes corresponding to both conditions are seen in the kidneys. In recent years, the rapid downhill course of many patients with malignant hypertension has been arrested by antihypertensive drugs. Maintenance of the blood pressure below the very high levels of malignant hypertension prevents the severe lesions of the interlobular arteries, fibrinoid necrosis of the afferent arterioles, and the consequent rapid destruction of nephrons. Accordingly the prognosis has improved, particularly if treatment is begun before there is extensive renal damage. This suggests that fibrinoid necrosis of the arterioles is attributable to severe hypertension, and this is supported by various experimental observations; for example, partial clamping of one renal artery prevents fibrinoid necrosis in the clamped kidney in animals with severe hypertension (p. 375).

The vascular changes of malignant hypertension occur also in the other viscera, although the effect is not usually so devastating as in the kidneys: an example of a lesion in the intestine is illustrated in Fig. 14.18, p. 374.

Secondary hypertension

As already indicated, the vascular changes and consequent renal injury observed in essential hypertension occur also in hypertension secondary to other conditions. Various grades of persistent hypertension result from certain renal diseases, and depending on the height of the blood pressure and the rate of rise, the renal changes described above for benign or malignant essential hypertension become superadded to those of the renal disease which has caused the hypertension. Such secondary hypertensive lesions are an important factor in hastening failure of the already damaged kidneys.

Other vascular diseases

Senile arteriosclerosis. Although arteriosclerosis and arteriolosclerosis, and their associated renal changes, are seen particularly in hypertensives, they occur also in some normotensive old people, and the kidneys present the same features as in benign essential hypertension.

Here also, the changes do not seriously impair renal function.

Atheroma occurs in the main renal arteries and their segmental branches, but is much less common than in other arteries of comparable size. Except in diabetes mellitus, it is rarely severe enough to interfere with the renal circulation: superadded occlusion by thrombosis is also rare. Disturbances arise more commonly from involvement and narrowing of the origins of one or rarely both renal arteries by aortic atheromatous plaques. This can lead to hypertension. presumably from ischaemia of one or both kidneys. Compared with essential hypertension, this is a rarity, but it is important to diagnose, for in some cases relief of the stenosis by a bypass operation, or removal of the ischaemic kidney, has resulted in cure of the hypertension. Such cases require careful investigation, including bilateral renal biopsy, for the non-ischaemic kidney may be damaged by hypertension or concomitant disease, e.g. pyelonephritis, and removal of the ischaemic kidney may then do more harm than good. The mechanism of hypertension in renal artery stenosis is discussed on p. 259.

Fibromuscular dysplasia of the renal arteries. This term includes several distinct abnormalities of the main renal arteries, affecting mostly the media, and including irregularities in thickness and in arrangement of the smooth muscle fibres and irregular fibrosis. The changes are rare, and occur predominantly in women over a wide age range. They can give rise to renal artery stenosis or to dissecting or true aneurysms; we have observed a case in which an aneurysm of 3 cm. diameter compressed the renal pelvis and resulted in hydronephrosis.

The renal changes in *diabetes mellitus* are described on p. 840, and those of *polyarteritis nodosa* on p. 832.

Glomerulonephritis

The term glomerulonephritis embraces a group of diseases in which the renal lesions are primarily glomerular, other changes in the kidneys resulting from the glomerular injury. Lesions due to infection of the kidneys (pyelonephritis) are not included in the group, and although no type of glomerulonephritis is fully understood, there is now very strong evidence that most types are due to injury caused by antigen–antibody complexes deposited in the walls of the glomerular capillaries. Much of this evidence is based on work with animals, and some of the more important experimental findings will be described before turning to human glomerulonephritis.

Experimental immunological glomerular injury

This is of two main types, one due to deposition of antigen–antibody complexes in the glomerular capillary walls (immune-complex glomerulonephritis), the other to the reaction of antibody with the glomerular capillary basement membrane (nephrotoxic-antibody glomerulonephritis).

Immune-complex glomerulonephritis

A basic knowledge of the features of immune-complex disease (pp. 152–6) is necessary to the understanding of the following account, which concentrates on the nature and pathogenesis of the glomerular lesions of experimental immune-complex disease.

When a single large injection of a suitable antigen is administered to an animal (e.g. bovine serum albumin to rabbits), antibody appears after a week or so and reacts with antigen still present in the plasma to form immune complexes. At first these are formed in gross antigen excess and consist of only 2–4 molecules: such small complexes remain in the circulation and do not appear to cause glomerular lesions. As antibody production increases, larger complexes are formed until, at antigen–antibody equivalence, the complexes form large insoluble aggregates (Fig. 5.6, p. 110) which are rapidly removed from the circulation by phagocytes and are not deposited in the walls of vessels. Between these two extremes there is a period of a few days during which **complexes of intermediate size** are formed (Fig. 6.7, p. 154):

these are deposited in the walls of blood vessels, especially the glomerular capillaries, where they induce lesions. In chronic immune-complex disease, in which multiple injections of antigen are administered at frequent, e.g. daily, intervals, chronic glomerular injury results in those animals in which the antibody levels and amounts of antigen injected are such that there is intermittent or continuous formation of intermediate-sized immune complexes in antigen excess over a long period.

The mechanism of immune-complex deposition has not been fully elucidated. For complexes to penetrate into the walls of capillaries and other vessels there must be an increase in endothelial permeability: this may be brought about by activation of complement by circulating complexes, with consequent formation of anaphylatoxins (p. 153), or a type I hypersensitivity reaction, mediated in the rabbit via basophils and platelets (p. 155), may be involved.

Why are the glomeruli involved? Not only are the glomeruli an important and sometimes the sole site of deposition of circulating immune complexes, but complexes deposited in this site persist much longer than those deposited elsewhere in the walls of blood vessels. It is likely that the predilection of the glomeruli for deposition is due to (a) the unusually high filtration pressure in glomerular capillaries and high renal blood flow, and (b) the relative thickness of the glomerular capillary basement membrane and its special function of filtering large volumes of plasma fluid. Partial clamping of one renal artery decreases the deposition of immune complexes in the glomeruli of that kidney in the experimental animal, and renal artery stenosis is similarly protective in human immune-complex glomerulonephritis. Susceptibility of the glomeruli is thus an unfortunate consequence of their specialised function of filtering large volumes of fluid.

The types and pathogenesis of glomerular injury. Three major types of glomerular lesion are seen in immune-complex disease. The first is a **diffuse inflammatory lesion** affecting all the glomerular capillaries. It consists of swelling and proliferation of endothelial or mesangial cells and variable infiltration of the capillary walls by polymorphs. It is accompanied by increased permeability of the capillary basement membrane with leakage of plasma proteins and escape of red cells and polymorphs into the uri-

nary space: these abnormal constituents appear in the urine. The second type of lesion is a **focal inflammation**, affecting only parts of some glomeruli. Both types of inflammatory lesion may occur in acute or in chronic immune-complex disease: both vary in severity from mild inflammation to necrosis. The acute diffuse lesion, unless unduly severe, will resolve. The focal lesions tend to result in scarring, as do chronic diffuse lesions. The third type of glomerular injury is termed **membranous change**. It occurs only in chronic immune-complex disease and consists of diffuse thickening of the glomerular capillary basement membrane but without associated inflammatory change. It is accompanied by increased permeability and proteinuria but usually without escape of cells.

Among the many factors which probably influence the nature and severity of the glomerular lesions, Germuth and Rodriguez (1973) have emphasised the importance of the size of the circulating immune complexes and the rate of their deposition in the glomerular capillaries, although the shape and surface charge of the complexes are also of importance. **The acute diffuse inflammatory lesion** develops when relatively small intermediate complexes are present in the plasma in high concentration. Immunofluorescence shows granular or irregular deposits of immune complex distributed diffusely in the capillary walls: at first they are scanty and sometimes even undetectable; later they may become more prominent and persist for some weeks before finally disappearing. Electron microscopy usually shows no more than occasional discrete deposits of immune complex on the epithelial side of the capillary basement membrane. If, as most workers believe, immune complexes are responsible for the acute inflammatory lesion, then it is likely that they are pathogenic when deposited in relatively small amounts in the inner part of the capillary wall, i.e. subendothelially. At this site the products of complement fixation are likely to cause direct injury to the capillary wall and also, by chemotactic activity, to attract polymorphs which phagocytose the complexes but in doing so release lysosomal enzymes and so cause tissue injury. Activation of the coagulation system with deposition of fibrin has also been shown to contribute to the glomerular injury. The small complexes diffuse through the basement membrane and form aggregates which, as noted above, may be visible in electron micrographs, and which account for the granular pattern on immunofluorescence microscopy.

Focal inflammatory lesions appear to result from *diffuse* deposition of relatively large intermediate complexes subendothelially (Fig. 22.12). Such complexes tend to be phagocy-

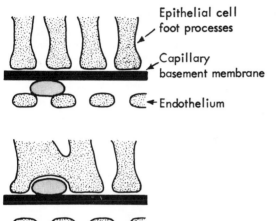

Fig. 22.12 The sites of deposition of immune complexes in the glomerular capillary walls. Larger complexes aggregate on the sub-endothelial side of the basement membrane (*above*). Smaller complexes are deposited on the epithelial side of the basement membrane (*below*).

tosed rapidly and so removed from this site by the mesangial cells and it is only when this clearance mechanism is overwhelmed that capillary lesions appear: failure of a mesangium is thus followed by an inflammatory focus in that lobule. This explanation is supported by the demonstration of immune complexes and complement in the mesangial cells and, when focal lesions are present, also in the adjacent parts of the capillary walls. These sites of complex deposition are confirmed by electron microscopy. Being relatively large, the complexes do not diffuse into the basement membrane. Mesangial-cell hyperplasia may be a prominent feature of the focal inflammatory lesions.

In chronic immune-complex disease, diffuse inflammatory lesions usually occur in those animals in which high plasma concentrations of relatively small complexes are formed. Low concentrations of small complexes are associated with gradual development of the **membranous change**. Immunofluorescence shows

very heavy discrete, 'granular' deposits of immune complexes and complement scattered diffusely along the capillary walls (Fig. 22.13), and electron microscopy shows these deposits to lie in the outer part of the capillary basement membrane (Figs. 22.12, 22.14). This results from prolonged but slow deposition of small complexes. At no time are they present in the inner part of the capillary wall in sufficient concentration to induce inflammatory change. The complexes gradually diffuse through the basement membrane and become arrested in its outer part. Although they appear to activate complement in this site, the activation products are liable to be carried away by the filtrate into the urinary space and thus do not cause inflammatory change.

In summary, the deposition of immune complexes in the glomerular capillary walls may produce focal or diffuse inflammatory lesions, both transient and progressive, and also membranous lesions. These different effects can be explained by the concentration and duration of

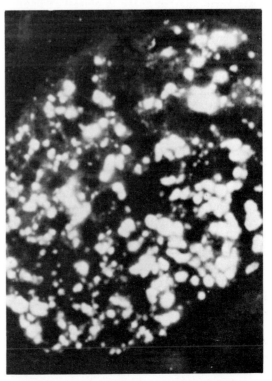

Fig. 22.13 Experimental foreign-protein glomerulonephritis. Irregular deposition of immune complexes in the capillary walls, shown by fluorescent antibody to IgG. (Professor R. Lannigan.)

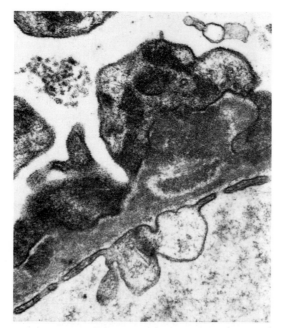

Fig. 22.14   Electron micrograph of segment of glomerular capillary wall in experimental immune complex glomerulonephritis, showing dense nodular deposits in outer part of basement membrane (capillary lumen below; urinary space above). × 25 000.

complexes in the blood, their size and rate of deposition. As will be seen later, the spectrum of human glomerulonephritis resembles that of experimental immune-complex disease, but often the human situation is more complex. For example, in systemic lupus erythematosus (SLE) auto-antibodies develop against DNA and various other cell constituents: accordingly, complexes of various sizes, forming in various antigen–antibody ratios, are likely to be present and to vary from time to time. It is thus not surprising that the glomerular lesions of SLE are complex and varied. A similar complexity of glomerular lesions is observed in the hybrid NZB/NZW mice which develop a disease remarkably like human SLE.

Nephrotoxic antibody nephritis

When a tissue preparation containing glomerular basement membrane (GBM) of one species (e.g. rat) is injected into animals of other species, e.g. duck or rabbit, the hetero-antibody to GBM which develops is capable of causing acute diffuse glomerulonephritis when injected into rats. This was first reported by Lindemann

in 1900 but is usually known as *Masugi-type nephritis*. The antibody becomes bound to the GBM, and is seen as a linear deposit on immunofluorescent staining (Fig. 22.15). Both polymorphs and complement appear to play a pathogenic role, but depletion of both does not completely prevent glomerular injury.

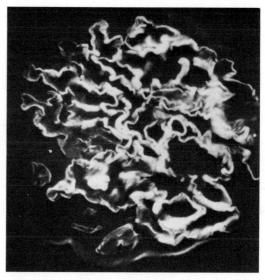

Fig. 22.15   Nephrotoxic-antibody nephritis; linear deposition of nephrotoxic antibody in the glomerular capillary walls, demonstrated by the immunofluorescence technique.

Masugi nephritis is complex, because development, by the test rat, of antibody to the foreign (duck or rabbit) Ig aggravates the renal lesion. The condition has been produced in various species, and has been shown to develop in sheep *actively* immunised by antigen of heterologous (e.g. human) GBM: the antibody reacts with the sheep's own GBM. This is of interest because a rare form of human disease (Goodpasture's syndrome) is now known to be caused by auto-antibody reacting with pulmonary and glomerular basement membrane. Otherwise, Masugi nephritis is worth noting because it demonstrated that glomerulonephritis could result from an immunological reaction.

Glomerulonephritis in man

Classification

The widespread practice of renal biopsy is now providing much information about the histological changes of glomerulonephritis and particularly about the early stages, while immunological studies are providing important aetiological clues. However, there is still much to be learned, and classifications of glomerulonephritis must still be regarded as provisional, in the knowledge that modifications will be necessary in the coming years.

As regards the recognition of different types of glomerulonephritis, a major contribution was made by Volhard and Fahr (1914) and has since formed the basis of most classifications of this group of diseases. More recent classifications by Longcope and by Ellis have proved useful, but are now known to be oversimplifications and have fallen into disuse.

In the classification of glomerulonephritis proposed below, we have selected, from the terms in common usage, those which seem to us to indicate best the major glomerular changes. Commonly used alternatives are given in italics.

It must be emphasised that this classification is not intended to be comprehensive. Moreover, some of the types include more than one disease entity. Certain other conditions, e.g. systemic lupus erythematosus, diabetes mellitus and amyloidosis, can give rise to glomerular lesions resulting in clinical syndromes resembling one or other type of glomerulonephritis, and it seems appropriate to discuss them together with or immediately after glomerulonephritis.

Acute diffuse proliferative glomerulonephritis

Clinical features. This relatively common type of glomerulonephritis occurs at all ages, but particularly in children and young adults. It affects males more often than females and usually follows an acute infection with Group A haemolytic streptococci—most often pharyngitis (including scarlet fever), but sometimes infections of the middle ear or skin. In many cases, the disease develops 1–4 weeks after the onset of the streptococcal infection: very often this has settled down and there is a latent period of apparent well-being before glomerulonephritis becomes apparent.

The presenting features include peri-orbital oedema (the eyelids appearing puffy), malaise, fever, and discoloration of the urine due to altered blood in it. The oedema is most marked in the morning and may involve the rest of the face and other lax tissues. The blood pressure is usually slightly or moderately raised. The demonstration of haematuria microscopically in otherwise well children following a streptococcal sore throat indicates that renal involvement is often subclinical.

Biochemical changes. There is usually a mild or moderate rise in the level of blood urea. The urine is diminished in volume, of high specific gravity, and commonly brownish and turbid ('smoky') from the presence of altered red cells. (The haematuria, together with oliguria and hypertension constitute *the nephritic syndrome*.) There is moderate proteinuria and, as in all types of glomerulonephritis, the protein is mainly plasma albumin. Quantitative analysis reveals that larger protein molecules, e.g. IgG, are also usually present in appreciable amounts and the proteinuria is thus not a highly selective albuminuria. Microscopy of the urine shows many red cells, moderate or large numbers of neutrophil polymorphs, and hyaline, granular or cellular casts (p. 808).

Course of the disease. Ninety-five per cent of children who develop acute diffuse glomerulonephritis recover completely after an illness lasting a week or two. In adults the condition tends to be more severe or persistent and only about 60–70 per cent of patients make a complete and permanent recovery.

CLASSIFICATION OF GLOMERULONEPHRITIS

Acute diffuse proliferative glomerulonephritis

Rapidly progressive glomerulonephritis
(*Crescentic glomerulonephritis*)

Diffuse membranous glomerulonephritis
(*Idiopathic membranous glomerulonephritis: epimembranous nephropathy*)

(*a*) Nephrotic stage
(*b*) Chronic stage

Membranoproliferative glomerulonephritis
(*Mesangiocapillary glomerulonephritis*)

Minimal-change glomerulonephritis
(*Minimal-change nephropathy: lipoid nephrosis; light-negative glomerulonephritis*)

Focal glomerulonephritis

Chronic glomerulonephritis

Some patients die in the acute stage from the effects of hypertension, e.g. acute heart failure, or from acute renal failure. In others the glomerular lesions and clinical features persist and get progressively worse, causing death from hypertension and renal failure within two years: these patients are correctly classified as *rapidly progressive glomerulonephritis* (p. 821). In a small proportion of patients proteinuria persists long after apparent recovery from the acute attack. Proteinuria for several months is consistent with complete recovery but when it continues for over a year, and particularly when there are also some red cells and leukocytes in the urine, it is very likely that the glomerular injury, although clinically silent, is progressing; such patients are liable to develop *chronic glomerulonephritis*, with hypertension and renal failure, at any time within the next twenty years or so.

Pathological features. In acute diffuse proliferative glomerulonephritis the cortex is pale and distinctly enlarged due to oedema. In fatal cases the cortex is up to twice the normal thickness, pale, and the glomeruli may be just visible with a hand lens as light grey dots projecting from the cut surface.

Microscopically, the appearances are similar in biopsy and necropsy material. The most conspicuous changes are diffuse enlargement and increased cellularity of the glomeruli (Fig. 22.16). The enlargement results in narrowing or obliteration of the capsular space. When a glomerulus happens to have been cut in the appropriate plane, part of the glomerular tuft can often be seen to have herniated into the lumen of the first part of the tubule. The capillary lumina appear narrowed, and the endothelial cells are swollen. It is not clear whether the increased capillary cellularity is due to increase in endothelial or mesangial cells. Neutrophil polymorphs are seen in the glomeruli but vary considerably in number from case to case (Fig. 22.17).

An additional change in the glomerular tufts is an increase in the number of strands of basement-membrane-like material demonstrable by electron microscopy in the mesangial regions. These strands are normally present between mesangial cells and are made more conspicuous by oedema. In cases which fail to resolve the material apparently increases considerably and contributes to the hyaline appearance of the

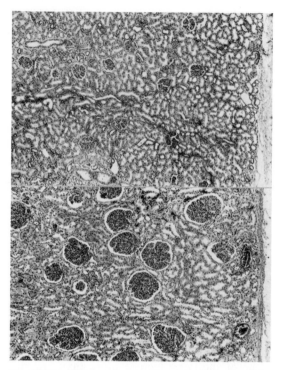

Fig. 22.16   The renal cortex in acute diffuse proliferative glomerulonephritis (*below*) compared with the cortex of a normal kidney (*above*). Note the gross enlargement and hypercellularity of the glomeruli. × 30.

glomeruli in the chronic stage of glomerulonephritis.

Electron microscopy shows localised deposits of granular material, mostly projecting from the outer surface of the basement membrane and giving it a 'lumpy' appearance (Fig. 22.18), while in some cases there are deposits also on the inner surface of the basement membrane.

The epithelial cells do not show widespread fusion of foot processes, although this may occur focally. Some proteinous debris, and occasionally red cells, may be seen in the narrowed capsular spaces. In most cases, the epithelium of Bowman's capsule appears normal, but here and there some proliferation may be seen. Epithelial crescents (p. 822) are few or absent in typical cases. The changes are represented diagrammatically in Fig. 22.19.

Changes in the rest of the kidney are secondary to the glomerular lesion: there is diffuse oedema, seen as an increase in the loose interstitial tissue between the tubules, and often accompanied by a light scattering of poly-

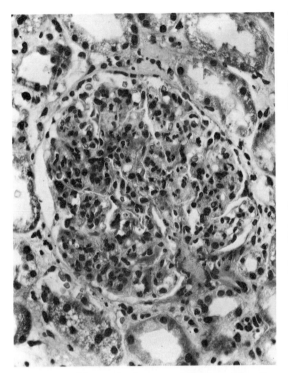

Fig. 22.17 Glomerulus in acute diffuse proliferative glomerulonephritis, showing swelling and increased cellularity of the glomerular tuft. × 200.

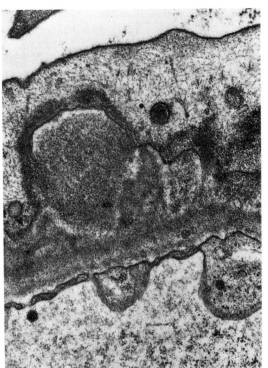

Fig. 22.18 Electron micrograph of part of glomerular capillary wall in acute diffuse glomerulonephritis, showing a large granular sub-epithelial deposit. Note also fusion of the foot processes (lumen below, urinary space above). × 25 000.

morphs or mononuclear cells. The tubules contain proteinous and cellular casts, including blood casts, and the epithelial cells of the proximal convoluted tubules contain hyaline droplets (p. 824). Occasionally there are foci of disruption of tubular epithelial cells, possibly attributable to ischaemia secondary to the glomerular changes. Hypertension is not usually sufficiently severe or prolonged to produce changes in the heart and blood vessels.

With recovery from the disease the glomeruli return to normal, although increased numbers of cells in the mesangial zones of the glomerular lobules may persist for months, and are regarded as a retrospective diagnostic feature.

Clinico-pathological correlation. In acute diffuse glomerulonephritis, light- and electron-microscopy show narrowing of the glomerular capillary lumina attributable to increase in number and size of endothelial or mesangial cells and infiltration of polymorphs. Some impairment of blood flow through the kidneys might be expected, and indeed the renal plasma flow has been shown to be reduced in some

cases, but is normal in others. However, the fraction of plasma filtered off by the glomeruli (the glomerular filtration fraction) is reduced, and hence *the total glomerular filtration rate (GFR) is also less than normal*. This largely explains the usual rise in the blood urea level, although ischaemic injury of the tubular epithelium may play a part by impairing the functional selectivity of reabsorption.

The factors concerned in the production of oedema and oliguria in acute diffuse glomerulonephritis are not yet fully understood. The point is made several times in this chapter that the *volume* of urine produced, and its *concentration*, are dependent mainly on tubular reabsorption and not on the GFR. Two important factors in tubular reabsorption are, firstly the concentration of solutes remaining in the lumen (i.e. not reabsorbed)—a high concentration of solute, e.g. urea, produces an osmotic diuresis by interfering with reabsorption of water (p. 837); secondly, the pituitary

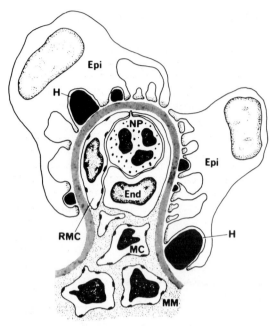

Fig. 22.19 Diagram of a glomerular capillary loop in acute diffuse proliferative glomerulonephritis, showing reduction of the lumen by endothelial cell (End), swelling and a reactive mesangial cell (RMC). The lumen is occupied by a polymorph (NP). Note the various-sized lumpy sub-epithelial deposits (H) and focal fusion of the foot processes of the epithelial cell (Epi). MC, mesangial cells; MM, mesangial matrix. (By courtesy of Dr. D. R. Turner and Churchill Livingstone.)

antidiuretic hormone, which increases reabsorption of water. It is not clear what part these and other factors play in the oliguria and oedema of acute diffuse glomerulonephritis: the subject is discussed more fully on p. 256. The transient hypertension is presumed to result from decreased renal blood flow.

Urine. It seems reasonable to assume that the appearance of protein, red cells and leukocytes in the urine is attributable directly to the glomerular lesion. It must be admitted, however, that the severity of the glomerular changes does not correlate closely with the amount of protein or numbers of cells escaping in the urine. It is probable that the basement membrane is the main crude filter in the glomerular capillary wall, in which case the glomerular lesion must result in increased permeability of the capillary basement membrane, the pathogenesis of which is discussed below.

In a small proportion of patients with acute diffuse glomerulonephritis, proteinuria is un-

usually heavy and the nephrotic syndrome (p. 823) results. At the other extreme are patients with the usual clinical and histological changes of acute diffuse glomerulonephritis but little or no proteinuria.

Unfavourable histological features. Thrombosis and necrosis of individual glomerular capillaries, glomerular haemorrhages, deposition of fibrin and the development of numerous large epithelial crescents are all indications of unusually severe glomerular injury and carry the risk of death in the acute disease. There is no sharp dividing line between such severe cases and rapidly progressive glomerulonephritis (p. 823).

Following acute diffuse glomerulonephritis, increase in the size and number of mesangial cells may persist for weeks or even months without serious sequelae. Increase in basement-membrane-like material in the mesangial areas is, however, a more serious feature; it is seen, together with persistent cellular increase, in those few cases which, after a latent period, develop chronic glomerulonephritis.

Aetiology. Immunofluorescence microscopy of renal biopsy material in cases of acute diffuse glomerulonephritis typically reveals granular deposition of immunoglobulin (usually mainly IgG) and components of complement in the glomerular capillary walls (Fig. 22.20).

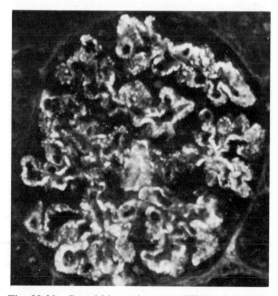

Fig. 22.20 Renal biopsy in acute diffuse glomerulonephritis. Immunofluorescence technique, showing granular and ill-defined deposition of IgG in the glomerular capillary walls. × 350.

These findings, together with the detection by electron microscopy of dense sub-epithelial deposits (Fig. 22.18), are strongly suggestive of the deposition of immune complexes, and the diffuse inflammatory glomerular changes also resemble those of experimental acute 'small-complex' glomerulonephritis (p. 814). As acute glomerulonephritis usually follows a streptococcal infection it is likely that antibodies to streptococcal products, appearing a week or so after the infection, combine with streptococcal antigens still present in the plasma, thus providing immune complexes which would, at first, be formed in the presence of antigen excess. Attempts to demonstrate streptococcal antigen in the glomerular deposits have provided conflicting results: in general, detection of antigen has been reported mostly in biopsy material obtained early in the course of the disease, and it is likely that, later on, the deposited antigen becomes coated, and thus obscured, by an excess of antibody. Still later, immunofluorescence microscopy may reveal complement components alone, the antibody, in turn, having apparently been obscured by complement. The difficulty in demonstrating streptococcal antigen in the glomeruli is not surprising because similar difficulty has been experienced in demonstrating antigen in experimental acute immune-complex glomerulonephritis, in which not only is the antigen known, but powerful antibodies are usually available to facilitate its detection by immunofluorescence microscopy. It is not understood why certain types of Group A streptococci, notably Griffiths types 12, 4, 1, 25 and 49, are nephritogenic, whereas other types and other micro-organisms are not.

As in the experimental condition, the mechanisms by which deposited immune complexes cause glomerular injury are not fully elucidated. The acute injury is probably due to the presence of complexes in relatively small amounts in the inner part of the capillary wall: the sub-epithelial aggregates appear at a relatively late stage of the disease and are unlikely to be of early pathogenic importance, as explained on p. 814. At an early stage, there is a fall in the level of serum complement (which is further evidence consistent with the presence of circulating immune complexes), and it is likely that local complement activation, polymorph activity and perhaps the clotting mechanism, all contribute to the acute capillary injury.

Rapidly progressive glomerulonephritis

This usually fatal condition may develop without known predisposing cause, or may follow a streptococcal infection. It can supervene also in patients with the focal glomerulonephritis associated with certain diseases (p. 830). It can occur at any age, and is commoner in males than females. The clinical features and urinary changes may be indistinguishable at first from those of acute diffuse glomerulonephritis (p. 817), but instead of regressing after a week or two, become progressively more severe, and without haemodialysis death usually results from uraemia and hypertension after a period of a few weeks to a year or so. Rarely, proteinuria may be severe enough to give rise to the nephrotic syndrome. In other cases, severe oliguria or even anuria lead to early death.

Rapidly progressive glomerulonephritis is much less common than acute diffuse glomerulonephritis, but because of its severity it makes an important contribution to the number of individuals dying of renal failure.

Pathological changes. The kidneys are normal in size or enlarged due to oedema: on section the cortex is pale, but may show petechial haemorrhages, and the glomeruli stand out conspicuously as grey dots, visible with a lens on the cut surface. In most cases, there is little or no gross scarring and the surface of the kidneys is smooth.

Microscopy shows the most important changes to be glomerular. As in acute diffuse glomerulonephritis, there is proliferation, probably of both endothelial and mesangial cells, with narrowing of the capillary lumina, and variable polymorph infiltration of the tuft (Fig. 22.21). Although all the glomeruli are affected, some glomerular lobules may be more severely involved than others, and there may be ruptures in the basement membrane, haemorrhages and necrosis and thrombosis of capillaries or lobules. There are conflicting reports on the therapeutic value of heparin.

A surprising feature of the disease is the rapidity with which glomerular scarring may occur: thus in cases with a history of only 2 weeks or so, biopsy may reveal sclerosis of lobules or whole glomeruli, and also fibrous adhesions between the tuft and Bowman's capsule (Fig. 22.22). There is thus a combination of glomerular proliferation, necrosis, thrombosis and

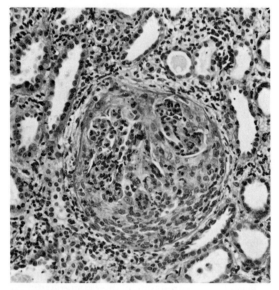

Fig. 22.21 Glomerulus in rapidly progressive glomerulonephritis, showing destruction and fibrosis of parts of the tuft, hypercellularity of the remainder, and formation of a large crescent around the tuft. × 200.

scarring, amounting to very severe glomerular injury.

A most characteristic histological feature is proliferation of the parietal epithelium of Bowman's capsule to form '*epithelial crescents*' (Figs. 22.21, 22.22) which occupy the capsular space and surround the tuft. (This change used to be known as *extracapillary glomerulitis* to distinguish it from changes in the glomerular tuft, which were termed *intracapillary*: the terms have now largely lost their usefulness). Formation of epithelial crescents occurs in other diseases, for example in subacute infective endocarditis, malignant hypertension, and in some cases of acute diffuse glomerulonephritis, but the crescents are neither so numerous nor so large as in rapidly progressive glomerulonephritis, in which they may fill and distend the capsular space of most glomeruli. In time, the epithelial crescents are usually replaced by fibrous tissue. Study of glomerular explants in tissue culture has led to a recent suggestion that the crescents are composed of macrophages (Atkins *et al.*, 1976), but most observers consider that they are epithelial, perhaps with an infiltrate of macrophages. Crescent formation is not understood, but fibrin deposits are usually demonstrable by im-

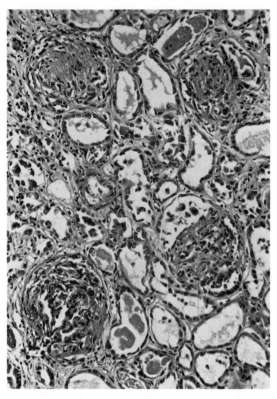

Fig. 22.22 Rapidly progressive glomerulonephritis. The four glomeruli show severe destruction; the lowest one shows crescent formation and the upper two have undergone rapid scarring. The tubules are dilated and there is extensive loss of epithelium. × 110.

munofluorescence in the crescents, and they are generally associated with severe glomerular injury. Depletion of fibrinogen by ancrod or administration of heparin largely prevent the formation of crescents in experimental glomerulonephritis and improve the prognosis.

The tubules may be dilated (Fig. 22.22), and usually contain hyaline and cellular casts and red cells, and proteinous droplets are present in the cells of the proximal convoluted tubules. There may be focal necrosis or irregular tubular atrophy and increase of intertubular connective tissue, presumably due to ischaemia resulting from the glomerular changes.

In some cases hypertension is severe, and the changes of malignant hypertension (p. 810) become superadded. There may also be left ventricular hypertrophy and changes associated with uraemia, e.g. fibrinous pericarditis, anaemia and superadded infections.

The glomerular changes result in severely impaired renal blood flow and consequent reduction in GFR. The clinical and biochemical changes are similar to those in acute diffuse glomerulonephritis, but becoming progressively more severe.

Aetiology. In some cases, rapidly progressive glomerulonephritis follows a streptococcal infection, and these represent the severe end of the spectrum of acute diffuse proliferative glomerulonephritis. They show granular deposition of Ig and complement and sub-epithelial deposits on electron microscopy. In other cases, there is no known preceding infection, and evidence of immune-complex deposition is sometimes absent. Thirdly, the condition can supervene in a group of systemic conditions which also give rise to the less serious focal glomerulonephritis (p. 830). Lastly, the same picture is caused by the development of auto-antibody to glomerular basement membrane in Goodpasture's syndrome (p. 832).

It is thus apparent that rapidly progressive glomerulonephritis can develop in a number of types of acute glomerulitis. Although the prognosis is poor, some cases recover, at least partially, after a period of haemodialysis. The outlook appears to be slightly better in post-streptococcal cases, and treatment by plasma-exchange and cytotoxic drugs has given encouraging preliminary results in those cases with Goodpasture's syndrome and in cases with immune complex deposition (Lockwood *et al.*, 1976, 1977).

The nephrotic syndrome

This is described here because it is an important feature of some of the types of glomerulonephritis dealt with below.

The syndrome occurs when prolonged and severe proteinuria results in **hypoalbuminaemia** and consequently in **generalised oedema**. The proteinuria is virtually always due to increased glomerular capillary permeability and amounts in adults to the daily loss of 10 g or more of plasma protein. As indicated below, it can be brought about by the glomerular lesions of many different diseases and diagnosis of the cause of the condition often requires renal biopsy. Conditions other than the renal disease which bring about hypoalbuminaemia, e.g. chronic malnutrition or protein-losing enter-

opathy, are similarly accompanied by generalised oedema.

The nature of the oedema and factors involved in its development have been discussed on p. 256. Another common feature of the syndrome is **hyperlipidaemia**, increase in levels of lipoproteins of lower density often being considerable. This biochemical change is unexplained and the evidence on its causation is conflicting.

Pathological changes. In addition to generalised oedema, including free fluid in the body cavities, there is a high risk of infections, and before the introduction of sulphonamides and antibiotics a high proportion of patients used to die of pneumonia, peritonitis or meningitis.

The kidneys show striking changes in the nephrotic syndrome. These include generalised enlargement and pallor due to oedema, and frequently a yellow, radial streaking of the cortex due to deposition of lipids (Fig. 22.23). The combination of increased glomerular capillary permeability (responsible for the heavy proteinuria) and hyperlipidaemia results in leakage of relatively large amounts of lipoprotein into the glomerular filtrate: some of this is reabsorbed and deposited in the tubular epithelial cells or in the interstitial tissue of the cortex (Fig. 22.24). There may be accumulation of 'foamy' lipid-laden macrophages and also

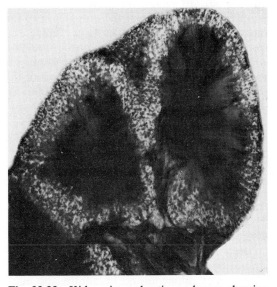

Fig. 22.23 Kidney in nephrotic syndrome, showing abundant cortical deposits of neutral fat and anisotropic lipids. (Photographed using crossed polarising filters.) × ⅘.

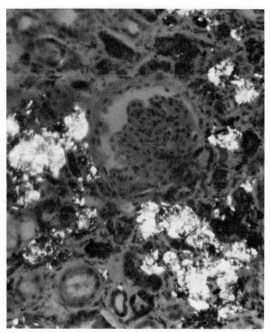

Fig. 22.24 Kidney in nephrotic syndrome, showing abundant anisotropic lipid with some sudanophil neutral fat (dark) in the interstitial tissue and tubules. (Photographed using crossed polarising filters.) × 150.

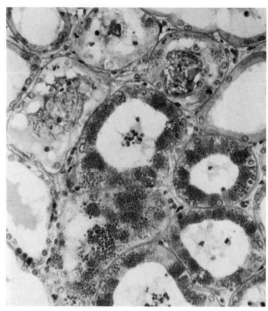

Fig. 22.25 Hyaline droplets in renal tubular epithelium resulting from reabsorption of protein from the filtrate. × 300.

giant-cell granulomas around crystals of cholesterol. Hyaline droplets due to reabsorption of protein are abundant, along with globules of lipid, in the cytoplasm of the lining cells of the proximal convoluted tubules (Fig. 22.25) and protein casts are present in the distal tubules.

The glomeruli in patients with the nephrotic syndrome show the pathological features of the causal disease. The only feature common to most cases is seen by electron microscopy and consists of loss of the foot processes of the epithelial cells, the cytoplasm of which is closely applied to the outer part of the glomerular basement membrane (Fig. 22.28): this is not specific for the nephrotic syndrome and experimental work suggests that it is a *result* of proteinuria and not its cause.

Causes of the nephrotic syndrome are numerous. In children, minimal-change glomerulonephritis is much the commonest cause, followed by acute diffuse glomerulonephritis and focal glomerulonephritis. In adults, the acute diffuse, membranous and minimal-change types of glomerulonephritis are about equally common, followed by membrano-proliferative

glomerulonephritis, renal amyloidosis, diabetes, systemic lupus erythematosus and focal glomerulonephritis.

In some reports, chronic glomerulonephritis is regarded as a relatively common cause of the nephrotic syndrome. This is probably a matter of nomenclature, for some forms of glomerulonephritis and other renal lesions manifest as the nephrotic syndrome, which may persist for years, and then progress to glomerulosclerosis with reduced renal blood flow and so diminished GFR, leading to renal failure: frequently the proteinuria diminishes as this stage develops and the nephrotic syndrome subsides, but in some cases there is a combination of nephrotic syndrome and chronic renal failure.

Diffuse membranous glomerulonephritis

Clinical features. This disease is commoner in males than females, and occurs over a wide age range, but more often in adults than in children. It presents as *the nephrotic syndrome*, i.e. heavy proteinuria, generalised oedema and hyperlipidaemia (see above). The oedema develops gradually, often being first noticed in the face and only partly influenced by gravity. It eventually becomes severe and generalised,

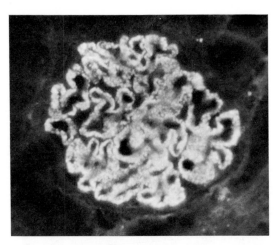

Fig. 22.31 Renal biopsy in membranous glomerulonephritis. Immunofluorescence technique, showing granular deposition of IgG in the glomerular capillary walls. × 250.

dense deposits in the outer part of the basement membrane seen by electron microscopy and the gradual uniform thickening of the capillary basement membrane, provide a close parallel to experimental immune-complex glomerular injury of the chronic 'small-complex' type (p. 815) and the nephrotic syndrome is a major feature of both conditions. The common termination of the human disease in a stage of glomerulosclerosis with chronic renal failure is seen also in those forms of the experimental condition which are progressive, i.e. when foreign protein injections are continued over a long period or in the auto-immune form of the disease in rats.

Although the evidence for immune-complex deposition in membranous glomerulonephritis is strong, the disease is still idiopathic in the sense that the nature of the antigen is unknown. In a few cases surface antigen of type B hepatitis virus (HBsAg) has been detected in the blood and in the glomerular deposits. Membranous glomerulonephritis can also result from immune responses to microbial infections, e.g. in quartan malaria and syphilis, and occasional cases have been associated with a cancer, removal of which has led to regression of renal symptoms. The auto-immune reactions involving DNA, etc. in systemic lupus erythematosus sometimes produce a closely similar condition (p. 832). Identification of the antigen(s) involved in the idiopathic condition might open the way to specific immunotherapy and is thus of practical importance.

Renal vein thrombosis is now regarded as a complication, rather than the cause, of membranous glomerulonephritis and other conditions associated with the nephrotic syndrome.

Membranoproliferative glomerulonephritis

This condition occurs at all ages but particularly in older children. Its presenting features may resemble closely those of acute diffuse proliferative glomerulonephritis, or there may be symptomless proteinuria or development of the nephrotic syndrome.

In general the outlook is poor. The disease continues over a period of years; at some stage the nephrotic syndrome is likely to develop and approximately 50% of patients die within ten years of chronic renal failure. Some patients do, however, appear to recover. Response to steroids, etc., has so far not been very encouraging, and if renal transplantation is performed the condition tends to recur in the transplant.

Pathological changes. At an early stage the glomeruli show diffuse proliferative change with increase in size and number of mesangial and endothelial cells; the mesangia in particular show increased cellularity and the lobular pattern of the glomeruli is accentuated (Fig. 22.32), the disease sometimes being termed lobular glomerulonephritis. The capillary lumina are reduced and there is irregular thickening of their walls. Silver stains show, here and there, a double basement membrane (Fig. 22.33). Electron microscopy shows extension of the cytoplasm of mesangial cells between the endothelium and basement membrane—mesangial interposition: in places, a second layer of basement membrane is laid down between the endothelium and mesangial cytoplasmic extensions, thus accounting for the double contour seen in silver-stained preparations (Fig. 22.34). In some cases, electron microscopy shows also discrete, irregular, dense deposits on the inner side of the (original) basement membrane: in others, dense material is deposited within the lamina densa, causing more diffuse thickening of the basement membrane, the density of which has sometimes led to use of the term *dense deposit disease* (Fig. 22.34). The two patterns of deposition are sometimes dis-

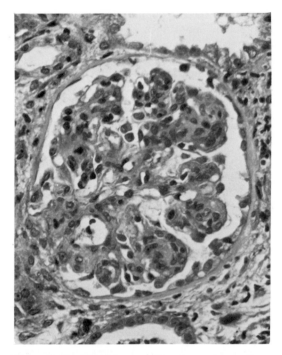

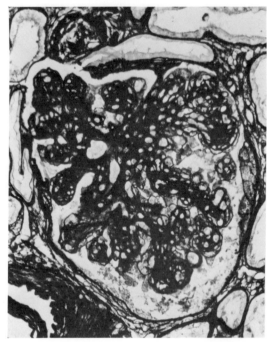

Fig. 22.32 Membranoproliferative glomerulone-phritis. The glomerular lobulation is accentuated, there is increased cellularity, and thickening of capillary walls. × 350.

Fig. 22.33 Membranoproliferative glomerulone-phritis. Stained by silver impregnation to show the thickening of the glomerular capillary basement membrane which has a double contour in some peripheral capillary loops. × 350.

tinguishable by light microscopy of very thin sections but are seen more readily by electron microscopy. In some cases, particularly with linear deposition, there is formation of small crescents in the capsule of occasional glomeruli.

As the disease progresses the mesangial cells diminish in number and hyaline material accumulates, while the capillaries become progressively thickened so that glomerulosclerosis and chronic renal failure usually result.

The aetiology of this condition is unknown. In cases with sub-endothelial deposits, components of complement and sometimes also immunoglobulin are detectable in the capillary walls (Fig. 22.35). In some such cases there appears to be good evidence of a preceding streptococcal or other acute infection and the disease could be an unusual form of immune-complex injury. In the type with linear deposition, neither complement components nor Ig is usually detectable, although there may be C3 in the mesangia. In both types, there may be depression of C3 in the plasma and activation of the alternative pathway (p. 143) has been suggested. A factor which acti-

vates C3 (*the nephritic factor*) has been detected in the serum in some cases and appears to be an immunoglobulin (Davis *et al.*, 1978).

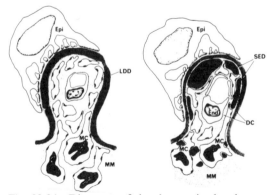

Fig. 22.34 Diagrams of the changes in the glomerular capillary loops in membranoproliferative glomerulonephritis with sub-endothelial deposits (SED) (*right*) and linear deposition (LDD) (*left*). End, endothelial cell; Epi, epithelial cell; MC, mesangial cell; MM, mesangial matrix. DC, double contour of basement membrane. (By courtesy of Dr. D. R. Turner and Churchill Livingstone.)

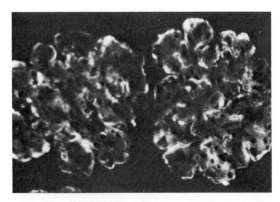

Fig. 22.35 Immunofluorescence staining of two glomeruli in a case of membranoproliferative glomerulonephritis, showing deposition of IgG at the margins of the lobules. × 200. (Dr. J. M. Vetters.)

Minimal-change glomerulonephritis

While this name is not altogether satisfactory, it is preferable to the more commonly used *lipoid nephrosis* because it indicates that the essential lesion is glomerular and that the structural changes are inconspicuous.

General features. The disease has a peak incidence in children between 1 and 4 years old, but occurs in children and adults of all ages. It is by far the commonest cause of the nephrotic syndrome in children. The oedema and proteinuria tend to fluctuate, spontaneous remission and recurrences being common. The blood pressure and blood urea are usually normal and tests of inulin clearance have confirmed that, in most cases, there is no detectable fall in glomerular filtration rate. As usual in the nephrotic syndrome (p. 823), there is a rise in the level of blood lipids, including cholesterol.

Formerly, there was a high mortality from superadded infections developing in the severely oedematous patient, but the outlook has been improved greatly by the use first of sulphonamides and later of antibiotics. Glucocorticoid therapy has also improved the prognosis, for it cuts short the disease by suppressing the proteinuria. Steroid therapy usually takes 2–3 weeks to show an effect, and the mechanism is quite unknown: there is a risk of relapse on stopping therapy, and at present there is no way of predicting the cases in which this will occur. The progress of large series of children has been observed for some years by Arneil and Lam (1967) and by others, and it appears that the prognosis is good, although a minority of patients eventually develop renal failure with uraemia and hypertension (see below).

The long-term prognosis in adults developing this disease is uncertain. The eventual development of chronic renal failure appears to be more common than in children.

The proteinuria is due to increased glomerular capillary permeability, and is usually highly selective, albumin being accompanied by only very small amounts of the plasma proteins of larger molecular size; this contrasts with the less highly selective proteinuria observed in most other renal diseases, with or without the nephrotic syndrome. The urine contains lipid-rich protein casts but few or no leukocytes or red cells.

Pathological changes. Some patients still die from infection supervening on the nephrotic syndrome and the kidneys show the usual features of this syndrome (p. 823).

Microscopically, the glomeruli look normal apart from an appearance of fixed dilatation of the capillaries; there is no thickening of the capillary walls and no increased cellularity of the glomerular tufts (Fig. 22.36). The most conspicuous glomerular change on electron microscopy is fusion of the foot processes of the epithelial cells, the basement membrane being covered externally by a layer of epithelial cell cytoplasm (Fig. 22.37): the epithelial cells also show increased vacuolation and in some cases the basement membrane is slightly thickened with loss of definition of the junction between its inner margin and the cytoplasm of the adjacent endothelial cells. As already explained (p. 824), fusion of the foot processes is probably a result, rather than the cause, of proteinuria. It appears that a reversible increase in the permeability of the capillary basement membrane, not reflected in any obvious structural change, is responsible for the heavy proteinuria and consequent changes in this disease.

Aetiology. The nature of this disease remains unknown. It may follow immediately on a respiratory infection, but does not show a definite relationship to any particular micro-organism. Immunofluorescence studies have failed to demonstrate deposition of immunoglobulin or complement in the glomerular capillary walls, and the aetiology is quite obscure, as is the mechanism of the beneficial effect of steroid therapy in curtailing the albuminuria.

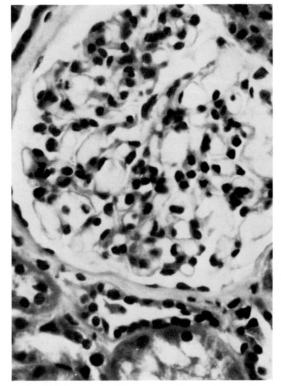

Fig. 22.36 Minimal-change glomerulonephritis. The glomerulus shows no obvious abnormality apart from dilatation of many of the capillaries. × 560.

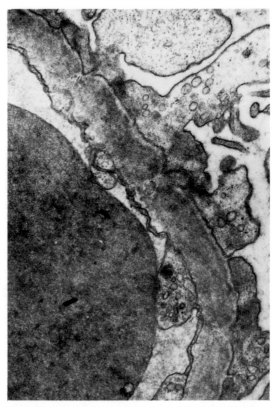

Fig. 22.37 Electron micrograph of glomerular capillary wall in minimal-change glomerulonephritis. The only abnormality is fusion of the foot processes. × 18 000.

Focal glomerulosclerosis. It is not yet known whether this condition, which was described by Rich in 1957, is a variant of minimal-change glomerulonephritis or a distinct entity. The clinical features are similar to those of minimal-change glomerulonephritis, but proteinuria is less selective and red cells are more commonly present in the urine. Although most of the glomeruli appear normal, those close to the medulla show sclerosis, consisting of deposition of hyaline material with consequent obliteration of capillaries: this change is at first focal but gradually destroys whole glomeruli and extends peripherally to involve more glomeruli. There is associated tubular atrophy. Renal biopsy is only diagnostic if it includes some of the deeper, affected glomeruli. The condition is resistant to steroid therapy and, although most series of cases are small, it is clear that the prognosis is relatively poor, there being a high risk of chronic renal failure. It is not clear whether those patients diagnosed as minimal-change glomerulonephritis who eventually develop chronic renal failure are really missed cases of focal glomerulosclerosis.

Congenital nephrotic syndrome is a rare familial condition which develops within a few weeks of birth, does not respond to steroids, and has a bad prognosis. The glomeruli may be mostly normal or show various abnormalities and there is usually marked dilatation of the proximal convoluted tubules. Immunological changes have been reported, but the nature of the abnormality is unknown.

Focal glomerulonephritis

This may be defined as a glomerulitis affecting only a proportion of the glomeruli. The lesions usually involve only part of the glomerular tuft, e.g. one or more lobules. In most cases the condition is 'idiopathic', i.e. of unknown cause, although sometimes the onset is associated with acute respiratory infections. It occurs also as a feature of certain specific diseases, notably sub-acute infective endocarditis (in which it was formerly considered to be embolic), systemic lupus erythematosus (SLE), anaphylactoid (Henoch–Schönlein) purpura, the microangiopathic form of polyarteritis nodosa, and the rare Goodpasture's syndrome. It must be emphasised that focal glomerulonephritis is not the only renal lesion which occurs in these conditions: rapidly progressive glomerulonephritis may develop in any of them, and is the common lesion in Goodpasture's syndrome. The type of membranoproliferative glomerulonephritis with sub-endothelial deposits (p. 827) may also occur in SLE, anaphylactoid purpura and subacute infective endocarditis.

Haematuria is the usual presenting feature of focal glomerulonephritis, but in some patients it gives rise to heavy proteinuria and the nephrotic syndrome.

Pathological changes. The glomerular lesion consists of a cellular proliferation, probably of mesangial cells, affecting the peripheral part of one or more lobules (Fig. 22.38), and in some cases accompanied by fibrinoid necrosis of capillary loops: within the lesions, individual capillary lumina may be obliterated by eosinophilic thrombus which blends with the necrotic capillary walls. Red cells may be present in the capsular space and in the tubules, and there may also be some proliferation of the epithelium lining Bowman's capsule, i.e. formation of small crescents (p. 822). Lesions may occur in only a small proportion of glomeruli, or may involve the majority. In patients with a long history, old scarred glomerular lesions are

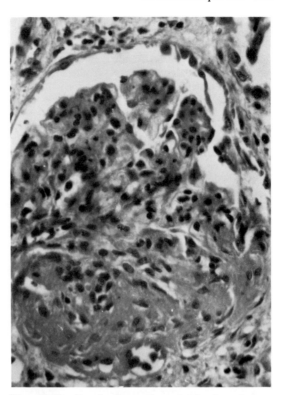

Fig. 22.39 Focal glomerulonephritis: late lesion. The lower part of the tuft is scarred and adherent to the capsule. × 350.

usually seen (Fig. 22.39), often adherent to the capsule. In cases developing the nephrotic syndrome, the renal changes consequent upon this condition (p. 823) may also be evident.

While this account is concerned mainly with focal glomerulonephritis, opportunity is taken below to outline also the additional renal lesions which occur in those diseases of which focal glomerulonephritis is a feature.

Idiopathic focal glomerulonephritis. When it occurs apart from specific diseases, focal glomerulonephritis is usually related to ill-defined respiratory infections, including pharyngitis, 'colds' and 'flu'. In contrast to acute diffuse glomerulonephritis, there is no special relationship with Group A streptococcal infections, and the interval between the respiratory infection and the onset of renal disease is only a day or so. Haematuria is often the presenting feature and is usually of not more than a few days' duration. In most cases, there is only mild proteinuria and the illness subsides with no evidence of residual impairment of renal function. Some patients are subject to recurrences, each associated with a respiratory infection, and these may occur over many years: there is evidence that chronic renal failure eventually super-

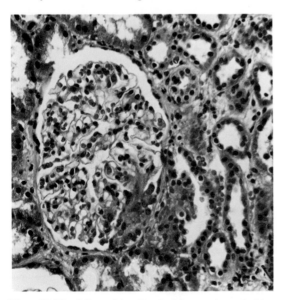

Fig. 22.38 Idiopathic focal glomerulonephritis: early lesion. Note the hypercellularity of the affected part of the tuft on the right. × 200.

venes in a minority of cases. Patients presenting with the nephrotic syndrome have been observed to recover without evidence of residual impaired renal function. The condition is not common: it occurs particularly in children and young adults, more often males than females. Its aetiology is discussed below.

Subacute infective endocarditis. Renal lesions are commonly present in this condition, but in most cases they do not lead to serious impairment of renal function and their practical importance lies mainly in the resulting haematuria, either gross or microscopic, which is of diagnostic value.

As in other organs, infarcts are common in the kidneys in subacute infective endocarditis and are usually non-suppurative. Focal glomerulonephritis occurs in about 50 per cent of cases, and tends to develop after some months. Most of the cases have been caused by *Streptococcus viridans* or *Haemophilus influenzae*. Macroscopically, the kidneys are usually of normal size, and show petechial haemorrhages visible on the subcapsular surface and scattered throughout the cortex. Microscopically, a minority of the glomeruli are usually affected, and the focal lesions show capillary thrombosis, fibrinoid necrosis and proliferative changes (Fig. 22.40). Blood is often seen in the capsular space and tubules, and there may be epithelial crescents. Bacteria cannot usually be seen in the glomerular lesions, but cultures have been positive in some cases.

In a minority of patients with subacute infective endocarditis, diffuse proliferative glomerulonephritis develops, and may progress to renal failure.

Polyarteritis nodosa. The necrotising arteritis which is the essential lesion of this condition usually

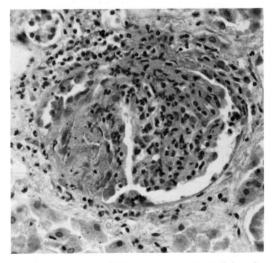

Fig. 22.40 Glomerulus in subacute bacterial endocarditis, showing a large focal necrotic glomerular lesion, with inflammatory infiltration around. × 200.

involves the larger arteries in the kidneys, with aneurysm formation and/or thrombosis, and renal infarcts are commonly present (Fig. 14.30, p. 381). In about one-third of cases, death results from renal failure with hypertension. In the *micro-angiopathic variant* of polyarteritis, the vascular lesions show the same features—fibrinoid necrosis and inflammatory changes—but involve mainly the interlobular arteries (Fig. 14.28, p. 381), afferent glomerular arterioles, and also the glomerular capillaries, giving rise to focal glomerulonephritis. As the disease progresses, most of the glomeruli may be involved and renal failure may develop, although hypertension is less common than in the classic form of the disease.

Anaphylactoid purpura occurs mainly in children, and gives rise to a skin rash, joint pains and colic with bloody diarrhoea due to a haemorrhagic exudate into the gut. In some cases there is a focal glomerulonephritis, with haematuria and proteinuria, but renal failure is either absent or mild and transient, and the kidneys usually recover completely, even after recurrent attacks. Rapidly progressive glomerulonephritis may, however, supervene, and in some other cases chronic renal failure develops after some years.

Goodpasture's syndrome. In this rare condition, haemorrhage from the alveolar capillaries gives rise to haemoptysis, accompanied by haematuria and proteinuria attributable to focal glomerulonephritis. Pulmonary haemorrhage may become increasingly severe and the renal lesion usually develops into rapidly progressive glomerulonephritis. The glomerular injury is caused by auto-antibody to basement membrane (see below). Although the prognosis is poor, treatment by repeated plasma-exchange and cytotoxic drugs has been reported to give encouraging results (Lockwood *et al.*, 1976).

Systemic lupus erythematosus (SLE). Clinically apparent renal disease occurs in over 50 per cent of patients with this disease, and carries a poor prognosis. The nephrotic syndrome may develop when proteinuria is heavy, and uraemia, with or without hypertension, is an important cause of death. The essential changes are in the glomeruli, which show a great variety of lesions. These include (1) focal glomerulonephritis which is indistinguishable from the proliferative and necrotising lesions described above except that haematoxyphil bodies (p. 941) are sometimes apparent; (2) a focal thickening of the capillary walls with a refractile eosinophilic appearance, known as the wire-loop lesion (Fig. 22.41); (3) hyaline thrombi in individual glomerular capillaries; (4) various combinations of diffuse proliferative and irregular membranous change; (5) diffuse membranous change resembling that seen in idiopathic membranous glomerulonephritis. The duration of these various lesions, and thus the degree of glomerular

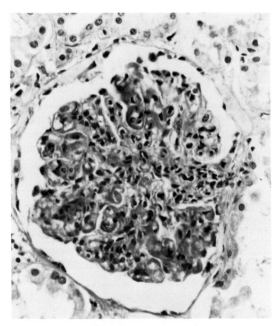

Fig. 22.41 A glomerulus in systemic lupus erythematosus, showing hyaline thickening of some of the capillaries—the 'wire-loop' lesion, and a more diffuse increase in cellularity. × 300.

sclerosis, also vary greatly. Immunofluorescence and electron microscopy provide strong evidence that these glomerular changes represent the spectrum of immune-complex injury as described on pp. 813–16. For example, the focal lesion is accompanied by deposition of immunoglobulin and complement in the mesangia and focally in the inner parts of the capillary walls: more extensive deposition of complexes in the inner parts of the capillary walls is seen in the combination of diffuse proliferative and patchy membranous change, while the diffuse granular pattern of deposition, much of it along the outer part of the basement membrane, is seen in the diffuse membranous lesion. Antibody to DNA has been eluted from the kidney tissue in SLE and there is good evidence that DNA is an important, although not the only, antigenic constituent of the pathogenic complexes. Curious tubulo-reticular structures are sometimes seen by electron microscopy in the endothelial cells. Originally thought to be viral, they are now considered to represent a response to injury by various agents, including virus infection. Although reported in other conditions, they are seen most often in SLE.

Depending on whether or not the nephrotic syndrome has been present and on the nature and duration of the renal lesions, the kidneys in SLE may be enlarged and pale, of normal size, or small and scarred. The degree of tubular atrophy and interstitial fibrosis will depend upon the nature of the glomerular lesions and there may also be changes resulting from hypertension.

Renal failure is the most important cause of death in SLE and attempts to arrest the glomerular lesions by corticosteroids, cytotoxic drugs and other agents have so far been only partially successful.

Aetiology of focal glomerulonephritis. Idiopathic focal glomerulonephritis is probably not a single entity. In some cases aggregates of immunoglobulin and complement are detectable by immunofluorescence microscopy in the mesangia and in the walls of occasional capillaries. These features are similar to the findings in the experimental focal glomerulonephritis associated with deposition of relatively large immune complexes (p. 815). In occasional cases the immunoglobulin is predominantly IgA (Berger's disease) and the significance of this is obscure: in others, immunofluorescence tests for Ig and complement are negative.

The available evidence suggests that the diseases which focal glomerulonephritis accompanies are attributable to abnormal immunological reactions. The evidence is strongest in the case of sytemic lupus erythematosus (see above). Anaphylactoid purpura, as its name suggests, is widely regarded as a hypersensitivity disease, and the antigens which may be concerned include streptococci and certain foods. Deposition of IgG and C3 is commonly demonstrable in the mesangia and focally in the glomerular capillary walls. Lesions resembling those of polyarteritis nodosa occur in serum sickness: fixed immunoglobulins, and in some cases HBsAg, have been observed in the early vascular lesions, although evidence for immune-complex deposition in the glomeruli is not convincing.

In subacute infective endocarditis the prolonged infection provides a possible basis for immunological injury from circulating antigen–antibody complexes, and the long-held view that the focal glomerular lesions of this condition are embolic is no longer widely accepted. Antibody to capillary basement membrane is demonstrable in Goodpasture's syndrome (Fig. 22.42).

While the above immunological findings suggest a possible common basis for focal glomerulonephritis, the pathogenesis of the lesions is still largely obscure.

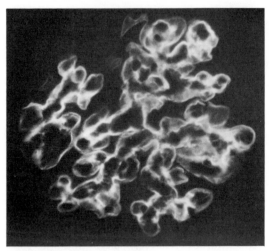

Fig. 22.42 Antibody to glomerular capillary basement membrane in Goodpasture's syndrome, showing the characteristic linear pattern of staining by the immunofluorescence technique.

Chronic glomerulonephritis

It is apparent, from the foregoing descriptions of the various types of glomerulonephritis, that an end stage may be reached in which total glomerular function is so reduced that chronic renal failure develops: this is characterised by uraemia and usually by hypertension. The time taken to reach this stage, and the rate of progression once it has developed, vary with the type of preceding glomerulonephritis, and also in individual cases. Hypertension, sometimes of the accelerated (malignant) type, usually develops and aggravates the renal tissue destruction, leading, if untreated, to end-stage renal failure which progresses rapidly to death. In cases where hypertension is absent or less severe, renal failure may progress more slowly, and the end stage may last for several years.

In over 70 per cent of patients with chronic glomerulonephritis, there is no history to suggest preceding renal disease, and the renal lesions have progressed silently until chronic renal failure develops. In such cases, it is often not possible to decide, even by histological examination of the kidneys, what type of glomerulonephritis has led up to the chronic stage. In other cases, there is a history of previous glomerulonephritis: this may have been an acute attack of post-streptococcal glomerulonephritis years before, or the patient may have had membranous, membranoproliferative or recurrent focal glomerulonephritis, which has progressed to the stage of chonic renal failure.

Pathological changes and pathogenesis. Both the kidneys are uniformly and equally reduced in size, sometimes only slightly so, but often to about one-third of normal (Fig. 22.43). In those kidneys which are greatly shrunken, the capsule is often firmly adherent and the subcapsular surface uniformly and finely irregular ('*granular contracted kidney*'). There is diffuse thinning of the cortex (Fig. 22.44), which accounts largely for the reduction in kidney size, while the medullary pyramids are also, although less markedly, shrunken. The amount of fatty tissue around the renal pelvis is increased. *In contrast to chronic pyelonephritis, the calyces and renal pelvis are not distorted.*

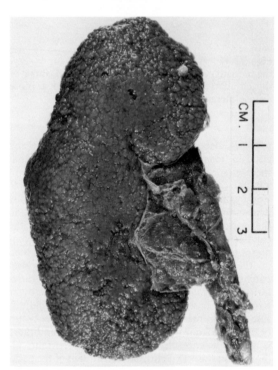

Fig. 22.43 Chronic glomerulonephritis. The kidney is uniformly shrunken, in this case to about half the normal size, and the surface is diffusely granular.

The renal arteries and their major branches show arteriosclerotic thickening, and in cases complicated by malignant hypertension the cortical mottling and haemorrhages of this condition are superimposed on the changes described above. The other organs and tissues

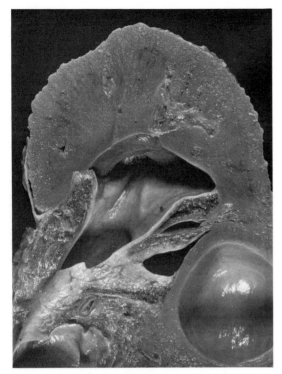

Fig. 22.44 The cut surface of the same kidney shown in Fig. 21.38, showing diffuse cortical thinning. The cyst is incidental. × 2.

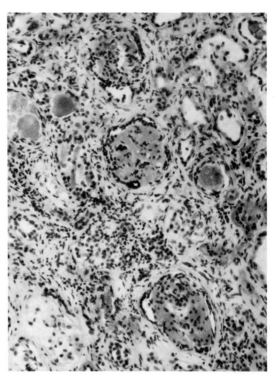

Fig. 22.45 Chronic glomerulonephritis, showing hyalinisation of glomeruli; the tubular epithelium is atrophic and there is interstitial fibrosis. × 100.

show the changes of chronic renal failure (p. 838).

Microscopically, in the small granular kidneys, it is common to find all degrees of hyalinisation of glomeruli. Many are completely hyalinised (Fig. 22.45) and some show partial destruction. A small percentage are normal or nearly so, and may be hypertrophied (Fig. 22.46). In cases in which the kidneys are not greatly shrunken the glomeruli are usually more uniformly damaged: this is seen in the chronic end stages of membranous and membranoproliferative glomerulonephritis.

The arcuate and interlobular arteries and the afferent arterioles show hypertensive changes which are likely, by causing ischaemia, to have contributed to the glomerular scarring. When malignant hypertension has supervened the consequent changes (Fig. 22.11, p. 812) are seen in those glomeruli which have not been destroyed already by the glomerulonephritic process.

The tubules show extensive atrophy, many being completely lost, and there is an increase

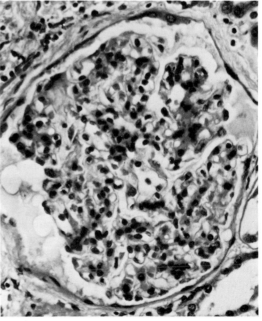

Fig. 22.46 A relatively healthy, hypertrophied glomerulus in chronic glomerulonephritis. × 250.

in the intertubular connective tissue and irregular interstitial aggregation of lymphocytes and usually small numbers of plasma cells. In cases with some near-normal hypertrophied glomeruli, the corresponding tubules are enlarged and conspicuous, and account for the elevations which give the sub-capsular surface its granular appearance. These surviving functioning tubules may show hyaline droplets in the epithelial cytoplasm and frequently contain protein casts (p. 808), features which relate to the proteinuria. When malignant hypertension has supervened, there may be blood in the capsular spaces and in functioning tubules.

In cases of chronic glomerulonephritis preceded by the nephrotic syndrome, the kidneys may still be enlarged, and lipid deposits may still be visible in the cortex by the naked eye. Although the glomeruli show advanced scler-

osis, their appearance may still suggest the type of glomerulonephritis responsible, e.g. membranous (see Fig. 22.30). All the glomeruli are affected to some extent, and the tubular atrophy is accordingly more uniform, without prominent enlarged tubules: for this reason, the surface of the kidney is often smooth and does not exhibit the granularity usually found in chronic glomerulonephritis.

Clinical features. Most patients developing chronic glomerulonephritis are between 10 and 50 years old. The clinical features and changes in other organs and tissues are those of *chronic renal failure* and are attributable to *uraemia*, usually accompanied by *hypertension*. Since chronic renal failure results also from various other diseases of the kidneys, a description common to all causes seems appropriate, and is given below.

Chronic Renal Failure

Chronic renal failure results when the functions of the kidneys have been so reduced by a chronic disease process that there is retention of nitrogenous waste products normally excreted mainly in the urine, and loss of the capacity of the kidneys to maintain homoeostasis of fluid and electrolytes and acid–base balance in the face of the normal variations of fluid and dietary intake and of physical activity. In most cases hypertension is superadded, and may be of the malignant type. Chronic pyelonephritis and chronic glomerulonephritis account for the majority of cases, but there are many other causes, including essential (primary) malignant hypertension, polycystic disease of the kidneys, systemic lupus erythematosus, diabetes mellitus, amyloid disease, nephrocalcinosis, gout, irradiation injury and analgesic nephropathy. The pathological changes characteristic of these diseases are described in the appropriate sections: in all of them, severe chronic renal injury may occur, but the resulting chronic renal failure presents biochemical, clinical and morphological changes which are sufficiently similar to warrant a common description.

Biochemical disturbances

Non-protein nitrogen retention. As only a small proportion of functioning renal tissue

remains in patients with chronic renal failure, it follows that renal blood flow and total glomerular filtration rate (GFR) are considerably reduced. When GFR falls below normal, the amount of urea removed from the blood falls below the normal level of urea production, and the level in the blood rises. If kidney function remains steady, the blood urea will stabilise at a level at which the normal amount is removed in the glomerular filtrate. To give an example, the normal GFR may be taken as 120 ml per minute and the blood urea level as approximately 30 mg per 100 ml (5 mmol/l). Since urea is very highly diffusible, the concentration in the glomerular filtrate will also be 30 mg per 100 ml, and the total amount of urea filtered off from the blood will thus be $120/100 \times 30$ mg, i.e. 36 mg per minute. Some re-absorption of urea takes place from the tubule, and the amount excreted is about 25 mg per minute (36 g daily). Consider now the patient with chronic renal failure and sufficient functioning nephrons to provide a GFR of, say, 12 ml per minute. Obviously, this will result in urea retention, which will be reflected in a high blood urea: when the level reaches 300 mg per 100 ml, the 12 ml of filtrate per minute will then contain 36 mg, i.e. the amount normally filtered, and provided that tubular reabsorption is not altered, the normal amount will be excreted. In fact, this is an over-simplification, for urea production varies with dietary protein intake, and there are also variations in the amount reabsorbed from the tubules. In chronic renal failure there is usually distinct polyuria and, as explained below, less reabsorption occurs from the tubules. In spite of these complicating factors, the level of the blood urea gives useful information in chronic renal failure, and is easy to estimate: provided certain precautions are taken, changes in the level reflect changes in renal function. The level of blood creatinine is less influenced by dietary factors and tubular reabsorption and provides a better indication of renal function, but its estimation is less simple.

Urea itself has little or no toxicity, but its retention is an indication of retention of various other non-protein nitrogenous metabolites, some of which are toxic.

Excretion of water. In normal circumstances, the kidneys play the major role in adjusting water loss to suit intake. This is effected by varying the volume of urine from approximately 400 ml to several litres daily. Within these limits, the excretion of urinary solutes is not affected significantly, and the specific gravity of the urine is inversely proportional to the volume, varying between 1·002 and 1·040. In chronic renal failure, the variability of urine volume is commonly lost, and provided sufficient water is taken in, the kidneys excrete daily approximately 2·5 litres of dilute urine of specific gravity approximately 1·010. If water intake is inadequate in this condition, production of dilute urine continues and dehydration results, with consequent fall in blood volume and blood pressure: renal blood flow and GFR are consequently diminished, the volume of urine falls and uraemia increases. If water intake is excessive, the urine volume is little affected, and the patient develops water intoxication and pulmonary oedema. The supervention of heart failure, a common complication of chronic renal failure with hypertension, results in further impairment of renal blood flow and fall in GFR, with consequent oliguria, increase in uraemia, and cardiac oedema (p. 255).

The **polyuria** of chronic renal failure is at first sight surprising in view of the small amount of glomerular filtrate produced, but it will be recalled that in the healthy individual, the volume of urine is controlled mainly by the degree of concentration taking place in the tubules, and not by variations in the glomerular filtrate. Obviously, in chronic renal failure the polyuria results from failure of the tubules to effect the normal variations in concentration, and the most likely explanation is that the high concentration of urea in the glomerular filtrate exerts an osmotic diuretic effect similar to that which occurs when a large amount of urea is administered to a normal individual. The effect is not peculiar to urea, and can be induced by giving any substance which diffuses readily into the glomerular filtrate and which is largely unabsorbed in the tubules, e.g. inulin. Normally, 80 per cent of the volume of the glomerular filtrate is reabsorbed in the proximal part of the tubule, but the fluid remaining in the lumen does not exceed isotonicity. In chronic renal failure, the high concentration of urea in the glomerular filtrate results in isotonicity being reached when much less than 80 per cent of the volume has been reabsorbed, and further concentration cannot be achieved in this part of the nephron. In the distal part of the tubule and the collecting tubule, the 'sodium pump' normally results in a high concentration of Na^+ in the adjacent medullary interstitial tissue, and this facilitates further concentration of the tubular fluid and production of a hypertonic urine. In chronic renal failure (and osmotic diuresis induced in a normal individual) failure to achieve the normal five-fold concentration in the proximal tubule results in a large volume of fluid passing into the distal tubule, and rapid absorption of water here dilutes the Na^+ in the interstitial fluid and so interferes with further urinary concentration.

Electrolyte disturbances. It is a remarkable fact that, in contrast to the blood urea, the plasma concentrations of sodium and potassium are virtually unaltered until the terminal stages of chronic renal failure. In the normal individual, the amounts of Na^+ and K^+ excreted in the urine vary considerably, depending on intake. In chronic renal failure, the range of excretion is limited, and extremes of intake are not well tolerated. Nevertheless, considering that in some cases few functioning nephrons remain, it is apparent that, to maintain homoeostasis, considerably more Na^+ and K^+ must be excreted per nephron than normally. This is brought about by the continuous state of osmotic diuresis, referred to above, which pertains in chronic renal failure, diuresis being accompanied by decreased reabsorption of various solutes, including Na^+ and K^+. **Deficiency of Na^+** is a common late effect, for the urinary loss is somewhat inflexible, and deficiency may result from restricted intake of salt or from vomiting and diarrhoea, attacks of which are common in uraemia. Na^+ deficiency in time leads to fall in plasma volume and blood pressure, and to oliguria: nitrogen retention increases and acidosis (see below) supervenes. In some cases of chronic renal failure due to pyelonephritis, sodium loss is severe, and the clinical features may be similar to those of adrenocortical insufficiency (Addison's disease). Correction of Na^+ deficiency in chronic renal failure must be carefully controlled, for administration of too much Na^+ and water can readily induce systemic or pulmonary oedema.

In chronic renal failure, **potassium retention** may arise from excessive intake or as a complication of dehydration and acidosis; in this state, dehydration results in oliguria and reduced K^+ excretion, while acidosis results in exchange of some intracellular K^+ for H^+; both effects raise the level of plasma K^+, and there is a risk of cardiac arrest. **Potassium deficiency** is uncommon in chronic renal failure, but can occur in certain cases of chronic pyelonephritis, where excessive loss of K^+ in the urine can result from secondary aldosteronism attributable, in turn, to excessive Na^+ loss, and producing a picture like Conn's syndrome (p. 1041).

Another effect of chronic renal failure is **acidosis**. To conserve acid–base balance, the kidneys must excrete 40–60 mmol of acid (H^+) daily. This is excreted in combination with urinary phosphate and organic acid radicles (e.g. creatinine), and by combination with ammonia as NH_4^+. For homoeostasis, therefore, the glomerular filtrate must provide sufficient dibasic phosphate and other available anions, and the cells of the distal convoluted tubules must produce and secrete an adequate amount of ammonia, which is normally derived by deamination of amino acids. In chronic renal failure, the diminished volume of glomerular filtrate does not contain the normal amount of dibasic phosphate, but tubular reabsorption is also reduced as a result of the continuous osmotic diuresis, and the net amount available for excretion of acid is not very much less than

normal until the late stages. Because relatively few functioning nephrons remain, total ammonia production and secretion into the tubules is reduced. There is also some loss of bicarbonate in the urine, whereas normally it is almost completely reabsorbed. As a result of these changes, the patient with chronic renal failure is prone to develop acidosis. In most cases, the **plasma phosphate** level is normal except in the late stages, but if lack of water or salt arises, either from deficient intake or from vomiting or diarrhoea, or if the glomerular filtration rate falls even further as a result of heart failure, phosphate excretion is diminished, the blood level rises and acidosis develops.

The level of **plasma calcium** tends to be slightly low in chronic renal failure, and is further depressed if the level of phosphate rises. In this state, however, acidosis is also likely, and this increases the proportion of plasma calcium in ionic form, with the result that frank tetany does not usually develop, although muscle twitching is common.

Hypertension

This develops in most cases of chronic renal failure, often before there is nitrogen retention, and is sometimes of the malignant type. The renal changes resulting from hypertension cause further injury to the already damaged kidneys, and progress of renal failure is hastened. Life can be prolonged by amelioration of severe hypertension by antihypertensive drugs and this is now an important aspect of treatment.

The cause of hypertension in chronic renal failure (and indeed in renal disease in general) is not well understood (p. 375).

Pathological changes

The disease processes most commonly responsible for chronic renal failure are noted on p. 836, and their pathological features are described in the appropriate sections. It remains to describe the pathological changes throughout the body which *result from* chronic renal failure, whatever the cause. These changes are neither constant nor specific. **Fibrinous pericarditis**, accompanied by little or no effusion, is common in the late stages, and also '**uraemic pneumonitis**', consisting of a sero-fibrinous exudate into the alveolar spaces, sometimes fanning out from the hila, and giving a butterfly shadow on x-ray. The changes resemble those of neonatal hyaline membrane disease (p. 452), but there is often partial organisation of the exudate. Inflammatory changes occur also in the **gastro-intestinal tract**, including haemorrhagic ulceration and also a pseudomembranous enterocolitis. The cause of these various inflammatory lesions has not been established. **Immunological depression**, with a tendency to infections, is known to occur in uraemia, but the fibrinous pericarditis is usually sterile and cannot be explained thus. In some cases, the fibrinoid necrosis of arterioles resulting from malignant hypertension may be responsible for some of the lesions (e.g. Fig. 14.18, p. 374). The **cardiovascular features of hypertension** are usually obvious in such cases, although cerebral haemorrhage is less common than in essential hypertension. The commonest lesion found in the brain at necropsy is **cerebral oedema**. Changes have also been described in the pancreas (p. 717).

Bone changes. Various bone changes may occur, and are termed collectively *uraemic osteodystrophy* (p. 888). In some cases, the plasma levels of ionised calcium and phosphate are sufficiently changed to induce increased function and hyperplasia of the parathyroid glands, with consequent bone changes (secondary hyperparathyroidism). In children, a condition bearing some resemblance to rickets, and termed *renal dwarfism* or *renal rickets*, may develop.

Haematological changes in chronic renal failure include a normochromic normocytic anaemia which is due to depressed erythropoiesis and is roughly proportional to the degree of uraemia. There may also be a microangiopathic haemolytic anaemia (p. 531) in those patients who develop malignant hypertension, this being one form of the haemolytic-uraemic syndrome (p. 852).

Clinico-pathological correlations

Many of the clinical features of chronic renal failure can be surmised from the foregoing account of the biochemical and structural changes. Polyuria may be the presenting symptom, and is most noticeable at night when it replaces the low volume of concentrated urine normally produced. Any of the clinical features of severe hypertension may be present, including heart failure, visual disturbances due to retinal involvement, and convulsions followed by fatal coma from hypertensive encephalopathy. If heart failure supervenes, the volume of urine diminishes and oedema of cardiac type develops (p. 255).

Urea itself is without serious toxic properties, but the retention of other, ill-defined nitrogenous compounds in uraemia gives rise to toxic effects characterised by vomiting and anorexia and by mental dullness: coma often supervenes, but may be long delayed. As already explained, the impairment of renal function renders the patient liable to dehydration and acidosis, with their corresponding clinical features, and in this state there is also a danger of muscular irritability due to fall in plasma calcium, and of hyponatraemia and hyperkalaemia. Excessive fluid and sodium loss, e.g. from vomiting and diarrhoea, must be corrected in order to avoid these serious biochemical disturbances, but care must also be taken to avoid therapeutic overloading with sodium and water, as this leads rapidly to pulmonary oedema. When uraemia is advanced, severe anaemia is commonly present, and contributes to the clinical picture. Hypertensive encephalopathy may accompany uraemia, with generalised convulsions which are believed to result from cerebral oedema due to vascular spasm (p. 374).

In most instances, the changes in the kidneys which have brought about chronic renal failure are irreversible, and the prognosis depends on the rate of progression and on the availability of, and suitability of the patient for, chronic dialysis or renal transplantation. In some cases of chronic pyelonephritis, however, renal function can improve, at least for a time, if the infection is active and can be suppressed. While it is therefore important to search for evidence of chronic pyelonephritis, it is even more important that this condition should be detected and eliminated before it has caused sufficient renal injury to result in chronic renal failure.

Miscellaneous Renal Diseases

Diabetes mellitus

Renal failure is an important complication of diabetes. It causes death in more than 10 per cent of all diabetics, and in over 50 per cent of those developing diabetes in childhood. The most important contribution to this high mortality is *diabetic glomerulosclerosis*, which can also give rise to the nephrotic syndrome. Hyaline thickening of the afferent glomerular arterioles is also very common in diabetes: it is similar to that already described in hypertensives and old people, but is more often very severe in diabetics, both with and without hypertension, and affects also the efferent arterioles much more severely than in non-diabetics (Fig. 22.47). Acute pyelonephritis is also unduly common in diabetics, and is particularly prone to be accompanied by papillary necrosis (p. 845).

Diabetic glomerulosclerosis. This consists of deposition of eosinophilic hyaline material in the mesangium of the glomerular lobules. The deposits may be discrete rounded nodules, sometimes laminated, situated near the tip of the lobule and therefore appearing peripheral in the glomerulus (Kimmelstiel–Wilson lesion). Such *nodular* deposition affects lobules and glomeruli unequally, and one or more nodules, of various sizes, may be seen in affected glomeruli (Fig. 22.48). The glomerular capillaries are seen around the margin of the nodules, and may long remain unaffected, but nodular glomerulosclerosis is usually accompanied by more diffuse deposition of hyaline material in the mesangium of all the glomerular lobules, with associated thickening of the glomerular capillary basement membranes (Fig. 22.47). This *diffuse* glomerulosclerosis may resemble membranous glomerulonephritis, but shows less uniform basement membrane thickening: it occurs together with the nodular lesion, and may eventually progress to obliteration of most of the capillaries and severe hyalinisation of the glomeruli. Ischaemic changes, including obliter-

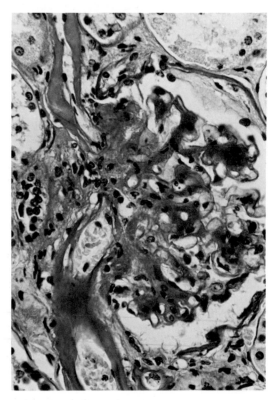

Fig. 22.47 Hyaline change in the afferent and efferent glomerular arterioles in diabetes. Note also the diffuse glomerulosclerosis. × 250.

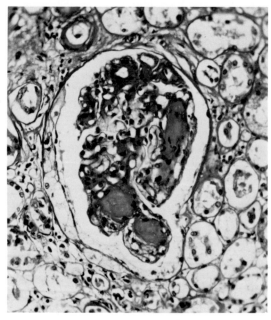

Fig. 22.48 Nodular glomerulosclerosis in diabetes (Kimmelstiel–Wilson lesion). × 205.

ation of the capsular space by collagen and glomerular collapse (Fig. 22.7, p. 810) occur, and are presumably related to hyaline thickening of the afferent arterioles. As a result of glomerulosclerosis, secondary atrophy occurs in the tubules, and the kidneys may be reduced in size with thinning of the cortex and a granular surface.

The pathogenesis of diabetic glomerulosclerosis is not understood, and electron microscopy has so far not contributed much to its elucidation. The deposited hyaline material is PAS-positive and has an electron-microscopic appearance similar to basement membrane. At present, Lendrum's suggestion that the material originates from exudation of plasma constituents (p. 809) seems the most likely explanation, both for the glomerulosclerosis and for the hyaline material deposited in the glomerular arterioles. The observed differences in staining reactions of these two lesions may be due to differences in their age. It has also been suggested that glomerulosclerosis in diabetes may result from an immunological reaction. Beef insulin is antigenic to man, and most diabetics receiving it develop circulating antibody; there is thus the possibility of circulating insulin–antibody complexes and of immune-complex nephritis (p. 813). In support of this possibility, Berns *et al.* (1962) have reported immunofluorescence studies which suggest that beef insulin and antibody to beef insulin are deposited in the glomerular capillary walls. However, this cannot be the sole cause, for diabetic glomerulosclerosis occurs in some diabetics not treated with insulin, and was recognised before the introduction of treatment by insulin. The possibility remains of auto-antibody, i.e. to autologous insulin, with consequent immune-complex deposition, but the evidence for this is not strong.

Diabetic glomerulosclerosis has been reported in 25–50 per cent of diabetics at necropsy. In most instances, the nodular and diffuse forms are combined, but in some the diffuse form occurs alone. It is worth while distinguishing between the two forms, for while the nodular lesion is highly characteristic of diabetes, the diffuse lesion is related much more closely with disturbances of renal function. In many cases, diabetic glomerulosclerosis is unsuspected during life, and may be clinically silent. It is commonly associated with protein-

uria, and when severe this may result in the nephrotic syndrome. It may also lead to chronic renal failure with the usual features of uraemia and hypertension. As already mentioned, glomerulosclerosis is especially common in early-onset diabetes; its incidence and severity increase with the duration of diabetes, and there is some evidence that poor control of the diabetic state is a contributory cause.

Other renal changes in diabetes. Atheroma is very common and often severe in diabetics. In non-diabetics the renal arteries rarely show severe narrowing from atheroma unless they are involved at their origins by aortic atheromatous plaques. In diabetes, however, severe atheroma does occur in the main renal arteries and their segmental branches and probably contributes to the high incidence of hypertension.

Other renal lesions occurring in diabetes have been referred to above, and include hyaline arteriolar thickening, pyelonephritis and papillary necrosis. The evidence for a high incidence of chronic pyelonephritis is not entirely convincing, but acute pyelonephritis, often with papillary necrosis, is common at necropsy in diabetics.

Amyloid

The kidneys are involved in nearly all cases of amyloidosis secondary to chronic infections, rheumatoid arthritis, etc., and are also commonly affected in primary amyloidosis. The most important site of deposition is around the glomerular capillary basement membrane (Fig. 22.49): this is accompanied by increased permeability, and proteinuria may be sufficiently heavy to cause the nephrotic syndrome. As the deposits increase, capillary narrowing and obliteration ensue, and the glomeruli may be largely replaced by amyloid (Fig. 22.50). Secondary atrophy of the tubules and interstitial fibrosis result from the glomerular lesion, and chronic renal failure gradually supervenes. The kidneys are firm and pale, may be of normal size, enlarged, or shrunken and granular, and the glomeruli are usually visible by naked eye after treating a slice of kidney with Lugol's iodine (Fig. 22.51). In cases with the nephrotic syndrome, the usual accompanying features are seen in the kidneys (p. 823).

Amyloid is deposited also in the walls of the

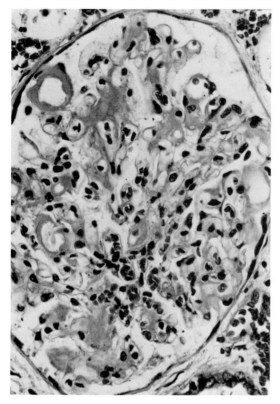

Fig. 22.49 Deposition of amyloid in the glomerular capillaries at a relatively early stage as compared with Fig. 22.50. × 250.

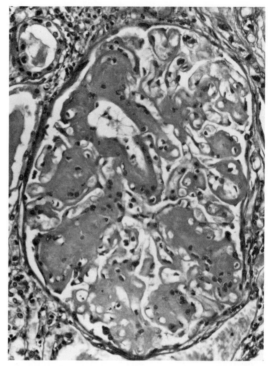

Fig. 22.50 Glomerular amyloidosis, showing thickening and hyaline appearance of capillary walls. × 350.

small blood vessels of the kidneys and upon the tubular basement membranes. The careful studies of Lendrum (1969) have revealed similarities in the pattern of amyloid deposition and hyaline change, e.g. in diabetes (p. 840), which have led him to suggest that amyloid may originate from an exudative process.

There is a tendency to thrombosis of the intrarenal veins in renal amyloidosis, sometimes extending to the main renal veins, and causing acute renal failure.

Gout

The main features of gout are described on p. 924. The excretion of increased amounts of urates by the kidneys may result in crystal formation in the medulla. The crystals are deposited mainly in the collecting tubules where they cause local destruction of the tubular wall and become surrounded by a giant-cell reaction and eventually by fibrous tissue. They are

usually at first needle-shaped, but tend to become amorphous. The destructive changes in the collecting tubules result in atrophy of the corresponding nephrons and the kidney may be reduced in size with a granular surface and scarring of the medulla. Urate stones may develop in the renal pelves and may cause renal colic, haematuria and obstruction.

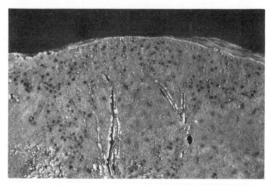

Fig. 22.51 Amyloidosis. A slice of the renal cortex has been treated with Lugol's iodine. The glomeruli contain sufficient amyloid material to be visible as darkly stained spots.

A moderate degree of hypertension is common in gout and is accompanied by the usual renal changes. Features suggestive of chronic pyelonephritis are also common at necropsy; polymorphs are often seen in the tubules, but do not necessarily indicate an infection, for it has been shown experimentally that acute inflammation, including polymorph infiltration, can occur around injected urate crystals without superadded infection, and this happens around urate deposits in the acute attack of gout.

In spite of the high frequency and variety of renal changes in gout, renal failure supervenes in only a small proportion of cases.

Kidney lesions in pregnancy

There is no doubt that the incidence of renal disease is increased during pregnancy. A factor which contributes to this is the tendency to dilatation of the ureters, attributable to the relaxation of smooth muscle which is a feature of pregnancy, and also to pressure effects of the enlarged uterus. It is probably as a consequence of these effects that urinary infection, including pyelonephritis, is a common complication of pregnancy.

Secondly, acute tubular necrosis (p. 847), and rarely renal cortical necrosis (p. 851), are encountered as complications of pregnancy, particularly in cases of retroplacental haemorrhage, infected abortion and post-partum haemorrhage.

Lastly, pregnancy increases the functional demands on the kidneys, and latent chronic renal disease (e.g. chronic glomerulonephritis) may first become clinically apparent during pregnancy. Essential hypertension may also be aggravated by pregnancy, during which the blood pressure may increase temporarily.

Toxaemia of pregnancy. Albuminuria is a common occurrence in pregnancy, particularly in the last trimester, and may be accompanied by some oedema of the ankles: these disturbances are not of serious significance unless there is also a rise in the blood pressure, when the combination of features is termed *pre-eclampsia* or *pre-eclamptic toxaemia*. This is usually mild, and the changes—oedema, proteinuria and hypertension—do not often increase to alarming degrees, and subside usually within a few days after parturition. But in some cases the features become progressively more severe during late pregnancy, and impaired renal function is reflected in a rise in the levels of blood urea. In such cases, hypertensive convulsions may occur, the condition then being termed *eclampsia*. Death may result from uraemia or hypertensive encephalopathy, and considerable judgement is sometimes required to decide whether pregnancy should be allowed to continue to term.

In patients dying from eclampsia, the kidneys are of normal size or slightly enlarged due to oedema: the cortex is pale and the glomeruli may be visible with a hand lens as grey dots projecting from the cut surface. Microscopy (of biopsy or necropsy material) shows diffuse enlargement of all the glomeruli, but without obvious increase in cellularity. The glomerular capillaries contain very few red cells: their walls appear diffusely thickened, eosinophilic and refractile, and special staining techniques show the thickening to be due to enlargement of the endothelial cells. Electron microscopy shows the endothelial cell cytoplasm to be increased in amount and vacuolated: the capillary basement membrane is usually normal, but in severe cases may show some thickening. The epithelial cells may also be enlarged, but do not show fusion of foot processes.

The clinical and histological features of pre-eclampsia indicate impaired renal blood flow with narrowing of the glomerular capillary lumina. The hypertensive convulsions of eclampsia are probably attributable to cerebral vascular spasm (seen also in the retinal arteries). There is evidence also of a reduced uterine blood flow in pre-eclampsia, probably due to arterial spasm, and sometimes resulting in retro-placental ischaemia. The causes of the glomerular changes, and of the vascular spasm, are not known, but the urinary output of aldosterone has been shown to be greatly increased.

Hypertension from any cause during pregnancy increases the risks of abortion, premature labour and retroplacental haemorrhage.

Interstitial nephritis

This term is applied to any acute or chronic inflammatory change involving mainly the interstitial tissue of the kidney. *Pyelonephritis* is mainly an interstitial infection, and inflammatory cellular infiltration of the kidneys is sometimes observed with acute infections elsewhere in the body. *Hypersensitivity reactions* to certain drugs can result in peritubular inflammation and acute tubular injury. The renal lesions of irradiation, of analgesic abuse, and a form of chronic renal disease known as *Balkan nephritis* can all be described as interstitial nephritis.

There is also evidence that tubular injury and interstitial nephritis can accompany immune-complex glomerulonephritis, complexes being deposited also in the tubular basement membranes. An autoimmune reaction to tubular basement membrane has also been reported as a cause of interstitial nephritis.

Drugs, chemicals and renal disease

Many drugs are excreted predominantly in the urine, and in patients with impaired renal function conventional dosage may result in toxic levels being attained. It is therefore necessary to modify the dosage of many types of drug in patients with acute or chonic renal failure.

Various drugs can cause renal lesions, either by a direct cytotoxic effect, or because the patient has developed a hypersensitivity to the drug. The production of acute tubular necrosis by drugs and chemicals is dealt with on pp. 848–51, and chronic renal disease due to analgesics opposite.

Lead poisoning is contracted most often in industry from inhalation of dust or fumes, or ingestion of lead compounds. In Queensland, Australia, lead paint was used up to 1930 for painting the wooden verandas of houses, and children playing on the verandas ingested paint powdered by the strong sunlight: acute lead poisoning was common, and follow-up studies have shown a high incidence of chronic renal failure, appearing often many years later and progressing very slowly. The kidneys are uniformly reduced in size with a finely granular surface, uniform cortical thinning and hypertensive changes—in fact, closely similar to the changes in chronic glomerulonephritis. Microscopically, the lesion differs from glomerulonephritis; there is marked tubular atrophy with interstitial fibrosis, and the glomeruli are spared for a long time. However, as in granular contracted kidneys from any cause, the specific diagnosis is often difficult. Characteristic inclusion bodies are seen in the nuclei of the tubular and other cells.

The relationship to excessive intake of lead many years before is convincing in the Queensland studies, and the incidence has fallen considerably since the introduction of legislation against lead paints. The use of lead paint for cots and toys has also been responsible for lead poisoning in childhood.

The renal lesion of potassium deficiency

In conditions of potassium depletion and lowering of the plasma potassium level, the kidneys exhibit a striking morphological change consisting of intense hydropic vacuolation of the cells of the proximal tubules (Fig. 22.52), chiefly in the descending straight portion. The lesion is associated with marked loss of concentrating power, but only trivial albuminuria and absence of urea retention.

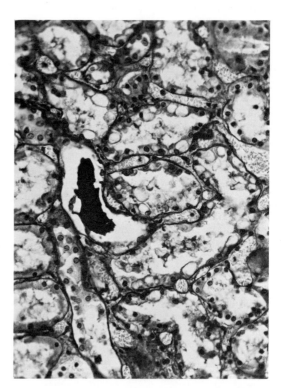

Fig. 22.52 The kidney in severe potassium depletion following prolonged diarrhoea in ulcerative colitis. The cells of the proximal convoluted tubules show gross cytoplasmic vacuolation. × 230.

It occurs most frequently in conditions which cause severe and prolonged diarrhoea, e.g. in ulcerative colitis, or induced by excessive purgation. It occurs also in primary hyperaldosteronism (p. 1041) and sometimes in Cushing's syndrome or during glucocorticoid therapy. It is a feature of some disorders of the renal tubules including the diuretic stage of acute tubular necrosis and can result from administration of diuretics. Less obvious, acute changes occur during recovery from diabetic coma under insulin therapy, when the plasma potassium falls because insulin promotes the cellular uptake of potassium. Serial biopsies of the kidney have shown the early changes to be completely reversible by restoration of normal potassium levels, and there is no evidence of permanent ill effects.

Papillary necrosis

This consists of necrosis of the distal parts of some or all of the papillae in one or both kidneys. It occurs acutely as a complication of *urinary tract obstruction* and *diabetes*, particularly when there is superadded *acute pyelonephritis*. It also occurs in more chronic form as the major renal lesion of *analgesic abuse*.

The kidneys frequently show changes of urinary tract obstruction or diabetes, commonly with superadded acute pyelonephritis. The necrotic distal parts of the papillae are usually yellowish-white and demarcated from the living tissue by a red line of congestion. The junctional zone with living tissue is congested and usually infiltrated with polymorphs. One or more necrotic papillae may have sloughed off, leaving an irregular ulcerated surface.

The clinical features are often dominated by urinary tract obstruction, pyelonephritis, etc. However, if necrosis occurs in most or all of the papillae in both kidneys, acute renal failure supervenes. There may also be haematuria and renal colic due to passage of a sloughed papilla.

Analgesic abuse. Chronic renal failure is now a well recognised cause of death in subjects taking large amounts of analgesic drug mixtures, usually containing aspirin and phenacetin, over a number of years. It seems likely that phenacetin is the important pathogenic constituent but this is unproved. Curiously, the incidence of renal failure from this cause is especially high in Australia, Switzerland and the Scandinavian countries, and relatively low in other West European countries and in North America. In Australia, the incidence is greater in Queensland, with its warm climate and relatively high urine concentration, than in the cooler Victoria. In most cases 0·5–1 kg of analgesic mixture has been taken annually for some years, either for painful chronic disease such as rheumatoid arthritis or for vague subjective illness.

It is now established that papillary necrosis is the primary change and that this leads to destructive changes in the rest of the kidney tissue. Symptoms may arise from the hypertension and uraemia of chronic renal failure or there may be recurrent urinary infection, polyuria, or renal colic due to the passage of sloughed papillae or phosphatic concretions. The urine may contain polymorphs and/or red cells.

Papillary necrosis appears to occur more gradually than in mechanical obstruction or diabetes and the necrotic papillae may remain attached or may sequestrate: frequently they become calcified. Atrophy of the overlying cortex ensues, so that the gross appearances of the kidneys come to resemble those of chronic pyelonephritis with large patches of cortical thinning and surface depression alternating with raised patches of more normal, sometimes hypertrophied renal tissue. The junction between the living and dead papillary tissue may be indistinct and microscopy may show a zone of partial necrosis. The cortex shows atrophy and loss of tubules, interstitial fibrosis and later, glomerular sclerosis.

Diagnosis is important, for striking improvement may result from stopping analgesics. Characteristic changes are sometimes seen in pyelograms.

Pathogenesis. The mechanism of papillary necrosis is not understood. The appearances, particularly in the acute form, are suggestive of infarction and the lesion tends to occur in middle-aged and old people with advanced arterial disease. The renal vascular lesions common in diabetes may be a contributory factor. The rise in pressure in urinary tract obstruction may also interfere with blood flow through the papillae. There is evidence that aspirin-type analgesics induce contraction of the efferent arterioles of juxtamedullary glomeruli, blood from which supplies the medulla. This effect may be due to suppression of prostaglandin synthesis (p. 56).

Renal tubular acidosis

Deficient tubular function is partly responsible for the acidosis which complicates chronic renal failure (p. 838). The term 'renal tubular acidosis' is, however, usually restricted to acidosis resulting from a tubular deficiency in the absence of chronic renal failure. It occurs in many conditions and traditionally is divided into two types.

In type I, function of the distal part of the tubule is impaired, with reduced capacity to produce urine of a low pH. This may occur as an inherited tubular defect, or as a result of tubular injury from pyelonephritis, hypercalcaemia, urinary tract obstruction or an auto-immune reaction.

In type II, there is impaired secretion of H^+ by the proximal tubule. This occurs in association with other tubular defects, e.g. amino-aciduria, renal glycosuria, cystinosis, hypophosphataemia.

In both types of tubular acidosis, there is hyperchloraemia, osteomalacia or rickets which is resistant to vitamin D, and a danger of deposition of calcium salts in the renal medulla (nephrocalcinosis) which may cause further renal damage. In type I cases, oral administration of alkali is effective, but in type II this is of little value.

Rejection of renal transplants

Renal transplantation has not only saved the lives of many thousands of individuals with renal failure, but has restored them to good health. The alternative of chronic haemodialysis is much less satisfactory for the patient and is considerably more expensive.

The general immunological aspects of renal transplantation and tissue typing are discussed on p. 167. Problems relating to the transplanted kidney include the technical difficulties involved in the vascular and ureteric anastomoses, acute tubular necrosis which results from the inevitable period of ischaemia when cadaver kidneys are used for transplantation, and immunological rejection of the transplant by the recipient.

Rejection is commonly classified clinically as immediate (hyperacute), acute and chronic. Apart from immediate rejection, however, these terms bear little relationship to the pathological changes, which are better classified as *immediate*, *cellular*, *vascular* and *glomerular*.

Immediate rejection, within minutes or hours of renal transplantation, occurs when the kidney donor's ABO blood group is incompatible for the recipient, or when, as a result of pregnancy, blood transfusion or a previous transplant, the recipient has developed cytotoxic HLA antibodies reactive with the donor's cells.

The kidney regains its normal pink colour and starts to produce urine when blood flow is established, but then rapidly becomes soft, cyanotic and anuric. Microscopy shows arrest of polymorphs along the walls of arterioles and venules and in the glomerular and peri-tubular capillaries. Platelets aggregate in the small vessels and thrombosis and haemorrhage occur; unless removed, the kidney becomes necrotic. The process is a type 2 or an Arthus (type 3) hypersensitivity reaction in which circulating antibody reacts with graft antigen.

Cellular rejection is most likely to occur within the first few weeks, when it is difficult to distinguish clinically from ischaemic tubular necrosis (see above); but can also occur much later. Lymphocytes, immunoblasts, plasma cells and macrophages aggregate among the tubules

and around the glomeruli, the kidney becomes oedematous and tubular necrosis develops with consequent acute renal failure. The reaction is seldom intense in immunosuppressed patients and is rapidly reversed by more intensive immunosuppression. It is a combination of the effects of cytotoxic antibody and delayed hypersensitivity reactions.

Vascular rejection may occur acutely, usually within the first few months. Endothelial swelling and hyalinisation of the media of arterioles and interlobular arteries is a common early change, and may accompany the cellular rejection described above. In more severe vascular rejection, plasmatic vasculosis (p. 809) may develop, with or without an inflammatory reaction which may progress to fibrinoid necrosis and thrombosis. These changes are indistinguishable from those of malignant hypertension, and in less acute vascular rejection there may also be intimal proliferation in the arteries, leading to narrowing or obliteration of the lumen (Fig. 22.53).

In some cases, usually after months or years,

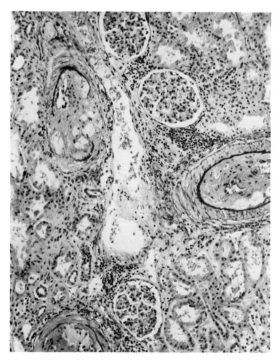

Fig. 22.53 Chronic vascular rejection of a human renal allo-transplant. Note the obliterative intimal changes and disruption of the artery walls. (Professor K. A. Porter.)

lipid-laden macrophages may accumulate in the intima of arteries, giving them a yellow appearance obvious to the naked eye and sometimes termed 'acute atheroma'.

These vascular changes result in renal ischaemia and failure, and are very difficult to reverse by immunotherapy.

'Glomerular rejection.' Glomerular injury may be secondary to the vascular rejection described above, or result from a direct rejection process. The glomerular changes of vascular rejection are the same as in malignant hypertension. The direct rejection injury of the glo-

meruli results in a slow deterioration of renal function, and may present several features in various combinations, including thickening of the capillary basement membrane, fusion of foot processes, sub-endothelial deposition of immune complexes, and mesangial hyperplasia and interposition (p. 827). Changes resembling a range of types of glomerulonephritis may thus be observed. In relatively few cases, the original form of glomerulonephritis which has caused renal failure develops in the transplant; the risk of this is greatest in membranoproliferative glomerulonephritis.

Acute Renal Failure

Renal function is impaired by any acute condition causing severe reduction in glomerular filtration. This occurs during the circulatory failure of shock following severe trauma and haemorrhage, and also as a result of marked dehydration (*pre-renal uraemia*). Complete obstruction of the urethra also causes fatal acute renal failure unless relieved in time: this condition is termed *post-renal uraemia*. Impairment of renal blood flow and glomerular filtration occurs in some degree in most cases of acute diffuse proliferative glomerulonephritis; in some cases, acute renal failure is severe with virtual anuria, particularly in the rapidly progressive variant of the disease.

The commonest form of acute renal failure is however the condition which, for want of a better name, is termed '*acute tubular necrosis*'. This has a number of causal agents, two of the most important being a state of shock and various toxic chemicals. Other causes of acute renal failure include renal cortical necrosis, renal papillary necrosis, and hypersensitivity reactions to certain drugs, but these are less common.

The functional disturbances of acute renal failure are described in the section on the clinico-pathological correlations of acute tubular necrosis (p. 849).

'Acute tubular necrosis'

In this condition there is a sudden onset of *anuria* or *severe oliguria* with consequent accu-

mulation of fluid and urinary waste products and disturbances of electrolyte and pH balance. If it is not fatal, this phase is followed by a *diuretic phase* and, in favourable cases, by *recovery* of renal function.

Causal factors

The mechanism of renal failure in acute tubular necrosis is not fully understood, and will be discussed later. At this point it is useful to note the main predisposing factors.

(a) Shock. During an acute state of shock from whatever cause there is a considerable reduction of blood flow through the kidneys and so impaired renal function. In 'acute tubular necrosis', acute renal failure with anuria or severe oliguria persists after the state of shock has passed off. This is liable to occur in cases of severe and prolonged shock, for example in association with major injury, prolonged and complicated surgical operations or extensive burns. Severe bacterial infection with endotoxic shock, the trauma of unskilled abortion, retroplacental haemorrhage and postpartum haemorrhage all carry a special risk of acute renal failure. In the bombing of cities in the 1939–45 war, individuals were commonly trapped for some hours under fallen masonry and developed traumatic and ischaemic necrosis of skeletal muscle, particularly in crushed limbs. After rescue, myoglobin and other constituents of muscle from the areas of crush injury diffused into the blood, and myoglobinuria developed. The high incidence of acute tubular necrosis in such cases (*crush syndrome*), and also in the rare condition of acute paroxysmal myoglobinuria, suggests that products of muscle breakdown have a special predisposing effect. Acute haemolysis, as in transfusion of incompatible blood, may also be followed, although much less commonly, by 'acute tubular necrosis'. Operations on the liver and biliary tract are particularly likely to be complicated by 'acute tubular necrosis' (*hepatorenal syndrome*), and although it is likely that shock and disturbance of fluid and electrolytes are at least partly responsible, there may be a special relationship between hepatic trauma and the renal lesion. The prognosis is appreciably worse in cases associated with severe trauma or surgery than in those following incompatible transfusion, complications of pregnancy or chemical poisoning (see below).

(b) Various chemicals are cytotoxic to the tubular epithelium and cause acute renal failure, often together with acute injury to the liver and other organs. Some of the more important examples include carbon tetrachloride, used extensively in the dry-cleaning of fabrics, trilene, ethylene glycol (antifreeze), carbolic acid (phenol), and organic mercurials used as diuretics. Metallic poisons are also important causes, including mercuric chloride and compounds of uranium, arsenic and chromium. Many other compounds have been implicated.

Pathological changes

In fatal cases, the kidneys are usually enlarged and the cut surface bulges, due mainly to dilatation of tubules and interstitial oedema. The cortical vessels contain little blood, and the cortex appears pale, with blurring of the normal radial pattern, while the medulla is often dark and congested. Occasionally there are petechial haemorrhages in the cortex.

Microscopically, the glomerular tufts appear normal. Usually there is some granular debris in the capsular space and the parietal cells lining Bowman's capsule may be unduly prominent and cuboidal. The tubular changes are variable and depend on the severity and duration, and on the particular causal agents involved. In many cases, however, the causation is complex, and specific changes cannot readily be attributed to particular causal agents. Also,

it is often difficult to identify, in histological sections, which parts of the tubules have been damaged. At necropsy, the lesion is often obscured by terminal ischaemic changes and postmortem autolysis.

In cases resulting from shock, etc. (group **a** above), both the proximal and distal convoluted tubules are commonly dilated and the epithelial lining is flattened with basophilia of the cytoplasm and mitotic activity (Fig. 22.54). These changes, which are seen as early as three days after the onset, appear to be a sequel to loss of tubular epithelium; the remaining cells become flattened and undergo proliferation, thus restoring epithelial continuity. In the distal convoluted and collecting tubules epithelial proliferation may be pronounced, the cells sometimes forming syncytial masses, particularly around casts (see below).

Tubular epithelial necrosis is not conspicuous and in many cases cannot be seen. In a minority there are foci of necrosis, most numerous in the distal convoluted tubule but also

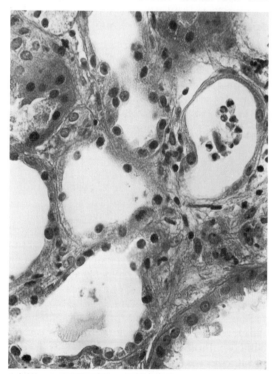

Fig. 22.54 Acute renal failure resulting from post-surgical hypotension. Note the tubular dilatation and flattening of the epithelial cells. Mitotic figures are seen and some cell debris is present in the lumen. × 320.

occurring in the proximal tubule. This change, which was described by Oliver *et al.* (1951) as *tubulorrhexis*, may be accompanied by disruption of the tubular basement membrane and an inflammatory reaction in the adjacent interstitial tissue. This may progress to scarring and in the event of recovery lead to tubular obstruction and so loss of function of the affected nephrons. The tubulorrhexic lesion and its site in the tubule were demonstrated by Oliver *et al.* by dissection of nephrons. The epithelial necrosis is not conspicuous and is readily obscured by post-mortem autolysis.

From the ascending limb of Henle's loop onwards, the tubules contain proteinous and brown granular casts, and in cases associated with haemoglobinuria or myoglobinuria brown pigment casts and rounded granules of pigmented material are particularly prominent.

Distension of the intertubular connective tissue by oedema fluid is conspicuous in some cases, but almost absent in others. The vasa recta of the medulla usually contain groups of nucleated cells which appear to represent erythropoietic foci, a feature which is sometimes seen in the hepatic sinusoids in liver cell necrosis.

The changes described above are seen in acute renal failure resulting from shock, trauma, etc. They occur also in those cases resulting from administration of the nephrotoxic poisons listed above, but in the poisoning cases there is, in addition, more extensive necrosis affecting mainly the proximal convoluted tubule of all or most of the nephrons and resulting from the direct effect of the toxic compounds or their metabolites. This *nephrotoxic change* is often conspicuous but, unlike tubulorrhexis, it does not involve rupture of the tubular basement membrane, and if the patient can be kept alive, e.g. by haemodialysis, it is often repaired by epithelial regeneration without leaving any residual damage or scarring.

Some variation is observed in the nephrotoxic lesions brought about by different chemicals. For example, mercuric chloride tends to affect the whole of the proximal convoluted tubule, and in some instances the necrotic part of the tubule rapidly becomes calcified, resulting in permanent injury. Carbon tetrachloride causes necrosis especially of the terminal part of the proximal tubule, and also perivenular hepatic necrosis. If ethylene glycol is ingested, a small proportion of it is converted into oxalate,

crystals of which form in the tubular lumina: in addition to tubular necrosis it may cause death from liver or brain injury or from acute heart failure.

Clinico-pathological correlations. Oliguria or anuria lasts from a day or two to about 4 weeks, and is followed by a diuretic phase of roughly the same period. **During the anuric phase**, renal blood flow and GFR are reduced (see below). Tubular function is also disturbed, so that most of the diminished amount of glomerular filtrate produced is re-absorbed non-selectively across the injured tubular epithelium or denuded basement membrane. Consequently there is oliguria (defined as less than 400 ml urine per day in adults) or anuria (less than 100 ml daily), and the urine comes to resemble in composition a protein-poor filtrate of the plasma. There is thus a progressive rise in urea and other nitrogenous metabolites, and unless fluid and electrolyte intake is carefully regulated, death will result from a combination of uraemia, generalised and pulmonary oedema, and electrolyte disturbances. Acidosis may result from breakdown of endogenous fat and protein, particularly in the crush syndrome or other severe injury. Protein catabolism will aggravate the uraemia and accordingly the most appropriate diet is one which is low in protein and provides sufficient calories to avoid excessive endogenous protein catabolism. One of the most important electrolyte disturbances is retention of potassium, particularly in cases with severe injury and tissue breakdown, and dietary potassium should be carefully controlled. The level of plasma Na^+ is often low, usually due to its dilution by fluid retention, but the urine, even though markedly reduced in volume, may contain excess Na^+, and Na^+ administration may become necessary. Plasma Cl^- is similarly lowered, and this may be aggravated by vomiting. The plasma level of phosphate tends to rise, with an associated fall of Ca^{++}, although this is rarely severe. Experience has shown that carefully controlled conservative therapy, including the use of osmotic diuretics such as mannitol, can prolong life in acute renal failure, and where the lesion is reversible, as in acute tubular necrosis, the prognosis has been greatly improved. However, in some cases haemodialysis is necessary. The blood pressure is commonly raised during the anuric phase.

A factor which has been suggested as contributing towards acute renal failure is leakage of tubular fluid into the interstitial tissue in tubulorrhexic lesions, with subsequent reabsorption into the blood. Obliteration of vessels by interstitial fluid is unlikely to be of importance, as oedema is sometimes minimal, and blockage of tubules by casts cannot always be a major factor, for casts are not always present. **During the diuretic phase**, large volumes of urine are produced but it continues to be very dilute, resembling a plasma filtrate and the levels of blood urea and creatinine may remain raised. There is a great danger of dehydration and loss of electrolytes and death may occur in this stage unless the urinary losses are made good. Renal concentrating power and homoeostatic mechanisms are gradually restored, sometimes over many months, but full renal function may not be achieved.

Aetiology

Two factors are of known importance in the aetiology of acute tubular necrosis. Firstly, the shock associated with trauma, incompatible transfusion, etc., and secondly, nephrotoxic chemicals. The part played by shock is by no means clearly defined: the most obvious possibility is ischaemic injury resulting from impaired renal blood flow, but experimental acute ischaemia of the kidney results in lesions particularly in the proximal convoluted tubules, whereas in those cases attributable mainly to trauma and shock the lesion in man (tubulorrhexis) is focal, and usually affects the distal convoluted tubules most severely. Because of this, and because tubulorrhexis is seen also in cases attributable to nephrotoxic chemicals, it may be that the lesion is produced by some endogenous mechanism which can be set in motion by various causal factors.

Although acute renal failure following the shock of severe injury, haemorrhage, or surgical operations, has long been attributed to tubular injury, there are unexplained discrepancies. For example, the extent of tubular necrosis does not correlate with the degree of renal failure (see Sevitt, 1959). Accordingly, it has been suggested that reduced glomerular filtration rate, attributable to diminished renal blood flow, is an important factor. There is no doubt that the renal blood flow is greatly diminished during the period of shock which precedes acute renal failure, but there is also evidence that the reduction in flow persists during the period of renal failure, and is largely responsible for it. Tubular injury, which is to be regarded as a consequence of the ischaemia of reduced renal blood flow, would thus be relegated to a secondary role in acute renal failure. These views have been advanced by Lever and his colleagues and other workers, who have provided strong evidence that persistent overactivity of the renin-angiotensin system is responsible for acute renal failure induced experimentally by administration of globin, glycerol or dichromate. By inducing arteriolar spasm, angiotensin impairs renal blood flow and glomerular filtration, and acute renal failure develops. It is of particular interest that antibody to angiotensin II minimised glycerol-induced acute renal failure although it did not prevent tubular necrosis.

Acceptance that increased activity of the renin-angiotensin system plays an important pathogenic role in acute tubular necrosis does not necessarily imply that the renal failure is due to reduced glomerular filtration. Recent investigations suggest that renal blood flow is reduced to about one-third of normal, which is no less than is encountered in heart failure *without* acute renal failure. Although tubular necrosis does not correlate well with acute renal failure, there is no doubt that the tubules are profoundly changed (see above), and it remains likely that their function is impaired. It seems most unlikely that the extensive tubular necrosis caused by various cytotoxic chemicals does not greatly impair renal function, and it is also very difficult to explain the diuretic phase of acute tubular necrosis on any basis other than impaired tubular function.

The part played by haemoglobin and myoglobin in acute renal failure is also obscure. In experimental studies, haemoglobin has not been shown to be nephrotoxic in otherwise healthy animals, although it has been shown to cause injury in conditions of dehydration, acidosis and renal ischaemia. Myoglobinuria has been shown to be more prone than haemoglobinuria to be accompanied by acute renal failure, particularly in crush injuries, and it may be that other products of muscle breakdown, in addition to myoglobin, are involved. The more extensive necrosis of the proximal tubules which occurs in cases attributable to various chemicals is more uniform, and is explicable as a direct toxic effect upon the tubular epithelium.

Disseminated intravascular coagulation (DIC)

Disseminated intravascular coagulation is a well recognised entity in which there is activation of the clotting system in the circulation and formation of thrombi in many small blood vessels (Fig. 9.35, p. 265), with consequent ischaemic damage in various organs. This widespread coagulation depletes the blood of platelets, fibrinogen and other clotting factors, and thus these patients develop *a haemorrhagic diathesis* despite the fact that the initial problem is one of excessive coagulation. Formation of fibrin also activates the plasma fibrinolytic system (p. 235) with consequent breakdown of the thrombi and remaining fibrinogen, and release of fibrin degradation products, which may be detected in the urine. The presence of fibrin strands within the small vessels causes deformity and damage of the red cells as they pass through the network and thus the patient develops a haemolytic anaemia associated with abnormal red cell morphology— *micro-angiopathic haemolytic anaemia* (p. 531). The major predisposing causes of DIC are as follows.

1. *Shock*, particularly septic shock due to Gram −ve bacteria, and less commonly other types of shock.

2. *Complications of pregnancy*, including retroplacental haemorrhage, eclampsia, amniotic fluid embolism and post-partum acute renal failure.

3. *Disseminated carcinoma.*

4. *Haematological disorders*, e.g. acute leukaemia, incompatible blood transfusion and thrombotic thrombocytopenic purpura.

5. *Systemic lupus erythematosus.*

6. *Malignant hypertension.*

7. *Renal transplant rejection.*

DIC varies considerably in the degree to which it affects different organs. It may have widespread effects, but often affects most severely a particular organ, usually the kidneys but sometimes the lungs, brain or adrenals. (Acute adrenal haemorrhage—p. 1043—is probably a manifestation of DIC.)

Renal changes. Many of the above predisposing causes are themselves responsible for renal lesions, on which the changes of DIC may be superimposed. It may, for example, aggravate the renal ischaemic changes of shock, resulting in tubular injury or cortical necrosis (Fig. 22.55). Renal injury in DIC results from obstruction of arterioles and glomerular capillaries by fibrin thrombi (Fig. 22.56). In addition, circulating non-polymerised fibrin and fibrin degradation products pass through the fenestrae of the glomerular capillary endothelium and aggregate subendothelially on the basement membrane and in the mesangia in the same fashion as intermediate-sized immune complexes in focal glomerulonephritis (p.815). There is mesangial hyperplasia and thickening of the basement membrane. Insudation of the walls of interlobular arteries with fibrin may also occur, and stimulate a proliferative endarteritis resembling that of malignant hypertension. The afferent

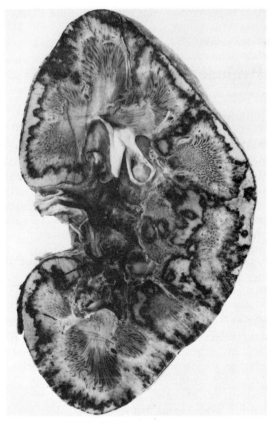

Fig. 22.55. Renal cortical necrosis from a case of eclampsia; the pale necrotic areas with haemorrhagic margins are well shown. × 0·7.

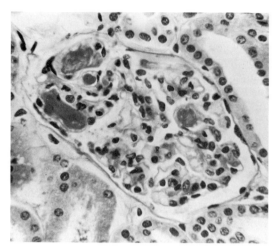

Fig. 22.56 The kidney in DIC. Some of the glomerular capillaries are occluded by fibrin. × 250.

arterioles may also be permeated by fibrin and undergo fibrinoid necrosis, which, as in malignant hypertension, may extend into the glomer-ular tufts with focal proliferative and necrotic changes.

Clinically, the features of renal failure are superimposed on those of the predisposing cause of DIC. Treatment of DIC poses a difficult therapeutic problem, for both the coagulation and plasmin systems are activated, and the difficulty lies in preventing further coagulation without aggravating the haemorrhagic state.

The term **haemolytic-uraemic syndrome** is sometimes used to describe cases of DIC in young children, in whom renal failure, thrombocytopenia and microangiopathic haemolytic anaemia are prominent, usually together with neurological and cardiovascular symptoms.

The Shwartzman reaction is an experimental model of DIC induced by administering two injections of bacterial endotoxin 24 hours apart. If the first injection is extravascular and the second intravascular, a localised lesion results. When both injections are intravascular, DIC is produced.

Pyelonephritis

Introduction

Pyelonephritis is a bacterial-induced inflammation of the renal pelvis, the calyces and renal parenchyma. It can occur in acute and chronic form and affects one or both kidneys, usually in a quite irregular, patchy fashion. Most cases are due to ascending infection of the urinary tract by *Escherichia coli* or less commonly other faecal bacteria, and for this reason urinary tract infection in general will be considered in the present account. Urinary tract infections, including pyelonephritis, are commoner in females at all ages than in males. Acute pyelonephritis causes death only when bilateral and very extensive. In less severe form, and particularly when recurrent, it may progress to chronic pyelonephritis, which is an important cause of chronic renal failure. In many instances of chronic pyelonephritis, however, there is no previous history indicative of acute attacks, nor indeed of urinary infection at all. There is evidence that asymptomatic bacteriuria in early childhood is followed in some instances by chronic pyelonephritis. Any structural or functional abnormality of the urinary tract, but particularly vesico-ureteric reflux of urine (see below) and lesions which cause chronic or intermittent obstruction, predispose to infection and in these circumstances the infection tends to be severe, to extend to the kidneys causing pyelonephritis, and to be difficult to eradicate.

Causal organisms. Initial acute episodes of urinary tract infection are usually caused by *Escherichia coli* or, less commonly, other faecal bacteria (Enterococcus, Pseudomonas, *Strep. faecalis*, etc.), any of which is often obtained in the urine in pure culture. Patients with recurrent urinary infections, who have usually received previous antibiotic therapy and who may have been subjected to instrumentation of the lower urinary tract, commonly have a mixed infection of these various faecal bacteria.

Bacteriuria. This is not synonymous with urinary tract infection, for the normal distal urethral mucosa is populated by coliform bacilli, *Proteus*, staphylococci, *Strep. faecalis*, etc. These may be washed off the mucosa by the stream of urine and thus be detectable in the collected sample; alternatively they may be carried into the bladder by a catheter or cystoscope and the 'catheter specimen' of urine may similarly contain bacteria. In neither instance is there a urinary tract infection although bacterial cultures of the urine will be positive. It is therefore necessary to assess the importance of bacteriuric states. Experience has shown that bacterial counts of over 100 000 organisms per ml. of urine usually indicate urinary tract infection but that counts of less than this number can result from contamination.

Asymptomatic bacteriuria. This implies significant bacteriuria in the absence of symptoms of urinary tract infection. It is encountered in approximately 1 per cent of healthy schoolgirls, only about one-quarter of whom have a history suggestive of a previous urinary tract infection. Tests on younger children suggest that bacteriuria often develops before the age of 3 years. Follow-up studies indicate that some children with symptomless bacteriuria eventually develop chronic pyelonephritis (see below). Symptomless bacteriuria is especially frequent (about 5 per cent) in pregnant women, but fears that it is commonly followed by chronic pyelonephritis appear to be largely unfounded.

Recurrent or persistent infection. The number of individuals who die from acute pyelonephritis in this country is very small, and the chief danger now is the recurrent or smouldering chronic types of infection, for these are often related to the development of chronic pyelonephritis with ultimate renal failure. Serial studies have usually shown that repeated attacks of urinary tract infection in subjects without any obvious predisposing cause are due to different strains of bacteria, suggesting an abnormal susceptibility to re-infection. There is no doubt that urinary tract infections are more liable to arise when there is obstruction of the urinary tract, and unless the obstruction can be relieved the infection is often difficult to eradicate and liable to recur. However, investigation of patients with recurrent urinary tract infection has failed to demonstrate an obstructive lesion in most of them.

Pathogenesis

Pyelonephritis may result from bacteria reaching the kidney either by the bloodstream or by an ascending infection of the urinary tract.

Blood-borne infection occurs in acute pyaemia or septicaemia (Figs. 8.9, p. 201 and 8.10, p. 202), and this is seen as a complication of staphylococcal infections, e.g. boils and carbuncles. The bacteria normally present in the distal urethra can also gain entrance to the blood during surgical procedures upon the urethra: in these circumstances, the possibility of blood-borne infection of the kidneys is increased if the lesion which has required urethral surgery has also brought about urinary obstruction, e.g. urethral stricture or enlarged prostate (see below). Blood-borne infection is not, however, the cause of the majority of cases of pyelonephritis.

Ascending urinary tract infection. The commonest site of infection of the urinary tract is the bladder, and it is likely that cystitis is the predisposing factor in most cases of pyelonephritis. As already explained, most attacks of 'spontaneous' cystitis are caused by *Esch. coli*, whereas cystitis following catheterisation is commonly a mixed infection. In normal circumstances, the uretero-vesical valves are competent, and radiological studies have shown that **vesico-ureteric reflux**, i.e. reflux of urine from the bladder to the ureters, is uncommon, but when present as an apparently congenital condition, it may cause renal injury leading to scarring. *The association of bacteriuria and vesico-ureteric reflux in young children is a dangerous combination, and often causes chronic pyelonephritis leading to scarring before the age of 5 years. It is very important that this should be detected and treated, for renal injury is otherwise likely to progress and eventually cause chronic renal failure. It is, however, not practicable to screen for vesico-ureteric reflux, except in children found to have bacteriuria.* There is also evidence that vesico-ureteric reflux may develop as a result of cystitis. The detection of such reflux requires urography during micturition, which shows that bladder urine may pass as far as the renal pelves, thus explaining how infections ascend the urinary tract.

When pyelitis has developed, the bacteria may spread into the kidney directly by the lumina of the collecting tubules, or by passing from the submucosa of the inflamed calyces into the interstitial tissue of the renal papillae. Here they proliferate, and an acute inflammatory response occurs, often with abscess formation, eventually involving the adjacent tubular lumina. From here, infection can spread peripherally to the cortex (Fig. 22.57)

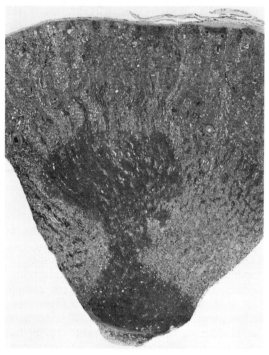

Fig. 22.57 Acute papillitis in pyelonephritis showing severe inflammatory infiltration of the renal papilla extending to the boundary zone. × 5.

via both the tubular lumina and the intertubular connective tissue spaces. Thus there develop linear streaks of suppuration with considerable tubular destruction. Since there is haphazard spread of bacteria from variably infected calyces, the renal lesion is not uniform and diffuse, but irregular and patchy. Significant bacteriuria can reflect inflammation at any level of the urinary tract and exact localisation is often clinically difficult. It is particularly important to determine whether or not bacterial inflammation has involved the renal parenchyma and two factors are often helpful in reaching such a conclusion. The first is the presence of a high titre of serum antibody to the bacterium cultured from the urine. If this is present renal involvement is highly probable. The second is the presence of cellular casts in the urine: pus cells in the urine (*pyuria*) can result from infection anywhere in the urinary tract, but their aggregation into cylindrical casts can only have happened in the renal tubules, thus indicating pyelonephritis.

Predisposing factors. *Vesico-ureteric reflux* is of major importance in the development of chronic pyelonephritis in early childhood (see above).

Urinary tract obstruction. Patients with an obstruction of the urinary tract are particularly liable to develop pyelonephritis, and this is attributable to four factors. Firstly, stagnant urine is a suitable culture medium for coliform and certain other bacteria which in normal circumstances would be washed out. Secondly, obstruction facilitates the upward spread of infection in the urinary tract by predisposing to vesico-ureteric reflux: this can occur intermittently even without gross structural change in the ureters, but in prolonged partial obstruction the ureters become permanently thickened and dilated, allowing free reflux to occur. Thirdly, there is convincing evidence that obstruction impairs the capacity of the kidneys to resist infection. Lastly, chronic urinary obstruction may cause uraemia, and thus lower the resistance to infections in general (p. 839).

Structural abnormalities of the urinary tract without obstruction also appear to predispose to infection.

In *diabetes mellitus*, there is a general susceptibility to infections, including cystitis, pyelitis and pyelonephritis (p. 184).

Age and sex. At all ages, the incidence of pyelonephritis, like urinary tract infections in general, is greater in females than in males. This may be due to the shorter, wider urethra and the turbulence of urethral flow, with peripheral eddying, in the female. As regards age, it is now firmly established that urinary tract infections, including symptomless bacteriuria, are more likely to be followed by chronic pyelonephritis when they occur in early childhood than in adult life.

Pregnancy produces a degree of ureteric dilatation and urinary stasis by virtue of the effect of the hormonal climate upon the musculature of the urinary tract and latterly the mechanical pressure of the enlarged uterus. Symptomless bacteriuria in early pregnancy is often followed by acute pyelonephritis later in pregnancy, but there is little evidence that it predisposes to chronic pyelonephritis. *Chronic hypokalaemia, gout,* and the ingestion of excessive amounts of *analgesics* (p. 845) over a long period can all produce renal histopathology similar to bacterial-induced chronic pyelonephritis. Accordingly, these conditions should be kept in mind in the differential diagnosis on chronic pyelonephritis in renal biopsy material.

Incidence

Acute pyelonephritis is a not uncommon disease in young females, including children, and is especially liable to occur during pregnancy. It is less frequent in the male unless there is a pre-existing urinary tract obstruction. The frequency of chronic pyelonephritis is very difficult to assess. Incidences as high as 15 per cent have been reported in general hospital necropsies, but this usually includes cases in which a few cortical scars are present as an incidental finding in otherwise normal kidneys. If the necropsy diagnosis is limited to those cases with severe chronic pyelonephritis, likely to have been of clinical significance, then the incidence is of the order of 1 per cent.

Pathological changes

Acute pyelonephritis

This consists of acute suppurative inflammation of the pelvis, calyces and parts of the kidneys, with pale linear streaks of suppuration bordered by a red rim of congestion, extending radially from the tips of the papillae to the surface of the cortex (Figs. 22.58, 22.59) where adjacent lesions may fuse to produce extensive abscesses. Microscopically, all the features typical of acute inflammation are present in the pelvis, calyces and kidney. Within the kidney the suppurating lesions cause very extensive but focal tubular destruction. In the cortex there is remarkable sparing of glomeruli and large blood vessels, even when these structures are directly surrounded by intense acute interstitial inflammation. All of these changes tend to be more florid and more extensive if there is obstruction in the lower urinary tract. Obstructed cases often, and very intensely inflamed non-obstructed cases sometimes, develop papillary necrosis (p. 845).

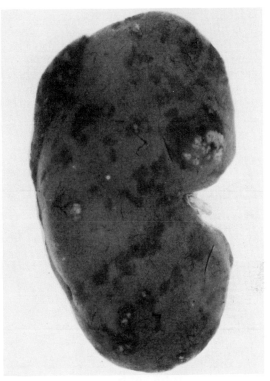

Fig. 22.58 Surface view of child's kidney in acute pyelonephritis, showing small abscesses and areas of haemorrhage. × 1.

Chronic pyelonephritis

The naked eye appearances of the kidney, calyces, and renal pelvis are of paramount importance in the differentiation of chronic pyelonephritic shrinkage from other varieties of scarred kidneys. The pelvic and calyceal walls are usually thickened and their mucosa may be either granular or atrophic: they are always distorted by scarring of the pyramids and the calyces are usually dilated (Fig. 22.60). Pyelography is therefore of great diagnostic value. The kidney is reduced in size and shows irregular patchy contraction in which the pyelonephritic process has largely destroyed the parenchyma and led to focal scarring and shrinkage. The intervening parenchyma may be normal or may show the changes of hypertension. The cortical surface is depressed over the contracted areas, the cortex and medulla both being consistently narrowed. The cortical surface depressions tend in most instances to be shallower than those produced by ischaemia but they may be very similar, and *the single*

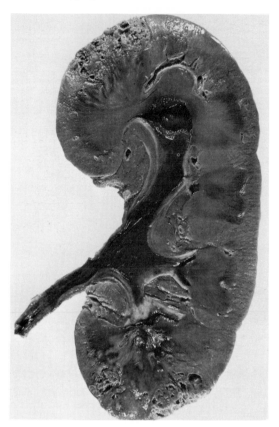

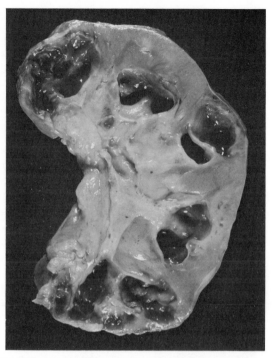

Fig. 22.60 Chronic pyelonephritis, showing dilatation and distortion of the calyces, over some of which the kidney tissue has been largely destroyed and now consists of a thin fibrous layer.

Fig. 22.59 Acute pyelonephritis. In this case the lesions are at the upper and lower poles. Note the cortical abscesses and the streaks of suppuration in the medulla. Note also the acutely inflamed pelvis and ureter.

most important diagnostic feature of the pyelonephritic scar is its close relationship to a deformed calyx. Microscopically the pelvic and calyceal mucosa may be thickened by granulation tissue and infiltrated by lymphocytes, plasma cells and polymorphs; lymphoid follicles sometimes form and are often responsible for the surface granularity of the mucosa. When the inflammation is florid, the surface epithelium may be lost, the pelves and calyces then being lined by granulation tissue. In cases where the inflammation has subsided, the walls of the pelvis and calyces are atrophic with some scarring.

As explained later, chronic pyelonephritic scarring may vary in extent from involvement of only a small proportion of the renal tissue to extensive renal destruction. When of lesser extent, it is usually an incidental finding at necropsy.

The scarred areas. There is extensive atrophy and loss of tubules, especially the proximal segments (Fig. 22.61), and this is a most important histological feature of chronic pyelonephritis. Tubular atrophy is often accompanied by gross thickening of the tubular basement membranes, and there is increase in fibrous tissue between the tubules. Commonly partial destruction of tubules results in survival of isolated segments; these become distended with inspissated eosinophilic secretion (presumably produced by the lining epithelium), and the epithelium becomes flattened: these changes occur in groups of adjacent tubules which come to resemble superficially thyroid acini (Fig. 22.62). The interstitial tissue is densely packed with lymphocytes, plasma cells and sometimes neutrophil and eosinophil polymorphs: in the late stages of the disease the inflammatory cell infiltrate is replaced by dense scar tissue. In such 'burnt out' pyelonephritis, there may be little evidence of active inflammation. The glomeruli are preserved for a very long time but eventually a spectrum of glomerular abnormalities appears,

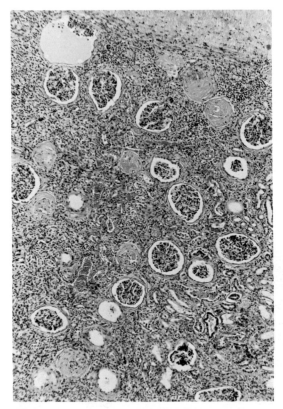

Fig. 22.61 Chronic pyelonephritis. The tubules are greatly atrophied and there is a marked interstitial inflammatory cell infiltrate. Many of the glomeruli still appear normal, but others are completely hyalinised. × 38.

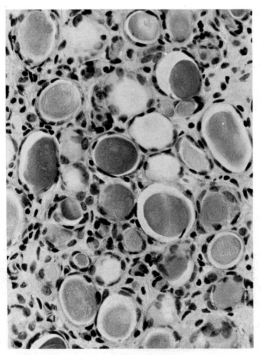

Fig. 22.62 Chronic pyelonephritis. Inspissated colloid-like material in sequestrated portions of renal tubules, presenting an appearance resembling superficially that of thyroid tissue. × 250.

the most specific of which is concentric periglomerular fibrosis around a thickened Bowman's capsule (Fig. 22.63). Other changes are ischaemic and resemble those in essential hypertension: they include gradual hyalinisation of the glomerular tuft and fibrosis within Bowman's capsule (p. 810 and Fig. 22.61). At an earlier stage some capillary tufts may show irregular proliferation of endothelial and mesangial cells. Arteriolar and glomerular capillary necrosis occurs only if malignant hypertension has supervened. The arteries show variable degrees of medial and intimal fibrous thickening.

The non-scarred areas. The glomeruli may show compensatory hypertrophy. Other glomerular and vascular changes often develop as a result of arterial hypertension.

The pyelonephritic nature of small, irregularly scarred kidneys which histologically show no evidence of active bacterial infection is doubtful, and this doubt is increased by the frequent absence of any history suggestive of previous urinary tract infection.

Clinical features

Acute pyelonephritis is usually accompanied by acute infection of the lower urinary tract, i.e. cystitis, so that there is frequency of micturition and dysuria. The features of pyelonephritis itself include fever, often with rigors, and pain and tenderness in the lumbar regions. The urine is heavily infected and contains large numbers of pus cells and often red cells. Microscopy may reveal cellular casts in which most of the cells are polymorphs: this finding is of particular diagnostic importance, indicating pyelonephritis and not just lower urinary tract infection.

In chronic pyelonephritis there is, in most cases, no preceding history suggestive of urinary tract infection. There may be a long history of vague ill-health with, in children, reduced rate of growth. Commonly, however,

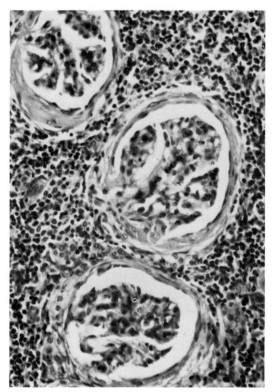

Fig. 22.63 Chronic pyelonephritis. There is periglomerular fibrosis, a heavy chronic inflammatory infiltrate, and almost complete loss of tubules. × 150.

the presenting features are attributable to the hypertension or uraemia of chronic renal failure. Depending on whether or not the infection is still active, the urine may contain significant numbers of bacteria (see above), pus cells and cellular casts. There is usually mild proteinuria. Perhaps because destruction of the tubules precedes that of the glomeruli, the urine tends to be of greater volume and more dilute than in chronic glomerulonephritis. Demonstration by intravenous pyelography of irregular coarse scarring and distortion of the calyces is particularly helpful in the diagnosis of chronic pyelonephritis.

Hypertension in chronic pyelonephritis. Approximately 70 per cent of patients with extensive chronic pyelonephritis develop hypertension, and in 15–20 per cent of these the hypertension is of the malignant type. There has been some controversy over the nature of the relationship between the two conditions, and it has been suggested that the association

might result from a predisposition of individuals with essential hypertension to develop pyelonephritis. We do not consider this a likely explanation, for it would not account for the occurrence of hypertension in young patients with chronic pyelonephritis. The obvious explanation is that chronic pyelonephritis, like other conditions giving rise to extensive scarring of the kidneys, commonly leads to hypertension of secondary (renal) type. Admittedly, the mechanism of production of the hypertension of chronic renal disease is not well understood (p. 375) but this seems no reason for doubting that it occurs in chronic pyelonephritis.

Tuberculous pyelonephritis

This results from blood spread of tubercle bacilli, e.g. from pulmonary lesions. Like other organs, the kidneys are studded with minute tubercles in acute miliary tuberculosis, but of more importance are the localised renal lesions of tuberculous pyelonephritis which may slowly extend to destroy the kidney(s). Other common sites of blood-borne metastatic tuberculous lesions in the genito-urinary tract are the epididymis in the male and the Fallopian tube in the female, and spread from these sites can give rise to tuberculosis of the bladder and ascending infection to involve the kidneys. Conversely, renal tuberculosis can spread to involve the ureters, bladder and other pelvic viscera.

Clinical features. Renal tuberculosis may produce vague illness, with weight loss and fever, or may present with local features such as lumbar pain, dysuria, haematuria or pyuria. *Myco. tuberculosis* can usually be detected in the urine, and pyelography may show distortion of one or more calyces. In most cases, there is neither evidence nor history of tuberculosis elsewhere in the body (although this must, of course, have been present), and even at necropsy active pulmonary tuberculosis is present in only a minority of cases. Renal tuberculosis occurs usually in adult life, and it may be that, as in the lungs, it can remain latent for many years and then flare up: this would account for its occurrence long after any primary lung lesion has healed.

The incidence of renal tuberculosis in Europe has declined along with tuberculosis in general, and it is now a rather uncommon condition: its main danger is the involvement of both kidneys to such an extent as to cause renal failure.

Pathological changes. The initial renal lesion results usually from blood-borne infection, mycobacteria becoming arrested in the cortex, with development of one or more tubercles: these enlarge, caseate and coalesce, while lymphatic and tubular spread leads to tubercles round about, and so the lesion grows as an enlarging patch of caseation. Spread through the adjacent papilla is common, and on reaching the renal pelvis the lesion may soften and discharge its contents, leaving a ragged cavity. Further tubercles develop in the walls of the renal pelvis caseate and ulcerate; from here infection spreads into other parts of the kidney, which may then develop multiple caseous lesions (Figs. 22.64, 22.65). The ureter or renal pelvis may become obstructed by tuberculous lesions in their walls, or by plugging with caseous material, and the urine (coming solely from the other kidney) may then be normal. Apart from this, renal pelvic involvement often results in haematuria and the renal lesions tend also to suppurate, giving pyuria.

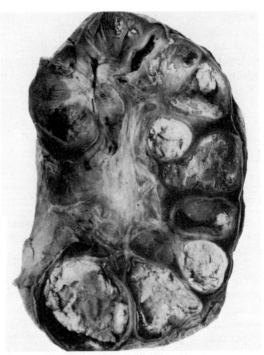

Fig. 22.65 Old tuberculosis of kidney, which has been largely replaced by caseous lesions enclosed by fibrous tissue.

Cytomegalovirus disease

This occurs in newborn infants as a localised or generalised condition, and also as an opportunistic infection at all ages in subjects with various forms of immunodeficiency or being

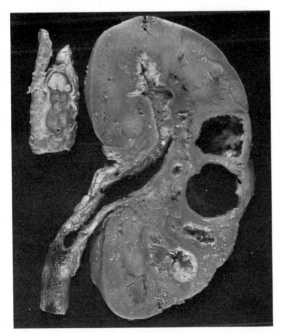

Fig. 22.64 Renal tuberculosis. The kidney contains several caseous lesions, which have discharged into the pelvis. The wall of the uppermost calyx is also caseous and the ureter and seminal vesicle (*inset*) are also involved.

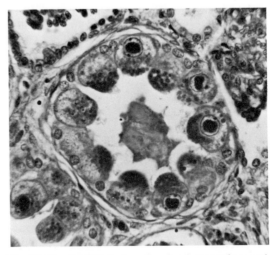

Fig. 22.66 Renal tubules, showing intranuclear and cytoplasmic inclusion bodies in the lining cells in cytomegalovirus disease in an infant. × 400.

treated with immunosuppressive drugs. Involvement of the liver and bone marrow in infants may cause changes resembling those of erythroblastosis fetalis. Serological evidence of infection has been reported in over 50 per cent of renal transplant patients. Colonised cells become greatly enlarged and often show nuclear or cytoplasmic inclusions (Fig. 22.66). Involvement of the renal tubules does not appear to have much affect on function but may allow the diagnosis to be made by detection of colonised cells in the urine.

Congenital Lesions

Congenital cystic kidneys

This occurs in two main forms, one of which does not usually cause illness until middle-age, while the other is usually fatal in infancy.

Adult polycystic disease is the least rare form of congenital cystic renal disease. The kidneys contain large numbers of cysts which enlarge throughout life. Rarely death from renal failure occurs in infancy or childhood, but more than 50 per cent of patients present in the 3rd to 5th decades with symptoms due to hypertension or uraemia, and most of the remainder die of unrelated causes.

In adult patients, the kidneys are greatly enlarged and occupied by numerous cysts of various sizes, while little kidney substance may be recognisable between the cysts. Prolonged survival presupposes, of course, the presence of enough functioning renal tissue, but this is gradually compressed by the slowly-enlarging cysts and secondary hypertension or chronic renal failure develops. Each kidney may weigh 1 kg or even more (Fig. 22.67) and be easily palpable. The cysts may be of any size up to 4–6 cm in diameter; they usually contain serous fluid, colourless or brownish, though it may be mucoid, especially in the smaller cysts. Occasionally the cystic change is practically restricted to one kidney. The condition may be the result of disturbance of normal development due to imperfect fusion between the kidney tubules proper and the collecting tubules, which grow up from the extremity of the ureter to meet them, but other embryological explanations have been proposed. The condition is inherited as an autosomal dominant trait, and there may be accompanying cystic change in the liver, although not sufficient to disturb hepatic function. There is also an association with aneurysms of the cerebral

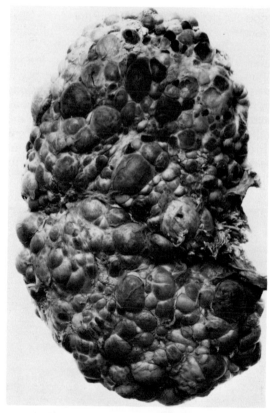

Fig. 22.67 Surface view of congenital cystic kidney, which weighed 1·5 kg.

arteries, and about 15 per cent of patients with polycystic kidneys die from subarachnoid haemorrhage.

Lesser degrees of cystic change are common in the kidneys, ranging from a few to many cysts, but with sufficient tissue remaining to avert renal failure. Occasionally a single cyst may reach such a size as to be palpable during life.

Infantile polycystic disease is rare and usually causes death shortly after birth. It may be due to an autosomal recessive trait. The kidneys contain multiple elongated radially arranged cysts lined by cuboidal or columnar epithelium. Renal enlargement may be sufficient to interfere with birth or, in live-born infants, with respiration. Occasional patients survive longer and develop fatal hypertension in childhood. The condition is associated with multiple hepatic cysts or abnormalities of the small bile ducts in the portal areas.

Sponge kidney (medullary cystic) disease consists of cystic dilatation of the collecting ducts in the papillae. It is usually bilateral and may affect any or all of the papillae in each kidney. Symptoms usually develop after the age of 30, and are due to the formation of stones composed of calcium salts in the cysts or to superadded pyelonephritis. The cysts are usually less than 5 mm in diameter and their epithelial lining may be single layered or squamous. The diagnosis may be apparent from intravenous pyelograms. The cause of this condition is unknown and its congenital nature uncertain.

There are now known to be several types of inherited congenital cystic disorders of the kidney, some of which can be detected *in utero* by ultrasonography. It is important to distinguish these from **congenital renal dysplasia**, which is not inherited, and in which abnormal mesenchymal tissues (cartilage, smooth muscle, etc.) develop in the kidneys.

Other congenital defects

These are numerous and some are comparatively common. Occasionally one kidney, usually the left, is absent—*agenesis*—and there is generally an absence of the ureter also. In such cases, the surviving kidney undergoes compensatory hypertrophy, and its weight may sometimes double: this occurs also in *hypoplasia* of one kidney, which appears usually as an irregular atrophic structure around the upper end of its ureter. Hypoplasia of both kidneys may occur to such a degree as to be incompatible with life; minor degrees of the condition may possibly lead to renal dwarfism. Sometimes the two kidneys are fused, and this most frequently occurs at the lower pole, so that the '*horseshoe kidney*' results: the pelves are directed somewhat forward and the two ureters pass in front of the connecting bridge. In rarer forms the fusion of the kidneys is more complete and an oval or somewhat irregular kidney results, which varies in position. Occasionally a kidney, more rarely both, may lie in front of the sacrum: its ureter is correspondingly short and the arterial blood supply comes from the lower end of the aorta or an adjacent large branch. In these various renal abnormalities the position of the adrenals is usually quite normal. The kidney is originally composed of five lobules and ordinarily their fusion is complete. Sometimes slight grooves on the surface mark the original lobules and the term *fetal lobulation* is applied; the condition is of no importance. The arrangement of the renal arteries is very variable. Division of a so-called accessory artery is likely to be followed by infarction of the tissue supplied by it.

Tumours

Benign tumours

These are not very rare, the commonest being a small *fibroma* in the medulla; it rarely reaches 1 cm in diameter. *Adenomas* occasionally occur, usually in the cortex, and some have a characteristic appearance with narrow bands of stroma and papilliform ingrowths (Fig. 22.68). They are usually benign, but carcinoma may supervene. In the renal pelvis *villous papillary tumours* are sometimes seen; they correspond to the papillary tumours of the bladder (p. 870) and are sometimes associated with them. *Angioma* is another uncommon benign tumour. It may occur in the pyramids or just underneath the lining of the pelvis, and, even when small, may lead to severe haematuria.

Malignant tumours

Malignant tumours are much less common in the kidneys than in several other organs, but two are of importance—*renal carcinoma* and *nephroblastoma*.

Renal carcinoma

Clear-cell carcinoma is the commonest type. It was formerly called *Grawitz tumour* or *hypernephroma*. This last term was based on a superficial resemblance of this type of tumour to adrenal tissue, which led Grawitz to suggest that it arose from adrenocortical tissue misplaced within the kidneys. However, it is now widely accepted that it originates from renal

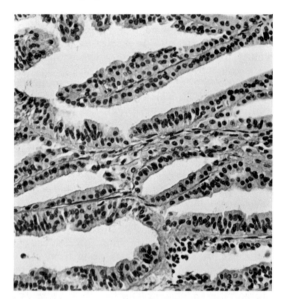

Fig. 22.68 Papillary adenoma of kidney, showing the delicate stroma and the appearances of the epithelium. × 140.

tubular epithelium, and accordingly the term hypernephroma is a misnomer.

Clear-cell carcinoma is often large, and may occasionally form an enormous mass. It may occur in any part of the kidney. On section, there are usually large areas of dull yellowish tissue (presenting a superficial resemblance to the adrenal cortex), interspersed with vascular, haemorrhagic and necrotic areas, and also broad bands and patches of connective tissue, somewhat mucoid or translucent in appearance (Fig. 22.69). Although the tumour may often appear to be encapsulated, like a benign tumour, it shows distinctly malignant properties. It commonly grows into the tributaries of the renal vein and forms thrombus-like masses within them; metastases may follow, especially in the lungs and bones. It may also burst through the capsule of the kidney or into the pelvis. Haematuria is common and often a prominent symptom.

On microscopic examination, such a tumour has, as a rule, a distinctly acinous arrangement in many parts, the spaces being lined by tall columnar epithelial cells: a papilliform type of growth also is sometimes present, and in other parts the arrangement of the epithelium is in solid masses. The tumour cells are large and often remarkably uniform, with abundant clear cytoplasm (Fig. 22.70) rich in glycogen and

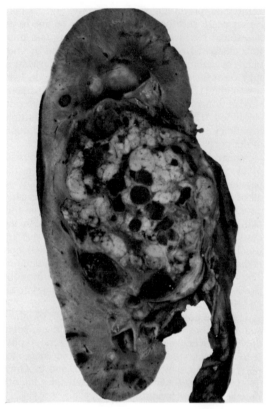

Fig. 22.69 Clear-cell carcinoma of kidney, growing from the central part of the kidney and compressing the renal pelvis. Note the haemorrhagic and gelatinous areas and rounded nodules of whitish tumour.

doubly-refracting lipid, and a relatively small round nucleus. There may, however, be greater variation in the cells, which may have an eosinophilic cytoplasm, or may be smaller and more anaplastic. As in other tumours, the prognosis depends on the degree of anaplasia, and invasion of the renal vein is not incompatible with long survival.

Tumours of purely adenocarcinomatous pattern occasionally occur in the kidney and papillary adenocarcinoma may arise both in the renal substance and in the pelvis, the two types being, however, quite distinct. In some renal carcinomas the cytoplasm of the tumour cells contains large homogeneous acidophil inclusions.

Papillary cystadenocarcinoma. This is a rather uncommon type of renal carcinoma: it consists of numerous cysts containing papillary processes, the stroma of which is often packed with foamy lipid-rich macrophages. It tends to

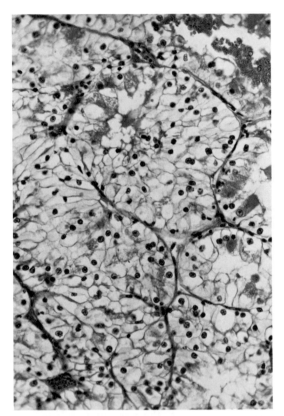

Fig. 22.70 Clear-cell carcinoma of kidney, showing typical empty-looking cells with well-defined walls and delicate stroma. × 205.

invade the regional lymph nodes, and carries a prognosis similar to that of clear-cell carcinoma.

Nephroblastoma is an embryonic tumour, which has the general appearance of a rapidly growing sarcoma. It may reach a large size and, though fairly well enclosed within the kidney capsule, rapidly invades blood vessels and so produces metastases, chiefly in the lungs. It occurs especially in the first three years of life, and is known also as 'embryoma', 'mixed tumour' or 'Wilms' tumour' of the kidney. Although rare, it is one of the commonest malignant tumours in childhood.

Microscopically, the tumour is composed of a spindle-celled tissue, with formation of acini and tubular structures, and apparent transitions may be seen between the spindle cells and those of epithelial type (Fig. 22.71). There may also be imperfect formation of glomeruli. This tumour is derived from the cells of the kidney rudiment. In some instances it has a more complicated structure, striped muscle fibres being present, and the tumour may have originated from cells of the mesoderm before the differentiation of the myotomes.

Spindle-cell sarcoma is a rare renal tumour.

Secondary carcinoma in the kidneys is not uncommon, although metastases are neither as frequent nor as numerous as might be expected in view of the very large blood supply of the kidneys.

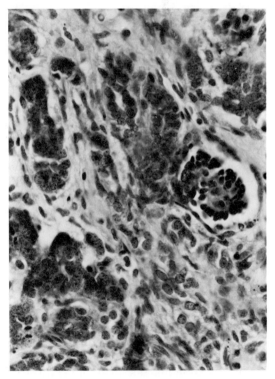

Fig. 22.71 Nephroblastoma, showing spindle-shaped tumour cells and differentiation into imperfect tubules and glomeruli. × 275.

Renal Pelves, Ureters and Bladder

The lesions of these structures are considered together, as they are so often involved in the same pathological process. Three main factors are concerned in the majority of these lesions, viz. (*a*) *obstruction to urinary flow*, (*b*) *infections* and (*c*) the *formation of stones*. Two or even all three of these conditions may be present at the same time. *Epithelial tumours* of the urinary tract are not uncommon and are mostly malignant, although often low grade.

Effects of obstruction

Serious mechanical obstruction to outflow of urine from the bladder is practically confined to the male sex, and is commonly produced by enlargement of the prostate or stricture of the urethra: occasionally severe phimosis, tumour or calculus are responsible. The chief effect on the bladder is the production of variable degrees of hypertrophy and dilatation. When the outstanding feature is hypertrophy, the muscular part of the wall is thickened and the bands of muscle, which have an interlacing arrangement under the mucosa, enlarge and form prominent ridges or bands with depressions between (Fig. 25.3, p. 992). Occasionally one of these depressions may become enlarged and form a large projecting diverticulum. When infection occurs, as is so often the case, pus may collect in such diverticula, and ulceration and even perforation may follow. Obstruction to the outflow from the bladder ultimately leads to dilatation of the ureters and pelves of the kidneys. The former may undergo considerable dilatation and their walls become somewhat thickened, and the pelves also become enlarged, so that there is a condition of bilateral hydronephrosis. The dilatation is sometimes more marked on one side than on the other.

Hydronephrosis

This means a dilatation of the renal pelvis and may occur on one or both sides.

Causation. Urethral obstruction, referred to above, is the commonest cause of **bilateral hydronephrosis**. It can result also from pressure of a tumour, or neoplastic infiltration, affecting both ureters. Such infiltration occurs commonly, for example, in cancer of the cervix uteri. Occasionally dilatation of the ureters and hydronephrosis are due to congenital abnormality in the posterior urethra, the mucosa of which forms valve-like folds; the resulting hydronephrosis may be accompanied by renal dwarfism (p. 839). Another cause of bilateral hydroureter and hydronephrosis is neurogenic disturbance of bladder control due to lesions of the spinal cord. In all these conditions of bilateral hydronephrosis the dilatation of the ureters and pelves is usually moderate. The most striking degree of dilatation is seen, however, in **unilateral hydronephrosis**. This can result from impaction of a calculus, usually at the upper end of the ureter, at the level of the brim of the pelvis, or at the entrance to the bladder. It may be produced also by a scar, which sometimes follows ulceration due to the passage of a stone, by a tumour of the ureter itself, or pressure of a tumour from outside. In many instances of unilateral hydronephrosis there is a severe narrowing of the ureter, usually just below the pelvi-ureteric junction, but without scarring. The cause of this is unknown; it may represent a congenital structural abnormality or result from some form of neuro-muscular dysfunction. As the renal pelvis dilates the ureter may become kinked at its origin, thus aggravating the obstruction. Kinking of the ureter by an aberrant renal artery to the lower pole of the kidney sometimes appears to be a convincing cause of hydronephrosis (Fig. 22.72), but often the ureter shows the non-scarred stricture described above, and kinking over the artery may occur *after* hydronephrosis has developed. Hydronephrosis is also observed occasionally in congenitally misplaced kidneys.

Structural changes. The effects of obstruction vary greatly. Sometimes a calculus may be firmly impacted, and there may be obvious distension of the pelvis and calyces (Fig. 22.73), or the whole pelvis and calyces may be distended by a branching calculus, though this is more common when infection has been superadded (p. 866). In such cases, fibrosis and atrophy of the kidney follow. In other cases, distension is so great that the dilated pelvis may become pal-

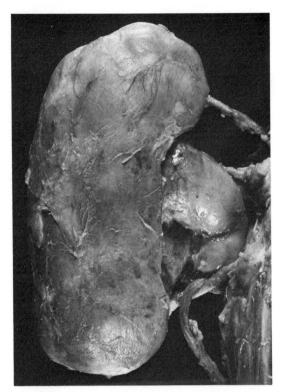

Fig. 22.72 Hydronephrosis with bending of the ureter around an accessory renal artery to the lower pole of the kidney.

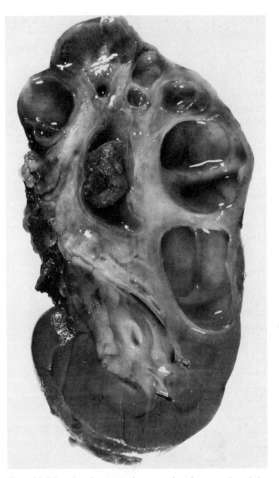

Fig. 22.73 An impacted stone in the renal pelvis, which has caused hydronephrosis and consequent atrophy of the renal tissue. The stone was in such a position that the lower part of the pelvis was not obstructed, and the lower pole of the kidney appears normal.

pable. As the distension progresses the calyces become flattened, the kidney substance becomes stretched over the dilated pelvis and ultimately may form a mere rind (*intrarenal hydronephrosis*) and the surface of the kidney usually develops a lobulated appearance. Atrophy of the kidney substance may be regular or irregular, so that parts of considerable thickness may be left while the rest is much thinned; the latter result apparently depends on the degree to which the vascular supply is impaired, and the microscopic appearances resemble those resulting from major artery stenosis, i.e. the glomeruli are relatively spared, but the tubules are atrophied. Sometimes the dilatation is mainly in the form of a sac projecting medial to the kidney and there is little effect on the appearance of the kidney—*extrarenal hydronephrosis*.

The results of obstruction of a ureter vary greatly. If it is sudden, complete and persistent, production of urine ceases almost immediately and the pelvis does not dilate very much. This

may result from impaction of a stone. If, however, obstruction develops gradually, or is partial or intermittent, the kidney continues to produce urine and the urinary tract above the obstruction becomes greatly dilated. This may result from pressure of, or infiltration by, a tumour, from movement of a stone or from a stricture or kinking of the ureter over a renal artery. When the kidney becomes greatly stretched and thinned, the tubules, and ultimately the glomeruli, become atrophied, and there ensues general overgrowth of the connective tissue. The contents of a dilated pelvis are, of course, at first urine; but, as the condition becomes chronic, the urinary constituents disappear, while proteins are added to the fluid by transudation from the wall of the sac.

Urinary tract infection

The commonest serious complication of urinary tract infection is extension to the kidneys, and accordingly the subject has already been discussed in the account of pyelonephritis (pp. 852–9). The main features of urinary tract infection are as follows:

(1) Normal urine is often contaminated by bacteria living in the lower urethra: normally, there are fewer than 100 000 bacteria per ml of urine, and greater numbers are suggestive of infection.

(2) Infection is much commoner in females of all ages than in males, possibly due to the shorter, wide female urethra.

(3) Infection is especially common in pregnancy because of the hormonal relaxation of smooth muscle and the pressure of the uterus on the urinary tract.

(4) Most infections are caused by bacteria gaining entrance to the bladder via the urethra, and the renal pelves may be involved, spread being either intra-luminal or in the interstitial tissue of the urinary tract.

(5) In the presence of cystitis, reflux of urine from bladder to ureters is likely to promote ascending infection which, in young children, is the major cause of chronic pyelonephritis.

(6) In patients without urinary tract obstruction, who have not been subjected to catheterisation or other instrumentation, urinary tract infections are usually caused by *Escherichia coli*. With obstruction or following instrumentation, mixed infections, including coliform bacilli, *Proteus* and staphylococci, are common.

(7) Urinary tract obstruction, including neurogenic disturbances of bladder control, is of major importance in predisposing to, enhancing and prolonging infection, and promoting its spread. This is especially so when the obstruction is chronic and has resulted in ureteric dilatation.

(8) Once infection has involved the renal pelves and calyces (pyelitis), direct spread into the renal papillae can occur, leading to pyelonephritis.

(9) Chronic infection, especially with *Proteus*, predisposes to formation of phosphate deposits

in the urinary tract by splitting urea and thus rendering the urine alkaline: the deposits can both obstruct the flow of urine and enhance the infection.

In the early stages of an acute urinary infection, the urine may contain a heavy concentration of bacteria with few cells, but pus cells soon appear; in some instances there may be sufficient haemorrhage from the inflamed mucosa to present clinically as haematuria.

The morbid anatomical changes in **cystitis** are usually classified as catarrhal, purulent and pseudo-membranous. Pseudo-membranous cystitis is found chiefly in association with chronic obstruction and hypertrophy of the bladder; there is superficial necrosis of the mucosa with fibrinous exudate, especially over the muscular ridges, and the necrotic mucosa is sloughed off in decomposing shreds. The most severe changes are usually observed when there is alkaline decomposition of the urine. Haemorrhages into the mucosa are common, and these may become greenish and almost black, while the surface is covered with pus and often a deposit of phosphates. Such an infection may ascend the dilated ureters, and produce a pyelitis with similar features, and the dilated pelvis may become ulcerated or filled with an accumulation of pus—**pyonephrosis**. Here also secondary deposit of phosphates may occur. Inevitably the infection extends to the kidneys and gives rise to pyelonephritis. Often only one pelvis is affected in this way, but both may be involved.

Pyonephrosis also arises when a hydronephrosis due to a calculus in the renal pelvis becomes infected. The presence of a renal calculus seems to predispose the pelvis to infection, and this leads in turn to alkaline decomposition of the urine. Phosphates are precipitated in the dilated pelvis and calyces and particularly on the pre-existing calculus, which develops into an irregular branching mass with bulbous ends extending into the calyces, the whole forming a rough cast of the pyonephrotic sac. This is known as a *staghorn calculus* (Fig. 22.75).

The urinary tract is not infrequently infected from the kidney by *typhoid bacilli* in the course of typhoid fever. Usually only a mild catarrhal inflammation is the result, and the condition may be almost a pure bacilluria. The bacilli may persist indefinitely, the patient becoming a 'urinary carrier' (p. 632); the establishment of the carrier state is facilitated by almost any anatomical abnormality in the urinary tract. In some cases of coliform infection also, there may be comparatively little inflammatory reaction. Cystitis may rarely be produced by the gonococcus in cases of *gonorrhoea*, and has usually the features of purulent catarrh. Coliform bacilli and the gonococcus do not render the urine alkaline, but infection by *Proteus* is quickly followed by ammoniacal decomposition owing to splitting of urea.

Malakoplakia. This is a rare condition found in some cases of chronic cystitis, and is characterised by the formation of numerous soft rounded elevations or plaques in the bladder wall, varying up to 1–2 cm. They have a pale, sometimes yellowish appearance surrounded by vascular areas, and tend to ulcerate on the surface and be invaded by bacteria. They are essentially composed of cellular granulation tissue in which there are numerous large cells which contain granules of various kinds and small hyaline spheres with concentric marking known as Michaelis–Gutmann bodies. These inclusions give a positive PAS-staining reaction: calcium salts may be deposited in them and they also stain positively for iron. The lesions are infiltrated with lymphocytes and plasma cells. Although it is clearly granulomatous, the cause of this condition is unknown.

Tuberculosis. Tuberculous disease of the bladder is, as a rule, the result of direct infection of its mucosa by tubercle bacilli in the urine. It occurs most often in cases of renal tuberculosis, though also in tuberculosis of the genital tract. The bacilli invade the mucosa and give rise to tubercles which then undergo ulceration. In this way, multiple small ulcers are formed, especially at the base of the bladder, and sometimes the orifices of the ureters are specially involved. The ulcers increase in size and form large areas by confluence. Sometimes there is a considerable amount of caseous thickening of the lining. Secondary invasion by other organisms sometimes occurs, and more acute inflammatory change is superadded.

Schistosomiasis (bilharziasis). The bladder is the most frequent site of lesions in this condition, which is caused by *Schistosoma haematobium*. It is very common in many hot countries, notably in Egypt. The adult parasites lie in the veins of the bladder, and the eggs laid by the female pass into the surrounding tissues, where their presence in large numbers induces the formation of abundant vascular granulation tissue which causes great thickening of the mucosa and submucosa. Nodular projections appear, and the interior of the bladder may be beset with rounded and somewhat pedunculated vascular polypi, which tend to become ulcerated. Haematuria is a common feature and the ova are readily found in the urine. Pyogenic infections may become superadded, and carcinoma develops in a proportion of cases in Egyptians, but very rarely in infected Europeans. Schistosomal lesions sometimes occur also in the ureters and renal pelves.

Schistosoma haematobium is a dioecious trematode. The adult male is about 13 mm long, the female about 20 mm; the female is thinner, and lies enclosed in the gynaecophoric canal of the male. The eggs are oval in form, about 130μm in length, and the shell has a distinct terminal spine; the embryo is visible within. When the urine becomes diluted on being mixed with water, the investing shell swells and bursts and a ciliated embryo or miracidium escapes. Further developmental stages take place within fresh-water snails, from which the free-swimming cercariae emerge: these enter the human host, chiefly through the skin but also through the mucous membrane of the mouth and pharynx. They pass by systemic veins to the lungs, through the pulmonary capillaries, and thence to the systemic arteries via the heart. Those reaching the liver mature into adult worms within the portal vessels. The young adults then pass against the blood stream to the portal radicles, especially those of the inferior mesenteric vein, and thence they reach the vesical plexus, where they settle and pair as described above. Occasionally the parasite remains in the liver and the eggs are discharged into the peri-portal connective tissue and give rise to hepatic fibrosis (p. 698). There are two other pathogenic species of schistosoma, *S. mansoni* and *S. japonicum*: they have similar life cycles to *S. haematobium*. The adult *S. mansoni* colonises the veins of the colon (p. 637), and *S. japonicum*, which occurs in the Far East, the veins of the small intestine. The ova of both species cause granulomatous reactions in the gut, with ulceration and melaena, and they may also colonise the liver, producing periportal fibrosis: the ova are found in the faeces.

Ureteritis cystica. Inflammation of the urinary tract may be followed by formation of multiple small cysts which contain clear fluid and project into the lumen (Fig. 22.74). Apparently foci of epithelium become sequestrated deep to the surface and form these cysts. The change occurs also in the renal pelves and bladder (*pyelitis* and *cystitis cystica*).

Calculi

Urinary calculi are formed by precipitation of urinary constituents, a small amount of organic

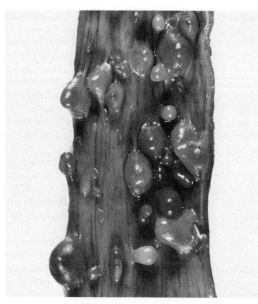

Fig. 22.74 Ureteritis cystica. The thin-walled cysts have formed in sequestered epithelium, but as they enlarged have come to project into the lumen. × 3.

material also being incorporated. Deposition is favoured by a highly concentrated urine, and by secretion of excessive amounts of one or other constituents (oxalate, urate, etc.). Calculi occur in the renal pelvis or ureter, or in the bladder, although some of the latter originate in the kidneys, and subsequently enlarge in the bladder.

There are 3 main types of urinary calculus composed respectively of (*a*) a mixture of uric acid and urates—uric acid stones, (*b*) calcium oxalate: both (*a*) and (*b*) are laid down in acid urines and stones may contain a mixture of both substances; (*c*) calcium carbonate and phosphate combined in the complex forms of carbonate-apatite and hydroxyapatite; these are laid down in alkaline urines and often form an outer laminated deposit upon other stones.

The commonest pure type of stone consists of calcium oxalate whereas only 6 per cent are of uric acid. Most stones consist principally of the apatites but contain also some oxalate and urate. It has long been supposed that calculi begin as minute deposits in the collecting tubules of the kidney and then pass to the pelvis where further increase in size takes place. Randall has shown that some stones develop by enlargement of plaque-like deposits attached to the apices of the pyramids. Carr has sug-

gested from radiographic evidence that the primary site of deposition is in the lymphatics of the renal papillae that normally remove particulate matter from this region. If this mechanism is overloaded or if the lymphatic pathway is obstructed by inflammation of the papilla, microliths accumulate and are extruded through the lymphatic lining into the calyx where they grow into small concretions by further deposition of urinary solids. The part in stone formation played by organic matter is uncertain, but Boyce and his co-workers have suggested that urinary mucoproteins attract and fix calcium ions which later, as a result of alterations of pH, are precipitated as crystalline salts to form the nuclei of stones: all the calcium-rich calculi except pure oxalate stones have a mucopolysaccharide binding agent. An increase in the urinary excretion of a particular substance is usually an important factor, as, for example, in hyperparathyroidism, where the increased excretion of calcium and phosphate in the urine very frequently leads to the formation of urinary calculi of the apatite variety.

Renal calculi. Stones in the renal pelvis may be single or multiple. They are sometimes particularly numerous when there is partial obstruction and dilatation. A single calculus may, however, grow to the size and shape of the dilated pelvis (Fig. 22.75).

A small calculus may pass along the ureter to the bladder, giving rise to renal colic with haematuria. It may be arrested temporarily, usually at the narrow lower end of the ureter. Permanent impaction, usually at the upper or lower ends of the ureter or at the level of the pelvic brim, produces hydronephrosis as already described, and when the obstruction is intermittent the hydronephrosis may be extreme. When the urine is infected with urea-splitting bacteria (e.g. *Proteus*) ammonia is produced and calculi or softer deposits composed of phosphates form in the alkaline urine and are precipitated in the inflamed pelvis. The condition may be accompanied by suppuration and ulceration. The large branching 'staghorn' calculi arise in this way and are composed largely of complex hydrated phosphates. A calculus in the renal pelvis, especially when it is movable, may give rise to metaplasia of the lining of the pelvis to stratified squamous epithelium. As a further result of the irritation, squamous carcinoma has occasionally

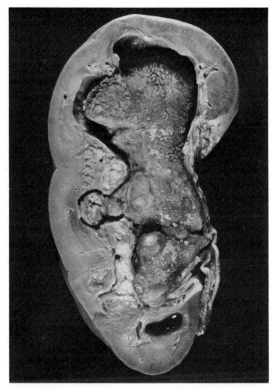

Fig. 22.75 A large 'staghorn' calculus occupying the dilated renal pelvis and calyces.

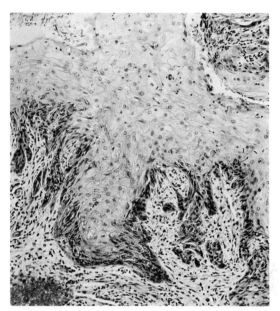

Fig. 22.76 Section through the renal pelvis in nephrolithiasis, showing squamous metaplasia of epithelium and early squamous carcinoma. × 65.

been found to arise, as is illustrated in Fig. 22.76.

Precipitation of sulphonamide drugs may occur in the renal tubules and pelvis unless the fluid intake is maintained at a high level to promote diuresis. If this is neglected, actual obstruction of tubules, pelves and ureters may result from masses of crystals of the drug or its acetylated form. Acute renal failure from this cause was encountered in the early days of sulphonamide therapy.

Bladder calculi may be single or multiple: they are sometimes numerous and like coarse sand. They are now relatively uncommon in Europe. In many cases calculi form first in the renal pelvis, especially uric-acid and oxalate calculi, and pass to the bladder where they increase in size; in other cases they are formed locally. The larger calculi vary greatly in composition and structure, but as a rule there is a nucleus of primary stone surrounded by concentric laminae. The primary stones are composed of urates and uric acid, or of calcium oxalate or calcium phosphate, rarely of cystine

or xanthine. The primary urate stone, seldom larger than a few mm, and often formed first in the renal pelvis, is rounded, hard and brown. The primary oxalate stone is small and very hard with irregular outline, and is often dark brown from altered blood pigment. Primary phosphatic stones are whitish, often friable, but sometimes hard. They occur in conditions causing hypercalciuria, e.g. hyperparathyroidism, chronic resorptive bone disease, immobilisation in bed, sarcoidosis and the milk-alkali syndrome. In many cases, however, hypercalciuria occurs without known cause. Any of these primary stones may have *secondary* deposits formed on their surface, and thus compound or laminated stones arise. The particular substance secondarily deposited, which need not be in a saturated state in the urine, depends not only on the composition of the urine but also on its pH. Examples of stones are shown in Fig. 22.77. As the state of the urine varies from time to time, the great variations in the composition of stones can be readily understood. Bladder stones sometimes grow to measure several centimetres, and may weigh over 300 g.

Stones may form without the presence of bacterial infection or inflammation, and lead to mechanical effects—pain and irritation with haematuria, intermittent obstruction, damage

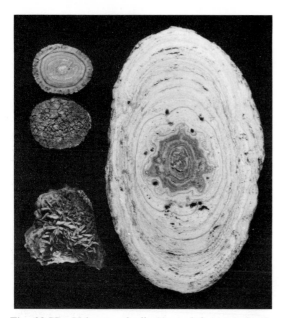

Fig. 22.77 Urinary calculi. *Upper left*, a renal calculus composed of uric acid and calcium oxalate, showing the inner lamellae and rough surface. *Lower left*, a renal calculus composed mainly of calcium oxalate. *Right*, a large bladder stone, which started as a urate stone, probably in the renal pelvis, and subsequently gained layers of phosphates while in the bladder. × 1.

to the bladder mucosa with ulceration, etc. When, however, there is secondary bacterial invasion, and ammoniacal decomposition of the urine occurs, then triple phosphates and ammonium urate separate out, often in large amount, and form a further deposit on calculi already formed. Deposits of these substances may occur also in cases of purulent cystitis (p. 866) without the previous occurrence of calculi, and form primary inflammatory calculi or irregular deposits.

Tumours

Nearly all tumours of the urinary tract arise from the transitional epithelial lining. There is evidence that chemical carcinogenesis is of aetiological importance, and, in accordance with this, it is not uncommon to encounter two or more tumours in the same individual, either simultaneously or over a period. It is not surprising that, having a relatively large surface area, the bladder should be a commoner site of tumours than the ureters or renal pelves, but the trigone appears to be particularly often involved.

It is difficult to adopt the usual classification of benign and malignant for urinary tract tumours, and the following classification takes into consideration the reported experience of the Institute of Urology of the University of London.

Benign papilloma. This is a pedunculated tumour, often less than 1 cm. in diameter, which projects into the lumen from a narrow stalk and is composed of fine branching fronds, each of which has a thin central core of vascular connective tissue and a lining which is 3–4 cells thick and resembles very closely the normal transitional epithelium of the urinary tract (Fig. 22.78). The cells are regular, and mitoses are few. Tumours showing this very high degree of differentiation are rare, and are benign.

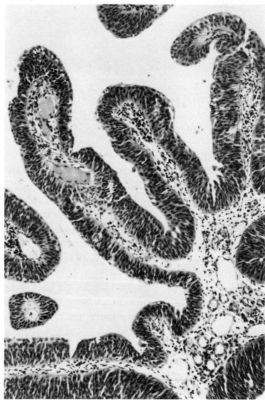

Fig. 22.78 Papilloma of bladder. Part of the tumour, showing the frond-like processes. Where the epithelium has been cut perpendicularly, it is 3–4 cells thick: in other places, oblique section gives a false impression of more cell layers. × 85.

Well-differentiated transitional cell carcinoma. These tumours may be papillary (Fig. 22.79) or solid, or may contain both types of structure. They comprise the majority of urinary tract tumours.

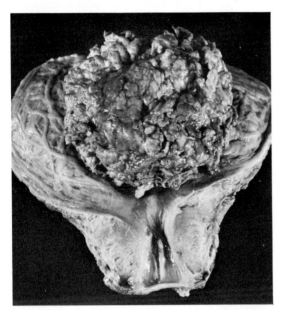

Fig. 22.79 A large papillary carcinoma of the bladder.

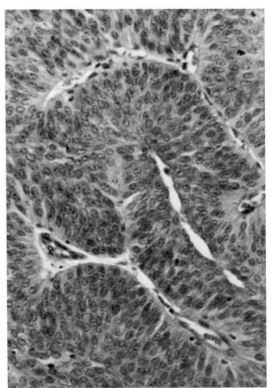

Fig. 22.80 Well-differentiated transitional-cell carcinoma of the urinary bladder. × 350.

(*a*) *Papillary.* Tumours of this type have a structure similar to the benign papilloma; they differ, however, in having a thicker epithelial lining composed of more layers of cells. Mitoses are more numerous, and the epithelial cell nuclei show variations in size, but tend to be larger and more deeply staining, giving the impression of crowding of cells. In spite of these appearances, the cells are sufficiently differentiated to be recognisably of transitional type. The base of the epithelium is not so regular as in the benign papilloma, and it extends more deeply into the underlying connective tissue. Careful search must be made for foci of invasion, and extension into lymphatics or venules. Even in the apparent absence of such changes, some of these tumours recur or behave as carcinomas, but the presence of invasion greatly worsens the prognosis.

(*b*) *Solid.* This has the appearance of a raised plaque attached to the surface by a broad base, and sometimes appearing lobulated or nodular. Microscopy shows solid sheets of epithelial cells with appearances similar to the cells of the papillary tumours (Fig. 22.80), but enclosed by bands of vascular connective tissue. The prognosis is similar to the papillary type, and the detection of invasion is again of great importance.

Some tumours are papillary in their superficial parts, but have a broad base of attachment and deeper solid elements.

Anaplastic carcinoma. This also presents as a plaque raised above the surface, but usually shows central necrosis and sloughing and thus appears as a sloughing ulcer with raised edges. The epithelium is in solid masses, and may have some resemblance to transitional cells but with obvious cell aberration and numerous and abnormal mitoses (Fig. 22.81). Foci of poorly differentiated squamous epithelium are often present. There is frank invasion into the underlying muscle, and lymphatic and venous extensions are often apparent. The prognosis is poor.

Squamous carcinoma also occurs in the urinary tract: in some instances it arises from squamous metaplasia attributable to the pre-

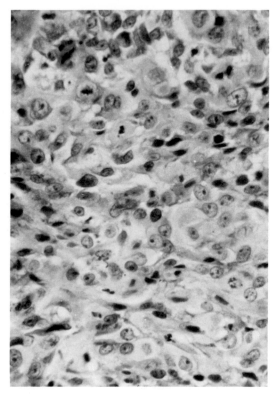

Fig. 22.81 Anaplastic carcinoma of the urinary bladder. × 350.

sence of calculi and chronic inflammation. In other cases, squamous cancer arises directly from transitional epithelium.

Adenocarcinoma is relatively uncommon. It may arise from transitional epithelium and occurs particularly in congenital extroversion of the bladder, when the epithelium undergoes metaplasia to mucus-secreting type. Another possible origin is from remnants of the urachus around the apex of the bladder.

Clinical features. Both benign and malignant tumours of the urinary tract tend to bleed, and haematuria is the common complaint. In some instances, infection is superadded, and recurrent cystitis is not unusual, particularly with ulcerated malignant tumours. Symptoms may also arise from local invasion or distant metastases.

Aetiology. Bladder tumours, and particularly the transitional cell types, are a well known industrial hazard in workers in the aniline dye industry, in which 2-naphthylamine has been incriminated (p. 299). There is also an increased incidence in workers in the rubber industry, and more recently there is evidence incriminating benzidine. The incidence is also increased in cigarette smokers. A high incidence of bladder tumours has been observed in Egypt, and is attributable to chronic schistosomiasis.

Other tumours. Myxoma and leiomyoma are occasionally encountered, and both leio- and rhabdo-myosarcomas, the last appearing as raised blunt processes.

Congenital abnormalities

Renal pelves and ureters. The ureter may be double in its upper part or in its whole length; in either case, a partial doubling of the pelvis is usually present. When the duplication is complete, the ureter from the upper part of the kidney opens separately into the bladder, or sometimes into the urethra or a seminal vesicle. Such a condition may be present on one or both sides. Narrowing of a ureter without scarring, possibly of a congenital nature (p. 864), is a common cause of unilateral hydronephrosis, and some cases appear to be due to an aberrant renal artery. Such abnormalities appear to favour the occurrence of infection and also its persistence when established.

The bladder. The most important abnormality is a defect of its anterior wall, accompanied by a corresponding median defect of the abdominal wall, the condition being known as *extroversion* of the bladder. The posterior wall of the bladder is thus exposed, and appears as an area of vascular mucous membrane, on which the ureters open. The epithelium of the exposed mucosa undergoes metaplastic alteration, in part into squamous epithelium and in part into a columnar mucus-secreting epithelium resembling that of the colon. In the male, the urethra remains open on its dorsal aspect, the condition being known as *epispadias*; in the female there is usually a split clitoris. The symphysis pubis is also usually deficient, though this may occur apart from extroversion of the bladder.

In the posterior **urethra** valve-like folds of the mucosa may cause obstruction with consequent hypertrophy of the bladder and bilateral hydronephrosis. Other abnormalities of the male urethra include epispadias (see above), and *hypospadias* in which it opens on the ventral surface of the penis.

References

Arneil, G. C. and Lam, C. N. (1967). Long-term assessment of steroid therapy in childhood nephrosis. *Lancet* **ii**, 819–21.

Atkins, R. C., Holdsworth, S. R., Glasgow, E. F. and Matthews, F. E. (1976). The macrophage in human rapidly progressive glomerulonephritis. *Lancet* **i**, 830–32.

Berns, A. W., Owens, C. T., Hirata, Y. and Blumenthal, H. T. (1972). The pathogenesis of diabetic glomerulosclerosis. II. A demonstration of insulin-binding capacity of the various histopathological components of the disease by fluorescence microscopy. *Diabetes* **II**, 308–17.

Boyce, W. H. and Sulkin, N. M. (1956). Biocolloids of urine in health and disease. III. The mucoprotein matrix of urinary calculi. *Journal of Clinical Investigation* **35**, 1067–79.

Carr, R. J. (1954). A new theory on the formation of renal calculi. *British Journal of Urology* **26**, 105–17.

Davis, A. E., *et al.* (1978). Heterogeneity of nephritic factor and its identification as an immunoglobulin. *Proceedings of the National Academy of Sciences* **74**, 3980–83.

Germuth, F. R. and Rodriguez, E. (1973). *Immunopathology of the Renal Glomerulus*, pp. 227. Little Brown, Boston.

Horster, M. and Thurau, K. (1968). Micropuncture studies on the filtration rate of single superficial and juxtamedullary glomeruli in the rat kidney. *Pfluger's Archiv.* **301**, 162–81.

Lendrum, A. C. (1969). The validation of fibrin and its significance in the story of hyalin. In *Trends in Clinical Pathology*, pp. 159–83. British Medical Association, London.

Lever, A. F. (1969). See Brown, J. J. *et al.* (1970). Renin and acute renal failure: studies in man. *British Medical Journal* **i**, 253–8.

Lockwood, C. M. *et al.* (1976). Immunosuppression and plasma-exchange in the treatment of Goodpasture's syndrome. *Lancet* **i**, 711–15..

Lockwood, C. M. *et al* (1977). Plasma-exchange and immunosuppression in the treatment of fulminating immune-complex crescentic nephritis. *Lancet* **i**, 63–7.

Oliver, J., MacDowall, M. and Tracy, A. (1951). The pathogenesis of acute renal failure associated with traumatic and toxic injury: Renal ischaemia, nephrotoxic damage and the ischemuric episode. *Journal of Clinical Investigation* **30**, 1307–1440.

Powell, H. R. (1976). The relationship between proteinuria and epithelial cell changes in minimal lesion glomerulopathy. *Nephron* **16**, 310–17.

Rich, A. R. (1957). A hitherto undescribed vulnerability of the juxtamedullary glomeruli in the lipoid nephrosis. *Bulletin of the Johns Hopkins Hospital* **100**, 173–86.

Sevitt, S. (1959). Pathogenesis of traumatic uraemia. A revised concept. *Lancet* **ii**, 135–40.

Vassilli, P. and McCluskey, R. T. (1971). The pathogenetic role of the coagulation process in glomerular disease of immunologic origin. *Advances in Nephrology* **1**, 47.

Volherd, F. and Fahr, T. (1914). *Die Brigtsche Nierenkrankheit*. Springer, Berlin.

Wirz, H. (1956). Der osmotische Druck in den corticulen Tubuli der Rattenniere. *Helvetia Physiologica et Pharmacologica Acta* **14**, 353–62.

Further Reading

Black, D. A. K. (1972). *Renal Disease*, 3rd edn., pp. 871. Blackwell Scientific, Oxford, London and Melbourne. (A clear account of the pathophysiology and clinical aspects of renal disease.)

Brewer, D. B. (1973). *Renal Biopsy*, 2nd end., p. 103. Edward Arnold, London.

Fleisch, H., Robertson, W. G., Smith, L. H. and Vahlensieck, W. (Eds.) (1976). *Urolithiasis Research*, pp. 582. Plenum Press, New York and London. (Reprint of a symposium.)

Heptinstall, R. T. (1974). *Pathology of the Kidney*, 2nd edn., pp. 1171. Little Brown, Boston.

Meadows, R. (1978). *Renal Histopathology*, 2nd edn., pp. 544. Oxford University Press, Oxford, New York and Melbourne.

Turner, D. R. (1979). Glomerulonephritis. In *Recent Advances in Histopathology*, No. 10, pp. 235–57. Ed. by A. A. Antony and N. Woolf. Churchill-Livingstone, Edinburgh, London and New York.

23

Locomotor System

Diseases of Bone

Normal bone structure

Bone is a specialised form of connective tissue important both for its mechanical properties and in the maintenance of mineral homoeostasis. Certain fundamental concepts of its normal anatomy and physiology are essential to an understanding of its pathology. *Normal bone* consists of cells (osteocytes) lying in small spaces (lacunae) in a matrix formed of collagen fibres, amorphous ground substance and mineral complexes. The mineral consists of calcium and magnesium in combination with phosphate and carbonate, in the complex known as bone apatite. Cell nutrition and respiratory exchange is maintained through this calcified matrix by the fine meshwork of canaliculi that contain extensions of the osteocyte cytoplasm.

Bone formation and resorption. Bone may be formed through the intermediate stage of cartilage (endochondral ossification) or directly from collagen (membranous ossification) but in both these circumstances the production of bone is thought to occur in two stages. Firstly, an uncalcified matrix, *osteoid*, is formed by osteoblasts and secondly, under normal conditions, this is rapidly mineralised. The removal of bone (resorption) is generally believed to occur in one stage, mineral and matrix disappearing together. The terms decalcification and demineralisation are therefore to be avoided as they give a false picture of the process in living bone. At sites of bone resorption the bone surface has scalloped edges, *Howship's lacunae,* and these often contain multinucleated giant cells (osteoclasts). Bone is not a static tissue and throughout life the two processes of bone formation and bone

resorption continue actively though at a slower rate in adult life than in childhood.

Types of bone. While all bone consists of cells, collagen fibres, ground substance and mineral, different types of bone may be formed depending on the arrangement of fibres and cells. Two main types are found in the human skeleton, woven bone and lamellar bone.

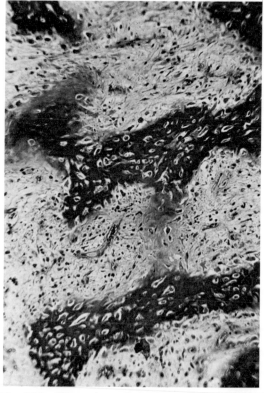

Fig. 23.1 Woven bone, from fracture callus, showing large, closely packed lacunae. × 190.

Woven bone consists of fibre bundles running in an irregular, interlacing pattern through a matrix rich in ground substance. The cells are large and closely packed (Fig. 23.1). It is formed whenever bone is rapidly laid down as in the embryonic skeleton, subperiosteally in a growing bone, in fracture callus, as reactive bone in relation to tumours, in Paget's disease, osteitis fibrosa and also in fibrous dysplasia. It is, however, an impermanent structure and, given time, is usually replaced by lamellar bone which is mechanically stronger.

Lamellar bone. The fibre bundles are fine and run in parallel sheets (Fig. 23.2), different sheets having different fibre directions and so giving the whole a stratified appearance. The

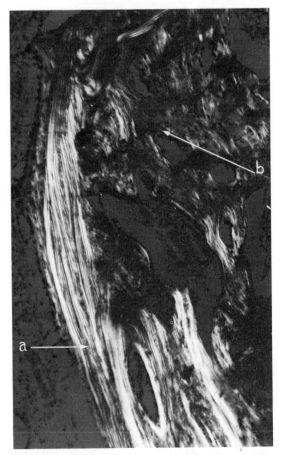

Fig. 23.2 Lamellar bone in polarised light showing **a** the orderly orientation of the bone lamellae. On the surface are some new formed trabeculae of woven bone, **b** showing lack of lamellar orientation. × 190.

cells are smaller and less numerous than in woven bone and have more frequent and delicate processes. The histological differences are most clearly demonstrated either by silver stains or by viewing the sections in polarised light. Lamellar bone usually replaces pre-existing cartilage or woven bone in the growing skeleton.

Transplantation of bone (bone grafting)

Bone grafting is a relatively common surgical procedure and the reparative processes are similar to those in the healing of a fracture (p. 87). Struts of cortical bone may be used to bridge a gap in a bone or chips of cancellous bone to fill a cavity. The graft becomes vascularised by the ingrowth from the 'host' bed of blood vessels which are accompanied by osteogenic cells. These cells lay down new woven bone trabeculae which join the graft bone to the surrounding host bone (Fig. 23.3). Gradually the graft bone and any dead host bone are resorbed by osteoclasts and replaced by new living woven bone. This is slowly remodelled to form normal lamellar cortical or spongy bone. The stored allograft or homograft from another human being contains no living cells and even when the patient's own bone is used only the more superficial cells survive to make a contribution to the healing process. Autogenous cancellous bone is, however, the most potent stimulator of host osteogenesis and the first choice in most clinical situations.

Aseptic necrosis of bone

The processes of revascularisation, laying down of new bone and gradual resorption of dead bone involved in the replacement of bone grafts also come into play in the replacement of aseptic necrotic bone whether this follows fracture (p. 87), caisson disease (p. 779), sickle-cell anaemia (p. 523), Gaucher's disease, the long-term administration of steroids or is of unknown aetiology. Necrosis involving the medullary cavity is symptomless. However in juxta-articular sites such as the femoral and humeral heads if revascularisation and reossification is incomplete or fails to occur, necrotic trabeculae may eventually collapse with resultant deformity of the joint surface and disabling secondary degenerative changes. Aseptic necrosis is thought to be the cause of a number of eponymous conditions affecting the epiphyses of children (*osteochondritis juvenilis*), the most important of which is Perthes' disease of the femoral head.

Fig. 23.3 Incorporation of a bone graft (after Ham). **a** The graft, seen in the centre, consists of cortex with some attached spongy bone trabeculae and marrow. Both the graft and the margins of the bony bed into which it is laid are dead (hatched). New living bone (black) is forming under the 'host' periosteum and around living (white) endosteal trabeculae.

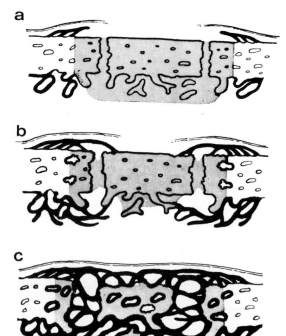

b The amount of new living bone has increased and the graft bone is now attached to the 'host' bone by new trabeculae which have formed partly on the surface of dead bone. Haversian canals in the dead 'host' bone have been revascularised and widened by osteoclastic resorption. Some living bone is also proliferating around the margins of the canals. Union has occurred between the 'host' bone and the graft.

c The remaining amount of dead graft bone is much diminished by osteoclastic resorption and there is also some resorption of the remaining dead bone of the 'host' bed. The dead graft is being replaced by living new bone.

The type of reaction illustrated occurs no matter the type of graft used. There tends to be rather more graft osteoblast contribution to the final amount of new bone when fresh autograft bone is used.

Pyogenic Infections of Bone

Acute osteomyelitis

Different terms are applied to inflammation of bone according to the site—periostitis, osteitis proper, and osteomyelitis—but these should not be taken as indicating separate conditions; one may lead to another, and sometimes all three are present together. Acute osteomyelitis is seen most often in childhood though its relative incidence is increasing in neonates and adults. The metaphyses adjacent to the more actively growing epiphyses of long tubular bones, i.e. lower end of femur, upper end of tibia, upper end of humerus and lower end of radius, are the sites usually involved, though vertebrae, pubis, clavicle and indeed any bone may be affected.

Aetiology

Bone infection may result from bacterial contamination of a compound fracture, from surgical operation, especially when metal implants are used, or by direct spread from an adjacent focus of infection (i.e. to the jaw from an apical tooth abscess). In most cases, however, it arises as a result of haematogenous spread of organisms and is initially an osteomyelitis, the organisms having settled first in haemopoietic marrow. Sometimes there is an obvious inflammatory lesion elsewhere such as a boil or paronychia, but frequently the source of infection cannot be traced and is probably some slight lesion of the skin or mucous membrane. While suppurative osteomyelitis may be produced by various organisms, by far the commonest cause is the *Staphylococcus aureus* which is often penicillin resistant (Fig. 23.4). Streptococci and *Haemophilus influenzae* produce occasional infections especially in infants, while other pyogenic organisms are rarely responsible. A mixed flora is characteristic of osteomyelitis involving the feet of elderly diabetics. An attack of *typhoid fever* may be followed, sometimes many years later, by osteomyelitis, usually in the long bones or

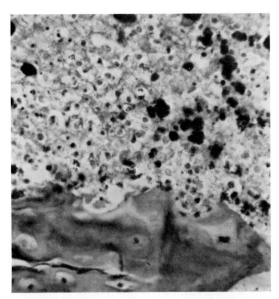

Fig. 23.4 Acute osteomyelitis, showing masses of staphylococci. × 250.

spine. Sickle cell anaemia in children and Gaucher's disease may be associated with osteomyelitis due to *Salmonellae*.

In about two-thirds of patients, organisms may be recovered by blood culture early in the disease but treatment should not be delayed either for the result of the culture or for the appearance of radiological changes, lest fatal septicaemia or irreparable damage to the bone results.

Macroscopic appearances

From the vascular spongy bone of the metaphysis the suppuration may spread widely, so that the medullary cavity becomes largely occupied by pus (Fig. 23.5). In children, because of the presence of the epiphyseal cartilage plate, extension occurs more readily in a transverse direction than onwards into the epiphysis. The infection, after breaking through the thin metaphyseal cortex, may reach the periosteum which during growth is often only loosely attached to the underlying shaft though more firmly anchored at the epiphyseal plate. A **subperiosteal abscess** thus forms which may spread extensively, bathing a large part or even the whole diaphysis in pus but usually sparing the epiphysis. The abscess may burst through the peri-

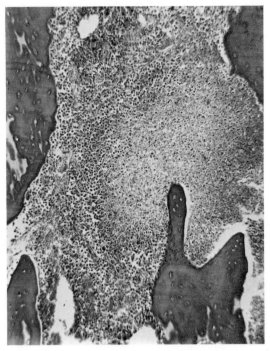

Fig. 23.5 Acute osteomyelitis showing necrosis of bone and marrow and an intense polymorph reaction. × 95.

osteum and lead to diffuse suppuration in the muscles and other soft tissues, and later, if the condition is not treated, may discharge externally. Suppuration leads to increased pressure in the medullary cavity and to thrombosis in blood vessels, which in turn lead to bone necrosis. Suppurative periostitis by itself results in necrosis of only a superficial layer of bone owing to the anastomoses with the endosteal vessels, while in the case of medullary suppuration also, the resulting necrosis, though varying in degree according to the amount of vascular involvement, may be limited. If, however, both lesions are extensive at the same time, the affected bone tissue is completely deprived of its blood supply and undergoes necrosis (Fig. 23.6). This is especially the case when, as may happen with a large accumulation of pus under the periosteum, the nutrient artery becomes involved and occluded by thrombus. In extreme cases, death of the whole diaphysis may result, and then the dead bone becomes separated from the epiphysis and forms a large **sequestrum** (Fig. 23.6). Towards its ends,

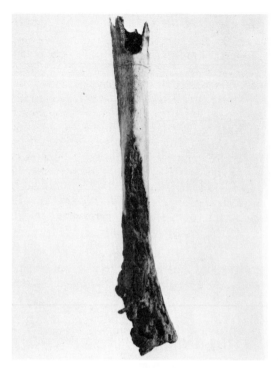

Fig. 23.6 Sequestrum of shaft of tibia from a case of acute suppurative osteomyelitis. Note the partial resorption of the bone at its ends.

the dead bone may become eroded by granulation tissue, and irregular resorption results; but the part actually bathed in pus undergoes little change and the surface remains smooth. Small sequestra may be completely resorbed by osteoclasis. As the infection becomes less acute, new bone is usually produced under the periosteum and this may form an encasing sheath to the dead bone, known as an **involucrum** (Fig. 23.7). This new bone is irregular and is often perforated by openings through which pus may track into the surrounding soft tissues and eventually drain to the skin surface, forming a discharging sinus. The above description applies to the severer forms of the disease which are still commonly seen in tropical countries where delay in treatment and mixed bacterial infections tend to lead to large sequestra and sinus formation. In developed countries, however, good host resistance and the early administration of appropriate antibiotics have reduced the incidence both of large sequestra and of abscesses requiring drainage (Fig. 23.8). Sometimes in-

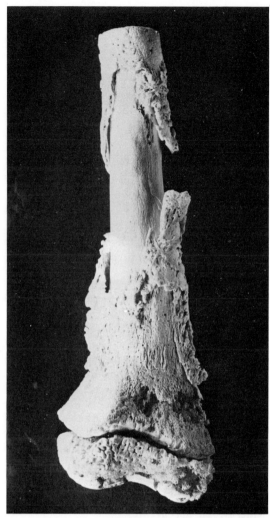

Fig. 23.7 Femur from a case of long-standing suppurative osteomyelitis and periostitis in a child, showing the irregular formation of an involucrum of new bone round the sequestrum.

fection is aborted before any radiological change becomes apparent.

Complications

Septicaemia or pyaemia. These complications are especially likely to arise in haematogenous osteomyelitis due to staphylococci, where, owing to the production of coagulase by these organisms, the delicate vascular sinusoids in the marrow commonly become thrombosed and suppurative softening of the thrombi allows the organisms to

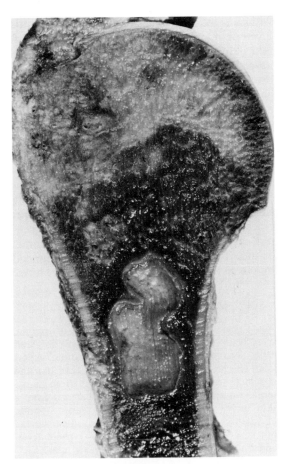

Fig. 23.8 A localised pyogenic bone abscess is seen in the upper end of the humerus of an elderly patient with rheumatoid arthritis treated with steroids. The abscess cavity is surrounded by a rim of granulation tissue. Proximally, the marrow is more diffusely involved.

invade the blood. Pyaemia with abscesses in the lungs, kidneys and myocardium and acute ulcerative endocarditis may result even when the osteomyelitis is not extensive or is at an early stage. The causal organisms may be obtained in blood culture. Pyaemic abscesses are less frequent in infections with other bacteria.

Septic arthritis occurs more commonly when the metaphysis is within the joint capsule. Although rare in children it is seen in infants especially when the osteomyelitis involves the femoral neck. *Metastatic blood borne arthritis* involving several joints may complicate infantile streptococcal or pneumococcal osteomyelitis.

Alteration in growth rate. Growth is sometimes retarded, especially in infants, when the epiphyseal cartilage plate has been damaged, but occasionally it is accelerated, probably due to increased vascularity of the metaphyseal side of the epiphyseal plate.

Chronic osteomyelitis. Acute osteomyelitis, particularly in adults, may become chronic with recurrent exacerbations of infection, repeated formation of abscesses with discharging sinuses and increasing patchy bone sclerosis (Fig. 23.9). Long continuing osteomyelitis with the discharge of pus may be followed by **amyloid disease** or occasionally by the development of **squamous carcinoma** in the epithelial-lined wall of a sinus.

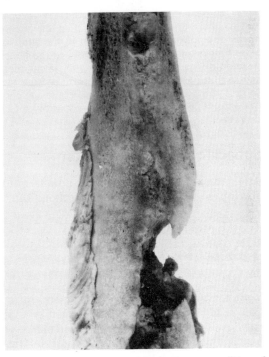

Fig. 23.9 Chronic suppurative osteomyelitis of femur. The lower part of the medullary cavity contains pus and granulation tissue; there is sclerosis of surrounding bone and the medullary cavity above is obliterated. Opening on right is surgical.

Neonatal osteomyelitis

Haematogenous osteomyelitis in the newborn presents a rather different picture from the disease in the older child. It may involve one bone only, often the maxilla, or many bones may be affected, so-called *generalised osteomyelitis of the newborn*. It arises sometimes in association with umbilical or other sepsis and is most commonly caused by *Staphylococcus aureus*, often of a penicillin-resistant strain and occasionally by *Streptococcus pyogenes* or *Strep. pneumoniae*. In the more severe cases associated with septicaemia there may be accompanying symptoms of pneumonia or gastroenteritis and the infant is desperately ill. The osteomyelitis itself is characterised by the tendency to form a massive involucrum which may be completely resorbed after recovery, by damage to the epiphyseal cartilage causing growth retardation, and by septic arthritis. Involvement of the cartilaginous epiphysis and the joint may be due to spread by the metaphyseal vessels which penetrate the epiphysis.

Osteomyelitis in the adult

This condition is relatively rare but may complicate injury or debilitating disease. It tends to involve the diaphysis of the bone rather than the metaphysis or epiphysis. The periosteum in the adult is more fibrous and adheres more firmly to the bone. Accordingly periosteal abscesses are uncommon and large sequestra do not usually form because the cortical blood supply is maintained. However, cortical erosion is common and chronic marrow infection almost invariable in the adult.

Subacute pyogenic infection

An increasing number of patients now seem to develop a subacute pyogenic infection, often with an insidious onset and relatively little fever or malaise. This may give rise to localised abscess formation of which **Brodie's abscess** is one type (see below). Vertebral osteomyelitis, sometimes due to coliform organisms and associated with urinary or pelvic organ infection, usually has a good prognosis, since bone destruction is soon followed by sclerosis and bony bridging between affected vertebrae.

Brodie's abscess. This is a form of localised, subacute or chronic pyogenic osteomyelitis which arises insidiously and is usually situated in the metaphysis of a long bone, especially the upper end of the tibia. The central cavity contains pus, which may be sterile, is lined by granulation tissue, and surrounded by reactive bone sclerosis.

Acute periostitis

Acute periostitis may occur as the result of trauma, there being inflammatory oedema with swelling and little accompanying leukocytic infiltration. Apart from this, it is produced by bacterial invasion and is sometimes suppurative. It may result from an external wound or from the spread of bacteria from a skin ulcer, or, in the jaws, from a carious tooth. Haematogenous infection of the periosteum is rare but is a well-known complication of **typhoid fever**, and it may appear months or even years later.

Tuberculosis of Bone

With the virtual eradication of bovine infection in advanced countries, the human type of bacillus is the chief cause of tuberculosis of bone. This condition is decreasing in frequency and now affects fewer children with a *relative* increase in adult cases. The disease most commonly involves the vertebrae, the metaphyses and epiphyses of long bones such as femur and tibia (in which it is often accompanied by tuberculous arthritis (p. 915)) and the small tubular bones of the hands and feet. Infection usually arises as a result of blood spread from a tuberculous lesion in lung, lymph nodes or elsewhere; occasionally there is direct or lymphatic spread to bone from an adjacent focus, e.g. to ribs from pulmonary lesions or to the spine from adjacent lymph nodes.

Structural changes. When tubercle bacilli settle in the spongy bone marrow, tubercles develop, followed by extensive caseation or by formation of granulation tissue. In either case bone destruction results (Fig. 23.10). The lesion usually progresses more slowly than pyogenic osteitis and new bone formation is scanty in the active stage. Large sequestra rarely form, although occasionally wedge-shaped areas of necrosis under the articular cartilage may result from interference with the blood supply, probably due to endarteritis. When healing does occur it is by fibrosis and at this stage some new bone formation may be seen. Tubercle bacilli may remain in these healed foci for a long time and the disease may later become active again.

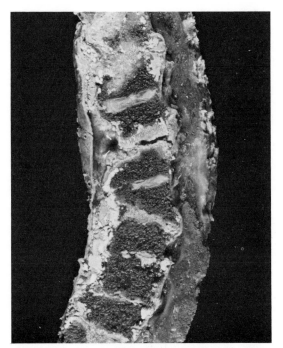

Fig. 23.10 Many thoracic vertebrae are affected by old caseating tuberculosis. Partially calcified caseating material is seen beneath the anterior longitudinal ligament (*on the left*). There is destruction of disc spaces and some vertebral body collapse.

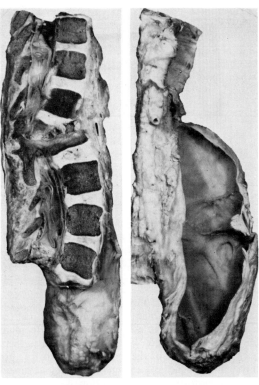

Fig. 23.11 Tuberculosis of spine (Pott's disease). Loss of intervertebral disc and collapse of T.12 and L.1 with paraplegia and formation of psoas abscess.

Tuberculosis in different sites

Pott's disease of the spine. This is usually a disease of childhood in developing countries, but apart from Asian immigrants it is now much commoner in adults in Britain. The thoracic, lumbar and cervical vertebrae are affected in that order of frequency. Often more than one vertebra is involved; they are usually adjacent (Fig. 23.10) but occasionally widely separated. The lesion commonly arises near the intervertebral disc, which soon becomes involved. When the infection begins in or spreads to the periosteum, the caseous material is invaded by polymorphonuclear leukocytes and converted into pus. This often extends to form a paravertebral abscess at the front and sides of the vertebra which may spread, especially under the anterior vertebral ligament, to infect other vertebrae. Later the pus sometimes penetrates the sheaths of muscles and tracks along their length (Fig. 23.11). In this way tuberculosis of the lumbar vertebrae may cause a *psoas* or *lumbar 'cold' abscess*, the pus tracking beneath the psoas sheath to point in the inner aspect of the thigh. When the cervical vertebrae are affected, a large collection of pus may form behind the pharynx—*retropharyngeal abscess*.

The cold abscess may burst through the skin with the formation of a sinus which tends to become secondarily infected. Such patients are especially liable to develop *amyloid disease*. Bone destruction may result in vertebral collapse anteriorly, and, especially when two adjacent vertebrae are involved, angulation of the spinal column (kyphosis) results (Fig. 23.11).

In Britain about a quarter of patients with vertebral tuberculosis develop **paraplegia**, usually as a result of compression of the cord by extradural abscess, granulation tissue, sequestrated bone or disc material. In less than 20 per cent of these patients the infection penetrates the dura to produce an intradural abscess or to involve the cord directly. Occasionally, the tubercle bacilli spread to the spinal subarachnoid space and tuberculous meningitis results. In immigrants, tuberculous paraplegia may occur *without* vertebral disease probably by extension from a blood borne focus of infection in the meninges.

Paraplegia arising years after the original infection may result from reactivation of the infection or from stretching of the cord over the apex of a severe kyphosis; in the latter case the prognosis is less good.

Tuberculous dactylitis may involve a single phalanx or rarely several phalanges of a hand or foot. The infection occurs in the medullary cavity and there is abundant formation of tuberculous granulation tissue which leads to resorption and also expansion of the bone, so that it may be reduced to a shell.

Tuberculous trochanteric bursitis usually arises in young adults. The bursa is replaced by a mass of tuberculous granulation tissue and caseating material which ramifies in the surrounding tissue planes. This is usually associated with tuberculous disease of the trochanter but the hip joint is not involved.

Other Bone Infections

Syphilis of bone

Bone lesions may occur in both congenital and acquired syphilis but are now rare in Britain.

Congenital syphilis. The commonest form of bone disease in congenital syphilis is *osteochondritis*. The metaphyseal surface of the growth plate is marked by a broad irregular yellowish band which consists of a trellis of unresorbed, patchily calcified cartilage. Bone formation is inhibited and the marrow spaces of the adjacent metaphysis contain fibrous and granulation tissue. In severe cases there may be separation of the epiphysis due to fracture through the delicate cartilage trellis at the metaphysis. *Periostitis*, with the formation of subperiosteal new bone, is sometimes seen. *Saddle nose* results from perforation, destruction and collapse of the nasal septum.

Acquired syphilis. Transient periostitis involving especially the tibia and skull bones occurs occasionally in the secondary stage. The bone changes of tertiary syphilis are also seen in congenital syphilis in older children and adults. These consist of periostitis which may be associated with the formation of gummas. The bone becomes irregularly thickened and sclerotic (Fig. 23.12) due to the formation of subperiosteal new bone while necrosis and bone resorption may also occur. The tibia, clavicle and skull are most often involved while perforation of the nasal septum occasionally follows a gummatous periostitis.

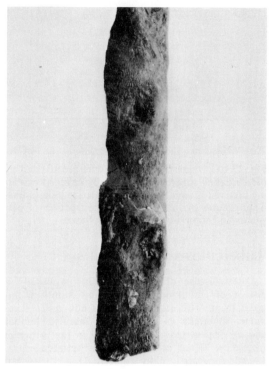

Fig. 23.12 Syphilitic disease of periosteum of tibia, showing nodular thickenings and eroded areas in the bone.

Actinomycosis

Bone involvement usually results from extension of suppuration of the soft tissues. For example, the jaw may be affected by spread from an oral focus or the pelvis from a lesion of the appendix or caecum. The infection is characterised by bone destruction and suppuration with the formation of multiple inter-connected abscesses and sometimes fistulae. Large sequestra are rare and there is usually little reactive new bone formation. *Madura disease* may be caused by a variety of actinomycetes or fungi which are soil saprophytes or plant pathogens. It usually affects the foot and results in multiple abscesses with discharging sinuses and extensive bone destruction.

Brucellosis (Undulant fever)

Bone involvement in *Brucella abortus* infections is not common but spondylitis occasionally occurs with back pain due to involvement of the lumbar or thoracic spine. As in tuberculosis, granulomas form and bone is eroded with early involvement of the adjacent intervertebral disc. Rarely small paravertebral abscesses appear. However, in brucellosis, reactive bone formation with the production of vertebral osteophytes occurs earlier: the disease may be self-limiting, healing occurring by bony fusion. Osteomyelitis of long bones is rare (see also pp. 563, 916).

Effects of Radiation on Bone

For a general description of the effects of radiation see pp. 32–8.

Excessive doses of radiation, whether from external sources or following ingestion of a radionuclide such as radium, may damage bone and cartilage cells directly as well as by obliterating small blood vessels. Bone may become necrotic and is more likely later to fracture or to become infected. For example, **pathological fracture** of the femoral neck may occur some years after irradiation for pelvic cancer, especially in women. **Osteomyelitis** is particularly likely to follow irradiation of the jaw. In children inclusion of the epiphyseal cartilage plate in the radiation field may damage the cartilage cells causing **retardation of growth** and sometimes premature closure of the epiphysis.

Neoplasia following irradiation

Leukaemia. External radiation of the skeleton tends to affect most severely the haemopoietic cells of the marrow and is a well-established cause of myeloid leukaemia (p. 548). Leukaemia, however, does not seem a common complication of ingested radium which is incorporated into bone.

Nasal carcinoma. A high incidence of carcinoma of the nose and nasal sinuses has been found up to 50 years after radium ingestion.

Bone sarcoma has occurred in as many as 20 per cent of survivors of those who ingested doses of radium or its salts, but is rare following external radiation. The latent period before development of bone sarcomas is usually from 5–20 years and may be even longer following internal radiation when the tumours may be found anywhere in the skeleton and are sometimes multiple. Post-radiation tumours are usually osteosarcomas or fibrosarcomas and are often rapidly fatal from pulmonary metastases.

External radiation of bone carries a relatively small risk of subsequent neoplasia, but due to variation in individual response the 'safe' dosage is uncertain. This small risk is accepted in the treatment of malignancy but, when possible, benign or non-neoplastic lesions, especially in children, are usually treated by other means.

Bone Changes Associated with Vitamin Deficiency or Excess

Vitamin D deficiency

Osteomalacia and rickets

Definition. Dietary osteomalacia in adults and rickets in infants and children are due to a deficiency in vitamin D which results in an increase in the amount of uncalcified bony matrix (**osteoid**) (Fig. 23.13) and <u>in addition in rickets produces defective mineralisation of the epiphyseal cartilage.</u> These changes may also result from causes other than simple vitamin deficiency. It should be noted that the term osteomalacia is applied not only to a disease process but also to the abnormal bone structure.

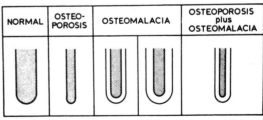

Fig. 23.13 Diagram of bone changes.

Sources and functions of vitamin D. Vitamin D is the name applied to all the sterols with pronounced antirachitic properties. This fat-soluble vitamin exists in two main forms. Vitamin D_2 (calciferol) is produced by irradiation of ergosterol. Vitamin D_3 is present in fish oil and egg yolks, in much smaller amounts in butter and milk and is synthesised by the action of ultra-violet light on 7-dehydrocholesterol in the human skin.

The antirachitic effect of sunlight depends on its angle of incidence so that both latitude and season are important, as is the clarity of the atmosphere. While it has been suggested that skin pigmentation may reduce the beneficial effects of ultra-violet rays, diet is another factor probably contributing to the increased incidence of rickets in Asian immigrants. Children brought up in northern cities with their smoky atmosphere and few hours of winter sunshine are especially liable to be dependent on their dietary intake of vitamin D to prevent rickets. The preventive dose is about 400 international units/day for the fair-skinned infant but there is considerable individual variation both in requirements and in sensitivity to toxic effects of hypervitaminosis. (One international unit has been defined as being equivalent to 0·025 μg of pure crystalline vitamin D.) Since naturally occurring sources of vitamin D are scanty, dried milk and cereals for infants and margarine are fortified either by added calciferol or by irradiation. The dietary requirement of the vitamin in adults is uncertain and probably less than 100 international units/day.

The steps in the conversion of vitamin D to its active metabolites are shown in Fig. 23.14. The metabolites are essential for the absorption of calcium from the small bowel, they probably also have a direct effect on bone, promoting resorption and act on the renal tubule to increase phosphate reabsorption. Some recent work suggests that they may also have a direct effect on muscle. The main physiological function of the most active metabolite, $1,25(OH)_2D$ appears to be under pituitary control and is to increase calcium absorption during the growth spurts of childhood and in pregnancy and lactation. The production of $1,25(OH)_2D$ is stimulated by a low level of plasma calcium (probably in the acute stage via the parathyroid gland) or by a low level of plasma inorganic phosphate: a number of regulatory mechanisms are probably involved.

Fig. 23.14 Vitamin D metabolism,

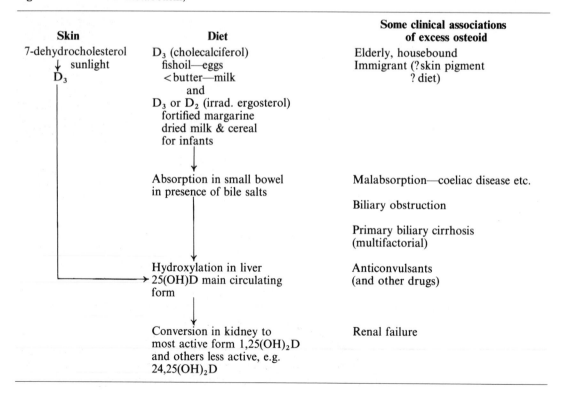

Skin	Diet	Some clinical associations of excess osteoid
7-dehydrocholesterol ↓ sunlight D_3	D_3 (cholecalciferol) fishoil—eggs <butter—milk and D_3 or D_2 (irrad. ergosterol) fortified margarine dried milk & cereal for infants	Elderly, housebound Immigrant (?skin pigment ? diet)
	Absorption in small bowel in presence of bile salts	Malabsorption—coeliac disease etc. Biliary obstruction Primary biliary cirrhosis (multifactorial)
	Hydroxylation in liver 25(OH)D main circulating form	Anticonvulsants (and other drugs)
	Conversion in kidney to most active form $1,25(OH)_2D$ and others less active, e.g. $24,25(OH)_2D$	Renal failure

The mechanism by which vitamin D promotes mineralisation of bone is not clear but whatever the cause, bone laid down after the onset of vitamin D deficiency is poorly calcified and the previously-formed calcified trabeculae are covered by osteoid borders of varying thickness. Both osteomalacia and osteoporosis may give rise to bone weakness clinically and to decreased bone density radiologically and it is important to grasp the fundamental difference between them. In osteomalacia and rickets a normal or even excessive amount of matrix is produced but it is not calcified. In osteoporosis the matrix is diminished in amount but its calcification is normal. In old people osteoporosis is common and is seen occasionally in association with osteomalacia (Fig. 23.13).

Osteomalacia

Osteomalacia, due to a low dietary intake of vitamin D combined with little exposure to sunlight, though rare is now being recognised more often in Britain. Old people, often housebound and living on restricted diets, the coloured immigrant population and food faddists are most often affected. Other causes of vitamin D deficiency and of excess osteoid formation are seen in Fig. 23.14 and discussed on p. 888.

Biochemical findings. Although vitamin D deficiency gives rise to failure of calcium absorption, the plasma calcium level is often not lowered. This is probably because the level is controlled by the parathyroids and a tendency to fall is corrected by release of the mineral from resorbed bone and by reduction of calcium excretion.

The most constant abnormality is a low plasma phosphate due partly to vitamin D deficiency and partly to parathyroid over-activity. Increased osteoclastic activity and fibrosis of the marrow is seen in bone biopsies of some osteomalacic patients and in a few the hyperparathyroidism is sufficiently marked for subperiosteal erosions to be recognisable radiologically (p. 891). Whenever the plasma calcium is low, tetany may occur. The failure of the parathyroids to respond to the hypocalcaemia in these cases may be due to unusually complete coverage of the bone surfaces by osteoid which inhibits osteoclastic resorption.

The serum alkaline phosphatase is often raised, indicating increased osteoblastic activity.

Clinical and radiological features and structural changes. The patient commonly presents with muscular weakness especially noticeable on climbing stairs and with a waddling, penguin gait. Pain is usually vague, aching and poorly localised so that a diagnosis of 'muscular rheumatism' may be suggested. Occasionally a fracture following a mild injury fails to produce radiological evidence of callus formation although uncalcified callus is present in abundance. An incomplete or greenstick fracture in an adult may also suggest the diagnosis. Sometimes **Looser's zones** or pseudo-fractures are seen and when present are almost diagnostic (Fig. 23.15). The radiological picture is of a linear zone of translucency, cutting across at right angles to and usually affecting only one cortex. Looser's zones

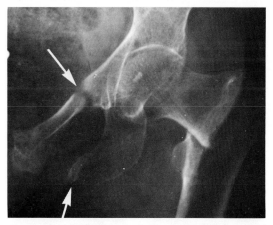

Fig. 23.15 Radiograph of a woman who developed osteomalacia and suffered a pathological fracture of her femur. The radiograph also shows Looser's zones in the pelvic bones (arrowed). (Mr. John Chalmers, FRCS.)

are painless and are most often found in the pubic rami, ribs, inner scapular borders, neck of humerus and femur, sometimes being bilateral and symmetrical and probably representing bony remodelling at areas of stress. There may be a generalised decrease in bone density, especially noticeable in the peripheral skeleton compared with the spine (c.f. osteoporosis, p. 893). In the more severe cases deformity may occur without any fracture, due to the weakening and softening of the bones.

The pubic rami may be buckled and pushed forward into a beak (*triradiate pelvis*) with consequent narrowing of the pelvic outlet; the limb bones may be bowed and the spine kyphotic. These severe deformities are seldom seen nowadays except very occasionally in coloured immigrants or in old people who suffered from severe, late-diagnosed rickets or osteomalacia in early life. It must be emphasised that some patients with osteomalacia may show no recognisable radiological abnormality.

Microscopic appearances. The osteoid matrix which is laid down after the onset of vitamin D deficiency fails to calcify (Fig. 23.16). The recognition of the osteoid borders covering the previously-formed mineralised bone is seen most readily in undecalcified sections stained by von Kossa's method (p. 286) in which calcified matrix is stained black and the osteoid remains unstained (Fig. 23.16). Osteomalacia can be diagnosed by bone biopsy

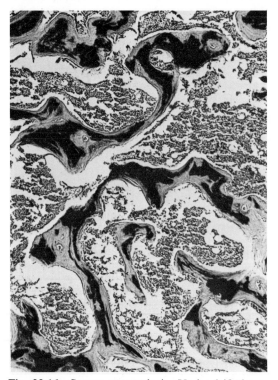

Fig. 23.16 Severe osteomalacia. Undecalcified sections stained by von Kossa's method. Only the bone stained black is calcified. There are wide seams of unstained osteoid. No secondary osteitis fibrosa is seen here. × 40.

preferably of a site containing both cortical and cancellous bone such as the iliac crest. Caution is necessary in the diagnosis of minor degrees of osteomalacia. In normal subjects, when bone is being rapidly formed, a thin border of osteoid may be present on the surface beneath the layer of osteoblasts and even in the slower process of physiological bone turnover in the adult skeleton an occasional narrow border of osteoid may be recognisable. Osteomalacia can be diagnosed either when more than half the trabecular surface is clothed by narrow osteoid seams bare of osteoblasts or, if osteoblasts are present, when osteoid seams are wide. In undecalcified sections of normal bone a haematoxyphilic line, the calcification front, can be seen in most places between calcified bone and any osteoid present. This line tends to be deficient in osteomalacia. The amount of matrix formed in osteomalacia is very variable. It is sometimes markedly increased and the trabeculae are broader than normal probably partly due to an increased amount of formation but also to a decrease in bone resorption. Occasionally, particularly in the elderly, the total amount of matrix is much diminished and the conditions of osteomalacia and osteoporosis exist together (see Fig. 23.13). Mild changes of osteitis fibrosa may be present (p. 891) with some marrow fibrosis and osteoclasis of bone not covered by osteoid.

The diagnosis of dietary osteomalacia may be difficult sometimes on clinical, radiological or biochemical grounds. In any suspected case bone biopsy should be done and undecalcified sections examined. The diagnosis is important because the condition rapidly responds to vitamin D administration.

Rickets

Rickets is the equivalent of osteomalacia in infancy and childhood. In addition to the failure of mineralisation of osteoid matrix as seen in osteomalacia there is failure of mineralisation of the cartilage of the epiphyseal growth plate.

Dietary rickets is chiefly a disease of infancy, being commonest from 6 months to 2 years though 'late' rickets is seen especially in immigrant adolescents, perhaps due to an increased demand for vitamin D during the growth spurt. Rickets is present at birth only in infants born to osteomalacic mothers. Prematurity predisposes to rickets partly due to increased growth rate and partly to defective hydroxylation of vitamin D in the liver. Prolonged breast feeding may also predispose because breast milk provides little vitamin D. A further group particularly at risk are infants in large low-income families who are weaned early from fortified dried milk to a share in the vitamin D-poor family diet.

Biochemical findings. As in osteomalacia, the plasma calcium level is normal or slightly low, but the plasma phosphate is usually between 0·3 and 1 mmol/1 (1–3 mg/100 ml) i.e. markedly lower than the normal value for infants (1·3–2·3 mmol/l or 4–7 mg/100 ml). The plasma alkaline phosphatase is frequently raised.

Clinical and radiological features. There are muscular hypotonia, skeletal changes, sometimes anaemia and especially in the early stages, tetany.

The ends of the long bones are swollen and this may be particularly noticeable at the wrists. Radiological examination shows wide, irregular, fuzzy, cupped metaphyses, thin bony cortices and the late appearance of epiphyseal centres which are often indistinct. There may be greenstick fractures with deficient callus on x-ray examination. Sometimes Looser's zones (pseudo-fractures) are seen (see p. 885). Deformity results from bending of the soft, poorly mineralised bone and antero-lateral bowing of the femur and tibia is characteristic.

The costochondral junctions tend to be swollen (Fig. 23.17) ('rickety rosary') and 'pigeon chest' due to indrawing of the ribs and protrusion of the sternum is sometimes seen. There may be flattening of the pelvis with constriction of the outlet (of importance during childbirth) and scoliosis may occur. The skull appears square and box-like with bossing of the frontal bones and the closure of the fontanelles is delayed. Dentition may be late.

Microscopic appearances. *In normal growth* of bones proliferation of cartilage cells at the epiphyseal plate is followed by mineralisation of the matrix, hypertrophy of the chondrocytes, vascularisation of the lacunae of these hypertrophic cells by metaphyseal vessels,

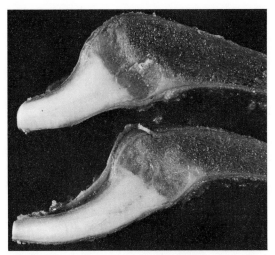

Fig. 23.17 Rickets. Section through two ribs shows marked swelling of the costochondral junctions. The child had a 'rickety rosary' during life.

laying down of osteoid on the surface of the mineralised cartilage and finally brisk calcification of the osteoid followed by metaphyseal remodelling. *In rickets* the primary change at the epiphyseal growth plate is failure of the normal mineralisation of the cartilage matrix. As a result the hypertrophic cartilage cells persist for an abnormally long time and as proliferation continues at the usual rate the epiphyseal plate becomes thicker. Patchy calcification leads to some irregular ingrowth of blood vessels but long tongues of cartilage remain projecting far down into the metaphysis (Fig. 23.18). The osteoid matrix which is laid down on the surface of the cartilage is not calcified and, since osteoid is less readily resorbed by osteoclasts, metaphyseal remodelling is also deficient. These microscopic changes account for the gross and radiological appearances of a wide, irregular growth plate with flared metaphyses. It must be emphasised that if the infant has ceased to grow because of other illness or malnutrition, the changes in the epiphyseal plate will not be seen though there will of course be osteomalacic change in the bone as in the adult. Osteoid matrix formed by intramembranous bone deposition also fails to calcify.

Administration of vitamin D leads to resumption of calcification: in the epiphyseal plate this occurs first in the region of those cartilage cells which have most recently

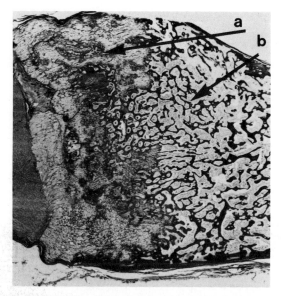

Fig. 23.18   Costochondral junction of rib in rickets. **a** The cartilage plate is thickened and irregular. **b** The spongy bone is partly uncalcified. × 6·5.

become hypertrophic. Since the amount of osteoid laid down is not usually diminished in rickets and its removal is impaired, the bones may become heavier than normal when calcification does occur. Deformities may become less marked but are not fully corrected so that the child with healed rickets may have permanently bent long bones with bow legs, knock knees or other abnormalities.

Non-dietary causes of osteomalacia and rickets

It is still uncommon to see dietary rickets or osteomalacia in Britain but failure of mineralisation, alone or associated with other bone abnormalities, may accompany a variety of conditions. The structural changes are as described above but they tend to be less severe and may be modified by other co-existent bone disorders. The more important conditions are as follows (Fig. 23.14).

A. Malabsorption syndromes. The association of rickets and osteomalacia with coeliac disease and other causes of malabsorption from the gut has been recognised for some time. It probably results from failure of absorption of vitamin D, though other factors may contribute. There is sometimes an associated osteoporosis.

B. Uraemic osteodystrophy, renal rickets. Bone changes which, in mild degree, are very common, may result from any renal disease which gives rise to prolonged uraemia.

In uraemic osteodystrophy the bones may show rickets (osteomalacia) and osteitis fibrosa (p. 891), alone or together and in any degree of severity. The changes of secondary hyperparathyroidism may be very striking (Fig. 23.21) and associated with a diffuse chief-cell or clear-cell hyperplasia of all the parathyroid glands. **In children** growth may be stunted and bony deformities of the rachitic type develop. The changes in the epiphyseal cartilage plates are rachitic but in addition there is often severe osteitis fibrosa, especially in the metaphyses. **In adults** there is usually no deformity though bone pain, decreased skeletal radiodensity, subperiosteal erosions and other abnormalities may be present. Occasionally osteosclerosis may be seen especially in the vertebrae, due to an increase of apparently normal bone or, more commonly, associated with osteitis fibrosa. When osteitis fibrosa is severe, metastatic calcification may occur in the soft tissues (p. 890).

Patients on chronic renal dialysis may develop similar bone changes, sometimes with loss of bone volume and a tendency to fracture. The pattern varies from one centre to another and from one patient to another.

Biochemical changes. The serum phosphate is almost always raised, the serum calcium low or normal and if bone disease is marked the alkaline phosphatase is raised.

Osteomalacia may result from failure of conversion of $25(OH)D$ to $1,25(OH)_2D$ in the damaged kidney while raised parathormone levels may not only follow hypocalcaemia provoked by phosphate retention and poor calcium absorption but be associated with frustrated attempts to increase $1,25(OH)_2D$ synthesis. Improvement may be brought about by massive doses of vitamin D, sometimes as much as 200 times the dose given to cure dietary osteomalacia. Treatment with $1,25(OH)_2D$ is easier to control.

C. Renal tubular osteodystrophy.

(1) *Hypophosphataemic vitamin D resistant rickets.* This condition, which is now known to be inherited by a sex-linked dominant gene, develops in early childhood and is associated with a tubular reabsorption defect of phosphate (and sometimes also glucose) with consequent hypophosphataemia. The condition may be indistinguishable from dietary rickets, leading to stunting and deformity, though muscle weakness is not seen. It is relieved by phosphate supplements along with vitamin D. It may regress spontaneously but there is a tendency for recurrence in middle age. Renal failure and secondary hyperparathyroidism do not occur. Occasionally non-sexlinked hypophosphataemic rickets may present *de novo* in adult life and in some cases is associated with the presence of a tumour whose removal is followed by cure.

(2) *Fanconi syndrome.* This disease occurs mostly

in children, is due to a recessive gene defect and is associated with impaired tubular reabsorption of phosphate, glucose, various amino acids and sometimes potassium. There may also be inability to form an acid urine and cystinosis—a metabolic defect of cystine metabolism (Lignac–Fanconi syndrome): patients with these additional defects tend to develop uraemia. Micro-dissection of the kidney had shown a long thin segment at the glomerulotubular junction associated with a short proximal tubule. The bone changes, which are initially rachitic, may later, especially in the uraemic cases, become complicated by osteitis fibrosa.

(3) *Distal renal tubular acidosis* is another cause of osteomalacia and rickets. This condition may present at any age and is not usually hereditary: it may follow ureterosigmoid anastomosis. The primary defect is an inability to form an acid urine and the chronic hyperchloraemic acidosis leads to an increased urinary excretion of phosphate and of fixed bases such as calcium and potassium. The patient may present with renal stones, hypokalaemic paralysis or bone disease. If treatment with alkali is given there may be little renal damage, but if untreated, nephrocalcinosis and progressive renal failure result. Secondary hyperparathyroidism may then occur.

D. Anticonvulsant drugs. Long-continued high dosage of several anticonvulsant drugs may lead to osteomalacia, probably by stimulating production of liver iso-enzymes which convert vitamin D to inactive metabolites.

Hypophosphatasia

In this condition, which clinically closely resembles rickets, there is a reduction in serum alkaline phosphatase and an increase in its substrate phosphoethanolamine in the urine. The disease is thought to be inherited as an autosomal recessive, the parents being clinically normal but having either or both of the biochemical abnormalities in lesser degree. The earlier the condition presents the more severe are the symptoms. Infants are ill as well as developing severe bone changes similar to rickets, often most noticeable in the skull vault. Children over six months are stunted with widespread rickets, early loss of deciduous teeth and sometimes premature ossification of cranial sutures with subsequent brain damage. The few patients first diagnosed in adult life present with an increased tendency to fracture. Unfortunately treatment with vitamin D is ineffective.

Vitamin D excess

Hypervitaminosis D

If doses of vitamin D several thousand times the usual therapeutic dose are administered there is an increase in the blood calcium due partly to increased intestinal absorption and partly to increased bone resorption. Increased excretion of calcium and phosphorus in the urine occurs and renal calculi may form. In addition, there may be widespread metastatic calcification in the kidney, arteries, myocardium and stomach.

Infantile hypercalcaemia

The relatively mild form of this condition was fairly common in Britain in the 1950s due probably to high vitamin D fortification of many infant foods and of cod liver oil. Individual susceptibility to the toxic effects of the vitamin is a factor since some infants develop hypercalcemia with doses which are harmless to others. Although the amount of vitamin D in fortified foods is now reduced, occasional sensitive babies are still affected. Infantile hypercalcaemia is characterised by a raised blood calcium, sometimes over 3·5 mmol/l (14 mg/100 ml), by anorexia, vomiting and failure to thrive. Deposition of calcium in the renal parenchyma (*nephrocalcinosis*), may lead to scarring and uraemia. Radiological examination sometimes shows dense epiphyses. In the severe form of the condition the babies may develop the additional features of mental retardation, cardiovascular abnormalities, goblin facies and osteosclerosis.

Vitamin C deficiency

Scurvy

Scurvy results from vitamin C deficiency and is now a rare disease in Britain, where it is seen chiefly in elderly people on a restricted diet and in neglected or mentally retarded infants. There is a defect in the synthesis of collagen since ascorbate is a cofactor in the hydroxylation of proline and lysine residues. This defect involves not only soft tissue collagen but that of bone matrix and dentine. Wound and fracture healing are impaired and there is a tendency to haemorrhage because of weakness of the capillary walls.

Bone changes in infants precede the haemorrhagic tendency and are due to failure to lay down bony matrix, associated with the persistence of an unabsorbed calcified cartilage lattice. In contrast to rickets there is no failure of calcification. The cartilage cells of the epiphyseal plate multiply and orientate themselves normally and the intervening matrix becomes calcified, but osteoblasts fail to lay down osteoid and the calcified cartilaginous matrix is only slightly and patchily resorbed (*scorbutic lattice*) so that the epiphyseal plate becomes widened and irregular. Spicules of the calcified cartilage fracture and a very irregular, radiologically dense zone arises at the junction of epiphysis and shaft. The metaphysis itself is weak because of failure of bone deposition, the marrow spaces contain much loose fibrous tissue, and separation of the epiphysis through this site is not uncommon. The pre-existing bony trabeculae in the shaft are thin and delicate (osteoporosis) probably because of continuing normal resorption without bone deposition.

Haemorrhagic tendency. There is a tendency to bleed spontaneously or from trivial injury. The gums are spongy and bleed readily and the teeth may be loosened. There may be haemorrhage into the skin, mucous membranes, joints or subperiosteally.

Subperiosteal haemorrhages cause the severely affected child to lie immobile and to be apprehensive of movement which causes pain. Radiological changes may not appear until subperiosteal new bone is laid down on the surface of the haematoma. Bleeding into the kidney, orbit, brain or adrenals occasionally complicates the picture. The exact cause of fragility of the capillaries in scurvy is not apparent even on electron microscopy.

Failure of healing. In scorbutic patients, skin and flesh wounds and fractures either fail to heal or do so more slowly than normal, and occasionally there have been reports of old wounds breaking down. The administration of extra Vitamin C to non-scorbutic individuals does not however increase the rate of healing.

Anaemia. Anaemia tends to occur due to deficiency of iron or folic acid (p. 557).

'Battered baby' syndrome

This syndrome may be confused clinically with scurvy and accordingly, although it does not arise from vitamin deficiency, is conveniently discussed here.

Subperiosteal haemorrhage with subsequent formation of an involucrum of new bone may be seen as a result of epiphyseal damage in infants who have been repeatedly assaulted. Several bones may be involved, the subperiosteal new bone formation being at different stages in different bones. The epiphyseal damage may be accompanied by multiple bruises, fractures of limb bones or more commonly of ribs or clavicle and with subdural haematoma or a head injury which may prove fatal. In this condition the bones are normal radiologically apart from the effects of trauma and there is no haemorrhagic tendency. It is important to make the diagnosis since if the infant is allowed to return home further assault, sometimes fatal, may occur.

Bone Changes in Endocrine Disorders

Primary hyperparathyroidism

This results usually from an adenoma of one of the parathyroid glands (Fig. 26.21, p. 1037); occasionally an adenoma may be present in two or more glands and very rarely hyperparathyroidism results from parathyroid carcinoma. Primary hyperplasia of the glands is also a cause of primary hyperparathyroidism but is less common than an adenoma. Hyperparathyroidism may be familial and associated with the multiple endocrine adenoma syndrome (p. 1034). Excess hormone may be produced intermittently. It appears to have a direct action on bone, stimulating resorption. It also inhibits the reabsorption of urinary phosphate and increases calcium absorption from the gut and the renal tubule perhaps by stimulating the synthesis of $1,25(OH)_2D$ (p. 884) in the kidney. The effect of the hormone is to mobilise calcium and raise the blood calcium from the normal level of 2·5 mmol/l (10 mg/100 ml) to 3 mmol/l (12 mg/100 ml) or more. The blood phosphorus falls to 0·7 mmol/l (2 mg/100 ml) or less and the alkaline phosphatase is increased. A rise in the urinary excretion of calcium follows so that these patients tend to develop *renal calculi* (p. 868). Sometimes when the bones are severely affected, *metastatic calcification* of the walls of blood vessels, soft tissues, kidneys and other sites may occur.

Bone changes. Though bone turnover is increased, easily recognisable gross bone changes are infrequent. They tend to be found in the 10 per cent or so with large tumours and high serum levels of parathormone. There is then evidence of increased bone resorption; osteoclasts and Howship's lacunae are prominent on the surface of the trabeculae which become surrounded by delicate, fibrillar fibrous tissue. There may also be 'dissecting resorption' of trabeculae, the central parts being replaced by fibrous tissue (Fig. 23.19). The picture is often one of active bone formation and resorption and the two processes may be seen on opposite sides of the same trabecula. At this stage radiology may demonstrate subperiosteal erosion of the phalanges and of other bones due to patchy replacement of subperiosteal cortical bone by fibrous tissue. As the condition increases in severity the marrow spaces become filled with fibrous tissue—hence the term **osteitis fibrosa**—and the normal structure of bone in both cortex and medulla is replaced by a meshwork of fine, irregular and delicate trabeculae. These often consist chiefly of normally calcified woven bone; narrow osteoid borders may be present beneath a row of plump osteoblasts as is sometimes observed in fracture callus and indicate only the rapidity of bone formation rather than a real deficiency of mineralisation. Radiology now shows loss of definition between cortex and medullary cavity, the whole bone having a fuzzy, mottled appearance, and because of the loss of normal structure it is more liable to fracture. The loose fibrous tissue is vascular and secondary changes may occur in it as a result of degeneration or haemorrhage. Cystic spaces may form and in areas of haemorrhage the resulting haemosiderin and the large numbers of multinucleated giant cells give rise to the '**brown tumour of hyperparathyroidism**' (Fig. 23.20). The differ-

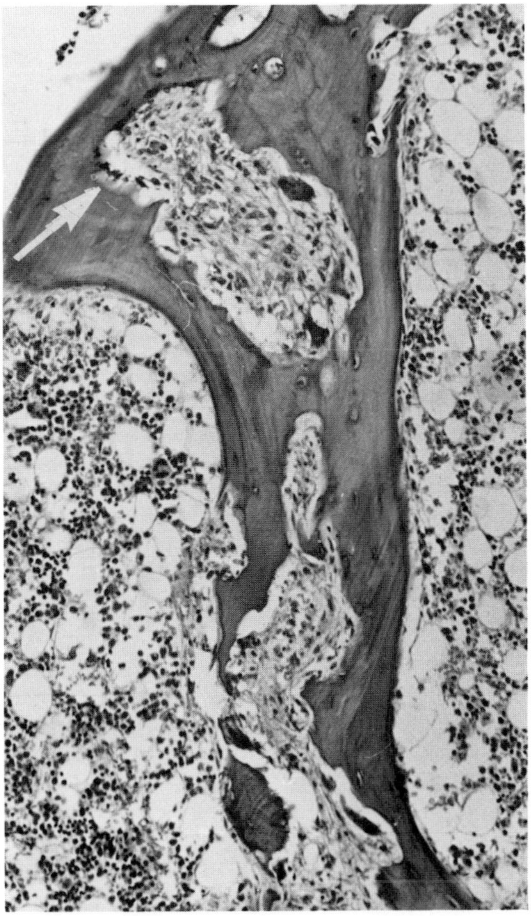

Fig. 23.19 Osteitis fibrosa of hyperparathyroidism. There is osteoclastic resorption of the central part of a bone trabecula with fibrous tissue replacement, so-called dissecting resorption. Some osteoblasts are also seen (*arrow*). × 100.

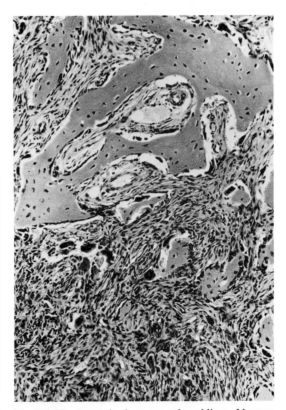

Fig. 23.20 Bone in hyperparathyroidism. Numerous multinucleated giant cells and spindle cells form a 'brown tumour'. Newly formed bone is seen in the upper part of the photograph. × 120.

entiation of this lesion from giant-cell tumour of bone may give considerable difficulty and the possibility of brown tumour should always be considered especially in a site unusual for giant-cell tumour such as jaw, skull or phalanges and above all when the lesions are multiple.

Pyrophosphate arthropathy (p. 925) is found in about 15 per cent of patients with hyperparathyroidism.

Effect of removal of the parathyroid tumour. Excision of the parathyroid tumour leads to a fall in the serum calcium level, and within a week bone biopsy may show diminution of osteoclast activity, the bone structure slowly returning to a more normal appearance. Failure of improvement may indicate the presence of a second tumour. In some instances tetany has followed immediately after removal of the affected parathyroid, but function of the remaining parathyroid glands, apparently suppressed by the tumour, soon returns to normal.

Secondary hyperparathyroidism

In dietary rickets, osteomalacia, pregnancy, chronic uraemia and some other conditions, there is a tendency to a fall in serum calcium levels and there may be a compensatory increase in parathyroid activity leading to enlargement of the glands. Of these conditions chronic uraemia especially may give rise to bony changes, slight or severe, mimicking those of primary hyperparathyroidism (Fig. 23.21). An autonomous adenoma (tertiary hyperparathyroidism) may develop in long-standing secondary hyperparathyroidism.

Excess of growth hormone

Before puberty (gigantism). There is increased growth of the whole skeleton and growth may continue for longer than normal because of delay in closure of the epiphyseal cartilage plates (retardation of skeletal maturity.)

After puberty (acromegaly). Bone enlargement occurs and is due partly to subperiosteal proliferation but possibly also to re-establishment of endochondral ossification of the articular cartilage and vertebral end plates. The bones of the hands and feet and the jaw are most strikingly affected.

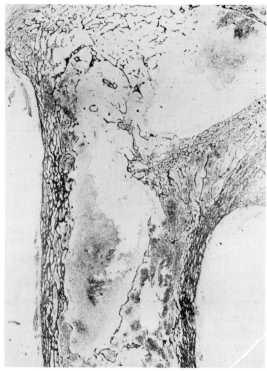

Fig. 23.21 Upper part of femoral shaft from a case of hyperparathyroidism secondary to chronic renal failure. There is osteitis fibrosa and osteoporosis, with severe cancellisation of the cortex. × 1·5.

Excess of corticosteroids (Cushing's syndrome)

Cushing's syndrome is associated with osteoporosis and has the usual clinical and morbid anatomical features (p. 894). The porosis is thought to be the result of a reduced rate of bone formation and perhaps also an increased rate of resorption though osteoclasts are not prominent in histological material. Identical skeletal changes are more frequently seen with prolonged cortisone therapy.

Thyroid deficiency in infants (cretinism)

Long-standing hypothyroidism in early life results in retardation of both growth and maturation of the skeleton with severe dwarfing. The epiphyses may be irregular, deformed, and radiologically stippled.

Excess of thyroid hormone (thyrotoxicosis)

Prolonged hyperthyroidism may cause osteoporosis. There is an increase of both resorption and bone formation but resorption exceeds formation.

Miscellaneous Bone Conditions

Osteoporosis

In osteoporosis there is a decrease in the amount of bone tissue but the matrix is normally mineralised (Fig. 23.13). It may result from decreased bone formation, increased bone resorption or a combination of both. Osteoporosis arises in a localised and a diffuse form following various unrelated disorders.

Disuse atrophy (immobilisation osteoporosis, disuse osteoporosis, localised osteoporosis). Disuse atrophy is found in immobilised or paralysed limbs, e.g. following poliomyelitis or in the course of treatment for bone tuberculosis. It may be recognisable within weeks and seems to be associated both with loss of muscle action and with loss of weight bearing. It is striking that in even the most severely affected bones cancellous trabeculae remain prominent along lines of stress. The bones become increasingly radiolucent; the trabeculae of spongy bone are scantier and more slender; the cortical bone becomes thinner and more porous due chiefly to opening up of Haversian spaces on the endosteal surface, so-called *cancellisation*. The changes of osteoporosis may be patchy and are usually first recognised radiologically in cancellous bone especially that in the metaphysis and subchondral articular regions, probably because bone turnover is more rapid in these sites. Focal radiological bone changes due to osteoporosis may be mistaken for extension of the local disease responsible for disuse.

An initial increase in resorption is thought to cause the porosis (Fig. 23.22) but later bone deposition and resorption may return to equilibrium. Once muscle activity is resumed there is an increase in bone production and especially in children the bone slowly returns to normal. Occasionally permanent deformity results from *premature epiphyseal fusion* in children. Generalised immobilisation may be complicated in the early stages by hypercalcaemia and the formation of renal calculi. Similar osteoporosis is said to have been found in the first astronauts, probably due partly to the enforced relative inactivity within the space capsule and partly to the weightless state.

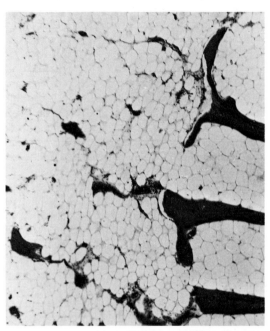

Fig. 23.22 Immobilisation osteoporosis. The articular surface is beyond the left hand border of the picture. The subchondral trabeculae to the left have almost completely disappeared and there is active osteoclasis spreading to involve the normal sized trabeculae on the right. × 45.

Generalised osteoporosis. Only a small proportion of people with osteoporosis suffer from known endocrine abnormalities such as Cushing's syndrome (p. 1039), thyrotoxicosis or hypogonadism. There is a much larger group of post-menopausal women and elderly men who have generalised bone atrophy causing vertebral collapse and a tendency to fracture. It is known that skeletal mass diminishes in both men and women from the third decade onwards and osteoporosis of the elderly may be regarded as an exaggeration of this age-related bone loss though the cause is uncertain. The increased incidence of osteoporosis after the female menopause and the association of oophorectomy with osteoporosis in younger women suggest that lack of oestrogens plays a part in some cases. In these younger women the bone loss may be prevented by continuing postoperative oestrogen therapy, though the possible risk of inducing endometrial cancer prevents its long-term prophylactic use in all postmenopausal women. Increased effect of parathyroid hormone, longstanding mild negative calcium balance, minor degrees of vitamin D deficiency with poor calcium absorption from the gut and relatively slender bones in young adult life have also been suggested as possible factors. Whatever the cause of the porosis, and probably many factors contribute to it, bone is lost and not replaced. Search should be made for any treatable hormonal factors, diet should contain adequate amounts of calcium, protein and vitamins D and C and the patient be encouraged to remain as active as possible.

The structural changes associated with osteoporosis, whether they arise in association with known endocrine disorders or with ageing, are essentially the same. Vertebral changes (Fig. 23.23) may be particularly striking with bulging of the intervertebral disc through the weakened end plate (Schmorl's nodes), increased concavity of the vertebrae, collapse with wedging, or less commonly uniform flattening (vertebra plana). These changes give rise to a loss of height, development of a thoracic hump or lumbar lordosis, and the compression fractures are frequently accompanied by pain. There is also a tendency to fracture of long bones from trivial injury, especially at the femoral neck, wrist and upper humerus and for the production of cough fractures in the ribs. The blood calcium, phosphate and alkaline phosphatase levels are usually normal. Bone biopsy may be necessary to exclude osteomalacia, osteitis fibrosa, myelomatosis or carcinomatosis before attributing radiological decreased vertebral density or collapse to osteoporosis.

Paget's disease of bone (Osteitis deformans)

This condition was first described by Sir James Paget in 1877. It was for many years confused with the osteitis fibrosa of hyperparathyroidism. Paget's disease, however, is not a generalised metabolic disorder but a chronic bone dystrophy of unknown aetiology and the blood biochemistry is usually normal apart from a raised alkaline phosphatase level, indicating increased osteoblastic activity. Urinary hydroxyproline, a measure of collagen break-

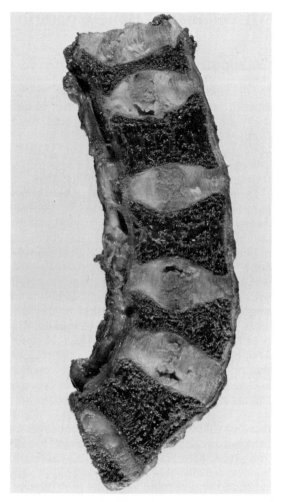

Fig. 23.23 The lumbar spine of this 74-year-old with severe osteoporosis shows bulging of the intervertebral discs and collapse of the vertebral bodies of L1 and L4.

down, is increased in parallel with the alkaline phosphatase. The condition is commoner in men than women and usually appears after the age of 40.

Sites of occurrence. The lumbar vertebrae and sacrum, skull and pelvis are the most frequently affected bones, though limb bones may also be involved. In about 10 per cent of cases only a single bone, often a vertebra, or even a part of a bone, is involved. The condition may be widespread but is always multifocal and not diffuse (cf. osteitis fibrosa).

Incidence. The condition is almost unknown in Scandinavia and Japan but in Germany and Britain necropsy series show Paget's disease in about 3 per cent of patients over 40 years of age. In only 5 per cent or 10 per cent of these does the disease give rise to symptoms such as bone pain, tenderness, bowing of the lower limbs or increase in skull size.

Macroscopic appearances. In the long bones, the shafts become thickened both subperiosteally and endosteally, so that the bone is enlarged and the medullary cavity is diminished. The femur and the tibia often show forward bowing and the neck of the femur becomes set more nearly at a right angle to the shaft (*coxa vara*). X-rays may reveal cystic spaces and stress fractures. The skull enlarges and the calvarium may be three or four times thicker than normal (Fig. 23.24). The distinction between diploë and the tables is gradually lost (Fig. 23.25), and the whole bone becomes fairly uniformly porous and so soft that it may be cut with a knife. (The form of localised rarefaction of the skull known as *osteoporosis circumscripta* is probably an early stage of Paget's disease.) Similar but less severe changes may be present in the bones of the

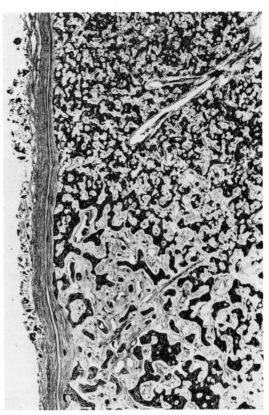

Fig. 23.25 Paget's disease of the skull, showing loss of distinction between the table and the diploë and the variable density of the bone. The marrow is fibrous and highly vascular. × 7·5.

face. When the vertebrae are involved they tend to collapse anteriorly so that a dorsal kyphus forms and the patient may come to have a crouching attitude.

Microscopic appearances. There is simultaneous and irregular resorption and regeneration of bone, with fibrosis and greatly increased vascularity of the intertrabecular marrow. The picture is often, especially in the early stages, one of intense activity, large osteoclasts and also osteoblasts being abundant. Due to the rapidity with which new matrix is laid down some bone is woven rather than lamellar, and osteoid borders may be seen beneath a covering of plump osteoblasts without there being any defect in mineralisation. To begin with, bone resorption is most marked and the bone is lighter than normal with a consequent tendency to fracture and bowing deformities. Later resorption de-

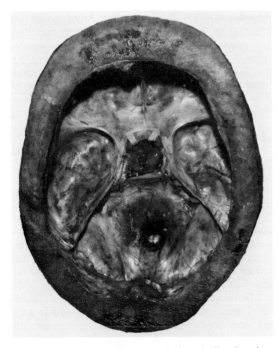

Fig. 23.24 Paget's disease of the skull, showing enormous thickening of the calvarium with loss of distinction of the tables. The sella turcica is much enlarged owing to the fortuitous presence of a chromophobe adenoma of the pituitary.

creases and the trabeculae are often thickened with the formation of a *mosaic pattern* of irregular cement lines indicating numerous previous phases of resorption and reconstruction (Fig. 23.26). At this stage the bone may be heavier than normal but because of the destruction of the cortical Haversian systems it remains structurally weaker.

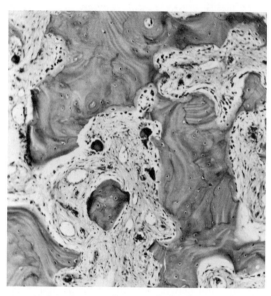

Fig. 23.26 Paget's disease of the femur, showing the typical mosaic structure of the bone, with both active osteoclastic resorption and osteoblastic formation. (Professor J. B. Gibson.) × 90.

Complications. (1) The weakened bones are liable to *fracture*, which in the long bones is often transverse and may be preceded by a stress fracture on the convex surface. There may occasionally be sequelae such as cord compression due rarely to vertebral collapse or more often to bony overgrowth with narrowing of the vertebral canal. Cranial nerves may be compressed and deafness is a common symptom.

(2) *Osteoarthritis* (p. 921) may result from unusual stress on joints caused by the bone deformities.

(3) *High output cardiac failure* may occur when the disease is extensive and there is greatly increased blood flow through the affected bones and the overlying skin.

(4) In Paget's disease there is a thirtyfold increase in the risk of developing *bone sarcoma* in one or more affected bones. The humerus is affected disproportionately often and vertebrae surprisingly seldom. Progressive localised pain should arouse the suspicion of malignant change. The tumours are almost invariably osteolytic and may be osteosarcomas, fibrosarcomas or occasionally chondrosarcomas, often very pleomorphic and with numerous tumour giant cells. The prognosis is very bad because of early pulmonary metastases. Occasionally a giant cell tumour (with a good prognosis) develops especially in the jaw, face or skull.

Fibrous dysplasia

Fibrous dysplasia is a benign fibro-osseous abnormality of bone of unknown aetiology. It is sometimes monostotic, less commonly polyostotic and rarely the polyostotic form is associated with patchy skin pigmentation and precocious sexual development (*Albright's syndrome*). In monostotic cases the lesions are commonly found in a rib (often symptomless), the jaw, femur or tibia, though any bone may be involved. Deformity and exophthalmos may occur when the maxilla or facial bones are affected. In polyostotic cases the femur and tibia are most frequently affected along with various other bones and often the condition is almost but not entirely unilateral. The lesions appear in childhood and new foci may develop even after puberty. When many bones are affected early in life the condition tends to progress with increasing deformity and multiple fractures. Malignant change to fibrosarcoma is very rare.

Macroscopic appearances. The normal bone is sharply demarcated from the whitish, gritty fibrous tissue, often containing cysts and small nodules of cartilage, which expands the bone. The epiphyses of long bones tend to be spared. The typical focus of fibrous dysplasia shows a ground-glass, finely mottled appearance on x-ray and can sometimes be cut with a knife, but lesions in the skull and jaw tend to be more densely bony and indeed often appear radiologically as areas of increased density.

Microscopic appearances. There is a loose, small spindle-celled fibrous stroma in which curving and 'lobster-claw' trabeculae of non-lamellar woven bone (Fig. 23.27), apparently devoid of osteoblasts, are scattered. These trabeculae are characteristic and repeated biopsy has shown that they fail to mature to lamellar bone. Groups of osteoclasts and occasional nodules of cartilage may be present.

granuloma with a preponderance of eosinophils, lipid-containing macrophages and some small multi-nucleated giant cells. It usually heals but is thought occasionally to progress to a more generalised granulomatosis of the Hand–Schüller–Christian type.

Digital clubbing and hypertrophic osteoarthropathy

Clubbing of the distal phalanges of the fingers and less commonly the toes occurs in association with various chronic lung diseases, notably persistent infections, emphysema, bronchial carcinoma and, more rarely, with other abnormalities such as cyanotic congenital heart disease, cirrhosis of the liver, ulcerative colitis and Crohn's disease. The phalanges are widened and thickened, whilst the nails are raised, curved, and often fibrous in texture. The clubbing is the result of thickening and fibrosis of the soft tissues, particularly under the nailbed, and is thought to be associated with vascular engorgement. Occasionally there is an increase in subperiosteal bone of the terminal phalanges.

Patients with **hypertrophic osteoarthropathy** develop, in addition to finger clubbing, a periostitis and sometimes also joint disease. Layers of subperiosteal new bone form first in the distal thirds of the shafts of the bones of the forearms and lower legs and later sometimes spread to involve the remainder of these bones and the femora and humeri. The condition is associated most frequently with pleural mesothelioma, bronchial carcinoma of adenocarcinomatous or squamous pattern, sometimes with metastatic lung tumours, rarely with non-neoplastic lung disease and very infrequently with other disorders. Hypertrophic osteoarthropathy may appear early in the course of the pulmonary disease and disappear after surgical resection of the diseased lung. Its cause is not known.

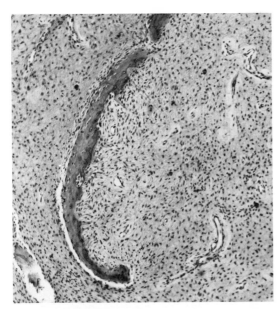

Fig. 23.27 Fibrous dysplasia of bone. The delicately cellular fibrous tissue contains a thin trabecula of woven bone. × 75.

Hand–Schüller–Christian disease

This condition, which usually occurs in children, is characterised by the formation of multiple osteolytic lesions, often affecting the skull and consisting of lipid-filled macrophages (containing mainly cholesterol esters) together with neutrophil and eosinophil polymorphs, plasma cells and lymphocytes and sometimes small multi-nucleated cells. As the lesion ages there is a tendency to fibrosis and formation of cholesterol clefts with foreign body giant-cell reaction. Its other features are described on p. 568.

Eosinophil granuloma of bone is usually solitary but sometimes multiple, and affects most often the skull, vertebrae and long bones in children and young adults. The histological picture is that of a

Generalised Developmental Abnormalities of Bone

Osteopetrosis, marble-bone disease (*Albers–Schönberg*). This disorder is characterised by excessive density of all the bones with obliteration of the marrow cavities and development of leuko-erythroblastic anaemia. It is associated with failure of resorption of the cartilaginous spongiosa and of bone remodelling. Involvement of the skull leads to narrowing of the foramina with deafness and impairment of vision. In spite of their increased density the bones are brittle and fractures occur from slight violence. The disease is a hereditary one, and is transmitted in young, severely affected patients as an autosomal recessive character and in a relatively benign form as an autosomal dominant.

Osteogenesis imperfecta. Osteogenesis imperfecta is a hereditary disease characterised by generalised osteoporosis with slender fragile bones. It may develop during intrauterine life (*osteogenesis imperfecta congenita*) and is then generally fatal, or in later childhood or adult life (*osteogenesis imperfecta tarda*) when the severity varies greatly.

In severe cases the long bones are thin with narrow, poorly formed cortices. Spontaneous fractures may be numerous and result in short, bowed, deformed bones especially in the lower limbs. Fracture and callus formation may occur *in utero*. Fractures usually heal without trouble but pseudarthrosis sometimes occurs and occasionally callus is very hyperplastic, forming tumour-like masses which may be difficult to distinguish microscopically from osteosarcoma. Severe spinal *osteoporosis* may give rise to markedly biconcave ('codfish') vertebral bodies, to collapse or to scoliosis. Narrowing of the pelvic outlet may occur. Membrane bones are also poorly formed. The skull is thin, bulging, particularly over the ears and with a mosaic pattern due to numerous Wormian bones. It forms little protection to the brain during birth and many affected infants die of intracranial haemorrhage.

Microscopically, in bones formed by endochondral ossification there seems to be no defect in the epiphyseal cartilage and invasion of regularly arranged cartilage columns by capillaries is normal but in severe cases little bone is laid down (Fig. 23.28). The bone which is formed, whether by endochondral or membranous ossification, consists of a spongy, open network of small delicate woven bone trabeculae with little production of cortical bone. The condition may be partly the result of failure of control of the type of collagen produced. A higher proportion of type III compared with type I is found and some of the type I fails to mature. The sclerae appear blue because they are so thin that the pigmented choroid shines through and the dentine of the teeth may be poorly formed. Herniae and joint hypermobility with lax ligaments may also be present. The skin is thin and translucent; it bruises easily and wounds heal poorly. Patients may become deaf due to defective conduction by the ossicles.

Osteogenesis imperfecta tarda is inherited as an autosomal dominant but it is likely that an autosomal recessive form exists, giving rise to the few nonsporadic cases of the congenital type of disease.

Achondroplasia. This remarkable condition, which is known also as *chondrodystrophia fetalis*, is brought about by failure of endochondral ossification. It is present at birth and may be diagnosed radiologically *in utero*. The head appears large, the forehead bulging and the root of the nose is indrawn or sunken; the limbs are short and stumpy,

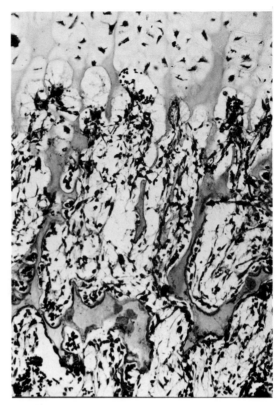

Fig. 23.28 Osteogenesis imperfecta showing poor formation of bone at the epiphyseal line. × 115.

sometimes curved, and as there is more growth of the soft tissues than of the bones, the skin of the limbs is in folds. There are vertebral abnormalities with narrowing of the spinal canal in the lumbar region. Obesity is common, and sometimes there is some oedema. The hands are broad with fingers of equal length (trident hands). While pathological studies have been few it appears that the characteristic changes depend on the failure of the process of bone formation in cartilage. At the epiphyseal line, the cartilage cells form only short rows, or are irregularly arranged, and there is little or no ossification, hence the failure of growth. The cartilaginous epiphysis is sometimes considerably broadened, and with the small shaft presents a mushroom-like appearance; there may be also areas of softening in the cartilage. The indrawing of the nose results from a shortening of the base of the skull, and this also is due to imperfect ossification, which is sometimes accompanied by premature union of the basisphenoidal and sphenoidal sutures. In fact, all the bones ossified from cartilage are small, whilst intramembranous ossification proceeds normally. There are varying degrees of the condition, and 80 per cent of affected infants are stillborn or die within the first year of life, usually of neurological complications such as hydrocephalus due to undue smallness of the skull base and posterior fossa. The less severely affected child may survive to adult life as a dwarf with short thick limbs, and a tendency to develop neurological problems. Achondroplasia is due to a dominant gene with a very high mutation rate; thus most cases are the result of a mutation in one or other parent, whose chance of producing a second affected child is no greater than that of other normal persons. Achondroplastic dwarfs who survive to adult life may produce normal and affected children in equal numbers when mated with normal persons.

Multiple osteocartilaginous exostoses (*diaphyseal aclasis*) and **multiple enchondromatosis** (*Ollier's disease*) are discussed with benign cartilage tumours (p. 904).

Tumours in Bone

Metastatic tumours in bone

Frequency. Metastatic tumours in bone are commoner than primary bone tumours and probably occur in as many as 70 per cent of cases of disseminated malignant disease. Bone, along with lungs and liver, is the most frequent site of secondary spread. An accurate assessment of frequency depends on meticulous post-mortem study. The true incidence of vertebral secondaries for instance is higher than suspected even from sophisticated radiological examinations.

Sites of occurrence. If metastases are present anywhere in the skeleton the vertebral column will almost certainly be affected, especially the thoracic or lumbar regions. Bony secondaries are commonly found in areas where haemopoietic marrow is normally present, i.e. the axial skeleton and the proximal ends of humerus and femur. Skeletal metastases are uncommon below the knee and very uncommon below the elbow. Tumour usually reaches the bone by arterial tumour-cell emboli but it has been suggested that retrograde spread along the vertebral venous plexus may account for the frequent involvement of lumbar vertebrae by tumours of the pelvic organs.

Common primary sites. Tumours which most often give rise to metastases in bone are carcinomas of breast, prostate, lung, thyroid, kidney, melanomas and, in young children, neuroblastomas.

Types of secondary tumours. Bone metastases are commonly *osteolytic* or destructive, and may result in pathological fracture. Resorption of bone trabeculae, especially in metastases from breast cancer, may be stimulated by prostaglandins produced by the carcinoma cells, while in myeloma some lymphoid cell lines may secrete an osteoclast activating factor. Hypercalcemia often results from extensive bone destruction and occasionally from the production of ectopic parathormone-like peptides by the primary tumour, especially in squamous carcinoma of the bronchus and renal carcinoma.

Sometimes infiltration of the marrow by carcinoma stimulates marked laying down of new bone by osteoblasts. In these patients the serum alkaline phosphatase may be raised due to the increased osteoblastic activity. These *osteoplastic or osteosclerotic* secondaries arise most commonly in association with prostatic carcinoma (Fig. 23.29) but carcinoma of breast, lung, stomach and various other sites may infrequently give rise to the same picture, as may lymphomas. Sometimes both osteosclerotic and osteolytic secondaries are present in the same patient. Where much of the bone marrow is encroached on by new bone formation (Fig. 23.30), a progressive anaemia may

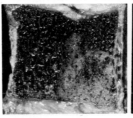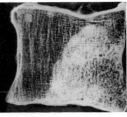

Fig. 23.29 The body of the lumbar vertebra is partially replaced by secondary prostatic carcinoma. The radiograph of a thin slice shows that this has provoked reactive bone sclerosis.

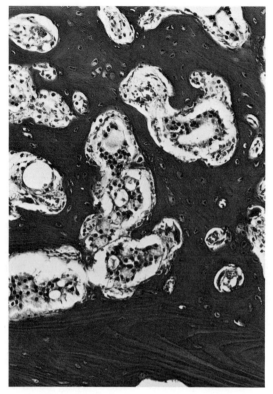

Fig. 23.30 Secondary prostatic carcinoma in bone with reactive new bone formation causing osteosclerosis. × 130.

result. This is often leuko-erythroblastic and is associated with splenomegaly due to extramedullary haemopoiesis (p. 565).

Occasionally there is widespread diffuse marrow replacement with little bony change.

Solitary secondaries. Metastatic tumours in bone sometimes present as solitary lesions and, while this is usually rapidly followed by the appearance of further secondaries, in a very occasional case of renal or thyroid carcinoma, the bony focus may remain the sole metastasis. Only very rarely is surgical resection of both primary and secondary tumour followed by worthwhile remission or by cure.

Primary tumours of bone

The precise diagnosis of certain bone tumours is so difficult that it is essential for the clinical and radiological features to be considered along with the naked-eye and microscopic appearances before a final decision is reached.

Classification also is not easy, for in some the histogenesis is obscure and in others the very nature of the lesion is uncertain (see Table 23.1).

Classification. *Firstly*, it may be difficult to decide whether one is dealing with a true tumour or a developmental abnormality, e.g. multiple osteocartilaginous exostoses is clearly a hereditary condition and possibly solitary exostosis is a *forme fruste* of this, but, since exostoses, whether single or multiple, may progress to malignancy, they are discussed in this section. *Secondly*, in many cases, although the tumour has a distinctive histological appearance, its histogenesis is uncertain; even osteosarcoma is best regarded as a tumour which produces bone or osteoid rather than one which arises from osteoblasts. The number of malignant mesenchymal tissues which may be found in an osteosarcoma points to its origin from a more primitive cell and serves as a reminder that the mesenchymal cell is capable of differentiation in different directions. In spite of these difficulties a classification is worthwhile because when it can be applied to a given tumour it allows a useful prediction of its behaviour.

In this section certain lesions are not discussed but they have been included in the table for the sake of completeness. Lesions of doubtful origin and non-neoplastic lesions simulating bone tumours have been mentioned in relation to the tumours with which they may be confused.

Osteoma

The term 'osteoma' is now almost entirely restricted to bony outgrowths of skull bones which sometimes protrude into the orbit or paranasal sinuses. These lesions may be formed of osteoblastic connective tissue and spongy bone trabeculae or of extremely dense compact bone or of a mixture of these components. They are benign but may cause pressure symptoms.

Osteoid osteoma

This is a benign osteoblastic lesion which is usually less than 1 cm in diameter. It occurs chiefly in the long bones of the lower limbs of adolescents or young adults although any bone

Table 23.1 Classification of bone tumours

Derivation or type of tumour	Benign	Malignant
Fibrous tissue	Non-ossifying fibroma Desmoplastic fibroma	Fibrosarcoma
Cartilage	Osteocartilaginous exostosis ———→ Enchondroma ————————→ Chondrosarcoma Benign chondroblastoma Chondromyxoid fibroma	
Bone	Osteoma Osteoid osteoma Benign osteoblastoma	Osteosarcoma (including some Paget's and post-irradiation sarcomas) Parosteal osteosarcoma
Unknown	Giant-cell tumour ———————→	Giant-cell tumour Ewing's tumour 'Adamantinoma' of long bones
Vascular tissue	Haemangioma Glomus tumour	Haemangioendothelioma Angiosarcoma
Fat cells	Lipoma	Liposarcoma
Haemopoietic	Solitary plasmacytoma ———————→	Myelomatosis Malignant lymphoma
Neural tissue	Schwannoma Neurofibromatosis ———————→	Neurofibrosarcoma
Notochordal tissue		Chordoma

The arrows indicate that these benign lesions may progress to malignancy

and age may be affected. The clinical history is of increasingly severe and unusually well-localised pain and tenderness, often relieved by salicylates. Radiology shows the lesion itself as a rounded zone of radiolucency (Fig. 23.31). If cortical, there is often massive sclerosis of adjacent bone whereas in cancellous bone sclerosis may be minimal. Macroscopically the osteoid osteoma is usually red and cherry-like and microscopic examination shows a very vascular nidus of osteoblastic tissue with a disorderly mass of irregular small trabeculae of osteoid or bone undergoing active remodelling (Fig. 23.32). Sometimes the central part of the nidus is more solid. If incompletely removed, symptoms may recur.

Osteosarcoma (osteogenic sarcoma)

Osteosarcoma is a malignant tumour in which osteoid or bone is formed directly by sarcoma cells and is thought to arise from cells of the primitive bone-forming mesenchyme. If myeloma is excluded it is the commonest primary malignant bone tumour and occurs more frequently in males than females. About 150 new cases of osteosarcoma are seen every year in Britain.

Age incidence. Osteosarcoma is rare under the age of 5 years and about 75 per cent of patients are between 10 and 25 years old. In more than half of the patients over 40 years old the tumour is associated with Paget's disease of bone. Some tumours follow radiation.

Sites of occurrence. The commonest site of osteosarcoma is in the metaphysis of long bones: about half the cases occur around the knee and many others at the upper end of femur and humerus. The tumour sometimes arises in vertebrae, pelvis and skull, especially when associated with Paget's disease. Osteo-

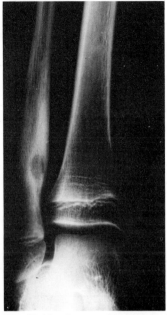

Fig. 23.31 An osteoid osteoma has given rise to an ovoid translucency in the lower end of the fibula. There is a little surrounding reactive bone sclerosis.

sarcoma is very uncommon in the small bones of the hands and feet. Multicentric tumours are occasionally reported, usually in association with Paget's disease.

Clinical features. Patients often give a fairly short history of increasingly severe pain, worse at night, and this may be followed by swelling, oedema, increase in local heat and dilated subcutaneous veins. Pathological fracture is relatively rare. The serum alkaline phosphatase may be raised. The patient is usually in good general health; if not, the presence of metastases should be suspected.

Radiological and macroscopic appearances. Osteosarcoma usually arises in the medullary bone in the region of the metaphysis or diaphysis. The epiphyseal cartilage plate may act as a barrier for a while but in about 75% of cases the tumour spreads to the epiphysis. The joint cavity is seldom involved. Osteosarcoma may spread quite rapidly through the bony cortex without either completely destroying or markedly expanding it and form a subperiosteal mass (Fig. 23.33)

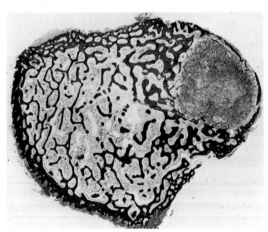

Fig. 23.32 A transverse section of the fibula shows the small bone trabeculae of the osteoid osteoma in the cortical bone with slight surrounding reactive sclerosis. × 6.

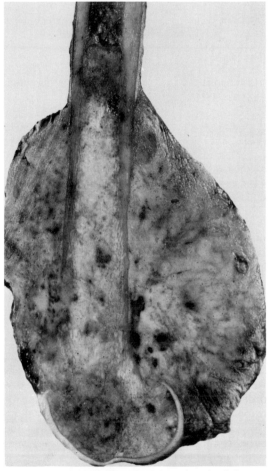

Fig. 23.33 Osteosarcoma of lower end of femur. The medullary tumour has permeated and partly destroyed the cortex, spreading outwards to form a large subperiosteal mass.

which, in its turn, may burst through the periosteum and infiltrate muscles. When the periosteum is raised spicules of new bone are laid down at right angles to the bone shaft (Fig. 23.34) giving rise radiologically to sunray spic-

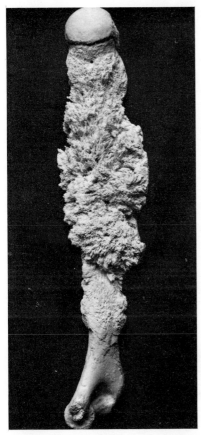

Fig. 23.34 Osteosarcoma of humerus. Macerated specimen to show the characteristic spiculation on the surface of the bone.

ulation. At the junction between raised and normal periosteum, Codman's triangle of reactive bone develops. Neither of these appearances is present in all cases of osteosarcoma, nor when present are they specific signs of osteosarcoma; the same appearances may be seen in metastatic carcinoma or even sometimes in infections. Biopsy material should not be taken from an area where reactive bone formation is active as this may greatly increase the difficulty of diagnosis. Apart from spread outside the bone there may be medullary extension of the tumour and this

is sometimes greater than is suspected radiologically. The gross appearances of the tumour vary according to the amount of tumour osteoid and bone which has been formed. Some tumours contain little bony matrix (*osteolytic*) and these tend to be soft, friable, vascular destructive lesions with areas of haemorrhage and necrosis. Others may contain much tumour bone (*osteosclerotic*) especially in their central areas: they are dense and of turnip-like consistence in their softer parts. The amount of tumour bone formation is not related to the age of the tumour nor does it appear to affect the prognosis.

Microscopic appearances. The essential criteria for the diagnosis of osteosarcoma are the presence of frankly sarcomatous malignant cells and the direct formation of tumour osteoid or bone from them. The histological pattern of osteosarcoma is, however, very variable. In addition to tumour bone, some osteosarcomas contain a large amount of cartilage and others much malignant spindle-celled fibrosarcomatous tissue. In the osteolytic type of osteosarcoma the tumour often contains pleomorphic and giant tumour cells with many aberrant mitoses and irregular vascular channels lined by tumour cells (Fig. 23.35). By contrast in the osteosclerotic type, such a mass of tumour bone may be laid down on and between pre-existing trabeculae that malignant cells within the mass of matrix are small and scanty except at the growing edge. Osteosarcomas in Paget's disease are almost invariably of the osteolytic type (Fig. 23.36) and are characterised by their extreme pleomorphism and by large numbers of tumour giant cells.

Metastatic spread. As in most sarcomas spread of the tumour is almost invariably by the bloodstream to the lungs and sometimes to other bones and viscera, lymph node metastases being unusual. Pulmonary metastases occur early and are often believed to have arisen before the patient appears for treatment although at that time they may not be visible radiologically. The prognosis in osteosarcoma is not good and five-year survival rates of only 5–20 per cent are reported. In some series the outlook is better in tumours of the distal skeleton and of the jaws. Attempts to increase the survival time after surgery are continuing with the administration of repeated courses of

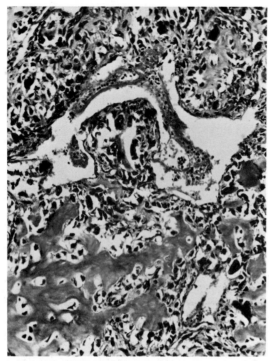

Fig. 23.35 Osteosarcoma. A highly vascular, cellular tumour with osteoid formation well seen in the lower part of the field. × 200.

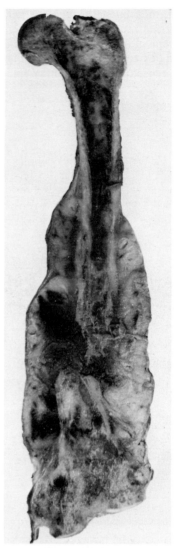

Fig. 23.36 Paget's disease of femur showing an osteolytic sarcoma with pathological fracture.

cytotoxic drugs and various forms of immunotherapy. Osteosarcomas arising in Paget's disease may be multicentric and have a worse prognosis than those arising in normal bone. Local recurrence or seeding of the tumour in the wound is unusual, in contrast with chondrosarcoma (p. 908).

Parosteal (juxtacortical) osteosarcoma. This is a rare tumour but worth distinguishing since it has a much better prognosis than medullary osteosarcoma. In most of the reported cases the tumour is metaphyseal and has arisen at the lower end of femur, upper tibia or humerus. It forms a broad-based swelling arising initially on the surface of the bone and sometimes growing to encircle the shaft, cortical penetration and medullary infiltration being late. Microscopically the tumour usually consists of well-formed bony trabeculae separated by atypical spindle cells; sometimes near the surface the bone is less well formed and there may also be islands of cartilage. The tumour grows slowly and tends to occur in a wider age group than osteosarcoma. If the lesion is inadequately dealt with it may recur or become frankly malignant and metastasise, sometimes within two years, sometimes not for twenty

years. If it is treated by radical surgery initially the outlook is usually good.

Benign cartilage tumours

Osteocartilaginous exostosis (osteochondroma, ecchondroma) is the commonest benign tumour of bone and consists of a bony excrescence. Its outer shell and medulla are continuous with that of the bone from which it arises and it is covered by a cartilage cap from the undersurface of which growth occurs by endochondral ossification (Fig. 23.37). The *ungual exostosis,* which is often painful, is not an exactly comparable lesion. It arises often following infection or trauma as a result of cartilaginous and osseous metaplasia of the fibrous tissue around the terminal part of the distal phalanx.

Enchondroma is a benign cartilage tumour arising within the medullary cavity, most commonly of the small bones of the hands and feet (Fig. 23.38). The cartilage tumours may be single or multiple and when multiple are thought to arise as a failure of normal endochondral ossification (*multiple enchondromatosis*). In multiple enchondromatosis the hands are almost invariably involved but there may also be lesions in long tubular bones associated with bowing and deformity, especially of the

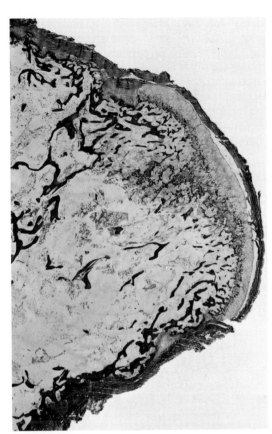

Fig. 23.37 Osteocartilaginous exostosis of humerus consisting of cancellous bone covered by cartilage and perichondrium. Endochondral ossification is occurring. × 8·5.

lesion may be single or multiple; when multiple the condition is familial and may be associated with some failure of bone remodelling (*hereditary multiple exostoses, diaphyseal aclasis*). Exostoses may arise in any bone formed by endochondral ossification but the metaphyses of long bones, especially the femur, humerus and tibia, are the commonest sites. The lesions are usually first noticed in childhood and adolescence and growth commonly ceases in adult life, the cartilaginous cap sometimes completely disappearing. Malignant change is rare in solitary exostoses but probably more than 10 per cent of patients with multiple lesions develop chondrosarcoma, usually in adult life. Exostoses of the axial skeleton or proximal limb bones are much more likely to become malignant than those in the peripheral skeleton (see chondrosarcoma for discussion). So-called *sub-*

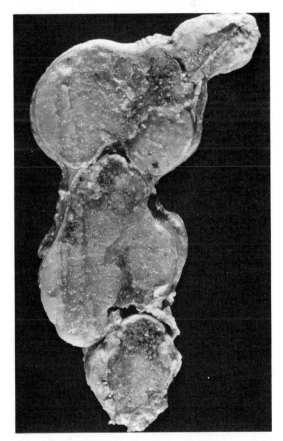

Fig. 23.38 Benign enchondromas of finger. The finger has been amputated just proximal to the metacarpal head. While the joint spaces remain intact each phalanx is replaced by a mass of hyaline cartilage. The cortices have disappeared but periosteum still surrounds the cartilage.

forearm. When the enchondromas are predominantly unilateral the condition is sometimes referred to as *Ollier's disease*. Solitary benign enchondroma may also occur in long tubular bones, particularly the humerus and femur. The tumour arises initially in the metaphysis and may spread into the shaft or occasionally into the epiphysis if the cartilage plate is closed. Radiologically the lesions are radiolucent, sometimes with spotty calcification and naked-eye examination of an enchondroma shows the usual appearance of cartilage though often more gelatinous than normal. Microscopic examinaton of the benign lesion shows small uniform cells with small and few double nuclei (Fig. 23.39). The lesions of the phalanges and metacarpals, especially in multiple enchondromas, may be unusually cellular without there being any sinister prognostic significance. The common clinical complaints, particularly in the phalangeal lesions, are of swelling or pathological fracture. Malignant transformation in cases of solitary enchondroma is probably rare but about a third of patients with multiple enchondromatosis develop chondrosarcoma. Pain unassociated with fracture, or the onset of enlargement in an enchondroma of the axial skeleton or long tubular bones in an adult should immediately raise the suspicion of malignant change.

Chondrosarcoma

Chondrosarcoma is a malignant cartilage tumour and may arise *de novo* or, in about 10 per cent of cases, from a pre-existing benign cartilage tumour. It may be situated within the bone (central) or outwith it (peripheral). The tumour is slightly less common than osteosarcoma and is twice as common in males as in females. In contrast to osteosarcoma, chon-

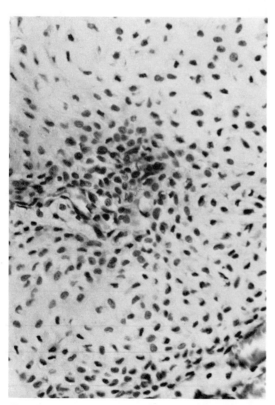

Fig. 23.39 Benign enchondroma from finger in multiple enchondromatosis. The cartilage is highly cellular but the cells are mononuclear and fairly uniform in size. × 250.

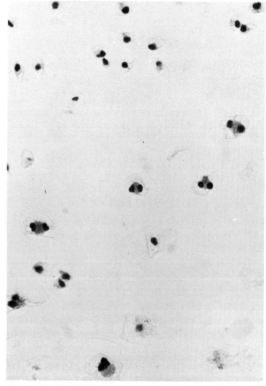

Fig. 23.40 This recurrent low grade chondrosarcoma killed the patient by local spread without metastases. The cartilage matrix is well formed and the tumour is not very cellular but there are numerous foci of chondrocytes with plump double nuclei. × 250.

drosarcoma is rare under the age of 30 years and most patients are in the 40–70 age group.

Sites of occurrence. About half the lesions arise in the pelvic girdle (Fig. 23.41) and ribs; the proximal femur is another common site. A careful watch should therefore be kept on all cartilage tumours of the axial skeleton, particularly in adults, and increase in size and pain should arouse the suspicion of malignancy. The incidence of malignant change is lower in chondromas of the distal part of the skeleton and is very rare in those of the bones of the hands and feet except for the os calcis and talus.

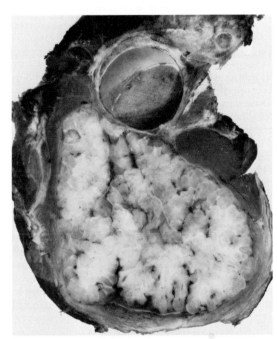

Fig. 23.41 Low-grade chondrosarcoma of pelvis showing the large cartilaginous tumour arising from the ilium.

Macroscopic appearances. *Central tumours.* A central cartilage tumour usually causes slight bone expansion and in slowly growing tumours there is often buttressing of the cortex in response to endosteal erosion. Not uncommonly, however, the cortex is broken through and the tumour is found growing in the adjacent soft tissue. Sometimes, particularly in large tumours which are especially prone to arise in pelvis and ribs, the exact site of origin becomes difficult to identify and the lobulated tumour is soft, slimy and cystic due to mucoid degeneration of the matrix. Spotty calcification may be present and

is sometimes extensive, an aid in the radiological diagnosis of these tumours.

Peripheral tumours may arise *de novo* or from previously existing osteocartilaginous exostoses; the cartilage caps are then much thickened and in the early stages the normally smooth surface may be covered with little nodules of proliferating cartilage. Later these tumours may become very large and undergo heavy calcification or myxoid degeneration.

Microscopic appearances. If the cells in a cartilage tumour are pleomorphic and there are abundant multinucleated tumour cells and moderate numbers of mitotic figures, the recognition of malignancy is easy (Fig. 23.42). In slowly growing tumours, however, it may be difficult. The generally accepted criteria of malignancy are the presence, even in only scattered areas, of many chondrocytes with plump nuclei and of moderate numbers of chondrocytes with two or more nuclei (Fig. 23.40). Failure to detect mitoses does not necessarily

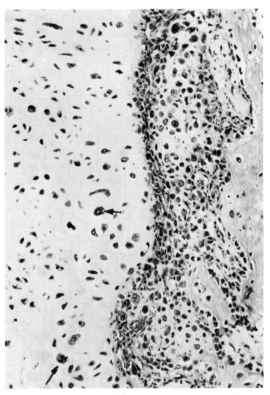

Fig. 23.42 Metastasising chondrosarcoma of ilium. The cartilage cells vary greatly in size and there are several mitoses, two of which are arrowed. × 100.

indicate that the tumour is benign. The best opportunity of assessing the tumour's likely behaviour is in studying material from the growing edge and every scrap of biopsy tissue must be examined microscopically. Biopsies from heavily calcified or degenerate cartilage are useless. Because of variations in histological malignancy in different parts of the same tumour a microscopic diagnosis of chondroma should be viewed with suspicion if clinical and radiological features suggest malignant change. It is particularly important in this tumour that the pathologist should be aware of the *age* of the patient and the *site* of the tumour. Minor changes from normality are much more alarming in cartilage tumours of the axial skeleton, where recurrences may not be resectable, but experience shows they may be largely discounted in growing cartilage tumours in children, in lesions of the small tubular bones and of the soft tissues of the hands and feet, in subperiosteal cartilage tumours and in synovial chondromatosis (p. 926).

Implantation. Cartilage cells have low nutritional requirements and this may explain their special tendency to implant and grow in soft tissues. This has great practical importance to the surgeon as it means that the site of biopsy must be carefully planned in a suspected case so that the whole of the tissue planes opened up may be excised at the time of definitive treatment. There is a very marked tendency to local recurrence after excision even when the original operation appeared to be clear of the tumour. In order to prevent this in sites where removal of a recurrent tumour would be difficult, such as chest wall or pelvis, a radical operation is often necessary in the first instance.

Course of the disease and prognosis. Chondrosarcoma runs, in contrast to osteosarcoma, a more prolonged course. The patients have often some years' history when they first come to hospital. Excision may be followed by local recurrences which may grow slowly for many years before the patient is finally killed by local involvement of some vital structure. Pulmonary metastases are a less common cause of death. These are tumours which respond most successfully to radical treatment in the first instance where this is surgically feasible. More malignant, rapidly-growing and metastasising chondrosarcomas may lead to death within

a few years but even they may persist for a surprisingly long time. Occasionally a low-grade chondrosarcoma may be associated with, and overrun by, an anaplastic, metastasising sarcoma. In adolescence primary chondrosarcomas are rare and have a poor prognosis. Chondrosarcoma metastasises by blood spread, frequently to the lungs and has a tendency to direct retrograde spread along veins. Lymph node metastases are rare. In the past the prognosis has been poor, partly as a result of the pathologist's under-diagnosis of the lesion and partly from inadequate initial treatment. However, with adequate surgery more than half the patients should be cured.

Chondromyxoid fibroma of bone

This is a rare benign tumour of bone, important only because of its tendency to be misdiagnosed as chondrosarcoma. It occurs chiefly in the metaphyses of long bones of adolescents and young adults, especially in the lower limb. It usually gives rise to a sharply defined, eccentric, osteolytic defect which bulges the periosteum. The tumour is commonly rather firm and rubbery and on naked-eye examination lacks the gelatinous, slimy features that one would expect from the histology. Microscopy shows relatively poorly cellular tissue separated into pseudolobules by curving strands or trabeculae of aggregated cells (Fig. 23.43). The cells of the lobules are spindle-shaped or stellate and lie in a myxomatous vacuolated matrix. The trabecular cells are similar but may show some hyperchromatism, pleomorphism and occasional mitotic figures—features which may lead to misdiagnosis of malignancy. Small multi-nucleated

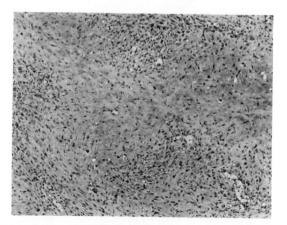

Fig. 23.43 Chondromyxoid fibroma of bone, showing the loose spindle-celled tissue with imperfectly formed cartilage. × 60.

giant cells may also be seen. The tumour is benign, and though it may recur, is usually cured by curettage.

Fibrosarcoma

This is a rare malignant tumour which may arise within the medullary cavity (endosteal) or beneath the periosteum (periosteal), usually in adults. **Endosteal fibrosarcoma** affects especially the bones around the knee joint, though other sites are not exempt. In long bones it commonly involves the metaphysis and sometimes the shaft. The tumour in general is osteolytic, and may break through the cortex and into the soft tissues. In parts, however, it tends to infiltrate between pre-existing medullary bone trabeculae without destroying them and sometimes stimulates new bone formation on their surfaces. This gives rise radiologically to a moth-eaten appearance of the bone with irregular areas of translucency and sclerosis. The extent of radiological destruction may thus not indicate the true extent of tumour spread in the medulla. Multiple bones may be involved when the patient is first examined. Microscopically, fibrosarcoma varies from a fasciculated spindle-celled tumour producing collagen in its more mature parts, to a highly pleomorphic tumour with little recognisable fibrous tissue. When present in the same tumour such variations can be misleading. Differentiation histologically from metastatic spindle-celled renal or squamous carcinoma, or from malignant melanoma, may be difficult.

The 5-year survival rate is around 28 per cent though a few patients develop metatases later. In some series prognosis has been linked to the degree of differentiation of the sarcoma.

Ewing's tumour

In 1921 Ewing described a primary malignant tumour of bone under the name of diffuse endothelioma and since its histogenesis remains uncertain the eponymous title is retained.

Age and sex incidence. Ewing's tumour is rare over the age of 30, and most common between the ages of 5 and 20 years; it is very rare in the first two years of life. Males are slightly more often affected.

Sites of occurrence. The long tubular bones are most frequently involved, e.g. femur, tibia, humerus and fibula but the pelvis and ribs are also affected.

Naked-eye appearances. The tumour appears to originate within the medullary cavity and in long bones may involve the metaphysis and permeate much of the shaft. It is usually osteolytic and perforation of the cortex with raising of the periosteum and formation of an extraosseous mass may occur early. This subperiosteal elevation may give rise to parallel layers of reactive new bone (onion skin ap-

pearance) and less frequently to strands of bone forming at right angles to the cortex (sunray spiculation).

The tumour is usually whitish; some are rather firm while others are very soft, almost puriform.

Microscopic appearances. Ewing's tumour is composed of fairly uniform rounded or polyhedral cells, often with pale nuclei due to the fine dispersion of chromatin. The cell boundaries are indistinct and the cells are arranged in syncytial sheets (Fig. 23.44) without a lobular pattern but divided by broad strands of collagen. Reticulin fibres are scanty and there is often much necrosis. Intracellular glycogen may be demonstrable. Here and there the cells may be arranged in clusters resembling rosettes but without clearly defined central fibrils. This very inconstant feature is probably the result of degeneration.

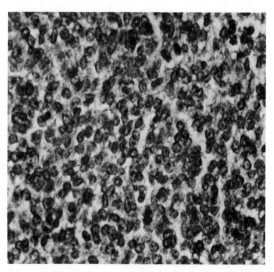

Fig. 23.44 Ewing's tumour of femur showing syncytial structure and uniform cell type. × 450.

Clinical features. Ewing's tumour usually presents with pain and swelling, often of some months' duration. Sometimes fever, anaemia and leukocytosis suggest low-grade osteomyelitis and the patients with these systemic symptoms have the worst prognosis. The tumour is at first radiosensitive, but frequently recurrence takes place later and secondaries appear especially in other bones and in the lungs. Some improvement in prognosis is expected when radiotherapy or surgery is supplemented by repeated courses of cytotoxic drugs.

Differential diagnosis. In the absence of clearly distinctive histological features leukaemic deposits, lymphoid neoplasms, myelomatosis, secondary carcinoma and, in young children, metastatic neuroblastoma must be considered in the differential diagnosis. The increased urinary excretion of catecholamine derivatives in many cases of neuroblastoma and their normal values in patients with Ewing's tumour helps to distinguish between these tumours. Occasionally the true diagnosis only becomes apparent at necropsy.

Malignant lymphoma of bone

In contrast to lymphoid and some other tissues, bone is a relatively uncommon site of primary lymphoma.

Age, sex incidence and site. Malignant lymphoma is rare in childhood (cf. Ewing's tumour). It is commoner in males and affects both the metaphysis and the adjacent shaft of long bones, and may arise also in flat bones and the axial skeleton.

Clinical features. Malignant lymphoma of bone presents with pain and swelling but fever is rare. X-ray often shows a fairly widespread, diffuse, moth-eaten area of patchy rarefaction. Periosteal new bone formation is not usually conspicuous but there may be patchy reactive bone sclerosis in the medulla. The radiological appearances may suggest a chronic osteomyelitis, and in small biopsies with much necrosis and secondary inflammatory cell infiltrate, considerable difficulty may also arise in making this histological differentiation. The tumour is radio-sensitive, and the prognosis after radiotherapy is distinctly more favourable than that in Ewing's tumour. About 45 per cent of cases are said to survive for five years and about 30 per cent for ten years. Involvement of regional lymph nodes may occur early or late and may be followed by infiltration in spleen and liver. The lungs tend to be affected only late in the disease. Occasionally leukaemia develops. In every patient with a presumed primary lymphoma of bone, search should be made for involvement of other bones or of lymph nodes since the relatively good prognosis does not apply if the bone lesion is simply the presenting sign of more generalised disease.

Macroscopic appearances. The tumour tends to affect chiefly the metaphyseal region and adjacent shaft, and it is osteolytic so that the bony cortex becomes mottled and rarefied. The tumour penetrates the cortex usually without eliciting any new reactive periosteal bone, and spreads into the adjacent tissues.

Microscopic appearances. The tumour is usually composed of a mixture of cell types including lymphocytes, lymphoblasts and larger round or polyhedral cells each with a folded nucleus and a prominent nucleolus. The cell boundaries are often well-defined and between the cells there is sometimes a rich reticulin network, a feature conspicuously absent in Ewing's tumour. Intracellular glycogen is usually absent.

In some cases the distinction between malignant lymphoma and Ewing's tumour may be difficult or even impossible on the initial, often inadequate biopsy. When, however, a group of such cases is surveyed retrospectively with the clinical course, radiological and pathological features fully available, they can often be separated into the two categories.

Giant-cell tumour of bone (osteoclastoma)

Giant-cell tumour is an osteolytic, eccentrically placed tumour arising most commonly in the end of a long bone of an adult.

Age. The lesion frequently arises in the 20–40 age group. The diagnosis should be regarded with suspicion at a site where the epiphyseal cartilage plate is still open as there are several benign lesions in children and adolescents which to some extent simulate giant-cell tumour. Some of these are discussed below.

Site of occurrence. Half of all the tumours occur in the lower end of femur or upper tibia (Fig. 23.45). Another common site is the lower end of radius. Although flat bones may be involved, giant-cell tumour is rare in the jaw and in the vertebral column above the sacrum. When the tumour occurs in a long bone it arises almost invariably in the bone end and the metaphysis is involved only later. Accordingly joint symptoms are common.

Macroscopic appearances. Giant-cell tumour

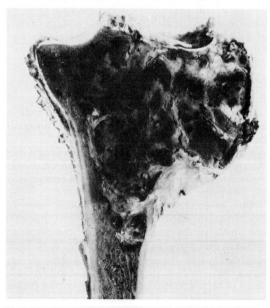

Fig. 23.45 Section of giant-cell tumour of upper end of tibia showing eccentric expansion of the bone end and much haemorrhage within the tumour.

is usually located eccentrically and often causes marked expansion of the bone end (Fig. 23.45). It is covered, initially, by a thin shell of subperiosteal bone which may be renewed on the surface as expansion progresses but this may later be breached by the tumour which then extends into the soft tissues. Invasion of the joint through the articular cartilage is uncommon. The tumour is entirely destructive and its cells do not form bone. As a result of its osteolytic propensities patients often present with a pathological fracture. There is none of the subperiosteal sunray bony spiculation seen in an osteosarcoma. The tumour is usually reddish-grey and commonly shows areas of haemorrhage and necrosis. If there has been a fracture or previous treatment by surgery or radiotherapy the picture may be complicated by callus formation, fibrosis and cystic degeneration.

Microscopic appearances. Giant-cell tumour consists of plump spindle or ovoid mononuclear cells abundantly interspersed with giant cells containing many nuclei, sometimes as many as 100 (Fig. 23.46). Fibrous tissue is

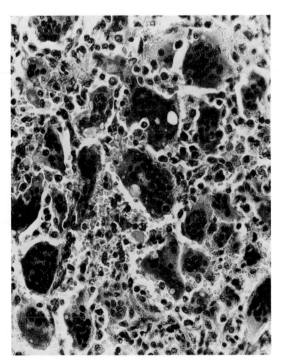

Fig. 23.46 Giant-cell tumour. The mononuclear tumour cells have the same characteristics as the scattered multinucleated cells. × 240.

usually scanty unless the tumour has previously fractured or been treated. Areas of necrosis, haemorrhage, lipid-containing macrophages and cholesterol are sometimes seen. Following surgical treatment there may be recurrence in the soft tissues; neither this nor the presence of tumour in periosteal veins is necessarily of sinister significance.

Prognosis. About half the tumours respond to thorough local removal, about a third recur and the remaining 15–20 per cent are liable to be malignant from the beginning or more often after recurrence, and to metastasise to the lungs. The tumour may recur as a fibrosarcoma or occasionally as an osteosarcoma. Some help in assessing the prognosis is given by the histology in that tumours which look frankly sarcomatous usually behave badly; however, very rarely, tumours which appear microscopically benign later metastasise.

Lesions likely to be confused with giant-cell tumour

Besides the differentiation of true giant-cell tumour from the benign lesions principally of childhood and adolescence described below, the lesion must be distinguished from **brown tumour of hyperparathyroidism** (p. 891). Since this may not be possible on histological grounds the blood chemistry should be investigated and a radiological search for subperiosteal erosions made, especially if the apparent giant-cell tumour is in the skull or jaw.

Aneurysmal bone cyst. This is probably not a true tumour but has been confused with giant-cell tumour. It is commonest in the long bone *metaphyses* or vertebrae of children or young adults and gives rise to an extremely eccentric osteolytic lesion which may balloon out the periosteum and sometimes involves contiguous bones. Within the thin bony shell the 'cyst' is found to consist of cavernous bloodfilled spaces separated by a brownish spongy meshwork of trabeculae: these are formed of vascular fibrous tissue, the larger ones reinforced by osteoid or bony strands. Giant cells are smaller and less evenly distributed than in giant-cell tumour (Fig. 23.47). The lesion is benign and is cured by surgery, sometimes even when removal has been incomplete. If untreated it may progressively increase in size, but sometimes appears to be self-limiting.

Benign chondroblastoma. This rare benign bone tumour of uncertain histogenesis is important because it may be mistaken for a malignant giant-cell tumour or occasionally a chondro- or osteo-sarcoma. Benign chondroblastoma occurs most often in adolescents and is usually located in the epiphysis of long bones, especially around the knee or in the

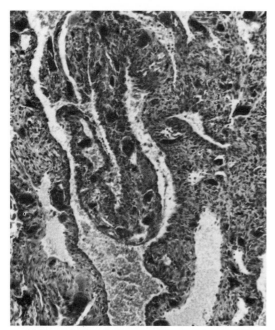

Fig. 23.47 Aneurysmal bone cyst. Vascular spaces lined by fibrous tissue with giant cells. × 45.

upper humerus. Radiologically there is a well-defined radiolucent area often with a narrow sclerotic border and sometimes with mottling due to spotty calcification. The tumour may spread across the epiphyseal plate into the metaphysis and rarely into the adjacent joint. Microscopically the lesion consists of fairly uniform small rounded or polygonal cells with a moderate sprinkling of multinucleated giant cells. A characteristic lacy pattern of intercellular calcification may be seen and this is thought to be followed by cellular necrosis and later transformation of necrotic areas to plaques of hyaline chondroid or osteoid-like material. The tumour is usually curable by curettage. It may recur but pulmonary metastases are very rare and usually not progressive.

Non-ossifying fibroma (non-osteogenic fibroma). This doubtfully neoplastic lesion was once thought to be a healing variant of giant-cell tumour. It sometimes appears to arise from a metaphyseal fibrous defect, a developmental lesion which is readily diagnosable radiologically as a small scalloped radiolucent area with a sclerotic edge hugging the metaphyseal cortex in the long bones, particularly the femur, of young children. These developmental abnormalities have the same naked-eye and microscopic appearances as do larger lesions involving the medullary cavity, which are described as non-ossifying fibromas and it seems probable that the larger ones are derived from the smaller. Macroscopically

the tissue is usually orange-yellow and microscopically shows whorled fibrous tissue with moderate numbers of small giant cells, haemosiderin and in some cases aggregates of lipid-containing macrophages. These lesions, whatever their derivation, are benign and heal after curettage.

Simple bone cyst. This is a benign non-neoplastic unilocular cystic lesion, probably related to some local disturbance of bone growth and commonly arising in the upper humeral or femoral metaphyses in children and adolescents. As the bone grows, the cyst appears to migrate down the shaft away from the epiphyseal line. It is commoner in males. Attention is frequently drawn to the lesion by pathological fracture and occasionally, following this, the cyst fills in. The appearances are of a smooth-walled cavity containing clear fluid and usually slightly expanding and markedly thinning the cortices. The lining consists of a meagre layer of rather acellular collagen. When fracture has occurred the fluid may be bloody and the lining transformed to a thick layer of granulation or fibrous tissue with areas of haemorrhage, cholesterol clefts, calcification, new bone formation, and osteoclast aggregates which sometimes have given rise to confusion with giant-cell tumour. The cysts, while perfectly benign, have a strong tendency to recur, particularly if they are near the epiphyseal plate when initially treated.

Chordoma

This tumour arises from notochordal remnants, and usually develops within or in close proximity to the axial skeleton. In post-natal life the notochord persists in the nucleus pulposus of the intervertebral discs. In addition, small remnants are found in the hollow of the sacrum and coccyx and as little gelatinous nodules in the region of the spheno-occipital synchondrosis (*ecchordosis physaliphora*); the latter are, of course, observed merely as incidental findings at necropsy. It is from these ectopic remnants rather than from the discs that most chordomas are thought to originate.

Sites of occurrence. Chordoma usually comes to notice in adult life and most commonly involves the sacrococcygeal region and the spheno-occipital part of the skull base. Cervical, dorsal and lumbar vertebral tumours are much rarer.

Clinical features. Chordomas are very slow-growing and commonly cause pressure on adjacent structures. In the sacral region they may become very large and press on the rectum; in the spheno-occipital site the symptoms are chiefly due to compression of cranial nerves but pituitary dysfunction may occur. The latter group are inevitably more quickly fatal. Radiological examination usually shows a lytic bone lesion with a soft tissue shadow and sometimes some patchy calcification. Death usually occurs from local extension of tumour rather than from metastasis.

Macroscopic appearances. The chordoma usually appears well circumscribed in its soft tissue mass but irregularly infiltrates adjacent bone. It is lobulated, greyish, semi-translucent and gelatinous with areas of haemorrhage and softening.

Microscopic appearances. Clusters or cords of cells are surrounded by a sea of mucin (Fig. 23.48). The most characteristic pattern is of cords of syncytial cells radiating towards the margins of the lobules. Some of these rounded or polyhedral cells may appear vacuolated due to intracytoplasmic droplets of mucoid material ('*physaliphorous cells*'). Some spheno-occipital chordomas contain nodules of cartilage. The histological differentiation between chordoma and chondrosarcoma or mucin-secreting carcinoma may be difficult and is better made on a careful assessment of the architecture than on the results of staining reactions.

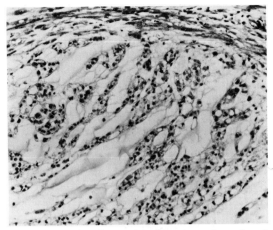

Fig. 23.48 Chordoma from sacrum. Strands of cells, many of them vacuolated, are seen lying in a background of mucinous material. × 140.

Diseases of Joints

Normal joint structure

Joints may be categorised as those without a joint cavity, the non-synovial *synarthroses* and those with a joint cavity, the synovial *diarthroses*. In a diarthrosis the bone ends are almost invariably covered by hyaline articular cartilage and the surfaces lubricated by synovial fluid produced by the synovial membrane which is supported by the fibrous joint capsule.

Articular cartilage. Normal articular cartilage forms a smooth, glistening, slightly elastic covering to the bone ends. It is bluish and translucent in the young, averaging 2–4 mm in thickness; in the old it becomes yellower and more opaque. The matrix consists partly of type II collagen fibres (p. 82) which run parallel to the surface in the superficial layer and in the deeper layer form an interlocking meshwork of coiled fibres. Smaller slender filaments lacking the characteristic banding of collagen surround the chondrocytes. The collagen meshwork entraps a gel of proteoglycans containing chains of chondroitin and keratan sulphate. These substances give cartilage its metachromatic staining.

The chondrocytes lie in lacunae in the matrix and have branching processes which extend into it. Those cells near the surface are flattened and horizontal, the deeper ones are arranged in columns. In the adult a wavy basophilic line marks the junction between the uncalcified cartilage and the small layer of calcified cartilage which is adjacent to the subchondral bone.

Articular cartilage is avascular and has a relatively low oxygen requirement. Its nourishment is derived from the synovial fluid and probably also, in growing animals, from blood vessels of the subchondral marrow. Exchange between the synovial fluid and cartilage is thought to be promoted by joint movement. Hyaline cartilage has little power of regeneration (p. 93).

Synovial membrane forms synovial fluid: it lines tendon sheaths and bursae and covers all the surfaces of joints except articular cartilage and menisci. The synovium may be smooth or folded and may form small villi especially at the joint margins. It is lined by a layer of ellipsoidal cells, one to four cells thick. These intimal cells are not separated by a basement membrane from the underlying tissues which may be areolar, dense fibrous or fatty in different parts of the joint. Two types of intimal cells are distinguished on electron microscopy. It is thought that Type A, the more numerous, acts as a macrophage while Type B synthesises hyaluronic acid.

The synovial membrane has a rich network of blood vessels, many of which run close to the surface. It is able to regenerate after synovectomy and a lining indistinguishable from synovium may form in adventitious bursae and pseudarthroses (false joints), presumably by metaplasia.

Synovial fluid is a dialysate of blood plasma with the addition of hyaluronic acid which gives the fluid its viscous property. The proportion of hyaluronic acid and hence the viscosity is said to diminish with age. The function of the fluid is twofold: to nourish the articular cartilage and to lubricate the joint surfaces. Under normal circumstances human joints contain less than 1 ml of synovial fluid. In healthy human joints the fluid contains up to $0.4 \times 10^9/l$ nucleated cells with few polymorphs, about 25 per cent lymphocytes, a few synovial cells and a majority of macrophages, perhaps derived from the synovium. In animals, and probably in man, the number of cells varies in one individual from one joint to another.

Albumin and globulin are present in lower concentration in the fluid than in plasma with a preponderance of albumin in the ratio of about $4:1$. Glucose levels are normally much less than in the blood.

Joint Inflammation of Known Cause

Acute infective arthritis

Since infections with pneumococcus, meningococcus, gonococcus or typhoid bacilli are usually promptly treated with antibiotics acute arthritis is now an uncommon complication. When it does occur it tends to be transient, non-suppurative and leaves little disability. While many different pyogenic bacteria, including *Streptococcus pyogenes* and *Haemophilus influenzae*, may give rise to suppurative (septic) arthritis, *Staphylococcus aureus* is most often the cause. The disease is commonest in infants, children and the aged, especially when the patient is debilitated or treated with bone marrow depressants or corticosteroids. The knee and hip are most often involved and, especially in infants, more than one joint may be affected.

Path of infection. Acute infective arthritis arises chiefly as a result of haematogenous spread and sometimes a focus of infection such as a staphylococcal boil or a septic throat is identifiable. Infection may spread from adjacent osteitis, especially when the affected metaphysis is within the joint cavity. It is a dreaded complication of reconstructive surgery and occasionally follows a penetrating wound or a compound intra-articular fracture.

Clinical features. There are the usual signs of acute inflammation, i.e. local redness, heat, pain, tenderness, oedema, joint effusion and limitation of movement, fever with rigors and often a polymorphonuclear leukocytosis and raised erythrocyte sedimentation rate. Difficulty in diagnosis may arise when, as sometimes happens, a pyogenic infection complicates pre-existing joint disease such as rheumatoid arthritis.

Early non-suppurative stage. The joint effusion contains a large increase of cells, mostly polymorphs. Synovial fluid and blood cultures should immediately be obtained in a suspected pyogenic arthritis, but are not always positive, and antibiotics should be administered thereafter without delay. The synovium at this stage is intensely red and congested and flecked with yellowish fibrin. Microscopically it shows the features of acute inflammation. If the disease is arrested at this stage the condition resolves with little residual joint damage.

Suppurative stage. If suppuration develops, within a few days, extensive cartilage destruction occurs probably as a result of the increase of proteolytic enzymes from polymorphs and of excess plasmin by bacterial activators. The exposed bone also undergoes necrosis (Fig. 23.49). An acute suppurative arthritis is entirely destructive but once the condition subsides into a subacute or chronic stage there is proliferation of granulation tissue within the joint, which is followed by ossification and bony ankylosis. Bony ankylosis occurs more commonly in untreated suppurative arthritis than in tuberculous or rheumatoid disease.

Gonococcal arthritis has become uncommon and is now seen more often in women than men. In the 2

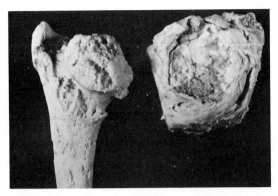

Fig. 23.49 Suppurative arthritis of hip joint. The articular cartilage of both the femoral head and the acetabulum is destroyed and there is erosion of the underlying bone.

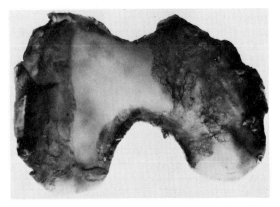

Fig. 23.50 Tuberculous disease of knee-joint. Note the spread of vascular tissue with tubercles over the surface of the cartilage.

per cent of patients with gonococcaemia, an acute arthritis involving first one and perhaps later several joints may develop. Tendon sheaths may also be affected. Blood cultures are often positive though the synovial fluid may be sterile. The arthritis usually subsides leaving little, if any, disability.

Tuberculous arthritis

Joint tuberculosis is decreasing in incidence. While no age in the indigenous population of Britain is exempt, the emphasis has slowly changed from children to the elderly: the hip and knee joints are the commonest sites. The disease is now usually the result of infection by the human strain of bacillus, which almost invariably has spread by the bloodstream from a primary or reactivated tuberculous focus elsewhere in the body, especially the lungs or lymph nodes. The synovium is frequently involved first. In some cases there may be secondary involvement by spread directly or by the periosteum from small or large tuberculous foci in adjacent bone.

Macroscopic appearances. There is often a moderate joint effusion, usually of clear or slightly turbid fluid, with 'melon-seed bodies' (p. 925). The synovial membrane is oedematous, hyperplastic and congested and may be studded with small greyish tubercles with yellowish caseating centres. If diagnosed and treated at this stage the lesion usually regresses leaving little residual damage. In untreated cases however, extensive joint destruction results. Soft gelatinous granulation tissue arising from the synovial membrane grows in from the

periphery of the joint to form a *pannus* (Fig. 23.50) creeping over and replacing the articular cartilage. In addition the articular cartilage may be destroyed by the ingrowth of subchondral granulation tissue which separates it in large flakes from the underlying bone. The cartilage may float free in the joint fluid or retain a tenuous attachment to bone. The exposed bone has an irregular surface with necrosis and fibrinous exudation. Occasionally caseous foci with suppurative softening form in the capsule of the joint and in the soft tissues outside, and pus may break through the skin surface giving rise to sinuses and allowing secondary infection to occur. Tuberculous arthritis heals by fibrosis, but the fibrous adhesions which form across the joint surfaces may later, if secondary infection occurs, become ossified with complete obliteration of the joint space by a bony mass which contains foci of pus or caseous material. It is now unusual to see, in Britain, joint tuberculosis proceeding to massive joint destruction with discharging sinuses and final spontaneous ankylosis, although these conditions may still be seen in countries where tuberculosis is unchecked by specific therapy.

Microscopic appearances. The histological diagnosis of tuberculosis from synovial biopsy may be made most readily if the synovium is studded with discrete tubercles showing the usual microscopic features. When the synovium is replaced by gelatinous granulation tissue, however, the condition may appear to be a non-specific inflammation with only a diffuse infiltrate of lymphocytes and plasma cells unless very careful search is made for the scanty and often ill-defined tubercle follicles. The pannus on the surface of the cartilage and the subchondral granulations are even less fruitful sites for diagnostic examination. Acid-fast bacilli are found in Ziehl–Neelsen stained tissue sections in rather more than half the cases and bacteriological culture of synovial tissue is positive in about the same proportion. When the superficial subchondral bone is also involved the marrow spaces may contain tubercle follicles with caseation and there may be some resorption and necrosis of bone.

The synovial fluid has a raised cell count and half or more of the cells may be lymphocytes. Melon-seed bodies and flakes of articular cartilage may also be present, the melon-seed bodies being formed usually of fibrin and sometimes of necrotic synovial fronds.

In patients with an undiagnosed monarthritis it is advisable to examine a synovial biopsy histologically in order to exclude tuberculosis rather than to rely on synovial fluid culture alone.

Tuberculous tenosynovitis. Tuberculosis may also affect the tendon sheaths, especially of the flexor tendons at the wrist. There is, as in joint tuberculosis, effusion of fluid into the sheath, the formation of melon-seed bodies and some-times proliferation of exuberant granulation tissue within the sheath. Here also extensive caseation with destruction of tendons is rarely seen except in untreated cases.

Syphilitic arthritis

In contrast to tuberculosis, syphilis comparatively seldom gives rise to important joint lesions.

Acquired syphilis. In the *secondary stage* there may be transient arthritis while gummas occasionally arise in the joint capsule in *tertiary* syphilis. Patients with tabes dorsalis sometimes develop neuropathic arthropathy (p. 923).

Congenital syphilis. There may be joint pain and swelling in infants and young children with syphilitic epiphysitis. Older children may develop chronic painless effusion, usually of the knees, with some synovial thickening which does not progress to severe joint damage (*Clutton's joints*).

Brucellosis (Undulant fever)

Joint symptoms are the presenting feature of about 25 per cent of cases of undulant fever, the joints being involved in the course of the septicaemia. The arthritis is transient and of non-specific inflammatory pattern. Sometimes granulomas similar to those of sarcoid or tuberculosis are seen (p. 563). Bursae may also be involved.

Joint Inflammation of Unknown Cause

Arthritis associated with rheumatic fever

Rheumatic fever usually follows a pharyngitis due to *Streptococcus pyogenes* and is characterised by pancarditis, fever and a reactive transient acute arthritis unrelated to rheumatoid arthritis. The large joints are usually inflamed, i.e. knees, ankles and wrists, and as the condition subsides in some joints others become affected.

In the acute stage there is usually a sterile joint effusion with a cell count around $10 \times 10^9/l$ (normal up to $0.4 \times 10^9/l$), most of these being polymorphs.

As the condition subsides the polymorphs diminish in the synovial fluid and lymphocytes become prominent. A diffuse chronic inflammatory cell infiltrate may be seen in the synovium but it lacks both the intensity and the accompanying proliferative changes seen in rheumatoid arthritis. Small granulomas resembling Aschoff bodies (p. 412) may be present in the synovium. The joint usually returns to normal, the inflammatory cell infiltrate disappears and the granulomas fibrose. Occasionally, especially when the capsule has been involved, there may be some residual pain and stiffness with persistent chronic inflammation and synovial thickening. In children small *subcutaneous nodules* up to 10 mm. in diameter may be found in groups at sites prone to minor trauma such as around the olecranon and ulnar border of the forearm and about the patella. These granulomas usually consist of small areas of degenerate collagen with histiocytes, chronic inflammatory cells and some proliferation of fibroblasts and capillaries. They become fibrotic and disappear within a few months. (Rheumatic fever is described more fully in Chapter 15.)

Rheumatoid arthritis

Rheumatoid arthritis is one of the connective tissue diseases (p. 937), and is characterised by a subacute or chronic non-suppurative arthritis usually affecting several joints. Its course is punctuated by spontaneous remissions.

Age and sex incidence. The disease usually begins in the years between 25 and 55 but may affect both older and younger people. *Still's disease* in children consists of rheumatoid arthritis with associated splenomegaly, lymphadenopathy and occasionally pericarditis. Rheumatoid arthritis affects about 3 per cent of the female and 1 per cent of the male population in this country: a small proportion of these patients become severely crippled.

Sites of occurrence. Any synovial joint may be affected but those of the hands and feet are most often involved, the disease often being bilateral and symmetrical. Temporomandibular, crico-arytenoid joints and those of the cervical spine are occasionally involved. Destructive spinal disease may produce instability and neurological complications.

Course of the disease. The onset is often insidious but sometimes acute. The condition may abate after a single attack but more commonly there are repeated relapses and remissions, the joint each time suffering further damage. Involvement of tendons, soft tissue swelling, muscle atrophy, and ligamentous and capsular laxity all contribute to increasing deformity. Sometimes the arthritis progresses to fibrous, occasionally to bony, ankylosis. The tendency is for the rheumatoid disease eventually to burn itself out but even then the joint disability may increase due to further damage from secondary osteoarthritis. During the active phase of polyarthritis tests for rheumatoid factor are usually positive (p. 939).

Clinical and macroscopic appearances. In the early acute stage or during relapses, the joints are hot, swollen and tender; the usual appearances of an acute inflammation. There is often general constitutional upset with fatigue, weight loss and fever; the ESR is raised, there is

a leukocytosis and sometimes a normocytic, normochromic anaemia. The swelling, which often gives the finger joints a spindle-shaped appearance, is partly due to synovial effusion which may be turbid but is sterile. There is an increase in cells, sometimes up to $50 \times 10^9/l$ with about 75 per cent polymorphs, and fibrin flakes may be present. The primary changes are in the synovium which is red and congested, oedematous, markedly frondose and frequently patchily covered by fibrinous exudate (Fig. 23.51), After the early stages it may be heavily pigmented with haemosiderin.

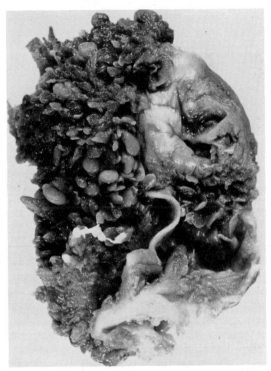

Fig. 23.51 Synovium from a rheumatoid knee joint. The synovial surface is markedly frondose and some of the villi are tipped with white fibrin.

Microscopic appearances. In the florid case there is marked villous hypertrophy of the synovium with synovial cell proliferation, fibrinous and polymorph exudate on the surface, lymphocytes in dense focal aggregates, sometimes with germinal centres, accompanied by a heavy and more diffuse plasma cell infiltrate (Fig. 23.52). These appearances may persist for an indefinite period after an acute attack. When these features are all pronounced, the

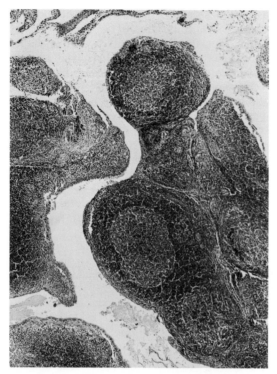

Fig. 23.52 Synovial membrane in chronic rheumatoid arthritis. The synovium shows villous hypertrophy and is extensively infiltrated with lymphocytes, amongst which occur poorly defined germinal centres. Plasma cells also are abundant. × 38.

diagnosis of rheumatoid arthritis may be suggested with fair, though not with absolute certainty. However, the synovium has only a limited range of response to different stimuli and less severe degrees of these changes may be seen in a wide variety of conditions, e.g. following trauma, in joints adjacent to tumours, in psoriatic arthritis, in various non-specific arthritides and in the late stages of osteoarthritis. Rarely the diagnosis may be confirmed by finding a typical 'rheumatoid nodule' (see below) in the subsynovial tissue.

While the changes in rheumatoid arthritis are confined to the synovium, the functional disability is reversible, but this is often followed by secondary irreversible changes in other joint structures. Subchondral erosions form at the joint margin and a thin layer of vascular granulation tissue (**pannus**) grows over the joint cartilage, which is eroded and destroyed by enzymes from the cells. If the underlying bone is exposed it may become pocketed by chronic granulations. In the later stage this granulation tissue may eventually become fibrosed with resultant adhesions across the joint space and later ossification sometimes converts fibrous to bony ankylosis, especially in the small joints of the carpus and tarsus.

While these changes are going on in the joint, *the bone* at an early stage may become markedly porotic due to hyperaemia and disuse. *The muscles* become atrophic and there is wasting and weakness especially of the interossei and sometimes also of the hand flexors. *Tendons* may also become infiltrated by rheumatoid granulation tissue and this leads to pain and disability and sometimes to rupture of the tendon with further deformity. As a result of muscle atrophy and tendon destruction, ligamentous and capsular laxity, the hand in particular comes to be greatly deformed with marked ulnar deviation, subluxation and dislocation of joints (Fig. 23.53b).

Non-orthopaedic features of rheumatoid disease. Rheumatoid nodules consisting of a central area of fibrinoid necrosis of collagen surrounded by palisaded fibroblasts (Fig. 23.53a) occur in the subcutaneous tissues over pressure sites in about 20 per cent of cases. These

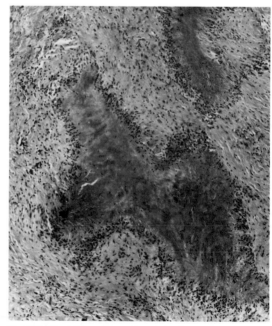

Fig. 23.53a Rheumatoid nodule from the region of the elbow-joint. × 90.

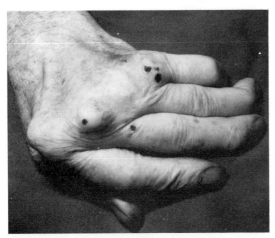

Fig. 23.53b The hand shows the typical severe deformity of rheumatoid arthritis with marked ulnar deviation of the fingers and muscle wasting. Ulcerated rheumatoid nodules are present over the metacarpo-phalangeal joints.

nodules persist throughout life and are a helpful clinical and histological diagnostic aid. They tend to occur in more severely affected patients and to be associated with a worse prognosis (Fig. 23.53b).

Similar nodules are occasionally found at other sites, including the lungs of coalminers with rheumatoid disease (Caplan's syndrome, p. 489), the pleura, the heart and pericardium, and the eye.

Inflammation of arteries and veins may occur and when severe gives rise to skin ulceration and occasionally gangrene, bowel perforation and myocardial infarction. Peripheral neuropathy may also result. The skin is often atrophic, thin and papery.

Reactive and hyperplastic changes occur in lymph nodes and spleen (pp. 562, 572). About 20 per cent of cases of chronic rheumatoid arthritis coming to necropsy have some evidence of amyloid disease affecting the spleen, liver and kidney, although symptoms attributable to amyloid are rare. Sjøgren's syndrome (p. 594) may accompany rheumatoid disease.

Aetiology. The cause of rheumatoid arthritis is not known. It presents features which suggest that the lesions in the joints and elsewhere are brought about by hypersensitivity reactions. In particular, *rheumatoid factors* are present in the serum of most cases: these consist of IgM or IgG which reacts with antigenic components of the Fc part of IgG, forming immune complexes. Accordingly, rheumatoid arthritis is commonly termed **seropositive arthritis** to distinguish it from a group of **seronegative arthritides**, in which rheumatoid factors are absent.

The aetiology of rheumatoid arthritis is discussed further with the connective tissue diseases on p. 939.

Seronegative arthritis

As is suggested by the name this group of diseases is characterised by negative tests for rheumatoid factor and by the absence of rheumatoid nodules. The different conditions within this group include ankylosing spondylitis, psoriatic arthritis, arthritis associated with ulcerative colitis and Crohn's disease and 'reactive arthritis'; that is an arthritis presumably of immunological origin associated with infection at a distant site such as the gut or urethra. There is often considerable clinical overlap between the different conditions. The features of the group, though not all are present in each disease, are a tendency to axial skeletal involvement (spondylitis) with radiological evidence of inflammation of the sacroiliac joints, an asymmetrical peripheral arthritis, inflammation of the uveal tract of the eye, an aortitis involving the aortic ring and ulceration of the mouth, intestine or genital tract. There is a tendency to familial aggregation of each of these diseases and for other seronegative conditions to occur within the family. Recently an association has been shown with HLA-B27 especially when there is spinal involvement.

HLA system and seronegative arthritis. The most striking relationship is between HLA-B27 and ankylosing spondylitis (see below). The individual with B27 is 300 times more likely to develop the disease than one without that antigen and 90 per cent of patients with ankylosing spondylitis have HLA-B27. The association between the HLA antigen and the disease has led to the recognition that spondylitis is much commoner than had been suspected, radiological changes affecting perhaps 1–2 per cent of the population and that often, and especially in women, it is a mild, self-limiting condition. Its features appear to be the same in the 10 per cent of patients who are B27 negative. Patients with ankylosing spondylitis may develop peripheral arthritis or attacks of acute anterior uveitis and these have been regarded as complications of the condition. However, both are probably genetically determined since there is a high incidence of B27 amongst patients with uveitis (40 per cent) and with seronegative peripheral arthritis (30 per cent) *without* spondylitis. (About 8 per cent of Europeans have B27 antigen and of these around 75 per cent have no evidence of ankylosing spondylitis.)

Of the groups of patients suffering from psoriasis, ulcerative colitis, Crohn's disease and bowel infections with *Shigellae, Salmonellae* or *Yersinia enterocolitica*, those with B27 antigen are more likely to develop arthritis or spondylitis. Similarly there is a high incidence of B27 antigen in Reiter's syndrome with arthritis (see opposite) whether this follows urethritis or dysentery.

Ankylosing spondylitis

Ankylosing spondylitis is a polyarthritis which in severe cases may lead to bony ankylosis of the sacroiliac, intervertebral, and costovertebral joints with ossification of spinal ligaments and the borders of intervertebral discs resulting in rigidity of the spine. Sometimes the sternoclavicular and hip joints are similarly involved. The classical form of the disease is much commoner in males than females and usually the onset is in adolescence or early adult life. It is sometimes familial.

Course of the disease. There is usually an insidious onset of stiffness in the back with clinical and radiological evidence of inflammation of the sacroiliac joints. The condition is often self-limiting but may progress with exacerbations and remissions until the patient is left with an absolutely rigid back showing the radiological appearances of *bamboo spine* (Fig. 23.54a). When the cervical spine is involved there is danger of atlanto-axial dislocation or vertebral fracture and care must be taken in the handling of the anaesthetised patient. During exacerbations the ESR is commonly raised. The hips may be involved transiently, or chronically with final bony ankylosis in the most severely affected patients. Although diminished chest expansion is common, respiratory complications are rare.

Structural changes. The synovial changes resemble those of rheumatoid arthritis. The characteristic extra-articular ossification is thought

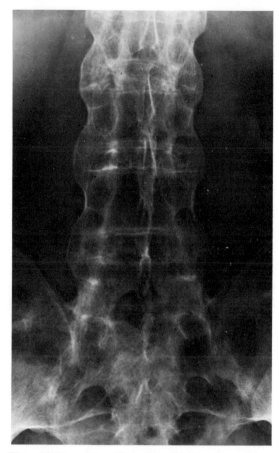

Fig. 23.54a A radiograph shows the typical 'bamboo' spine of late severe ankylosing spondylitis.

to result from healing of inflammatory foci at the site of attachment to bone of ligaments, joint capsule or the outer fibres of the annulus fibrosus. This marginal ankylosis may be followed by endochondral ossification of remaining cartilage (Fig. 23.54b).

Aortic lesions. A few patients with longstanding ankylosing spondylitis may develop aortic valvular incompetence due to changes in the aorta indistinguishable from those of syphilis, but limited to the immediate vicinity of the aortic valve and sinuses of Valsalva. Serological tests for syphilis have been consistently negative and this appears to be a non-syphilitic lesion.

Leukaemia. Irradiation of the spine in ankylosing spondylitis includes a large volume of the haemopoietic marrow and this increases tenfold the chance of the patient developing chronic (less commonly acute) myeloid leukaemia.

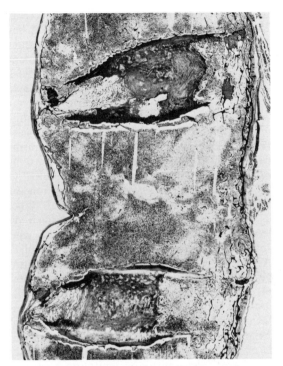

Fig. 23.54b Bone bridges the lumbar intervertebral discs anteriorly (*on the left*). As a result of endochondral ossification much of the disc has been replaced by bone. There is very severe porosis of the vertebral bodies. (Reproduced by permission from Applied Surgical Pathology, Blackwell Scientific Publications.)

Psoriatic arthritis

Patients with psoriasis, especially those with involvement of the nails, have a tendency to develop a remittent arthritis which has a predilection for the distal joints of the hands and feet. While the synovium shows much the same non-specific picture of hyperplasia with lymphocytic and plasma cell infiltrate as in the less florid cases of rheumatoid arthritis, the clinical and radiographic features and the negative test for rheumatoid factor serve to make the distinction. While deformities of the hands and feet may result, the condition is usually less disabling than rheumatoid arthritis. A small number of patients develop spondylitis, of these about 65 per cent are HLA-B27 positive; uveitis may also occur.

Reiter's syndrome

This consists of 'abacterial' urethritis, conjunctivitis and arthritis, sometimes following diarrhoea. It may be due to chlamydial infection (p. 988) and occurs most frequently in adult males. The knee, ankle, small joints of the hands and feet and sometimes the spine are involved in a transient polyarthritis which in contrast to gonococcal arthritis may not respond to penicillin therapy. While often there is no permanent disability there may be recurrences with a tendency to destructive changes in the feet and sacroiliac joints. The incidence of HLA antigen B27 (p. 919) is high in such cases. The mouth may be involved and skin lesions affect especially the soles and palms.

Degenerative Arthropathies

Osteoarthritis or degenerative arthritis

Osteoarthritis is the commonest form of chronic joint disease and is characterised clinically by the insidious but progressive onset of joint pain and stiffness. In spite of the name it is not an inflammatory or systemic disease but results from destructive and degenerative changes in the articular cartilage of joints. While any joint may be affected, disease of the hip or knee is most frequent and most disabling.

Osteoarthritis is found chiefly in the elderly. In younger patients there is usually an obvious predisposing cause. This 'secondary' osteoarthritis may be the result of intra-articular abnormalities such as congenital dislocation of the hip, of damage to the cartilage by fracture or loose bodies, or by previous inflammation. Extra-articular abnormalities which throw unusual stress on the joint, such as malunion of a fracture, bowing of the legs or scoliosis also predispose to osteoarthritis. The cause of 'primary' osteoarthritis developing in a normal joint is not known though excessive physical activity or misuse appear to play a part.

Structural changes. *Articular cartilage.* The first abnormality recognised by light microscopy is loss of metachromasia in the surface layers. Whether this results from rupture of the superficial collagen network or from depletion of the proteoglycan ground substance following release of enzymes from damaged chondrocytes remains speculative. It is associated with the development of tangential flaking of the surface and this may progress to deeper fissuring or fibrillation. Proliferation of chondrocytes and increased production of ground substance adjacent to the fissures fails to produce healing and loss of the cartilage substance follows so that the subchondral bone may be exposed (Fig. 23.55) with diminution of the width of the joint space radiologically.

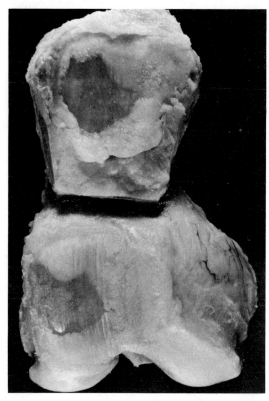

Fig. 23.55 Osteoarthritis of the knee joint has caused complete loss of articular cartilage with exposure of the bone on opposing surfaces of the patella (*above*) and the femur. There is parallel scoring of the joint surfaces.

The distinction between age changes and osteoarthritis is difficult. Studies of the hip joint suggest that fibrillation in some sites may be a self-limiting age change while in the load bearing area it is the forerunner of progressive destructive changes.

Bone. While these changes are occurring in the articular cartilage the subchondral bone

trabeculae become greatly thickened (Fig. 23.56). When this dense bone is exposed it becomes polished and eburnated, sometimes grooved in the direction of joint movement (Figs. 23.55, 23.59). The superficial osteocytes are usually dead. Fibrocartilaginous metaplasia tends to occur in any exposed marrow spaces.

Marked bone remodelling results in change in the shape of the joint surface. This is particularly obvious in the flattening and mushrooming of the load-bearing surface of the femoral head in osteoarthritis of the hip joint (Fig. 23.56). Another result is the formation of radiological 'cysts' in the subchondral bone. These are areas devoid of bone but filled by loose rather degenerate fibrous tissue and sometimes surrounded by new bone trabeculae. At the joint margins small excrescences form, giving first an appearance of beading and later of lipping of the joint. These osteophytic outgrowths form by proliferation of cartilage, followed by endochondral ossification (Fig. 23.56), but the stimulus to cartilage production is not fully understood. The osteophytes may give rise to deformity and limitation of movement. Spontaneous ankylosis does not occur in uncomplicated osteoarthritis.

Synovium. In the early stages the synovium appears normal but when disintegration of the joint surfaces take place there is absorption of

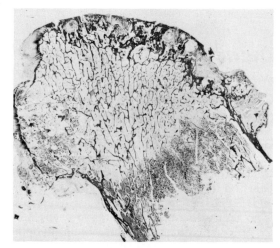

Fig. 23.56 Osteoarthritis of hip joint. The load-bearing surface of the femoral head is flattened and mushroomed and the articular cartilage has largely disappeared. The exposed bone is dense, small osteoarthritic 'cysts' are present and there are peripheral osteophytes.

abraded fragments of cartilage and bone, associated with villous hypertrophy and followed by subsynovial fibrosis. Chronic inflammatory cell infiltrate may then be seen.

Synovial fluid. Synovial effusion tends to be associated with synovitis, apparently a reaction to debris in the joint. The cell count is slightly raised and only about 15 per cent of cells are polymorphs.

Heberden's nodes. These are small bony elevations on the terminal phalanges of the fingers near the joint line. They may give rise to some deformity and limitation of movement. Some are the result of osteoarthritis; others result from post-traumatic ossification of para-articular tissues.

Primary generalised osteoarthritis sometimes has a familial incidence, affects multiple joints often in relatively young patients and is almost invariably associated with Heberden's nodes.

Chondromalacia patellae is a condition arising in young people and giving rise to pain, effusion, loss of movement and crepitus of the knee joint. A history of trauma to the patella is often given. The naked-eye and microscopic changes in excised patellae are those of localised degeneration in the articular cartilage.

Neuropathic arthropathy (Charcot's joint)

Neuropathic arthritis is an accelerated form of degenerative arthritis resulting from the progressive disorganisation of an insensitive joint when subjected to trauma. It was first described by Charcot as occurring in tabes dorsalis and has since been found in many other neurological conditions. The commonest cause nowadays is probably *diabetic neuropathy*, the joints of the feet most often being involved.

The condition can be attributed to continued use of an analgesic joint with associated proprioceptive loss. A cycle of events may occur in, for instance, the knee joint in a case of tabes dorsalis. The ataxia leads readily to some minor or major trauma to the joint which results in effusion; the swelling and muscular hypotonia increase the instability of the joint and its liability to further damage. Because the joint is painless the patient fails to guard it and continued use leads to repetition of the cycle. The structural changes in this condition are basically those of an extremely severe, and often rapidly progressive, osteoarthritis. The cartilage is destroyed, the bone ends grossly

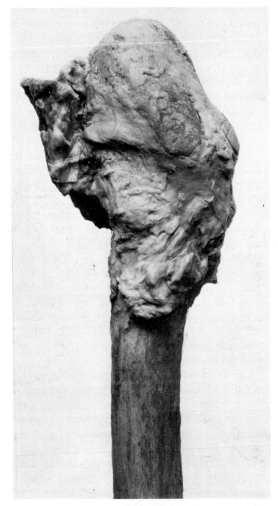

Fig. 23.57 Upper end of femur in neuropathic arthropathy of the hip joint in a patient with tabes. Note the irregular absorption of the head and the new formation of bone below.

distorted (Fig. 23.57) partly by remodelling and partly by the early formation of very large osteophytic outgrowths which may fracture and cause further damage. Fracture of the joint surface may also occur and the pathology of neuroarthropathy may be complicated by hyperplastic callus formation. The gross and bizarre radiological changes contrast with the relative lack of pain.

Arthritis associated with gout

Gout is a disease with a hereditary tendency, associated with an incompletely understood disorder of purine metabolism. It results in repeated attacks of acute arthritis which may be followed by chronic degenerative joint changes. Most patients with gout have hyperuricaemia, i.e. a serum urate level of more than 0·42 mmol/l (7 mg/100 ml) in males; 0·36 mmol/l (6 mg/100 ml) in females. Hyperuricaemia is much commoner than clinical gout and the higher the serum urate level the greater the likelihood of the patient eventually developing symptoms.

So-called **secondary gout** may arise in the treatment of neoplastic conditions, e.g. leukaemia, with cytotoxic drugs; the hyperuricaemia results from the increased nucleoprotein breakdown. Occasionally secondary gout complicates uraemia, the decreased renal output leading to a raised blood uric acid level.

Age, sex and site incidence. The first attack usually occurs over the age of 40; the disease is much commoner in males, females seldom being affected until after the menopause. In more than half the cases the metatarso-phalangeal joint of the great toe is first affected, but the ankle, knee, elbow, wrist and other toe and finger joints may be involved.

The acute attack. In the susceptible subject an acute attack of gout may be precipitated by many factors such as trauma, surgery, overexertion, alcoholic or dietary excess, certain diuretics and purgation. Some of the drugs given to gouty patients to promote urinary excretion of uric acid may produce an acute attack since they free some of the acid which is bound to plasma proteins and so increase the amount of diffusible uric acid. Acute gout is sometimes ushered in by pyrexia, leukocytosis and a raised erythrocyte sedimentation rate. The onset is sudden, may be nocturnal and there is excruciating pain in the affected joint, often the great toe (podagra) or its associated bursa, which shows all the signs of an acute inflammation. Needle-like strongly negative birefringent crystals of monosodium urate may be recognised in the synovial fluid, often within polymorphs (cf. pseudo-gout, p. 925). The polymorphs which have taken up the crystals release a chemotactic substance which attracts other leukocytes. The ingested crystals damage the membrane-limited phagolysosomes in which they lie, hydrolytic enzymes are released into the cytoplasm and the cell dies, releasing the crystal. Cells in the synovial fluid may increase to $14 \times 10^9/l$ with 70 per cent or more

polymorphs. The attack lasts usually for a few days or weeks and is followed by remission, though hyperuricaemia may persist. The prompt beneficial effect of colchicine which is thought to block the release of, and alter the response to, the chemotactic factors, may be used as a therapeutic test of acute gout.

Chronic gout is associated with the formation of crystalline deposits of sodium urate, often with cholesterol and calcium salts, in relatively avascular collagen, hyaline and fibro-cartilage. These deposits are known as **tophi** and may be found in the fibrocartilages of the ear, in bursal walls, especially the olecranon and prepatellar bursae and in the articular cartilage of joints (Fig. 23.58). Tophi are less frequent since drug therapy has become more effective. They may occur at sites of previous acute gouty arthritis or appear insidiously. Tophi are not significantly radio-opaque.

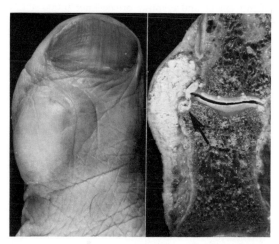

Fig. 23.58 A gouty tophus is seen in the subcutaneous tissue overlying the interphalangeal joint of the great toe. The tophus has produced a little resorption of bone at the joint margin (*arrow*). The articular cartilage is also flecked with white crystalline material.

Microscopic examination of alcohol-fixed material from a tophus shows sheaves of urate crystals, with a surrounding very marked foreign-body giant cell and granulomatous reaction (Fig. 10.17, p. 289).

In joints, the urate deposition occurs first in the superficial articular cartilage where it can be seen as opaque white spots like paint. The crystalline deposits are accompanied by degenerative changes in the articular cartilages which may cause some of the disability of chronic gouty arthritis. Later, urates may be precipitated in the subchondral and subperiosteal bone giving rise to bone destruction and punched out defects which are radiologically diagnosable. Tophi may occur in relation to synovium or para-articular tissues and may sometimes reach great size and destroy cartilage, bone, synovium and capsule, leaving a totally disorganised joint. (Purine metabolism and the aetiology of gout are described on p. 289 and the renal changes on p. 842.)

Pyrophosphate arthropathy (Articular chondrocalcinosis; pseudo-gout)

In recent years a condition with only a slight male preponderance has been described, chiefly in the middle-aged and elderly. It is characterised clinically by episodes of acute or subacute inflammation of one or more large joints, especially the knees. Involvement of the big toe is rare. During the acute stage (*pseudo-gout*) 'rod' and 'tablet' crystals of **calcium pyrophosphate** may be identified in the synovial fluid, mostly within polymorphs. The mechanism of production of the acute inflammatory response is similar to that in gout. Calcification may appear in the menisci of the knee, the articular disc of the distal radio-ulnar joint, the annulus fibrosus of the intervertebral discs, the symphysis pubis and also in articular cartilages, ligaments, tendons and joint capsules (*chondrocalcinosis*). Chronic degenerative joint disease may follow. While about a third of patients have hyperuricaemia and an occasional one has clinical gout, the condition should be distinguished from true gout by the involvement of large joints, the distinctive radiological findings and the characteristic crystals which exhibit a faint positive birefringence in polarised light. Once the diagnosis of pyrophosphate arthropathy is made, predisposing causes such as hyperparathyroidism, haemochromatosis or diabetes should be sought.

Mixtures of crystals are sometimes found and recently the tiny crystals of *hydroxyapatite* have been recognised by electron microscopy in the joint fluid and synovium of some osteoarthritic joints. It remains uncertain whether apatite crystals or free pyrophosphates are important in the production of osteoarthritis.

Haemophilic arthropathy

Acute haemarthrosis, especially in the knee, is a common finding in haemophilia and the joint may become greatly distended by blood which is gradually resorbed. The synovium becomes deeply pigmented with haemosiderin. After repeated haemarthroses there is often some destruction of the articular cartilage, probably partly the result of subchondral haemorrhages. Where damage to cartilage has occurred osteoarthritic changes may supervene.

In addition, organisation of intraosseous haemorrhage may lead to bone resorption and the formation of bone 'cysts', while subperiosteal haematomas may simulate scurvy.

Miscellaneous Joint Conditions

Intra-articular loose bodies

Multiple soft loose bodies are sometimes known as '*rice or melon-seed*' bodies. They are usually formed from fibrin or necrotic synovial tissue and are found in tuberculosis and rheumatoid arthritis. Symptoms are those of the accompanying arthritis.

Hard loose bodies may be caused by:

(1) Osteochondritis dissecans. Here the loose body is derived from part of the articular cartilage and underlying bone which for some reason separates from the surrounding tissue. When completely separated, the cartilaginous part of the body remains viable and may proliferate: the bone dies. Usually one, occasionally several, loose bodies may be present, the medial condyle of the femur being most frequently affected.

(2) Osteoarthritis. The fracturing of marginal osteophytes is a rare occurrence. It is said to occur more commonly in the severe osteoarthritis associated with neuroarthropathy.

(3) Fracture of the articular margins. Occasionally fracture of the articular margins results in one of the fragments of the fracture entering the joint and acting as a loose body, i.e. in fractures of the lower end of the humerus the medial epicondyle may, in spite of its muscle attachments, form a loose body in the elbow joint.

(4) Synovial chondromatosis or osteochon-

dromatosis. In this condition the synovial membrane shows cartilaginous metaplasia. These very numerous cartilaginous nodules may then ossify: some may become detached to lie free in the synovial fluid.

Clinically, hard loose bodies may give rise to episodes of locking of the joint. Damage to the articular cartilage may result in osteoarthritis (Fig. 23.59).

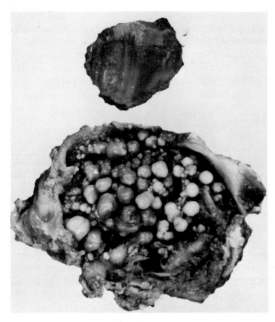

Fig. 23.59 Chondromatosis of synovium of the knee joint. Osteoarthritis of patella.

Pigmented villonodular synovitis

Pigmented villonodular synovitis is an uncommon condition of unknown aetiology, thought to be reactive rather than neoplastic which may affect joints, bursae or tendon sheaths in a localised or in a diffuse form. Males between the ages of 20–50 years are most commonly affected and the knee or hip joint is often involved. The diffuse synovitis gives rise to pain, a blood-stained serous effusion, and sometimes to locking of the joint.

Macroscopic appearances. The diffuse form has a most striking appearance. In the early stages the synovium looks like a tangled red-brown beard; matting together of the hyperplastic, pigmented villi later gives rise to a spongy orange and brown pad of great com-

plexity. There may also be firm nodules, sessile or pedunculated, and one of several of these may be present in the localised form of the disease. Occasionally, and especially when the hips or fingers are affected, adjacent bone is infiltrated by the pigmented tissue and the extra-articular soft tissue may be involved. Regional lymph nodes may become pigmented with haemosiderin.

Microscopic appearances. The villi are enlarged, the synovial lining cells increased and prominent, macrophages and chronic inflammatory cells and sometimes small multinucleated giant cells are abundant (Fig. 23.60). Much haemosiderin is present partly in macrophages and synovial lining cells and also lying free in the tissue. There may also be xanthomatous areas with foamy lipid-laden macrophages. When the villi become matted together clefts lined by synovial cells are seen and may give an appearance alarmingly similar to synovial sarcoma. The nodular projections often are more hyalinised with dense collagen, little pigment and many giant cells.

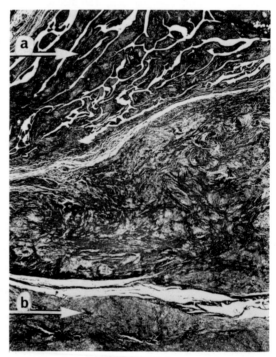

Fig. 23.60 At **a** there is diffuse pigmented villonodular synovitis while at **b** a solid mass containing abundant lipid macrophages and haemosiderin has developed. × 10.

Prognosis. In its diffuse form this condition is difficult to eradicate completely and there is a tendency to recurrence. In spite of recurrence, its occasional involvement of bone, its liability to spread into extra-articular tissue and its sometimes alarming histological appearance, no carefully documented case has been known to metastasise and the differentiation between this lesion and synovial sarcoma is of the first importance if needless amputation is to be avoided. The localised form, whether occurring as nodules within joints or associated with tendon sheaths (see below), is more readily cured by excision.

Bursae. The popliteal bursa is the most frequently involved. A tumour-like mass forms, and the gross and histological appearances are the same as in joints.

Tendon sheaths. Very rarely there is widespread diffuse involvement of a tendon sheath but the common finding is of multinodular masses in close proximity to the extensor tendons of the hands (Fig. 23.61). The histological appearance of these nodules is identical with those of the sessile or pedunculated lumps sometimes seen as part of the diffuse form of the disease. Careful dissection sometimes shows a little diffuse villous involvement of an adjacent tendon sheath or small joint. The nodules have formerly been described as benign giant-cell tumours of tendon sheath, and while the aetiology and nature of pigmented villonodular synovitis is still undecided it is probably immaterial which label is used.

Synovial tumours

Benign, giant-cell tumour of tendon sheath

This condition is considered to be the localised form of pigmented villonodular synovitis and is discussed above (Fig. 23.61).

Synovial sarcoma (malignant synovioma)

Synovial sarcoma is a rare and highly malignant tumour usually found adjacent to but outside a joint. Though it occurs most often in young adults there is a wide age range. The tumour is most common in the lower limb especially around the knee or ankle.

Macroscopic appearances. This malignant tumour, like many soft tissue sarcomas, often has a falsely reassuring appearance of en-

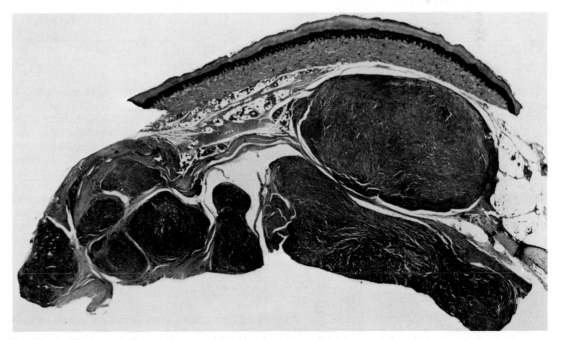

Fig. 23.61 Pigmented villonodular synovitis of tendon sheath. Multiple nodules of pigmented giant-cell tissue are loosely attached to a tendon of the ring finger. × 5·5.

capsulation due to compression of surrounding tissue. It may be white or pinkish-grey, sometimes with areas of haemorrhage and frequently with spotty calcification which may be sufficient to be seen radiologically.

Microscopic appearances. The tumour consists of both fibrosarcomatous and pseudo-epithelial elements, either of which may predominate without altering the prognosis. In the fibrosarcomatous tissue there are clefts or gland-like spaces sometimes containing mucinous material and lined by cuboidal or columnar cells (Fig. 23.62). Branching strands of hyaline collagen with a superficial resemblance to osteoid are sometimes a feature and may be patchily calcified. Invasion of blood vessels is sometimes seen.

Prognosis. Metastases develop in lungs, lymph nodes and other organs. There is a 5-year survival of between 25 per cent and 50 per cent of patients though some die later of their disease.

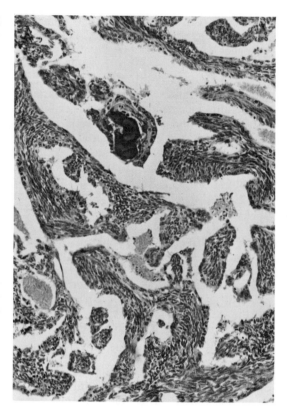

Fig. 23.62 Synovial sarcoma showing fibrosarcoma-like spindle cells and clefts lined by cubical cells. There is a focus of calcification. This tumour metastasised. × 115.

Miscellaneous Disorders of the Para-articular Tissues

Ganglion. Ganglia occur in the soft tissue around joints or tendon sheaths. The commonest site is the dorsum of the wrist, but they may also be found on the palmar aspect and around the knee. They usually develop by myxoid change and cystic softening of the fibrous tissue of the joint capsule or tendon sheath and sometimes have a direct connection with a joint cavity. Rarely they are found within nerve sheaths and may give rise to symptoms of nerve compression. They consist commonly of a thin, fibrous-walled sac, often rather gelatinous due to the patchy mucoid change, and not lined by synovium. A ganglion contains clear glairy fluid.

Similar lesions occasionally arise in the periosteum, particularly of the tibia and also sometimes within bone, beneath a normal articular surface.

Cyst of semilunar cartilage. The cyst arises in relation to the external semilunar cartilage (lateral meniscus) of the knee and has naked-eye and histological features identical with those of a ganglion. Often it appears to arise in the loose fibrous tissue adjacent

to, rather than actually within, the fibrocartilage of the meniscus.

Bursitis. A bursa is a synovial-lined sac and is found chiefly over bony prominences. It may communicate with a joint and is subject to many of the same disorders. Inflammation may arise as a result of repeated trauma as, for instance, in prepatellar bursitis (*housemaid's knee*). The bursa becomes distended with fluid, often with much fibrin, and the synovial lining may show villous hyperplasia or may be replaced by granulation and later by fibrous tissue. Loose bodies of the melon-seed type may form. *Baker's cyst* arises in the popliteal space by herniation of the synovial membrane through the joint capsule. The connection to the articular cavity may be closed by scarring.

Tumoral calcinosis. In this condition radio-opaque calcium phosphate forms small discrete nodules or larger masses around joints, especially the hip, or in soft tissues. Young Africans are particularly likely to be affected. The condition is usually initially painless though later there may be pressure on nerves. The overlying skin may ulcerate with discharge of chalky fluid or granular white material. Microscopically the deposits of calcium are often surrounded by macrophages, foreign-body giant cells and dense collagen. Plaques of degenerate collagen may be seen near the deposits. The patients are usually healthy and biochemical changes in the blood are inconstant. The aetiology remains uncertain. It has been suggested that the deposits may be the result of traumatic fat necrosis or of an abnormality of phosphate metabolism.

Dupuytren's contracture is a painless hereditary condition involving the palmar fascia and resulting in flexion contracture of the fingers. It occurs most commonly in middle-aged males and is often bilateral. The fifth, fourth and third fingers tend to be affected in that order of frequency. The fascia becomes thickened, contracted and sometimes nodular. In the active phase, microscopy shows a whorled pattern of very marked fibroblastic proliferation which may give rise to alarm on account of its cellularity (Fig. 23.63). It progresses, however, to extremely dense hyalinised collagen and is entirely benign. Usually a mixture of fibroblastic and hyalinised areas is seen. A similar condition (*plantar fibromatosis*) may be present in the sole of the foot, causing nodules in the plantar fascia without contracture. This also is benign, though often locally recurrent and difficult to eradicate surgically.

Fibrositis and panniculitis. The clinical syndrome of muscular pain and localised tenderness may be accounted for by a variety of conditions from cervical spondylosis to Coxsackie virus infection. There is considerable doubt as to whether 'fibrositis' itself exists though tender fibrofatty nodules have been described associated with oedema, a mild chronic inflammatory cell infiltrate and followed by fibrosis. Acute pain of sudden onset may sometimes be due to herniation of a fatty lobule through a small aperture in the investing fibrous tissue and this is termed panniculitis. When associated with obesity the condition may be designated *adiposis dolorosa* or *Dercum's disease*.

Relapsing febrile nodular panniculitis (Weber–

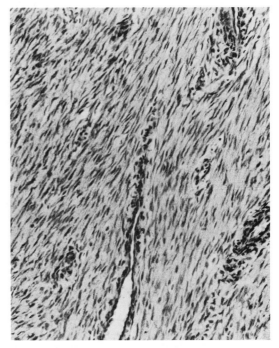

Fig. 23.63 Dupuytren's contracture, showing the highly cellular fascial tissue. × 130.

Christian syndrome). In this condition successive attacks of weakness and muscular pains are followed by bouts of fever in which tender nodules appear in the subcutaneous and other adipose tissues. These consist of foci of subacute inflammation with areas of secondary fat necrosis and granulomatous reaction. Rarely suppuration may occur and ulceration of the skin then follows, but micro-organisms have not been found in the lesions. The cause is unknown.

Polymyalgia rheumatica. This clinical syndrome, which usually affects the elderly, consists of pain, stiffness and tenderness of the muscles of the shoulder and pelvic girdles, with a raised erythrocyte sedimentation rate. There is a mild and often transient non-specific synovitis and about half the patients have evidence of giant-cell arteritis (p. 382).

Diseases of Skeletal Muscle

Normal muscle structure

A muscle consists of bundles of muscle fibres bound together by fibrous tissue, the epimysium. This fibrous sheath penetrates between the muscle bundles as the perimysium and each muscle fibre is surrounded by a delicate tenuous sheath of endomysium. Fat cells normally may lie between the muscle bundles but not within them. The muscle or sarcolemmal nuclei in the human lie at the periphery of the fibre under the cell membrane or sarcolemma except in the ocular muscles and at tendinous insertions. Cross-striation, which is recognisable under the light microscope, results from the parallel arrangement of myofibrils with alternating series of interdigitating myosin (thick) and actin (thin) protein filaments. During contraction these filaments are thought to slide into one another.

Each muscle fibre is a single, elongated, multi-nucleated cell, varying in length and diameter both within a muscle and from one muscle to another. Each fibre has one neuromuscular junction or motor end plate which lies at the midpoint. A motor unit consists of all the muscle fibres which are innervated by a single anterior horn cell. The number of muscle fibres in a motor unit varies. The more delicate the function to be performed the fewer the fibres in the unit and the smaller the individual fibre diameter. In any one muscle there are two distinct types of muscle fibre, the relative number of each varying from muscle to muscle. Type I fibres, the slow or red fibres, have a high mitochondrial enzyme activity as shown by various histochemical methods, e.g. the succinic dehydrogenase or NADH tetrazolium oxidoreductase techniques. They also contain relatively large amounts of lipid but little glycogen. Type II fibres, the fast or white fibres, have low mitochondrial dehydrogenase activity but a high ATPase activity. They contain little lipid and large quantities of glycogen.

Sensory organs in muscles are numerous, the most common type being the muscle spindle, though other varieties concerned chiefly with stretch and pressure are found in the tendinous insertions. The muscle spindle consists of a long ovoid fibrous capsule containing several thin striated muscle fibres with numerous nuclei in their centres. Sensory endings connected with cells in the posterior root ganglia are present and the fibres receive their motor supply from small cells in the anterior horn. About a third to a half of myelinated fibres in nerves supplying muscle are of sensory origin.

Muscle biopsy. Artefacts produced in the processing of muscle biopsies are common, sometimes confusing and may be minimised by allowing the biopsy to lie unfixed for a minute or two on a piece of card, to which it readily adheres, and then dropping it into fixative. Both longitudinal and cross-sectional blocks should be taken when fixation is complete.

Muscle diseases. Most lesions in skeletal muscle fall into two distinct groups—focal lesions due to trauma, or to inflammatory or circulatory disturbances, and more generalised diseases of muscle. The latter are of three principal types: (i) intrinsic metabolic and often genetically determined diseases of muscle known as the *muscular dystrophies*; (ii) diseases of muscle which are thought to be related to the collagen diseases known as *polymyositis*; and (iii) atrophy of muscle secondary to disease of the lower motor neuron known as *neurogenic atrophy*. Neurogenic atrophy may be a local phenomenon if it is caused by damage to one particular nerve.

General disorders of muscle are characterised by progressive muscular weakness and often pose considerable clinical problems, special investigations such as electromyography, the measurement of nerve conduction velocity, and muscle biopsy often being required to establish the diagnosis. The examination of a muscle biopsy is now a highly specialised field requiring histological, enzyme histochemical, ultrastructural and often immunopathological techniques. The interpretation of these investigations is beyond the scope of this brief account of diseases of muscle. One particular problem with regard to conventional histological examination is that muscle displays a relatively restricted range of histological abnormalities, and many of these are non-specific. Thus it is often very difficult to distinguish between the early stages of dystrophy and polymyositis while the late stages of dystrophy, polymyositis and neurogenic atrophy may be remarkably similar.

A. Traumatic and circulatory disturbances

Ischaemic necrosis of the flexor muscles of the forearm may follow injuries around the elbow and later give rise to a characteristic deformity with clawing of the fingers (*Volkmann's ischaemic contracture*). Attempts at muscle regeneration are abortive; phagocytosis of dead muscle is followed by the ingrowth of cellular fibrous tissue which later becomes densely collagenous (Fig. 23.64). The inclusion of peripheral nerves, especially the median, in the ischaemic area leads to atrophy of surviving muscle and to sensory abnormalities.

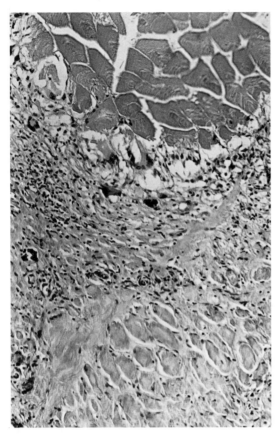

Fig. 23.64 Volkmann's ischaemic contracture. Dead muscle fibres undergoing phagocytosis are seen at the top. In the lower part muscle tubes have been colonised by fibroblasts, and the sarcoplasm replaced by collagen. × 100.

Similar ischaemic necrosis followed by fibrosis sometimes occurs in the anterior tibial muscles following unaccustomed exercise, the swollen muscles being compressed in the relatively unyielding compartment (*anterior tibial syndrome*).

Massive ischaemic necrosis of muscle is seen in cases of 'crush syndrome' where compression of a limb has resulted in prolonged arterial obstruction. On release of pressure and re-establishment of the circulation, large portions of muscle may fail to recover. From these necrotic muscles the myoglobin and other substances are absorbed and excreted in the urine and acute renal tubular necrosis may result (p. 848). The affected muscles become pale and soft—so-called fish-flesh appearance—and if the patient recovers, they undergo fibrous replacement.

Congenital torticollis. This is a condition of fibrosis and contraction of the sternomastoid muscle which develops in the early years of life. The head tends to be inclined to the affected side, and asymmetry of the face and skull may result.

The torticollis used to be ascribed to the results of fibrous repair of necrotic, ischaemic muscle following a birth injury. However, histological evidence of such a pathogenesis is lacking and the condition is now usually regarded as an example of fibromatosis (p. 342).

Myositis ossificans is a localised benign lesion in which about half the patients have a history of a single injury or of repeated minor trauma. Adolescents and young adults are most often affected and the commonest sites are the muscles of the upper arm and thigh. At first an ill-defined tender mass forms with very active proliferation of undifferentiated and sometimes pleomorphic mesenchymal cells. Then, first at the margin of the lesion, metaplastic cartilage and osteoid are produced. The osteoid usually calcifies and after a few weeks radiographs may show a well-defined ovoid shell of bone within muscle or, if close to a bone surface, a veil-like shadow of bony reaction adjacent to the periosteum; this may be difficult to distinguish from a parosteal osteosarcoma. In the early stages the lesion may readily be misdiagnosed histologically as a sarcoma but the more advanced maturation of the bone at the margins is helpful in arriving at the correct diagnosis (Fig. 23.65).

Heterotopic ossification may occur in soft tissues following fracture, dislocation or surgical operation. In paraplegics the hip or knee joint may occasionally become completely fixed by pararticular bony bridges.

Progressive myositis ossificans is a very rare disease of unknown aetiology, not hereditary but sometimes associated with other congenital abnormalities, in which there is progressive ossification of various muscles in the body, in some cases almost the whole skeleton being immobilised by the newly-formed bone. The affection starts in early life, usually in infancy, and involves the neck, back and shoulders; the disease then extends to other muscles, those of mastication not infrequently being involved. The first indication of the disease is the formation of doughy and sometimes painful swellings in the muscles, and when the swellings subside ossification takes place in the areas of fibrosis. In this way strands and plates of bone of an irregular form are

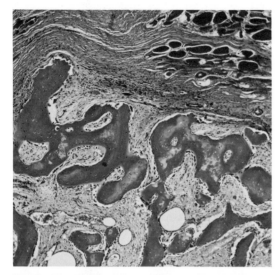

Fig. 23.65   Well-formed bone trabeculae around an area of haemorrhage in muscle.

produced in the muscles. The disease advances by a series of attacks rather than by steady progression, and the exacerbations are sometimes accompanied by fever.

B. Inflammatory diseases of muscle

Skeletal muscle becomes secondarily implicated by acute and chronic inflammation of the interstitial tissue. The changes vary according to the nature of the inflammatory lesion. Thus in acute inflammation, oedema and necrosis of the muscle followed by phagocytosis are prominent features, while in chronic inflammation there is fibrosis with atrophy and disappearance of the muscle fibres.

Bacterial myositis

Gas gangrene is an important acute lesion of muscles lacerated by severe trauma and contaminated by soil and often by foreign bodies such as fragments of clothing. If there is sufficient deprivation of oxygen in the wound, the muscles are invaded by anaerobic organisms, the commonest of these being *Clostridium welchii*, which spreads within the sarcolemmal sheath, causing oedema and necrosis of the fibres throughout their length and in all the tissues adjacent to the wound through the effects of its α-toxin. The muscle fibres show coagulative necrosis and vacuolation and con-

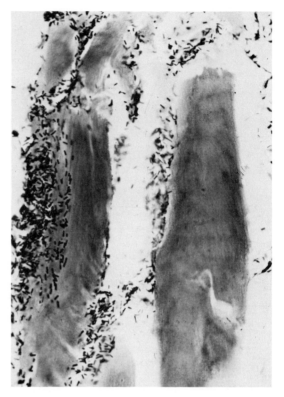

Fig. 23.66   Gas gangrene, showing necrosis and oedema of muscle with numerous *Cl. welchii* but virtually no leukocytes. × 400.

tain, as do the interstitial tissues, large numbers of Gram + ve bacilli (Fig. 23.66). At the margins of the infection, oedema, haemorrhage and vascular damage are seen, and there is some leukocytic infiltrate which, owing to the leukocidins produced, is abundant only in mild infections and the less severely damaged areas (see p. 203).

Suppuration in muscle is usually the result of direct extension from other suppurative lesions, especially of joints and bones. The metastatic type, due to haematogenous infection associated with *Staphylococcus aureus*, is very uncommon in Great Britain and occurs in the tropics, and particularly in West Africa, when it may have an association with filarial infection.

Zenker's degeneration (pp. 94, 632), a form of focal coagulative necrosis, is sometimes seen in the abdominal muscles in typhoid fever, and occasionally in epidemic influenza. The affected muscles may sometimes be recognised by the naked eye by their pale hyaline appearance.

Viral myositis

Epidemic myalgia (pleurodynia, Bornholm disease) is an acute transient febrile illness due to Coxsackie B virus and involving the muscles in the costal region, back and shoulders. The affected muscles are tender and painful on movement and in some cases biopsy has shown acute myositis. In the CSF there is pleocytosis and a raised globulin level.

Parasitic myositis

Trichinosis. This affection is produced in the human subject usually by the ingestion of uncooked pork containing the embryos of *Trichinella* or *Trichina spiralis*. It is rare in this country, except for an occasional epidemic. When an infested muscle, e.g. a portion of trichinous 'measly' pork, is examined, whitish oval specks may be seen with the naked eye. On microscopic examination, it is found that these represent small oval cysts, containing embryonic trichinellae. A number of the cysts may be calcified, and when the parasites die, they also become calcified. When infested muscle is eaten by another animal, the cyst walls are dissolved by the gastric juice and the embryos are set free. In the bowel they reach full sexual maturity, and the impregnated females bore their way into the wall of the small intestine. The young trichinellae are discharged and migrate by lymphatics to the thoracic duct and circulating blood, from which they penetrate the muscles, especially those of the abdominal and thoracic walls, the diaphragm, muscles of the pharynx, tongue and eye, though the heart and limb muscles may also be affected. The larvae encyst, probably in the interfascicular fibrous tissue, and the adjacent muscle fibres become swollen, lose their striations and are destroyed.

The symptoms which occur during the passage of the young parasites from the intestine to the muscle vary in intensity according to the number of the parasites; when the infestation is heavy there may be fever, muscle pains, difficulty in swallowing and breathing. Oedema of the face, especially around the eyes, is a common symptom. Death occasionally follows due to myocarditis or involvement of respiratory muscles, with bronchopneumonia. There is marked eosinophilia in the acute phase of invasion.

C. Generalised diseases of muscle

1. Muscular dystrophies

The muscular dystrophies are hereditary conditions, usually of insidious onset, characterised by progressive muscular weakness and wasting and due to an intrinsic defect in the muscle itself.

The differentiation between the various types of muscular dystrophy is mainly a clinical problem since the histological findings are similar in each type. Each muscle fibre is affected as an individual unit and this leads to a very intimate admixture of muscle fibres of all sizes, a few of normal size, many in varying stages of atrophy and some of increased diameter. The atrophying fibres lose their polygonal shape on cross-section and become rounded and may be further diminished in size by longitudinal splitting. Degenerative changes such as increased eosinophilia, loss of cross-striation, flocculation and phagocytosis of sarcoplasm are seen, often associated with an interstitial cellular infiltrate (Fig. 23.67). Transverse sections of muscle

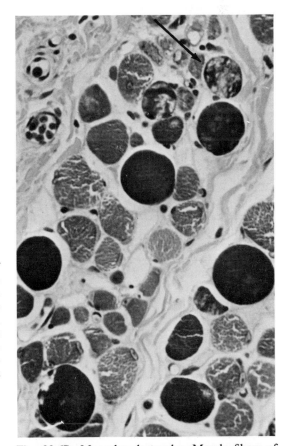

Fig. 23.67 Muscular dystrophy. Muscle fibres of all sizes are intermixed. Enlarged fibres are conspicuous. A group of fibres in the upper right corner (*arrowed*) are undergoing floccular degeneration. × 200. (Dr. A. McQueen.)

sometimes show that nuclei, instead of being confined as normally to the peripheral sheath, are present within the sarcoplasm—*central migration of nuclei*. Infiltration of fat between individual fibres may be notable and endomysial rather than perimysial fibrosis occurs.

Duchenne type of muscle dystrophy (*Pseudohypertrophic muscular dystrophy*). This form of muscular dystrophy is inherited as a sex-linked recessive, is almost exclusively found in males and usually arises insidiously about the age of 5 years, though occasionally older patients are affected. The wasting and loss of power begin symmetrically in the thighs and pelvic girdle, the calf muscles may be enlarged and the shoulder girdle is sometimes later involved. The child waddles, has difficulty in standing up, rising from sitting and climbing stairs. Tendon reflexes are reduced. The disease progresses inexorably without remission and the patient often dies in adolescence from intercurrent infection. The affected muscles, including the 'hypertrophic' calves, in the terminal stage of the disease are almost entirely replaced by fat, only a few scattered muscle fibres remaining though the muscle spindles are unaffected. The activity of creatine phosphokinase in the serum is usually markedly increased.

Facio-scapulo-humeral dystrophy. This disease, which usually begins in adolescence, may arise earlier or later, the more delayed the onset the better the prognosis. Both males and females are affected and there is often a family history. The initial stage is insidious. There is asymmetric involvement of the muscles of the shoulder, arms, trunk and face, which may progress to affect the lower limbs. Pseudohypertrophy is not seen. The dystrophy is very chronic, slowly progressive but with long remissions, and seldom gives rise to total disablement. In the later stages there is often some fatty infiltration but not to the same extent as in the Duchenne type of muscular dystrophy and endomysial fibrosis may be marked.

Dystrophia myotonica. This muscle dystrophy, which occurs in both sexes, usually in adult life, is inherited as a Mendelian dominant. It is associated with premature cataract, gonadal atrophy and sometimes other endocrine disturbances, and is accompanied by myotonia. When a voluntary movement is performed by a patient with myotonia, especially when cold and tired, the muscular contractions take place more slowly and last longer than normal. A similar prolongation of contraction occurs following mechanical or electrical stimulation. The muscles commonly affected by myotonia are those of the tongue, giving rise to dysarthria, and of the hand and forearm resulting in difficulty in releasing any object held in the hand. There is also muscle weakness followed by atrophy of the distal muscles of the

upper limb, the face and sternomastoids and sometimes later of the distal muscles of the lower limb. The disease is progressive and disabling, death usually occurring in late middle age.

Microscopically a striking feature may be the presence of long rows of central nuclei.

Other forms of muscular dystrophy are the limb-girdle type which usually begins in adolescence and starts in the shoulder-girdle, and distal myopathy which commonly does not manifest itself until adult life.

2. Polymyositis

This condition presents usually as an acute progressive disease of muscle but subacute and chronic types are also encountered. In acute cases there is often involvement of the skin, the process then being referred to as *dermatomyositis*. The skin shows a diffuse erythema with oedema and sometimes also, in the arteriolar walls, multiple foci of fibrinoid degeneration resembling those lesions found in systemic lupus erythematosus and other connective tissue diseases (p. 938). *Polymyositis* usually begins in adult life and is often rapidly progressive. Unlike muscular dystrophy and the neurogenic atrophies, there may be periods of spontaneous remission. Other cases are more slowly progressive and clinically may be very similar to muscular dystrophy. Muscular weakness, sometimes with tenderness, is an early feature, the proximal muscles being most often affected and in contrast to the dystrophic pattern the bulbar musculature is not infrequently involved with consequent dysarthria and dysphagia. Muscle wasting with diminished tendon jerks follows. The disease may be rapidly fatal due to involvement of the heart or respiratory muscles and in these cases myoglobinuria may result from severe muscle destruction. In less severe cases spontaneous remission may occur at any stage, but is not uncommonly followed by further exacerbation leading to increasing muscle weakness and disability. Occasionally the disease runs a chronic course from the outset.

Microscopic appearances are those of an acute degeneration of muscle fibres with increased eosinophilia, increase in sarcolemmal nuclei, patchy loss of cross-striation and floccular change. In the interstitial tissue a diffuse or focal infiltrate of chronic inflammatory cells, macrophages, neutrophil and eosinophil polymorphs occurs. The muscle fibres show varying degrees of atrophy and some are hypertrophied. There may be attempted muscle regeneration as shown by the presence of thin basophilic muscle fibres sometimes with sarcolemmal giant cells. Even in the later stages endomysial fibrosis is seldom marked. The histological differentiation between dystrophy and polymyositis becomes increasingly difficult the less acute the lesion and in the later stages or in the chronic form of polymyositis may be almost impossible.

3. Neurogenic atrophy

This is secondary to disease of the lower motor neuron and the histological changes in muscle are similar irrespective of whether the abnormality is in the nerve cell body, the spinal nerve root or the peripheral nerve. Probably the commonest cause of widespread neurogenic atrophy is motor neuron disease (p. 776). Only those fibres atrophy which have lost their nerve supply and this leads to small or large groups of atrophic fibres lying adjacent to groups of normal unaffected fibres (Fig. 23.68). The atrophied muscle fibres may be 5–10 μm in diameter and there is an apparent increase in sarcolemmal nuclei due to shrinkage of sarcoplasm, which, however, retains its cross-striations and normal staining reactions. Sometimes the sarcolemmal sheaths are empty but there is little interstitial cellular infiltrate. Later there may be

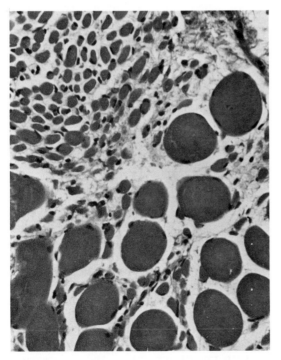

Fig. 23.68 Muscle following neural atrophy. A group of small atrophic fibres in the upper left hand corner is seen adjacent to normally sized fibres. × 320. (Dr. A. McQueen.)

fibrous tissue proliferation around atrophic muscle groups, and a considerable increase in fat. The unaffected muscle fibres usually show little if any compensatory hypertrophy.

Anterior poliomyelitis is a good example of an acute neural atrophy and here it is common to find, within an atrophic motor unit, between one atrophic unit and another and even in different muscles, that muscle fibres are in much the same stage of atrophy. When there is severe and widespread loss of motor neurons in the spinal cord an entire muscle may atrophy. In diseases of less acute onset, such as motor neuron disease (p. 776) and in the various types of polyneuropathy (p. 779), the fibres show a greater variation of size within the motor unit as though all did not undergo atrophy at the same rate. A particularly characteristic feature in progressive neurogenic atrophy is the occurrence of collateral and ultraterminal axonal sprouting and the formation of new motor end plates (p. 780). Later, groups of muscle fibres may become more uniform in size but there is still variation from one group to another and it is only in longstanding disease that uniform atrophy is seen.

Peroneal muscular atrophy of Charcot-Marie-Tooth. This is a hereditary disease, commoner in boys and usually developing in children or young adults. Weakness and atrophy, often symmetrical, first develop in the extensor and abductor muscles of the feet, giving rise to pes cavus; later all muscles below the middle of the thigh and sometimes the hand and forearm muscles may be involved. The muscular atrophy is thought to be secondary to degeneration of the lower motor neurons, but there may also be changes in the spinal cord similar to those seen in Friedreich's ataxia (see p. 777).

Miscellaneous disorders of muscle

Muscle weakness associated with carcinoma

Muscle weakness and wasting in patients with carcinoma may be due to nutritional factors, to neurogenic atrophy which is attributable to compression or involvement of nerves or spinal nerve roots by tumour or to carcinomatous neuropathy (p. 771), and also possibly to a primary affection of the muscle. In the latter group the weakness may be associated with myasthenia and usually involves the proximal muscles. This condition is most commonly associated with bronchial and pancreatic carcinoma and a striking feature is that the severity of the myopathy does not parallel the extent of the malignant disease. The myopathy may be apparent many months before the carcinoma is diagnosable clinically, or may remit when the patient is dying from the neoplasm.

Histological changes in the muscle may be non-specific, being those of simple atrophy with an increase of sarcolemmal nuclei. In other cases the changes resemble those in polymyositis, with flocculation and vacuolation of the sarcous substance and pronounced cellular infiltration between the fibres, some of which show longitudinal splitting (Fig. 23.69). A clear understanding of this condition has not yet been achieved.

Myasthenia gravis

This is a specific muscular disease characterised by the development of abnormal weakness in

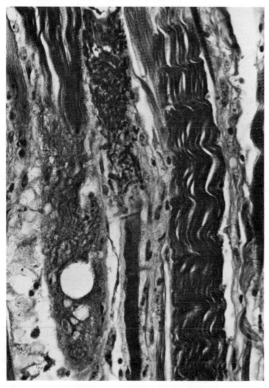

Fig. 23.69 Carcinomatous myopathy showing splitting of muscle fibres, flocculation and loss of striation. × 400.

voluntary muscles, particularly after repetitive activity or prolonged tension. There is usually recovery of motor power after a period of inactivity or lessened tension. Thus muscle function may be normal early in the day but, with continuous use, weakness develops later. The most common, and usually the earliest, muscles involved are those of the eyelids, the extraocular muscles, the bulbar muscles, the neck muscles and the proximal muscles of the limbs. The upper eyelids droop, and to counteract this the head is often tilted backwards in a characteristic posture. In the late stages of the disease there is often permanent muscle weakness and moderate atrophy of muscle is not uncommon. The most common age of onset is about 20, when the disease is much commoner in females than in males. When the onset is later in life, however, the sex incidence is about equal.

Aetiology. It has long been known that the underlying cause of myasthenia gravis is a defect in neuromuscular transmission, and pharmacological confirmation of the diagnosis is usually easy, as drugs with anticholinesterase activity produce temporary improvement. There is also an increased sensitivity to curare. There is now little doubt that myasthenia gravis is an organ specific auto-immune disease, and that *antibodies to acetyl choline receptors* (AChR) play a central role in impairing neuromuscular transmission. AChR can be demonstrated in the serum of most patients with myasthenia gravis, while they have rarely, if ever, been demonstrated in normal subjects or in patients with other types of neuromuscular disease. The titres of AChR correlate well with the clinical severity of myasthenia, and they tend to be higher in these patients with a thymoma (see below). Transplacental transfer of these antibodies probably accounts for the temporary neonatal myasthenia observed in some infants of mothers with myasthenia gravis; this only persists up to 8 weeks. Removal of AChR probably accounts for the clinical improvement in myasthenia gravis that may be brought about by plasma exchange combined with immunosuppressive therapy.

The thymus is abnormal in nearly every patient with myasthenia gravis, and this suggests that it is the site of auto-immunisation. The commonest abnormality is the presence of germinal centres. About 10 per cent of patients, however, have a thymoma, but in cases developing in middle-age the incidence of thymoma is about 30 per cent. The thymoma is usually of the mixed epithelial and lymphocytic type. Even in patients with a thymoma, however, there are usually germinal centres in the thymic tissue around the tumour. Thymectomy is often beneficial if it is undertaken in the early active stages of the disease but it is of no value in the later stages when the response to anticholinergic drugs also tends to diminish.

In the early active stages of the disease, there is probably immunological damage to the neuromuscular junctions with the result that they have a diminished sensitivity to acetylcholine, and in muscle biopsy specimens from patients with myasthenia gravis it has been possible to demonstrate IgG bound to acetylcholine receptors in the neuromuscular junctions. Other structural abnormalities have been described in motor end plates; they become elongated, their expansions are reduced in size, and there may be increased terminal arborisation. The muscle may appear normal but so-called lymphorrhages are not uncommon: these consist essentially of collections of lymphocytes in the interstitial tissue but they sometimes include plasma cells. Occasionally there may be foci of muscle necrosis and regeneration, while in the late stages of the disease there may be undoubted neurogenic atrophy.

A dramatic deterioration is not uncommon in the early active stage of the disease. This usually takes the form of a 'myasthenic crisis' when paralysis of the respiratory muscles may be fatal unless artificial ventilation is instituted. Overdosage with anticholinesterase drugs may produce a 'cholinergic crisis' due to persisting depolarisation of motor end plates. The disease may progress rapidly, with death in a few months, or slowly over many years. In some patients there are remissions of months or years, and in others the disease may remain stationary, with some fluctuations in severity, for many years. The commonest cause of death is aspiration pneumonia due to respiratory muscle weakness.

Periodic paralysis

Muscular activity requires that the intracellular potassium concentration be maintained at normal levels but if the plasma potassium is depleted, e.g. by diuretics, gastro-intestinal fluid loss, in some renal diseases, or on recovery from diabetic coma, weakness of the voluntary muscles and cardiac irregularity may develop and the former may amount to temporary muscular paralysis. The rare familial disorder known as *periodic paralysis*, inherited as an autosomal dominant, is associated with intermittently low levels in the plasma potassium concentration and attacks of muscle weakness may be precipitated by rest following exercise, and by the ingestion of large amounts of carbohydrate. The cardiac irregularity is curiously slight in contrast to the findings in other states of potassium depletion.

Myotonia congenita (Thomsen's disease)

This rare congenital and hereditary disease was described by Thomsen who suffered from it himself. It is commoner in males and first appears in childhood, muscular contraction either voluntary or on electrical stimulation being delayed in onset and slower in performance than is normal. Myotonia may be localised or widespread and the affected muscles are hypertrophied and more powerful than normal. The tendon reflexes are not abnormal. The myotonia may diminish with advancing age and in any case life is not shortened. Occasionally involved muscles may eventually become somewhat atrophic. Histologically the muscle fibres may be enlarged with some central nuclei, and striation is poorly marked.

The Connective Tissue Diseases

The concept that the connective tissues of the body comprise a system, subject to its own specific diseases, led Klemperer and his colleagues to introduce the term *diffuse collagen disease*. It has subsequently become apparent that in most types of disease affecting the connective tissues, collagen is not solely nor primarily involved, and accordingly the term *connective tissue disease* is to be preferred. The diseases most commonly included under this heading are rheumatoid arthritis (RA), systemic lupus erythematosus (SLE), rheumatic fever, progressive systemic sclerosis, scleroderma, polyarteritis nodosa and dermatomyositis. The group of diseases is also referred to, somewhat loosely, as the *rheumatic diseases*. They are now classed together not because they are clear-cut examples of diseases affecting primarily the cells or matrix of the connective tissues (which is doubtful), but because they present associations with one another, suggesting common aetiological and pathogenic factors. Many other conditions—mostly rare and of unknown aetiology—could be regarded as connective tissue diseases, but this simply increases the size and heterogeneity of the group.

General features. Little is known of the aetiology of the connective tissue diseases. There are, however, certain features which are generally applicable to the group: these are as follows:

(1) *Sex incidence.* As a group, these diseases affect females more often than males, with the exception of polyarteritis nodosa which predominantly affects young adult males.

(2) *Overlap between diseases.* Although readily distinguishable from one another in typical cases, the connective tissue diseases show considerable overlap. For example, patients presenting mixed features of systemic lupus erythematosus (SLE) and rheumatoid arthritis are not uncommon, while polyarteritis nodosa may complicate either of these conditions and develops also in some patients with progressive systemic sclerosis.

(3) *Hereditary factors.* Epidemiological studies suggest that rheumatoid arthritis tends to occur with undue frequency among the blood relatives of cases. However, this familial tendency is not strong, and moreover it is not known whether it is dependent on genetic predisposition, environmental factors (e.g. a transmissible agent), or both.

(4) *Immunological features.* The serum level of IgG is commonly raised in patients with SLE, less commonly in rheumatoid arthritis and the other diseases. Of more interest is the presence in the serum of various auto-antibodies. The best known of these are rheumatoid factor and antibodies to deoxyribonucleoprotein and other constituents of cell nuclei. Rheumatoid factor (see below) is present in a high proportion of patients with RA, and a high titre is usually associated with this

condition. However, it is not always present in RA, and low titres are quite common in apparently healthy individuals. The incidence and titres of rheumatoid factor are increased in the other connective tissue diseases. Antinuclear antibodies (p. 164), particularly antibody to deoxyribonucleoprotein, are virtually always present in the serum of patients with active SLE, and are frequently demonstrable in the other diseases. Like rheumatoid factor, antibody to deoxyribonucleoprotein is not uncommon in low titre in apparently normal individuals, especially in the middle-aged and elderly. Various other auto-antibodies to cellular constituents have been described in the serum of patients with connective tissue diseases: like antinuclear antibodies, they react with antigens common to a wide variety of cells and are not 'organ-specific'.

(5) *Pathological changes.* The lesions of the connective tissue diseases vary considerably in appearance, and the differences are due to the occurrence, in various combinations, of fibrinoid change, necrosis, acute and chronic inflammation and dense fibrosis. The changes occur focally in the connective tissues in various parts of the body, and also in the walls of small blood vessels. Vascular involvement is of particular importance, because it leads to ischaemia and thus to secondary changes, not only in the connective tissues, but also in the parenchyma of various organs and in the skin. Since none of these pathological changes is specific, morphological diagnosis of the connective tissue diseases depend upon the appearance and site of the individual lesions, e.g. the polyarthritis of RA, the glomerular and skin lesions of SLE, and the necrotising inflammatory arterial lesions of polyarteritis nodosa. The major pathological features of the individual diseases are described in the appropriate systematic chapters, and the following brief accounts are intended simply to summarise the various manifestations of each disease.

Rheumatoid arthritis. This disease is described on pp. 917–19. It usually occurs alone but may accompany overt SLE, or be complicated by the incomplete picture of SLE, e.g. a positive LE-cell test (see below). Anaemia is common in RA; usually it is of dyshaemopoietic nature, but occasionally autoimmune haemolytic anaemia develops.

Seronegative polyarthritis clinically resembling RA, but usually relatively mild, complicates some cases of psoriasis, and typical RA is a common feature of Sjøgren's syndrome (p. 594). Pain in the joints, usually without progressive structural changes, is common in rheumatic fever, progressive systemic sclerosis and polyarteritis nodosa.

Aetiology. The cause of rheumatoid arthritis remains unknown. Features suggesting an immunological disturbance include (1) a marked hyperplasia of the cortical germinal centres of lymph nodes, suggestive of an antibody response; (2) the common occurrence of rheumatoid factor and antinuclear antibodies; and (3) the heavy lymphocytic and plasma-cell infiltration of the synovia of affected joints.

Rheumatoid factors. The serum of most cases of RA contains rheumatoid factors. These consist of IgM or IgG which behaves as an antibody to components of the Fc part of IgG. Although they form loose complexes with IgG in the plasma, rheumatoid factors react most strongly with IgG which has been modified by reacting (as antibody) with an antigen, or by heat-aggregation. Accordingly, the factor is best demonstrated by means of IgG which has been heated or combined with inert particles, e.g. erythrocytes or latex. In the Waaler–Rose test, dilutions of the patient's heat-inactivated serum are tested with sheep erythrocytes sensitised with rabbit IgG antibody. Agglutination in a significantly higher serum dilution than occurs with unsensitised sheep erythrocytes indicates a positive result. The rheumatoid factor may be present at an early stage or appear only later in the disease. As detected by these methods, the absence of rheumatoid factors is, in general, associated with less severe cases. However, more sensitive techniques have demonstrated their presence in virtually all cases of the disease.

Recent work has demonstrated the complicated nature and heterogeneity of rheumatoid factors. Two factors may be present, one reacting with both rabbit and human IgG, the other only with human IgG. Moreover, rheumatoid factors which react specifically with genetically determined human IgG allo-antigens (termed Gm factors) have been detected, and in some instances the patient's serum has contained such a factor which reacts with an allo-antigen absent from her/his own IgG.

Rheumatoid factors in the serum of RA patients are mainly of IgM class, and have been shown by means of aggregated labelled IgG to be produced in the lymph nodes. Rheumatoid factor can also be shown to be formed in approximately 50 per cent of the plasma cells in the synovium and pannus of the rheumatoid joint, and is mainly of IgG class; being an antibody to Fc of IgG, it acts as both antigen and antibody and itself forms complexes (Fig. 23.70) within the plasma cells producing it. These complexes are also present in the inflamed synovium and in the joint fluid. They activate complement and thus induce inflammation with migration into the joint of

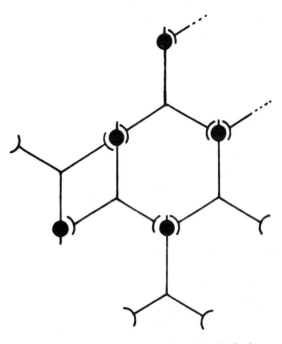

Fig. 23.70 Formation of complexes by IgG rheumatoid factor which acts as both antibody and antigen. The antigenic determinant of the Fc is shown as the solid black areas.

neutrophil polymorphs and monocytes. These, together with macrophages in the synovial lining and pannus, phagocytose the complexes and in doing so release their lysosomal enzymes and cationic proteins which aggravate the inflammation and contribute to the enzymic injury to the articular cartilage. There may also be development of an auto-immune reaction to collagen altered by enzymic injury within the joint, but this is uncertain.

The factors responsible for initiating RA, and for inducing the production of rheumatoid factors, remain unknown. Rheumatoid factor develops in some chronic infections, notably subacute bacterial endocarditis, and can be induced experimentally in rabbits by immunising injections of autologous IgG antibody complexed with antigen. It thus seems reasonable to suggest that RA may be initiated by an infective agent in the joints which stimulates an antibody response, and that rheumatoid factor develops in response to the IgG antibody complexed to antigen of the infective agent. However, although isolation of various micro-organisms from rheumatoid joints has been reported, there have been no consistent findings. Once the local production of IgG rheumatoid factor in the synovium has been initiated, the IgG complexes themselves might provide the necessary antigenic stimulus for its continued production. The extra-articular lesions, including rheumatoid nodules and vasculitis, might also be mediated by rheumatoid-factor complexes.

Cell-mediated immunity. The lymphocytes in the synovium of joints affected by RA include some T cells, and T-cell lymphokines have been detected in the joint fluid. Also, seronegative chronic arthritis closely resembling RA occurs in boys with congenital agammaglobulinaemia (p. 170). It has also been reported that the recirculating T lymphocytes in RA include cells which are cytotoxic for synovial lining cells in culture and that RA is improved by thoracic-duct drainage. Finally, it has been reported that the lymphokines released by T cells include a factor which activates osteoclasts thus enhancing bone resorption: this is not perhaps surprising because osteoclasts apparently belong to the macrophage system (p. 74).

It may thus be that T lymphocytes play a pathological role in RA.

Genetic factors. Although the importance of genetic factors in RA has not been established (see above) it is nevertheless suggested by the observation that the incidence of RA in individuals possessing the HLA antigen DRw4 is seven times greater than in others.

Systemic lupus erythematosus. This is an uncommon condition, affecting mostly adolescent females and young women. It may run an acute course with fever, and if untreated is often fatal in months or years, the commonest cause of death being renal failure. The clinical features and pathological changes show great individual variation. The tissues most often involved are the skin (p. 1067), the kidneys (p. 832), the endocardium (p. 424), and the serous membranes, but any organ may be affected. There may be arthritic pain, pleurisy, albuminuria, haematuria and the nephrotic syndrome. Fibrinoid change is seen in the small vessels—arterioles, capillaries and venules—in the various tissues. This may have important effects by causing ischaemia, but fibrinoid change occurs also in avascular connective tissue, e.g. in the heart valves. Necrosis, a granulomatous reaction and fibrosis are also common features.

Patients with SLE have a strong tendency to develop hypersensitivity to various drugs. Haematological features include leukopenia, sometimes thrombocytopenia, and less commonly auto-immunological reactions. Auto-antibodies to nuclear and other cellular constituents occur with greater frequency in SLE than in the other connective tissue diseases. In the LE-cell test, examination of the patient's leukocytes following incubation of whole blood at 37 °C shows phagocytosis of homogeneous basophilic material by neutrophil polymorphs (Fig. 23.71). These so-called LE cells result from the reaction of auto-antibody to deoxyribonucleoprotein with the nuclei of degenerate leukocytes, with subsequent fixation of complement and phagocytosis of the altered nuclear material. The test is positive in patients with a high plasma level of antibody to deoxyribonucleoprotein ('LE-cell factor'). It is not positive in all cases of SLE, and is positive in a small proportion of patients with RA or other connective tissue diseases. The lesions of SLE commonly exhibit patchy basophilia, the so-called haematoxyphil bodies, due to deposition

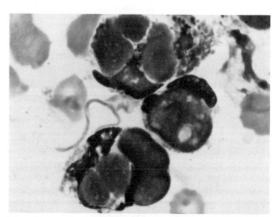

Fig. 23.71 LE cells from a case of disseminated lupus erythematosus. × 600. Three cells are shown with characteristic ingested masses of altered nuclear material. (From a preparation kindly lent by Dr. J. M. Robertson.)

of deoxyribonucleoprotein complexed with antibody. Serological tests for syphilis, e.g. the Wassermann reaction, are commonly positive in SLE; this is due to auto-antibodies which cross-react with antigenic constituents of cardiolipin.

There is now good evidence that the glomerular lesions are due to a type III hypersensitivity reaction (p. 833) resulting from deposition of immune complexes composed of auto-antibodies and the corresponding auto-antigens, in the glomerular capillary walls. Fibrinoid lesions in the skin and elsewhere may be of similar nature. The cause of the predisposition to develop auto-antibodies and hypersensitivity to drugs is, however, not known. Investigations on NZB/NZW mice, which develop spontaneously a disease resembling SLE (p. 164) suggest the possibility that virus infection may play a pathogenic role, but virological studies in SLE have so far been inconclusive.

Progressive systemic sclerosis. The main features of this rare chronic disease are intimal thickening of small arteries and arterioles, patchy loss of specialised tissue, and replacement fibrosis. In addition to the skin lesion (p. 1068), the gastro-intestinal tract, heart, skeletal muscles, kidneys and lungs are most often affected. Clinical features include dysphagia from fibrosis and loss of smooth muscle of the oesophagus, disturbances of the gastro-intestinal tract, respiratory insufficiency and repeated infections resulting from progressive pulmonary fibrosis. The interlobular renal arteries are narrowed by severe concentric intimal fibrosis resembling closely that of malignant hypertension: patchy renal ischaemia results, and there may be associated hypertension. Vascular involvement and shrinkage of the skin bring about ischaemia of the extremities, often with Raynaud's phenomenon (p. 384), and sometimes progressing to ulceration and gangrene. There may also be subcutaneous calcification. Cardiac function may be impaired by myocardial fibrosis, hypertension and lung involvement.

The aetiology of progressive systemic sclerosis is quite unknown. Antinuclear auto-antibodies may be present in the serum, and the condition may be accompanied by rheumatoid arthritis or lesions suggestive of SLE.

The major features of *scleroderma* (p. 1069), *polyarteritis nodosa* (p. 380) and *dermatomyositis* (p. 934) are described in the appropriate systematic chapters.

Rheumatic fever (p. 415) is characterised by transient polyarthritis, myocardial injury, focal fibrinoid and inflammatory lesions of the connective tissues of the endocardium and of the myocardium, a fibrinous pericarditis and lesions of small vessels. It differs from the other connective tissue diseases in being a complication of a specific infection, namely a pharyngitis due to *Streptococcus pyogenes*. The pathogenesis is not fully understood, although the cross-reaction of streptococcal antibodies with myocardium, and the demonstration of such antibody attached to myocardium (p. 416) provide strong evidence for the participation of a cytotoxic (type 2) immunological reaction (p. 150).

There is little association between the connective tissue diseases and the organ-specific auto-immune diseases (p. 161) except in Sjögren's disease, in which features of both groups are commonly demonstrable.

Further Reading

Bethlem, J. (1970). *Muscle Pathology: Introduction and Atlas*, pp. 132. North Holland Publishing Co., Amsterdam.

Dahlin, David C. (1978). *Bone Tumors*, 3rd edn., pp. 445. Charles C. Thomas, Springfield, Illinois.

Dent, C. E. and Stamp, T. C. B. (1978). Vitamin D, Rickets and Osteomalacia, pp. 237–305. In *Metabolic Bone Disease*, Vol. I, pp. 447. Edited by L. V. Avioli and S. M. Krane. Academic Press, New York.

Gardner, D. L. (1965). *Pathology of the Connective Tissue Diseases*, pp. 456. Edward Arnold, London.

Sissons, H. A. (1979). Bones; Diseases of Joints, Tendon Sheaths, Bursae and Other Soft Tissues, pp. 2383–2489 and 2491–2522. In *Systemic Pathology*, 2nd edn. Edited by W. St. C. Symmers. Churchill Livingstone, Edinburgh and London.

Smith, Roger (1979). *Biochemical Disorders of the Skeleton*, pp. 293. Butterworths, London.

Walton, J. T. (Ed.) (1974). *Disorders of Voluntary Muscle*, 3rd edn., pp. 1149. Churchill Livingstone, Edinburgh and London.

24

Female Reproductive Tract

The Vulva

The skin of the vulva is part of the body integument and is therefore subject to all the diseases that can afflict the skin elsewhere in the body, such as, for example, psoriasis, pemphigus or lichen planus. Dermatological conditions developing in the vulva tend, however, to be modified by the effects of local heat and moisture, by the easy access afforded to gut flora and by the changes induced in vulvar skin as a result of its sensitivity to ovarian hormones.

Infections

Many vulvar infections, especially those occurring in debilitated women, are of mixed nature but some are due to streptococci or staphylococci, the latter occurring with increased frequency in diabetics as do also monilial infections. The features of the various sexually transmitted diseases which involve the vulva are described for both male and female in Chapter 25 (pp. 987–9).

Atrophy

Thinning of the vulval epithelium is a common factor in a number of otherwise unrelated conditions. Of these, the most frequently encountered is **simple atrophy**, some degree of which occurs as a physiological response to oestrogen withdrawal in all postmenopausal women but which is sometimes sufficiently marked to cause narrowing of the introitus. Another moderately common cause of vulval atrophy is **lichen sclerosus et atrophicus** (Fig. 24.1), a chronic progressive lesion which can be found anywhere in the skin but which occurs unduly frequently in the vulva in middle-aged women.

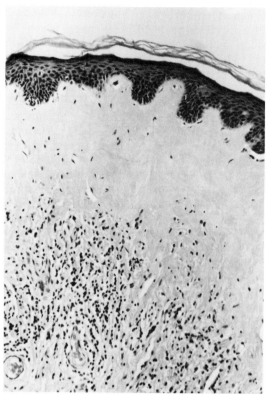

Fig. 24.1 Lichen sclerosus et atrophicus of the vulva. The upper dermis is hyalinised whilst in the deeper part of the dermis there is a non-specific chronic inflammatory cell infiltration. The epidermis is atrophic. × 150.

This is commonly characterised by thinning of the epidermis, flattening of the epidermodermal junction and hyalinisation of the upper third of the dermis: the end stage of this disease is indistinguishable from severe simple atrophy. The epidermis is also thinned in some vulvas with intra-epithelial malignant change and it is unfortunate that all forms of vulval atrophy are often grouped together under the heading of '*kraurosis*', a clinical term which, in a pathological context, is devoid of meaning and should not be employed.

Premalignant disease

Malignant vulvar tumours usually evolve from skin that is already showing changes of a premalignant nature. These are characterised by the presence, within the vulvar epidermis, of cells which show varying degrees of atypia, which fail to mature normally and which have hyperchromatic nuclei and an increased nucleo-cytoplasmic ratio. Mitotic figures, often of abnormal form, are seen with some frequency in these cells which do not, however, invade the dermis. The whole question of premalignant change in squamous epithelium is discussed more fully in the section on the cervix but it may be mentioned here that if abnormal cells occupy less than the full thickness of the vulvar epithelium the condition is considered to be a *dysplasia*, whilst if the full thickness of the epithelium is replaced by such cells the lesion is classed as *carcinoma-in-situ*. These distinctions are largely artificial for both dysplasia and carcinoma-in-situ can evolve into an invasive tumour, and it would probably be best to class all these various grades of abnormality together as **intra-epithelial neoplasia**. It should not be thought, however, that development of invasive cancer is a necessary consequence of vulvar premalignant disease, for many cases either remain stationary or regress.

It is regrettable that premalignant vulvar disease has been encumbered by a variety of names which are largely meaningless; thus, the relatively minor degrees of intra-epithelial abnormality are known variously as vulvar dysplasia, vulvar dystrophy and vulvar dermatosis whilst carcinoma in situ is also frequently called Bowen's disease or erythroplasia of Queyrat; furthermore, premalignant changes in the vulva are often classed as *leukoplakia*, a clinical observational diagnosis denoting whitening of the vulvar skin but one that has, in the pathological sense, no specific meaning and which should be shunned by pathologists.

Tumours

A variety of benign skin neoplasms, such as papillomas, fibromas and lipomas, occur in the vulva and this is a site at which benign sweat gland tumours (hidradenomas) are particularly prone to develop.

Malignant vulvar neoplasms are uncommon and most are **squamous cell carcinomas**; these tumours usually develop in elderly women and almost invariably in skin which already shows premalignant intra-epithelial change. The tumour may present as an indurated plaque, an ulcer with hard rolled edges or as a warty mass, most commonly on the labia majora; histologically it is usually, though not invariably, well differentiated. The tumour spreads first to the inguinal lymph nodes and, because of anastomoses between the lymphatics of the two sides, it is by no means unusual for bilateral inguinal node involvement to occur: later spread is to femoral, iliac and para-aortic nodes. The prognosis for vulvar carcinoma is rather poor, patients with lymph node involvement having a 5-year survival rate of between 40 and 60 per cent.

Rare primary malignant neoplasms of the vulva include *adenocarcinoma of Bartholin's gland*, *malignant melanoma* and *basal cell carcinoma*; metastatic deposits of endometrial adenocarcinoma or choriocarcinoma are also sometimes encountered.

The Vagina

Infection

Vaginal infections are common but many are non-specific in nature and due to lowered vaginal resistance to bacterial invasion, as occurs for instance in vaginal epithelial atrophy resulting from oestrogen deficiency. Specific infections may be due to organisms such as *N. gonorrhoeae*, mycoplasma, herpes virus, chlamydia or cytomegalovirus, whilst monilial infection, predisposed to by the high glycogen content of the vaginal epithelium, is common; sexually transmitted infestation with the protozoal parasite *Trichomonas vaginalis* also occurs with considerable frequency.

Adenosis

This is characterised by the presence of small glands or cysts in the submucosa of the upper third of the vagina; the epithelium in these may be endocervical, endometrial or tubal in type. This usually asymptomatic congenital abnormality is particularly common in girls whose mothers received synthetic oestrogen therapy during pregnancy and, although innocuous in itself, predisposes to the development of an adenocarcinoma.

Tumours

Squamous cell carcinoma of the vagina is uncommon; it usually occurs in the upper part of the vagina in elderly women and presents as an indurated plaque: the tumour is often poorly differentiated and tends to invade the cervix, paravaginal tissues, rectum and bladder, the 5-year survival rate being only about 30 per cent.

Adenocarcinoma of the vagina was, until a decade ago, of exceptional rarity but in recent years a considerable number of clear-celled vaginal adenocarcinomas have occurred in girls aged between 15 and 25, mostly in North America. Common to virtually all of these cases has been pre-existing vaginal adenosis and a history of prenatal exposure to synthetic oestrogens, particularly diethylstilboestrol.

The Cervix

Cervicitis

Cervical infection is common, possibly because the complex deep folds of the endocervical crypts offer a relatively protected haven in which micro-organisms can flourish. The inflammatory response to infection may be either acute or chronic, the histological characteristics of the inflammatory process being exactly the same as those seen in comparable infections elsewhere in the body. Many cervical infections are of a non-specific, and probably polymicrobial, nature but specific infection with *N. gonorrhoeae*, herpes virus, chlamydia, mycobacteria, *Tr. vaginalis.*, *Myco. tuberculosis* and *Treponema pallidum* can occur.

Cervical ectopy

This term is applied to a red area on the ectocervix which surrounds the external os (Fig. 24.2): this abnormality was previously known as a cervical *erosion* and this term is, indeed, still often used by gynaecologists who tend to regard this as an inflammatory or ulcerative process. An ectopy is, however, usually a physiological change consequent upon an increase in cervical bulk, as occurs at puberty or in pregnancy; this causes an unfolding of the cervix

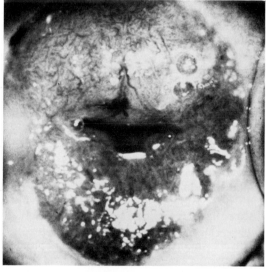

Fig. 24.2 Cervical ectopy as seen through a colposcope. The external os is circumferentially surrounded by thin endocervical epithelium through which the sub-epithelial vessels are clearly visible.

with eversion of the distal endocervix out into what is anatomically the ectocervix. The thin endocervical columnar epithelium is relatively transparent and hence the sub-epithelial vessels impart to an ectopy its characteristic redness. The exposure of the delicate endocervical epithelium to the acidity of the vagina results in its undergoing *squamous metaplasia*, the squamous cells differentiating from pluripotential basal reserve cells which are normally present in endocervical epithelium. Squamous metaplasia can therefore be seen as a protective mechanism in which the relatively fragile endocervical epithelium is replaced by more robust stratified squamous cells and when this process is complete the ectopy is said to be '*healed*'. This area of squamous metaplasia is often known as the '*transformation zone*' and is of considerable importance in so far as most cervical carcinomas appear to originate at this site.

Premalignant disease of the cervix

It is now recognised that a squamous cell carcinoma of the cervix does not arise abruptly in otherwise normal cervical squamous epithelium but evolves over a number of years, probably 10–15, from an epithelium which shows progressively severe degrees of abnormality. The early, or premalignant stage of cervical carcinoma is characterised by the presence within the squamous epithelium of cells showing a failure of maturation, loss of polarity, excessive and abnormal mitotic activity, an increased nucleo-cytoplasmic ratio and both nuclear and cytoplasmic pleomorphism. Until recently, considerable stress was laid upon both the degree and extent of these intra-epithelial abnormalities. Epithelia in which the cells showed only a minor or moderate degree of abnormality or in which the abnormal cells did not occupy the full thickness of the epithelium were considered as **dysplastic** and those in which the full thickness of the epithelium was occupied by abnormal cells were said to show **carcinoma-in-situ** (Fig. 24.3), a lesion differing from a frank carcinoma only by its confinement within the epithelium and its lack of any stromal invasion. These terms are still widely used but it has become increasingly apparent that the abnormal cells in a dysplastic epithelium are identical in all respects to those in a carcinoma in situ and that the progression from dysplasia to carcinoma in situ is a single continuous process, the division between the two types of intra-epithelial abnormality being both subjective and arbitrary. Hence the term **cervical intra-epithelial neoplasia** (CIN) has

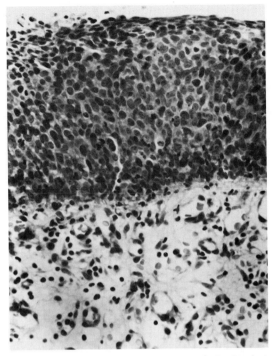

Fig. 24.3 Cervical intraepithelial neoplasia Grade 3 (carcinoma *in situ*) of the uterine cervix. The cells in the cervical epithelium show a complete lack of maturation, are pleomorphic and have an increased nucleocytoplasmic ratio. × 275.

become fashionable to cover the whole spectrum of 'premalignant' change in cervical epithelium, abnormalities previously classed as mild or moderate dysplasia now being called CIN 1 and CIN 2 respectively and both severe dysplasia and carcinoma-in-situ being classed together as CIN 3. *It should not, however be assumed that all examples of CIN 1 or 2 progress to CIN 3 or that CIN 3 will invariably proceed to an invasive carcinoma.* Many cases of CIN, at any stage in the evolution of this abnormality, either remain stationary or regress with probably no more than one third of cases of CIN 3 advancing to the invasive stage; indeed, it is almost certain that some, probably many, examples of CIN 1 and 2 are not truly neoplastic in nature but represent an atypical cellular response to factors such as viral infection. Currently, however, *there are no available methods for distinguishing a reactive lesion from one which is truly neoplastic or for the recognition of those cases of CIN which will progress to invasive cancer.* Hence all cases of CIN have to be regarded as potentially invasive: fortunately these epithelial lesions, though asymptomatic, are readily detected by cytological examination and their treatment and eradication, by techniques such as cryocautery and laser therapy, are relatively simple. Widespread cytological screening and prompt treatment of intra-epithelial abnormalities appear to have reduced markedly the incidence of invasive cervical carcinoma.

Malignant neoplasms of the cervix

Ninety-five per cent of malignant cervical tumours are squamous carcinomas and nearly all of the remaining 5 per cent are adenocarcinomas.

Squamous cell carcinoma

Aetiology and pathogenesis. Epidemiological studies have demonstrated an association between squamous cell carcinoma of the cervix and early marriage, early pregnancy, a high number of pregnancies, sexual promiscuity, divorce, sexually transmitted diseases, prostitution and low socio-economic status. These findings clearly suggest a correlation with a particular life-style but it is virtually certain that the one common factor linking these various factors is early onset of sexual activity. It is believed that a carcinogen is transmitted sexually by the male at a time when the epithelium of the cervix is in an unstable state, i.e. when the transformation zone is undergoing squamous metaplasia during late adolescence (see above). The nature of this carcinogenic agent remains uncertain but it is unlikely to be smegma and suspicion has fallen particularly on *Herpesvirus type 2* and spermatozoal DNA. Certainly the role of sexual transmission is indicated by the fact that barrier methods of contraception are associated with a lowered incidence of cervical carcinoma and by the apparent proneness of some men to be 'carcinogenic', their sexual partners having an unusually high risk of developing cervical cancer. Various racial and ethnic factors which were formerly thought to be significant in the aetiology of this neoplasm are now thought to be related principally to the sexual mores of those particular groups.

Macroscopic features. The growth pattern of a cervical squamous cell carcinoma may be predominantly *exophytic*, (i.e. it grows out from the surface as a bulky, friable, papillary or polypoid mass—Fig. 24.4), or *endophytic* so that it infiltrates deeply into the cervix, converting it into a hard bulky, nodular mass which eventually ulcerates.

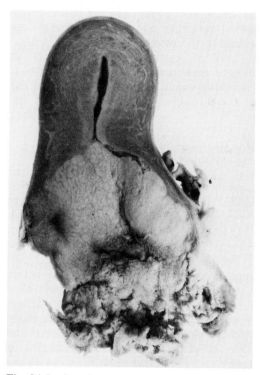

Fig. 24.4   An advanced squamous cell carcinoma of the uterine cervix.

Microscopic features. The tumour tends to infiltrate as irregular sheets of epithelial cells, sometimes with pointed or spiky margins (Fig. 24.5). Formation of epithelial pearls and keratin is unusual but does occur rather more commonly in those neoplasms showing an exophytic mode of growth. A proportion are extremely poorly differentiated.

Spread and prognosis. The tumour invades locally into the uterine body, vagina, parametrial tissues, bladder and rectum; of particular importance is involvement of the ureters, either by direct invasion of their walls or by compression from extrinsic tumour masses. Lymph node spread occurs at an early stage to pelvic, inguinal, iliac and aortic nodes but blood borne spread, principally to liver, lungs and bone, does not occur until a late stage. Death is most

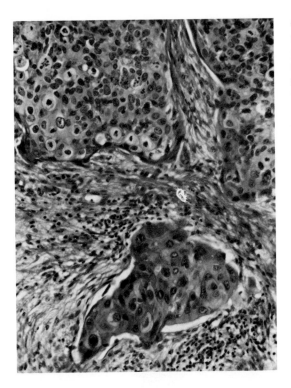

commonly due to uraemia consequent upon ureteric obstruction. The 5-year 'cure' rate for patients in whom the tumour is confined to the cervix is, with modern therapy, about 85 per cent, falling to between 50 and 75 per cent for those cases with pelvic invasion.

Adenocarcinoma

The factors linked aetiologically with cervical squamous cell carcinoma do not apply to cervical adenocarcinoma and, indeed, this neoplasm tends to be associated with nulliparity. Some adenocarcinomas of clear cell type occur in young girls exposed prenatally to diethylstilboestrol.

The tumour grows in the endocervix and is commonly well differentiated: it tends to spread upwards into the myometrium and outwards into the pelvis but the 5-year 'cure' rate is approximately 70 per cent.

Fig. 24.5 Squamous carcinoma of the cervix uteri, showing infiltrating masses of tumour cells without cell-nest formation. Note the numerous mitotic figures. × 165.

The Endometrium

The endometrium is that part of the uterine lining above the level of the internal os and consists of a basal layer, which is largely unresponsive to hormonal stimulation, and a superficial functional layer which is markedly sensitive to ovarian hormones.

Endometrial morphology during the menstrual cycle.

An awareness of changing endometrial morphology during the menstrual cycle is basic to an understanding of much of endometrial pathology. The menstrual cycle is divided into three stages; the *pre-ovulatory*, during which the developing Graafian follicle is secreting oestrogens, the *postovulatory*, throughout which the corpus luteum is producing both oestrogens and progesterone, and the *menstrual*. During the pre-ovulatory stage the endometrium regenerates and grows under the influence of oestrogen and is said to be in the **proliferative phase** (Fig. 24.6); the glands are straight and narrow, the stroma is compact and cellular and mitotic figures are seen in both the glands and stroma. After ovulation, which usually occurs about the 14th day of the cycle, the endometrium enters the **secretory phase**, the first morphological evidence of which is the appearance of subnuclear glycogen-containing vacuoles in the glandular epithelial cells (Fig. 24.7); these appear about 36–48 hours after, and are strong presumptive evidence of, ovulation. As the secretory phase progresses the vacuoles disappear, the epithelial nuclei return to a basal position, the glands become increasingly dilated and tor-

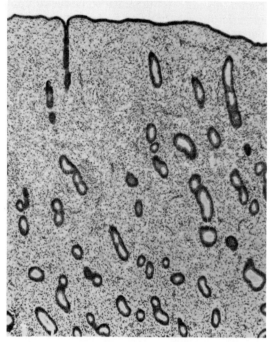

Fig. 24.6 Section of the endometrium on the 10th day of the cycle, showing the appearances of the proliferative phase. The glands are relatively small. × 60.

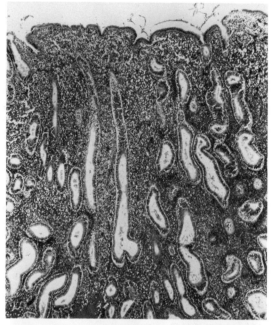

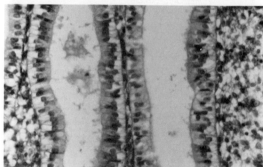

Fig. 24.7 Post-ovulatory endometrium on the 15th day of the cycle. The glands have increased in size and show basal vacuolation. *Above*, × 30; *below*, × 245.

tuous and secretions appear in their lumina (Fig. 24.8); because oestrogens increase endometrial intracapillary hydrostatic pressure the stroma becomes markedly oedematous during the mid part of the secretory phase. When the corpus luteum begins to degenerate there is a precipitous fall in oestrogen levels, a rapid regression of the stromal oedema and a sudden decrease in thickness of the endometrium with buckling of the spiral vessels, vascular stasis and ischaemic necrosis of the functional layer. As the oedema regresses the stroma becomes compact and the stromal cells take on a decidua-like appearance. Shortly before breakdown of the endometrium the stroma becomes infiltrated by polymorphonuclear leukocytes and these harbingers of overt necrosis are soon followed by crumbling and haemorrhage, the menstrual phase of the cycle now having been reached. Most of the functional layer is lost during menstruation but the basal layer persists to give rise to the regenerative phase of the next cycle.

The menstrual cycle is a recurrent priming of

the endometrium for the reception of a fertilised ovum, but menstruation is not an essential biological component of this process. Endometrial necrosis, and hence resultant menstrual loss, is due solely to the very rapid rate at which oestrogen levels fall as the corpus luteum degenerates; in some species oestrogen values decline at a much slower rate and endometrial necrosis, and hence menstruation, is avoided, although only at the cost of lengthening the menstrual cycle. Menstruation is therefore the price that women pay for the shortening of their menstrual cycle which allows for a greater

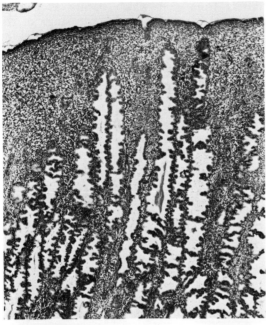

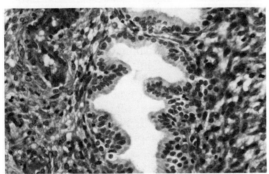

Fig. 24.8 Secretory-stage endothelium on the 25th day of the cycle. The glands contain secretion and are convoluted, presenting a 'saw-tooth' appearance. *Above,* × 30; *below,* × 245.

number of possible conceptions during their limited years of fertility.

Factors altering endometrial morphology

Pregnancy. The normal cycle will be interrupted if a fertilised ovum implants in the endometrium; when this occurs the corpus luteum persists, the stromal oedema fails to subside completely, the stromal cells become large, plump and polygonal with abundant cytoplasm, the glands enlarge and glandular secretion increases. An unusual endometrial response to placental tissue, whether this be in an intra-uterine or ectopic site, is the **Arias–Stella reaction** in which one or more glands are lined by tall cells with clear cytoplasm and, often, hyperchromatic nuclei; the glandular epithelium shows budding, multilayering and some degree of pleomorphism and these appearances may be mistaken for an adenocarcinoma. The cells in an Arias–Stella reaction are endometrial glandular cells in a hyperactive secretory state.

Oral contraception. The use of oral steroid contraceptives markedly alters endometrial morphology. The type of pattern seen depends upon the dosage and the type of preparation used, but a very characteristic pattern with the combined type of regime is one of endometrial atrophy in which the glands are small, relatively few, and largely inactive, with a compact stroma showing a variable degree of decidua-like change (Fig. 24.9). Occasionally the stromal cells become spindle-shaped and may

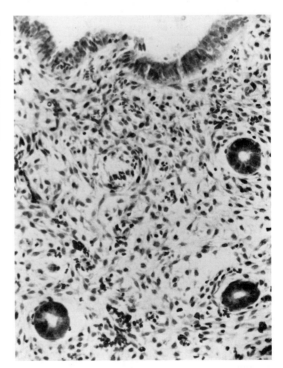

Fig. 24.9 Endometrium from a woman taking a steroid contraceptive pill. The stroma is abundant whilst the glands are reduced in number, small and inactive. × 200.

appear sufficiently pleomorphic to suggest a sarcoma, but this change is very rare with modern low dosage contraception. The endometrium rapidly reverts to normal after stopping oral contraceptives.

Intra-uterine contraceptive devices. The effects on the endometrium vary with the type of device used but focal atrophy and fibrosis are commonly seen; foci of haemorrhage and squamous metaplasia may be present whilst there is frequently a mononuclear cell infiltration of the stroma. Cyclical changes continue in the endometrium but the secretory phase tends to be accelerated.

The Menopause. Some slight proliferative activity may occur in the endometrium for a year or two after the menopause but the postmenopausal endometrium undergoes a progressive atrophy and the glands eventually become quite inactive. Stromal fibrosis is not uncommon and this often leads to obstruction of the necks of many of the glands, which tend to become cystically dilated; the cystic glands are lined by a thin, inactive epithelium and they thus differ strikingly from those seen in cystic glandular hyperplasia (see opposite).

Endometritis

The endometrium is relatively resistant to infection, partly because of the excellent natural drainage which it enjoys, and partly because it is difficult for an infection to become established during reproductive life in a tissue which is regularly shed.

Acute endometritis

An acute inflammation of the endometrium occurs most commonly after an abortion or parturition, especially if fragments of placenta or membranes are retained in the uterus; a variety of organisms, including streptococci, staphylococci, *Esch. coli* and *Pseudomonas*, may be implicated. An acute sterile inflammation can also occur with certain types of intra-uterine contraceptive device and may also complicate irradiation of the uterus.

The inflamed endometrium is reddened and boggy whilst histologically there is oedema, congestion, a varying degree of ulceration and tissue destruction and a polymorphonuclear leucocytic infiltration. The cellular infiltrate differs from that which occurs as a physiological event during the late stage of the menstrual cycle by being present not only in the stroma but also in the glands where small intraluminal abscesses are commonly seen.

A virulent infection may spread to involve the myometrium and parametrium but complications such as septic pelvic venous thrombosis, pyaemia and septicaemia are nowadays very uncommon.

Non-specific chronic endometritis

A chronic inflammation of the endometrium may follow an acute endometritis but is more commonly chronic from the outset. Macroscopically the endometrium may be somewhat thickened but often appears normal. There has been much dispute over the criteria for the histological diagnosis of chronic endometritis, largely because occasional lymphocytes are normally present in the endometrium. Chronic inflammation in this site is, however, characterised by the same features as elsewhere in the body and the diagnosis rests upon the finding of a chronic inflammatory cell infiltration of the stroma; the infiltrate must be of more than trivial degree and although occasionally purely lymphocytic in type there is usually an admixture with, and sometimes a predominance of, plasma cells. Some degree of fibroblastic and vascular proliferation may be present but the inflammatory process is limited to the stroma and does not involve the glands; the normal cyclical changes may continue undisturbed, be accentuated or absent.

Chronic endometritis may follow abortion or childbirth and can occur in association with an intra-uterine contraceptive device, chronic salpingitis or endometrial adenocarcinoma; furthermore, endometrial tuberculosis can masquerade as a non-specific inflammation. Hence, although there do appear to be a very small number of cases of chronic endometritis of apparently idiopathic origin, this diagnosis should not be entertained until all these factors have been eliminated as aetiological possibilities.

Specific endometrial infections

Tuberculosis of the endometrium is nearly always secondary to tubal tuberculosis and is now uncommon in Western countries. The disease is often accompanied by infertility but this may well be because of the accompanying tubal lesions rather than a result of endometrial damage, for the normal cyclical changes are not usually interrupted by a tuberculous endometritis. Continued menstrual shedding of the endometrium prevents the disease proceeding to the stage of caseation and in premenopausal women the characteristic histological finding is of a few small scattered tubercles with little or no central caseation. The tubercles are maximally developed, and so most obvious, in the later stages of the menstrual cycle and diagnostic biopsy in suspected cases should always be undertaken at this time. Occasionally tubercles are absent and the findings are of a non-specific chronic endometritis. The presence of neutrophil polymorphs and eosinophilic debris in the lumen of occasional glands should arouse suspicion. In all suspected cases, culture and/or guinea pig inoculation should be undertaken.

In postmenopausal women endometrial tuberculosis is rare but when it does occur there is no obstacle to its progression to caseation. In such cases the endometrium may appear as a thickened whitish-yellow, shaggy lining to the uterine cavity and sometimes the latter is itself filled with caseous material; histologically the endometrium will show confluent caseating tuberculosis.

Schistosomiasis of the endometrium is common in areas where this disease is endemic, e.g. Africa, and can cause infertility. Ova are deposited in the endometrium and these usually, but not invariably, elicit a macrophage granulomatous reaction.

Actinomycosis of the endometrium, though rare, is sometimes found in association with an intra-uterine contraceptive device.

Endometrial polyp

The term 'polyp' is a purely descriptive one and does not denote any specific pathological process; it is, however, usually applied to a focal overgrowth of the endometrium which protrudes into the uterine cavity. Such polyps are common: they may be pedunculated or sessile and are characteristically pink and fleshy with a smooth surface. Histologically a polyp is covered by columnar epithelium and contains endometrial stroma and glands; the latter are commonly either inactive or show patchy irregular cyclical changes but are, in some cases, resistant to the effects of progesterone and thus show a cystic glandular hyperplasia (see below). A pedunculated polyp may undergo torsion whilst ulceration of the tip of the polyp may cause bleeding. Malignant change is extremely uncommon.

Endometrial hyperplasia

Two quite separate conditions are included together under the general term endometrial hyperplasia and a diagnosis of hyperplasia without specification of the type is of no value.

(a) Cystic glandular hyperplasia

In this condition the uterus is moderately enlarged whilst the endometrial lining is vascular and thickened, often appearing polypoidal. Histologically the endometrium is diffusely involved and the distinction between functional and basal zones is lost. The endometrial glands are straight and cylindrical but of very variable calibre, some being unusually small but invariably a number are considerably larger than normal (Fig. 24.10). The glands are lined by columnar cells with basophilic cytoplasm; some multilayering may be present but there is no pleomorphism or cellular atypia. The stromal cells are plump and closely packed thus giving a hypercellular appearance. Mitotic figures are common both in the stroma and the glands and there may be foci of haemorrhage or necrosis.

Cystic glandular hyperplasia is due to prolonged, unopposed oestrogenic stimulation of the endometrium, the commonest cause of which is *a succession of anovulatory cycles*. These occur most frequently in the perimenopausal years but are not uncommon during the menarche and are characterised by the development of a succession of Graafian follicles which mature, fail to release their ova, persist for weeks or months and then degenerate; the consequent fluctuations in plasma oestrogen levels lead to intermittent breaking down of the hyperplastic endometrium and irregular, heavy bleeding. Cystic glandular hyperplasia can also be produced by *prolonged oestrogen therapy* and by *oestrogen-secreting ovarian tumours*; these should always be considered as possible aetiological factors in post-

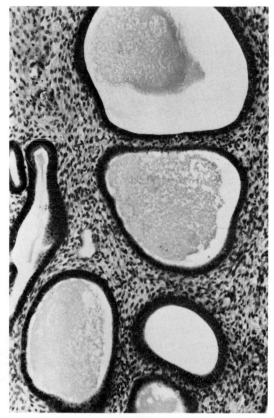

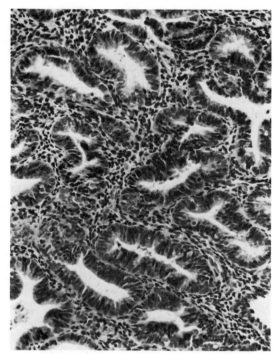

Fig. 24.11 Atypical hyperplasia of the endometrium. Note the crowding of the glands which are of irregular shapes and show evidence of multilayering. × 190.

Fig. 24.10 Cystic glandular hyperplasia of the endometrium. The glands, many of which are greatly enlarged, are lined by tall darkly staining cells. × 100.

menopausal women who develop this form of hyperplasia. Cystic glandular hyperplasia is associated with only a minimally increased risk of the eventual development of an adenocarcinoma and does not merit consideration as a pre-malignant condition.

(b) Atypical endometrial hyperplasia

This may be combined with, or occur independently of, cystic glandular hyperplasia; this form of hyperplasia is, however, typically focal rather than diffuse and is not simply a late stage of cystic glandular hyperplasia. Atypical hyperplasia is characterised by irregular glandular proliferation without any accompanying stromal proliferation (Fig. 24.11). The glands are increased in number and crowded together, in severe cases being in direct apposition with each other to give a 'back-to-back' appearance:

they are irregular in outline and are lined by tall cells with eosinophilic cytoplasm, the epithelium often being multilayered and forming intraluminal buds. Varying degrees of cellular and nuclear atypia are present and mitotic figures are common and occasionally of abnormal form. In the most extreme cases of atypical hyperplasia the distinction from a well differentiated adenocarcinoma may be almost impossible.

Atypical hyperplasia tends to occur under the same circumstances as does cystic glandular hyperplasia and is most common around the time of the menopause; the focal nature of the abnormality suggests that whilst cystic glandular hyperplasia is the normal response to prolonged oestrogenic stimulation, atypical hyperplasia represents an abnormal tissue response to this hormonal stimulus. *Atypical hyperplasia, unlike cystic glandular hyperplasia, is associated with a high risk of progression to an endometrial adenocarcinoma*; the degree of risk is related to the severity of the atypia and in severe cases is in the region of 50 per cent.

Malignant tumours of the endometrium

Adenocarcinoma of the endometrium

The vast majority of malignant tumours of the endometrium are adenocarcinomas: such neoplasms have been increasing in incidence over the last 15 years and occur most commonly between the ages of 50 and 60.

Aetiology and pathogenesis. Nulliparous women are particularly prone to develop an endometrial adenocarcinoma: an association between this neoplasm and the triad of obesity, hypertension and diabetes mellitus has also been often canvassed but the evidence is contradictory.

The aetiological role of oestrogens has been much debated but there is now little doubt that such hormones *can* contribute to the development of endometrial adenocarcinomas, as shown by the frequent occurrence of such neoplasms in women with oestrogenic ovarian tumours and their greatly increased incidence in women receiving long-term oestrogen therapy. Most patients who develop an endometrial adenocarcinoma do so, however, in the absence of such factors and have a normal urinary output of total oestrogens; fractionation of plasma oestrogens in these patients has, however, shown that oestrone, which is the most carcinogenic of the natural oestrogens, forms an unusually high proportion of the total, this being apparently due to an increased capacity for converting androstenodione, of adrenal origin, into oestrone in the body fat.

Atypical endometrial hyperplasia can, and often does, evolve into an adenocarcinoma; this is often cited as further evidence of the causal role of oestrogens in the genesis of adenocarcinoma but cystic glandular hyperplasia, which is equally oestrogen dependent, is not a precursor of carcinoma and most adenocarcinomas arise from an atrophic endometrium: rarely an adenocarcinoma may develop in an endometrial polyp.

Macroscopic appearances. The tumour may appear as a localised nodule, plaque or polyp, usually in the upper part of the uterus, but more commonly it presents either as a diffuse nodular or polypoid thickening of the uterine lining (Fig. 24.12), often with superficial ulceration and bleeding, or as a bulky, friable, par-

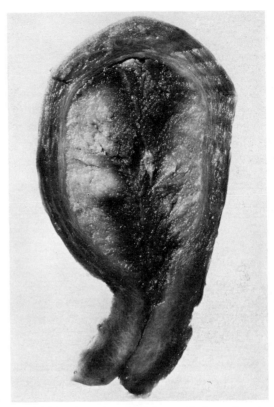

Fig. 24.12 An adenocarcinoma of the endometrium. The tumour is filling and distending the uterine cavity.

tially necrotic mass which may fill, or even expand, the uterine cavity.

The uterus may be slightly or moderately enlarged, whilst the myometrium, although usually focally thinned by invading tumour, is occasionally diffusely thickened by widely infiltrating neoplastic cells.

Microscopic appearances. The neoplasm is commonly a well differentiated adenocarcinoma (Fig. 24.13) but solid areas, a cribriform pattern and papillary formations are common and sometimes dominant. Foci of intraglandular squamous metaplasia are frequent, and if these are extensive the tumour is sometimes described as an *adeno-acanthoma*; definition of the extent of metaplasia necessary for this diagnosis is subjective and arbitrary and there is little justification for regarding an adenocanthoma as a separate or specific entity. Some endometrial adenocarcinomas are, however, admixed with malignant squamous tissue and such tumours, known as **adeno-squamous**

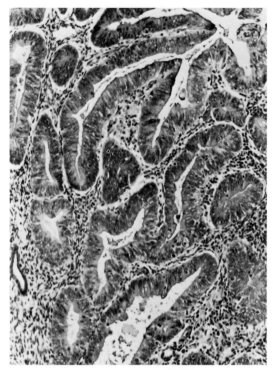

Fig. 24.13 A well-differentiated endometrial adeno-carcinoma. × 150.

carcinomas, do merit specific identification for they have an unusually poor prognosis. In most endometrial adenocarcinomas scattered foci of cells with clear cytoplasm are found and occasionally such cells, which are of secretory endometrial type, predominate.

Spread and prognosis. Endometrial adenocarcinoma invades the myometrium at an early stage but, because of the thickness of this muscular barrier, tends to be confined to the uterus until late in the course of the disease. Eventual penetration of the myometrium leads to parametrial infiltration and tumour deposits in the pelvic peritoneum and pouch of Douglas, whilst extension along the lumen of the tube, a particular feature of growths arising in the cornu of the uterus, can result in implants in the ovaries and broad ligament. Vaginal metastases occur by venous or lymphatic dissemina-tion but spread to the hypogastric, obturator and para-aortic lymph nodes occurs late. Distant metastases to liver and lung are uncommon and death is usually due to the effects of neoplastic infiltration of the pelvis, including uraemia from ureteric involvement.

The prognosis is related to the degree of differentiation of the tumour and to the clinical stage at the time of diagnosis. The overall 5 year survival rate is in the region of 66 per cent.

Sarcomas of the endometrium

Endometrial sarcomas arise from undifferentiated mesenchymal cells which not only retain their embryonic potentiality to develop into endometrial stromal and glandular cells but also have a capacity to differentiate into connective tissue cells of a type foreign to the uterus, e.g. cartilage, fat, striated muscle. Sarcomas containing only endometrial-type tissue are known as 'homologous' whilst those in which extra-uterine cell types occur are called 'heterologous'. Further, the neoplastic cells may differentiate along only one cellular pathway to give a 'pure' sarcoma or into a variety of cell types to form a 'mixed' sarcoma.

Thus a sarcoma formed solely of malignant endometrial stromal cells is a *pure homologous sarcoma* whilst a uterine rhabdomyosarcoma is a *pure heterologous sarcoma*. A neoplasm containing both endometrial stromal sarcoma and endometrial adenocarcinoma is a *mixed homologous sarcoma*, and is usually known as a *carcino-sarcoma*, whilst the presence, in such a tumour, of malignant foci of cartilage or striated muscle indicates a *mixed heterologous sarcoma*, commonly known as a *mixed mesenchymal tumour*.

All endometrial sarcomas are rare but the carcino-sarcoma and the mixed mesenchymal tumour are the least uncommon: both usually develop in elderly women and form large polypoid tumour masses which expand the uterine cavity and extend through the endocervical canal to present in the vagina. The prognosis is very poor.

Endometriosis

Endometriosis is a condition in which tissue identical in all respects to the endometrium is found in sites distant from the uterus (Fig. 24.14). The ectopic tissue occurs most com-

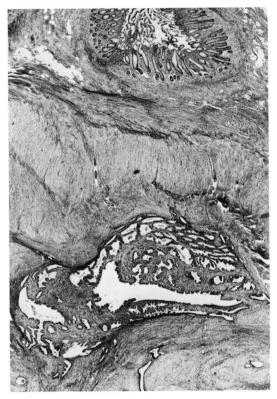

Fig. 24.14 Endometriosis of the appendix and caecum. A focus of endometrial glands and stroma and showing cystic change is present in the muscular coat of the caecum close to the appendix (*see above*). × 12.

monly in the ovaries, Fallopian tubes, pouch of Douglas, uterine ligaments, rectovaginal septum and the bowel; occasionally foci of endometriosis are encountered in laparotomy scars, at the umbilicus or in the skin, whilst exceptional instances of lesions occurring in lymph nodes, limbs, pleura and lung have been recorded.

The pathogenesis of this disorder is still far from clear but one possible mechanism for its development is the reflux of viable fragments of endometrial tissue through the tubes during menstruation with subsequent implantation on, and growth in, the ovaries and pelvic peritoneum: certainly, scar endometriosis appears to be due to implantation of endometrial tissue during uterine surgery. A further possibility is that endometriosis arises ectopically as a result of endometrial metaplasia of the peritoneal serosa; this is a feasible hypothesis and it may be that, in fact, such metaplasia is induced by regurgitated fragments of endometrial tissue which, after initiating the process, subsequently die. The occurrence of endometriosis in distant sites cannot, however, be explained except by invoking haematogenous or lymphatic dissemination and it is probable that there is no single pathogenetic mechanism which applies to all cases of this condition.

Macroscopically, pelvic endometriosis is seen as small bluish nodules, often with surrounding fibrosis. In the ovaries the endometriotic lesions are commonly cystic and contain altered blood; these may reach a considerable size, and, because of the dark colour of their contents, are often referred to as '*chocolate cysts*'. Ovarian endometriosis is frequently associated with dense adhesions, the ovaries being bound down to the broad ligament or the bowel. Tubal lesions may occur on the serosa or in the wall and, although these often lead to some distortion of the tube, there is virtually never tubal occlusion.

Histologically the lesions of endometriosis consist of both endometrial glands and stroma. The endometrium is, however, usually functional and hence menstrual type bleeding occurs and often obscures and distorts the original histological appearances; indeed the epithelial component is frequently destroyed and a presumption that the lesion was originally one of endometriosis is then only made possible by the presence of stroma containing many haemosiderin-laden macrophages.

It is the hormonal sensitivity of the endometriotic lesions that is responsible for their role in producing symptoms; recurrent swelling causes pain and repeated bleeding leads to fibrosis. Hence the commonest complaints are of pelvic pain just before and during the menstrual period, deep pain on sexual intercourse and rectal discomfort. Infertility is often noted but the basis for this is obscure; as already remarked, it is not due to tubal occlusion but may result from a disturbance in either tubal motility or ovarian function. The symptoms tend to improve dramatically during gestation in those patients who do become pregnant.

The Myometrium

The myometrium is the thick muscular wall of the uterus and is capable of marked alterations in size, capacity and contractility during pregnancy and labour.

Adenomyosis

This common condition, often misleadingly referred to as '*internal endometriosis*', is characterised by the presence of abnormally sited endometrial tissue within the myometrium, well below the base of the endometrium (Fig. 24.15). The nodules of ectopic tissue may be distributed diffusely, in which case the uterus shows a roughly symmetrical enlargement, or they may be focal, causing a poorly delineated tumour-like asymmetrical thickening of the myometrium. Histologically, foci of adenomyosis are not encapsulated and consist of typical endometrial glands and stroma; the glands are commonly of basal type and hence inactive but cyclical changes and menstrual bleeding sometimes occur. The myometrial lesions can cause dysmenorrhoea and irregular, excessive bleeding with symptoms usually starting during the fourth decade and persisting until the menopause.

Adenomyosis is due to a downgrowth of basal endometrium into the myometrium and continuity of the ectopic tissue with the endometrium can be demonstrated by serial sectioning; the condition is not a form of, and is unrelated to, endometriosis.

Benign tumours

Leiomyoma. Uterine leiomyomas originate from, and are tumours of, the smooth muscle cells of the myometrium; there is commonly an intermingling with fibrous tissue and these neoplasms are often called '**fibroids**'. Myometrial leiomyomas are extremely common, being found in at least 20 per cent of women above the age of 35; they are usually multiple (Fig. 24.16) and vary in size from tiny 'seedlings' to huge masses which fill the abdomen. They may be within the wall, i.e. *intramural*, in a *submucosal* site immediately below the endometrium, or lie just beneath the peritoneum to form a *subserosal* tumour. The submucosal leiomyomas bulge into and distort the uterine cavity and the overlying endometrium is stretched and thinned; these neoplasms may become pedunculated and form a polypoid mass within the uterine cavity which can even extend through the cervix into the vagina. The subserosal tumours grow out from the uterine surface, occasionally into the broad ligament,

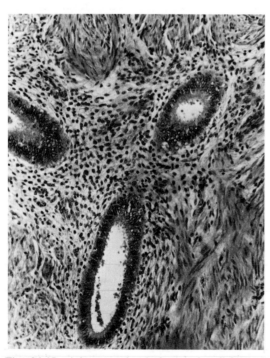

Fig. 24.15 Adenomyosis. A focus of well-formed endometrial glands and stroma lies deep within the myometrium. × 150.

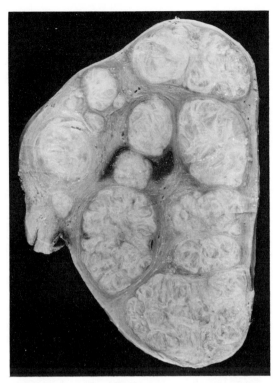

Fig. 24.16 A uterus containing many intramural leiomyomas. The cervix is seen on the left.

and may also become pedunculated; very rarely such a tumour becomes attached to the omentum or pelvic peritoneum and loses its stalk to become a 'parasitic leiomyoma'.

Leiomyomas have a well-defined, regular outline and a surrounding capsule of compressed muscle fibres; they are firm and their cut surface has a white whorled appearance. Histologically the neoplasms are formed of interlacing bundles of smooth muscle fibres arranged in twists or whorls; some, known as *cellular leiomyomas*, contain densely packed spindle cells with elongated nuclei: rarely the smooth muscle fibres are rounded with central nuclei and clear cytoplasm, tumours containing such cells being variously called *epithelioid leiomyomas*, *clear cell leiomyomas* or *leiomyoblastomas*. In all except the smallest tumours the appearances are altered to a variable degree by degenerative changes which are due to the neoplasm outgrowing its blood supply and thus fibrosis, hyaline change, calcification, patchy necrosis or fatty change are common. Infarction of a leiomyoma is uncommon but a pedun-

culated tumour may undergo torsion, whilst a specific form of necrosis, known as *red degeneration*, occurs particularly, but not only, in pregnancy and is characterised by a dull beefy red appearance of the whole tumour; this change may be accompanied by pain and fever and the presence of thrombosed vessels indicates that it is probably due to haemorrhagic infarction of an extensively hyalinised neoplasm. Cells near an area of necrosis may contain large, bizarre hyperchromatic nuclei and form multinucleated giant cells; such a finding is not an indication of malignant change unless mitotic figures are also present.

Uterine leiomyomas appear to be, at least partially, under hormonal control, for they occur almost entirely during the reproductive years, enlarge during pregnancy and in women on oral contraceptives, and tend to regress after the menopause; nevertheless attempts to relate them to a hormonal disturbance have been unsuccessful.

Many small leiomyomas are asymptomatic but large tumours can cause pressure effects with pelvic discomfort and urinary frequency, and complaints of heavy prolonged menstrual bleeding, dysmenorrhoea and reduced fertility are common. Malignant change is rare (see below).

Other benign tumours. Fibromas, lipomas and haemangiomas occur infrequently in the myometrium but **adenomatoid tumours** are less uncommon. They appear as small subserosal nodules, usually in the cornual region, and consist of numerous small channels lined by endothelial-like cells and set in a connective tissue stroma: they are always benign and are probably derived from the serosa, resembling in their fine structure a benign mesothelioma or adenomatoid tumour of the epididymis.

Malignant tumours

Leiomyosarcoma. Myometrial leiomyosarcomas are rare and may arise either in a pre-existing leiomyoma or directly from the myometrium. They are less well defined in appearance than leiomyomas, often show areas of haemorrhage or necrosis, and are characterised histologically by their cellularity, pleomorphism and mitotic activity, this latter feature being the only one that offers definitive evidence of malignancy. Leiomyosarcomas occur most commonly during the sixth decade and have a poor prognosis.

Endolymphatic stromal myosis. This condition, also known as *stromal endometriosis*, is one in which sheets of benign-appearing endo-metrial stromal cells permeate the myometrium and infiltrate the myometrial lymphatics. Local recurrence, and occasionally metastases, can occur and this lesion is best considered as an *endometrial stromal sarcoma* of low-grade malignancy.

The Fallopian Tube

The Fallopian tube plays a vital role in sperm and ovum transport and damage to the tube often results in infertility.

Salpingitis

Classical accounts of **acute salpingitis** from the pre-antibiotic era described two varieties of this disease: an **endosalpingitis**, due usually to a gonococcal infection ascending via the uterine cavity to produce an acute inflammation of the tubal mucosa, and **interstitial salpingitis**, due commonly to post-abortal or puerperal strepto-coccal infection in which the organisms reach the tube via the uterine lymphatics to establish an acute inflammatory lesion within the wall of the tube.

Acute salpingitis today is virtually always due to an infection which ascends via the uterine cavity and hence takes the form of an endo-salpingitis. The disease may occur after abortion, parturition or uterine instrumentation and has a rather high incidence in patients with an intra-uterine contraceptive device; nevertheless most cases occur in the absence of such factors and are commonly polymicrobial, due usually to a mixture of aerobic and anaerobic organisms of enteric type. *Neisseria gonorrhoeae* is now an uncommon cause of acute salpingitis and indeed the ability of this organism to cause an acute tubal inflammation is doubted by many, who consider that gonococcal salpingitis is usually only transient but inflicts sufficient minor damage to pave the way for the subsequent establishment of a polymicrobial infection. *Mycoplasma, Herpesvirus* and *Chlamydia* are now emerging as important causes of acute salpingitis.

In acute salpingitis both tubes are usually involved; they are congested, perhaps slightly swollen, and pus may be seen oozing from the fimbrial ostia, the fimbriae themselves being often swollen, congested and matted. Histologically there is swelling and congestion of the mucosal folds (plicae) which are infiltrated with polymorphonuclear leukocytes; the lumen often contains pus.

Many cases of acute salpingitis resolve but a proportion pass into a chronic stage with poly-morphonuclear, lymphocytic and plasma-cell in-filtration (Fig. 24.18) and fibrosis; adhesions between the plicae become established and a

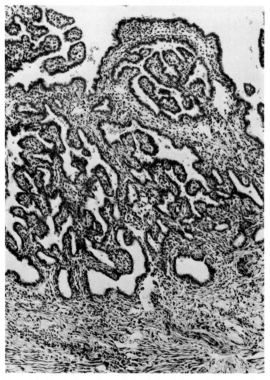

Fig. 24.17 Chronic salpingitis. There is extensive fusion of the plicae, producing blind-ending crypts in the mucosa. × 130.

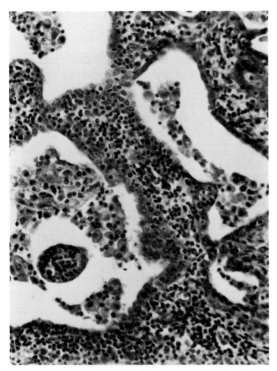

Fig. 24.18 Chronic gonococcal salpingitis. The plicae are fused, thickened and infiltrated with inflammatory cells. Purulent exudate containing polymorphs and macrophages is present in the lumen. × 200.

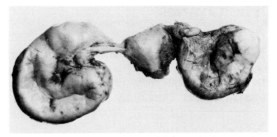

Fig. 24.19 Bilateral hydrosalpinx. Both tubes are extremely dilated and flask-shaped; they are distorted further by adhesions.

complex cribriform pattern often results, this being known as **follicular salpingitis**. The chronic inflammatory cell infiltrate may persist but often subsides leaving a legacy of residual scarring and deformity (Fig. 24.17).

An acute salpingitis may also result in a **pyosalpinx** in which the fimbrial ostia become occluded and the tube distended by pus; such a condition may persist but more commonly infection is eliminated and a **hydrosalpinx** results (Fig. 24.19), in which the tube is thin walled, greatly distended and contains clear watery fluid. The pathogenesis of a hydrosalpinx is not fully understood for the isthmic end of the tube remains patent and there seems no good reason why the fluid should not drain into the uterus.

Tuberculous salpingitis. The Fallopian tubes are usually the first part of the female genital tract to be involved in tuberculosis, tubal infection being almost invariably secondary to extragenital disease and reaching the tube via the blood stream.

The infected tubes are usually moderately or markedly thickened and the tube deformed and bound down to the ovary by dense adhesions: in the less common exudative form of the disease the tube becomes grossly distended to resemble an ordinary pyosalpinx. Histologically there is a diffuse non-specific chronic inflammatory cell infiltration of the mucosa and tubercles, usually few in number, are found scattered in the mucosa and submucosa; central caseation is usually apparent in the tubercles and foci of caseation often become confluent and rupture through the mucosa into the lumen. The mucosa itself is commonly markedly hyperplastic and may sometimes show a degree of atypia, features that can lead to a mistaken diagnosis of carcinoma.

Tumours of the tubes

Benign tumours such as fibroma, adenoma, haemangioma and leiomyoma, are sometimes encountered but malignant neoplasms are rare. Adenocarcinoma is bilateral in a considerable proportion of cases, is sometimes associated clinically with a characteristic watery vaginal discharge, and has a poor prognosis. Choriocarcinoma can develop in the tube as a sequel to a tubal pregnancy.

The Ovaries

Inflammation. Acute inflammation of the ovary occasionally complicates acute salpingitis and this combination may progress to a **tubo-ovarian abscess**. Oophoritis is, however, rare.

Non-neoplastic cysts

Cystic change occurs with some frequency in Graafian follicles and corpora lutea. **Corpus luteum cysts** are usually solitary, contain either altered blood or clear amber fluid, are lined by luteinised granulosa and theca cells and, although usually asymptomatic, can rupture and bleed into the peritoneal cavity. **Follicular cysts** are found in the cortex and are small and unilocular; their smooth lining is formed of flattened granulosa cells and the clear fluid within the cyst cavity often contains oestrogens which can inhibit pituitary FSH secretion and lead to anovulatory cycles with consequent endometrial hyperplasia. Multiple follicular cysts occur in a variety of conditions to give the picture of a *polycystic ovary*; when multiple cysts are associated with thickening of the ovarian capsule, hyperplasia and luteinisation of thecal cells and anovulation there is often an accompanying clinical triad (expressed either partially or fully) of infertility, obesity and hirsutism which is known as the **Stein–Leventhal syndrome.** The exact pathophysiology of this condition is obscure but it appears that this particular type of polycystic ovary secretes, possibly because of an enzyme defect, an excess of androstenedione.

If the ovaries are subjected to excessive gonadotrophic stimulation, as occurs in patients with a hydatidiform mole and in some women receiving gonadotrophin therapy, cysts, known as **theca-lutein cysts**, may develop in the luteinised granulosa cells of atretic follicles.

Tumours of the ovaries

The many different ovarian tumours are classified on the basis of their cell or tissue of origin, it being believed that these neoplasms arise from undifferentiated cells in mature tissues which retain the same potentiality for differentiation as is possessed by the embryonic cells which are the precursor of that tissue.

A simplified form of the complex classification of ovarian tumours defines five main groups:

I. Tumours derived from the surface epithelium.
II. Tumours of sex cord-stromal origin.
III. Tumours derived from germ cells.
IV. Miscellaneous tumours.
V. Metastatic tumours.

I. Tumours derived from the surface epithelium

Approximately 60 per cent of all ovarian tumours, and 90 per cent of those which are malignant, are derived from the surface epithelium: they are collectively known as the **common epithelial tumours**. The ovarian surface epithelium is derived from, and is the mature equivalent of, the coelomic epithelium which in embryonic life overlies the gonadal ridge and from which are derived the Müllerian ducts and the tissues to which these give rise, i.e. the tubal, and endocervical epithelia and the endometrium. Neoplasms arising from indifferent cells in the surface epithelium retain this embryonic potential for Müllerian differentiation. In some, the tumour epithelium differentiates along an endocervical pathway, producing the *mucinous* neoplasms; others differentiate into a tubal type of epithelium, forming the *serous* group of tumours, while a third group differentiate along endometrial lines to produce the *endometrioid* neoplasms. Surface epithelial tumours also have a potential for differentiating along Wolffian lines to form uro-epithelium, neoplasms containing such epithelium being eponymously called *Brenner tumours*. Finally, it must be borne in mind that all these neoplasms, arising as they do from serosa, are in essence mesothelial, though their true nature is obscured by varying degrees of Müllerian or Wolffian differentiation. Some neoplasms show little or no such differentiation and are, because of a historical misinterpretation of their nature, known as *mesonephroid tumours*.

All these epithelial neoplasms can exist in benign and malignant forms and those which are malignant are often grouped together as **ovarian adenocarcinomas**. These are increasing in incidence: they are the commonest fatal tumour of the female reproductive system and form bulky masses which tend to infiltrate locally into the pelvic tissue and seed tumour implants on to the omentum, but they rarely metastasise to distant sites. Patients with ovarian adenocarcinoma have a 5-year survival rate of only 30 per cent and little is known of the aetiology of this form of neoplasia; it is thought that recurrent ovulation, which repeatedly inflicts minor trauma on the surface epithelium, and exposure to exogenous ascending material, such as talc or asbestos, may possibly be of aetiological significance.

In addition to the benign and malignant forms a third category of **tumours of borderline malignancy** or **tumours of low malignant potential** is recognised for epithelial neoplasms. These resemble macroscopically the benign forms but are characterised histologically by changes in their epithelium which suggest malignancy, i.e. multilayering, irregular budding, cellular atypia and mitotic activity, without, however, any evidence of stromal invasion. Most, but not all, such neoplasms behave in a benign fashion.

Benign mucinous tumours (mucinous cystadenomas) are common and form large cysts with a smooth outer surface; they are usually multilocular and contain clear mucoid material (Fig. 24.20). Histologically the cyst epithelium is formed of tall mucin-secreting columnar cells which in most cases are identical to those lining the endocervix (Fig. 24.21). In a minority, however, the epithelium is of gastro-intestinal type and contains argyrophil and Paneth cells; neoplasms containing this enteric type of epithelium are probably not derived from the surface epithelium and are thought to be teratomas which have developed along only one tissue line. Benign mucinous cysts may attain a huge size and distend the abdomen; torsion may occur, and occasionally the cyst ruptures

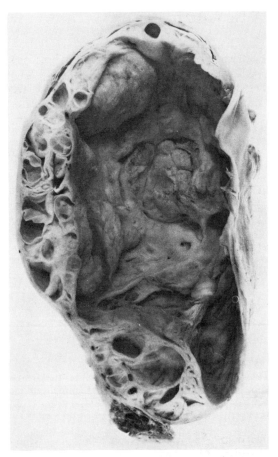

Fig. 24.20 A benign cystic mucinous tumour of the ovary: the multiple locules contained thick mucoid material.

and the contents escape into the peritoneal cavity, where tumour cells may become attached and form seedling growths which continue to secrete mucin (*pseudomyxoma peritonei*). This condition is likely to cause death from matting together and obstruction of the intestine by masses of mucin undergoing organisation.

Malignant mucinous tumours (mucinous cystadenocarcinomas) are often partially solid.

Benign serous tumours commonly occur as thin-walled unilocular cysts (**serous cystadenomas**) though in some the inner surface shows papillary projections into the lumen. Histologically the epithelium of these cysts is identical to that of the Fallopian tube (Fig. 24.22). Serous tumours may also grow as a papillary warty outgrowth on the surface of the

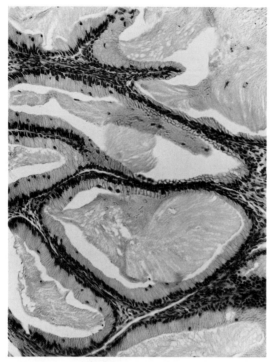

Fig. 24.21 Mucinous cystadenoma of the ovary, showing acini lined by tall columnar epithelium and containing mucous secretion. × 130.

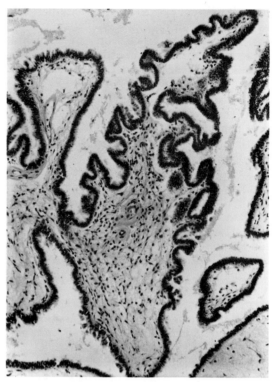

Fig. 24.22 Serous cystadenoma of the ovary, showing papillary processes which are lined by tubal-type epithelium and project into the lumen. × 100.

ovary (Fig. 24.23) and such a neoplasm *may* give rise to seedling deposits on the omentum and pelvic peritoneum which may prove fatal. Although the original warty outgrowth and the seedlings individually have the features of benign tumours, such behaviour places them in the malignant category.

Malignant serous tumours are usually cystic (**serous cystadenocarcinomas**) but contain numerous soft papillary ingrowths and are frequently solid in some areas.

Endometrioid tumours are nearly always malignant, benign and borderline forms being very rare. The tumours, usually solid with areas of haemorrhage, are commonly histologically identical with endometrial adenocarcinomas but any type of endometrial neoplasm can occur in the ovary as a form of endometrioid tumour, e.g. mixed mesenchymal sarcoma. Although most endometrioid neoplasms originate from the surface epithelium, a minority arise from foci of pre-existing ovarian endometriosis.

Brenner tumours are usually small, solid and benign; histologically they consist of rounded

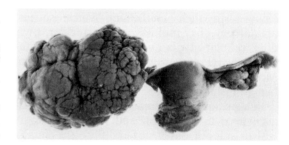

Fig. 24.23 A benign serous surface papillary tumour of the left ovary.

islands of transitional-type epithelium embedded in a dense fibrous stroma (Fig. 24.24).

'**Mesonephroid tumours**' (p. 961) are invariably malignant and show a complex papillary pattern intermingled with sheets of clear cells.

II. Tumours of sex cord stromal origin

During the early embryonic stages of gonadal development, cords of cells, possibly derived

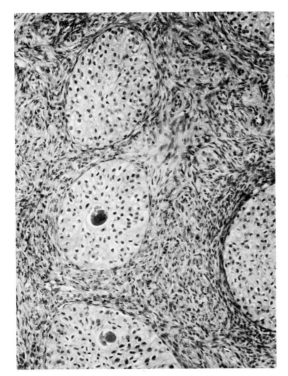

Fig. 24.24 Brenner tumour of the ovary. × 150.

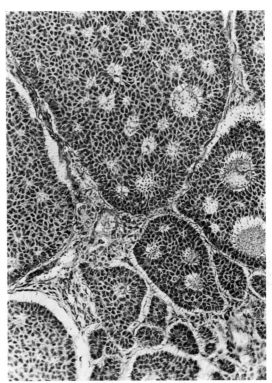

Fig. 24.25 Granulosa-cell tumour of the ovary, showing the characteristic masses of cells containing Call–Exner bodies. × 225.

from the surface epithelium and known as *sex cords*, envelop the germ cells: at this stage the primitive gonad is capable of developing into either an ovary or a testis and the cells derived from the sex cords can differentiate into either the granulosa cells of the Graafian follicle or the Sertoli cells of the seminiferous tubules. There is an interaction between the sex cords and the adjacent primitive gonadal stroma, cells from the latter differentiating into either thecal cells or Leydig cells. Tumours derived from tissues of sex cord-stromal origin retain this bisexual embryonic potentiality and can differentiate into any of these various cell types, either singly or in any combination.

Granulosa cell tumour is the commonest representative of this group of neoplasms. It is usually small, solid, and formed of cells of granulosa type arranged in follicles, trabeculae, islands or sheets; the solid groups of cells often contain tiny cystic spaces filled with eosinophilic fluid and nuclear debris, known as *Call–Exner bodies* (Fig. 24.25). Granulosa cell tumours frequently secrete oestrogens and can be responsible for signs of precocious puberty in

young girls: in older patients the effects of prolonged oestrogenic stimulation of the endometrium, i.e. hyperplasia and sometimes adenocarcinoma, lead to complaints of menorrhagia or postmenopausal bleeding. Granulosa cell tumours are of low grade indolent malignancy and may recur after many years: the histological features offer no guide to prognosis but the larger the neoplasm the greater is the risk of recurrence.

Many granulosa cell tumours are pure but some contain an admixture of thecal cells and pure **theca cell neoplasms** are sometimes encountered: these present as solid, yellowish masses and are formed of plump, lipid-containing, spindle-shaped cells. Theca cell tumours are often oestrogenic and thus produce symptoms similar to those of granulosa cell tumours; they are, however, almost invariably benign.

Neoplasms composed of Sertoli cells, Leydig cells, or any combination of these cells are known collectively as **androblastomas**. Pure

Sertoli cell tumours, which are formed of well differentiated tubules, and pure Leydig cell neoplasms, formed of sheets of acidophilic Leydig cells and derived either from the stroma or from pre-existing hilar cells, are rare and always benign. Mixed Sertoli-Leydig cell tumours (Fig. 24.26) are slightly more common and show a very wide range of differentiation, most behaving in a benign fashion but a minority pursuing a malignant course; the histological features are of little prognostic value. Pure Sertoli cell tumours are sometimes oestrogenic but all other types of androblastomas often secrete androgens and produce some degree of virilisation, breast atrophy, facial hirsuties, clitoral enlargement, amenorrhoea, deepening of the voice and temporal recession of head hair being quite commonly noted.

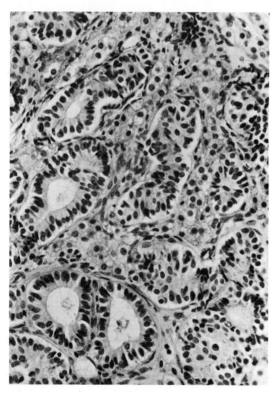

Fig. 24.26 Androblastoma of the ovary showing tubules lined by Sertoli cells and Leydig cells in the stroma. × 220.

III. Tumours of germ cell origin

Tumours derived from germ cells may show no evidence of either embryonic or extra-embry-onic differentiation; such undifferentiated germ cell neoplasms are known as **dysgerminomas** and are histologically identical in all respects to the seminoma of the testis, sharing with this neoplasm also the attributes of early dissemination to the para-aortic lymph nodes and a marked degree of radiosensitivity.

A germ cell tumour may, however, differentiate along extra-embryonic pathways into either placental tissue, resulting in the rare and highly malignant **ovarian choriocarcinoma**, or into yolk sac tissue to produce the equally uncommon and malignant **yolk sac carcinoma**: the latter, also known as an **endodermal sinus tumour**, occurs in young girls and has a complex histological structure which resembles that of primitive yolk sac, a similarity further accentuated by the ability of these neoplasms to secrete alpha-fetoprotein. These tumours were until recently invariably fatal but many now respond to chemotherapy.

Teratoma results from differentiation of a germ cell tumour into embryonic tissues. The embryonic tissues within a teratoma may be fully mature, i.e. resemble histologically those seen in adult tissues, in which case the neoplasm is benign, or may resemble immature embryonic tissue in which case the tumour tends to behave in a malignant fashion. The majority of ovarian teratomas are of the mature variety and most of these are cystic. The **mature cystic teratoma** (Fig. 24.27), often misleadingly called a 'dermoid cyst', accounts for 15–20 per cent of all ovarian neoplasms. It usually takes the form of a large thick-walled cyst containing hairs and pultaceous matter; the cyst is lined by a stratified squamous epithelium and skin adnexae, such as hair follicles, abound; within the wall of the cyst a variety of tissues may be found amongst which cartilage, bone, teeth, thyroid tissue, gastrointestinal or respiratory epithelium and neural tissue are the most common. Malignant change supervenes in about 1 per cent of mature cystic teratomas, and usually takes the form of a squamous cell carcinoma.

Teratomas containing immature tissues, are usually solid and occur in children and young adults; although malignant, these tumours are now being successfully treated, in many cases, by chemotherapeutic methods.

Although teratomas classically contain a mixture of tissues, some appear to develop

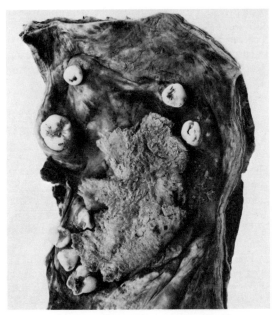

Fig. 24.27a Part of the wall of a mature cystic teratoma ('dermoid cyst') of the ovary, showing irregular growth of teeth from the inner surface of the cyst.

along only one tissue line; thus some, known as *struma ovarii*, contain only thyroid tissue whilst others are formed solely of gastrointestinal epithelium and constitute one form of mucinous tumour (p. 961).

IV. Miscellaneous tumours

Placed in this group are a number of extremely rare tumours of unknown histogenesis, primary malignant lymphomas of the ovary and tumours derived from the non-specialised tissues of the ovary. Amongst the latter group, which includes haemangiomas, lipomas and leiomyomas, is the **fibroma** which merits special attention partly because it is common and partly because this neoplasm can be associated with ascites and hydrothorax (Meig's syndrome) which resolve after removal of the ovarian neoplasm.

V. Metastatic tumours

The ovary is a common site for metastatic tumour, especially from the uterus, breast and gastrointestinal tract. A particular type of

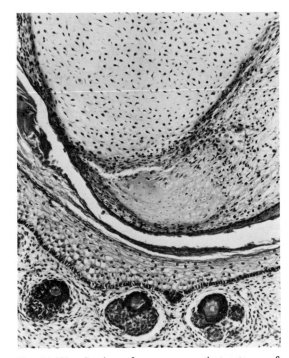

Fig. 24.27b Section of a mature cystic teratoma of the ovary. The cyst cavity is lined by squamous epithelium and shows hair follicles. Note also the nodule of cartilage. × 120.

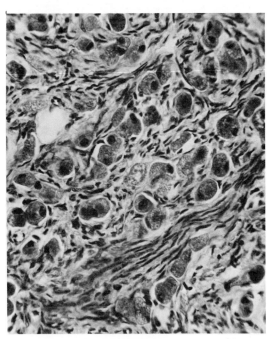

Fig. 24.28 Krukenberg tumour of the ovary, secondary to a primary carcinoma of the stomach. Note the abundant fibroblastic stroma and the large mucin-containing carcinoma cells. × 315.

metastatic lesion is the **Krukenberg tumour** (Fig. 24.28): this is due to transcoelomic spread of a gastric or colonic adenocarcinoma and is characterised by the presence of mucin-containing 'signet-ring' cells scattered in a fibrous stroma which is extremely cellular and resembles a sarcoma. This florid stromal reaction is seen before the menopause. Metastases in postmenopausal ovaries usually have the same appearances as elsewhere.

Abnormalities Related to Pregnancy

Only a few of the more important aspects of the complex subject of obstetrical pathology will be considered here.

Hydatidiform mole

This is an abnormal conceptus in which an embryo is absent and the placental villi are so distended by fluid that they resemble a bunch of grapes.

Gross and microscopic appearances. The placental mass is often unduly large and distends the uterine cavity: the villi appear as clusters of tense, translucent, fluid-filled vesicles which commonly measure up to 1 cm, and exceptionally as much as 2 cm, in diameter (Fig. 24.29). No trace of an embryo, amniotic sac or umbilical cord is apparent.

Histologically the stroma of the villi is markedly oedematous (Fig. 24.30), often to a degree of complete liquefaction, and no fetal vessels are present. A constant feature is the presence of villous trophoblastic hyperplasia

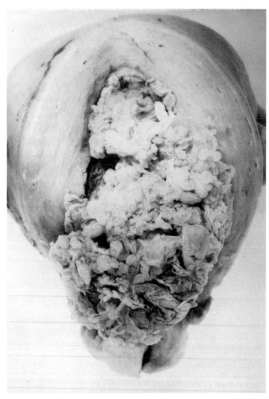

Fig. 24.29 An Opened uterus containing a hydatidiform mole. (Dr. C. W. Elston.)

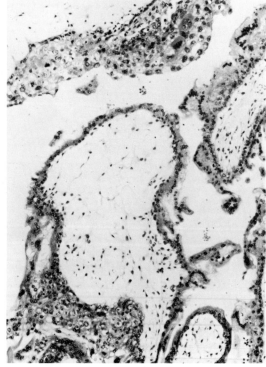

Fig. 24.30 A hydatidiform mole; the placental villi are avascular and markedly oedematous. There is a moderate degree of trophoblastic hyperplasia. × 100. (Dr. C. W. Elston.)

which is variable in degree and involves both the cytotrophoblast and the syncytiotrophoblast; some pleomorphism is often apparent but it has to be borne in mind that the proliferating trophoblast of the normal early placental villi is often moderately pleomorphic.

Epidemiology. Hydatidiform mole occurs most commonly in women aged less than 18 or more than 40; it also shows a striking geographical variation in incidence, being uncommon in Europe and North America, rather more common in Australia and of frequent occurrence in the Far East and parts of Africa, India and Central America. Attempts to explain this regional variation in terms of socio-economic status or ethnic group have met with little success. There is also a clear cut relationship between hydatidiform mole and choriocarcinoma (a highly malignant neoplasm of trophoblast), for about 50 per cent of choriocarcinomas occur in women who have previously had a hydatidiform mole.

Aetiology. In the past a hydatidiform mole was often thought to be a non-specific consequence of fetal death but it is now realised that it represents an abnormal development of trophoblast. Some light on the cause of this abnormality has been shed by the discovery that all true moles have an XX chromosomal constitution, both X chromosomes being of paternal origin; accordingly, it is postulated that moles arise from the formation and replication of a diploid cell derived from a single sperm that has penetrated a dead or dying ovum (Y sperm replication probably being lethal). How this extraordinary phenomenon results in a mole is far from clear but there is a widespread tendency to regard a mole as an expression of atypical trophoblastic proliferation, probably hyperplastic but possibly neoplastic in nature.

Course and prognosis. A mole leads inevitably to abortion, often preceded by unduly rapid uterine enlargement and haemorrhage. After the uterus has been emptied a woman with a mole has a 5 per cent risk of eventually developing a choriocarcinoma but unfortunately the histological features of any individual mole offer no guide to eventual prognosis, no relationship existing between the degree of trophoblastic hyperplasia and the later occurrence of a choriocarcinoma.

Both hydatidiform moles and choriocarcinoma secrete large amounts of the placental hormone human chorionic gonadotrophin (HCG) and *patients who have had a mole should be periodically assessed by estimation of their urinary HCG output.*

Invasive mole

In most hydatidiform moles the abnormal villi do not invade the myometrium but in a proportion, between 5 and 10 per cent, the villi not only invade but may even penetrate through the uterine wall; in such cases the myometrial vessels may be breached and emboli of hydatidiform mole transported to distant sites as 'metastases'. Despite this local invasion and distant spread this form of mole is not malignant; after removal of the mole the 'metastases' will spontaneously regress and there is no increased risk of eventual choriocarcinoma.

Partial mole

This term is applied to placentae in which only a minority of the villi show hydatidiform change, the distended vesicular villi being scattered amidst otherwise normal placental tissue; a partial mole is often accompanied by a fetus, albeit one that is usually grossly abnormal. Histologically the vesicular villi in a partial mole differ from those in a true mole by containing fetal vessels and by the absence of trophoblastic hyperplasia. A partial mole is not simply a variant of a true mole but is invariably associated with, and is an expression of, a chromosomal abnormality in the fetus, most commonly a triploidy but sometimes a trisomy.

Choriocarcinoma

This is a malignant tumour of trophoblast and is formed of both cytotrophoblast and syncytiotrophoblast; it is a unique neoplasm in that, being of purely fetal origin, it is a neoplastic allograft in the mother. The aetiology is unknown but the tumour has a geographic pattern of distribution similar to that of hydatidiform mole, being rare in Great Britain where it occurs no more than once in 40 000 deliveries. The tumour follows a hydatidiform mole in 50 per cent of cases and an unremarkable abortion in a further 25 per cent: the remainder develop,

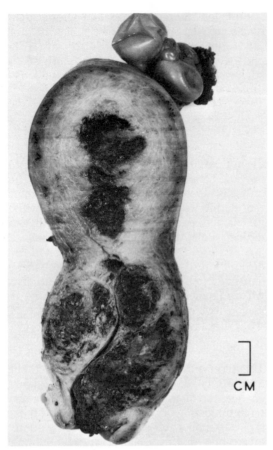

Fig. 24.31 A bisected uterus containing multiple dark haemorrhagic nodules of choriocarcinoma. (Dr. C. W. Elston.)

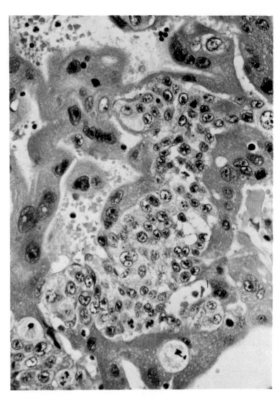

Fig. 24.32 A choriocarcinoma containing both cytotrophoblastic cells and multinucleated clumps of syncytiotrophoblast. × 300. (Dr. C. W. Elston.)

often after a period of months or years, as a sequel to an apparently normal pregnancy, arising presumably from retained fragments of placental tissue.

Because trophoblast has an inherent capacity for invading and eroding blood vessels the neoplasm is seen within the uterus as a soft, largely haemorrhagic mass (Fig. 24.31). Histologically a choriocarcinoma mimics the appearances of an early implanting blastocyst with central cores of mononuclear cytotrophoblast surrounded by a rim of multinucleated syncytiotrophoblast; the trophoblast shows a variable degree of pleomorphism and mitotic activity but no true villi are present (Fig. 24.32).

Choriocarcinoma invades rapidly and deeply into the uterine wall but penetration is principally by infiltration into venous sinuses rather than by destruction of myometrium. Because of this extensive vascular permeation, blood borne spread occurs at an early stage, principally to the lungs, liver, brain and vagina; metastasis via the lymphatics is uncommon. Despite this pattern of early spread there have been few neoplasms for which the prognosis has been altered so dramatically by the advent of chemotherapy; until recently it was always rapidly fatal, but at least 80 per cent of patients are now permanently cured by treatment with cytotoxic drugs.

Ectopic pregnancy

An ectopic pregnancy is one in which a fertilised ovum implants and begins to develop before it reaches its natural site in the uterus. An extra-uterine gestation can develop in the ovary or in the peritoneal cavity but such cases are of extreme rarity and 97 per cent of ectopic pregnancies occur in the Fallopian tubes, most commonly in the ampullary portion. Within the tube the developing placental tissue evokes an inadequate decidual response and not only invades the muscular wall but also erodes the intramural vessels. Erosion of a large vessel may lead to a haematosalpinx and separation of the conceptus from the tubal wall by haemorrhage; furthermore, the invading trophoblast weakens the tubal wall which may rupture, often with considerable intraperitoneal bleeding. Clinically these complications are usually accompanied by severe pain and other symptoms of an 'acute abdomen' demanding surgical treatment. Following tubal rupture the conceptus may implant on to the peritoneum and continue to grow as an intra-abdominal pregnancy, but this is distinctly unusual. Despite this range of dramatic complications it is probable that some tubal gestations quietly abort and are resorbed without causing any symptoms.

Many cases of tubal pregnancy are clearly due to tubal obstruction, usually as a consequence of tubal or pelvic infection, whilst some appear to result from the ovum lodging in a tubal diverticulum. Nevertheless some tubal pregnancies occur in the absence of these factors and suggested aetiological factors in such cases include increased tubal 'receptivity', because of endometriosis, delayed ovulation with washing back of the fertilised ovum by menstrual reflux, and transmigration of the ovum, i.e. an ovum released from the ovary traversing the peritoneal cavity to enter the contralateral tube. The incidence of ectopic pregnancy (about 0·7 per cent of all pregnancies) is increased to about 5 per cent in women who become pregnant in spite of the presence of a contraceptive intra-uterine device.

Congenital Abnormalities of the Female Genital Tract

During normal female embryogenesis **the internal genitalia** develop from the two Müllerian ducts which fuse distally to form the uterus and upper part of the vagina and remain separate proximally to form the Fallopian tubes. The lower part of the vagina develops from the urogenital sinus. The Wolffian ducts make no contribution to the female genital tract and atrophy.

This female type of development will occur in neuter embryos and is independent of the presence of functioning ovarian tissue; it is, however, radically altered by the presence of a testis which secretes a substance (not testosterone) that inhibits development of the Müllerian ducts and promotes that of the Wolffian ducts; this substance has a purely local action and thus a left-sided testis will only influence development of the reproductive tract on the left side of the body. **The external genitalia** will always develop along female lines unless virilisation is induced during embryonic life by their exposure to testosterone.

Hence malformations of the female genital tract fall into two broad groups, depending on whether the gonads are normal or abnormal.

Malformations in women with normal ovaries

These patients have normal ovaries and external genitalia and, usually, a normal chromosomal constitution.

i. Müllerian duct fusion defects. A total failure of Müllerian duct fusion will result in a reduplication of the uterus and vagina (uterus didelphys) whilst lesser degrees of failure can result in a single vagina with double uterus (uterus bicollis bicornis) or a single vagina and cervix with two uterine bodies (uterus unicollis bicornis). The lesser forms of fusion defect are compatible with a normal capacity to become pregnant but are associated with a high incidence of abortion, premature delivery and abnormal labour.

Genetic factors contribute to fusion defects which probably result from a very slight physical separation of the two Müllerian ducts at a critical stage of embryogenesis, possibly because of an altered shape of the embryonic pelvis.

ii. Müllerian duct aplasia. Total aplasia is very rare and found only in infants that are also otherwise grossly malformed; unilateral aplasia is slightly more common and results in a hemi-uterus with a single Fallopian tube.

iii. Failure of fusion of Müllerian ducts with urogenital sinus. A failure of fusion between the two structures that make up the vagina leads to a vaginal atresia; the uterus may be normal but is more commonly hypoplastic or absent (the Rokitansky–Küster–Hauser syndrome).

iv. Persistence of Wolffian ducts. Remnants of these ducts are often to be found in the broad ligament and lateral walls of the cervix and vagina and these may give rise to cysts or, very occasionally, neoplasms.

Malformations in women with abnormal gonads

Women of this type, though phenotypically female, often, though not invariably, have an abnormal chromosomal karyotype; if any testosterone-secreting tissue is present the external genitalia will show some degree of virilisation and are often classed as being 'ambiguous'.

Patients with a **pure gonadal dysgenesis (XO Turner's syndrome)** have bilateral streak gonads (a strand of undifferentiated stroma on the back of the broad ligament); both their external and internal genitalia develop along normal female lines but will remain infantile throughout life. Individuals with **mixed gonadal dysgenesis** have a streak gonad on one side and a testis on the other; Müllerian development occurs normally on the side with a streak gonad but is inhibited on the other, the external genitalia being ambiguous. **True hermaphrodites** (p. 1003) with an ovary on one side and a testis on the other are very rare: they show a pattern of genital development identical to that occurring in a mixed gonadal dysgenesis.

Some phenotypic females are in fact males with a normal karyotype and normally developed internal male genitalia; their external genitalia are, however, female. These patients have bilateral testes which are capable of producing the factor inhibiting Müllerian development; these individuals suffer, however, either from a defect in testosterone biosynthesis, an inability to convert testosterone to dihydrotestosterone in target tissues or a complete organ insensitivity to androgen effect, this latter syndrome being known as '**testicular feminisation**' (p. 1003).

The Breast

Inflammations

Acute infections

Acute inflammatory conditions of the female breast may be non-suppurative or suppurative, and these have widely different results.

An apparent acute inflammation occurs in connection with lactation, but although accompanied by pyrexia, it is mainly a condition of congestive swelling and oedema, and is essentially hormonal in origin from failure to establish satisfactory lactation: a galactocele may result.

The nipple is a not uncommon site for molluscum contagiosum infection, and a rare site for a syphilitic chancre. Fungal infections are also very rare in temperate climates, but must be considered in tropical countries.

Acute pyogenic mastitis. The most important form of suppurative mastitis is also related to lactation and is the result of infection via the ducts or through some abrasion of the nipple. It is usually caused by staphylococci acquired in hospital from the mouth of the suckling infant which has been colonised by the prevalent strain of *Staphylococcus aureus*: less commonly it is due to *Strep. pyogenes* (Fig. 24.33), and a spreading cellulitis may result. Unless effectively treated, staphylococcal mastitis may cause a loculated breast abscess, and extensive destruction and fibrous scarring of the breast may result. Abscess formation may also occur superficial to or deep to the mammary gland.

The neonatal infant may frequently show milk secretion caused by transplacental passage of the mother's hormones. This so-called 'witches milk' is not evidence of inflammation.

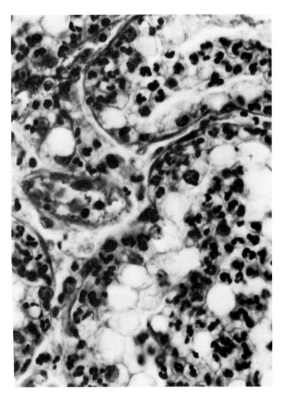

Fig. 24.33 Acute puerperal mastitis showing the secreting mammary acini, heavily infiltrated with polymorphonuclear leukocytes. × 500.

Chronic inflammatory mastitis

A group of hyperplastic and cystic conditions of the breast was formerly termed 'chronic mastitis'. These are not, however, inflammatory: they are probably hormonal effects and are described on pp. 973–6. True chronic inflammatory mastitis is a localised lesion which usually follows acute mastitis or difficult lactation, when there has been some infection, e.g. from cracked nipples, resulting in chronic low grade infection and a macrophage granulomatous reaction. It may also develop insidiously, without an obvious acute stage.

Mammary duct ectasia

This condition of progressive dilatation of the mammary ducts commences in the subareolar lactiferous sinuses and extends peripherally to the parenchymal ducts. Rarely, it is palpable, like a 'bag of worms'. Neutral fat and cellular debris accumulate in the ectatic ducts leading to a pale or coloured nipple discharge which may be confused clinically with that from a duct papilloma; microscopy, however, shows the discharge to contain only foamy macrophages in duct ectasia, while in duct papilloma red blood cells and tumour cells are usually seen.

Microscopic examination. The dilated ducts show marked elastic hyperplasia with thickening of their walls (Fig. 24.34), and usually a

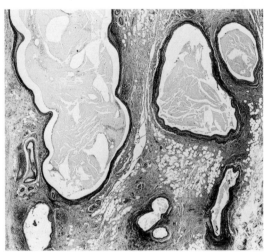

Fig. 24.34 Mammary duct ectasia. The ducts are dilated and filled with fatty material. Their walls show hyperplasia of the elastic tissue. × 13.

surrounding cuff of lymphocytes and plasma cells. Fibrosis of the ducts may lead to retraction of the nipple and arouse suspicion of breast cancer. Low grade infection within the ducts leads to ulceration and liberation of lipids into the surrounding connective tissue resulting in a chronic inflammatory reaction (Fig. 24.35) with many giant cells and macrophages. This has sometimes been mistaken for tuberculosis. These changes may be accompanied by a marked plasma cell reaction (*plasma-cell mastitis*) indicating an immune response. Plasma-cell mastitis may be mistaken clinically for carcinoma, and frozen-section examination is of value in its diagnosis. It appears to be less common nowadays.

Recurrent areolar infection

Some women suffer repeated inflammation, scarring and fistula formation in the subareolar

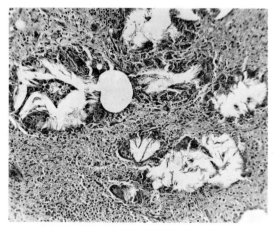

Fig. 24.35 Granulomatous reaction due to duct ectasia. Foreign-body giant cell reaction around fatty material, giving rise to a hard, palpable mass. × 50.

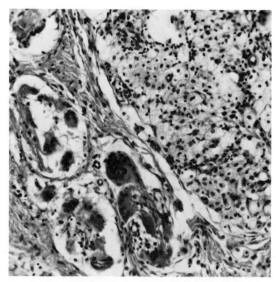

Fig. 24.36 Traumatic fat necrosis of breast, showing lipophages and foreign-body giant cells. × 150.

and juxta-areolar tissues; this may be associated with mammary duct ectasia. Sometimes a fistula lined by granulation tissue communicates with a subareolar duct with a squamous lining which may be due to metaplasia but in some cases is congenital, with pilo-sebaceous units in its wall. This is called a *mammillary fistula*. Removal of the sector containing all the affected duct system is necessary for cure.

Traumatic fat necrosis

This lesion in the fatty tissue of an obese and pendulous breast is caused by trauma (often forgotten by the patient). It gives rise to a localised firm or even hard mass which may underlie and be adherent to the skin and may easily be mistaken clinically for carcinoma. The appearances vary at different stages but there is often a central cavity containing brown oily fluid. This is surrounded by a broad zone of dull yellowish-white tissue with scattered areas of similar appearance in the outer part. At the periphery there is a fibrous capsule. Microscopic examination shows the presence of rounded foamy cells containing small fatty globules and multinucleated giant cells which may form large collections (Fig. 24.36). Many of the giant cells contain crystals of fatty acid and at places a number of them may be arranged around masses of crystals. Macrophages containing iron pigment are usually also present. The lesion represents the

result of traumatic rupture of fat cells followed by a slow lipolysis along with phagocytosis and other reactive changes. Similar appearances are sometimes seen after minor surgical operations on the breast. Traumatic fat necrosis is less commonly seen now, perhaps because there are fewer excessively obese breasts around.

Insertion of materials to increase the size of the breasts in women, or to simulate breasts in transvestite males, may produce a somewhat similar histological appearance. The nipples may also be damaged by piercing for the wearing of rings or other jewellery.

Tuberculosis

Tuberculosis of the breast is now rare. It may be the result of haematogenous infection, or it may be due to lymphatic or direct spread from caseous axillary lymph nodes or tuberculosis of the pleura or ribs. It may cause a large caseous swelling which may simulate tumour; in other cases, it is a more diffuse infiltration with nodular thickenings, a form of true chronic interstitial mastitis. In untreated cases, the caseous material may discharge through the skin with formation of a chronic sinus. *In view of the histological similarity of various non-tuberculous lesions (e.g. duct ectasia; fat necrosis), the diagnosis of mammary tuberculosis should not be made without proof that tubercle bacilli are present in the lesion.*

'Mastopathy'

It is difficult to find a comprehensive term to cover the various pathological changes commonly seen in the breasts that are neither inflammatory nor truly neoplastic. The changes include *hyperplasia, metaplasia* and *cyst formation*, and either inflammation or neoplasia may subsequently complicate the picture. The noncommittal term '**mastopathy**' is a convenient one for this group of changes. The term '**fibroadenosis**' is sometimes applied, but we prefer to restrict its use as described below.

Generalised cystic mastopathy

Generalised mastopathy is commoner in nulliparae and is sometimes associated with menstrual irregularity. The incidence increases towards the menopause, but it may occur in severe form early in the third decade. Although the changes may at first be local they tend to extend progressively and eventually affect much of the parenchyma of one or both breasts.

Structural changes. These are various and complex, but can best be considered under the headings, (*a*) fibrosis, (*b*) cyst formation, (*c*) adenosis and (*d*) epitheliosis.

The breast tissue is firmer and more nodular than usual and the lobules may be visible on section as groups of small elongated yellowish-brown foci in the white rubbery collagenous stroma. Cysts of 2–10 mm diameter frequently occur in clusters: less commonly one or more larger cysts of bluish appearance, containing a thin mucoid or dark brownish fluid, are present.

Microscopic examination reveals a great variety of structural changes. When the changes are limited to fibrosis, adenosis, sclerosing adenosis and cyst formation, the name **simple cystic disease** is applied; but when epithelial hyperplasia (*epitheliosis*) is marked in ducts and acini the condition is better termed **hyperplastic cystic disease**. This distinction is important since only in the latter condition is there evidence of transition to neoplasia.

Some **fibrosis** accompanies most cases of mastopathy but is difficult to assess; the normally fibrous breast of young women persists even after the menopause in thin women,

whereas in obese women the fibrous tissue of the breast may be extensively infiltrated with fat, and as age advances the fibrous mammary stroma becomes hyaline and relatively acellular while the epithelial elements atrophy. It is this collagenisation of pre-existing stroma rather than renewed fibroblastic activity that leads to fibrosis of the breast. Occasionally in heavy pendulous breasts this process leads to the appearance of an indurated mass in the upper outer quadrant.

Local dilatation of ducts, terminal ductules or acini results in **cyst formation**, and is presumably due to duct obstruction. Mammary duct ectasia may also occur (p. 971). Some cysts show metaplasia of the epithelial lining cells; these become large, columnar and eosinophilic with a feathery outline and at their apices may contain granules resembling those seen normally in apocrine gland epithelium (Fig. 24.37. Cyst formation is more frequent at about the time of the menopause or thereafter

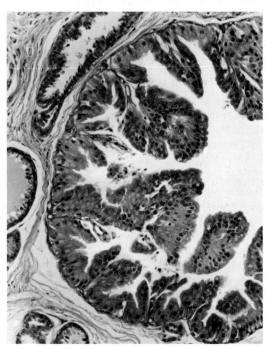

Fig. 24.37 Generalised cystic mastopathy, showing a cyst lined by apocrine-type glandular epithelium and with papillary projections into the lumen. × 120.

and tends to affect both breasts. It is probably an involutional effect related to changes in hormone production.

Lobules begin to appear in the female breast at puberty; before that, male and female breasts are similar and contain only ducts. After puberty, formation of new breast lobules and/or enlargement of pre-existing lobules occurs and is termed **adenosis**: the lobules retain their usual histological pattern (Fig. 24.38) and there is no intraluminal prolifera-

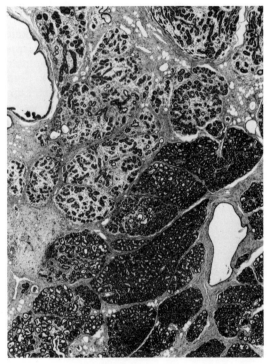

Fig. 24.38   Adenosis. There is a marked increase in the size and number of the lobules. Cystic dilatation of occasional ductules is present. × 22.

tion of cells to fill the acini, as occurs in pregnancy. A mild degree of adenosis occurs in the second half of each normal menstrual cycle, and the mammary hyperplasia of pregnancy begins as adenosis; during lactation secretory phenomena are super-added. Rarely there is incomplete involution after lactation and lactating lobules may still be seen in the breasts of women up to the 8th decade. This is not to be confused with the prolonged secretion of milk seen in elderly acromegalic women under the stimulation of excessive prolactin secretion.

Adenosis is accentuated in mastopathy and almost certainly results from hormonal stimulation. Adenosis plays no part in the development of carcinoma of the breast but may be prominent in the breast parenchyma around fibro-adenomas.

A perversion of adenosis, termed **sclerosing adenosis**, may occur as an isolated phenomenon producing a palpable rubbery greyish discoid mass in the breasts of young women. Commonly it follows incomplete involution after an interrupted pregnancy or lactational failure. Sclerosing adenosis also occurs in microscopic foci in the breasts of women of widely different age groups and may be present along with epithelial proliferative lesions, e.g. papillomas. As in simple adenosis the changes are always lobular but lack the simple acinar pattern seen in adenosis. Sclerosing adenosis proceeds through a sequence of changes beginning with an early florid, confused picture of proliferation of both epithelial and myoepithelial elements (Fig. 24.39). Mitotic activity

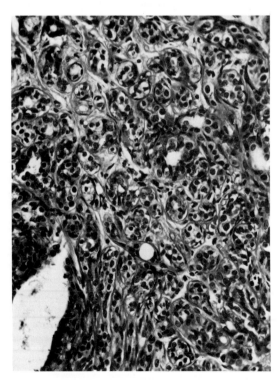

Fig. 24.39   Sclerosing adenosis in the florid phase; many small acini and solid cords of cells with much myo-epithelial hyperplasia. × 200.

may be high at this stage. Later the true epithelial elements atrophy and the myo-epithelial cells produce a corded appearance which simulates infiltrative carcinoma. Eventually the myo-epithelial elements undergo collagenisation which increases the resemblance to scirrhous carcinoma. *Sclerosing adenosis has no significance as a precursor of carcinoma; its importance lies in the possibility of misdiagnosis as cancer, especially on immediate section at the time of operation.* Such errors are best avoided by careful low-power examination which reveals the typical *lobular* nature of the change. Sclerosing adenosis may rarely be seen in perineural lymphatics and this must not be mistaken for evidence of malignancy. It is often accompanied by small papillomas and sometimes by microscopic foci of calcification which may be troublesome in mammography.

The term **epitheliosis** was coined by Mrs. E. K. Dawson to describe the condition in which hyperplasia of the epithelium of ducts and acini

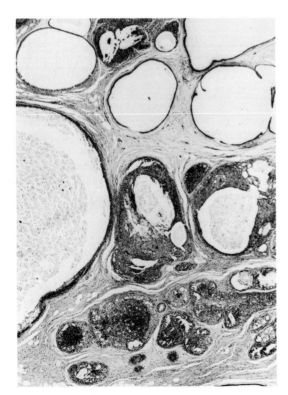

Fig. 24.40 Epitheliosis of breast. Some of the ducts are filled with masses of epithelial cells and others are dilated with granular secretion. × 22.

results in the heaping up of lining cells which may eventually fill the lumina of ducts and acini more or less completely (Fig. 24.40). This hyperplasia may take three forms (*a*) *a solid type* in which the ducts are solidly filled, (*b*) *a cribriform variety* in which there is a tendency to acinar arrangement without stroma formation, and (*c*) *a papillary arrangement* in which the exuberant epithelial ingrowths are usually less well provided with fibrovascular cores than are true papillomas. Epitheliosis is an important condition and, unlike adenosis and sclerosing adenosis, may possibly be associated with the development of carcinoma, although many patients with epitheliosis escape this change. The presence of epitheliosis is the essential feature that distinguishes hyperplastic cystic disease from simple cystic mastopathy.

Localised hyperplastic cystic disease

While all the changes enumerated above may occur in generalised mastopathy, local areas of epitheliosis are more likely to cause a clinically detectable lesion. Localised hyperplastic disease begins during the reproductive period and leads to an irregular induration or discrete swelling of the breast which demands surgical excision for exclusion of malignancy. Pain is not usually a feature and consequently hyperplastic disease often escapes notice. Necropsy studies have shown significant epithelial hyperplasia in about 25 per cent of unselected women. In a similar proportion of breasts presenting with carcinoma, hyperplastic cystic disease is found to coexist with the tumour. In this localised form of disease cyst formation is often slight or absent. The epitheliosis present may be severe and in any combination of patterns, affecting few or many ducts or duct and acinar systems. Examination of a large number of amputated breasts suggests a picture of progressive dedifferentiation of the proliferative cells. Even within the same breast an evolutionary sequence from obviously benign to obviously malignant cells may be traced within the ducts and may, although less frequently, extend to the acini. Ultimately the ducts and acini are filled partially or completely by masses of cells with hyperchromatic and aberrant nuclei to which the terms **intraduct carcinoma**, and **intra-acinar** *or* **lobular carcinoma** are suitably applied. From either lesion malignant cells may invade the surrounding stroma as an ordinary infiltrative carcinoma.

Nevertheless, in many infiltrative breast cancers, neither epitheliosis nor intraduct cancer can be found. Some authorities do not believe that there is a causal relationship and suggest that epitheliosis and cancer represent different responses to the same aetiological agents, but others regard mastopathy as a significant risk factor, particularly when it is associated with a late natural menopause.

Aetiology. The cause of hyperplastic cystic disease and its significant component of epitheliosis is still obscure. Inflammation plays no part and the commonly used synonym 'chronic mastitis' is quite unjustified. The changes seem likely to represent an endocrine effect, either from excess of oestrogen, which in certain species has been shown to bring about mammary hyperplasia and neoplasia, or from failure to achieve the normal balanced action of the sex hormones. Hyperplastic cystic disease in adolescents is sometimes accompanied by endometrial hyperplasia and menorrhagia.

'Hypertrophy' of the female breast

This must not be confused with the gross mammary adiposity still sometimes observed in obese middle-aged women. It usually develops soon after puberty although occasionally it may follow pregnancy. The breasts enlarge progressively and may eventually weigh several kilograms. The condition is usually bilateral but development may be unequal. The term hypertrophy is not really apt since the breast enlargement is due mainly to increase in soft oedematous connective tissue, and sometimes also of adipose tissue. Glandular tissue is not much increased and often appears scanty. The cause of hypertrophy is usually obscure, but rarely it accompanies various hormone-secreting tumours. Treatment by partial excision with preservation of the nipple and areola is often successful.

Tumours of the Breast

Benign tumours

Fibroadenoma

This is by far the commonest benign tumour of the breast and arises from the whole anatomical unit of the lobule. It is a mixed tumour with both stromal and epithelial neoplastic elements, and occurs chiefly in young women. Sometimes in young girls the fibrous component is inconspicuous and the tumour is then termed a simple *adenoma*. Fibroadenomas are small, well-circumscribed, elastic, round or ovoid masses which may occasionally attain a diameter of up to 7 cm. Rarely, they are multiple in one or both breasts. Although apparently encapsulated, they should not be enucleated by the surgeon's finger, for satellite portions of the tumour may be left behind from which recurrence takes place.

Two forms of fibroadenoma are usually distinguished but many tumours show both types of structure in different areas (Fig. 24.41). In young adults the so-called *pericanalicular type* occurs, in which the epithelial arrangement corresponds roughly to that in the normal breast lobule with an investment of loosely fibrillary connective tissue. The predominantly *intra-canalicular* type seen usually in older women shows numerous curved and branching clefts lined by epithelium and produced by the pressure of blunt rounded projections of cellular fibrous tissue upon ducts and acini. Growth of the lining epithelium merely keeps pace with that of the stroma and the characteristic clefting is produced. When cut across, the surface of an intracanalicular fibroadenoma often appears irregular and granular.

The site of origin of fibroadenoma is within the periductal elastic tissue; usually this is not obvious on cursory examination but occasional tumours present as intraduct lesions reminiscent of intraduct papilloma. In such cases bleeding from the nipple may occur. Multiple small fibroadenomatous areas sometimes occur in association with cystic disease (**fibroadenosis**)

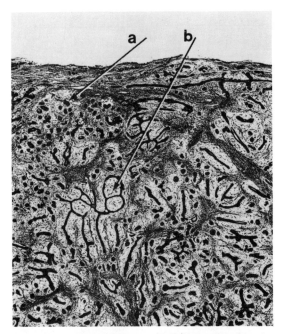

Fig. 24.41 Fibroadenoma of breast, showing the loose periacinar stroma. In places the tumour has a pericanalicular structure **a**, at other parts an intracanalicular arrangement **b**. Transitions are seen between the two types. × 16.

suggesting an intermediate phenomenon between hyperplasia and neoplasia. Fibroadenomas grow not only by proliferation of the actual tumour but also by incorporating at their periphery altered lobular units showing such fibroadenomatous change (*fibroadenomatoid hyperplasia*). Some intracanalicular tumours contain large amounts of smooth muscle in their stroma: we have seen no convincing evidence that this originates from myo-epithelium and in some cases it appears to be derived from vein walls. Commonly in the bitch and infrequently in the human female metaplastic bone or cartilage may be seen in the stroma of fibroadenomas. This must not be mistaken for tumour bone or cartilage. During pregnancy a fibroadenoma may show secretory activity.

Giant intracanalicular fibroadenomas. In older women large fibroadenomas tend to recur after removal (especially if 'shelled out') and the recurrent tumour may show a highly cellular and often a distinctly myxoid stroma. In some cases, especially after repeated recurrence, stromal proliferation is so marked that the epi-

thelial elements may be quite inconspicuous and the tumour merits the designation of **myxo-sarcoma** (Fig. 24.42). The old term *Brodie's serocystic sarcoma* is best avoided. Simple mastectomy or very wide local excision is the treatment of choice. Such tumours should not be designated as sarcoma unless the stromal cells show the morphological changes of unequivocal malignancy; the development of frankly sarcomatous change is discussed further below. Rarely carcinoma develops in a fibroadenoma.

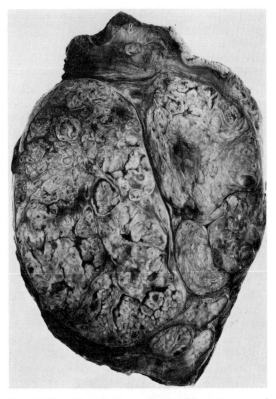

Fig. 24.42 Giant intracanalicular fibroadenoma of the breast. The stroma was very cellular and showed sarcomatous change. × 0·5.

Papillary cystadenoma

This benign tumour is much less common than fibroadenoma. Cysts of varying size are present and within these there is epithelial proliferation. Often these epithelial tumours have a somewhat papilliform pattern but they are composed of acini and do not show fibrovascular cores lined by epithelium as in a papilloma. Papillary cystadenoma may become large and, if not removed, may ulcerate through the skin and present as papillary masses on the breast surface. Most are benign but occasionally cystadenocarcinoma supervenes. Although this is usually of low-grade malignancy and requires only local excision, occasional cystadenocarcinomas are aggressive and may already have metastasised to lymph nodes at the time of diagnosis. Those in which the infiltrative component is of squamous-cell type appear to be the most dangerous.

Duct papilloma

Duct papilloma occurs most often as a rounded pedunculated tumour which forms within and eventually distends a lactiferous sinus, in or close to the nipple (Figs. 12.5, p. 325; 24.43). A papilloma comprises a branching fibrovascular stromal core clothed by a double-layered cuboidal or columnar epithelium (Fig. 24.44), which is sometimes apocrine-like. In time, the epithelium may atrophy and hyalinisation occur. The tumour may be solitary and attain a size of more than 10 mm but sometimes multiple tumours are present throughout the duct

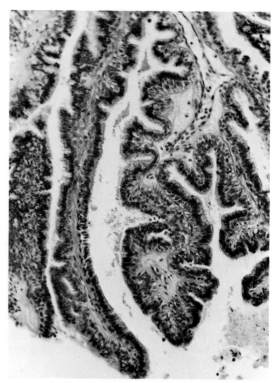

Fig. 24.44 Duct papilloma of breast, showing branching papilliform processes covered by epithelium mainly of columnar type. × 130.

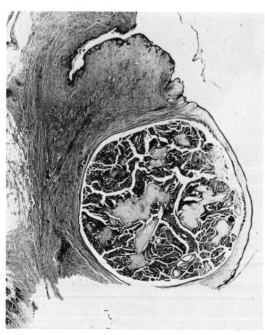

Fig. 24.43 A rounded duct papilloma distending a lactiferous sinus within the nipple. × 9.

system of the breast. The larger tumours are often accompanied by nipple discharge and those in the lactiferous sinus may present with frank bleeding from the nipple. Microscopic examination of such discharges usually shows red blood cells and tumour epithelial cells and often permits distinction from the coloured discharges present in mammary duct ectasia. Sometimes florid papillomas in young women may undergo considerable involution and hyalinisation so that incomplete removal may be followed by apparent cure even when several pregnancies and lactations follow.

Some papillomas of the lactiferous sinuses resemble papillary hidradenoma of the vulva, perhaps reflecting the developmental similarity of the breast to a sweat gland. Another rare lesion of the nipple is the so-called adenoma: double-layering of the epithelium helps to identify it as benign despite stromal distortion.

Papillary forms of epitheliosis occur in hyperplastic cystic disease and it is difficult to draw a clear line between them and papillomatosis; the presence of well-formed fibro-vascular stromal cores suggests multiple neoplasms. When such small papillomas are numerous, multicentric carcinoma occasionally develops. Carcinomatous change is rare in a solitary papilloma, and only local excision is necessary.

Other benign tumours

These are uncommon but fibroma, myxoma, lipoma, angioma and chondroma are recorded. Granular cell myoblastoma occasionally occurs in the breast and clinically may simulate carcinoma.

Malignant tumours of the breast

Carcinoma

This is among the commonest of human cancers. While it occurs more often in later adult life it is by no means rare in the third and fourth decades: for this reason all lumps in the breast, whatever the age of the patient, must be regarded clinically as possibly malignant until proved otherwise by histological examination. Immediate histological examination of frozen sections at the time of operation is of value in enabling the surgeon to decide upon the type of treatment required. Screening procedures involving clinical examination, mammography, xeroradiography and thermography are being applied to the detection of breast cancer at an early stage. Recent reports suggest that two-yearly screening in women over the age of 50 may indeed have some value in increasing survival rates.

Carcinoma of the breast is at least two hundred times more common in women than in men; it is more common in nulliparous than in multiparous women. Although it was for many years believed that several successful lactations decreased the risk of development of breast cancer, more critical studies have not confirmed that nursing histories have much to do with such development. Low rates in countries like Japan, where nursing is prolonged, apply to male as well as female breast cancer. Early maternal age at first birth of a child may, however, have some protective influence. Family aggregations of breast cancer, sometimes thought to be genetic, might only reflect similarities in reproductive histories or other environmental factors. Recently it has been suggested that high fat intake and obesity may be associated with an increased risk not only of ovarian and endometrial but also of breast cancer.

Varieties of breast cancer

Several types of breast carcinoma are described but this should not obscure the important fact that they are all manifestations of one disease process.

Scirrhous carcinoma. This is the commonest form of breast cancer; it produces an indurated mass of irregular outline and the resulting fibrosis of the stroma causes contraction and shrinkage rather than obvious enlargement of the breast (Fig. 24.45). Fibrosis is most marked

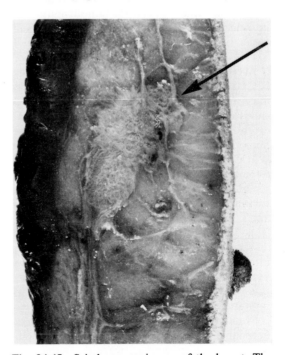

Fig. 24.45 Scirrhous carcinoma of the breast. The skin of the breast, including the nipple, is seen on the right and the pectoral muscles on the left. The cancer is seen on the cut surface (*arrow*) as an irregular paler area, lying in the breast tissue which is mainly fatty.

in the atrophic scirrhous carcinoma, which may remain less than 1 cm in diameter. When cut with a knife a scirrhous cancer gives a creaking sensation and the cut surface shows small yellow areas due to degeneration of tumour cells; this 'unripe pear' appearance is very characteristic of a scirrhous cancer. In the late states distortion or retraction of the nipple or puckering and indrawing of the skin may occur depending on the site of the tumour, which may be in any part of the breast, including the axillary tail, but is most frequent in the upper outer quadrant. Microscopy shows groups and cords of spheroidal carcinoma cells (Fig. 12.18, p. 331) between bands of fibrous tissue which are more hyaline at the centre while at the periphery this change is less advanced. In recent years, workers in several centres have published biochemical and ultrastructural evidence suggesting that collagen is produced by the tumour cells, and have cast doubt on the older assumption that the fibrous stroma represents a desmoplastic reaction.

The scirrhous carcinoma of the breast was recognised as early as Hippocratic times and the appearances of a central tumour mass with infiltrating prongs (Fig. 24.46) originally suggested the words *cancer* and *carcinoma* (i.e. crab-like).

Encephaloid carcinoma. This tumour is less common than scirrhous cancer; it forms a large mass or masses, of brain-like softness (hence *encephaloid*) and with ill-defined margins and extensive areas of necrosis and haemorrhage. Sometimes necrosis and ulceration through the skin occurs. Microscopically a scanty cellular stroma, often containing many lymphocytes, separates large collections of spheroidal tumour cells among which cellular aberration and frequent, often multipolar mitoses are seen (Fig. 12.19, p. 332).

The tumours with a heavy lymphocytic infiltrate (*medullary carcinomas*) have been reported to have a relatively high 5-year survival rate, and the lymphocytes may represent an immunological reaction to the cancer cells.

Mammary carcinoma in pregnancy and lactation may grow very rapidly and be accompanied by hyperaemia, warmth, sometimes pain and fever. The whole picture may thus suggest an acute mastitis. This type of breast cancer is sometimes very diffusely infiltrative, so that the whole breast is swollen, hard and

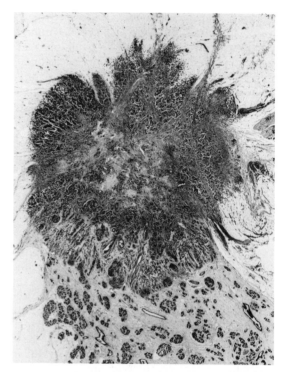

Fig. 24.46 Small scirrhous cancer of breast. The tumour has originated at the periphery of the breast and is invading both the breast tissue and the surrounding fat. Note the claw-like extensions. × 5·5.

hyperaemic with no discrete lump; consequently it looks clinically more like a cellulitis than a malignant tumour.

Histological appearances of breast carcinoma

In most scirrhous and encephaloid carcinomas the cells are quite anaplastic, spheroidal and arranged in irregular clumps (Fig. 12.16, p. 331). Less commonly the cells retain a certain polarity and a recognisably adenocarcinomatous pattern results. Such adenocarcinomas are said on statistical evidence to have a slightly better prognosis than anaplastic spheroidal cell tumours. Prognosis is also said to be better when pronounced elastosis is elicited by breast carcinomas or, as already stated, when tumours show a marked lymphocytic reaction. Rarely breast carcinomas are composed of masses of closely applied cells between which there are small circular spaces, sometimes containing mucoid material (Fig. 24.47): this pattern (*cribriform carcinoma*) is most readily seen in in-

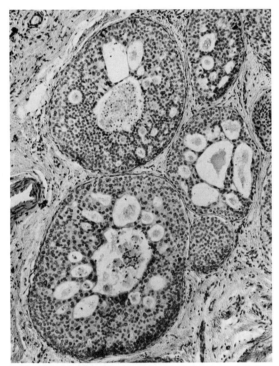

Fig. 24.47 'Cribriform carcinoma', showing masses of carcinoma cells among which are small circular spaces. The growth is still contained within ducts. × 100.

traduct cancer, and is usually less obvious and often absent in infiltrating parts of the tumour. These observations are of importance in tracing the evolutionary sequences from epitheliosis through intraduct cancer to anaplastic infiltrative tumour.

Rare tumours of low-grade malignant behaviour and identical in appearance with *adenoid cystic carcinomas* of salivary or sweat glands remind us that the breast has a histogenesis similar to these glands. Another rare carcinoma of apocrine type has similar connotations.

Mucous carcinoma (p. 330) is uncommon in the breast. It is usually bulky and often, but not always, less malignant than the commoner varieties, with delay in lymph nodal metastasis.

Focal mucoid change is seen in some breast cancers, and the cells of some spheroidal-cell cancers contain mucin, particularly those in which columns of cancer cells, in 'single file', invade the stroma, often encircling ducts: most of these arise from lobular carcinoma in situ.

Squamous carcinoma. Areas of squamous metaplasia sometimes occur in anaplastic carcinoma; the two histological variants may infiltrate together through the breast tissue and metastasise to lymph nodes. Occasional carcinomas are apparently entirely of squamous-cell type. A further interesting variant is the fibrosarcoma-like squamous carcinoma in which the bulk of the tumour is spindle-celled; only careful search reveals that these cells are undoubtedly derived from squamous carcinoma which is recognisable in occasional areas. Such tumours are sometimes misdiagnosed as carcinosarcoma.

Spread of infiltrative carcinoma

Unfortunately, at the time of first diagnosis breast cancer is often already widely disseminated. This explains the observation that age-adjusted death rates have remained remarkably stable and that different therapeutic approaches, e.g. radical or local mastectomy, or even simple 'lumpectomy' have little influence on survival.

The axillary lymph nodes are involved at an early stage by lymphatic dissemination and in many cases the internal mammary lymph nodes are also affected. Later the local skin lymphatics may be permeated leading to either focal nodularity or wider-spread involvement known as *cancer-en-cuirasse*. If the skin lymphatics are blocked, lymph-drainage is impaired and the skin becomes oedematous and swollen except where it is tacked down by hair-follicles; this produces the characteristic *peau d'orange* appearance of advanced breast cancer. Further lymphatic spread occurs through the connective tissues to the pectoral fascia and muscles and thence to the pleural cavities. In all of these situations microscopy may be required to reveal collections of malignant cells along the lymphatic pathways. It is upon these observations that the operation of radical mastectomy, now virtually abandoned, was based. As noted above, even before operation there is often already further spread by lymphatics (and possibly by the bloodstream) to other sites. Viscera and the thoraco-lumbar spine are frequently affected, the latter possibly by retrograde venous spread. Oöphorectomy, adrenalectomy and hypophysectomy (p. 983) have also revealed microscopic metastases in these organs. Metastatic spread to the opposite breast is not uncommon. Second primary carcinomas in the other breast also occur and may be identified as such by the presence of intraduct cancer (see below). Lymphatic dissemination of tumour occurs as rapidly in the atrophic scirrhous as in the fast-growing encephaloid variety.

Intraduct carcinoma (carcinoma-in-situ)

Intraduct carcinoma is a malignant prolifera-tion of epithelial cells within the ducts of the breasts, i.e. it is a pre-invasive neoplasm which has not yet broken through the walls of the duct system (Fig. 24.48). In the larger ducts it can be recognised macroscopically and is readily seen with a hand-lens. The ducts are filled with cylindrical masses of cells and de-generate fatty material which can sometimes be expressed like toothpaste from a tube; this is termed *comedo carcinoma*. Intraduct cancer may be relatively localised to one area or may affect the duct system extensively. Localised fibrosis (see below) may result in parts of the affected tissue becoming firm and palpable.

Microscopic examination shows rounded or polyhedral cells with a vesicular and often hyperchromatic nucleus, packed closely to-gether or arranged in a cribriform pattern (Fig. 24.47). Both cells and nuclei may show con-siderable aberration. The condition spreads slowly along the ducts towards the nipple and also deeply into the acini, and may long remain confined within the basement membranes. Local obliterative changes with fibrosis and elastosis sometimes occur with local healing of the lesion but this sclerosing process is never generalised.

Carcinoma-in-situ may occur also in the acini (*lobular* or *intra-acinar carcinoma*—Fig. 24.49) either alone or, more commonly, with intraduct carcinoma. Lobular carcinoma is most often found incidentally in a breast biopsy performed because of cystic disease, and empirical biopsies have shown that it is not uncommonly bi-lateral. The appearances must not be confused with those of lobular adenosis and a useful diagnostic feature is *expansion* and *total filling* of the acini by malignant cells, sometimes of the signet-ring type (see p. 617). Lobular car-cinoma may long remain confined to the acini, but when infiltration does occur the prognosis is poor. The infiltrating cells tend to form trains of single cells, whorling round ducts or

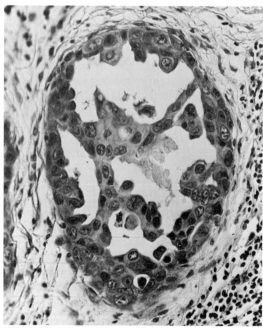

Fig. 24.48 Section of intraduct carcinoma of breast, showing collections of carcinoma cells of characteristic appearance in a duct. × 285.

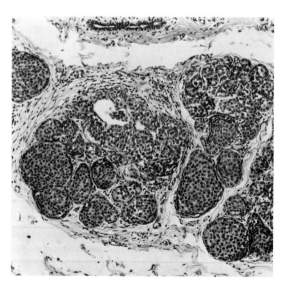

Fig. 24.49 Lobular or intra-acinar carcinoma, showing groups of acini filled with anaplastic car-cinoma cells without any break-through into the adjacent stroma. × 75.

lobules: the cells of both the lobular and infiltrating elements are almost always muci-carminophilic.

Hormone dependence

In 1896 Beatson in Glasgow first showed that bilateral oòphorectomy was followed by prolonged remission in some cases of advanced breast cancer and he postulated that such mammary cancers required for their continuing growth some influence from the ovaries. Later it also became evident that artificial induction of the menopause before the age of 35 years considerably reduces the risk of subsequent development of breast cancer. These observations led to the realisation that some breast cancers depend on hormones, e.g. oestrogens (p. 310). Some post-menopausal women with breast cancer continue to secrete oestrogens and in an attempt to remove all sources of oestrogen, oophorectomy was undertaken, followed by adrenalectomy and hypophysectomy when cortisone became available for maintenance treatment. Paradoxically, administration of oestrogens or androgens is sometimes beneficial in cases unsuitable for surgery.

In a small proportion of cases such procedures are successful in relieving symptoms, notably pain from skeletal metastases, but after a variable period the malignant cells resume their uncontrolled growth, i.e. the tumour becomes *hormone-independent*. No histological differences have been demonstrated by which hormone-dependent tumours can be recognised under the microscope and at present therapeutic trial is necessary to determine which cases will respond to endocrine ablation. Hormones other than oestrogen may be implicated, including progesterone, androgens and mammatrophic prolactin. Large-scale prospective studies are being carried out which may throw light on this problem, and the surface receptors of cancer cells for hormones are being studied in order to develop techniques of predicting hormone-dependence. Currently it appears that the number of oestrogen receptors may be a guide in predicting response to endocrine therapy and also that recurrence of breast cancer may be associated with absence of oestrogen receptors.

Despite the clinical remission obtained in cases of hormone-dependent cancer by such procedures there is only minimal evidence of tumour-cell destruction in most instances and only temporary arrest of tumour growth, but without doubt these drastic surgical procedures sometimes relieve pain.

There is no evidence that the use of oral contraceptives has any influence on the development of breast cancer (p. 309). It has even been suggested that they may confer some degree of protection.

Paget's disease of the breast

In this condition, first described clinically by Sir James Paget in 1874, part or all of the nipple and areola becomes reddened and excoriated and has a florid eczematous appearance with oozing of clear fluid. The tissues of the nipple are often firmer than normal. Paget observed that this state might persist for years but that eventually invasive cancer commonly developed, often deep in the breast parenchyma and separated from the nipple by apparently normal tissue.

Microscopic examination reveals *Paget cells* within the affected epidermis: there has been much debate concerning their nature. They occur singly or in groups, mostly in the deeper epidermal layers where they may form blunt processes projecting down into the dermis (Fig. 24.50). Actively proliferating Paget cells are large, round or oval cells with pale cytoplasm and vesicular, often hyperchromatic nuclei, with prominent nucleoli. Mitotic figures are sometimes seen. They resemble the cells of an undifferentiated carcinoma of glandular origin. They infiltrate and displace the cells of the Malpighian layer which become drawn out or flattened between them (Fig. 24.51). Many Paget cells undergo degeneration, i.e. their nuclei become irregular and pyknotic and their cytoplasm has a rather shrivelled appearance. When many of the cells show this change their recognition may be difficult. Paget cells may receive melanin from adjacent melanoblasts and sometimes they contain a small amount of mucin. The epidermal cells around groups of Paget cells undergo compression atrophy, and may appear to form a dense capsule-like structure. Paget cells never invade the underlying dermis but the latter shows reactive changes, e.g. plasma cell infiltration, formation of new capillaries, hyperaemia and serous exudation. It is these changes in the dermis which cause

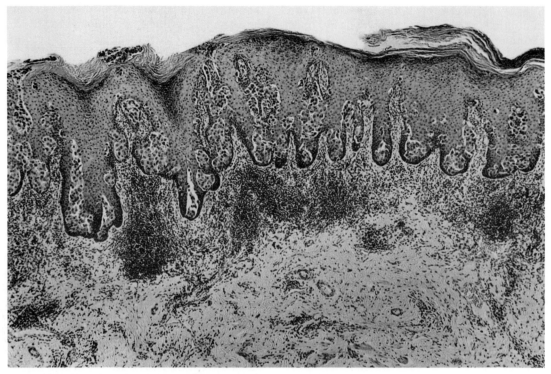

Fig. 24.50 Skin of nipple in Paget's disease, showing scattered Paget cells in deeper part of epidermis. Note marked lymphocytic infiltration of dermis. × 45.

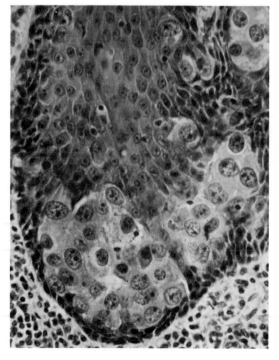

the characteristic clinical eczematous appearance of the nipple and areola.

Paget's disease is always accompanied by intraduct carcinoma in the ducts of the nipple (Fig. 24.52) and frequently direct continuity may be traced between the cells in the ducts and those in the epidermis. Intraduct carcinoma may be complicated by Paget's disease and/or by infiltrative carcinoma of the breast. Accordingly, *Paget's disease indicates the presence of intraduct carcinoma which may invade the breast stroma if it has not already done so.* Simple mastectomy is therefore essential. Whether intraduct carcinoma is followed by Paget's disease or by ordinary infiltrative carcinoma depends upon whether the affected ducts are in the nipple or deeper in the breast

Fig. 24.51 Paget's disease of nipple. Epidermal rete ridge invaded by cancer cells—'Paget cells'. The cells are particularly well preserved and show a marked contrast to the epidermal cells which are being stretched and atrophied. × 345.

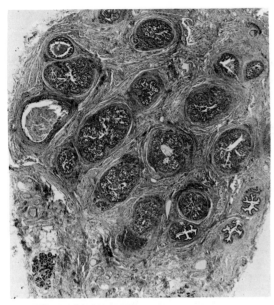

Fig. 24.52 Transverse section through the lactiferous ducts below the nipple in a case of Paget's disease, showing intraduct carcinoma in the ducts. × 12·5.

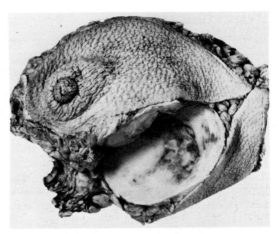

Fig. 24.53 Sarcoma of the breast. The tumour appears sharply circumscribed, and the cut surface shows central necrosis. × 0·6.

parenchyma. Occasional mastectomy specimens show that Paget's disease is commencing in an apparently normal nipple, or that intraduct neoplasm is nearing the epidermis.

Extramammary Paget's disease of the skin may occur in the vulva, perianal region, axilla, etc., by intra-epithelial spread of carcinoma of the sweat glands.

Primary intra-epithelial tumours occasionally arise in the epidermis of the nipple. Bowen's disease of the skin and malignant lentigo of the nipple may also produce widespread intra-epithelial growth, but in neither case is there intraduct carcinoma. Squamous carcinoma of the nipple is rare. An even rarer form of benign hyperkeratosis, usually bilateral, may also cause confusion.

Other malignant tumours of the breast

Sarcoma. This is much less common than carcinoma. It may arise *de novo* or more commonly supervene in giant intracanalicular fibroadenoma of middle-aged or elderly women especially after inadequate resection. It is usually well-defined (Fig. 24.53) and spindle-celled, myxomatous or pleomorphic. The degree of malignancy is related to cellular aberration and mitotic activity. Some sarcomas show metaplasia with formation of chondroid and osteoid and may resemble an aggressive osteoblastoma, osteosarcoma or giant cell tumour of bone. In these cases the prognosis is bad and death from pulmonary metastases is the rule. The rare malignant haemangio-endothelioma tends to occur especially in the breast and gives rise to very widespread metastases.

Lymphomas. Hodgkin's disease and other lymphomas and leukaemias may all affect the breast. Rarely, enlargement of one or both breasts may be the presenting symptom in leukaemia or Hodgkin's disease. As the axillary lymph nodes are likely also to be affected the clinical diagnosis may be difficult. Breast cancer and chronic lymphocytic leukaemia may co-exist.

Secondary carcinoma in breast. Spread to the contralateral breast may occur by lymphatic spread from a primary breast cancer. Carcinomas in other organs, e.g. bronchus, may also occasionally metastasise to the breast.

Congenital abnormalities

The absence of one or both of the breasts—*amazia*—is rare; in some instances it has been associated with a corresponding defect of one or both of the ovaries. *Athelia*, or congenital absence of the nipple, is less uncommon and usually bilateral. Hypoplasia of the breasts occurs in association with a similar condition of the ovaries and other parts of the genital system. There may be additional mammary glands (*polymastia*), which are capable of secretion, although they sometimes lack a nipple. They occur anywhere along the mammary line, but most often below the breasts. The term *polythelia* signifies the presence of multiple nipples.

The Male Breast

Hypertrophy (gynaecomastia). The male breast is essentially similar to that of the female until the onset of the secondary sex characters at puberty; in some adolescent males one or both breasts may then enlarge. This is known as **pubertal hypertrophy** and is rarely marked, but may cause pain or discomfort. It is due mainly to increase in stroma and of ducts, but without lobule formation. The hyperplastic duct epithelium may be surrounded by a zone of oedematous, fibrillary stroma. It tends to regress and operative removal is rarely necessary. Similar changes may occur in old age. Both pubertal and senile hypertrophy are due to changes in levels of sex hormones.

Gynaecomastia sometimes complicates cirrhosis of the liver, due to failure of the liver to metabolise and break down oestrogens. Hypertrophy also follows prolonged administration of diethylstilboestrol in the treatment of prostatic cancer, and less commonly other drugs, e.g. digitalis. It has been reported in workers manufacturing stilboestrol. In cases of prostatic cancer on oestrogen therapy, the stimulated breast is sometimes the site of metastases.

Occasionally hypertrophy results from an underlying endocrine disease such as a feminising tumour of the adrenal cortex. Less often testicular injury is causal. In chromatin-positive *Klinefelter's syndrome* (p. 1002) the enlarged breasts show lobules comparable with those of the normal female breasts. Lobule formation is excessively rare in other forms of enlargement, but is seen occasionally after prolonged administration of oestrogens.

Tumours are rare. Carcinoma may be of anaplastic spheroidal-cell type or adenocarcinomatous. Prognosis is often poor because of early spread to lymph nodes and to the chest wall. The possibility that genetic factors are involved or that there is an association with gonadal abnormalities or with exposure to x-irradiation remain unproved. Paget's disease of the male breast is very rare. Metastatic carcinoma, e.g. from bronchus, occasionally occurs and the male breast, like that of the female, may be involved in generalised lymphoid neoplasms and the leukaemias.

Further Reading

Blaustein, A. (Ed.) (1977). *Pathology of the Female Genital Tract*, pp. 897). Springer-Verlag, New York, Heidelburg and London.

Fox, H. and Langley, F. A. (1976). *Tumours of the Ovary*, pp. 312. Heinemann Medical, London.

Jordan, J. A. and Singer, A. (Eds.) (1976). *The Cervix*, pp. 529. Saunders, Philadelphia, London and Toronto.

Novak, E. R. and Woodruff, J. D. (1979). *Novak's Gynecologic and Obstetric Pathology*, 8th edn. pp. 975. Saunders, Philadelphia, London and Toronto.

25

Male Reproductive System

Sexually transmitted (venereal) diseases

Many aspects of these infections are dealt with separately, but it seems appropriate to review them here, between the female and male reproductive systems. The diseases usually classed as venereal are six in number and, although their features are diverse, they have two main characteristics in common.

(*a*) The organisms concerned are poorly adapted to other modes of transmission, being incapable of survival outside the body for any length of time or of passing through any intermediate host, and so requiring intimate contact, usually though not necessarily in coitus.

(*b*) They produce at some stage lesions about the genitals from which the infective agent is discharged.

Note that many other diseases, from the common cold upwards, can be transmitted to the sexual partner but are not on that account called venereal. Leishmaniasis, for instance, can be so transmitted and has been misdiagnosed as syphilis; diphtheria during the 1914–18 war was usually acquired by British soldiers in French brothels; infectious mononucleosis in students has a well-known association with kissing. But all these diseases are usually transmitted in other ways.

Syphilis

This was formerly the most important venereal disease but the continued susceptibility of *Treponema pallidum* to penicillin fortunately means that, while it has by no means vanished, it is now relatively infrequent in many countries and with antibiotic therapy hardly ever progresses beyond the secondary stage. Since about 1960 classical major lesions of late syphilis—aortic aneurysms (p. 385), gummas, tabes

dorsalis and general paralysis of the insane (p. 753) have all but vanished from the postmortem room tables of this country. A general account of the lesions and stages has been provided on pp. 217–21. The primary sore or chancre (Fig. 8.22, p. 218) which develops at the portal of entry on the genitalia (or occasionally the mouth) is still seen, and so are the secondary lesions—skin rashes, enlarged lymph nodes and infective mucosal lesions ('snail-track' ulcers): the warty genital lesions, condylomata lata, are especially important because of their high infectivity.

Under conditions of poverty and overcrowding, *Tr. pallidum* can spread, chiefly in the tropics and among children, in the relatively mild and non-venereal form known as *bejel*. (*Yaws* and *pinta* are similar diseases caused by closely related treponemes.) It is probable that a disease known in Scotland by the name of *sivvens* which persisted well into the last century was a form of bejel.

Gonorrhoea

The gonococcus (*Neisseria gonorrhoeae*) has shown enough resilience in the face of antibiotics to have increased again considerably after a period of suppression, and remains the commonest venereal agent, with a particularly high prevalence in some parts of tropical Africa. It has two important differences from most other pyogenic bacteria: (*a*) it survives well within polymorphs, producing a very characteristic appearance (Fig. 7.3, p. 181) and (*b*) it dies rapidly in all but the most favourable environments, being unable to survive even on mucous surfaces except those of the urethra, genital tract and conjunctiva.

Gonorrhoea is essentially a disease of the urethra and periurethral glands in the male, while in the female the glands of the vulva and vagina are also involved, infection being directly by the urethral discharge in coitus, with the sole significant exception of transfer to the infant's conjunctiva during delivery. Stricture of the urethra is the most important local complication. Spread to the bladder is rare: spread to the internal genitalia (prostate, seminal vesicles and epididymis in men, Fallopian tubes in women) is relatively common, and may result in sterility. Blood spread to joints (p. 915) occurs occasionally, and infective endocarditis is a rare complication. In a few African areas of very high incidence, chronic urethral lesions occasionally lead to carcinoma of the urethra.

Abacterial urethritis and Reiter's syndrome

In an increasingly large proportion of untreated cases of acute purulent urethritis of venereal origin (generally of only moderate severity) no bacteria can be found. *Chlamydiae* can be isolated from most but not all of these cases. The presence in these cases of any of the following additional lesions constitutes *Reiter's syndrome*, (*a*) purulent conjunctivitis (sometimes with uveitis), (*b*) mild polyarthritis (p. 921) and (*c*) rare skin lesions, especially of palm and sole. There is an association with HLA antigens (p. 920).

The causative chlamydia belongs to the same group (TRIC) as in trachoma and inclusion keratitis (pp. 223, 796) and there are echoes here of the relationship of syphilis to the Bejel/Pinta group (see above). The characteristic form of trachoma, with severe eye damage, is believed to occur only in conditions favouring repeated heavy reinfection, and it may well be that the apparently wide difference between the relatively mild conjunctivitis of Reiter's syndrome and the major lesions of trachoma reflect only the fact that the former is the result of a single mild infection.

Soft chancre (Chancroid)

The last three of these venereal diseases are usually associated with poor general hygiene and cleanliness and are seen now most often in the tropics, though they appear to be less rare in the U.S.A. than in Europe. Soft chancre is a relatively acute and self-limiting disease caused by Ducrey's bacillus, *Haemophilus ducreyi*. One or more ulcers, often painful, develop about the genitalia: there is active inflammation and considerable necrosis but little of the induration characteristic of the syphilitic chancre (hence *soft* chancre). The inguinal lymph nodes are often involved but there is no wider spread. The organism may be recognised in smears or sections but reliable diagnosis is best made by culture.

Lymphogranuloma inguinale (Lymphogranuloma venereum)

Though sometimes seen in relatively acute and short-lived form, this is usually a chronic disease involving the area of local lymphatic drainage around the inconspicuous primary genital lesion. The organism is another *chlamydia*, this time related to the psittacosis group. The inguinal nodes are usually persistently enlarged and show characteristic microscopic changes in the acute phase (Fig. 18.4, p. 569). There is massive proliferation of macrophages which often have an epithelioid appearance: the resemblance to tuberculosis may be marked, but a distinction may be readily made by the presence of numerous plasma cells and eosinophils in the infiltrate. Necrosis and suppuration to form stellate abscesses are conspicuous at first but are overtaken by fibrosis later, and at this late stage plasma cells may be the only indication of activity.

In the female the inguinal lesions, though rarely absent, are often less conspicuous than in the male, and instead, presumably because of the different lymphatic drainage from primary lesions in the vagina, the main chronic lesions may be peri-vaginal or in adjoining areas. The old name 'esthiomene' refers to granulomatous lesions of the vulva in this disease. Vaginal stricture and vulval elephantiasis may follow and in addition, and often more important, *stricture of the rectum*.

Laboratory diagnosis may be made (*a*) on histology of a biopsy; (*b*) by demonstration of intracytoplasmic inclusion bodies in a smear; (*c*) by culture in hen's eggs; (*d*) by a complement fixation reaction, or (*e*) by the Frei test. This last is a delayed hypersensitivity reaction developing at the site of intradermal injection of the killed causal agent: originally the material used was obtained from an active lesion but a culture of chlamydia is now the preferred source. Like the tuberculin test, a positive Frei test indicates either previous or present infection.

Granuloma venereum (Donovanosis)

This is often confused with lymphogranuloma inguinale (see above). Clinically and epidemiologically they have a good deal in common and the usual names are confusingly similar ('inguinale' and 'venereum' have often been interchanged). The use of the newer name Donovanosis is therefore to be encouraged. The organism *Donovania granulomatosis* is a small Gram−ve bacillus commonly seen intracellularly and difficult to culture.

The primary lesion differs from all other venereal 'primaries' in persisting for a long time, during which it develops into an irregular mass up to 40 mm across, which often ulcerates deeply. Satellite lesions may form in the neighbourhood, commonly in the groin, although the lymph nodes are not especially involved: spread to the uterus and ovaries is not unusual. When not complicated by ulceration and secondary infection, the lesions show active fibroblastic proliferation, plasma cell infiltration

with occasional foci of polymorphs and, most characteristically, scattered large macrophages containing the small donovania. Laboratory diagnosis rests chiefly on demonstration of these organisms either histologically or in smears. The long-term effects of the disease are limited to the consequences of local scarring and destruction (which may be considerable) but include local elephantiasis and (like lymphogranuloma) a small but significant incidence of scar cancers.

Minor infections

There are a number of infections which are much commoner in the sexually promiscuous than in the general population and could well be called venereal diseases, but escape that label probably because of their lesser clinical importance. Chief are colonization of the vagina and urethra with the flagellate protozoon *Trichomonas vaginalis*, cervical infection with the virus of *Herpes simplex* (Type 2 especially, with a possible association with cervical cancer—p. 305), and viral warts (*condylomata acuminata*) of the genitalia, thought to be due to a different strain of papovavirus from that which causes ordinary warts.

Penis, Urethra and Scrotum

Congenital defects

Hypospadias is the commonest lesion of any importance. The urethra fails to reach the end of the penis, opening usually on its inferior surface or even in the perineum.

Congenital valvular obstruction of the urethra by thin membranous flaps in the prostatic portion is a rare but important cause of urinary obstruction in neonates.

Infections

The most important are the venereal lesions already described, with various sores on the penile skin, and urethritis in gonorrhoea and Reiter's syndrome.

Balanitis is an acute non-specific pyogenic

infection of the space between the glans penis and the foreskin, the usual causes being a tight foreskin, poor personal hygiene or both. Its prevention is the sole useful short-term benefit of circumcision, though in the long-term the risk of cancer of the penis is also reduced.

Urethritis other than venereal is rare in the male (the male's relative freedom from urinary infection is roughly balanced by the female's freedom from urethral obstruction) and when it occurs is usually a minor complication of cystitis.

Stricture of the urethra is usually a late complication of gonorrhoea, repeated reinfection, inadequate treatment and persistent suppuration in the periurethral glands of the membranous urethra being major factors: urinary obstruction with all its complications is a result. Traumatic damage to the urethra, by falls astride the perineum or complicating a fracture of the pelvis, usually affect the relatively immobile membranous part, and may also be followed by stricture.

Tumours of the penis

Papillomas are the least rare **benign tumours** occurring on the penis, usually involving the glans or prepuce. The commonest is the *condyloma acuminatum*, attributable (like the common wart) to a papovavirus. They are reddish papillary growths, sessile or pedunculated, and may become very large. A sessile giant papilloma, which has not been proved to be caused by a virus and shows some cellular aberration, is much less common. Condyloma latum, the flat raised infective lesion of secondary syphilis, may also occur on the glans and prepuce, but is not a true tumour. *Pigmented naevi* may also occur on the penis.

Malignant tumours. *Bowen's disease* may affect the epidermis of the penis, and also a rare variety of uncertain status termed *Queyrat's erythroplasia*, consisting of an irregular hyperkeratotic overgrowth with a heavy inflammatory cellular infiltration of the dermis. Both are regarded as premalignant conditions. **Squamous carcinoma** is also uncommon. It usually develops on the glans or prepuce. As elsewhere, it varies in appearance from an indurated, ulcerating nodule to a large cauli-

flower-like growth. It is uncommon in Europe and North America, but the incidence varies greatly and is relatively high in some parts of Africa. It occurs chiefly in the uncircumcised. Among people practising ritual circumcision within a few days of birth it is virtually unknown, but circumcision around puberty, as practised by Moslems, only partly reduces the incidence. Apart from this factor, the marked geographical and socio-economic variations in incidence probably reflect mainly standards of cleanliness. Inspissated smegma beneath the prepuce may be a causal factor. *Malignant*

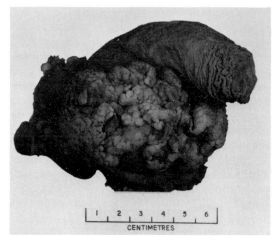

Fig. 25.1 Squamous carcinoma of the scrotum showing ulcerated papillary growth.

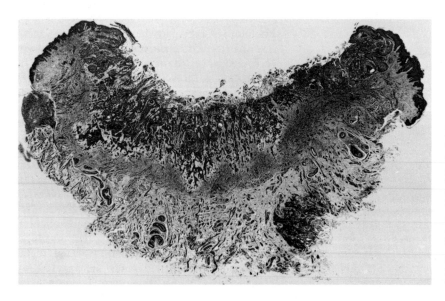

Fig. 25.2 Squamous carcinoma of the scrotum in a foreman in a sheep-dip works who was exposed to powdered arsenic trioxide and failed to wear the prescribed protective clothing. The tumour is large and has ulcerated: it must have been obvious for months.

melanoma may also occur on penile skin and presents the usual features.

Squamous carcinoma of the scrotum

Most of the many varieties of skin tumour can occur in the scrotal skin, but apart from the quasi-venereal condylomata acuminata (see above) are not common. A particular interest attaches, however, to *occupational squamous carcinoma* at this site, for Pott's description of its occurrence in chimney sweeps in 1775 was the first occupational cancer to be recognised and provided the first hint that a cause for any cancers might be found. The localisation appears to depend on the ability of the rugose skin of the scrotum to retain dirt. Tumours were formerly seen regularly not only in chimney sweeps (Fig. 11.5, p. 298) but also in machine-tool operators, gas-retort workers and men handling arsenic (Figs. 25.1 and 25.2). Precautions to prevent soiling of the scrotal skin with carcinogenic chemicals have greatly reduced the incidence of the condition, but it still occurs.

Prostate, vas deferens and seminal vesicles

Apart from infection, the vas and seminal vesicles are seldom the site of pathological changes. In gonorrhoea and urinary-tract infections, the organisms may cause suppuration of the seminal vesicles and spread by way of the vas to involve the epididymis. *Tuberculosis* may extend in either direction along the vas, depending on whether the initial site of infection of the genital tract is by haematogenous involvement of the epididymis, or by extension from the kidney to the urinary bladder and hence to the prostate and vas.

Obstructive lesions of the vas are considered in relation to infertility on p. 1003.

Prostatitis

Acute inflammation of the prostate is usually produced by spread of organisms from the urethra in either gonorrhoea or septic cystitis. In the latter, *Esch. coli* and the various other bacteria which infect the urinary tract are responsible. Gonococcal prostatitis may pass into a chronic state in which the organism persists for a long time in the tubules, the secretion of which remains infective. In septic cystitis, acute inflammation of the prostate is often followed by multiple foci of suppuration, or a large abscess may form and the prostate may be extensively destroyed. Chronic persistent infection may also result.

In *chronic prostatitis* there is a diffuse scarring of the gland, leading to diminution in size. Like prostatic hypertrophy, it may lead to urethral obstruction. A *granulomatous prostatitis*, with eosinophils, epithelioid cells and giant cells, like that in the testis, is a rare lesion of unknown cause. It must be distinguished from tuberculous prostatitis which results from spread from the urinary bladder or epididymis.

Benign nodular hyperplasia of the prostate (BNH)

This is also known as simple prostatic enlargement or hypertrophy. It is not neoplastic, but is comparable to such conditions as nodular goitre and cystic hyperplasia of the breast in which there is irregular overgrowth of many areas of an organ with obvious enlargement but a lack of the progressive proliferation to form a discrete mass that marks the true benign tumour. This condition is so common in minor and usually asymptomatic form in the elderly as to suggest that it is an exaggeration of a normal ageing process. In older men the central periurethral glands of the prostate tend to become hyperplastic and compress those at the periphery, and it is this process that appears to be exaggerated.

There is some evidence that these central glands are stimulated by oestrogens, and the peripheral glands by androgens: hence the normal moderate drop in androgens in old age, by altering the androgen/oestrogen ratio, might account for the prostatic enlargement. So far from being specially liable, however, eunuchs never develop BNH, though this may relate more to the failure of normal development at puberty than to the hormonal status in later decades. Animal experiments give results that are very inconclusive.

The mass of tissue that a surgeon removes by a standard 'prostatectomy' consists almost entirely of the hyperplastic central part of the gland, the remaining peripheral tissue, which is flattened against the capsule, being left behind. The mass so removed varies in size, but is usually between 50 and 100 g and is not often over 200 g, though 800 g has been recorded. The mass usually has its greatest bulk on each side of the urethra (so-called 'lateral lobes') but in many cases there is a localised hyperplasia of the tissue just behind the urethra to form a rounded lump (the so-called 'middle lobe') which projects into the bladder just behind the

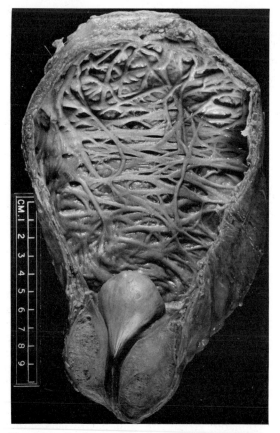

Fig. 25.3 Benign nodular hyperplasia of prostate. The 'middle lobe' is prominent, but the main mass is on each side of the urethra ('lateral lobes'). The compressed peripheral part of the prostate can just be detected as greyer areas in places. Though the urethra is not narrowed, the dilated bladder with prominent muscle bundles provides clear evidence of obstruction. × 0·5.

urethral orifice (Fig. 25.3). The tissue is usually firm, and its cut surface is white and more or less nodular. It may occasionally show areas of inflammation, abscess formation or infarction.

Effects. Though the urethra in its prostatic segment is greatly distorted, it is not usually much constricted, and the effects on bladder function result from a complex disturbance of the bladder sphincter mechanism by the obtruding prostate rather than simply from obstruction. Accordingly the symptoms of 'prostatism' are more diverse than those of simple obstruction, and the severity of the symptoms is not closely related to the size of the prostate. The pathological consequences, however, are very similar to those of obstruction—hypertrophy and dilatation of the bladder, followed in time by dilatation of ureters (hydroureter) and renal pelves (hydronephrosis). If unrelieved, these changes may impair renal function and chronic uraemia may result. *Esch. coli* or mixed bacterial infection of the urinary tract, including pyelonephritis, is often superadded (p. 854), and spread of infection to the prostate may precipitate acute retention of urine.

Patchy infarction of the enlarged prostate is common, and this may also result in acute retention.

Microscopically there is usually increase of both the glandular elements and stroma (Fig. 25.4). The glands are arranged chiefly in acini lined by columnar cells, and there may be small papilliform ingrowths into the lumina (Fig. 25.5). Often some of the acini are dilated and occasionally small cysts are formed: small concentric concretions or *corpora amylacea* are common. The connective tissue stroma usually contains a substantial proportion of smooth muscle fibres. Muscle hyperplasia is most marked in the earlier stages of the process, and muscle may form a very large proportion of smaller lesions. The hyperplastic acini are usually lined by a single epithelial layer, but there may be small foci of more active hyperplasia with the formation of masses of cells, and a cribriform pattern may develop. The relationship between prostatic hyperplasia and carcinoma is considered below.

Carcinoma of the prostate

Even when 'latent' cancer (discussed below) is disregarded, this is now one of the commonest

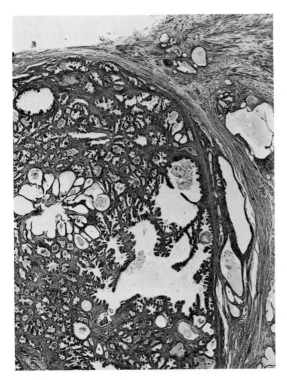

Fig. 25.4 Benign nodular hyperplasia of the prostate. The large adenoma-like nodule that fills most of the field shows predominantly glandular overgrowth, with small cysts. In the less actively growing area at top right, glands are hyperplastic but the stroma, with numerous smooth muscle fibres, is much more prominent. × 10.

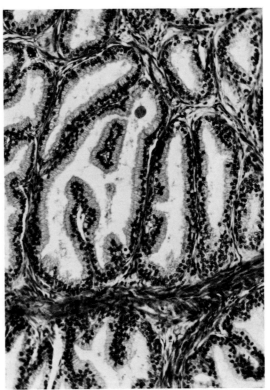

Fig. 25.5 Section of an enlarged prostate, showing hyperplasia of the glandular epithelium. × 130.

cancers of internal organs of males in the developed countries, usually being exceeded only by carcinomas of the bronchus, stomach and large intestine. The increase is probably entirely due to the increased number of old men in the population, for this tumour has its principal incidence later in life than most common cancers. Because so many cases are geriatric patients already suffering from other disabilities, the high frequency tends to be disregarded.

The tumour arises anywhere in the prostate, but often in the periphery of the gland (outside the area chiefly affected by BNH) and especially on the posterior surface. The relation to BNH has been much disputed; some carcinomas certainly arise within hyperplastic lesions, but on the whole the evidence suggests that the prior presence of BNH is

associated with little if any increase in cancer: neither the presence of BNH itself, nor 'prostatectomy' for BNH as usually practised (leaving behind the chief cancer-bearing area), either reduce or increase the incidence of carcinoma.

Histologically the lesion is an *adenocarcinoma* (Fig. 25.6), characteristically with relatively small cells surrounding small lumina ('micro-acinar'). The cells produce some mucin, and acid phosphatase can usually be demonstrated in them histochemically. A rare variant with larger acini, larger cells and a papillary intra-cystic pattern probably arises from periurethral glands.

Mode of spread. The tumour spreads within the gland, and often (but not by any means always) surrounds or invades the prostatic urethra, producing all the effects of prostatic obstruction. Because it often arises peripherally, it soon spreads also outside the gland, and has very often metastasised widely and silently before urinary symptoms appear. Spread may be (*a*) *lymphatic*, initially to pre-sacral,

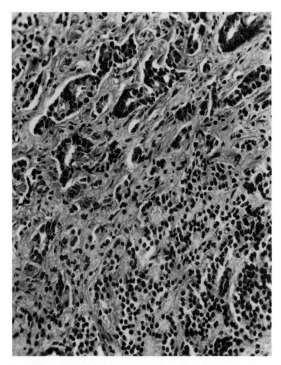

Fig. 25.6 Carcinoma of the prostate. The growth is of scirrhous type, consisting of poorly formed micro-acini (*above*) with transitions to a fine permeation of the tissue by rows of small darkly stained cells (*below*). × 225.

iliac and para-aortic lymph nodes, but often extending widely, (*b*) *retrograde venous*, to the lumbar and sacral spine, by the special mechanism discussed on p. 336 or (*c*) *blood spread* to anywhere in the body, with possibly a predilection for the skeleton. Growth and spread of these metastases is usually slow. A substantial proportion of patients first present with symptoms related to bone secondaries: the bone metastases (whether lumbar or elsewhere) are usually *osteoplastic* (i.e. with bone formation more prominent than destruction), and so appear dense in x-rays.

'Latent' cancer. Microscopic foci of apparent cancer are revealed surprisingly often by careful search of BNH prostatectomy specimens, or of prostates obtained at post-mortem from men dying of unrelated diseases. The changes are very like those in Fig. 25.6—groups of closely packed small acini, invading surrounding prostatic tissue, and sometimes apparently permeating perineural lymphatics within the prostate.

The incidence of latent cancers depends largely on the thoroughness of the search, but some workers have found them in 50 per cent of prostates of men in their 50s, and in practically 100 per cent in those over 75 years old. Their significance is very doubtful. If they were genuine cancers, one would expect a substantial proportion to have spread and proved fatal; in fact the rate of development of frank cancer in those in whom the lesions have been discovered accidentally is little or no more than in the population as a whole (Byar, 1972). There is some recent electron-microscopic evidence that the perineural cells are not in fact within lymphatics. On the whole, one must conclude that these lesions are of more interest than practical importance. However, it should be noted that even substantial nodules of frank cancer (too obvious to call latent) carry a good prognosis if they are removed when tumour is still confined to the gland: the poor prognosis of prostatic cancer relates chiefly to the large proportion which have spread outside the gland when first diagnosed, and the incidental finding of a latent cancer in a surgically removed prostate is not an indication for anti-cancer therapy or more extensive surgery.

Oestrogen effect. About 80 per cent of prostatic cancers show very marked remission of symptoms, often with demonstrable regression of tumour growth, on treatment with oestrogen—a more nearly constant and useful result than in any other form of hormone therapy of cancer, although most cases ultimately relapse. It has been claimed that while oestrogen relieves the pain of bone secondaries, etc., it does not prevent or even postpone the final death of the patient from the disease. However, the usually slow progress of prostatic cancer, the number of these elderly patients who die of intercurrent disease, and the small but definite risk of death due to oestrogen-induced thromboses of various sorts, render the statistical determination of this point very difficult.

Acid phosphatase. Like the normal prostatic epithelium, prostatic cancer cells secrete acid phosphatase. A rise in the enzyme can be detected by sensitive and highly specific radio-immunoassay methods in many cases even in the earliest stages, but a rise to the levels detectable by the usual chemical methods, which are less sensitive, occurs only with spread outside the prostate, and a 'raised acid phosphatase' as ordinarily reported nearly always means that metastases are already present. There is very little evidence on the effect of treatment of the early asymptomatic cases detectable by radioimmunoassay. The rise of *acid* phosphatase must not be confused with the rise of *alkaline* phosphatase that often occurs at the same time, and is a non-specific result of the presence of bone lesions.

Testis and epididymis

It is convenient to consider together these two organs which, along with the tunica vaginalis and lower end of the spermatic cord, make up the testicle (i.e. the contents of the scrotal sac). The epididymis is subject to various infections. Most clinically evident disease of the testis is due to infection, tumour or congenital defect. Many cases of testicular defect are, however, only discovered during the investigation of infertility: the chief conditions concerned are described on p. 1000 *et seq.*

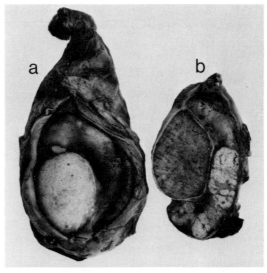

Fig. 25.7 Bilateral epididymal tuberculosis; in **a** the irregularly swollen epididymis is seen above the testis; in **b** caseation in the other epididymis is shown on section. × 0·7.

Inflammatory lesions

Acute epididymitis is usually a complication of gonococcal urethritis or urinary tract infection and results in both instances from spread of the infection along the vas. It may be unilateral or bilateral. In most instances, infection is relatively mild and is eliminated without much tissue destruction, but in some cases suppuration develops, followed by stenosis of epididymal tubules and sometimes sterility. The infection does not usually spread to the testis, but when it does, extensive destruction and scarring may result. The bacteria involved in urinary infections are given on pp. 852–3.

Tuberculous epididymitis. Tuberculosis of the male genital tract is now uncommon in developed countries. Blood spread to the epididymis from a distant lesion, nearly always in the lungs, results in tuberculous epididymitis with extensive caseation and destruction (Fig. 25.7): if untreated it may involve the scrotal wall and chronic discharging sinuses may develop. Extension to the seminal vesicles, prostate and base of the bladder may occur, and the vas may be focally obliterated. The testis is usually either unaffected or only develops lesions late and usually limited to the tissue immediately adjacent to the epididymis.

Acute orchitis. The commonest cause of this is the virus of **mumps**, which reaches the testis during the acute viraemia and in about 30 per cent of adult patients causes an acute orchitis. By contrast, it is a rare complication of mumps before puberty. The lesion is a diffuse orchitis with inflammatory oedema and a mixed inflammatory cellular infiltration. It may be followed by atrophy and fibrosis and, if bilateral, infertility. Occasionally the acute lesion is more severe with necrosis and infiltration of polymorphs. Orchitis may complicate smallpox and other viral diseases, and suppurating orchitis sometimes complicates acute bacterial epididymitis.

Syphilitic orchitis. Apart from the primary sore, the only important site of syphilis in the male genital tract is the testis, which is involved by tertiary lesions more often than any other tissue except the aorta. The commonest lesion is a gumma, which causes a hard, painless enlargement of the testis, and on section (Fig. 25.8) is seen as dull yellowish necrotic patches enclosed in greyish translucent granulation tissue or denser fibrous tissue. A diffuse chronic orchitis without gummatous necrosis but with formation of granulation tissue infiltrated with lymphocytes and plasma cells, and showing the characteristic periarteritis and endarteritis, also occurs in syphilis; it was sometimes seen in inadequately treated patients. The result of both types of lesion is a small fibrosed testis.

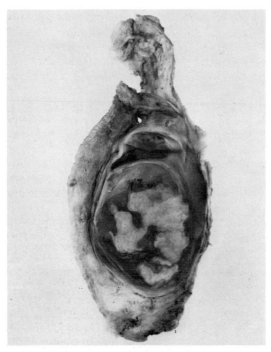

Fig. 25.8 Gumma of the testis, showing a large irregular central pale area of necrosis surrounded by darker granulation tissue. The upper pole of the testis is not yet involved. × 0·8.

Chronic granulomatous orchitis presents clinically as a unilateral painful swelling of the testis, usually in middle-aged men. After a few weeks this subsides leaving an indurated organ with diminished sensitivity to pressure. The lesion is characterised by interstitial inflammatory infiltration of lymphocytes, plasma cells and sometimes eosinophils, and formation of granulation tissue. Destruction of the germinal epithelium is accompanied by infiltration of the tubules with inflammatory cells including many giant cells. Microscopically it bears a superficial resemblance to tuberculosis because the granulomatous reaction within the tubules produces a follicular pattern, but caseation is absent and tubercle bacilli have not been demonstrated. It is regarded by some as a low-grade infection by coliform bacilli; others have suggested, with little supporting evidence, an auto-immune pathogenesis.

Congenital defects

Apart from the germ cell lesions and the intersexes, discussed under infertility, there are two important and relatively common defects.

(*a*) **Undescended testis** (cryptorchidism). Either one or both testes may be arrested at any point along the track marked by the testicular artery and vein from their origin near the kidneys down through the inguinal canal into the scrotum. Minor degrees with temporary arrest are common, the descent into the scrotum being completed by the age of four. Descent after that age is unusual. If the testis is otherwise normal there is still some hope of normal function if it can be brought down surgically into the normal cooler environment of the scrotum. In about half the cases, however, there is a marked deficiency of germ cells, and no hope of fertility in that testis. The risk of tumour in the undescended organ (see later) is sufficient to justify removal of any testis that cannot be brought into the scrotum after the age of ten, particularly if there is a functioning testis on the other side.

(*b*) **Congenital inguinal hernia.** In this, the fetal connection between peritoneal sac and tunica vaginalis remains patent (*persistent processus vaginalis*).

Rare congenital defects include bifid scrotum, absence or duplication of the testis (five have been recorded in one scrotum) and various types of congenital stricture, atresia or absence causing blockage of the outflow pathway via the epididymis and vas.

Miscellaneous lesions

Hydrocele. This is a collection of clear fluid (usually straw-coloured) within the tunica vaginalis. It can usually be distinguished from testicular enlargement by transillumination. Hydrocele may be part of a general oedema, may result from (and conceal) lesions of the testicle such as inflammation or tumour, and occasionally has no identifiable cause. Pus may also collect within the tunica vaginalis, usually following epididymal infection, and bleeding (*haematocele*) may result from trauma or testicular tumours.

Torsion of the testicle occurs usually during sleep and without obvious cause, and produces a twist of the cord at the inguinal ring. The testicle becomes hard and swollen and extremely painful. Obstruction of the vein results in gross congestion and interstitial haemorrhage and, unless it is corrected, infarction occurs.

Cysts are uncommon except in the epididymis. A **spermatocele** is a small cyst containing clear or opalescent, usually colourless, fluid in which spermatozoa can be found; it results from obstruction of an epididymal tubule. Other small cysts may arise from embryological remnants. **Serosal cysts** of the spermatic cord may arise from partial persistence of the processus vaginalis. For **varicocele** see p. 392.

Tumours

Tumours of the testis are not very common: they cause well under 1 per cent of all cancer deaths— a mortality rate less than a tenth of that from ovarian tumours. But their unusual peak incidence in early adult life, during which they are the cause of one-seventh of all cancer deaths in males in Europe and North America, enhances their importance. The spectacular results of early diagnosis and treatment of the commonest form (seminoma) and the many controversies concerning their causation and interrelations also add to their interest. Most are germ cell tumours, including *seminoma* (40%), *teratoma* (32%), combined seminoma and teratoma (14%): *lymphoma* (7%) is the only important exception.

Seminoma

This is the commonest malignant tumour of the testis. It is almost unknown before puberty, becomes important in the 20s, has a peak in the 30s and falls sharply in the 50s: this is, of course, in striking contrast to the rise in incidence of most other tumours after 50 years of age. It presents nearly always as a simple

enlargement of the testicle: local spread is minimal, the scrotal skin and the inguinal lymph nodes being rarely involved. The first metastases are usually noted in the para-aortic lymph nodes at renal level. The lungs are often the next site of major involvement. Tumour can often be seen microscopically in the lymphatics of the spermatic cord (and occasionally in the veins also).

Macroscopically the tumour usually forms a fairly well-defined rounded mass replacing and expanding the whole or part of the testis. It has a characteristic appearance on section, being uniformly pale and opaque, almost white in colour (Fig. 25.10a), often described as potato-like, although much softer than a potato. Histologically (Fig. 25.9), it is composed of relatively large cells with pale cytoplasm and central nuclei, in fairly well-defined solid sheets and strands. (They look sufficiently like spermatogonia to support an origin from those cells.) The tumour generally contains more lymphocytes than is usual in carcinomas, and in about 20 per cent they are very abundant: sometimes sarcoid-like granulomas are also present. An uncommon variant is the *spermatocytic seminoma*, important only because

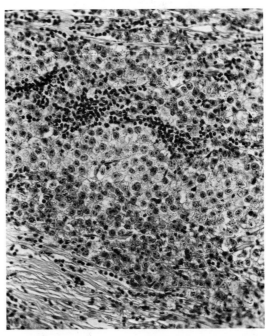

Fig. 25.9 Seminoma of the testis. The tumour consists of large round cells with vesicular nuclei. Note also the lymphocytic infiltration. × 210.

the larger darker-staining tumour cells give it an appearance of increased malignancy, while prognosis is, in fact, better than in the ordinary form.

Seminomas are remarkably radiosensitive, more so probably than any other highly malignant tumour. Provided spread is limited to the usual para-aortic lymph nodes, orchidectomy and radiotherapy cure as many as 90 per cent, and even cases with lung metastases have a good prognosis.

Teratoma

A general account of these tumours has been given on pp. 355–6. In the main, their behaviour in the testis is much like that of seminomas, *clinical* differences between them being relatively unimportant except for the absence of the seminoma's great radiosensitivity, which means that even relatively well-localised teratomas of average differentiation have a 5 year survival rate little better than 50 per cent. In general, they occur in younger patients, with a few cases in early childhood, the peak in the late 20s, and a marked drop in the 40s.

In the details of their appearance, however, differences are marked. The cut surface of a teratoma rarely shows the uniform pattern of a seminoma: areas of haemorrhage and necrosis are usually prominent (Fig. 25.10b), and cysts

are usually seen in the better differentiated examples (Fig. 25.10c). Histologically they fall into several distinct groups, and there is much dispute about their classification and names (the alternative names in brackets are those of the World Health Organisation classification, which will be discussed later).

(*a*) **Differentiated teratoma (Mature teratoma).** These show a variety of well-differentiated tissues (Fig. 25.11), similar to that of the common benign ovarian teratomas, though without assuming the form of a dermoid cyst. These are rare, and mostly occur before puberty. A significant proportion of such tumours metastasise.

(*b*) **Teratoma of intermediate differentiation (immature teratoma).** These consist wholly or chiefly of obviously malignant tissues (Fig. 25.11) which, however, retain sufficient differentiation to be recognisably of several different types. Often there is a mixture of anaplastic and relatively well-differentiated tissues. Areas of extra-embryonic fetal tissues—trophoblast and yolk sac—may be present.

(*c*) **Anaplastic teratoma (embryonal carcinoma).** These consist entirely of poorly differentiated tumour, resembling the more malignant-looking parts of the intermediate forms.

(*d*) **Choriocarcinomatous teratoma (choriocarcinoma).** This consists entirely of malig-

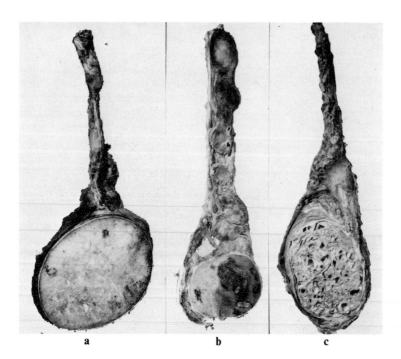

Fig. 25.10 Tumours of the testis. **a** Seminoma: typical solid 'potato' appearance. × 0·7. **b** Poorly differentiated teratoma, mainly solid and haemorrhagic. **c** Unusually well-differentiated teratoma (but still malignant) with multiple cysts. × 0·5.

a   b   c

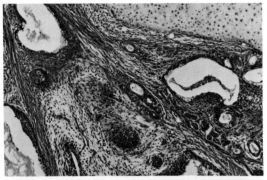
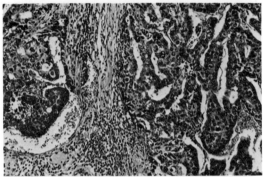
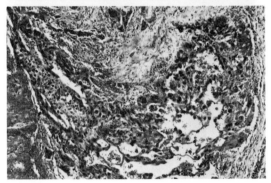

Fig. 25.11 Teratomas of the testis. *Top.* Well differentiated, showing cartilage, fibrous tissue, well-formed acini and epithelial-lined spaces. × 45.
Middle. Poorly differentiated showing papillary adenocarcinoma. × 70.
Bottom. Poorly differentiated anaplastic tumour invading the spermatic cord. × 70.

nant trophoblast (see Fig. 24.32, p. 968). Though it secretes gonadotrophins, it behaves more like a highly malignant teratoma than a uterine choriocarcinoma, lacking the high sensitivity to chemotherapy and the occasional spontaneous regression of the latter tumour.

The classification and the names given above are a simplified version of the United Kingdom Testicular Tumour Panel's recommendations (Collins and Pugh, 1963) which have been generally accepted in this country. The World Health Organisation names (Sobin *et al.*, 1978) reflect an unwillingness to include the anaplastic tumours and choriocarcinoma under the name teratoma, the original definition of the latter requiring the presence of multiple tissue types. In almost every category of malignant tumours there exists a spectrum whose far end is too anaplastic to show any significant resemblance to the original tissue, and the evidence that the anaplastic tumours are simply this end of the teratoma spectrum is so strong that the perpetuation of the old name of embryonal carcinoma seems quite unnecessary. It is less certain that the trophoblastic tumours are simply teratomas overgrown by their most malignant element, but this is the simplest way of accounting for them.

Tumour secretions

Gonadotrophin levels are high in practically all the choriocarcinomatous tumours of the testis, and also in a high proportion of intermediate and anaplastic teratomas. Surprisingly, they are also raised in many cases of seminoma. *Alphafetoprotein* is raised in a large proportion of teratomas, and is ascribed to the presence of yolk-sac elements.

Combined seminoma and teratoma

Elements of seminoma and teratoma are seen together in the testis in 14% of tumours. They may occur as separate nodules or be intermingled. The teratomatous element may be of any degree of malignancy. One can deduce from this that, whatever aetiological factors produce these tumours, some of them at least are capable of producing both types.

Relation to undescended testes

Of various possible aetiological factors, maldescent of the testis has been implicated with certainty. About 5 per cent of testicular tumours arise in undescended testes, some of them in testes that have earlier been successfully brought down to the scrotum by the surgeon (especially if this is done after the age of 10), and there is also a significantly increased risk of tumour in the normally descended testis on the other side. It has recently been shown that premalignant changes can be recognised by biopsy of undescended testes, and this may prove to be a useful procedure in determining whether to remove a maldescended testis. The incidence is higher in abdominal testes than in lesser degrees of maldescent, including cases of testicular feminisation and other major anomalies. As many as 30 per cent of pseudohermaphrodites (p. 1003) with undescended testes have been reported to develop tumours. It is tempting to associate carcinogenesis with injury to spermatogonia, as indicated by the partial loss of these cells seen in many undescended tests, but there is no direct evidence for this at present. Cases of Klinefelter's syndrome (XXY) with similar germinal cell deficiency are not specially liable to testicular tumours unless they also have maldescent.

Other tumours of the testicle

Apart from *lymphoma*, these are all uncommon. One of the most interesting is the rare childhood tumour formerly called an *orchioblastoma*, but now believed to be a *yolk-sac tumour* (Fig. 25.12): it is moderately malignant. Tumours of *Sertoli cells* and of *Leydig cells*, fairly common in dogs, are rare in man. They are often hormonally active, the Sertoli cell tumours usually producing oestrogens. Surprisingly, the Leydig cell tumours produce oestrogens at least as often as androgens. A benign glandular *adenomatoid tumour* is seen occasionally in the epididymis.

   Lymphoma. Malignant lymphoma sometimes presents as a testicular tumour, and may at least appear to remain localised there for some time. It occurs chiefly in the elderly, and above

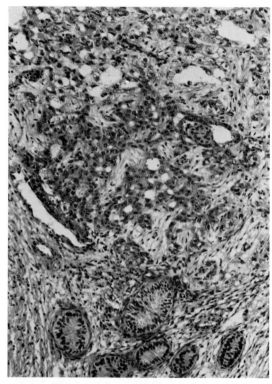

Fig. 25.12 Yolk-sac tumour of the testis of an infant. Surviving non-neoplastic testicular tubules lined by Sertoli cells are seen below. The papillary structure of the tumour (*above*) is not prominent here, but the uniform cell type is well seen. × 11·5.

the age of 65 becomes the commonest tumour of the testis. Histologically the tumours are mostly of highly malignant, diffuse type, and the prognosis is even poorer than for teratomas.

Infertility in the male

At least 10 per cent of married couples are infertile. Though the figures are not very reliable, the responsible partner is generally said to be male or female in roughly equal numbers, with a small group in which both partners have partial defects which combine to prevent conception. This suggests that about 5 per cent of males and of females are infertile. Some cases are psychological, endocrine or drug-induced, but most are due to lesions of the genital tract, chiefly in the testis and fallopian tubes.

   Sperm count. Laboratory examination of a specimen of semen is necessary in most cases of suspected male infertility; it should be delivered to the laboratory within 3 hours. The normal volume is 1 ml or more, averaging 4 ml. The normal sperm count is over 50 million per ml (5×10^9/litre) and is usually well over 100 million per ml. At least 60 per cent, and usually 80 per cent, of the spermatozoa should be motile and of normal morphology. While it is obvious that absence of sperm (*azoospermia*) indicates infertility (provided that it is not temporary—see below) it is remarkable that counts below 50 million per ml (*oligospermia*) are associated with greatly reduced fertility. With counts below 10 million, fertility is rare and below 1 million it is almost unknown.

Testicular biopsy is often necessary. Practical points are the need for a skin incision large enough to allow inspection of the testis and accurate measurement of its size, a biopsy not too small and the use of an acid fixative such as Bouin's or Davidson's.

Testicular lesions

Scarring

Gross destruction of testicular tissue by granulomatous orchitis, severe mumps orchitis, gumma or torsion, is, of course, followed by extensive scarring and atrophy and, if the lesion is bilateral, azoospermia. None of these is common however, especially in bilateral form, and the fibrosis found in cases of sterility generally consists of multiple scattered small scars, each involving only a few tubules, in an otherwise normal testis. The cause is usually unknown, but is presumably some mild unrecognised infection in childhood. The production of azoospermia or severe oligospermia by such inconspicuous scarring may seem surprising but it must be remembered that each of the 600 tubules in the testis is nearly a metre long and almost without anastomoses. Within each of the dozen or so sectors, the tubules are very intricately coiled together. With numerous small scars scattered through the testis, the chance of any one tubule having any substantial length free from obstruction is therefore small. The lesion is thus an intra-testicular obstruction.

Defective spermatogenesis

The extraordinary activity of the normal spermatogenic epithelium is very readily interfered with, and a fall in sperm count or even azoospermia follows: however, in most such cases depression of spermatogenesis is usually reversible. Possible causes of partial or complete arrest of spermatogenesis are very numerous: the following are the more important.

(*a*) **General causes.** Fever, malnutrition, many poisons, uraemia or indeed almost any severe illness will depress spermatogenesis.

(*b*) **More specific damage** is caused by cadmium, local x-rays and anti-mitotic drugs. In high dosage these cause destruction of the stem cells (the spermatogonia) and so permanent damage: in lesser doses, x-rays at least can cause germ cell mutations, though the evidence for this is based largely on animal work.

(*c*) **Temperature.** Spermatogenesis ceases at normal body temperature. Hot baths and tight pants depress spermatogenesis only enough to matter in men with low sperm counts already, but the vascular abnormality called *varicocele* (p. 392) can certainly produce azoospermia, and of all causes of impaired spermatogenesis this is the one in which surgical intervention is most likely to cure sterility.

(*d*) **Endocrine disorders.** In the embryo and in the adult, the tubules depend on androgens derived locally from the Leydig cells. These in turn depend on the pituitary. In the adult, LH is the main stimulus to Leydig cell activity. Both Leydig cell androgens and FSH are necessary for tubule activity. Spermatogenesis therefore ceases in most forms of pituitary failure. Most often this is caused by oestrogen excess, which suppresses LH and FSH. Oestrogen given in the treatment of prostatic cancer is an obvious example, but *cirrhosis of the liver* provides a more striking one, the rise in endogenous oestrogen seen in many relatively moderate cases of liver damage (p. 694) having a very marked effect on the testis. Leydig cells vanish, spermatogenesis ceases (spermatogonia, however, remain, and can resume activity), and there is, in addition, deposition of hyaline material round the tubules between epithelium and basement membrane, which eventually causes irreversible damage.

Germ cell defects

Absence or near-absence of germ cells is usually congenital. The effect is to produce tubular atrophy without loss of Leydig cells, and a rise of pituitary FSH presumably due to the absence of the feed-back hormone *inhibin* (not yet positively identified) which is apparently produced by active spermatogenic epithelium, and normally suppresses FSH (but not LH). Pituitary activity sometimes produces gynaecomastia. This combination was identified by

Klinefelter in 1943. His name, however, is generally used only for the first of the two main forms (below) of germ-cell defect.

(1) Klinefelter's syndrome (of XXY type). This, one of the commonest of chromosomal disorders, is the result of the presence of a Y chromosome (which ensures the formation of a testis and masculine development generally) together with a second X, which prevents normal development of the testis. The usual abnormal pattern is thus XXY, but variants such as mosaics are not rare and even an apparent pure XX (probably with some part of the Y translocated to another chromosome) may be found. A moderate increase in frequency of mental defect is the only important non-genital consequence. A eunuchoid body-build is frequent: FSH levels are high and androgens are usually moderately reduced. There may be gynaecomastia, and carcinoma of the breast is commoner than in normal males. The rare cases with three or four X chromosomes (XXXY, etc.) have a high incidence of congenital defects.

The testis in these cases is very small (5 g or less). The bulk appears to be made up of irregular masses of Leydig cells: among them are occasional tubules lined by Sertoli cells only (similar to those seen in the next group) but most of the recognisable tubules are inconspicuous and hyalinised ('ghost' tubules). In a few cases germ cells persist in an occasional tubule, and localised spermatogenesis occurs. A single well-authenticated case of a fertile man with XXY presumably represents an extreme example of this.

Diagnosis in these cases is made easy by the sex chromatin test; this is the only condition of any frequency in which it is positive in males (Figs. 25.13 and 25.14). Using this test, it has been shown that 1 in 200 male births are XXY.

The defect in the testis is not strictly congenital: the testes develop normally until about the time of birth; germ cells then disappear, but tubules remain normal until puberty, when active destruction takes place. The mechanism of this is quite unknown. XXY individuals have been found in all mammals in which such chromosomal abnormalities have been sought, and the effects are much the same in all of them.

(2) Germ-cell aplasia (non-chromosomal). (Also called *chromatin-negative Klinefelter's* or

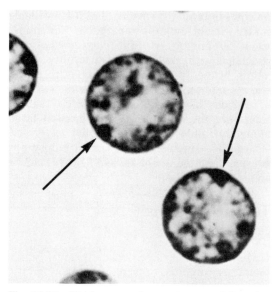

Fig. 25.13 Nuclear sex chromatin, resembling that of normal females, in the Leydig cells of a case of XXY Klinefelter's syndrome. Testicular biopsy. × 1500.

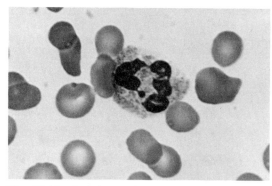

Fig. 25.14 A polymorphonuclear leukocyte showing the typical female sex-chromatin drumstick. × 1500.

the *del Castillo syndrome*.) Here there is absence or near-absence of the germ cells in the testis, of unknown cause but presumed to be congenital. The effects are similar to those of XXY, but are (except for the infertility, which is nearly invariable) less pronounced. There is no associated mental defect and eunuchoidism is less common. The testes are not so small, and the histology is less grossly altered: the tubules are well preserved but reduced in size, and are lined entirely by tall, pale-staining Sertoli cells with no germ cells. Between the tubules there is an apparent excess of Leydig cells. Many cases are partial, with some fertile tubules, producing oligospermia rather than azoospermia.

Leydig cells in testicular atrophy

The normal adult has about 0·9 ml of Leydig cells in each testis, and this quantity remains remarkably constant so long as the normal pituitary stimulus is present. If the tubules in both testes are atrophic, the proportion of the testis occupied by Leydig cells becomes proportionately increased (it may be over 50 per cent in an XXY testis) and it is easy to mistake this for hyperplasia. (True Leydig cell hyperplasia is very rare in man.) When only one testis is atrophic, the Leydig cells appear to be readjusted between the two testes, and little apparent hyperplasia occurs on the affected side.

It is worth remembering that apparent *excess* of Leydig cells in a biopsy in man is nearly always an illusion, produced by tubular atrophy, while *deficiency* is nearly always a sign of pituitary depression.

Causes of infertility outside the testis

These are numerous and sometimes treatable, but account for fewer cases than testicular lesions. They include the following.

(*a*) **Impotence** (i.e. inability to achieve orgasm). This is usually psychological, but may be drug-induced, endocrine (androgen failure, excess of oestrogen or prolactin), neural (spinal cord lesions especially) or vascular. Impotence due to vascular lesions occurs in the Leriche syndrome (p. 366). Recently, over half of one series of renal transplant patients were found to become impotent after a *second* graft, and this turned out to be due to use of both internal iliac arteries to supply the grafts.

(*b*) **Abnormalities which interfere with coitus.** These include penile deformities and extreme obesity.

(*c*) **Obstruction of the outflow pathway.** Part of the **vas** may be congenitally absent, or it may be interrupted by trauma or during operations, usually for hernia. The operation of vasectomy must be included here: its occasional failures illustrate the remarkable ability of some tubular structures to re-establish continuity spontaneously after division. Obstruction of the tubules of the **epididymis** may follow any of the epididymal infections described above. Some

lesions of the proximal **urethra**, for example stricture or the trauma of prostatectomy, may result in discharge of the semen into the bladder. This is the usual cause of *aspermia* (total absence of ejaculate). In bilateral obstructions of the vas or epididymis or tubular atrophy, the secretions of the seminal vesicles and prostate usually produce an ejaculate even though there is azoospermia.

Surprisingly enough, obstructive lesions have very little effect on the testis itself, no matter how long the duration. The finding of azoospermia with a normal testicular biopsy usually means obstruction, which can sometimes be corrected. Spermatozoa continue to be produced, and collect in the tubules of the epididymis, in time giving rise to 'sperm granulomas' with clumps of sperm heads and macrophages full of brown pigment.

Intersexes

Intersexes are individuals who present some degree of intermingling of the characters of both sexes. Apart from the psychological intersexes, homosexuality and transvestism, with which we are not concerned, the principal varieties are the following.

(*a*) **Chromosomal intersexes.** The commonest varieties are XXY Klinefelter's syndrome, considered above, and XO Turner's syndrome (p. 970). In both of these, and in contrast to the next group, the general anatomy is far less intersexual than the chromosomal picture.

(*b*) **Hermaphroditism.** This term is properly confined to the rare individuals who possess both testis and ovary: there may be an ovary on one side and a testis on the other, or various mixtures of the two. Intermediate forms of sexual development are a natural consequence. Most often the external genitalia are predominantly male at birth and internal genitalia correspond to the gonad nearest to them. Breast development or other signs of feminisation appear at puberty. In most cases the cause is obscure, but some are true *mosaics*—mixtures of XY and XX cells. There is strong evidence that this can result from double fertilisation, and can be regarded almost as an extreme case of Siamese twinning, with total fusion at the cellular level. These XX/XY mosaics should not be confused with XX/XY *blood cell chimeras*, in which exchange of blood occurs, and immunological tolerance develops, between dizygotic twins *in utero*: chimerism is limited to the haemopoietic tissue and cells of the blood and has no effect on sexual development (cf. chimeric cattle, p. 132).

(*c*) **Adrenal virilism** (p. 1042). In this, excessive androgenic hormone synthesis leads to virilisation of the external genitalia in females: the condition is of special importance because, if recognised early, it can often be treated effectively.

(*d*) **Male pseudohermaphroditism.** In this, male external genitalia are imperfectly developed, presumably as a result of temporary failure of testosterone output from the testis *in utero*. In its lesser degrees it fades away into such minor conditions as bifid scrotum and hypospadias.

A child of doubtful sex at birth is usually a case of adrenal virilism or a male pseudohermaphrodite: the sex chromatin test distinguishes reliably between them.

(*e*) **Testicular feminisation** is an interesting though rare form of intersex in which there is a metabolic defect of the target cells of the male sex hormones which renders them insensitive to testosterone. The effect is one of externally complete feminisation, though the patients are XY and possess (undescended) testes. The defect is determined by a gene on the X chromosome, heterozygous females acting as asymptomatic carriers. Offspring of these carriers have equal chances of belonging to any one of the four classes of normal males, normal females, carrier (but otherwise normal) females and affected sterile XY females.

References and Further Reading

Byar, D. P. (1972). Survival of patients with incidentally found microscopic cancer of the prostate: results of a clinical trial of conservative treatment. *Journal of Urology* **108**, 908–13.

Collins, D. H. and Pugh, R. C. B. (1964). Classification and frequency of testicular tumours. In *Pathology of Testicular Tumours*, pp. 1–11. Churchill-Livingstone, Edinburgh and London.

Pugh, R. C. B. (Ed.) (1976). *Pathology of the Testis*, pp. 487. Blackwell Scientific, Oxford and London.

Sobin, L. H., Thomas, L. B., Percy, Constance and Henson, D. E. (Eds.) (1978). *A Coded Compendium of the International Histological Classification of Tumours*, pp. 116. World Health Organisation, Geneva.

26

The Endocrine System

The clinical features of most endocrine disorders are attributable to the secretion of too much or too little hormone. Such disturbances can arise in various ways. For example, diminished secretion of thyroid hormone can result from chronic inflammatory destruction of the thyroid, usually due to auto-immune thyroiditis; it can result also from any lesion of the pituitary which interferes with the production and secretion of thyrotrophic hormone (TSH). The secretion of TSH is, in turn, influenced by the secretion of a TSH-releasing hormone (and possibly also by a release-inhibiting hormone) by the hypothalamus. Accordingly, hypothalamic or pituitary-stalk lesions can interfere with thyroid function. This possibility of lesions in various sites having a similar endocrine effect applies also to the functioning of the adrenals and the gonads, which, like the thyroid, are controlled largely by pituitary trophic hormones.

It must also be emphasised that complex functional interrelationships exist between the endocrine glands and between the effects of various hormones. Thus the effects of insulin on sugar metabolism are very largely antagonistic to those of growth hormone, thyroid hormone, glucocorticoids and catecholamines, and the control of glucose metabolism represents a balance between these various factors. Indeed, the normal endocrine status depends on the balanced functioning of the various endocrine glands with their feed-back mechanisms and complex interrelationships.

The relationships between the brain and pituitary are particularly important. The neurohypophysis acts as a store of hormones produced in the basal nuclei, while the release of the hormones synthesised in the adenohypophysis is influenced, as mentioned above, by low molecular weight polypeptide hormones secreted by the hypothalamus.

The pituitary has long been regarded as the 'conductor of the endocrine orchestra': it might now be added that the hypothalamus calls the tune.

The successful production of antibodies to many hormones in experimental animals has allowed the application of two types of immunological technique which are now making major contributions to endocrinology. The first is the use of antibodies to detect the presence of hormones in individual cells, e.g. growth hormone in pituitary cells, by means of fluorescent labels or peroxidase (p. 111 and Fig. 26.1). Some of these immunocytological techniques are not yet completely reliable nor suitable for routine use. For example, there is some

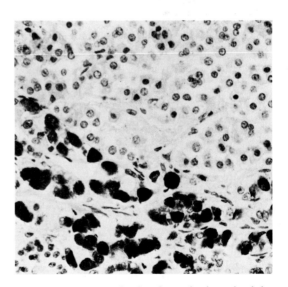

Fig. 26.1 Section of adenohypophysis stained by the immunoperoxidase method, using antibody to growth hormone. The cytoplasm of cells containing growth hormone is stained black. The field includes the edge of a chromophobe adenoma (*above*), the cells of which are devoid of growth hormone (Professor R. B. Goudie.)

overlap between gonadotrophins and cortico-trophin; demonstration of prolactin and growth hormone is, however, fairly reliable. Secondly, it is now possible to assay the low concentrations of many hormones in plasma, urine, etc., by radio-immunoassay techniques: this is of great value both in diagnosis and in endocrinological research. Problems do, how-ever, arise over breakdown products of hor-mones, which may be biologically inactive and yet retain some of the antigenicity of the intact hormone.

Most of the endocrine glands have consider-able functional reserve, and so can often con-tinue to function apparently normally when partially destroyed by disease. They also have a high capacity for hyperplasia, and can enlarge to meet an increased work load or to overcome some functional defect. For example indivi-duals who are deficient in iodine (an essential component of thyroid hormone) develop thy-roid hyperplasia, sometimes visible as enlarge-ment (goitre), and by increasing the rate of iodine turnover the hyperplastic gland

may be able to maintain relatively normal function.

In general, endocrine glands are not subject to bacterial infections, an exception being tuberculosis and some other chronic infections of the adrenals. Only a few viral infections are known, e.g. involvement of the gonads, pan-creas, and occasionally the thyroid, in mumps. An important group of endocrine disorders re-sults from the organ-specific auto-immune dis-eases, which cause destructive inflammation of the thyroid, adrenal and parathyroid glands, and rarely of the endocrine components of the gonads. The common form of hyperthyroidism (Graves' disease) is also of auto-immune nature.

Lastly, all the endocrine glands are subject to neoplasia, the frequency varying for the differ-ent glands and in different communities. Endocrine tumours are of special importance because they frequently secrete hormones in uncontrolled fashion: they may also, by com-pressing or invading the surrounding glandular tissue, lead to hypofunction.

The Pituitary

The adenohypophysis (anterior lobe)

Introduction

Despite its importance, the pituitary is a re-latively tiny organ which weighs about 500 to 900 mg in the male and often rather more in the female. There is a significant increase in size during pregnancy. The adenohypophysis de-velops from an upgrowth from the roof of the embryonic oral cavity which becomes contigu-ous with a downgrowth from the developing brain destined to become the neurohypophysis. The blood supply to the adenohypophysis is peculiar in that, except for the tissue im-mediately beneath the capsule, there is no direct arterial supply, blood passing from the capillaries in the hypothalamus into venous portal channels which traverse the stalk and break up into the sinusoids of the adenohy-pophysis. This arrangement allows hormonal factors secreted by the hypothalamus to influ-ence adenohypophyseal function (see below): it

also renders the adenohypophysis liable to isch-aemic injury, e.g. during the circulatory col-lapse of shock, and permits almost complete destruction of the gland by deliberate surgical interruption of the stalk.

The adenohypophyseal hormones include (1) *growth hormone* (GH) or *somatotrophin*, a glob-ular protein of molecular weight 44 000, which has been isolated in crystalline form; (2) *lac-togenic hormone*, or *prolactin*, also a globular protein; (3) *gonadotrophic hormones* (FSH and LH), which are glycoproteins; (4) *thyroid stim-ulating hormone* (TSH), also a glycoprotein; (5) *corticotrophin* (ACTH), a polypeptide; and (6) *melanin-stimulating hormone* (MSH), also a polypeptide.

The hormone-secreting cells

The anterior pituitary hormones listed above are synthesised and secreted by cells of the adenohypophysis. Although different types of cell can be distinguished by their morphological and staining properties, it has proved difficult to determine which cell secretes which hormone(s). Initially, the cells were classified by the presence or absence of basophilic or acidophilic (eosinophilic) cytoplasmic granules into basophil (13 per cent), acidophil (37 per cent) and chromophobe cells (50 per cent), the last containing neither type of granule. Subsequently, it was shown by Pearse's tri-PAS stain that all basophils, some acidophils and some chromophobes contain PAS-positive granules. Some cells were shown to contain large numbers of these; others were sparsely granular, and were termed *gamma cells*, acidophils being called *alpha cells* and basophils subdivided into *beta* and *delta cells* on the basis of staining differences. The relationships of eosinophil and basophil cell adenomas with acromegaly (or gigantism) and Cushing's syndrome respectively suggested acidophil cells as the source of growth hormone and basophils as the source of ACTH. Chromophobe adenomas were usually unaccompanied by evidence of excessive hormone secretion, and accordingly the chromophobe cells were regarded as inactive, possibly precursor cells. These early observations have been largely confirmed, but it has been shown by immunological techniques that heavy granulation indicates storage of hormones, while cells that are actively secreting are sparsely granulated. It has been demonstrated, for example, that some 'chromophobe' cells secrete both ACTH and MSH.

Electron-microscopy has contributed to the recognition of cell function. For example, secretory granules of growth hormone are large, spherical, and fairly regular (300–400 nm in diameter); granules of prolactin are also large and spherical, but vary more in size, and TSH granules are much smaller.

The use of immunofluorescence techniques to detect intracellular hormones has shown that: (1) growth hormone is synthesised by acidophil cells lying mainly in the lateral parts of the gland; (2) prolactin is also produced by acidophil cells, but they are different from the GH cells; (3) LH is produced by singly-scattered triangular basophil cells, while the source of FSH has not yet been firmly settled owing to the difficulty in developing specific antibody to FSH; (4) TSH is produced by tall basophil cells lying mainly centrally in the adenohypophysis; (5) ACTH is produced by basophil cells which are also situated centrally in the gland and adjacent to the neurohypophysis—it is likely that the same cells also secrete MSH; and (6) approximately 25 per cent of adenohypophyseal cells contain no detectable hormone, although secretion granules are demonstrable by electron-microscopy.

Control of adenohypophyseal function

Secretion of each of the adenohypophyseal trophic hormones—FSH, LH, TSH and ACTH—is controlled by a negative feed-back system in which the hormone secreted by the target organ inhibits secretion of the trophic hormone. For example, TSH is suppressed by a high level of thyroid hormone in the plasma. This control appears to work partly by the direct effect of thyroid hormone, cortisol, etc., on the appropriate cells in the adenohypophysis, but it is also partly under the control of the hypothalamus, which releases from the median eminence oligopeptide hormones which are carried by the hypophyseal portal vascular system to the sinusoids in the adenohypophysis and there influence the secretion of the trophic hormones. Releasing-hormones for TSH (TRH), LH and FSH (LH/FSH–RH) and GH (GRH) have been analysed and synthesised and TRH and LH/FSH–RH are already being used in clinical diagnosis. ACTH-releasing factor (CRF) has not been characterised and may be of several types. Release-inhibiting factors have also been detected, and growth-hormone release-inhibiting hormone (GHRIH or somatostatin) has been shown to be a tetradecapeptide, produced mainly, but perhaps not only, in the hypothalamus. Unlike the releasing hormones, somatostatin has been shown not only to affect pituitary function, but also to inhibit secretion of insulin and glucagon. It also inhibits secretion of prolactin, but this is not surprising in view of the close association of somatotrophin and prolactin secretion. Some workers, however, claim that there is a specific prolactin release-inhibiting hormone (PRIH).

In view of the number of adenohypophyseal hormones and the complexity of their control and interrelationships, it is not surprising that disorders of the pituitary have complex and varied results. Their complexity is further increased by the situation of the organ in the bony sella, for an adenoma of one cell type may secrete excess hormone and yet lead to compression and destruction of the normal pituitary tissue, with consequent deficiency of the other hormones. Moreover, a lesion in or above the sella may produce various effects on the complex functions of both the pituitary and the hypothalamus.

The adenohypophyseal hormones

Growth hormone (GH) is essential, together with thyroid hormone and insulin, for a normal rate of growth. Its somatotrophic effect has been demonstrated by replacement therapy in dwarf hypophysectomised animals. It may be assayed biologically in hypophysectomised rats by measuring its stimulating effect on the incorporation of [^{35}S]-sulphate into chondroitin sulphate or its effect on the thickness of the epiphyseal plates. One of the effects of GH is to stimulate protein synthesis. It exerts its hormonal effects by production of an intermediate factor, **somatomedin**. The human pituitary gland is a surprisingly rich source from which GH has been purified: on injection into patients with hypopituitarism, in doses of up to 10 mg daily, it reverses the negative nitrogen balance, and stimulates growth in hypopituitary dwarfs. Although it has a diabetogenic effect, this is not readily demonstrated in man except in hypophysectomised diabetic patients, in whom it greatly aggravates the diabetes.

Radio-immunoassay of human GH correlates moderately well with bio-assay and has the advantage of much greater sensitivity. By its use, the plasma level in adults is found to be usually below 3 μg/litre. Rapid rise of plasma GH follows exercise, ingestion of amino acids or injection of insulin, and these stimuli are enhanced by oestrogens. Its secretion is also stimulated by the effect of β-adrenergic receptor blockade on the hypothalamus, and by L-dopa.

Prolactin (lactogenic hormone) is concerned in the initiation and maintenance of lactation in breast tissue primed by oestrogen, progesterone, corticosteroids and insulin. It can be assayed by its lactogenic effect on explants of mammary tissue from pregnant mice, but a more rapid, accurate and sensitive method has been provided by radio-immunoassay. The plasma levels of prolactin in normal men and women are not very different, and yet its only known role is in lactation. In animals, however, it plays a part in growth, metamorphosis, gonadal function, parental care and electrolyte balance. Pituitary enlargement during pregnancy is attributable mainly to an increase in prolactin-producing cells in the adenohypophysis: the plasma prolactin level rises progressively but its lactogenic action is held in check by the high levels of oestrogen and progesterone which persist until after delivery. Mammary stimulation is followed by a sharp rise in plasma prolactin, the high levels of which inhibit ovulation and thus explain the usual temporary state of sterility during lactation. Human TSH-releasing hormone also appears to release prolactin. The hormone-dependence of some mammary tumours may involve prolactin.

Gonadotrophic hormones. Maturation and function of the gonads in both males and females is dependent on the two adenohypophyseal gonadotrophic hormones, **follicle-stimulating hormone (FSH)** and **luteinising** or **interstitial cell stimulating hormone (LH** or **ICSH)**. FSH is essential for the growth of the Graafian follicle and for ovulation, and LH for luteinisation of the follicle following ovulation. Under the influence of these hormones the Graafian follicle secretes oestrogen, which induces endometrial proliferation, and the corpus luteum secretes progesterone, which inhibits further ovulation and induces endometrial secretory change.

In males, FSH stimulates spermatogenesis and LH stimulates the Leydig cells to secrete testosterone.

Rare cases of infertility in both men and women result from gonadotrophin deficiencies. Excessive production of LH may also give rise to the syndrome of polycystic ovaries and infertility.

Thyrotrophic hormone (TSH) stimulates thyroid epithelium by activating adenyl cyclase and thus increasing intracellular cAMP (p. 144). It induces enlargement and proliferation of thyroid epithelium and increases secretion of thyroid hormone into the blood. Thyroxine exerts a negative feed-back on TSH secretion, partly directly and partly via the hypothalamus. Plasma TSH can now be determined by radio-immunoassay: it is undetectable in about 10 per cent of normal subjects, is always elevated in patients with untreated primary hypothyroidism, and is suppressed by administration of thyroxine. As explained later, the form of hyperthyroidism known as Graves' disease is due to an abnormal thyroid stimulator, and TSH secretion is suppressed by the high levels of thyroid hormone.

Adrenocorticotrophic hormone (ACTH) is essential for the secretion of glucocorticoid steroid hormones, e.g. cortisol and cortisone. These steroids operate a negative feed-back effect, partly directly on the adenohypophysis and partly via the hypothalamus, which secretes an ACTH-releasing factor (CRF) and possibly also a release-inhibiting factor. ACTH stimulates adrenocortical cells by activating adenyl cyclase. Hypophysectomy or administration of cortisol results in adrenocortical atrophy.

Reliable radio-immunoassay techniques have now been reported for ACTH and it has been shown that the plasma levels, usually below 50 μg/litre in normal adults, have a circadian rhythm, and that the hormone is secreted in short 'pulses'. The level rises in individuals exposed to stress and may exceed 500 μg/litre: high levels are also to be expected, and are observed, in Addison's disease (primary adrenocortical insufficiency) and in patients with 'inappropriate' secretion of ACTH, e.g. by a bronchial carcinoma.

ACTH consists of 39 amino-acid residues of which only the first 24 are necessary for its hormonal effect. It has been synthesised and can be administered repeatedly without development of a refractory state. Its administration causes adrenocortical hyperplasia and increased excretion of glucocorticoid hormones, resulting in gluconeogenesis, atrophy of the thymus and lymph nodes and lymphopenia. The secretion of the adrenal cortical hormone most active in controlling sodium and potassium—aldosterone—does not appear to be under anterior pituitary control; the factors controlling its release are not fully understood, but one of them is renin, produced by the granular cells of the juxta-glomerular apparatus (p. 258).

The importance of ACTH has been emphasised by the therapeutic effects of glucocorticoid hormones on various diseases, including some attributable to hypersensitivity reactions, and others of unknown aetiology.

Melanin stimulating hormone (MSH) is a polypeptide with a structure similar to part of the ACTH molecule, and indeed there is some doubt as to whether it is a separate hormone in man, or simply a fragment of ACTH. Some workers believe that it exists in two forms, α and β. Most antibodies to human ACTH prepared in animals react also with human MSH, but production of more specific antibodies said to distinguish between the two hormones has now been reported. It is probable, however, that ACTH and MSH are secreted by the same pituitary cells, and their relationship is still obscure.

When the adrenals are destroyed by disease, the output of MSH in the urine is increased, because increased pituitary secretion results from lack of inhibition by adrenal hormones. This is probably responsible for the increased pigmentation in Addison's disease (q.v.), and chloasma of pregnancy is probably also due to increase in MSH secretion.

Adenohypophyseal hyperfunction

Acromegaly and gigantism

These conditions are both due to prolonged and excessive secretion of growth hormone, usually by a pituitary adenoma (Fig. 26.2) but occasionally associated with an increase of GH-secreting cells without a tumour. The adenoma is most commonly of acidophil-cell type but sometimes chromophobe: electron-microscopy shows the characteristic growth hormone

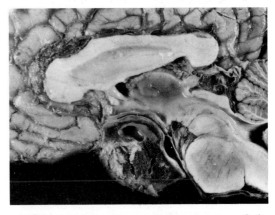

Fig. 26.2 A large chromophobe adenoma of the pituitary which had compressed the optic chiasma. The tumour is haemorrhagic and shows cystic change.

(GH) secretory granules (p. 1007), and immunohistology demonstrates the presence of GH in the tumour cells.

In both conditions there is excessive growth of bone and soft tissues and enlargement of most of the internal organs, e.g. liver, kidneys, heart, thyroid and adrenals. Initially, excessive growth hormone secretion is accompanied by normal or occasionally increased secretion of the other adenohypophyseal hormones. The reason for this latter is not fully understood; there may be great muscularity and abnormal strength, sexual precocity in children and increased libido in adults. Glucose tolerance is diminished and in 10 per cent of cases there is frank diabetes mellitus. The blood pressure is often raised and the heart hypertrophied. As the tumour enlarges, however, it compresses and destroys the surrounding adenohypophysis and lack of the hormones other than GH gradually supervenes. Muscle wasting, weakness and asthenia develop and glucose tolerance increases. In some instances the tumour undergoes infarction, cystic change and fibrosis, ceases to secrete excess of GH, and changes in bone and elsewhere then become inactive. At necropsy, it may appear as a thin-walled cyst lined by scanty acidophil cells. The enlarging tumour may also compress the inner parts of the optic nerves, resulting in bitemporal hemianopia sometimes progressing to blindness. The hypothalamus may also be compressed with various consequences, sometimes including diabetes insipidus.

Acromegaly means enlargement of the extremities. It results when the GH-secreting tumour develops after fusion of the epiphyses so that the bones cannot elongate but can grow thicker by periosteal ossification. The hands and feet are increased in size, especially in width. The increase is at first mainly in the soft tissues though thickening of bone occurs later. The face is enlarged, especially the nose, which is widened, and the lower jaw is lengthened and its angle widened (Fig. 26.3) so that the teeth project beyond those of the upper jaw. The lips become thickened and there is enlargement of the tongue. The skin is thickened and somewhat warty and the hair is coarse and wiry. In the skeleton generally there is often an increase of bony prominences and there may be roughening of the surface of the bones. Irregular bone growth distorts the joint surfaces and

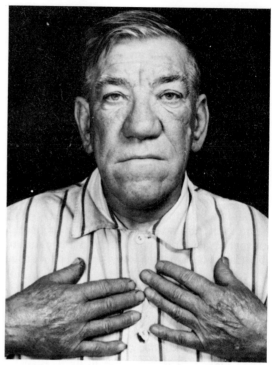

Fig. 26.3 Acromegaly, illustrating the thickening of the nose and enlargement of the lower jaw.

crippling osteoarthritis commonly results. Kyphosis is often present due to irregular vertebral atrophy and hypertrophy. Pain and paraesthesias may result from compression of nerves by bone or soft tissue, e.g. the carpal tunnel syndrome. The plasma prolactin level is raised in about 25 per cent of acromegalics, and in women may cause galactorrhoea which may be sufficiently troublesome to justify removal of the pituitary or radiotherapy.

Plasma levels of GH are usually raised, sometimes only slightly, e.g. 5–10 μg/litre, sometimes greatly, e.g. 1 mg/litre. Where the diagnosis is in doubt it may be confirmed by demonstrating failure to induce the normal fall in plasma GH by oral administration of glucose. Gross acromegaly is rare; lesser degrees are more common and sometimes accompany adenomas of chromophobe type. In either case the condition may become inactive due either to infarction of the tumour or in some cases to development of resistance of the various tissue cells to GH. If mild, such 'fugitive' acromegaly may be difficult to diagnose but enlargement of the sella, demonstrable radiographically, will often confirm the diagnosis. The paranasal sinuses may also be seen to be enlarged as part of the effect of GH on the bones. There is an increased mortality rate in active acromegaly, mostly from heart failure attributable to hypertension, often extensive atheroma, and sometimes to a form of cardiomyopathy with interstitial fibrosis. Other features of acromegaly occur also in gigantism and are as described above. Bromocriptine, a dopamine agonist, is now used with success in the treatment of acromegalics and has been shown to cause shrinkage of acidophil adenomas.

Gigantism is much rarer than acromegaly. It results when excessive GH secretion develops before the epiphyses have fused. A considerable increase in height, sometimes to over 8 feet (2·4 m), may result. Growth is proportionate, so that the bones are both long and thick, the thoracic cage enlarged, etc. Epiphyseal fusion is delayed but occurs eventually. If GH secretion is still excessive, the features of acromegaly then become superadded.

The hormonal changes are as described in acromegaly, and the glucose test described above may be necessary to distinguish between unusually rapid but physiological growth and mild or early gigantism. The stage of adenohypophyseal compression and insufficiency usually develops around early adult life and unless treated most patients die from infections or various effects of hypopituitarism. As in acromegaly, there is, in most cases, an eosinophil adenoma, but in 10 per cent a chromophobe adenoma. Small eosinophil adenomas are sometimes found at necropsy with no evidence of previous hyperfunction.

Hyperprolactinaemia. As mentioned above, this occurs in some cases of acromegaly. Some pituitary chromophobe adenomas secrete mainly prolactin ('prolactinomas'). In women, hyperprolactinaemia causes amenorrhoea: in men it is a rare cause of impotence, possibly by gonadal suppression. Bromocriptine is used in the treatment of hyperprolactinaemia. Some drugs, including hypotensive agents, antidepressants and oral contraceptives, can induce hyperprolactinaemia.

The pituitary in Cushing's syndrome

Cushing described a remarkable clinical picture which he attributed to the presence of a small basophil adenoma of the adenohypophysis. It is now known that the condition is due to excessive secretion of glucocorticoids by the adrenal glands, hyperplasia or neoplasia of which is invariably present. Most of the cases with adrenal hyperplasia are attributable to excessive secretion of ACTH by the adenohypophysis, either by an adenoma or as a result of increased secretion of CRF (p. 1009) by the hypothalamus. Some cases are caused by 'inappropriate' secretion of ACTH by a non-pituitary tumour, usually a bronchial carcinoma. The causes and types of Cushing's syndrome are discussed more fully on p. 1040.

In Cushing's syndrome, Crooke observed cells scattered around the periphery of the adenohypophysis showing a peculiar hyaline change (Fig. 26.4): this was the only pituitary lesion common to all cases. The change, which has since been observed by many workers, is a consequence of high levels of glucocorticoids for it is seen not only in association with adrenal hyperplasia but also in those with autonomously secreting adrenal cortical tumours and also after prolonged therapeutic administration of ACTH or cortisone. The hyaline material does not react with antibody to ACTH and electron-microscopy has shown it to be due to increase in micro-tubular material.

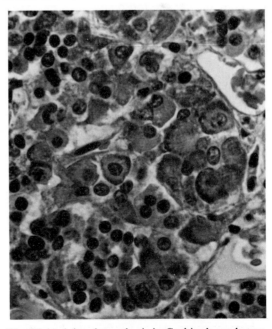

Fig. 26.4 Adenohypophysis in Cushing's syndrome, showing cytoplasmic hyaline change in the basophils. × 500.

Adenohypophyseal hypofunction

This may occur from an unknown cause, as a result of lesions arising in the pituitary itself, or from pressure and destruction by adjacent lesions. Pituitary lesions include adenomas, postpartum ischaemic necrosis, trauma, various infections and macrophage granulomas of unknown nature. Auto-immune destruction occurs rarely in association with the organ-specific auto-immune diseases.

The adenohypophysis has large functional reserves and destruction must be extensive to cause deficiencies. In progressive panhypopituitarism, deficiency of growth hormone and gonadotrophins appears first, followed by deficiency of ACTH and of TSH. Occasionally isolated deficiency of any one of the pituitary hormones occurs, the cause being obscure.

The clinical and pathological features of panhypopituitarism are described in the syndromes outlined below. Diagnosis may be confirmed by radio-immunoassay of adenohypophyseal hormones in the plasma. *Low plasma corticosteroids with a normal response to ACTH is virtually diagnostic.* If the plasma corticosteroid levels are borderline, TSH or growth hormone may be assayed.

The following are the best-known examples of hypofunction of the adenohypophysis.

Simmonds' disease (Sheehan's syndrome)

This is the commonest and most important example of adenohypophyseal hypofunction. Although first described by Simmonds, Sheehan elucidated the clinical and pathological features, and corrected the misconception that marked wasting was a feature.

Aetiology. The condition occurs in women and is nearly always the result of extensive ischaemic necrosis of the adenohypophysis associated with childbirth. Predisposing factors are the enlargement of the pituitary which occurs during pregnancy (p. 1008), the low-pressure portal vascular supply of the adenohypophysis, and the development of hypotensive shock as a result of difficult labour, often with trauma and excessive haemorrhage.

Clinical features. The first noticeable sign following the causal delivery is failure of lactation, which is due to deficiency of prolactin. Other symptoms develop slowly and in some cases are first noticed a few years after the childbirth presumably responsible for the pituitary deficiency. They include total loss of axillary and pubic hair, amenorrhoea, sterility and absence of libido.

Later, hypersensitivity to cold and other features of hypothyroidism develop, and ACTH deficiency leads to asthenia, hypotension, debility and sometimes fatal collapse. There may be a normochromic anaemia. The fasting blood sugar is usually below normal because the action of insulin is unopposed by growth hormone, corticosteroids and thyroxine, but 'compensatory' fall in insulin secretion usually occurs and averts serious hypoglycaemia. Nevertheless, patients are extremely sensitive to an injection of insulin.

Pigmentation of the skin, as in Addison's disease, does not occur: in fact, the pigment decreases, and the skin has a waxy or alabaster appearance. There is no serious loss of salt and water control, since the secretion of aldosterone is largely independent of the pituitary (p. 1038). There does seem to be some mineralocorticoid disturbance, however, for *when general metabolism is increased by administration of thyroxine, symptoms of serious adrenal insufficiency, including water and salt loss, may develop.* The neurohypophysis is not usually affected and its function is maintained.

Structural changes. In patients dying soon after the delivery responsible, Sheehan demonstrated extensive necrosis of the adenohypophysis, which he explained by ischaemia resulting from the causal factors noted above. In patients surviving longer, the necrotic tissue is organised and replaced by fibrous tissue.

Other structural changes include atrophy of the thyroid, adrenals, ovaries, uterus and mammary gland tissue.

The diagnosis may be confirmed by assay of the plasma levels of the pituitary hormones, or the demonstration of suppressed adrenal function and a normal response to ACTH (see above).

Some of Simmonds' cases exhibited generalised wasting and were probably examples of *anorexia nervosa* which is psychogenic and reversible. The distinction is an important one, as adult patients with panhypopituitarism require life-long treatment with thyroxine, corticosteroids and sex hormones.

Fröhlich's syndrome

This condition, described by Fröhlich in 1901 as *dystrophia adiposogenitalis*, occurs in children. Its main features include obesity and failure of sexual maturation. Boys develop a feminine distribution of fat over the breasts and buttocks, and tend to be wide-hipped.

In some cases, lesions are found in the vicinity of the pituitary or hypothalamus, apparently involving both; the least rare is a craniopharyngioma (Fig. 21.88, p. 792) but chromophobe pituitary adenoma, meningioma and glioma have also been found. A condition resembling the syndrome can be induced experimentally in animals by injury to the median eminence and adjacent nuclei: such injury probably interferes with the hypothalamic gonadotrophin-releasing hormone (p. 1007) which stimulates release of both FSH and LH.

Cases of Fröhlich's syndrome due to a detectable lesion are rare. Most obese children with delayed maturation have no detectable lesion and eventually attain sexual maturity.

A condition resembling Fröhlich's syndrome also occurs in adults of both sexes, with obesity, particularly of the trunk, sterility and reduced libido. Occasionally a causal lesion has been found, least rarely an adenohypophyseal chromophobe adenoma, which may have interfered with hypothalamic and adenohypophyseal function. Other pressure effects may include headache and increasing restriction of the field of vision, as with any expanding lesion in this vicinity.

Pituitary dwarfism (Lorain–Levi syndrome)

This results from a severe deficiency of growth hormone in childhood. In most cases, there is deficiency of the other adenohypophyseal hormones, but sometimes GH alone is deficient: some of these latter cases are familial.

In approximately one-third of cases, the condition is due to a pituitary tumour or a craniopharyngioma. Rarely there are multiple adenohypophyseal abnormalities, but more often than not the cause is unexplained.

Impaired general growth is usually noticed after one year of age, sometimes much later: although small, the child is well proportioned (cf. achondroplasia, p. 898) and is not obese (cf. Fröhlich's syndrome). Attacks of hypogly-

caemia may occur (cf. adults with hypopituitarism). The mental state is normal for age and so, being small, the child may seem unusually clever.

If GH alone is deficient, puberty is delayed but eventually occurs normally: the majority, however, also lack gonadotrophins, etc., and do not mature. GH is used in treatment, but some children develop resistance to it.

Diagnosis can be confirmed by plasma GH assay before and after provocation by arginine or L-dopa. Conditions which must be distinguished include gonadal dysgenesis (p. 970), cretinism (p. 1021) and also simple neglect of a child, which may be reflected in greatly stunted growth. There is also a condition of dwarfism in which plasma GH is high but somatomedin (p. 1008) is low.

Adenohypophyseal changes in other diseases

The changes in *Cushing's syndrome* have already been described (p. 1011). In untreated *primary myxoedema*, increased functional activity by the TSH-secreting cells is associated with their enlargement, loss of secretory granules, and development of PAS-positive inclusions (Fig. 26.5) seen by electron-microscopy to be in cisternae in the endoplasmic reticulum. There are no characteristic pituitary changes in *hyperthyroidism*. In *Addison's disease*, there is an increase in poorly granulated basophils believed to be active in secreting ACTH (p. 1045).

Adenohypophyseal tumours

Minute tumours of the adenohypophysis are often found incidentally at necropsy, but clinically significant tumours are rare. The least uncommon are *adenomas* which may cause symptoms by local pressure effects and/or by secretion of hormone.

Traditionally adenomas are classified into *chromophobe*, *acidophil* and *basophil* cell types. Those occurring in pluriglandular adenomatosis are usually of chromophobe or acidophil type.

Chromophobe adenomas do not usually secrete excessive amounts of hormone, and cause symptoms by pressure effects on the adenohypophysis (progressive panhypopituitarism), the optic chiasma (bitemporal hemianopia which

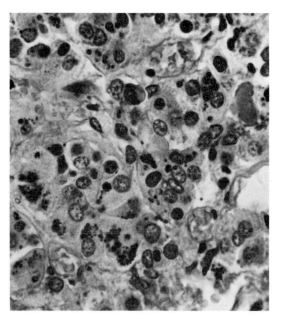

Fig. 26.5 Adenohypophysis in primary myxoedema. The PAS-positive inclusions in the basophil cells show up here as black granules and globules. × 500.

may progress to blindness) and the hypothalamus (diabetes insipidus, fever, etc.). Occasional chromophobe adenomas secrete excess of growth hormone, prolactin or ACTH, with consequent acromegaly (p. 1009), etc. During pregnancy, a chromophobe adenoma may enlarge rapidly and become clinically apparent.

Acidophil adenomas are asymptomatic when small, but when larger cause acromegaly or gigantism (p. 1011). Like chromophobe adenomas, they may grow very large and cause extensive local destruction. Some produce mainly prolactin.

Basophil adenomas are rarer than the others, usually remain small, and occasionally cause Cushing's syndrome (p. 1040). They tend to develop also in patients with Cushing's syndrome treated by total adrenalectomy.

Pituitary adenomas are soft, brown tumours, usually well-encapsulated, and often showing extensive infarction or fibrosis. They may compress and destroy the surrounding pituitary tissue, enlarge the sella and rupture its diaphragm. Occasionally they may erode into the nasopharynx, but this is more typical of the much rarer **pituitary carcinoma**.

Histologically, adenomas have a solid or occasionally papillary structure: the cells resemble closely one or other of the adenohypophyseal cell types, but some tumours are of mixed cell type, e.g. chromophobe and acidophil. More precise classification of adenomas depends on further experience with immunohistological techniques to demonstrate intracellular hormones and hormonal assay of tumour extracts.

Other tumours and cysts

The commonest **primary tumour** outside the pituitary to cause anterior lobe deficiency by pressure is the **craniopharyngioma**, which is derived from Rathke's pouch, i.e. from the craniopharyngeal upgrowth from which the hypophysis is developed. It is usually suprasellar in position and is often cystic (Fig. 21.88, p. 792). Cystic tumours or cysts occasionally arise also from the pars intermedia and the cysts may be lined by ciliated epithelium. These are also of Rathke pouch origin and they may cause atrophy of the rest of the gland. Rarely tumours resembling granular cell myoblastomas (p. 594) occur in the neurohypophysis: they are sometimes termed *choristomas* or *pituicytomas*. **Metastases** from carcinoma of the breast or bronchus are not uncommon, and pericapsular deposits occur in some cases of leukaemia. Extra-pituitary tumours in the suprasellar region may involve the nuclei of the hypothalamus and lead to disturbances of fat metabolism and obesity or to polyuria.

The neurohypophysis (posterior lobe)

This is composed of irregular fusiform cells of neural origin, among which are numerous nerve fibres which come from the hypothalamus. Two hormones, *vasopressin* and *oxy-* *tocin*, are synthesised in the hypothalamic nuclei and transmitted by modified nerve fibres to the neurohypophysis, where they are stored and released as required. The two molecules are octapeptides and are stored in combination with a common large storage molecule called *neurophysin*.

Antidiuretic hormone (ADH) or vasopressin controls water balance by increasing the permeability of the renal collecting tubules, thus allowing increased re-absorption of water and a more concentrated urine. The name vasopressin is a bad one, for only in very high dosage does it raise the blood pressure. If the plasma osmolarity increases, osmoreceptors in the anterior hypothalamus initiate a neural stimulus which releases neurohypophyseal-stored ADH into the blood. Conversely, ADH secretion is suppressed by lowered osmolarity of the plasma.

Diabetes insipidus. This is due to deficient secretion of ADH. It is usually caused by a hypothalamic lesion, e.g. head injury, glioma, metastatic cancer or encephalitis. Destruction of the neurohypophysis or high transection of the pituitary stalk do not normally cause diabetes insipidus, as sufficient ADH escapes from the severed neurohypophyseal tract.

The main feature of diabetes insipidus is excretion of a very large volume of dilute urine—often over 10 litres/24 hours. This is accompanied by polydipsia and, if drinking is restricted, the concentration of the urine increases only slightly and severe dehydration results. Onset of the condition is often surprisingly sudden. Apart from inconvenience, the polyuria has little harmful effect unless drinking is prevented. In *psychogenic polyuria*, withholding of fluid results in a concentrated urine without dehydration. Confirmation of the diagnosis of diabetes insipidus is provided by a response to a dose of ADH or of a recently synthesised analogue which is also valuable in treatment.

Oxytocin causes contraction of uterine smooth muscle and expulsion of milk during lactation. It may play a physiological role in uterine contraction during and after pregnancy, and was formerly widely used to initiate labour and to contract the uterus in post-partum haemorrhage, etc.

Women with diabetes insipidus, and therefore presumably deficiency of both ADH and oxytocin, can have a normal labour and lactation, and oxytocin has no known function in males.

The Pineal Body

The function of this minute structure, situated above the posterior part of the third ventricle, is very largely obscure. There is evidence that it secretes hormonal factors, one of which, *melatonin*, is derived from serotonin, and appears to antagonise the effects of MSH. Melatonin may also inhibit gonadal maturation and function.

The least rare lesions of the pineal are tumours which occur mainly in childhood. They include gliomas, teratomas and also tumours indistinguishable from seminomas. Effects are produced by pressure on neighbouring structures; thus hydrocephalus, ocular paralyses and deafness from implication of the corpora quadrigemina, also cerebellar effects, giddiness, etc., may result. In young boys precocious puberty may accompany a pineal tumour of any type. In other cases of pineal tumour such effects have been absent, and a similar group of changes has been observed in other lesions in the neighbourhood, such as tumour in the floor of the third ventricle, hydrocephalus, etc. The syndrome is probably not a pineal effect but rather the result of disturbance of nerve tracts possibly related to the pituitary.

The Thyroid Gland

The thyroid gland produces three hormones, **thyroxine, tri-iodothyronine** and **calcitonin**. Calcitonin is a polypeptide which lowers the concentration of calcium in the blood by causing increased deposition of bone crystal, but its physiological and pathological importance is still uncertain: it is secreted by specialised epithelial cells (C cells) which lie between the thyroid acini.

Thyroxine (tetra-iodothyronine, or T_4) and

tri-iodothyronine (T_3) are iodinated amino acids with a hormonal effect of influencing heat production in the tissues of the body by uncoupling oxidative phosphorylation, i.e. increasing oxygen utilisation relative to the rate of formation of high energy phosphate bonds, two processes which are closely linked in the economy of the cell. T_3 and T_4 are essential for normal physical and mental development and in the metabolism of protein, carbohydrate and fat. Excessive secretion of these thyroid hormones causes the serious disorder known as **thyrotoxicosis** or **hyperthyroidism** while inadequate secretion results in **hypothyroidism** which also has severe pathological consequences. Important physiological mechanisms have evolved to ensure that the amounts of T_3 and T_4 released into the circulation are appropriate to the varying bodily requirements in differing circumstances (e.g. environmental temperature), and, within limits, to compensate for suboptimal intake of dietary iodine.

Iodine metabolism in the thyroid gland. Iodine ions are concentrated in thyroid cells by a special concentrating or *trapping mechanism* which can be inhibited by perchlorate or thiocyanate ions. Iodide within thyroid epithelium is rapidly *oxidised* by a thyroid peroxidase to an active form which readily enters *organic combination* with the tyrosine present in the glycoprotein, thyroglobulin. This latter is synthesised by thyroid epithelium and stored extracellularly in the colloid within the acini. The organic binding of oxidised iodine results in the formation of mono- and di-iodotyrosine within the thyroglobulin molecule and the synthesis of the iodothyronine is accomplished by *coupling* of two appropriate iodotyrosines to give T_3 or T_4. (The antithyroid drugs thiouracil and carbimazole diminish the organic binding of iodine and the coupling reaction by inhibiting thyroid peroxidase which catalyses both of these reactions.) The hormones, still part of the thyroglobulin molecule, are thought to be stored within the colloid until required in the circulation. Thyroglobulin is then digested by a cathepsin, T_3 and T_4 are released and transported through the acinar epithelial cells to the vessels within the stroma of the gland. Hormonally inactive iodotyrosines which have not taken part in iodothyronine formation are also released from digested thyroglobulin but these are deiodinated by a *dehalogenase* enzyme and

the released iodide is available for re-oxidation and re-organification.

Due to inborn errors of metabolism one or other of these steps is sometimes defective and this leads to the condition of **dyshormonogenesis**. Thus failure of the iodide-trapping mechanism, defective organification of iodide due to peroxidase deficiency, secretion of abnormal iodoprotein, and dehalogenase deficiency each constitutes a different form of dyshormonogenesis and results in a tendency to hypothyroidism.

Control of thyroid secretion. The secretion of thyroid hormone is mainly controlled by TSH. Inadequate plasma levels of T_3 and T_4 cause release of TSH from the pituitary by a feedback mechanism and this activates adenyl-cyclase activity of thyroid epithelium and, by increasing cAMP stimulates all the processes of thyroid hormone formation and release described above. If prolonged, such stimulation by TSH causes important structural changes in the thyroid: in particular a change of the epithelium from cubical to columnar, proliferation of epithelial cells to form new follicles, and diminution of the volume and concentration of the colloid stored within the acini. These changes may result in **goitre**, i.e. enlargement of the thyroid. When the plasma level of thyroid hormone exceeds the physiological requirements of the body, the production of TSH by the pituitary is suppressed and the thyroid reverts to its resting state with diminished hormone production, diminished secretion and increased storage of hormone within the eosinophilic colloid which accumulates within the acini.

Hypothyroidism. The effects of subnormal secretion of T_4 and T_3 vary depending upon the severity of thyroid hormone deficiency and the age of onset of the disorder. Infantile hypothyroidism is called **cretinism** and is described on p. 1021.

In the adult the syndrome is called **myxoedema**. In severe cases there is lethargy, slowing of speech and impaired intellectual function sometimes associated with frank psychosis. The hair, brittle and lustreless, tends to fall out. Hydrophilic mucoprotein ground substance accumulates in the dermal connective tissue causing coarsening of the features (Fig. 26.6) and firm non-pitting oedema of the supraclavicular fossae and dorsum of the hands.

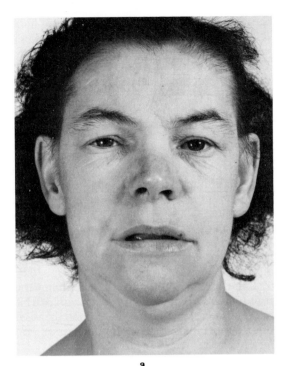 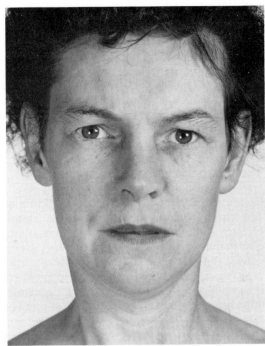

a
                                                b

Fig. 26.6 Myxoedema, (**a**): before treatment, (**b**): the effects of administration of thyroxine.

Similar mucinous deposits around nerves may impair peripheral nerve function and cause, for example, carpal tunnel syndrome or deafness, while involvement of tongue and larynx causes a characteristically slurred croaking voice. Despite a poor appetite the patient gains weight. The pulse is slow, the basal metabolic rate is lowered, and the patient suffers from constipation, feels cold and is unduly prone to develop hypothermia.

Biochemical abnormalities include a raised serum cholesterol level due to reduced rate of catabolism, but most significant is the low thyroid secretion rate of T_4 and T_3, the concentrations of which in the blood can be shown by radio-immunoassay to be abnormally low, while the serum protein-bound iodine is also low.

Secretion of TSH is increased, even in patients with early or subclinical thyroid failure, and this is reflected in the appearance in the anterior pituitary of mucoid cells which contain only a few prominent storage granules (vesiculate mucoid cells—Fig. 26.5). There is diminished sexual function and menorrhagia is common due to failure of ovulation and continued endometrial proliferation. All of the above changes, except, of course, the low thy-

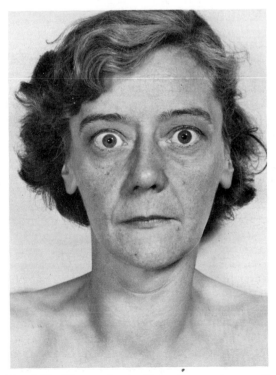

Fig. 26.7 Thyrotoxicosis. Note the prominence of the eyes and the diffuse thyroid enlargement.

roid hormone secretion rate, are reversed by therapy with T_4 or T_3.

Causes. By far the most common cause of hypothyroidism is primary myxoedema (the atrophic form of auto-immune thyroiditis—see below) but hypothyroidism with goitre is found in Hashimoto's disease, dyshormonogenesis, severe iodine deficiency and as a result of drugs with antithyroid effects. Extensive surgical resection of the thyroid, therapy with radioiodine, and hypopituitarism with diminished TSH secretion are other causes.

Hyperthyroidism (*syn.* **thyrotoxicosis**) results from excessive secretion of thyroid hormone and causes clinical features which are almost the opposite of those found in hypothyroidism. The patient, though weak, is restless, hyperkinetic and emotionally unstable. The appetite is increased but the patient loses weight. There is increased nitrogen excretion, and sometimes impaired glucose tolerance and glycosuria. The skin is warm and sweating, the pulse rapid and bounding and the cardiac output is increased.

Cardiac arrhythmia, particularly atrial fibrillation, may occur, especially in older patients and cardiac failure may be the presenting feature. Osteoporosis affecting cancellous bone may be present, associated with increased calcium excretion in urine and faeces. Many of the above features are attributable to the raised basal metabolic rate which is, in turn, due to the effects of excessive amounts of thyroid hormone on the tissues. The serum levels of T_3, less often T_4, and of protein-bound iodine are raised. Pituitary TSH secretion is inhibited. In the common clinical form of hyperthyroidism, **Graves' disease**, there is unexplained prominence of the eyes (*exophthalmos*) (Fig. 26.7) which cannot be attributed to the action of T_3 and T_4.

Most cases of thyrotoxicosis are due to an auto-antibody to thyroid epithelium (pp. 1026–7). Less often autonomous hyperfunctioning thyroid tumour-like nodules are responsible, while in very rare cases, hyperthyroidism is the result of excessive pituitary TSH production in acromegaly.

Nontoxic goitre (simple goitre)

Nontoxic goitre is the name given to various non-inflammatory conditions which result in enlargement of the thyroid gland without hyperthyroidism. All forms of nontoxic goitre are probably preceded and for a time accompanied by a phase of impaired thyroid hormone synthesis due to inadequate supply of iodide or to impaired thyroid enzyme activity, the result of genetic defect or exogenous toxic substances. To counteract the diminished secretion of thyroid hormone in these circumstances more TSH is produced and there is increased activity of the thyroid epithelium, which becomes hyperplastic. These compensatory changes may increase T_4 and T_3 secretion enough to prevent hypothyroidism, but the defect may be so severe that goitrous hypothyroidism results, a condition which some authors would not include under the heading of simple or nontoxic goitre.

Morphologically, the following varieties of nontoxic goitre are recognised; (*a*) **parenchymatous goitre**, showing hyperplasia of the type illustrated in Fig. 26.8 with little colloid storage; (*b*) **colloid goitre**, in which there is marked accumulation of colloid (Fig. 26.10). Both types may occur in a *diffuse form* in which the gland is generally involved or in a *nodular form* in which increase occurs in scattered rounded nodules of various sizes.

Epidemiology. Goitre may occur sporadically in any locality. Before the introduction of iodised salt, it was unduly common in certain districts (**endemic goitre**), notably in the valleys of Switzerland, the Pyrenees, the Himalayas and in New Zealand; in England in the Derbyshire hills; in parts of Southern Ireland, and in North America in the region of the Great Lakes. Where deficiency of iodine was great, as in the mountainous regions, e.g. the Alps, the goitre was usually parenchymatous, diffuse at first and becoming nodular later. Thyroid deficiency and cretinism were common, especially where the disease was very prevalent and of severe type. In goitrous districts in Switzerland the average weight of the thyroid at birth was often double the normal and occasionally a congenital parenchymatous goitre was present.

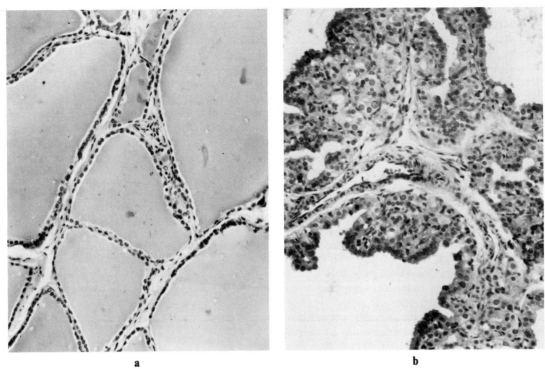

a   b

Fig. 26.8 Normal thyroid tissue (**a**) and thyroid showing the effects of chronic stimulation with TSH (**b**). Note the hypertrophy and hyperplasia of the thyroid epithelium and diminished colloid storage. × 185.

In North America, goitre was usually of the colloid type, either diffuse or nodular.

Aetiology. The causation of endemic goitre is not fully understood, but it is known that deficiency of iodine is the chief factor in its production. In remote communities where little food is imported, lack of iodine in the soil and water and in locally produced food is the basic defect. There may be contributory factors which render unavailable any iodine present, such as pollution of water supplies by sulphur-containing organic matter or the presence of much calcium or fluoride. In goitrous districts, rats, sheep and other animals are also affected. When iodine deficiency is severe, goitre appears in childhood; when it is moderate, goitre is not only less common but also appears later, occurring especially at puberty and during pregnancy and lactation, when there is a drain on the iodine supply. Males are affected less frequently than females. In the early stages especially, treatment by iodine may arrest the thyroid enlargement or cause it to regress. In the region of the Great Lakes and in Switzerland, the administration of small quantities of iodine

to school children has resulted in remarkable diminution in the incidence of goitre. In New Zealand and certain other districts the results have been less striking, perhaps because of the presence of iodine inhibitors.

Sporadic nontoxic goitre, i.e. that occurring in areas where goitre is not endemic, appears to have three main causes: (1) iodine deficiency due to faulty dietary habits; (2) dyshormonogenesis due to one of a group of inherited defects of thyroid hormone synthesis or secretion (see pp. 1016, 1022); (3) the action of chemicals which interfere with thyroid hormone synthesis: excluding antithyroid drugs used in treating thyrotoxicosis, perhaps the most important of these is large doses of iodine given in the form of iodopyrine, or less commonly simply as iodide, as expectorants in asthma or chronic bronchitis. In idiosyncratic subjects this inhibits the iodination of tyrosine; there is a fall in thyroid hormone release, and patients with 'iodide goitre' frequently become hypothyroid. Resorcinol, *para*-aminosalicylic acid and sulphonylureas are other drugs which occasionally cause nontoxic goitre.

Parenchymatous goitre. The initial changes are enlargement of the acinar cells to columnar type and formation of many small colloid-deficient acini. The tissue of the enlarged gland lacks normal thyroid translucency and looks more like pancreas to the naked eye. The changes are at first diffuse, affecting the entire gland, but if the iodine lack persists, foci of excessively active iodine uptake appear, while other parts of the gland become refractory and fail to take up and store iodine; this can be shown by autoradiography of thyroids excised after a dose of radioactive iodine. The hyperactive foci enlarge and compress the adjacent parenchyma so that the gland becomes nodular.

In nodular nontoxic goitre the appearances vary greatly. There may be only one or two nodular masses, or the gland may be studded with them, the parenchyma between becoming atrophied. Following the initially diffuse parenchymatous hyperplasia, the subsequent development of hyperplastic nodules probably depends on the severity of the continuing iodine deficiency, however brought about.

Colloid goitre. In diffuse colloid goitre the whole gland may be affected (Fig. 26.9), or one lobe may be chiefly involved. The affected tissue is tense and firm, and on section presents a translucent brownish appearance due to the accumulation of dense, firm colloid. Indeed, very large acini filled with colloid may be present. Dark red or brown areas due to haem-

orrhage may be seen, and in places there may be fibrosis, sometimes with calcification of the stroma. On microscopic examination, the acini are, in general, enlarged and distended with deeply-staining colloid, and the epithelium may be flattened (Fig. 26.10). Cysts may be formed by the confluence of acini. Colloid goitre is much commoner in women than in men, usually appears first at puberty or in pregnancy, and may be dependent on a less severe degree of iodine lack than that associated with parenchymatous goitre. This seems to hold generally with regard to the disease in low-lying countries.

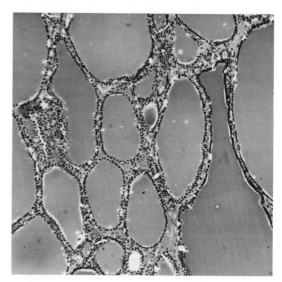

Fig. 26.10 Colloid goitre, showing accumulation of colloid in the acini and flattening of the acinar epithelium. × 40.

Effects. In nontoxic goitre, thyroid function often appears clinically normal, though minor disturbances are not so rare as was once supposed. The enlarged gland may occasionally cause pressure effects on a recurrent laryngeal nerve, the oesophagus, or on the trachea, and even death by suffocation. Pressure effects are more common when the goitre extends retrosternally. In mountainous regions the thyroid enlargement in children, usually of the nodular type, may be associated with cretinism, the result of severe deficiency of the thyroid hormone. In America, colloid goitre has been associated with some degree of thyrotoxicosis.

Despite much study, it is uncertain whether nontoxic goitre predisposes to the development of carcinoma.

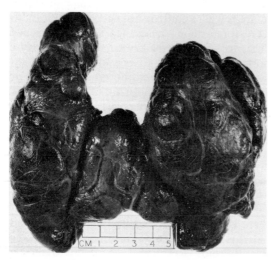

Fig. 26.9 Diffuse colloid goitre, showing general thyroid enlargement.

Cretinism

Severe hypothyroidism beginning in infancy is called *cretinism*. Cretins usually seem normal at birth, having received maternal thyroid hormone while *in utero*, but within a few weeks or months it becomes apparent that mental and physical development are retarded. The characteristic cretin is a dwarf with severe mental defect, disproportionately short limbs, coarse dry skin, deficient hair and teeth, a large protruding tongue (Fig. 26.11) and pot belly with umbilical hernia. The skeletal changes of cretinism are mentioned on p. 892. Unless replacement therapy with T_3 or T_4 commences early, the changes, especially the mental defect, become irreversible, though there may be some improvement in physical appearance.

Endemic cretinism occurred almost exclusively in mountainous districts such as Switzerland, where iodine deficiency was severe and endemic goitre common. It is said rarely to appear in a goitrous family until the second or third generation, and cretins of this type are nearly always the offspring of goitrous mothers. Unexplained deaf-mutism is very often present as an additional feature.

The thyroid. In most cases of endemic cretinism a goitre is present, although in some instances the thyroid is atrophic and fibrous. The goitre is nearly always nodular, the parenchyma between the nodules being compressed and atrophic. The appearances are similar to those seen in the nodular goitres of long-standing iodine deficiency.

Sporadic cretinism. This condition, due to congenital absence or hypoplasia of the thyroid tissue, is encountered from time to time in all localities and the causation is unknown. In some cases no trace of thyroid may be found, although there may be small nodules of atrophied thyroid tissue near the foramen caecum

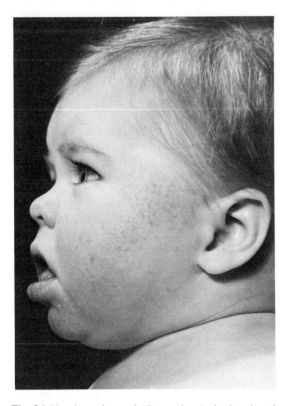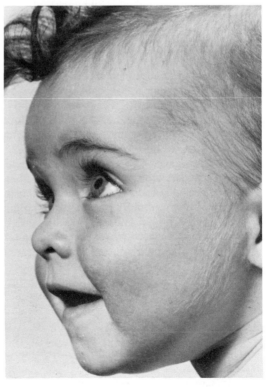

Fig. 26.11　A cretin aged 17 months. *Left*, showing the enlarged, protruding tongue, coarse dry skin and dull expression. *Right*, showing the effects of thyroxine treatment for two months. (Professor J. H. Hutchison.)

at the root of the tongue. In other cases the thyroid is small and shrunken, sometimes containing cysts. The thymus is usually atrophic, but the parathyroids are not affected and occupy their usual position.

Dyshormonogenesis. Goitre in sporadic cretinism is very rare, but it occurs as a familial recessive abnormality manifested by congenital absence of some essential enzyme system. In one variety, studied by McGirr and Hutchison in a family of Scottish tinkers, absence of the dehalogenase enzyme, which normally removes iodine from iodotyrosine, allows mono- and di-iodotyrosine to escape from the thyroid into the blood, from which they are excreted in the urine, thus leading to gross iodine deficiency. In another type iodide accumulates in the gland but thyroid peroxidase deficiency results in failure to oxidise iodide to free iodine which is therefore not available in the thyroid to combine with tyrosine. Accordingly iodinated hormone synthesis fails. In some congenital goitrous cretins deaf-mutism is present, an interesting finding in view of its unexplained frequency in endemic goitrous cretinism.

The thyroid is often greatly enlarged and nodular, and on microscopic examination the epithelial hyperplasia of parenchymatous goitre is found.

Less severe genetic defects of thyroid metabolism also occur: in some, the thyroid hyperplasia may compensate sufficiently to prevent or reduce the degree of hypothyroidism.

Auto-immune thyroiditis

In this condition there is infiltration of the thyroid by lymphocytes and plasma cells associated with abnormalities of the thyroid epithelium and, in many cases, thyroid-specific auto-antibodies in the serum.

Three main variants are encountered: (1) **Hashimoto's disease (lymphadenoid goitre)**—a diffuse and massive lesion causing goitre; (2) **primary myxoedema**, in which the thyroid is shrunken and the epithelium atrophic; (3) **focal thyroiditis** in which patchy lesions occur in an otherwise normal or hyperplastic gland.

Gross appearance. Areas of thyroid affected by auto-immune thyroiditis appear solid and white or peach coloured, lacking the translucent appearance normally presented by colloid stored in the acini. In Hashimoto's disease the gland is firm and there is enlargement, usually symmetrical and of moderate degree; the cut surface has a solid lobulated appearance resembling pancreas on section, and in most cases the capsule is not adherent to surrounding tissues. The shrunken thyroid of primary myxoedema is firm and white while in focal auto-immune thyroiditis ill-defined white patches of about 1 mm in diameter are seen on the cut surface of the gland.

Microscopic appearance (Fig. 26.12). The basic lesion common to all forms is the presence of small acini lined by large cubical epithelial cells with granular cytoplasm and large nuclei which are frequently bizarre in shape. These cells, known variously as Askanazy cells, Hürthle cells, oxyphil cells or oncocytes, owe their eosinophilic (pale pink to bright red) cytoplasmic granularity to the presence of numerous large mitochondria.

The colloid is scanty, usually densely eosinophilic and may contain macrophages or multi-nucleated giant cells. Surrounding the abnormal acini, and sometimes invading them, is an infiltrate of plasma cells and/or lymphocytes, accompanied by a variable amount of fibrous tissue.

In *Hashimoto's disease* (Fig. 26.12) the epithelium is all abnormal and increased in amount. The lymphoid infiltrate is massive and true germinal centres may be present. Mitotic figures are very infrequent. The amount of fibrous tissue is variable. Most of the gland in *primary myxoedema* consists of fibrous tissue (Fig. 26.13) containing sparse clusters of small acini lined by Askanazy cells and islets or cysts of epithelium sometimes of squamous type (a feature also seen occasionally in Hashimoto's disease). The lymphocytic and plasma cell infiltration is usually slight and situated mainly around the surviving epithelium. *Focal auto-immune thyroiditis* (Fig. 26.14) differs from both these conditions by the presence of greater or smaller areas of normal or hyperplastic thyroid tissue. The more severe examples, however, approach Hashimoto's disease in extent. It is very common in middle-aged women.

Clinical features. In *Hashimoto's disease* the patient, usually a middle-aged female, has a firm goitre of moderate size. Hypothyroidism is present in about half the cases, and is the rule if partial thyroidectomy is undertaken. The thyroid uptake of iodine is reduced and organification is impaired. An abnormal iodinated thyroprotein, which differs from serum protein-

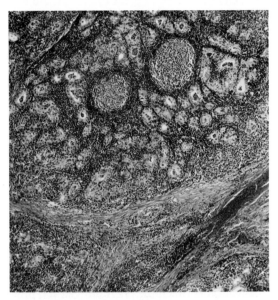

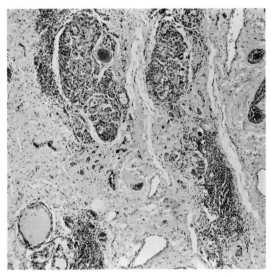

Fig. 26.13 The thyroid in primary myxoedema. Islands of thyroid tissue, showing the changes of chronic thyroiditis, are embedded in fibrous tissue containing wide vascular channels. × 50.

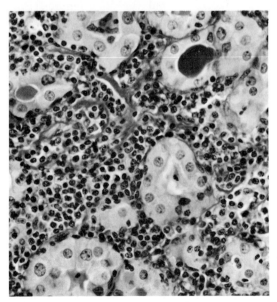

Fig. 26.12 Hashimoto's thyroiditis. *Above*, showing the diffuse lymphoid cell infiltrate, germinal centres, fibrosis and small thyroid acini. × 50. *Below*, showing the lymphocytic and plasma cell infiltrate and change in the epithelium to Askanazy-cell type. × 320.

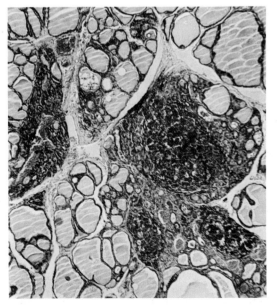

Fig. 26.14 Focal chronic thyroiditis. × 20.

bound T_4 in being insoluble in butanol, is sometimes found in the serum.

Primary myxoedema is characterised by hypothyroidism in the absence of goitre. *Chronic focal thyroiditis* is usually asymptomatic. It is, however, usually present in patients with Graves' disease, and the risk of developing hypothyroidism after partial thyroidectomy is greater if there is extensive focal thyroiditis.

Aetiology. Auto-antibody against thyroglobulin and antibody against a lipoprotein of the membrane of the endoplasmic reticulum ('microsomes') of thyroid epithelial cells are found in high titre in the serum of most, but not all, patients with Hashimoto's disease. The frequency and titre of such antibodies is lower in primary myxoedema and lower still in focal thyroiditis. There is evidence that most of the auto-antibody is formed by the plasma cells which are usually a conspicuous feature of the inflammatory infiltrate of the gland.

Experimental auto-immune thyroiditis can be produced in various animals, including primates, by injecting thyroglobulin in Freund's adjuvant emulsion (p. 114) which enhances immunological responsiveness. The experimental lesions are, however, transitory and their severity, which varies greatly, is related to the genotype, particularly at the histocompatibility loci, of the animal. The lesions parallel the development of cell-mediated immunity to thyroglobulin. Transfer of the disease to normal animals has been accomplished with difficulty using serum or very large numbers of lymphoid cells from affected animals. Mice depleted of T cells by thymectomy and x-irradiation develop persistent auto-immune thyroiditis spontaneously (i.e. without injection of thyroglobulin and adjuvant) and in this model there is a better correlation with thyroglobulin antibody. It has been suggested that loss of suppressor cells is important, and this may explain also the enhancement by thymectomy of the spontaneous auto-immune thyroiditis which occurs in an obese strain of chickens. Although of great interest, these findings have not established the aetiology of human 'auto-immune' thyroiditis: defective function of suppressor T cells may help to explain auto-immunisation but the pathogenic importance of delayed auto-hypersensitivity and/or auto-antibodies is not yet firmly established (see also pp. 163–4).

Patients with auto-immune thyroiditis are unduly prone to have in addition auto-immune gastritis (p. 605) (sometimes accompanied by pernicious anaemia), or auto-immune adrenalitis (idiopathic Addison's disease, p. 1044). In all these conditions there is also cell-mediated immunity to mitochondrial antigens which are not entirely organ-specific and which may account for their co-occurrence in the same individual. The occurrence of all these diseases within certain families suggests that the basic predisposition is inherited. There is a close association between the HLA antigen B8, primary myxoedema and the other organ-specific auto-immune diseases, but curiously this does not apply to Hashimoto's disease.

It remains to be discovered what event triggers the auto-immune process, why the disease occurs mainly in females, what factors determine whether the lesion is focal or diffuse and whether the epithelium becomes atrophic as in primary myxoedema or hyperplastic as in Hashimoto's disease. It is also not known why non-toxic goitre is unduly frequent in the relatives of patients with auto-immune thyroid disease.

Other forms of thyroiditis

Thyroiditis due to causes other than auto-immunity is very rare in Britain. Multiple small abscesses may be found in the thyroid in pyaemia and acute thyroiditis is said sometimes to complicate influenza and typhoid fever.

Giant-cell (de Quervain's) thyroiditis. This variety of subacute thyroiditis begins with the distinctive features of fever and pain in the neck with tenderness. There is a neutrophil leukocytosis and a raised ESR. Elevation of the protein-bound iodine with reduced thyroid iodide uptake is said to be pathognomonic of the disorder. Microscopically, there is polymorphonuclear infiltration followed by lymphocytes and plasma cells; destruction of acini with formation of epithelioid cells and giant cells gives a pseudotuberculous appearance. Israeli workers have recovered a virus having the properties of mumps virus from two cases and have shown the presence of neutralising and complement-fixing antibodies to mumps virus in others.

Riedel's thyroiditis. This very rare disease is characterised by enlargement of the thyroid by fibrous tissue of extremely hard consistency; the condition usually affects only one lobe and involves adjacent muscles. Microscopically, the fibrous tissue may be more or less cellular, and in the affected part the acini become atrophic and disappear. Hypothyroidism is unusual. The nature of the disease is unknown; a few cases have been associated with retroperitoneal fibrosis (p. 658); other supposed cases may be more properly classified as sclerotic thyroid adenomas or as fibrous variants of Hashimoto's disease.

Hyperthyroidism (thyrotoxicosis)

Excessive secretion, by the thyroid, of T_3 and usually T_4, occurs in three conditions. (1) **Graves' disease**, the most common, is characterised by diffuse thyroid hyperplasia apparently due to the presence of an inappropriate thyroid stimulator in the blood. Protrusion of the eyeballs (exophthalmos) and certain other features of the disease cannot be ascribed to thyroid hormone excess alone. (2) **Toxic adenoma** is a relatively uncommon condition, in which an autonomous thyroid tumour produces thyroid hormone in excess of the requirements of the body. (3) **Toxic nodular goitre**, in which excessive hormone is produced in multiple discrete foci within the thyroid, supervenes in older patients who already have a nontoxic nodular goitre. The main features of hyperthyroidism have already been outlined on p. 1018.

Graves' disease (exophthalmic goitre)

In this disease the **thyroid** shows hyperplasia which is characteristically diffuse though sometimes one lobe is larger than the other. On section the parenchyma is less brown and less translucent than normal owing to diminished colloid storage and the gland resembles salivary tissue, being dull greyish-pink in colour and lobulated. However, even in untreated cases some parts may contain a considerable amount of colloid and the surface may be slightly nodular. The gland is moderately firm and succulent, though if thyroiditis is marked (see below) there may be some fibrosis. The surface veins and arteries may be enlarged but the organ as a whole does not look especially vascular after surgical removal or at necropsy. The appearances may be much modified by treatment.

On microscopic examination, hyperplasia of the epithelium and diminution in the amount of the colloid stored are constant (Fig. 26.15). The epithelial cells of the acini are increased in size and more columnar in type. Numerous small acini are formed, while in the larger ones papilliform ingrowths are often present: both of these factors lead to a great increase in the epithelial surface area. What little colloid remains stains palely and appears watery. These changes reflect increased formation of hormones, which are, however, not stored in thyroglobulin but passed on to the bloodstream. In many cases there is focal auto-immune thyroiditis with lymphocytic infiltration (Fig. 26.14), and sometimes the formation of lymphoid follicles. When such infiltration is widespread, the lesion comes to resemble Hashimoto's disease (p. 1022), and in such cases hypothyroidism commonly follows partial thyroidectomy.

The alterations described are usually fairly uniform throughout the gland but in places there may be quiescent acini which contain a considerable amount of colloid, especially when, at a later period, the acute symptoms are beginning to subside. The picture may thus be one of hyperplasia and subsequent involution irregularly distributed, even with fibrosis in places.

The administration of iodine tends to reverse the hyperplastic changes in the thyroid; the epithelium becomes more cubical, and colloid accumulates in the acini (Fig. 26.15). These changes after iodine therapy bring about only temporary improvement in the symptoms, and the mode of action of iodine is uncertain. The anti-thyroid drugs derived from thiourea used in the treatment of hyperthyroidism prevent the synthesis of thyroxine and this leads to a striking reduction in the thyrotoxicosis although the epithelial hyperplasia is undiminished or even exaggerated. The histological effects of iodine and of thiouracil on the thyroid are thus an-

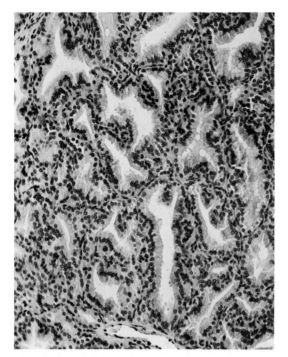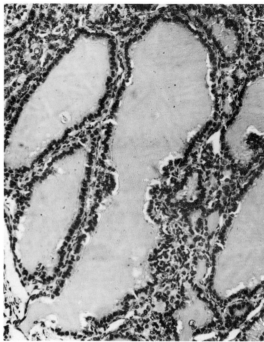

Fig. 26.15   The thyroid in Graves disease. *Left*, untreated: the epithelial cells are columnar and there is virtually no colloid. *Right*, after treatment with iodine for 10 days. The epithelial cells are cuboidal and some colloid has accumulated. × 125.

tagonistic and when both are administered before thyroidectomy the histological picture in the excised gland is complex.

Other organs. The thymus shows distinct enlargement in three-quarters of the cases, and the thymic lymphoid tissue is increased in amount and contains in its medulla lymphoid follicles with germinal centres. There may also be some enlargement of the lymph nodes. Some observers consider that these lymphoid changes are proportionate to the severity of the disease; they may reflect the auto-immune response of Graves' disease and the usually-associated focal thyroiditis, or they may be due to lowered adrenal cortical function resulting from the accelerated inactivation of cortisol found in thyrotoxicosis. Hypertrophy of the heart occurs in most cases of thyrotoxicosis. There may be neutropenia with relative lymphocytosis. Occasionally, however, there is an absolute lymphocytosis, and this is thought by some to occur in the more severe cases.

Occasionally bilateral patches of myxoedematous thickening appear on the anterior (pretibial) aspects of the lower leg, even while

thyrotoxicosis is active. Before partial thyroidectomy was rendered relatively safe by premedication with antithyroid drugs, it was recognised that in a few cases spontaneous thyroid involution might culminate in hypothyroidism.

Orbital changes. Exophthalmos in mild cases is attributable to fatty infiltration of the extrinsic muscles of the eye. When proptosis is severe there is, in addition, increase in amount and oedema of the orbital tissue, and marked lymphocytic infiltration of the extrinsic eye muscles and perivascular connective tissue.

Aetiology. The disease is most common in females, particularly during the reproductive period, and sometimes runs in families, especially in those in which there is an abnormally high incidence of organ-specific auto-immune diseases, e.g. Hashimoto's disease and pernicious anaemia.

It is now apparent, largely from the work of Dr. Duncan Adams, that Graves' disease is due to an auto-antibody which reacts with the thyroid epithelial cell surface receptor for TSH (see Adams, 1977). This thyroid-stimulating antibody is detectable in the blood of most untreated patients by an *in vitro* test in which the binding of labelled TSH by human thyroid cell membrane preparations is competitively inhibited by the patient's serum. In some cases, the thyroid-stimulating antibody can cross-react with mouse or guinea-pig thyroid epithelium and causes thyroid stimulation in these animals *in vivo*. In fact this is how the antibody (originally termed *long-acting thyroid stimulator* or *LATS*) was first demonstrated. Thyroid-stimulating antibody has been shown to be quite distinct from TSH.

The auto-immune nature of Graves' disease is supported also by the frequent presence of focal auto-immune thyroiditis and other organ-specific auto-immune diseases (p. 162), such as pernicious anaemia. Thyroid-stimulating antibody explains the failure to demonstrate TSH in the serum of patients with Graves' disease, and the failure of administered T_3 to suppress thyroid activity in these patients—findings which indicate that pituitary TSH production in Graves' disease is fully suppressed by the inappropriately high blood levels of thyroid hormone. Further support is obtained from the correlation between the presence of maternal thyroid-stimulating antibody and the occurrence of temporary thyrotoxicosis in the neonate.

Thyroid-stimulating antibody correlates also with pretibial myxoedema and, to some extent with exophthalmos. The pathogenesis of exophthalmos in Graves' disease is unknown. According to Kriss *et al.* (1975), thyroglobulin-antithyroglobulin complexes bind preferentially to the membranes of the extrinsic muscles of the eye, which they may reach by the lymphatic drainage of the thyroid and which they may damage by an antibody-dependent lymphocytotoxic reaction (p. 152).

Toxic adenoma

Approximately 1 per cent of thyroid adenomas give rise to hyperthyroidism, usually mild and not accompanied by exophthalmos or thyroid-stimulating antibody in the serum.

The tumours are usually single adenomas more than 3 cm in diameter and are composed of small acini resembling those seen in Graves' disease. Towards the centre of the adenoma stromal oedema and fibrosis may separate the vesicles. Haemorrhage may occur into the tumour and destroy so much of the epithelium that the hyperthyroidism subsides.

Scanning the neck following administration of radio-iodine shows marked radio-iodine uptake by the tumour, and, because of the autonomous nature of the growth, this cannot be suppressed by T_3. The remainder of the gland does not concentrate iodine since the hormone produced by the tumour results in diminished secretion of TSH by the pituitary.

Toxic nodular goitre

This disorder usually affects patients over 50 years of age who have had nontoxic goitre for many years. The thyrotoxicosis which subsequently develops is usually mild as judged by thyroid iodine uptake studies and hormone levels in the blood. Cardiac arrhythmias and failure may cause the presenting symptoms. Exophthalmos is uncommon.

The macroscopic and histological features are similar to those described in nontoxic nodular goitre (p. 1020). Autoradiography shows in some cases one or two hyperfunctioning nodules (in effect, and perhaps in fact, toxic adenomas) with complete suppression of radio-iodine uptake by the remainder of the goitre. In other cases multiple small groups of hyperplastic acini concentrate radioactive iodine though much of the gland is inactive, the appearances suggesting the effect of some extrinsic thyroid stimulator on a gland part of whose tissue is refractory. Thyroid microsomal antibody is found in the serum of such cases with the same frequency as in Graves' disease, but it remains to be seen whether thyroid-stimulating antibody is also demonstrable.

Tumours of the thyroid

Thyroid adenoma (Fig. 12.7, p. 325) is comparatively common. It has a fibrous capsule, compresses the surrounding gland, and is more often multiple than single. These tumours present varying appearances depending on the extent of degenerative change and the amount of colloid storage. Thus they may be haemorrhagic or cystic and, in the absence of degeneration, they may have the brown honeycomb appearance of colloid goitre on section or be composed of pale, fawn, soft, fleshy tissue. Microscopically some are composed of strands and cylinders of epithelium without acinar structure; others consist of very small acini containing little colloid (Fig. 26.16)—such tumours have been called '*fetal adenomas*', but they do not seem to be due to developmental errors. In yet others there may be considerable colloid storage. *It is not possible to distinguish between circumscribed hyperplastic changes constituting the nodules in nodular goitres and true adenomatous tumours.* Thyroid adenomas usually present clinically merely as localised swellings in the gland; those of the more cellular type are sometimes associated with hyperthyroidism. Some adenomas may possibly become malignant in the later years of life. It is often difficult to distinguish clinically and histologically between adenoma and carcinoma in the absence of metastases; *solitary tumours of the thyroid in children and young adults should be regarded with suspicion.*

Parathyroid adenomas occasionally occur in the substance of the thyroid. Simple connective tissue tumours such as fibromas and osteochondromas are rare.

Malignant tumours

Carcinoma of thyroid causes about 0·5 per cent of all deaths from cancer in this country. It invades surrounding structures, including the trachea and recurrent laryngeal nerves and death is commonly due to asphyxia. Its incidence is said to be higher in regions with endemic goitre but this is doubtful. It is known to result in some cases from x-irradiation of the neck in childhood, which was formerly used to treat haemangioma or supposed thymic enlargement. Some of the better differentiated human carcinomas may be TSH-dependent; treatment with thyroxine, which suppresses TSH production, has resulted in regression of established metastases in some cases and is thought to have prevented metastases in others. Also there are records of rapid growth of metastases following total thyroidectomy or the administration of anti-thyroid drugs. A noteworthy feature of well-differentiated thyroid carcinomas, especially in young patients, is the prolonged survival and well-being of the patient despite the presence of metastases.

In well-differentiated tumours, thyroglobulin can usually be demonstrated immunohistologically; this is sometimes helpful in patients presenting with metastatic tumour deposits and a clinically normal thyroid.

Papillary adenocarcinoma is the form most commonly encountered and is sometimes seen in children and young adults, in whom there is often a history of local x-irradiation (see above). The tumour is not well encapsulated, is sometimes only a few millimetres in diameter, and despite its relatively innocuous micro-

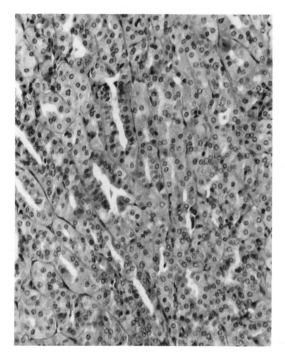

Fig. 26.16 Adenoma of the thyroid of follicular pattern, but with virtually no colloid. × 185.

scopical appearance it frequently spreads to the cervical lymph nodes, particularly of the side affected (Fig. 26.17). Indeed *all papillary tumours of the thyroid should be regarded as potentially malignant*. It was previously erroneously thought that cervical lymph-node metastases of this tumour were 'lateral aberrant thyroid'. Pulmonary and skeletal metastases are rarely found.

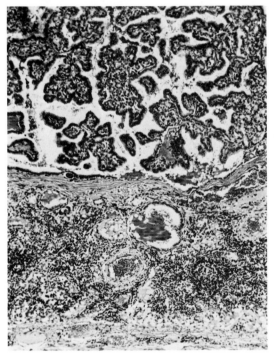

Fig. 26.17 Papillary cystadenocarcinoma of the thyroid in the cervical lymph nodes. × 65.

Follicular adenocarcinoma. Certain encapsulated tumours, with the gross appearance of adenomas, are carcinomas composed of glandular acini. The best differentiated examples closely resemble normal thyroid but more often there are mitotic figures and aberrant cells; in many cases solid sheets of tumour cells are also present, sometimes of eosinophilic 'Hürthle' type. Malignancy is recognised by invasion of the fibrous capsule and blood vessels, and metastasis is particularly common to bone and lung. Some of these tumours take up ^{131}I, which can be used therapeutically.

Occasionally squamous carcinoma is seen, possibly arising from the thyroglossal duct.

Anaplastic tumours. Anaplastic tumours of various types—round-cell, spindle-cell and giant-cell—are relatively common and the majority are probably anaplastic carcinomas rather than sarcomas. They cause respiratory obstruction from rapid enlargement of the gland. Tumours having the general appearance of poorly-differentiated lymphomas are sometimes difficult to distinguish from the more extreme examples of Hashimoto's disease, a difficulty accentuated by the fact that some have responded to radiotherapy and have not recurred, whereas others, histologically indistinguishable, behave as unequivocal malignant tumours. Brewer and Orr proposed the term *struma reticulosa* for this group and drew attention to the frequency of multiple growths of similar structure in the lymphoid tissues of the small intestine.

Medullary carcinoma. This tumour consists of solid masses of neoplastic C cells set in a hyaline stroma which in places contains amyloid and is sometimes calcified. Despite its rather anaplastic appearance the mitotic rate is usually low and survival for many years is common. The blood calcitonin level is usually abnormally high (especially after calcium infusion), making diagnosis possible in familial cases even before the tumour is palpable. No clinical syndrome of calcitonin excess has been recognised but medullary carcinoma, being a tumour of apud cells (p. 1034), is sometimes associated with diarrhoea, carcinoid syndrome or Cushing's syndrome. In a familial form of the disease there may be associated bilateral adrenal phaeochromocytomas and parathyroid adenomas (i.e. a special form of multiple endocrine adenoma syndrome) sometimes associated with neuromas of the buccal and conjunctival mucosae (Sipple syndrome).

Other thyroid disorders

Degenerative changes. Excluding changes in nodular goitre and tumours, degenerative changes in the thyroid are comparatively rare and of little importance. Evidence of damage produced by toxins is found in infections, and there may be actual necrosis of the epithelium. Amyloid disease may affect the thyroid either alone or as part of widespread amyloidosis. When well marked, it causes thyroid enlargement (*amyloid goitre*). Amyloid is found in the stroma of medullary carcinoma of the thyroid (see above). Hyaline change, calcification, etc., are often present in the stroma of chronic goitres.

Congenital abnormalities. The isthmus of the thyroid is formed by a downgrowth of a tube of epithelium from the base of the tongue (for-amen caecum). The upper portion of this tube above the hyoid bone is lined by squamous epithelium. If this persists and if the buccal end is obstructed, it may give rise to a 'lingual dermoid'. The lower part of the duct below the hyoid bone is lined by columnar ciliated epithelium. Thyroglossal cysts may take origin from this part when it does not undergo involution. Such a cyst may rupture on the skin surface, forming a median cervical fistula. In the walls of these cysts portions of thyroid tissue are sometimes found. Occasionally a mass of thyroid tissue is found in the base of the tongue, the so-called 'lingual thyroid', and the thyroid may then be absent from its normal site. Congenital absence and hypoplasia of the thyroid are among the causes of sporadic cretinism.

The Endocrine Pancreas

The lesions of the exocrine pancreas have already been described (p. 716) leaving for consideration here the disorders of the endocrine pancreas, i.e. the islets of Langerhans. The islets are more abundant in the body and tail than in the head. They consist of small cuboidal cells with a large vesicular nucleus, arranged in cords. Cell types include the *β cell* which produces insulin, the *α cell* which produces glucagon, the *δ cell* which produces somatostatin and cells which possibly secrete other polypeptide hormones. Insulin and glucagon are important in the intermediate metabolism of carbohydrates, fats and proteins; insulin increases the storage of these dietary components, whereas glucagon promotes their catabolism, and thus the two hormones have reciprocal functions. Insulin lack, either absolute or relative, causes diabetes mellitus, but in this disease and in normal carbohydrate intermediate metabolism, complex inter-relationships exist involving a number of different hormones. Somatostatin (originally regarded solely as a growth hormone release-inhibiting factor) is found not only in the *δ* cells of the pancreas, but also in the hypothalamus and other parts of the brain and in the D cells of the stomach, duodenum and jejunum. It inhibits insulin and glucagon release, probably by a local paracrine reaction. Deficiency of somatostatin may be responsible for unexplained neonatal hypoglycaemia.

Hyperfunction of the islets produces a spectrum of disorders dependent on which cell type is involved.

Diabetes mellitus

In diabetes there are varying degrees of failure to store and metabolise carbohydrates, with consequent hyperglycaemia and glycosuria. Insulin lack results in a failure of transport of glucose into muscle and adipose tissue. In the liver, insulin lack results in a failure to convert glucose to glycogen and in a failure to modulate hepatic gluconeogenesis (p. 1031). Consequently the blood sugar rises. Normally, the fasting blood glucose level is 4·5–5·5 mmol/litre (80–100 mg/100 ml), and the level does not rise above 10 mmol/litre (180 mg/100 ml) after oral glucose or a meal. In diabetes there is always hyperglycaemia after ingestion of carbohydrate, the glucose level reaching 22 mmol/litre (400 mg/100 ml) or more, and glycosuria results; the fasting blood sugar is usually raised but in mild diabetics may be within the normal range.

Glucose tolerance tests. When 50 g of glucose is given to a fasting normal person the blood sugar rises to a maximum level of about 8·3 mmol/litre (150 mg/100 ml) in about half an hour. In spite of continuing absorption from the gut, a comparatively rapid fall then occurs and the blood sugar reaches a normal level again within two hours. The rapid fall is due to stimulation of the β-cells of the pancreatic islets by the rise in the level of glucose; secretion of insulin is increased, and this enhances the utilisation of glucose.

The blood sugar curve of a diabetic patient after 50 g of glucose is quite different. It is absorbed normally from the gut and the blood level rises rapidly as before, and continues to do so for three or four hours, though the curve becomes less steep, and then there is a gradual fall which may go on for some hours. This shows that there is a deficiency in the normal metabolism of glucose. If the blood glucose in a normal subject is raised above 10 mmol/litre (180 mg/100 ml), glycosuria occurs, but in established cases of diabetes the renal threshold is raised and glycosuria does not occur until the blood sugar is substantially higher. Glucose tolerance tests are not required for diagnosis in frank diabetes, but are of great help in the diagnosis of doubtful cases, where slight or transient glycosuria is found on routine examination in the absence of overt symptoms. *Diabetes is excluded by a normal rise followed by the normal fall.* In some such cases, the glycosuria is due to the renal threshold value being abnormally low, e.g. about 7·2 mmol/litre (130 mg/100 ml), so that when glucose or much carbohydrate is administered and the blood sugar rises above this level, glucose is excreted by the kidneys. Such a condition is usually known as **renal glycosuria**. The condition is without serious effects. The result of a glucose tolerance test in which the 30 and 60 minute specimens show marked elevation of the blood sugar, often with glycosuria but with a normal 2-hour value, the so-called *lag curve*, is usually due to over-rapid absorption of glucose from the intestine without impairment of ability to metabolise glucose. Occasionally this type of curve is seen in persons who show a mild degree of impairment of glucose metabolism, and some of these eventually develop diabetes.

Clinical and biochemical changes

The disease is characterised by polyuria, polydipsia, polyphagia and weight loss. The principal biochemical manifestation is hyperglycaemia. When the normal renal capacity for glucose reabsorption is exceeded there is glycosuria and an osmotic diuresis with an accompanying loss of Na^+ and K^+. An increase in plasma osmolarity occurs, causing thirst and polydipsia. The loss of weight in spite of polyphagia results from the failure to utilise glucose, and from a compensatory increase in catabolism of proteins and fats.

Insulin normally stimulates the transport of amino acids into muscle and their synthesis into proteins. In insulin lack this protein synthesis is impaired, there is an accelerated rate of amino-acid catabolism to CO_2 and H_2O via the citric acid cycle, and in addition a marked increase in the rate of conversion of amino acids to glucose in the liver—gluconeogenesis. Glucagon, which is relatively increased in diabetes, helps to stimulate gluconeogenesis thus adding to the hepatic glucose which cannot be converted to glycogen, and so contributing to the hyperglycaemia.

In diabetes there is also an acceleration of fat catabolism. Increased amounts of free fatty acids are released from fat deposits. Normally they are catabolised to acetyl-CoA, which may be synthesised into new fatty acids, converted into ketone bodies, or completely catabolised via the citric acid cycle to CO_2 and H_2O. In insulin lack, increased amounts of acetyl-CoA are formed, and cannot be adequately catabolised because of the intracellular depletion of the carbohydrate components of the cycle. They are therefore preferentially converted into ketone bodies: two acetyl-CoA moieties are formed and in turn are converted into acetoacetic acid, which, together with its metabolites, acetone and β-hydroxybutyric acid, enter the circulation to produce ketosis. These 'ketone bodies' dissociate to yield hydrogen ions, and produce a metabolic acidosis (*keto-acidosis*) with a fall in plasma pH.

The metabolic acidosis (i) stimulates the respiratory centre, resulting in hyperventilation (Kussmaul breathing) which reduces the plasma HCO^-_3; (ii) results in acidification of the urine, excretion of the acidic ions of acetoacetate and β-hydroxybutyrate being accompanied by an increased excretion of NH_4^+ and later of Na^+ and K^+; this further aggravates the cationic loss which accompanies the glucose-induced osmotic diuresis. The total body Na^+ and K^+ are thus depleted; the serum Na^+ level falls, but the serum K^+ level is maintained at the expense of intracellular K^+, in part due to the acidosis and in part due to the lack of insulin, the movement of K$^+$ into cells being dependent on insulin and glucose.

This complex of metabolic disturbances produces hyperosmolarity, hypovolaemia, acidosis and electrolyte imbalance which have serious effects on the functions of neurons and result in **keto-acidotic coma**. In addition to this type of diabetic coma it has become recognised recently that there are two others. Firstly, **hyperosmolar non-ketotic coma**—approximately 15 per cent of diabetic coma admissions are of this type—in which there is massive dehydration and profound hyperglycaemia, usually in excess of 55 mmol/litre (1000 mg/100 ml) but with minimal or no keto-acidosis: this tends to develop slowly over a period of some weeks or months, usually in mild diabetics. The mechanism is not clear, but it is postulated that there is insufficient insulin for normal intracellular transport but sufficient to inhibit the increased lipolysis necessary to produce ketosis. Secondly, **lactic acidosis**, due to tissue anoxia, usually accompanies diabetic keto-acidosis: in a very small percentage of (usually mild) diabetics, severe lactic acidosis may *per se* produce coma. Some of the oral hypoglycaemic agents, notably phenformin, may produce this pattern, but the mechanisms are uncertain.

In addition to these forms of diabetic coma, **hypoglycaemic coma** is liable to occur when insulin therapy is not accompanied by adequate calorie intake.

Aetiology

The aetiology of diabetes remains unknown. Clinically, two 'primary' forms are recognised, type I or insulin-dependent diabetes and type II or non-insulin-dependent diabetes.

Type I or **insulin-dependent diabetes.** Formerly known as *juvenile* or *early-onset diabetes*, this appears to have a hereditary tendency of complex and probably multifactorial type. There is an increased incidence in individuals with any of the following HLA antigens: A1 or 2; B8, 15, 18 or 40; CW3; DW3 or 4; DRW3 or 4. The risk is further increased by the presence of two of the B locus alleles in the above list. Certain antigens, notably B7, DW2 and DRW2, are associated with a reduced incidence. These observations suggest considerable complexity of genetic factors in the aetiology of the disease.

Antibodies to islet cells have been detected in the serum of 70 per cent of patients tested soon after the onset: they subsequently decline and are detected in less than 10 per cent of patients 10 years after the onset: these persistently positive patients often have thyroid and gastric auto-antibodies, indicating an association with the organ-specific auto-immune diseases. The islet-cell antibodies react with all islet cells; they are not specific for β cells nor do they react with insulin. It seems probable that they develop following islet-cell injury and before the onset of clinical diabetes. There is a seasonal variation in onset, which is relatively common in autumn and winter, and virus infection is now suspected as the causal agent of the initial islet-cell injury.

Pancreatic changes. Morphometric studies have demonstrated that the β-cell mass is reduced in early-onset diabetes, and histological examination shows β-cell degranulation, the degree of which correlates with a reduction in extractable insulin. Extracellular deposition of hyalin, amyloid-like material (Fig. 26.18), fibrosis, lymphocytic infiltration, and, in untreated cases, hydropic degeneration due to glycogen accumulation in the islet cells, have all been observed, but are often inconspicuous at necropsy.

Type II or **non-insulin dependent diabetes** usually develops insidiously and occurs predominantly in older people—hence the former terms *maturity* or *late-onset diabetes*. There is a

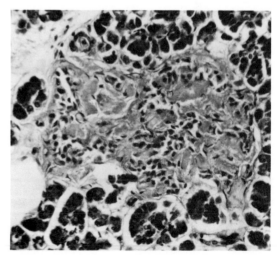

Fig. 26.18 Islet of Langerhans showing hyaline degeneration in a case of Type I diabetes. $\times$ 240.

female preponderance and the patients are frequently overweight. This type of diabetes has not been shown to be associated with particular HLA antigens. The hyperglycaemia can usually be controlled either by diet alone or by diet together with oral hypoglycaemic agents. In some of these patients there is apparent over-secretion of insulin, and the disease is thought to result from 'target cell' resistance, of un-known nature, to the hormone. In those pati-ents controllable by diet alone, the incidence of islet-cell antibody (approx 0·5 per cent) is scar-cely greater than in non-diabetic subjects, but about 10 per cent of those patients requiring oral hypoglycaemic agents or insulin have anti-body.

Other causes of diabetes. Secondary diabetes may complicate chronic pancreatitis, haem-ochromatosis, acromegaly, hypercortisolism (Cushing's syndrome or corticosteroid or ACTH therapy), glucagon-secreting tumours and phaeochromocytoma. Lesions of the brain can also cause hyperglycaemia and glycosuria, pos-sibly by hypothalamic disturbance. Acute hyperglycaemia can also occur in acute pan-creatitis.

In 1942 Shaw Dunn made a major experi-mental contribution to the study of diabetes by demonstrating that it could be induced per-manently in animals by administration of allo-xan. This compound causes a highly selective necrosis of the β-cells. It appears to attack cer-tain sulphydryl compounds and a rapid fall in the glutathione content of the blood follows. Injection of glutathione or cysteine before the injection of alloxan prevents the selective nec-rosis of islet cells.

Pathological changes

Apart from the changes in the pancreas dis-cussed above, diabetes predisposes to cardio-vascular disease, infections and various other complications.

Cardiovascular complications. Vascular dis-ease is one of the most serious complications of diabetes. Combined cardiovascular disease and diabetic glomerulosclerosis account for most deaths in diabetic patients. It is now customary to speak of a *diabetic macroangiopathy* involv-ing the large muscular arteries, and a *diabetic microangiopathy* most commonly affecting capillaries, but sometimes small arteries and arterioles. These complications appear not to be influenced by insulin control of the hyperglycaemic state and consequently have become progressively more important as deaths from keto-acidosis and infection have become less common.

In **diabetic macroangiopathy**, *atheroma* is the principal disease, but *Monckeberg's sclerosis* also shows an increased incidence. In general, atheroma develops early and becomes severe in diabetics of either sex, and consequently *myo-cardial and cerebral infarction and ischaemia* are unduly common.

Much recent and current interest has been focused on **diabetic microangiopathy**. In this, two types of lesion have been described: (*a*) a thickening of the basement membrane or an accumulation of basement membrane-like material in capillaries, and (*b*) endothelial cell proliferation together with basement mem-brane thickening affecting small arteries, arter-ioles and occasionally venules. The cause of the microangiopathy is uncertain. It is, however, of considerable importance in producing and con-tributing to peripheral vascular disease, dia-betic retinopathy (p. 800), diabetic glomerulo-sclerosis (p. 840), and possibly diabetic neur-opathy (p. 782) secondary to involvement of the vasa nervorum. Hypophyseal ablation sometimes arrests diabetic retinopathy, and there is some evidence that growth hormone may be implicated.

Infections. There is an increased susceptibility to bacterial and fungal infections, possibly due to glycogen deficiency in polymorphs (p. 184). Boils, carbuncles, urinary tract infections with pyelonephritis and renal papillary necrosis are of frequent occurrence and may precipitate diabetic coma. Diabetics have an increased incidence of tuberculosis, especially of the lungs, and unless treated the disease tends to progress rapidly.

Other pathological effects. Trophic disturb-ances such as ulceration or Charcot's joints may develop as complications of the diabetic neuropathy. Diabetic mothers show an in-creased liability to pre-eclamptic toxaemia and pregnancy aggravates the diabetic state. The babies of diabetic mothers are usually much above normal weight, and are flabby and oede-matous with a degree of erythroblastosis. A succession of unduly large children is strongly suggestive that the mother is diabetic or will later become so.

Hyperfunction of the endocrine pancreas

This results either from a hormone-secreting adenoma or carcinoma of islet type, although in occasional cases hyperplasia of the islets has been reported. The cells of the islets of Langerhans belong to that part of the endocrine system which has been called the **APUD** (**A**mine **P**recursor **U**ptake and **D**ecarboxylation) cell series. This series comprises the cells of the anterior pituitary, the C or parafollicular cells of the thyroid, various endocrine-secreting cells of the gastro-intestinal tract, including the gastrin-secreting G cells of the stomach and those cells which produce secretin and enteroglucagon, and probably also cells of the bronchi. These cells all secrete polypeptide hormones and have similar ultrastructural and histochemical properties. Tumours arising from them have been called **apudomas**.

It is now known that an apudoma may produce more than one hormone. This may be attributable to their containing more than one cell type.

Islet-cell tumour (nesidiocytoma)

This is a discrete, usually solitary mass, most often in the body or tail of the pancreas. There may be more than one such tumour, and sometimes associated tumours in the thyroid, parathyroid or pituitary—the *multiple-endocrine-adenoma* or *pluriglandular-adenoma syndrome*. Histologically, the component cells closely resemble normal islet cells, forming cords or clusters, and with a small amount of fibrovascular stroma. In some cases there is local deposition of amyloid material in the stroma (Fig. 26.19). A diagnosis of malignancy can seldom be made histologically, but apparently some 10 per cent of islet-cell tumours metastasise.

Islet-cell tumours may give rise to a number of syndromes by their secretory activity: these are outlined below. Others are nonfunctional.

Insulin-secreting tumours are of predominantly β-cell type and are associated with recurrent attacks of hypoglycemia, which may result in confusion, mania, somnolence, dizziness, loss of consciousness and other nervous symptoms: these effects can be prevented by taking glucose. Long intervals of freedom from symptoms may occur spontaneously, but prolonged episodes of hypoglycemia may lead to

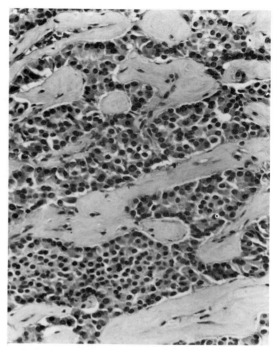

Fig. 26.19 A pancreatic islet-cell tumour showing the cords and clusters of tumour cells. The stroma contains amyloid material. × 230.

irreversible brain damage (p. 745). These tumours are rarely malignant.

Gastrin-secreting tumours cause persistent hypersecretion of acid gastric juice, producing multiple peptic ulcers which are refractory to medical treatment and may occur even in the jejunum. This combination constitutes the *Zollinger–Ellison syndrome* which tends to be slightly more common in males. More than half of these tumours are malignant. This syndrome may also arise from residual gastrin-secreting cells present in the pancreas in childhood. There may also be severe diarrhoea and also steatorrhoea from inhibition of lipase.

Other islet-cell tumours have been described which produce one or more of the following hormones. (i) **Glucagon**, resulting in diabetes and accompanied by peculiar skin manifestations. (ii) **Vasoactive intestinal peptide (VIP)**: these patients have watery diarrhoea, hypokalaemia and achlorhydria—the *'WDHA'* or *Verner–Morrison syndrome*. (iii) **Somatostatin**, with clinical hypochlorhydria, steatorrhoea and impaired (diabetic) glucose tolerance. (iv) **Inappropriate (ectopic) hormones** resulting in the *carcinoid syndrome, Cushing's syndrome*, etc.

The Parathyroids

The parathyroids, of branchial pouch origin, usually number four. They are small, yellowish-brown, and difficult to find at necropsy. Usually they are situated in the neck, posterior or postero-lateral to the thyroid but one or more may lie in the upper mediastinum. The majority of cells are *chief* and *water-clear* cells, which may represent differences in functional activity of a single cell type. With age, increasing numbers of *oxyphil cells* appear: their cytoplasm is rich in eosinophilic granules shown by electron-microscopy to be mitochondria. During childhood, fat cells appear in the parathyroids and increase up to middle-age.

Parathyroids secrete an essential hormone, *parathormone* (PTH), which is a single-chain polypeptide composed of 84 amino-acid residues: hormonal activity resides in the N-terminal sequences. The hormone is of vital importance, together with vitamin D, in regulating plasma calcium levels: the role of calcitonin (p. 1015) in human physiology remains uncertain. The mode of action of parathormone is not completely understood. It is known to stimulate resorption of bone and to promote excretion of phosphate by decreasing its reabsorption by the renal tubule: it may also promote reabsorption of calcium by the renal tubule and absorption of calcium from the gut. These latter possible effects may be due to the role of PTH in regulating the synthesis of the most active vitamin D metabolite, 1,25-DHCC (p. 884). Vitamin D derivatives may, in turn, exert a feed-back control on PTH secretion, which is stimulated by a fall in the level of ionised calcium in the plasma. Alkalosis or a raised plasma phosphate concentration may, by causing a fall in ionised calcium, also stimulate parathormone secretion, and in chronic renal failure phosphate retention may result in hyperplasia of the parathyroid glands.

PTH appears to exert its effect on target cells by activating adenyl cyclase (p. 144).

Parathyroid hyperfunction

This may be classified into *primary* and *secondary hyperparathyroidism*. In primary hyperparathyroidism excessive parathormone secretion occurs in the absence of any known physiological stimulus and various harmful effects result. Secondary hyperparathyroidism occurs when the glands are exposed to increased stimulation, as in the example of chronic renal failure mentioned above.

Primary hyperparathyroidism is usually due to a parathyroid adenoma (p. 1037) but occasionally to carcinoma or to primary hyperplasia of the chief or water-clear cells affecting all four glands. It may also result from 'inappropriate' production of parathormone by unrelated tumours (see below). Primary hyperparathyroidism may occur in as many as 1 in 1000 of the adult population although it is diagnosed much less frequently because the classical presenting features are often absent. It can occur at any age but is commonest in middle age and especially in post-menopausal women.

Presenting features and effects. The presenting features vary considerably depending on whether the symptoms and signs are mainly due to its effects on the kidney or bones or to hypercalcaemia, which may give rise to generalised muscle weakness, tiredness, anorexia, thirst and polyuria. *More than half the patients with primary hyperparathyroidism present with symptoms relating to renal stones*, which are rich in calcium salts and therefore detectable radiologically. Only a small proportion of patients with urolithiasis have hyperparathyroidism, but nevertheless its detection in this group is important. Metastatic deposition of calcium salts may occur in the walls of blood vessels, the lungs and gastric mucosa. Deposition in and around the renal tubules (nephrocalcinosis) is of special importance and may be visible radiologically. It leads to fibrosis, tubular injury and loss of nephrons; it is often complicated by pyelonephritis, and is likely to bring about chronic renal failure. *Symptoms relating to the bone changes (p. 890) are not frequent and overt radiological changes in the bones are recognisable in only about 10–20 per cent of patients, though most have some minor degree of microscopic abnormality.* Obvious bone changes tend to occur in those patients with relatively large and rapidly growing tumours and high levels of calcium and parathormone in the plasma. Patients presenting with renal stones tend to have smaller, slower growing tumours and less obvious increases in plasma calcium and parathormone.

Associated lesions include duodenal ulceration and chronic pancreatitis. Duodenal ulceration occurs in approximately 15 per cent of patients with hyperparathyroidism and is usually due to the enhancing effect of hypercalcaemia on gastrin. In some instances, however, there is more extensive peptic ulceration due to the association of a parathyroid adenoma with an islet-cell gastrin-secreting tumour (pluriglandular adenomatosis—p. 1034). The increased incidence of pancreatitis is unexplained.

Hyperparathyroidism also occurs in *Sipple's syndrome* (phaeochromocytoma associated with medullary thyroid carcinoma) and is usually due to parathyroid hyperplasia and rarely to an adenoma. When exploring the thyroid for a medullary carcinoma, opportunity should be taken to examine the parathyroids.

Diagnosis and sequelae. In suspected cases, repeated plasma calcium assays will usually confirm the diagnosis, but in occasional cases radio-immunoassay of PTH may be necessary. Removal of a functioning parathyroid adenoma is often followed by hypocalcaemia due to suppressed function of the remaining parathyroid glands; this is usually mild and lasts for only a few days. However, in those patients with marked bone changes hypocalcaemia may be more severe and persistent with tetany and psychotic disturbances; this is thought to be due to the avidity of the healing bone for calcium. Treatment with large calcium supplements, vitamin D and restriction of phosphate is necessary. Persistence of hypercalcaemia after removal of a parathyroid adenoma is usually due to the presence of a second, undetected adenoma (approximately 5 per cent of cases) or rarely to metastases from a parathyroid carcinoma. *If possible, all four parathyroids should be identified at operation to exclude the possibility of more than one adenoma.* In some instances no adenoma is present but all four glands are enlarged and hyperplastic. They may, however, differ considerably in size and unless the other glands are inspected an enlarged hyperplastic gland may be mistaken for an adenoma.

Hypercalcaemia is commonly observed in patients with cancer, and in some instances is due to 'ectopic' production of PTH or closely similar compounds with PTH activity. PTH production has so far been demonstrated in some squamous carcinomas of lung and elsewhere, and in some renal carcinomas. In other instances, hypercalcaemia results from tumour products quite different from PTH. Curiously, some carcinomas of lung and of breast secrete calcitonin.

Secondary hyperparathyroidism is compensatory to hypocalcaemia and occurs, for example, in chronic renal failure and in untreated malabsorption syndromes with osteomalacia. An additional factor in renal insufficiency may be failure of the kidney to convert vitamin D to its active metabolite (p. 884).

Occasionally in secondary hyperparathyroidism a parathyroid adenoma may develop, presumably in consequence of the hyperplasia. The hyperparathyroidism is then no longer compensatory: it is sometimes called **tertiary hyperparathyroidism**, and is characterised by a rising serum calcium level.

Hypoparathyroidism

Deficiency of parathormone secretion results in a fall in plasma ionised calcium and a rise in plasma phosphate. Hypocalcaemia increases the excitability of sensory and motor nerves, with various effects depending on the severity.

Causes. The commonest cause is *accidental removal of the parathyroid glands* during thyroidectomy. The condition sometimes develops following removal of a functioning parathyroid adenoma and it may then be mild and temporary or more severe and prolonged (see above). Thirdly, there is the so-called *idiopathic hypoparathyroidism* which, in some instances, is one of the organ-specific auto-immune diseases. *Congenital parathyroid deficiency* may also occur, for example in the DiGeorge syndrome (p. 170).

Effects. If severe, hypoparathyroidism results in overt **tetany**. The tone of the skeletal muscles is increased and there may be spasm of the hands and feet in characteristic positions, twitching and jerking movements, and painful cramps of the limb muscles. There may also be generalised convulsions resembling epileptiform fits. These manifestations of motor hypersensitivity are usually accompanied by paraesthesias, often by psychotic disturbances and sometimes even by dementia. In less severe parathormone deficiency, muscle tone may be increased but without obvious twitching, spasms or convulsions. Such latent tetany may be demonstrated by increased responsiveness of neuromuscular junctions to electrical stimuli and by various tests depending upon irritability of the nerves to mechanical stimuli. The nails tend to be brittle and there is a high incidence of cataract formation.

Idiopathic hypoparathyroidism. There is a rare acquired form of idiopathic hypoparathyroidism; it is commoner in women than men, and in many cases antibody to a cytoplasmic constituent of parathyroid epithelium is demonstrable in the serum by the immunofluorescence technique. The condition is an organ-specific auto-immune disorder (p. 162), and is sometimes associated with other disorders of this group, notably primary adrenocortical atrophy, pernicious anaemia, chronic thyroiditis or thyrotoxicosis. Another association is with moniliasis of the fingers and toes. There is no detectable PTH in the plasma and hypocalcaemia with detectable levels of PTH is most likely to be due to pseudohypoparathyroidism, assuming that rickets has been excluded.

Pseudohypoparathyroidism. A familial hereditary disorder, with the clinical and biochemical features of hypoparathyroidism, skeletal defects and metastatic ossification, has been described and given the above title because the abnormalities are not responsive to parathormone, and the parathyroids are actually hyperplastic. The disorder is therefore not due to lack of secretion but to failure to respond to it.

Other causes of tetany

Tetany used to be seen in children with **rickets**, in which there is deficient absorption of calcium from the intestine, although in many cases a compensatory hyperplasia and over-activity of the parathyroids is observed and may prevent tetany. Calcium deficiency may also result from the increased loss during **pregnancy and lactation** and this may lead to tetany. Thirdly, **alkalosis** may lower the level of ionic calcium in the plasma, and tetany is thus seen occasionally in patients with pyloric stenosis and repeated vomiting of acid gastric juice; indeed, even the alkalosis induced by hyperventilation may bring about or aggravate tetany.

Tumours

The commonest form of tumour is the adenoma, and in most cases this has been associated with hyperfunction as described above. It may exceed 5 cm in diameter but is usually much smaller: it is of yellowish-brown colour, occurring most often in the lower glands.

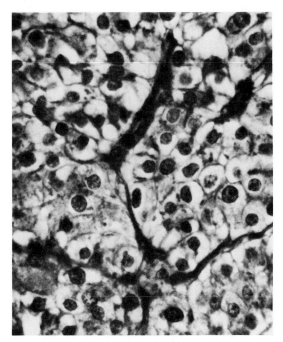

Fig. 26.20 Adenoma of parathyroid from a case of generalised osteitis fibrosa (p. 891). Both pale oxyphil and water-clear cells are present. × 500.

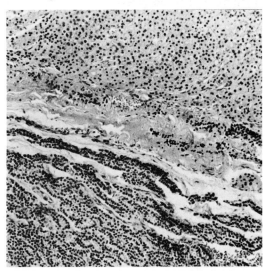

Fig. 26.21 Parathyroid adenoma, showing parathyroid tissue (*below*) separated by a thin capsule from the adenoma (*above*). × 100.

Microscopic examination shows that the cells of the tumour are similar to those of the normal gland—chief, water-clear and oxyphil cells in various proportions (Fig. 26.20). In spite of the richness of oxyphil cells in enzymes and mitochondria, pure oxyphil-cell adenomas seldom secrete excess of hormone. The cells are often larger than the normal cells and their nuclei may be very large in parts of the tumour; this does not indicate any tendency to malignancy. Also a stretched rim of normal parathyroid is often seen at the periphery of the adenoma (Fig. 26.21). These features are not seen in parathyroid hyperplasia. Cells of columnar form may occur and a papillary type of growth may be present in an adenoma, which may be incorporated in the substance of the thyroid. As noted earlier, adenomas may occur in two or more parathyroid glands. Carcinoma may arise in a parathyroid but is very rare; unless it causes hyperparathyroidism, its histogenesis is usually in doubt.

The Adrenals

Introduction. The adrenal glands are complex organs, the cortex being mesodermal and the medulla of neural origin. The cortex is the site of synthesis and secretion of a number of steroid hormones termed **corticosteroids**, which have various important effects on water and electrolyte balance, carbohydrate, protein and fat metabolism, immune responses and inflammatory reactions. The adrenal cortex is essential to life, mainly because of its control of fluid and electrolytes.

The adrenal medulla may be regarded as an effector organ of the sympathetic nervous system, for it secretes the **catecholamines**. By their secretions, both the cortex and medulla play major roles in the response to mental or physical stress, e.g. injury, shock, infections, severe illness and emotional disturbances. Also the medullary hormone adrenaline stimulates release of ACTH by the pituitary, which in turn increases the output of cortisol and related steroid hormones by the adrenal cortex.

The adrenal cortex

Adrenocortical hormones

These are all steroids and fall into three physiological groups, the *mineralocorticoids, glucocorticoids* and *cortical sex steroids*.

Mineralocorticoids are so-called because they play a major role in the homeostasis of sodium, potassium and water. The most important one is **aldosterone**, of which, under normal conditions, 80–100 μg is secreted daily into the blood. Aldosterone is synthesised and secreted by the cells of the *zona glomerulosa*, i.e. the peripheral part of the cortex. Its synthesis and release are largely independent of pituitary control, and are stimulated by the renin-angiotensin system (p. 258) so that a low sodium concentration in the renal tubule or low renal perfusion pressure, as in hypovolaemia, leads to secretion of aldosterone which increases renal tubular reabsorption of sodium and chloride and so reduces their loss in the urine. The consequent rise in osmolarity of the blood results in secretion of ADH (p. 1015) so that there is oliguria and fluid retention. Aldosterone also increases the tubular secretion of potassium, thus promoting potassium loss in the urine. Conversely, a rise of plasma (or tubular) sodium or increase in blood volume inhibits secretion of renin and so of aldosterone, with the result that renal loss of salt and water increases. Aldosterone also has a very weak glucocorticoid effect.

Glucocorticoids. These, like aldosterone, are C21 steroids. In man, **cortisol (hydrocortisone)** is the most important, about 20–30 mg being secreted daily; the others of physiological significance are cortisone, corticosterone and 11-dehydrocorticosterone. Synthesis and secretion of glucocorticoids is controlled by ACTH which, in turn, is regulated by a feed-back mechanism (p. 1009).

Glucocorticoids have a number of effects, of which the following are particularly important; (1) they stimulate production of glucose from protein (*gluconeogenesis*), with consequent rise in blood glucose, and deposition of glycogen in the liver; (2) they inhibit protein synthesis and increase protein catabolism in many tissues, including the muscles and skin; (3) in large dosage, glucocorticoids (*a*) have an anti-inflammatory effect, partly by interfering with emigration of polymorphs and macrophages and by stabilising the lysosomes of these cells, but they probably exert several other anti-inflammatory effects, (*b*) have a cytotoxic effect on lymphocytes, with consequent atrophy of the thymus and other lymphoid tissues and suppression of immune responses, particularly cell-mediated immunity, (*c*) inhibit somatic growth by suppressing secretion of growth hormone, and (*d*) result in deposition of subcutaneous fat in the face and trunk. Glucocorticoids also have mineralocorticoid activity, but this is very much weaker than that of aldosterone.

Glucocorticoids are synthesised and secreted by cells of the wide intermediate *zona fasciculata* and the narrow inner *zona reticularis* of the adrenal cortex. Their output is largely proportional to the concentration of circulating ACTH. In histological and other investigations on necropsy material from patients dying shortly after acute injury, etc., Symington and others (1955) equated certain changes in the pituitary with ACTH secretion and observed a correlation with loss of lipid from the cells of the zona fasciculata of the adrenals and with increase in RNA and various enzymes in the zona fasciculata and zona reticularis: these adrenal changes, formerly regarded as indicating functional exhaustion, were considered to reflect *increased* functional activity. As would be expected, destruction of the adenohypophysis is followed by very severe atrophy of the zona fasciculata and reticularis, but persistence of the zona glomerulosa, which continues to secrete aldosterone.

The adrenal sex hormones are **ketosteroids**: their physiological role is obscure, for the amounts of androgen and oestrogen secreted by the adrenals are insignificant compared with the

endrocrine activity of the gonads. In the pathological conditions, excessive secretion of adrenal ketosteroids can, however, cause premature puberty, virilism in females and very rarely feminisation in males.

Adrenocortical hyperfunction

As stated above, adrenal cortical hormones are of three principal types, the glucocorticoids regulating the intermediary metabolism of carbohydrate, fat and protein, the mineralocorticoids controlling electrolyte balance, and the ketosteroids which have androgenic and oestrogenic effects.

Three corresponding types of adrenal cortical hyperfunction are known to exist.

Cushing's syndrome (chronic hypercortisolism)

Cushing's syndrome results from excessive secretion of cortisol by the adrenal cortex or a cortical tumour. Although its natural occurrence is uncommon, it is important to recognise it as in most cases treatment can relieve an otherwise potentially fatal condition. Closely similar features are observed in patients on prolonged treatment with high doses of glucocorticoids or ACTH.

Clinical features. Cushing's syndrome occurs most often in women over a wide age range but is seen also in men and children. *In all instances the main features are due to cortisol excess although there is frequently in addition excessive androgen secretion resulting in virilism.*

In a severe case, i.e. with grossly excessive cortisol secretion, the features include: (1) *painful adiposity* of the face, neck and trunk which contrasts with the relatively thin limbs (Fig. 26.22); (2) *increased protein breakdown*, with consequent thinning of the skin, generalised osteoporosis and wasting and weakness of the skeletal muscles. The face is highly coloured and the weakened skin becomes stretched along lines of stress, e.g. where fat has accumulated in the abdomen, resulting in purple striae in which the small vessels are visible through the stretched skin. Osteoporosis is particularly important in the spine and may result in collapse of vertebral bodies, with kyphosis, etc. Muscle weakness and wasting are usually prominent features; (3) *systemic hypertension* in most cases; (4) *diminished glucose tolerance,*

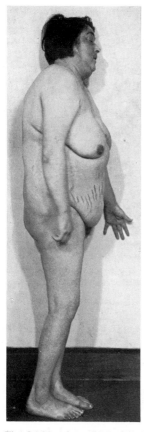

Fig. 26.22 A patient with Cushing's syndrome, subsequently cured by irradiation of the pituitary. Note the characteristic obesity of the face, neck and trunk, dusky cyanosis and facial hair, and striae of the abdominal skin.

which is usually only apparent following ingestion of carbohydrate, but in approximately 20 per cent of patients is more severe with a high fasting blood glucose level and glycosuria; (5) an increased tendency to *bacterial infections* and poor healing of wounds, and (6) *arrest of growth in affected children*. Mental confusion and psychoses are also common.

All the above features are explicable on the basis of excessive cortisol secretion. In addition, women with Cushing's syndrome usually show some features of virilism, e.g. masculine distribution of hair, acne, oligomenorrhoea, and sometimes enlargement of the clitoris and deepening of the voice. The changes in the pituitary resulting from hypercortisolism have already been described (p. 1011).

Unless treated, Cushing's syndrome is likely to result in death from the effects of hyperten-

sion, from bacterial infections or from suicide.

Diagnosis is based on the observation of abnormally high levels of plasma cortisol in evening specimens of blood (when the level is normally lowest), together with excess of 17-hydroxysteroids (excretory products of cortisol) in 24-hour urine specimens.

There is commonly increased excretion of 17-hydroxysteroids in obese individuals, and an association between common obesity and Cushing's syndrome has long been suspected. However, the demonstration of normal plasma levels and urinary excretion of cortisol has now ruled this out.

Causation and types. There are three major types of Cushing's syndrome and effective treatment depends on differentiating between them. Firstly, there may be **a cortical adenoma** which secretes cortisol in uncontrolled fashion. In such cases the high cortisol level suppresses ACTH secretion and so the cortisol hypersecretion is wholly resistant to dexamethasone (which suppresses ACTH secretion). About 5 per cent of cases of Cushing's syndrome, including most cases in childhood, are due to a *cortical adenoma*, which often exceeds 30 mm in diameter. Excision is curative. There may be *multiple micro-adenomas* necessitating bilateral adrenalectomy. Only 1 per cent of cases are due to adrenal carcinoma.

Secondly, Cushing's syndrome may be due to **excessive secretion of ACTH by the adenohypophysis**. An adenohypophyseal adenoma of basophil or sometimes chromophobe cell type can be detected in only 20 per cent or so of cases; this form of Cushing's syndrome is sometimes confusingly called *Cushing's disease*.

The plasma level of ACTH is raised and high doses of dexamethasone will, by suppressing ACTH secretion, reduce the output of cortisol. The adrenals show cortical hyperplasia (Fig. 26.23), although they may be depleted of lipid and so not necessarily enlarged. This is the commonest form of Cushing's syndrome in adults and treatment consists of reducing the excessive secretion of ACTH. This can usually be achieved by microdissection of the pituitary or irradiation, e.g. by a cyclotron, and it is often possible to relieve the condition without inducing hypopituitarism. Results of irradiation are, however, poor when the pituitary is obviously enlarged and it is now believed that in most of the adult cases without a pituitary

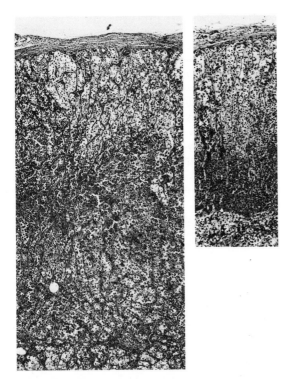

Fig. 26.23 Hyperplasia of the adrenal cortex in Cushing's syndrome (*left*) compared with a normal adrenal (*right*). The zona reticularis is greatly thickened and the cells of the zona fasciculata appear compact. In this instance, the adrenals were appreciably enlarged. × 45.

tumour the primary disturbance is in hypothalamic function. Treatment by adrenalectomy is sometimes followed by hyperpigmentation of the skin.

Thirdly, Cushing's syndrome may result from the **inappropriate secretion of ACTH by a nonpituitary tumour**—the *ectopic ACTH syndrome*. This is most commonly due to an oat-cell bronchial carcinoma but various other tumours including carcinoids, thymic, pancreatic and even adrenal tumours may be responsible. The clinical features of this form of Cushing's syndrome are often not conspicuous and wasting and weakness, etc., are likely to be attributed to malignant cachexia. The plasma level of ACTH is high and cortisol secretion is not suppressed by dexamethasone.

Where other methods of treatment are inappropriate there is the possibility of administering drugs which are cytotoxic to adrenal cortical cells.

Iatrogenic Cushing's Syndrome. The prolonged administration of high doses of glucocorticoids or ACTH results in the development of the features of Cushing's syndrome and the decision to use such therapy obviously requires careful judgement. Glucocorticoid therapy and certain forms of Cushing's syndrome are followed by a period of adrenocortical insufficiency (p. 1045).

Primary aldosteronism (Conn's syndrome)

This syndrome, first described by Conn in 1955, is due to uncontrolled and excessive secretion of aldosterone, usually by an adrenal adenoma. It differs from secondary aldosteronism in which the excessive adrenal activity is in response to angiotensin (p. 258).

Excessive secretion of aldosterone results in retention of sodium, and so of fluid, and increased excretion of potassium. The sodium and water retention results in *hypertension* which is usually moderate but may be severe and even malignant (accelerated). *Hypokalaemia* is usual but not invariable: if severe it may disturb cardiac rhythm, sometimes causing attacks of syncopy, and there may also be attacks of muscular weakness and hypokalaemic *alkalosis* associated with tetany, cramps and paraesthesias. Hypokalaemia also impairs renal concentrating capacity, resulting in nocturia and polyuria. The plasma sodium concentration is usually raised or in the upper normal range.

Diagnosis of the syndrome in patients with hypertension depends on the demonstration of an increased rate of secretion (or excretion) of aldosterone in spite of a high sodium intake, and a low level of plasma renin during a period of sodium restriction. Both of these criteria are essential as many patients with 'essential' hypertension have a low plasma renin and increased aldosterone secretion occurs commonly as a secondary effect in various conditions. Hypokalaemia can occur from various causes in any type of hypertension.

Primary aldosteronism is usually due to a single adrenal cortical tumour, most commonly an adenoma, rarely a carcinoma. In some cases, however, there is no tumour but bilateral hyperplasia of the zona glomerulosa with or without multiple nodules. Excision of the offending tumour is curative. If no tumour is found removal of one adrenal and part of the other may effect a cure or, if not, facilitate control by drugs, e.g. spironolactone.

Hypersecretion of adrenocortical sex steroids

The adrenals normally secrete much smaller amounts of sex steroids than the gonads, but clinical sexual disturbances can result from adrenocortical hyperfunction. Least rare is the virilism which is usually a feature of *Cushing's syndrome* in women. Secondly, some *adrenal tumours* secrete excess of sex steroids, more commonly androgen than oestrogen, and so may bring about precocious puberty in males and virilism in girls and women. In such cases, there will be an increase in urinary excretion of 17-ketosteroids unaccompanied by hypercortisolism and resistant to suppression by dexamethasone. An ovarian androblastoma has similar effects. Adrenal virilism may result from an adenoma (Fig. 26.24) or a carcinoma. Feminising adrenal tumours are very rare.

Thirdly, adrenal virilism can arise from *deficiency of 21-hydrolase*, one of a group of enzyme defects described below.

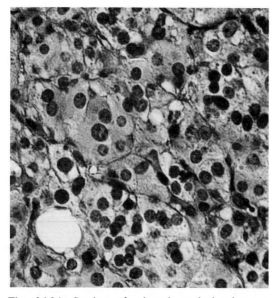

Fig. 26.24 Section of adrenal cortical adenoma associated with virilism, showing trabecular structure with tendency to variation in the size of cells. × 375.

Adrenocortical enzyme defects

There is a group of conditions due to autosomal recessive traits, in each of which there is deficiency of one of the enzymes necessary for steroid hormone biosynthesis.

In one condition, 20-hydrolase is deficient and steroid synthesis in the adrenals and gonads stops at the cholesterol stage. The adrenals become hyperplastic and greatly enlarged due to accumulation of cholesterol. The external genitalia are of female appearance (in both genetic males and females) and the affected infants usually die.

The least rare member of the group is *deficiency of 21-hydrolase*, which is necessary for synthesis of both cortisol and aldosterone. This results in increased secretion of ACTH (and probably also renin), with consequent adrenocortical hyperplasia. The defect varies in severity in different families. In severe cases, deficiency of glucocorticoids and mineralocorticoids results in features resembling those of Addison's disease. There is, however, an increased secretion of precursor steroids, which do not suppress ACTH secretion. They include the androgen dehydroepiandrosterone (DHEA), which causes masculinisation, so that the female infant is born with partially fused labia and clitoral enlargement and resembles a cryptorchid male with hypospadias ('*female pseudohermaphroditism*'), while precocious puberty occurs in affected males. Less severely affected females may present in childhood with virilism or later because of failure of puberty. In many cases, the defect is not severe, and the adrenal hyperplasia may result in sufficient cortisol and aldosterone production, so that the sex disturbances are the main feature.

Others in this group of enzyme defects include: (i) a condition similar to 21-hydrolase deficiency; (ii) deficiency of sex hormones and of cortisol together with excess mineralocorticoid secretion, resulting in sexual infantilism and hypertension; (iii) cortisol deficiency with increased secretion of androgens and mineralocorticoids, resulting in virilism and hypertension.

Early diagnosis of these conditions is very important, for it provides the opportunity to administer the deficient steroid(s), thus restoring the functional balance. In 21-hydrolase deficiency, for example, cortisol therapy (with extra salt and fluorocortisone if necessary) suppresses ACTH, and so reverses the adrenal hyperplasia and excessive androgen secretion: affected females treated early are sexually normal and fertile.

Primary adrenocortical hypofunction

The function of the adrenal cortex is partly dependent on normal production and secretion of ACTH and gonadotrophic hormones by the adenohypophysis, and, as already explained, pituitary failure results in depression of cortisol production by the adrenals, thyroxine by the thyroid, etc. In contrast to such *secondary* failure, primary adrenal hypofunction occurs in spite of normal pituitary function, i.e. the defect lies in the adrenals.

Primary adrenocortical hypofunction can occur as an acute condition in states of severe toxaemia, or it can develop from gradual adrenocortical destruction, usually due to an auto-immune reaction or to tuberculosis.

Acute adrenocortical insufficiency

The fatal effects of bilateral adrenalectomy in experimental animals are due to loss of cortical tissue: death can be delayed by giving salt and prevented by corticosteroids. The same applies to man, in whom bilateral adrenalectomy is performed in the treatment of selected cases of breast cancer, cortical hyperfunction or hypertension.

Acute adrenocortical insufficiency occurs also in some cases of septicaemia, particularly meningococcal, and in severe endotoxic shock: the adrenals become grossly haemorrhagic—'adrenal apoplexy' (Fig. 26.25). The cortex, which in fatal cases is largely necrotic, may be visible as a thin yellow layer stretched over the grossly swollen, haemorrhagic medulla. This condition is known also as the **Waterhouse–Friderichsen syndrome** and requires immediate and vigorous therapy.

Other toxic infections, e.g. diphtheria, may be associated with marked congestion and small haemorrhages in the adrenals, but these changes are now regarded as consistent with increased cortical activity and do not indicate failure.

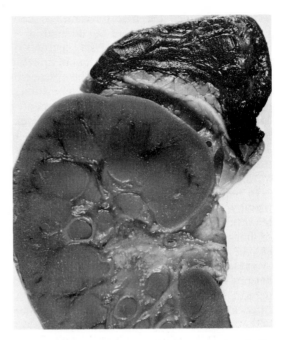

Fig. 26.25 Acute haemorrhagic necrosis of the adrenals in a child who died of meningococcal septicaemia. The adrenal lesion was bilateral.

The symptoms and biochemical changes of acute adrenocortical insufficiency are due mainly to deficiency of mineralocorticoids and glucocorticoids.

Deficiency of mineralocorticoids results in inadequate function of the distal convoluted tubules: there is failure to re-absorb salt and to secrete potassium, so that *salt deficiency, hyperkalaemia* and *dehydration* (p. 1038) result. Death is due to a combination of hypovolaemic shock and electrolyte disturbances. Loss of medullary function, which is important in adaptation to hypovolaemia (p. 261), is likely to aggravate the condition. These effects can, however, be prevented and reversed by administration of fluid, salt and mineralocorticoid.

Deficiency of glucocorticoids results in failure of gluconeogenesis with consequent *hypoglycaemia* and greatly *increased sensitivity to insulin.* Another effect is *vomiting* which increases the fluid and electrolyte disturbances.

Chronic adrenocortical insufficiency—Addison's disease

Addison's description, in 1855, of this condition and its relationship to lesions of the adrenals provided the first fundamental contribution to the pathology of the adrenals.

Clinical features. The outstanding features of Addison's disease are weakness, loss of appetite and weight, and hypotension. In the absence of these features the diagnosis is unlikely. Libido is usually diminished and the skin pigmented (p. 277), particularly the exposed parts, the external genitalia and scars; the pigmentation is increased by skin irritants and in mild cases may be the most noticeable feature. Sometimes, however, it is inconspicuous.

In the absence of high salt intake or steroid therapy, failure of reabsorption of salt in the renal tubules results in *hyponatraemia*, a finding of diagnostic value, and this is accompanied by *chronic dehydration.*

These features result from the combined deficiency of mineralocorticoids and glucocorticoids. Mineralocorticoid deficiency, as indicated above, results in loss of salt and water, with consequent hypovolaemia, hypotension, weakness and some weight loss. Chronic glucocorticoid deficiency contributes listlessness, mental confusion, hypoglycaemia, increased secretion of ACTH and MSH, impaired pressor response to catecholamines and poor reaction to stress. Anorexia, nausea, sometimes vomiting, and so weight loss and increased chloride deficiency, are also attributable to lack of glucocorticoids.

In addition to these chronic symptoms and signs *there also occur in Addison's disease acute exacerbations or* **crises**, *which are among the gravest emergencies in medical practice, demanding energetic investigation and therapy to prevent death.* In these there occur severe vomiting, which aggravates chloride loss, fall in blood pressure and extreme asthenia with hypoglycaemia terminating in collapse. Such a crisis may be precipitated by even minor infections, indiscretions in diet, or by vomiting or diarrhoea, in fact by anything which depletes still further the blood sodium level. As in acute adrenocortical insufficiency (see above) there is acute salt deficiency, dehydration and pre-renal uraemia, and death is liable to result from hypovolaemic shock and electrolyte disturbances.

Pathological changes. The commonest cause of Addison's disease in Europe was formerly destruction of the adrenals by chronic tuberculosis, which converts both glands into fibrocaseous masses. Where tuberculosis has declined, more cases of Addison's disease are now due to atrophy of the adrenal cortex accompanied by lymphocytic and plasma-cell infiltration (Fig. 26.26). The medulla is relatively un-

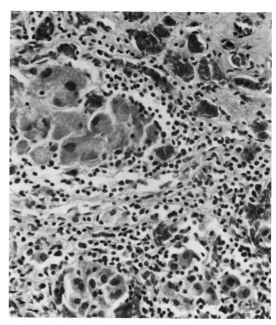

Fig. 26.26 Primary adrenal atrophy (auto-immune adrenalitis) in Addison's disease. Most of the cortical cells have been destroyed and the cortex consists of vascular fibrous tissue. In places there are foci of enlarged cortical cells with associated lymphocytic and plasma cell infiltration. × 320.

affected and this shows that loss of the cortex is the main cause of the symptoms of Addison's disease. Antibodies to adrenocortical tissue were first detected in this laboratory in 1957 (see Goudie *et al.*, 1968), in the serum of two patients with non-tuberculous Addison's disease, and their presence in over 50 per cent of cases has since been confirmed by various workers. They have been shown to react with lipoprotein of the endoplasmic reticulum of the cortical cells, and are not formed in cases of tuberculous Addison's disease. This finding, and the well-established associations of 'idiopathic' Addison's disease with chronic thyroiditis, thyrotoxicosis, atrophic gastritis and idiopathic hypoparathyroidism, indicate that it is one of the organ-specific auto-immune diseases (p. 162). Less commonly, fungal infections or amyloidosis of the adrenals result in Addison's disease, while rarely destruction of the glands by metastatic tumour is the cause. In all cases the syndrome of Addison's disease depends upon loss of 90 per cent or more of the cortical tissue.

It was also demonstrated by Anderson *et al.* (1968) that, while the adrenal antibodies of Addison's disease usually react specifically and solely with adrenocortical cells, in occasional cases antibody is present which reacts also with other steroid-producing cells, i.e. the theca-lutein and true lutein cells of the corpus luteum, the theca-interna cells of the Graafian follicle, placental trophoblast, Leydig cells and hilus cells of the ovary. In some female patients with Addison's disease accompanied by amenorrhoea and sterility, Irvine *et al.* (1968) demonstrated the presence of this steroid-cell antibody, and described destructive inflammatory changes in the ovaries.

In tuberculous Addison's disease the adrenals are enlarged, firm and irregular. They are changed into masses of putty-like caseous material, with dense fibrous tissue surrounding it (Fig. 26.27); calcification is frequent and may be detectable radiographically.

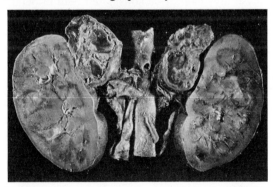

Fig. 26.27 Adrenal glands in tuberculous Addison's disease, showing extensive caseation and enlargement.

In some cases there are no obvious tuberculous lesions in the lungs or lymph nodes.

Apart from the adrenal lesions the main necropsy finding in Addison's disease is marked wasting of the muscles and adipose tissue. Atrophy of the heart is also striking; it is often more marked than in other wasting diseases, perhaps because of the low blood pressure. The gonads and breasts are also atrophic.

In Addison's disease there is a decrease of heavily-granulated basophil cells in the adenohypophysis with increase in sparsely granulated basophils: the latter are believed to secrete

ACTH. Acidophil cells are also diminished. The disturbance of carbohydrate metabolism results in a marked decrease in liver glycogen, the patients are highly sensitive to insulin and attacks of hypoglycaemia are fairly common.

In mild cases of Addison's disease, oral glucocorticoids and a high salt diet may be satisfactory, but in more severe cases the weak mineralocorticoid activity of glucocorticoids is inadequate and mineralocorticoids must be given.

Diagnosis of Addison's disease is readily confirmed by measuring the plasma levels and urinary output of corticosteroids before and during an infusion of ACTH. The distinction between auto-immune and tuberculous adrenalitis in Addison's disease is based on the history and appropriate tests (see above).

Assay of plasma ACTH levels readily distinguishes primary from secondary adrenal insufficiency.

Adrenocortical hypofunction from 'disuse'

The prolonged high dosage of glucocorticoids now used to treat various conditions results in suppression of ACTH secretion and so atrophy of the fasciculate and reticulate zones of the adrenal cortex. This occurs also in Cushing's syndrome due to an adrenal adenoma. Following removal of the tumour or cessation of prolonged glucocorticoid therapy it may take some months for full restoration of cortical function and reserve, and it may be necessary to administer corticosteroids in gradually diminishing dosage, with increased dosage to cover additional stress imposed by infections, surgical operations, etc.

Secondary adrenocortical insufficiency

This results from pituitary failure with diminished secretion of ACTH and consequently of adrenocortical steroids, particularly glucocorticoids. The condition has been considered earlier in relation to hypopituitarism.

Adrenocortical tumours

The commonest cortical tumours are **adenomas**. They occur in the form of comparatively small, rounded nodules, well defined, and usually of yellow colour, owing to the large amount of fat and steroids in the cells; they are sometimes multiple. In the smaller adenomas the cells are arranged in trabeculae and resemble closely those of the zona fasciculata; but particularly in the larger examples the cells may become large, often contain more than one nucleus, and all transitions to distinctly aberrant forms occur. The tumour rarely becomes malignant.

A cortical adenoma may be associated with abnormal sexual development as described above, causing either precocious puberty or virilism, or Cushing's syndrome, or it may, more rarely, secrete aldosterone in excess (p. 1041). It is becoming increasingly apparent that most cortical adenomas synthesise and secrete hormones, although most often in amounts insufficient to give rise to clinical abnormalities. The secretory activity of cortical adenomas may fluctuate considerably, even in those which produce clinical effects, and this may add greatly to the difficulties of diagnosis. Sometimes carcinoma is bilateral, although one may be a metastasis. Excessive hormone secretion may persist in spite of much cellular aberration.

The adrenal medulla

Sympathetic nerve endings and chromaffin cells (so named because they reduce chrome salts, producing brown reduction products) secrete catecholamines. Sympathetic nerve endings are the main source of the noradrenaline in the blood, while the adrenal medulla is responsible for intermittent secretion of adrenaline. The blood level of both of these catecholamines is increased almost instantaneously by stressful situations, e.g. by emotion, injury or shock. Part of the stimulus is neural, but histamine, bradykinin and various drugs have a direct stimulating effect. Secretion of adrenaline by the adrenal medulla is in some way dependent on a normal functional cortex, the blood from which is rich in corticosteroids and perfuses the medulla. In turn, adrenaline stimulates secretion of ACTH and so indirectly influences cortical function.

The binding of catecholamines to α- and β-receptors has a profound influence on the function of many types of tissue cell, and its elucidation is not only throwing considerable light on control of cellular function, but has also provided opportunity to develop drugs which activate or block α- or β-receptors and thus influence cell functions in various ways. Stimulation of β-receptors activates adenyl cyclase activity and so increases the intracellular cyclic AMP (p. 144), the effect of which depends on the type of cell stimulated and on the additional effects of various other hormones on it. Stimulation of cholinergic receptors activates guanyl cyclase with consequent increase in intracellular cyclic GMP, which usually produces the opposite effect to a rise in cAMP. The mechanism by which α-receptor stimulation influences cell functions is obscure.

This profoundly important aspect of cell physiology cannot be considered here in detail, but it must be emphasised that increased secretion of catecholamines in conditions of shock (p. 261) is of great importance in maintaining the blood pressure by causing vasoconstriction in the skin and splanchnic circulation: noradrenaline has the greater effect, because it causes vasoconstriction also in skeletal muscles.

In spite of these adaptive effects of adrenal medullary function, the most important effects of adrenal failure are due to deficiency of corticosteroids.

Hypersecretion of catecholamines is observed in patients with a functioning tumour of the adrenal medulla or of chromaffin cells elsewhere, i.e. a *phaeochromocytoma*, the features of which are described below.

Tumours of the medulla

These are of three types. Two of them take origin from nerve cells, namely the **ganglioneuroma**, a simple growth containing ganglionic nerve cells and nerve fibres, and the **neuroblastoma** or **sympathicoblastoma** composed of embryonic nerve cells or neuroblasts. These tumours are described elsewhere (pp. 787–9). Neuroblastoma is much the commoner growth; it occurs particularly in infants and children. It may reach a large size, is composed of soft cellular tissue, and is very haemorrhagic. Secondary growths are often widespread and occur both in other organs and in the bones, the skull often being affected. Similar tumours may arise also from other parts of the sympathetic system. Such tumours may secrete catecholamines other than adrenaline and noradrenaline, especially dopamine, which appears in the urine chiefly as vanillin mandelic acid (VMA) and homovanillic acid.

Phaeochromocytoma

This third variety of tumour takes origin from the chromaffin cells. It can arise also from chromaffin cells in other sites (see below) and is then sometimes called a *paraganglioma*. It is composed of polyhedral cells, many of which give the chromaffin reaction, staining a brownish-yellow colour with chrome salts, and rich in glycogen (Fig. 26.28). When placed in formol-saline it imparts a brown colour to the fixative. The cells are arranged in solid groups enclosed in a fine vasular stroma. Cell aberration is common, but the tumour is usually benign.

Clinical features arise from excessive although usually intermittent secretion of cate-

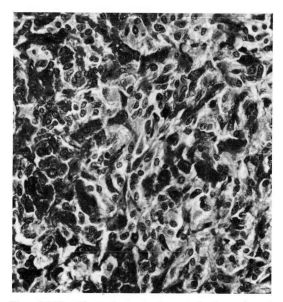

Fig. 26.28 Phaeochromocytoma of the adrenal medulla. The darkly stained elements are cells giving the chromaffin reaction. × 200.

cholamines. Symptoms include excessive sweating, nervousness, tremors and sometimes psychoses, attacks of blanching or flushing, headache and palpitations; also loss of appetite and weight.

There is hypertension, at first paroxysmal but sometimes becoming continuous; there may also be postural hypotension. The fasting blood sugar is usually raised and the basal metabolic rate increased. Obviously a phaeochromocytoma can mimic various other conditions. In most cases the diagnosis can be confirmed by demonstrating that the daily urinary excretion of vanillin mandelic acid (VMA, a metabolite of catecholamines) is more than doubled. The response to the α-blocking agent phentolamine is also of diagnostic value.

The hypertension is associated with arteriosclerosis even in young subjects. Occasionally death has occurred from cerebral haemorrhage. Neurofibromatosis has been present in 5 per cent of cases. Some families have a high incidence of phaeochromocytomas, often bilateral, occurring either alone or as part of the Sipple syndrome, a form of multiple endocrine adenoma syndrome whose other features may include medullary thyroid carcinoma, parathyroid adenoma, and neuromas of the buccal mucosa and conjunctiva (p. 1029). Early surgical removal of the tumour relieves the symptoms. Paragangliomas causing similar hypertension occur in chromaffin tissues outside the adrenal, e.g. in the organ of Zuckerkandl, but the majority are devoid of excessive hormonal activity. Rarely, phaeochromocytomas are malignant and metastasise.

Other adrenal tumours

These include *lipoma*, *myelolipoma* annd *haemangioma*, all of which are rare. *Melanomas* also occur, as a rule bilaterally. *Carcinomatous metastases* are often present in the adrenals, particularly in bronchial carcinoma, in which both glands may be implicated, the ipsilateral gland being first involved and usually the larger.

Congenital abnormalities

Absence of both adrenals is a rare abnormality, incompatible with life; or one (the right only) may be absent. These abnormalities, and also adrenal hypoplasia, are intimately related to gross defects of the central nervous system, such as micrencephaly or anencephaly.

Accessory adrenals are comparatively common; they are small masses of cortical tissue which can be readily recognised by their brownish-yellow colour. They occur in the surrounding tissues, on the surface or occasionally in the substance of the kidney or liver, and in the region of the ovary or testis, and very frequently at the apex of congenital hernial sacs. Rarely a tumour arises from them.

References and Further Reading

Adams, Duncan (1977). Auto-immune disease of the endocrine glands and stomach. In *Immunology in Medicine*, pp. 373–430. Edited by E. J. Holborow and W. G. Reeves. Academic Press, London.

Anderson, J. R., Goudie, R. B., Gray, K. and Stuart-Smith, D. A. (1968). Immunological features of idiopathic Addison's disease: an antibody to cells producing steroid hormones. *Clinical and Experimental Immunology* 3, 107–117.

Conn, J. W. (1955). Primary aldosteronism. *Journal of Laboratory and Clinical Medicine* 45, 661–664.

Goudie, R. B., McDonald, E., Anderson, J. R. and Gray, Kathleen (1968). Immunological features of idiopathic Addison's disease: characterization of the adrenocortical antigens. *Clinical and Experimental Immunology* 3, 119–131.

Gould, R. P., (1978). The apud cell system. In *Recent Advances in Histopathology*, No. 10, pp. 1–22. Edited by P. P. Anthony and N. Woolf. Churchill-Livingstone, Edinburgh, London and New York.

Hall, R., Anderson, J., Smart, G. A. and Besser, M. (1974). *Fundamentals of Clinical Endocrinology*, 2nd edn. pp. 494. Pitman Medical, London. (Deals mainly with mechanisms and clinical aspects of endocrine disorders.)

Howanitz, P. J. and Howanitz, J. H. (1979). Evaluation of endocrine function. Chapter 14 in *Clinical Diagnosis and Management by Laboratory Methods*, Vol. 1, pp. 1170. Edited by J. B. Henry. Saunders, Philadelphia, London and Toronto.

Irvine, W. J., *et al.* (1968). Immunological aspects of premature ovarian failure associated with idiopathic Addisons's disease. Lancet ii, 883–887.

Kriss, J. P., Konishi, J. and Herman, M. (1975). Studies on the pathogenesis of Graves' ophthalmopathy (with some related observations regarding therapy). *Recent Progress in Hormone Research* 31, 533–566.

O'Riorden, J. L. H. (Ed.) (1978). *Recent Advances in Endocrinology and Metabolism*, pp. 282. Churchill-Livingstone, Edinburgh, London and New York. (Reviews of selected topics in endocrinology.)

Symington, T., Currie, A. R., Curran, R. C. and Davidson, J. N. (1955). The reaction of the adrenal cortex in conditions of stress. *Ciba Foundation Colloquia in Endocrinology* 8, 70–84. Churchill, London.

Symmers, W. St. C. (Ed.) (1978). *Systematic Pathology*, 2nd edn., Vol. 4, Chapters 29–33, pp. 1863–2074. Churchill-Livingstone, Edinburgh, London and New York. (Chapters on the endocrine system, by various authors.)

Williams, R. N. (Ed.) (1974). *Textbook of Endocrinology*, 5th edn., pp. 1138. Saunders, Philadelphia, London and Toronto. (An authoritative multi-author text.)

27

The Skin

Skin pathology is often regarded as so specialised a subject that it is not suitable for inclusion in a general textbook. But the tissue responses in the diseased skin are basically the same as those that occur in other organs, and it is an ideal organ in which to study the correlation of naked-eye appearances with microscopic changes, especially as the evolution of a lesion may be readily followed by repeated biopsy.

The major functions of the skin include sensory perception, protection against mechanical trauma, UV light and infection (p. 175), insulation and temperature control (p. 188), conservation of fluid, biosynthesis and excretion and, of course, its aesthetic function. Such functional complexity is reflected in the morphology of the skin which, although at first sight simple, varies considerably depending on site, sex, age, race and environment.

Skin biopsy. In selecting the site for biopsy, it must be appreciated that very early or late lesions often yield less useful information than a fairly early representative lesion. The most satisfactory biopsy is taken by ringing the selected lesion and adjacent normal skin with adrenaline-free local anaesthetic and excising an ellipse containing affected and normal skin. The tissue should not be grasped with forceps but use of a Gillies hook is helpful to raise and maintain gentle tension on the skin during its removal. Excision should be accomplished with minimum trauma; use of a high-speed punch produces artefacts which often spoil the histology. Orientation of the excised skin is essential, and it is helpful to press it gently, undersurface down, on to blotting paper before placing it in fixative (usually 10 per cent neutral formol saline): this prevents distortion during fixation. After 12–24 hours in fixative the tissue is bisected transversely and processed.

Reactive changes in skin disease

The range of responses of the skin to pathogenic agents is limited and many causes can result in similar changes. This is particularly true of inflammatory changes, in which topical therapy, particularly with potent fluorinated corticosteroid preparations, may also alter significantly the clinical picture and obscure the diagnosis. For these reasons, it must be emphasised that while the histopathologist can diagnose with confidence some diseases of the skin, only too often the clinical history and naked-eye appearances of the lesions must be taken into account before reaching a definitive diagnosis. This chapter is intended to cover a representative selection of dermatological conditions, particularly those which have characteristic patterns of tissue reaction.

The following terms are in common use to describe pathological changes in the epidermis and require to be defined.

Acantholysis. Loss of cohesion between epidermal cells (keratinocytes) with consequent formation of intra-epidermal spaces containing oedema fluid and detached, rounded epithelial cells.

Acanthosis. Thickening of the epidermis, either focally or diffusely, due largely to increase of the stratum malpighii.

Dyskeratosis. Premature, abnormal or individual keratinisation of epidermal cells: the cells lose their prickles and become rounded off, and the nucleus becomes pyknotic. This is seen in some rare benign conditions but more commonly in pre-malignant lesions and carcinoma of the epidermis.

Hyperkeratosis. A thickening of the horny layer, usually accompanied by increase also in the granular layer. As the horny layer normally varies greatly in thickness in different sites, some experience is needed to assess minor degrees of hyperkeratosis.

Parakeratosis. The orderly but abnormal keratinisation of cells so that the keratin layer consists of plump nucleated keratinised cells instead of anuclear squames. It is associated with thinning or loss of the granular layer and is usually seen in diseases of increased cell turnover, whether inflammatory or neoplastic.

Spongiosis. Intercellular oedema, seen as increased width of the space between epidermal cells and leading, if severe, to formation of vesicles in the epidermis.

Vesication. The formation of fluid-filled spaces (*vesicles* or *blisters*) either within the epidermis or at the dermo-epidermal junction. A vesicle of 3 mm or more across is arbitrarily termed a *bulla*.

Hereditary and Congenital Conditions

There are some conditions in which skin involvement results from a known genetically-determined metabolic defect: examples include damage to the skin caused by UV light (*a*) as a result of photosensitivity in some forms of *porphyria*, and (*b*) in *xeroderma pigmentosum*, in which there is failure to correct abnormalities induced in epidermal-cell DNA by UV light because of deficiency of an endonuclease (p. 296).

In the conditions described below, there is good evidence of genetic factors, although the nature of the basic defect has not been elucidated.

Ichthyosis. At least six forms of this condition have been described and it also occurs as a feature of several syndromes. Two forms are important—*ichthyosis vulgaris*, which is determined by an autosomal dominant factor, and a *sex-linked recessive form* confined to males. **The autosomal dominant form**, which is relatively common, develops a few months after birth. Scaly lesions appear on the extensor aspects of the extremities; in unusually severe cases they are large and their appearance has led to the term 'fish scale disease'. The flexures are spared and elsewhere the scales are smaller, like flakes of bran. All grades of severity occur and in some cases the condition accompanies atopic dermatitis. The characteristic feature is hyperkeratosis accompanied by thinning or absence of the granular layer: this is an exception to the general rule that hyperkeratosis is associated with thickening of the granular layer. Electron microscopy shows the hyperkeratosis to be due to undue persistence of the desmosomes which bind the epidermal cells together, while deficiency of the granular layer may be due to delayed formation of keratin. Treatment is of no avail except in rare cases with a defect of vitamin A metabolism; in such cases treatment with retinoic acid is helpful.

In the rare **sex-linked recessive form**, the disease starts shortly after birth and may involve most of the skin, including the flexures, but the palms of the hands and soles of the feet are spared. Histologically there is hyperkeratosis, thickening of the granular layer and acanthosis, with occasional mild perivascular infiltration of the dermis with lymphocytes and plasma cells. In very severe forms, the disease may be rapidly fatal: in other cases it may persist for life, but may become less severe.

A non-inherited form of ichthyosis occurs in some patients with a lymphoma or carcinoma. The only histological changes are hyperkeratosis and increase in the granular layer, and such changes occurring alone should raise the suspicion of an internal neoplasm.

Darier's disease (Keratosis follicularis). A familial occurrence of this disease is now widely recognised. Though relatively rare, it is included here because of its characteristic histological features and its confusion with other conditions. The epidermis shows considerable hyperkeratosis and acanthosis, and is thrown into folds. This causes oblique cuts in the preparation of sections and gives rise to the appearance of a core of dermis surrounded by a single layer of epidermal cells, the so-called papillomatosis. Owing to the process of acantholysis, clefts (lacunae) appear in the epidermis and in properly orientated parts of the section these are found just above the basal layer. The two most striking features are, however, the presence of dyskeratotic cells in the epidermis called *corps ronds* and *grains* (Fig. 27.1). *Corps ronds*, which are enlarged keratinocytes,

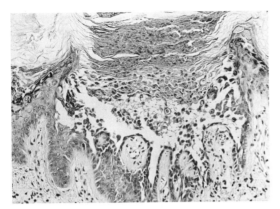

Fig. 27.1 Darier's disease. The corps ronds are seen in the upper layers of the epidermis and the grains underlying the central hyperkeratosis. × 150.

are seen mainly in the upper epidermis in the region of the granular layer. They are easily recognised by their large size (two to three times that of the surrounding keratinocytes) and in haematoxylin and eosin-stained sections by their hyaline-looking eosinophilic cytoplasm (premature keratinisation). Grains are found in the horny layer and differ only in size and shape from the plump keratinised cells in ordinary parakeratosis. These changes are focal and may involve only very small areas of the epidermis.

This form of benign dyskeratosis must be differentiated from its malignant counterpart which is seen in some types of intra-epithelial neoplasm.

Benign familial pemphigus. The essential feature of all forms of pemphigus is acantholysis with consequent formation of bullae, seen as raised fluid-filled blebs. Microscopically, benign familial pemphigus resembles keratosis follicularis (above) in showing acantholysis and papillomatosis (Fig. 27.2). The acantholysis is much more widespread and the epidermis has been aptly likened to a dilapidated brick wall. Dyskeratosis may be seen but is not so severe as in Darier's disease. Areas of grain-like parakeratosis are found overlying the acantholytic epidermis. In cases lacking dyskeratosis, differentiation from pemphigus vulgaris (see below) may be impossible on purely histological grounds.

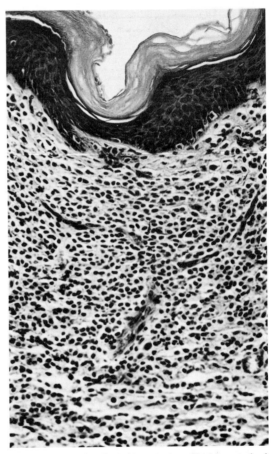

Fig. 27.3 Urticaria pigmentosa. Closely packed mast cells occupy the upper dermis. × 200.

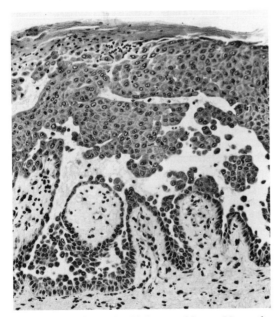

Fig. 27.2 Benign familial pemphigus. Note the acantholysis and 'papillomatosis'. × 175.

Urticaria pigmentosa. This disorder is usually congenital, but may appear first in adolescence or adult life. No familial background has been established. It usually presents clinically as widespread pigmented macules which urticate, i.e. develop into pale vesicles with surrounding erythema: occasionally the entire skin surface is involved. The congenital form tends to become gradually milder and may regress completely after puberty.

Histological examination (Fig. 27.3) reveals a normal epidermis apart from an increase in melanin pigmentation of the basal layer. Depending on the severity of the condition part or all of the dermis contains closely packed mast cells. In routine haematoxylin and eosin preparations these are seen as polygonal or hexagonal cells with abundant eosinophilic cytoplasm and well defined dense oval nuclei. Staining by toluidine blue or polychrome methylene blue brings out their typical granular appearance. A few eosinophil leukocytes are also seen. In the urticated phase oedema is evident and may at times be sufficiently severe to cause a subepidermal bulla.

In adults, the intensity of mast cell aggregation varies greatly. In some instances, particularly in the adult form, there may also be aggregation of mast cells in the internal organs, e.g. the spleen, liver and bone marrow, but progression to the fatal systemic mast cell disease is rare.

Adenoma sebaceum. In tuberous sclerosis (p. 772), a familial condition of autosomal dominant inheritance, multiple papules are seen on the face, and the name 'adenoma sebaceum' was given to what was mistakenly believed to be late developing 'pilosebaceous naevi'. The lesions are, in fact, angiofibromatous in nature, and there is no abnormality of the pilosebaceous apparatus in this condition.

Virus Diseases

Virus infections of the skin fall into two distinct groups. Firstly, those caused by DNA viruses which integrate into the epidermal cell genome and behave as tumour viruses, producing verrucas (warts). Secondly, those in which the virus replicates within the cell, exerting a cytolytic effect.

Verrucas (warts) and similar lesions

These common viral lesions of the skin usually affect the hands, feet, knees and face, and are seen particularly in children. They also occur in the genital region.

The four main types of warts are (*a*) verruca vulgaris and verruca plantaris, (*b*) verruca plana, (*c*) condyloma acuminatum and (*d*) molluscum contagiosum.

Verruca vulgaris and verruca plantaris may be considered together because they are caused by related strains of the papilloma virus group of DNA papovaviruses and have closely similar features. They consist of flat disc-like, sessile papillary lesions raised above the surface of the skin (except verruca plantaris which occurs on the sole of the foot and, because of pressure, is often flush with the skin surface).

Histologically, the epidermis is thickened and thrown into papillary folds: the rete ridges are elongated and those at the periphery curve inwards giving the lesion in section a cup-shaped appearance. There is hyperkeratosis alternating with parakeratosis.

Studies of iso-enzymes (p. 368) have demonstrated that verrucae arise from a clonal proliferation of epidermal cells and virus particles cannot be detected by electron microscopy in the proliferating cells in the basal part of the lesion. In the older lesions, the nuclei of the more superficial cells are vacuolated (Fig. 27.4) and contain densely basophilic inclusions shown by electron microscopy to consist of aggregates of virions. Both the nucleus and cytoplasm of the more superficial cells contain eosinophilic inclusions which are non-viral in nature.

The histological features of verruca vulgaris and verruca plantaris are very similar, but the latter often shows greater hyperkeratosis. In both types of wart, the DNA virus appears to integrate into a basal cell which is transformed and proliferates to produce the lesion. As the tumour cells age, they become permissive, i.e. support replication of the virus, which results in their death and release of virions. These feat-

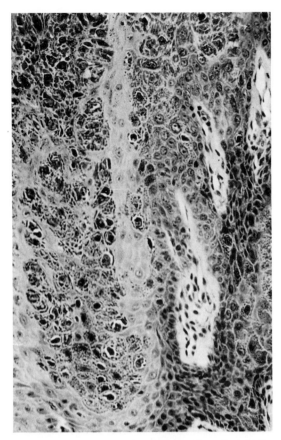

Fig. 27.4 Verruca vulgaris. Margin of a lesion showing the eosinophilic cytoplasmic inclusions and coarse basophilic nuclear inclusions. × 200.

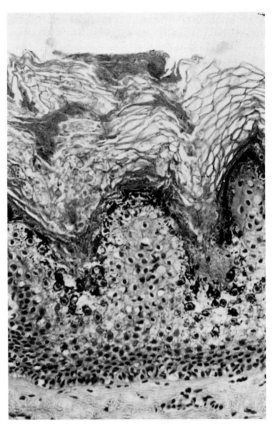

Fig. 27.5 Verruca plana. Vacuolated cells are seen in the upper layers of the acanthotic epidermis. Note the basket weave appearance due to vacuolation of cells of the stratum corneum. × 150.

ures resemble closely those of the papillomas produced in domestic rabbits by the Shope papilloma virus (p. 304).

Growth of these human warts is largely controlled by host resistance: they eventually regress, but fresh crops may develop. They do not become malignant, but may be seen in unusually florid form in immunosuppressed patients, e.g. following renal transplantation.

Verruca plana occurs most commonly on the hands and face. It presents as a papule with less obvious papillary folding and there is hyperkeratosis but no parakeratosis. The hyperkeratosis has a 'basket-weave' appearance (Fig. 27.5), and there is a corresponding increase in the cells of the granular layer, many of which may be vacuolated. Intranuclear inclusions are not usually seen.

Condyloma acuminatum. The moist regions of the vulva, the penis, and in and around the anus are the sites where condylomata acuminata develop as soft polypoid nodules which can achieve considerable growth into cauliflower-like masses. With irritation and bacterial infection, ulceration may develop, and clinical suspicion of carcinoma may be roused. Histologically, hyperkeratosis is not prominent, but parakeratosis is usually seen with an associated depletion or absence of the granular layer. There is a remarkable degree of acanthosis with fusion and broadening of the rete ridges resulting in marked papillomatosis. A characteristic feature is the presence of large cells with vacuolated cytoplasm and distinct nuclei, some of which may exhibit mitotic activity so that a picture of pseudo-epitheliomatous hyperplasia is seen. However, the cells retain an orderly arrangement and this, together with the appearance of pale cells greatly swollen by intracellular oedema, is helpful in diagnosis. These tumours are believed to be caused by a strain of papovavirus different from that responsible for the common wart, and infection is sexually transmitted. Very rarely they may become malignant.

Molluscum contagiosum is a common contagious lesion caused by a member of the poxvirus group. It occurs mainly in children but also in adults. The lesions are usually multiple, each consisting of a discrete waxy skin-coloured papule, which may grow to about 5 mm in diameter, with a central depression from which a little paste-like material can be expressed. The lesions can occur anywhere on the skin, but are commonly seen on the face and trunk.

Microscopically, a typical lesion consists of a sharply localised overgrowth of epidermis projecting above the surface but mainly downwards into the dermis, which it compresses to form a pseudocapsule (Fig. 27.6). The proliferating basal cells are free of inclusions but the cells just above this level each contain a small intracytoplasmic eosinophilic inclusion known as a molluscum body. As the cells progress towards the surface, this rapidly enlarges and becomes basophilic, forming the Henderson–Paterson body which compresses the cell nucleus into a thin marginal rim (Fig. 27.6). Electron microscopy has shown the basophilic bodies to consist of enormous numbers of large virions. In the centre of the lesion the colonised cells break down to form the paste-like material which discharges on to the surface, thus accounting for the central dimple. Without treatment, the lesions may become numerous but eventually they regress. The appearances are consistent with transformation of a basal cell by integrated virus, with resultant clonal proliferation and replication of virus in the older, more superficial and central epidermal cells. This has not yet, however, been confirmed by virological studies.

Cytotoxic virus infections

These include a group of conditions in which the predominant effect of the virus is to repli-

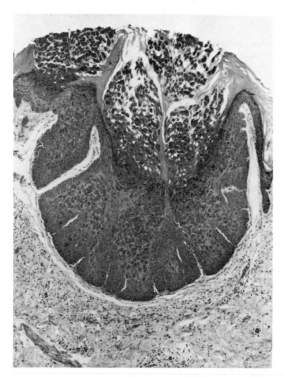
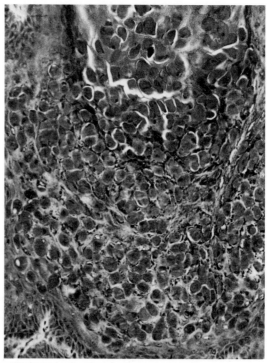

Fig. 27.6 Molluscum contagiosum, showing the whole lesion (*left*, × 70) and the central part (*right*, × 300). The lesion is a sharply localised epithelial proliferation with enlargement and eventual disintegration of the epidermal cells by the Henderson–Paterson bodies.

cate within and destroy epidermal cells. Examples are *variola* (smallpox) and *vaccinia*, both of which are caused by DNA viruses of the poxvirus group, and *varicella* (chickenpox), *zoster* (shingles) and *herpes simplex*, all of which are caused by *Herpesviruses*. Although these conditions are clinically very different, the individual lesions of them all show many similarities and may conveniently be considered together. In varicella, variola and primary herpes simplex, the original infection is via the upper respiratory tract or mouth, and in varicella and variola this is followed by a viraemic phase before colonisation of the skin to produce the characteristic lesions. Clinically, the lesions pass through macular, papular, vesicular and sometimes pustular stages. Histologically, in the early stages there may be some increased epidermal proliferation and formation of large cells with a single large or two or three nuclei. However, the major effect is cytotoxic: intracellular oedema results in swelling of the deeper epidermal cells (balloon degeneration) progressing to rupture of the cells to produce a vesicle or bulla (Fig. 27.7). The greatly swollen

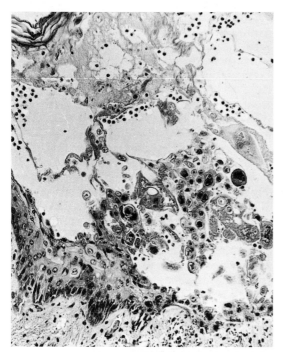

Fig. 27.7 Zoster. Multilocular intra-epidermal bulla, showing large swollen cells (balloon degeneration) and strands of cell walls traversing the bulla (reticular degeneration). × 350.

epidermal cells lining the space become detached and drift into the vesicular fluid. When cell death is rapid, neighbouring cell walls may persist as sheets and strands traversing the vesicle and giving it a multilocular appearance, a feature termed *reticular degeneration*. This is usually pronounced in smallpox, but is seen also in the other conditions.

Variola and vaccinia. Variola has apparently been eradicated, largely as a result of vaccination. The last reported case occurred in 1978 and was related to a laboratory holding stocks of the virus. The lesions progress through macular, papular, vesicular and pustular stages: they occur all over the body but have a centrifugal distribution, i.e. are most numerous on the head, hands and feet. All the lesions appear within a day or so and they progress at the same rate; pustulation is usually severe, with consequent scarring.

The severity of smallpox is usually related to the number and size of the skin lesions. In some cases, however, severe prostration, and sometimes death, occurs very early in patients showing only a few haemorrhagic spots or tiny macules with an erythematous halo. Lesions occur also in the mouth, pharynx and oesophagus, and widely in the internal organs. There may be viral encephalitis, and bacterial pneumonia is common. Smallpox in previously vaccinated individuals is often relatively mild and may be difficult to diagnose clinically. Definitive diagnosis depends on morphological identification of the virus, preferably by electron microscopy on scrapings of an early lesion, or by immunofluorescence, immunodiffusion or complement fixation tests on material from lesions, using anti-variola or anti-vaccinia antibodies.

The lesions of **vaccinia** are similar, but nearly always remain localised to the skin around the vaccination site.

Varicella and zoster are both caused by *Herpesvirus varicellae*. In varicella, which usually occurs in childhood, the lesions are widespread, but tend to occur in successive crops, so that the different stages are seen at the same time. They also differ from those of variola in having a centripetal distribution, being fewer on the extremities than on the trunk and proximal parts of the limbs. They cannot be distinguished with certainty by traditional histological examination from smallpox, although reticular degeneration and pustulation are often less marked and usually they heal without permanent scarring. In immunodeficient or immunosuppressed subjects the lesions may be very numerous and florid and there may be widespread visceral involvement, including a mild virus pneumonia and occasionally mild encephalitis. The virus can persist for years in the posterior root ganglia without causing symptoms, and zoster results (usually in adults) from a recrudescence of this latent infection (Fig. 21.43, p. 757). The virus reaches the skin, presumably via the sensory nerves, and produces a crop of lesions which are often preceded and accompanied by severe pain in the area supplied by the individual nerves—most commonly the trunk, face or arm. In immunodeficient individuals, zoster skin lesions may become widespread and there may be visceral involvement.

Herpes simplex is a ubiquitous infection. Most people acquire it asymptomatically in childhood via the oral mucosa: thereafter the virus (*Herpesvirus hominis*) remains latent, but may become active (usually during an incidental febrile illness) and produce the typical skin lesions around the lips, etc. Occasionally, more severe lesions occur, usually as part of the original infection, including neonatal generalised herpes, keratoconjunctivitis and an acute necrotising encephalitis (p. 756) which is often fatal.

Herpes simplex shares with vaccinia virus the capacity to colonise areas of dermatitis in children, producing in both cases a condition known as **Kaposi's varicelliform eruption**.

Inflammatory Conditions

Many different conditions, some of known and others of unknown aetiology, are arbitrarily grouped under the heading of inflammatory diseases. This is not so irrational as it may seem because those varied diseases show different degrees and facets of the changes of inflammation.

Dermatitis

Much confusion has been caused by the rather indiscriminate use of the terms *dermatitis* and *eczema* to describe similar conditions. It is now widely accepted that the two terms are synonymous, and in this text dermatitis will be used. The term covers the inflammatory response of the skin to a wide variety of pathogenic agents ranging from contact with external primary irritants to a hypersensitivity reaction to various antigens, both exogenous and endogenous.

The external primary irritants such as strong acids or alkalis produce an acute inflammatory response similar to that seen in other tissues and the dermatitis subsides once the irritant has been removed.

The hypersensitivity group is complex and imperfectly understood. Many chemicals which cause dermatitis following contact with the skin are haptenic (p. 104) and require to combine with an epidermal protein to become immunogenic. The hypersensitivity, which is of delayed type (p. 156) is termed contact dermatitis and may resolve on preventing contact with the hapten, but in some cases becomes self-perpetuating.

Dermatitis caused by drugs and other haptenic or antigenic material after absorption by mouth or some other route may be of atopic type (p. 146) or the result of immune-complex deposition (p. 152).

Various other clinically recognised disorders are of unknown cause, e.g. pompholyx, seborrhoeic dermatitis, lichen simplex chronicus (formerly neurodermatitis) and exfoliative dermatitis.

In all these conditions, various degrees of itching, erythema, exudation and scaling characterise the clinical picture. Whatever the cause, the basic microscopic picture is similar, and it is convenient to speak of the *dermatitis reaction* which, like any inflammatory process, may be acute, subacute or chronic. The pathologist can only report on the type of dermatitis reaction and can rarely suggest the aetiology without having recourse to the clinical history and findings.

Acute dermatitis. The earliest change is spongiosis (intercellular oedema) which separates the keratinocytes; this is followed by infiltration of the epidermis by polymorphs, macrophages and lymphocytes. Focal degeneration and lysis of keratinocytes occurs, with consequent formation of vesicles which may enlarge into bullae (Fig. 27.8). Depending on the stage at which biopsy is performed, the vesicles may contain cell debris, fibrin, neutrophil polymorphs and lymphocytes. Disordered keratin formation may result in focal parakeratosis which, together with dried inflammatory exudate and cell debris, forms loose or firmly adherent surface crusts. Depending on the severity of the reaction, the dermis may be hyperaemic and oedematous with perivascular aggregation of eosinophil and neutrophil polymorphs and lymphocytes.

As with other vesicular or bullous lesions, an early typical lesion should be selected for biopsy. The histological picture is similar in the acute phase of any clinical form of dermatitis including, for example, the lesion of **pityriasis rosea**, a common condition with typical clinical appearances.

Subacute dermatitis. As the acute stage subsides the lesions become less vesicular and although spongiosis and vesiculation may persist, they are usually less obvious. The epidermis becomes acanthotic with deepening and then fusion of the rete ridges. There is also parakeratosis with formation of surface crusts which include a mixture of fibrin, degenerating leukocytes and bacteria. Occasionally a vesicle may rupture on to the surface, leaving a naked dermal papilla covered by fibrin and debris (Fig. 27.9) and forming the so-called *dermatitis pit*. There is less oedema and vascular congestion in the dermis, but it is more heavily infiltrated with inflammatory cells, mainly lym-

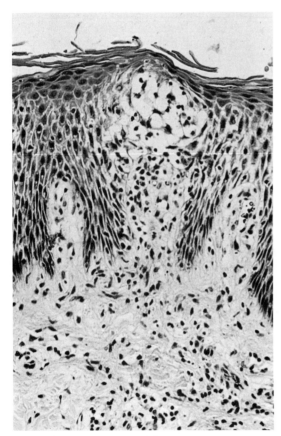

Fig. 27.8 Acute dermatitis, showing an intraepidermal vesicle containing leukocytes and degenerate epithelial cells. × 200.

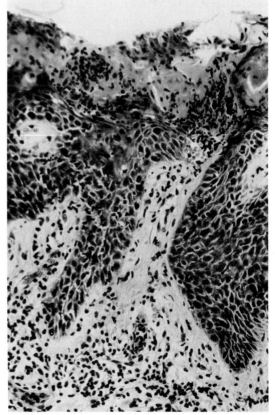

Fig. 27.9 Subacute dermatitis. Note the tip of the dermal papilla in contact with the serous exudate and debris on the surface. × 300.

phocytes and macrophages with only an occasional neutrophil leukocyte. **Nummular dermatitis** is the classical example of this stage of dermatitis although it occurs also as a phase of others, particularly atopic dermatitis. Stasis dermatitis, associated with impaired venous return from the lower limbs, may show the same changes with, in addition, scattered deposits of haemosiderin in the dermis.

Chronic dermatitis. An outstanding feature of this stage is marked acanthosis with elongation of the rete ridges. Hyperkeratosis with areas of parakeratosis are evident and there is a corresponding patchy thickening of the granular layer. Small foci of spongiosis may be seen but no vesicles (Fig. 27.10). The upper dermis is infiltrated with moderate numbers of lymphocytes, macrophages, fibroblasts and occa-

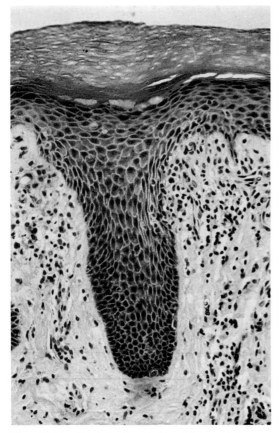

Fig. 27.10 Chronic dermatitis. There is hyperkeratosis, elongation of the rete ridges and a perivascular inflammatory infiltrate in the upper dermis. × 300.

sional eosinophil leukocytes. The walls of the small blood vessels often show hyaline thickening with reduction of their lumina, and there may be scarring of the dermis. These changes correspond to the clinical picture of thickened, leathery skin referred to as 'lichenified', seen in many types of chronic dermatitis. The most characteristic clinical condition is, however, **lichen simplex chronicus**.

The prognosis of dermatitis is variable. Acute and subacute phases can be quickly controlled by the use of appropriate topical treatment and, in the case of contact and irritant dermatitis, by removing the patient from the source. Chronic dermatitis, particularly of the hands and feet, is often extremely resistant to treatment and may persist for life, varying in intensity but never regressing completely.

Some conditions, e.g. chronic superficial dermatitis ('parapsoriasis'), erythema multiforme and annular erythema, are not regarded clinically as examples of dermatitis, and yet at some stage in their evolution they may show the histological features of dermatitis. Similarly, chronic indolent psoriasis and some atypical cases of lichen planus may be indistinguishable from chronic dermatitis.

Generalised exfoliative dermatitis (generalised erythroderma), a striking and serious clinical entity, has the histological features of subacute or chronic dermatitis. In some cases it is an adverse drug reaction, but 25 per cent of cases without known cause eventually develop a lymphoma, and diagnosis of this at an early stage may require repeated biopsies.

Acne vulgaris

This is very common in adolescents of both sexes. It begins about puberty, varies greatly in severity and duration and eventually subsides, although sometimes not until the mid-twenties. Acne affects mainly the face, chest and upper back but may extend to the deltoid regions and down to the buttocks.

The earliest structural change is blockage of the opening of the pilosebaceous follicle by a mass of keratin: this is seen as a **comedo** (blackhead) which is dark because of melanin deposition. Secretion of sebum continues in the blocked follicle until the sebaceous gland undergoes pressure atrophy. Meanwhile the follicle may become grossly dilated with keratinous debris and sebum (*cystic acne*). More commonly blockage is followed by suppuration, the pus discharging on to the surface (*pustular acne*). The skin commensal *Propionibacterium acnes* appears to thrive in the blocked follicle: it splits neutral fats of sebum into free fatty acids which are intensely irritating. Sometimes the wall of the distended follicle is disrupted and the contents escape into the dermis where they induce a macrophage granulomatous reaction with foreign-body giant cells. Granulation tissue is formed and permanent scarring results which occasionally progresses to keloid formation.

Extensive investigation has failed to elucidate the basis of acne: the influence of androgens on sebum production may be important, and the tissue reaction is probably aggravated by the fatty acids produced by bacterial enzymic activity on sebum. The use of long-term low-dose oral tetracycline therapy has done much to alleviate acne and reduce the tissue reaction and scarring.

The bullous diseases

These comprise pemphigus, pemphigoid, dermatitis herpetiformis and erythema multiforme.

It is possible to separate the pemphigus group from the others by histological examination but only if an early representative biopsy is taken. Secondary infection and degenerative changes rapidly alter the histological features. Ideally a small lesion should be taken within 12 hours of its appearance. Pemphigoid, dermatitis herpetiformis and some types of erythema multiforme may all show subepidermal bullae and immunofluorescence studies may be necessary (see below) for accurate diagnosis.

Pemphigus

Three major types of pemphigus are recognised: *pemphigus vulgaris*, *pemphigus vegetans* and *pemphigus foliaceous*. In the latter two types bullae may not be detectable clinically although histological examination will reveal the characteristic changes at the edge of the lesion. Pemphigus is a serious disorder and the vulgaris and vegetans types, if untreated, will cause death. Systemic corticosteroids and immunosuppressant drugs have greatly improved the prognosis. Pemphigus foliaceus is more benign and can often be satisfactorily controlled by one of the more potent topical corticosteroid preparations.

The bulla of pemphigus is intra-epidermal and arises as a result of acantholysis of epidermal cells which produces a horizontal plane of cleavage in the epidermis.

Pemphigus vulgaris is an uncommon disease of the middle-aged. It is characterised by the development of rather flaccid bullae of the skin: they appear in crops, soon rupture and leave a raw surface which does not granulate.

In this condition (Fig. 27.11), the cleavage takes place above the basal layer, this layer remaining intact due to its attachment to the dermis by cytoplasmic processes. The bulla contains serum and somewhat condensed, rounded-off keratinocytes. A few polymorphonuclear leukocytes and eosinophils may also be present within the bulla. The underlying dermis shows slight oedema and a sparse infiltrate of polymorphs and eosinophils.

Pemphigus vegetans. In pemphigus vegetans the early lesion is identical with that of pemphigus vulgaris. As the disease progresses, however, the epithelium proliferates and the characteristic acantholysis is not seen. There is marked acanthosis of a verrucose type and intra-epidermal 'microabscesses' composed almost entirely of eosinophil leukocytes (Fig. 27.12). The inflammatory infiltrate in the upper dermis includes many eosinophil leukocytes and is much more pronounced than in pemphigus vulgaris.

Pemphigus foliaceus. In pemphigus foliaceus the acantholysis occurs high in the epidermis, usually just below the stratum corneum (Fig. 27.13), and if the biopsy is not carefully taken or the tissue is roughly handled the superficial layer may be lost, making the diagnosis difficult. Careful examination of the surface, however, will reveal acantholytic cells.

Mucosal lesions of pemphigus. While all forms of pemphigus are usually regarded as skin diseases, many cases begin as 'ulcers' of the mouth or genitalia. These may precede the skin lesions by as long as two years. The histological changes in mucous membranes are similar to those in the skin, viz. acantholytic bullae (Fig. 27.11a). However, because of the moist conditions within the mouth or on the vulva, maceration occurs rapidly and the roof of the bulla is quickly lost, making histological diagnosis extremely difficult. The demonstration

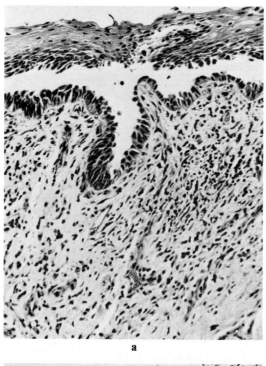

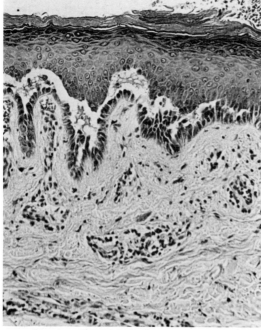

Fig. 27.11 Pemphigus vulgaris. **a** Acantholytic bulla in buccal mucous membrane. × 150. **b** Intra-epidermal bulla containing acantholytic cells, best seen just above the basal layer of the epidermis. × 150.

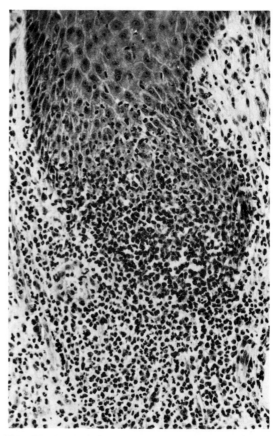

Fig. 27.12 Pemphigus vegetans. An early intra-epidermal abscess composed of eosinophil leukocytes at the tip of an elongated rete ridge. × 300.

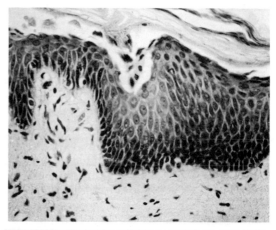

Fig. 27.13 Pemphigus foliaceus. Subcorneal bulla containing occasional acantholytic cells and some leukocytes. × 200.

that patients in the active stages of pemphigus have serum antibodies to an intercellular antigen of squamous epithelium, demonstrable by indirect immunofluorescence staining, has contributed greatly to the accurate diagnosis of the condition. (Fig. 27.17 and p. 1063.)

Dermatitis herpetiformis. This chronic condition usually appears after the age of 30. It presents as grouped crops of extremely itchy urticarial papules and vesicles, most commonly on the shoulders, lips, nose, external genitalia and over the sacrum. The early lesion is a subepidermal vesicle (Fig. 27.14) which rapidly enlarges into a bulla. There is no acantholysis. Difficulty may arise if an older lesion is biopsied as the epithelium regenerates rapidly and grows along the floor of the bulla which thus appears intra-epidermal. The subepidermal bulla is filled with serous exudate and con-

tains leukocytes, a high percentage of which are eosinophils. The underlying dermis is oedematous and there is a considerable leukocytic infiltration with a prominent eosinophil content. A useful diagnostic feature is the 'eosinophil abscesses'—oedematous dermal papillae packed with eosinophil leukocytes at the margins of the bullae (Fig. 27.15). Their detection may require examination of multiple sections.

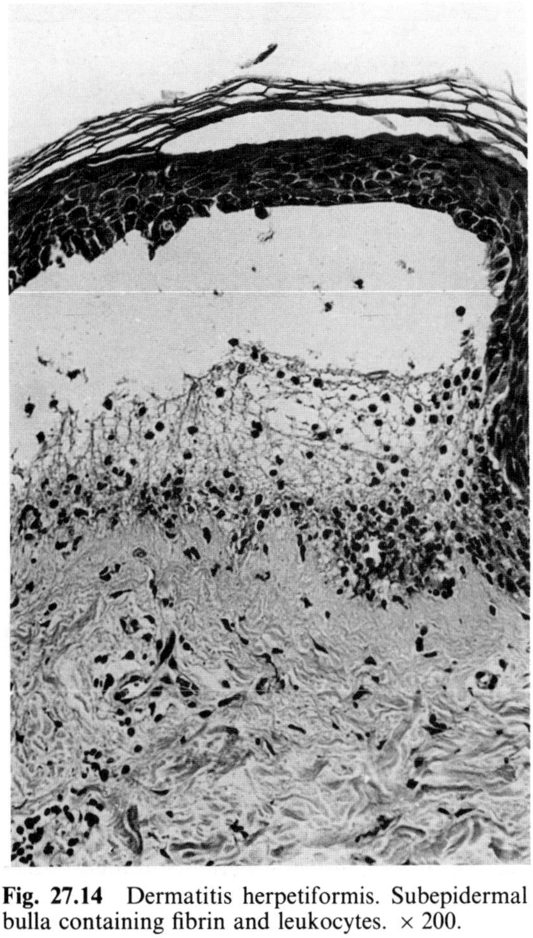

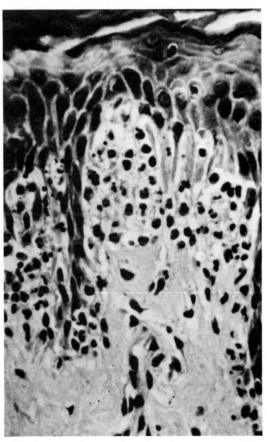

Fig. 27.15 Dermatitis herpetiformis. 'Eosinophil abscess' in an oedematous dermal papilla at the margin of a bulla. × 350.

In the majority of patients there is also a gluten-sensitive enteropathy with jejunal villous atrophy: this is usually mild and sometimes subclinical. Symptomatic relief of dermatitis herpetiformis can often be obtained by administration of small doses of sulphapyridine. The enteropathy (but not the dermatitis) responds to a gluten-free diet.

Fig. 27.14 Dermatitis herpetiformis. Subepidermal bulla containing fibrin and leukocytes. × 200.

Pemphigoid

This consists of a bullous disease which may affect mainly the skin (*bullous pemphigoid*) or the mucous membranes (*benign mucosal* or *cicatricial pemphigoid*). The early lesion, as in dermatitis herpetiformis, consists of a subepidermal bulla which contains relatively few inflammatory cells, including some eosinophils, and which soon becomes intra-epithelial as a result of extension of epidermal cells over the base. There is usually little dermal involvement until later, when neutrophil and eosinophil polymorphs aggregate both in the bullae and in the adjacent dermal papillae.

Bullous pemphigoid presents as an itchy erythema with development of large tense bullae, particularly in the flexural aspects of the limbs. After a few days the blisters burst and healing usually occurs. The condition, which is seen mostly in the elderly, is recurrent but often subsides after some months or years. It responds to systemic corticosteroid therapy. Its distinction from dermatitis herpetiformis is helped by antibody studies (see below).

Benign mucosal pemphigoid affects the mucous membrane of the mouth, the genitalia and the cornea and conjuctiva. The lesions resemble those of bullous pemphigoid and there may be some skin lesions. Scarring of the cornea and conjunctiva may seriously affect vision.

Erythema multiforme

This is an acute disorder seen at all ages and is sometimes recurrent. As the name suggests, there is a variety of clinical and histological appearances; in some the cause may be known, e.g., drugs or infections, while in others it is obscure. Typically the eruption involves the face, hands, forearms, and nose. It may appear as a number of 'target lesions', each consisting of a circular erythematous area of skin with a pale centre. The lesions vary greatly in severity and size: there may be macules, papules, blisters or pustules and haemorrhagic necrotic areas. A severe, sometimes fatal, form is the *Stevens–Johnson syndrome* in which extensive erosive lesions occur on the skin and mucous membranes.

Histologically, in the classical type of erythema multiforme, a diagnostic picture of an area of coagulative necrosis of the epidermis is seen, and this area may be raised above the underlying dermis by bulla formation (Fig. 27.16). The dermis shows oedema and there may be haemorrhage, with an acute necrotising capillaritis or vasculitis. More commonly there is a scattered perivascular cellular infiltrate consisting of varying numbers of neutrophils, eosinophils, lymphocytes and histiocytes. A frankly bullous form occurs without necrosis of the overlying epidermis, and differentiation from other causes of subepidermal bullae may not be possible histologically.

In the severe forms of erythema multiforme, including the Stevens–Johnson syndrome, early and intensive systemic corticosteroid therapy may be life-saving.

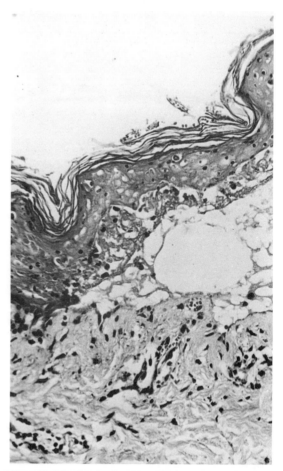

Fig. 27.16 Erythema multiforme. Subepidermal bulla roofed by necrotic epidermis. Regenerating epidermis can be seen at the left of the picture. × 200.

Immunofluorescence tests in the bullous diseases

In recent years, application of immunofluorescence (IF) tests (p. 111) has contributed greatly to the differential diagnosis of the bullous diseases. In the *indirect IF test*, a suitable fresh tissue substrate, such as rabbit or preferably (in our experience) baboon oesophagus, is treated successively with the patient's serum and fluorescein-labelled anti-immunoglobulin. In the *direct IF test*, unfixed cryostat sections of the patient's skin are treated with fluorescent-labelled anti-immunoglobulins and antibodies to complement components.

In the *pemphigus group*, circulating antibody (of IgG class) to a constituent of the intercellular substance of squamous epithelium is demonstrable, during active phases of the disease, by the indirect IF test (Fig. 27.17). The titre reflects the severity of the disease and may be used to monitor therapy. The direct IF test shows antibody and complement bound to the intercellular substance.

In *dermatitis herpetiformis* the direct IF test shows small granular deposits of IgA on the basement membrane in the prevesicular lesion and the adjacent skin. Antibody is not detectable in the serum.

In *bullous pemphigoid*, specific circulating antibodies may be demonstrated by direct and indirect IF testing. They bind to the basement membrane zone of stratified epithelium as homogeneous linear deposits principally of IgG (Fig. 27.18), and they also fix complement. In *benign mucosal pemphigoid*, fixed immunoglobulin, usually IgG, rarely IgM, together with complement, or sometimes IgA, is demonstrable on the basement membrane in many cases, while in some patients antibody reacting with basement membrane is detectable in the serum. Neither in bullous pemphigoid nor in benign mucosal pemphigoid can the titre of circulating antibody be used as an indicator of the severity of the disease or as a monitor of therapy, since such antibodies may be demonstrated in many cases long after clinical resolution has occurred.

In *erythema multiforme* the IF findings are inconstant and not diagnostic. Occasionally deposits of IgG and/or C3 are detectable in the walls of the small dermal vessels.

Immunofluorescence studies in lupus erythematosus are described on p. 1067.

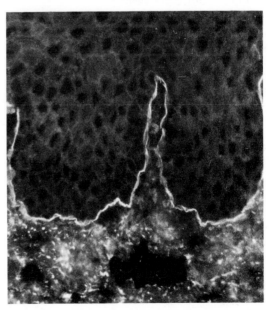

Fig. 27.18 Bullous pemphigoid. Homogeneous linear immunofluorescence of basement membrane. Direct immunofluorescence technique. × 300.

Scaling disorders

Psoriasis. This common, extremely chronic disorder is estimated to affect about two

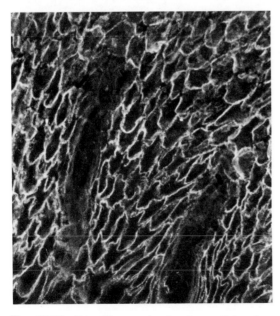

Fig. 27.17 Pemphigus vulgaris. Intercellular immunofluorescence staining in squamous epithelium. Indirect immunofluorescence technique. × 300.

per cent of the population. It usually appears first between the ages of 15 and 30 years. The lesions are slightly raised, sharply demarcated, red or pink, round or oval plaques with a fine scaly surface, varying in diameter from millimetres to centimetres. They may occur anywhere on the skin, including the scalp, but are commonest on the nose, elbows and over the sacrum. About 25 per cent of patients show a peculiar pitting of the finger and toe nails and about 5 per cent develop a chronic polyarthritis with absence of rheumatoid factor.

Characteristically there is parakeratosis with marked thinning of the epidermis over the dermal papillae which are oedematous and broadened at their tips. The rete ridges are greatly elongated and club-shaped (Fig. 27.19). There is usually a light chronic inflammatory cellular infiltration of the dermis. A characteristic feature of the early lesion is migration of neutrophil polymorphs into the epidermis, where they accumulate in and beneath the parakeratotic horny layers to form scattered '*Munro microabscesses*'.

Lichen Planus is an uncommon disease which often has a sudden onset and tends to persist: it affects both skin and mucous membranes. The skin lesions are intensely itchy: they consist of violaceous papules with a shiny surface which is often umbilicated, and the chronic lesions show various degrees of hyperpigmentation. Characteristic sites for the eruption are the wrists, trunk, external genitalia, legs and buccal mucosa. Delicate networks of white lines (Whickham's striae) are seen on the surface of the lesions and are said to be due to alterations in the reflection of light due to the thickened granular cell layer seen in this disorder.

The papule of lichen planus has characteristic microscopic features (Fig. 27.20). There is marked hyperkeratosis with focal increase in the granular layer. The epidermis is acanthotic and the rete ridges assume a pointed outline, giving a

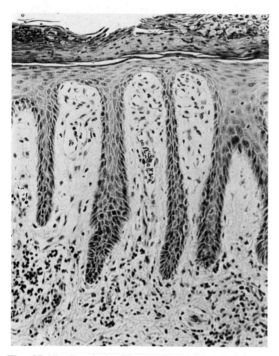

Fig. 27.19 Psoriasis. The surface is covered by a parakeratotic scale containing numerous polymorpho-nuclear leukocytes. The rete ridges are elongated and the suprapapillary epidermis is narrowed. × 150.

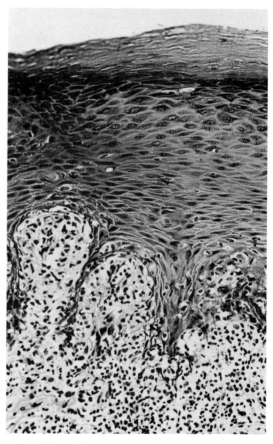

Fig. 27.20 Lichen planus. Note the hypertrophy of the granular layer and the saw-tooth appearance of the rete ridges. × 200.

saw-tooth appearance. There is often some swelling and disintegration (liquefaction degeneration) of the basal layer of the epidermis, and colloid bodies, probably derived from effete basal cells, may be seen in the lower epidermis and also in the upper dermis, which is heavily infiltrated with lymphocytes and occasional macrophages. The upper border of this infiltrate is in contact with the epidermis and may actually invade the basal layers, causing the dermo-epidermal junction to be indistinct. Lesions in the mucosa present a similar appearance although the hypertrophied granular layer is not so obvious. (Normally there is no granular layer in some areas of mucous membranes). The mucosal lesions may be diagnosed clinically as 'leukoplakia'.

Vascular Disorders

Erythema nodosum, nodular vasculitis and erythema induratum (Bazin's disease)

These three conditions are all characterised by nodular lesions of the subcutaneous fatty tissue of the lower extremities. While there are differences in aetiology and clinical course they cannot be clearly distinguished histologically and the appearances vary with the age of the lesion. They all produce tender subcutaneous nodules or thickenings of the legs, sometimes with reddening of the overlying skin. The lesions consist of areas of inflammation and fat necrosis with subsequent repair. In the early stages there is an infiltrate of polymorphonuclear leukocytes and lymphocytes in the subcutaneous fat. Inflammatory infiltration of the walls of small veins, which may be the basic lesion, is seen and in the more severe cases endothelial proliferation and thrombosis may occur (Fig. 27.21). As the nutrition of the fat is impaired, foci of epithelioid cells and giant cells appear in response to liberated fat. In severe cases necrosis resembling caseation is seen. These changes gradually subside and at a later stage the process of healing with fibrosis is observed.

It will be appreciated that the extent of the histological changes will be dependent on the severity or acuteness of the condition. In erythema induratum the fat necrosis may be so extensive that the lesion ulcerates, discharging caseous material on the surface.

Cutaneous Angiitis—anaphylactoid (Henoch–Schönlein) purpura; necrotising or allergic vasculitis

Until recently it was customary to consider such disorders as anaphylactoid purpura and

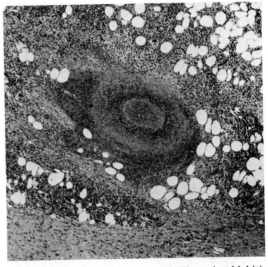

Fig. 27.21 Erythema nodosum. Thrombophlebitis of subcutaneous vein with surrounding inflammatory reaction in adipose tissue. × 30.

allergic vasculitis, etc., as separate entities. It is, however, now generally accepted that these are all variations on a single theme based on the deposition of immune complexes and complement in or around the vessel walls and the consequent Arthus-type inflammatory reaction. The majority of the small dermal vessels involved in this process are venous channels and it therefore seems appropriate to use the term angiitis rather than the previously used term of arteritis.

These conditions must be distinguished from the small haemorrhagic areas of bleeding into the skin (purpura) seen in association with increased venous pressure (stasis) or in deficiency states such as scurvy. In such cases histological examination will show merely extravasation of red cells into the dermis with perhaps some swelling of the capillary endothelium. Later the red cells disintegrate and collections of haemosiderin-laden macrophages indicate the site of previous haemorrhage.

In true angiitis there are conspicuous changes both in the vessel wall and in the tissues surrounding the vessels. The cutaneous lesions of angiitis tend to occur in dependent parts of the body where there is some slowing of the venous return. The lower limbs are particularly affected where, in addition to a certain amount of slowing of the venous return due to the site, there is further slowing of the blood flow due to cooling which increases the viscosity. The combination of slowing of the circulation and increased viscosity is thought to favour the deposition of immune complexes which initiate the pathological changes. In the early stage activation of complement by deposited immune complexes attracts neutrophil leukocytes in and around the walls of the small cutaneous vessels. Many of these neutrophils

disintegrate, releasing proteolytic enzymes which further damage the vessel wall. At this stage the endothelium is swollen and there is dense perivascular polymorphonuclear leukocytic infiltration which invades the vessel wall. Much nuclear dust is seen from the disintegrating polymorphs and at this stage the term *leukocytoclastic angiitis* is often used (Fig. 27.22). The damage to the vessel wall allows red cells to escape into the tissue (purpura) and deposition of various amounts of fibrin. The vessel wall finally undergoes necrosis and becomes surrounded by a mixture of fibrin and polymorphonuclear leukocytes (Fig. 27.23)— *necrotising angiitis*. Despite the extensive involvement of these small cutaneous vessels, ulceration of the overlying epidermis occurs only rarely (*purpura necrotica*). This immune complex angiitis may be seen following acute bacterial infections, adverse reactions to drugs, as a manifestation of systemic lupus erythematosus and as a cutaneous manifestation of visceral malignancy.

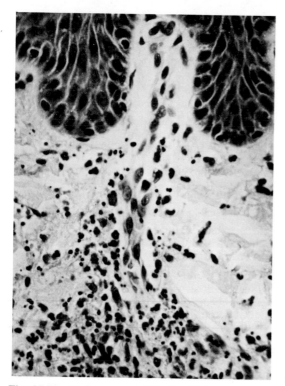

Fig. 27.22 Cutaneous angiitis. Small dermal vessel showing polymorphonuclear infiltration in and around the wall. × 350.

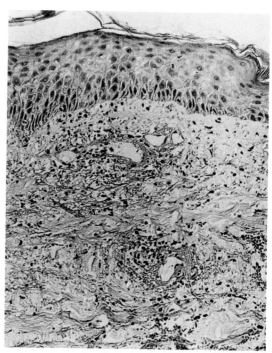

Fig. 27.23 Cutaneous angiitis showing fibrinoid necrosis of dermal vessels. There is haemorrhage under the epidermis and a marked perivascular inflammatory infiltrate. × 200.

Connective Tissue Diseases

Lupus erythematosus

Two basic types of this condition are recognised: (1) chronic discoid lupus erythematosus (CDLE), which is confined to the skin and is benign, and (2) systemic lupus erythematosus (SLE), in which visceral vascular lesions predominate (see p. 940) and which may be fatal, usually from renal involvement (p. 832). It may run its entire course without cutaneous manifestations. Intermediate forms between these extremes are encountered and transition from one type to another occurs, but is rare: the danger is increased if patients with chronic discoid lupus erythematosus receive drugs which cause photosensitivity.

Histologically, it is not usually possible to distinguish unequivocally between the two forms of lupus erythematosus, for many features are common to both. There is hyperkeratosis with plugging of follicular orifices (Fig. 27.24), liquefaction degeneration of the basal

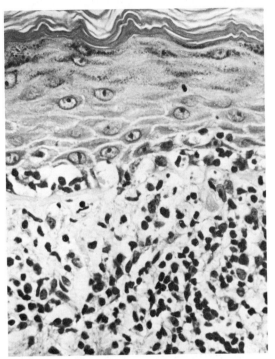

Fig. 27.25 Chronic discoid lupus erythematosus. Liquefaction degeneration of the basal layer of the epidermis. × 300.

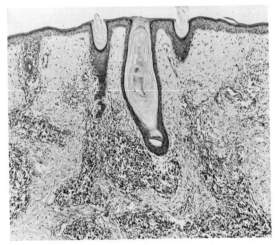

Fig. 27.24 Chronic discoid lupus erythematosus. Flattening of rete ridges, follicular plugging and focal lymphocytic infiltration of the dermis are seen. × 40.

layer and epidermal thinning (Figs. 27.25, 27.26). In the dermis there is lymphocytic infiltration, particularly around the dermal appendages, focal oedema and occasionally haemorrhages: colloid bodies may be present in the upper dermis. A diagnosis of lupus erythematosus should not be made in the absence

of liquefaction degeneration which, together with various degrees of the other features described, may provide a picture suggestive of the diagnosis. Similar findings may, however, be seen in lichen planus, and the clinical history and findings must be taken into account in interpreting a biopsy. Immunofluorescence tests are helpful in diagnosis and distinguishing between the two types of lupus erythematosus. In both conditions, direct IF tests (p. 1063) reveal in most cases granular deposition of immunoglobulin (usually IgG and IgM) and complement components in the vicinity of the basement membrane of *affected* skin. In most cases of SLE a positive result is observed also in areas of clinically *normal* skin from *exposed* areas, whereas such areas are negative in CDLE.

In SLE the LE-cell test (p. 940) is often positive, particularly in untreated patients with active disease, and antinuclear antibodies, usually in high titre, are almost always de-

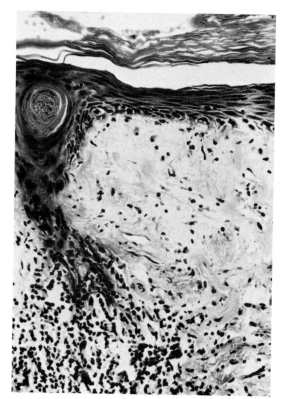

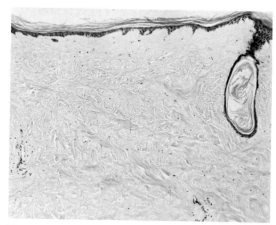

Fig. 27.27 Morphoea. Note the flattening of the rete ridges and the increase in thickness of the dermal collagen. Dermal appendages are absent. × 40.

Fig. 27.26 Systemic lupus erythematosus. Liquefaction degeneration of the basal layer with oedema and fibrinoid change in the collagen of the upper dermis. × 200.

monstrable by immunofluorescence. Rheumatoid factor is also sometimes present in SLE, 'standard' serological tests for syphilis (p. 220) often give (false) positive reactions, and occasionally auto-antibodies to red cells or platelets develop. Indeed, SLE is notable for the high incidence and variety of auto-antibodies (p. 164). In CDLE, the incidence of auto-antibodies is much lower.

Morphoea (scleroderma) and systemic sclerosis

Much confusion has been caused by the use of the term scleroderma to describe two different diseases, *morphoea* and *progressive systemic sclerosis*. Progressive systemic sclerosis (p. 941) is a generalised condition, involving the skin and other organs. Scleroderma should be used only as an alternative name for morphoea, which consists of areas of hardening of the skin and does not affect the viscera. Both are chronic

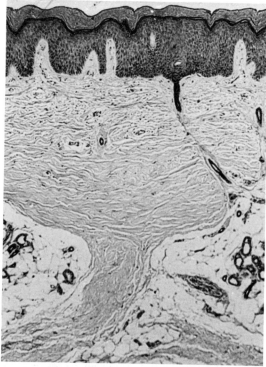

Fig. 27.28 Progressive systemic sclerosis. The microanatomy of the skin is maintained but the sweat glands and subcutaneous fat are much nearer the surface. Although from different regions of the skin, this figure and Fig. 27.26 are taken at the same magnification, illustrating the difference between systemic sclerosis and morphoea. × 40.

diseases, developing most often in the 3rd–5th decades, and affect both sexes.

Morphoea (scleroderma) consists of localised patches or larger areas of thickening and hardening of the skin. In the early stages, an erythematous halo is seen at the margin of the lesion. Microscopy shows thickening of the dermal collagen extending into the subcutaneous tissue, together with a light chronic inflammatory cellular infiltrate. The lesions spread for a variable period and then regress with depigmentation and thinning of the epidermis and loss of rete ridges, sweat glands and hair follicles and their surrounding fatty tissue (Fig. 27.27). The dermal collagen fibres appear swollen and coarse elastic fibres can be seen lying parallel with the surface.

Progressive systemic sclerosis. The picture is quite different from morphoea. It consists of atrophy of the skin and its appendages, but with maintenance of the normal architecture (Fig. 27.28), so that the appearances are those of 'skin in miniature'. Hardening of the skin does not occur unless infection and ulceration become superadded, with resultant fibrosis.

Granulomatous Diseases of the Skin

The skin is affected by many of the granulomatous diseases described in earlier chapters, notably tuberculosis, leprosy, sarcoidosis, syphilis, deep fungal infections and leishmaniasis. The skin is also exposed to injury, with lodgement of foreign material which stimulates a granulomatous reaction, as also does the escape of squames from ruptured 'sebaceous cysts' and fatty acids, etc. from dilated pilosebaceous follices in acne. Some of the skin diseases already described have a granulomatous component or result in chronic ulceration and secondary infection.

Three further granulomatous skin lesions, lupus vulgaris, granuloma annulare and necrobiosis lipoidica, require a brief description.

Lupus vulgaris. Tuberculosis of the skin is rare nowadays, but occasional examples of lupus vulgaris are still seen. It presents as one or more reddish-brown patches, usually on the skin of the face, in which small yellow-brown macules ('apple-jelly nodules') may be discerned by viewing the lesion through a glass slide pressed onto the skin. The nodules consist of well-defined tubercles with little or no caseation. The lesion lies in the dermis and often extends up to the epidermis through which it may eventually ulcerate. The condition progresses slowly and results in scarring with atrophy of the skin and disfigurement. Tubercle bacilli are rarely detectable in suitably stained histological sections.

Granuloma annulare and necrobiosis lipoidica. These two conditions form what are known as *palisading granulomas*. Granuloma annulare is seen mainly in children and young adults, as varying numbers of non-itchy, raised annular papules, often on the fingers and the backs of

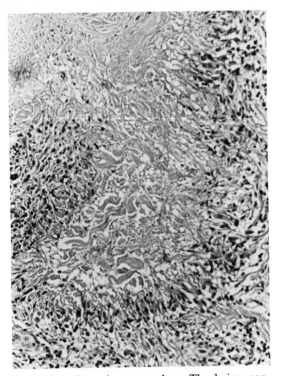

Fig. 27.29 Granuloma annulare. The lesion consists of a central acellular area of necrosis which is surrounded by a palisade of macrophages and, more peripherally, a mixture of chronic inflammatory cells. × 150.

the hands. It may also affect the subcutaneous tissue and is then closely similar to rheumatoid nodules (p. 918). Necrobiosis lipoidica has been associated traditionally with diabetes, but may also occur in non-diabetics. The lesions appear most often in the legs, as reddish patches which slowly spread and have a yellow centre. Scarring occurs and ulceration is occasionally seen.

In both conditions a central area of collagen degeneration is surrounded by an infiltrate of macrophages (Fig. 27.29). Multinucleated giant cells may be present and differentiation of the two conditions may depend on clinico-pathological correlation.

Lichen sclerosus et atrophicus. This is a dis-ease of unknown cause, affecting primarily the dermal connective tissue, and is conveniently described here. It is seen in the vulva as white patches which clinically may simulate malignancy, but it also occurs elsewhere in the skin in both sexes. Histological examination shows a characteristic picture of hyperkeratosis over a thinned epidermis which shows liquefaction degeneration of the basal layer. In typical cases, a split is seen at the epidermal–dermal interface, and the upper dermis has a pale hyaline appearance (Fig. 24.1, p. 942) with virtual absence of elastic fibres. A linear band of lymphocytes and histiocytes is present at the upper margin of the reticular dermis.

Lymphomas

The skin may be involved in both Hodgkin's disease and non-Hodgkin lymphomas. The histology of the skin lesions is that of the parent condition, except that the classical Reed–Sternberg cells of Hodgkin's disease are only rarely seen in the skin lesions. Non-specific pruritic eruptions may also occur during the course of Hodgkin's disease as well as in the leukaemias, but the histology is that of an inflammatory response and is not diagnostic. Occasionally leukaemic infiltration of the skin is the presenting feature of chronic leukaemias, but since pseudoleukaemic lesions may also occur in the skin from various causes, the diagnosis should not be made on skin histology alone.

Mycosis fungoides. Mycosis fungoides is a T-cell lymphoma which primarily involves the skin but after many years disseminates to lymph nodes and other organs in a high proportion of patients who do not die from other diseases. The characteristic histological changes may be preceded for many years by pruritic eruptions with non-specific histological appearances in which only an occasional atypical cell raises the suspicion of its true nature. Serial biopsies may be necessary before the histological diagnosis can be made despite strong clinical suspicion of mycosis fungoides.

During the second and third stages of the disease, i.e. the stages of induration of the skin and the development of nodules of tumour respectively, skin biopsy usually shows characteristic changes. These consist of infiltration of the upper dermis by atypical lymphoid cells which usually vary considerably in size, shape, staining characteristics, nuclear appearances and mitotic activity. The lesions may contain also variable numbers of lymphocytes, plasma cells, plasmacytoid cells, free red blood cells, macrophages and occasional neutrophil polymorphs. There is a tendency for these mononuclear cells to infiltrate the epidermis and accumulate within epidermolytic spaces. In

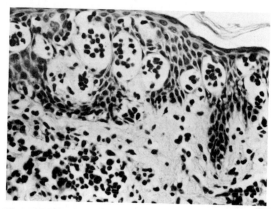

Fig. 27.30 Mycosis fungoides. Several Pautrier 'microabscesses' are seen in the epidermis. In the upper dermis there is a pleomorphic cellular infiltrate. × 265.

such situations they are known as 'Pautrier microabscesses' (Fig. 27.30), (a misnomer because they do not contain pus). While not invariably present, their presence is of considerable help in differentiating longstanding dermatitis from mycosis fungoides, and should always be sought by examination of multiple sections.

Tumours of the Skin

The skin is a large and complex organ in which the epidermal cells are labile and thus continuously dividing. They are also directly exposed to many carcinogenic agents in the environment and it is therefore not surprising that epithelial tumours are numerous. The skin is the site, above all others, where many malignant tumours which would otherwise prove fatal can be treated effectively by early detection and excision.

Skin tumours can be classified readily according to cell type. Epithelial tumours may arise from the epidermis, sweat glands or hair follicles: dermal tumours may arise from the fibrous, vascular, nervous or lymphoreticular elements and a third group arises from melanocytes. Some of the most important tumours, such as squamous carcinoma, have been dealt with already in Chapter 12 as local representatives of more general types, but many other tumours are peculiar to the skin.

Epidermal tumours

Embryological studies have revealed that the keratinocytes of the skin undergo specific differentiation at an early stage in development; three distinct cell lines are produced and form the surface epidermis, the pilo-sebaceous complexes and the sweat apparatus. This probably explains the differing biological behaviour of tumours arising from the epidermis and its appendages.

Two sharply distinct types of tumour arise from the surface epidermis, the *squamous group* and the so-called *basal-cell group* which includes basal-cell papilloma (verruca senilis) and basal-cell carcinoma (rodent ulcer). Tumours of the sweat glands form a heterogeneous group and are discussed later.

Basal-cell papilloma (verruca senilis) is a common benign warty growth seen most often on the trunk of older people. It appears as a

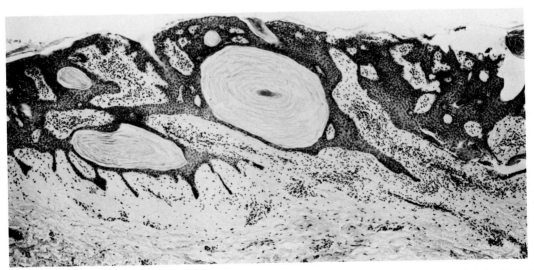

Fig. 27.31 Basal-cell papilloma. A flat papillary tumour composed of basal-like epidermal cells. Note the several 'pearls' of keratin formation within the epithelium. × 50.

soft, raised, flattened, sessile, brown patch, usually with a rough surface, Microscopically it consists chiefly of basal-like cells, with relatively little differentiation into keratinised cells unless irritated: keratin is however formed, often in fairly large amounts, characteristically in spherical masses (horn cysts) within the epithelium and sometimes reaching the surface (Fig. 27.31). Melanocytes are usually present among the basal-like cells and melanin is often abundant, accounting for the pigmentation which may cause clinical confusion with malignant melanoma. Mitoses are usually absent, growth is slow and malignancy so rare that cases can mostly be explained as coincidences or mistaken diagnoses. The name **seborrhoeic keratosis**, sometimes applied to these tumours, indicates their common occurrence on so-called seborrhoeic sites (forehead, chest and back).

'Squamous' group

These tumours consist of stratified squamous epithelium, and their mode of growth is clearly based on the ordinary process of growth of the epidermis. Neoplasia usually originates in the relatively undifferentiated basal cells, and the tumour cells show various degrees of differentiation towards squames. In the benign tumours, the undifferentiated basal layer is only one cell thick, and the differentiated cells and the keratin more conspicuous than in normal skin, but with increasing malignancy the undifferentiated cells become more numerous and keratin formation diminishes, though in skin tumours it hardly ever disappears altogether.

Squamous papilloma is the benign member of this group. Most are viral in origin, and seen usually on the hands of children (**juvenile warts**), on the soles of the feet of those who use communal changing-rooms (**plantar warts**), and about the genitalia of those exposed to venereal infection (**condylomata acuminata**). If one excludes viral tumours, and the keratoses dealt with in the next section, the squamous papillomas (Fig. 12.2, p. 323) are probably very rare. Malignant change in a skin papilloma is extremely rare, though occasionally genital tumours show an exuberant growth hard to distinguish from malignancy.

Squamous keratosis. This is the best name for the premalignant lesions of this group. When the aetiology is known, such terms as *actinic* or *arsenical keratoses* are commonly used, and in old people they may be called *senile keratoses*, but the lesions are identical. They are typically dry, rough-surfaced thickenings, arising usually in an area of skin which shows, by its thinness (Fig. 27.32), inelasticity and irregular pigmentation, the effects of pro-

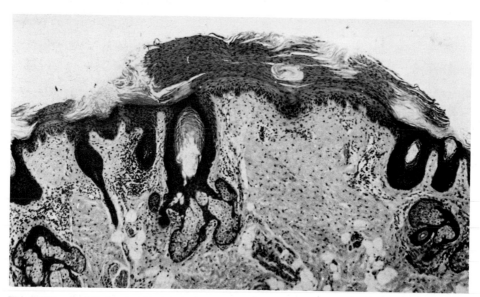

Fig. 27.32 Actinic keratosis, showing a patch of epithelial atrophy with dysplasia, hyperkeratosis and parakeratosis. × 25.

longed exposure to sunlight or other carcinogens: the face and the back of the hands are the usual sites.

Histologically one sees all stages from the slightest thickening and irregularity of the epidermis to large lesions with gross irregular hyperplasia of the epithelium, a massive overlying layer of keratin, and greatly enlarged rete ridges the cells of which appear to be on the brink of invasion. The hallmark of these lesions is the presence of alternating columns of hyperkeratosis and parakeratosis. Nuclear pleomorphism, frequency of mitoses and disordered, irregular cellular differentiation usually increase in parallel with the above changes. Sometimes, severe cytological changes occur in the presence of relatively minor general hyperplasia, and the term *carcinoma-in-situ* of the skin might reasonably include this condition.

Bowen's disease. Although this is an epidermal hyperplasia which may progress to squamous carcinoma, it is a very different lesion from squamous keratosis. It may arise anywhere in the skin, but nearly always in non-exposed areas. While squamous keratosis blends into surrounding skin, which is itself abnormal, Bowen's disease is sharply circumscribed from normal skin, forming rounded, reddish patches which spread slowly over a period of years. The epidermis in the affected area shows marked hyperplasia, with deep but fairly regular rete ridges and usually not much keratin: cellular de-differentiation is prominent, and large cells with multiple large clumped nuclei are a characteristic feature (Fig. 27.33). The importance of recognising Bowen's disease, which is another form of carcinoma-in-situ, is twofold. First, it may look like (and is often treated for years as) a patch of psoriasis or other chronic skin disease. Secondly, defective and irregular differentiation of the epidermis, which in a squamous keratosis showing carcinoma-in-situ would mean imminent invasion, in Bowen's disease is compatible with many years of continued limitation to the surface—even though ultimate invasion may occur.

Squamous carcinoma. The description of squamous carcinoma in Chapter 12, and the discussion on its aetiology in Chapter 11, make it unnecessary to say much of this important tumour of the skin. The great majority are better differentiated than the average mucosal squamous carcinoma: this, combined with accessibility, makes for a relatively good prognosis. Dissemination, when it does occur, is by the same routes of local, lymph and blood spread as with other carcinomas. It may arise anywhere on the body surface, but in most countries the face, the pinna of the ears and the backs of the hands are the commonest sites.

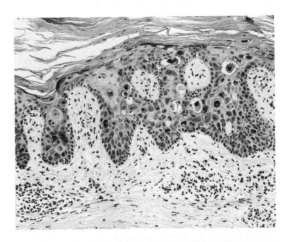

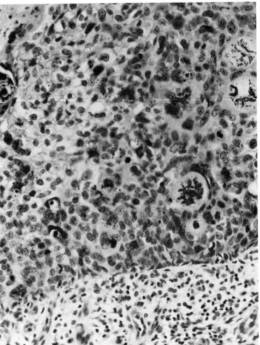

Fig. 27.33 Bowen's disease of the skin. *Above*, showing the large, abnormal cells in the epidermis. × 60. *Below*, showing more cellular detail, including enlarged and clumped nuclei and aberrant mitoses. × 160.

The muco-cutaneous junctions are also important sites, but the tumours mostly arise on the mucosal side of the junction: thus, most lip tumours arise from the red margin, most anal tumours within the canal, and most penile tumours from the glans. In the vulva, however, most squamous carcinomas arise in the true skin of the labia majora, the modified skin of the labia minora being a less common site.

The tumours of the exposed surfaces presumably arise chiefly from the effect of ultraviolet light in sunlight. Industrial exposure usually produces tumours of the hands and forearms, but with carcinogens which penetrate the clothes, such as the lighter mineral oils and dusts like soot (Fig. 11.5, p. 298) and powdered arsenic, the scrotum becomes an important site probably because its rugose surface traps dirt. The relation of circumcision to cancer is a particularly interesting one (p. 990). The majority of penile cancers are associated with an intact foreskin and a low standard of personal hygiene.

There is a small but clinically important group of squamous carcinomas which arise in areas of old scars caused by burns, at the edges of long-standing ulcers (the so-called *Marjolin's ulcer*) and in sinuses, presumably as a result of hyperplasia following prolonged attempts at healing.

Basal-cell carcinoma (rodent ulcer)

The typical basal-cell carcinoma begins as a slow-growing, flattened nodule of the skin of the face. The centre breaks down, forming a shallow ulcer, but the periphery of the nodule persists to form a smooth, slightly raised margin to the ulcer which, as the tumour grows, illustrates well the characteristic raised, 'rolled' edge of ulcerated malignant tumours. If not successfully treated, the ulcer spreads slowly, and ultimately erodes deeper and destroys the underlying structures of the face. Death results, if at all (for nowadays treatment is rarely so unsuccessful), from destruction of mouth and nose, or from invasion of the cranial cavity, most often via the orbit.

Neither lymph spread nor blood spread is seen except as the greatest of rarities. This is the only common malignant tumour other than those within the cranial cavity (where conditions are exceptional) which shows this extreme disinclination to metastasise, a finding that remains entirely unexplained.

Histologically, the tumour begins with groups of small dark basal-like cells, apparently sprouting from the undersurface of intact epidermis (Fig. 27.34). These cell groups

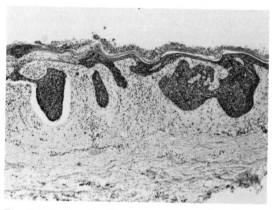

Fig. 27.34 Basal-cell carcinoma, showing the apparently multicentric origin from the base of the epidermis. × 32.

enlarge and grow down into the dermis, forming clumps with an outer layer of columnar cells which resemble the basal layer of the epidermis. Instead, however, of the keratinocytes which one would expect to see arising from this basal layer, the centre of each clump is occupied by a solid mass of darkly-staining spheroidal cells (Fig. 27.35). The term basal-cell carcinoma indicates the similarity of the tumour cells to the basal-cell layer of the surface epithelium, but should not be taken to imply that they originate from the basal layer of the surface epidermis.

Continued proliferation of the cell masses beneath the epidermis gives rise to a nodule: breakdown of the overlying epidermis and central part of the tumour results in ulceration and infection (Fig. 27.36). The characteristic rolled border is due to lateral invasion of the tumour under the intact epidermis.

The detailed histology of these tumours varies considerably, but the well-defined single peripheral columnar layer ('palisading'—one of several different uses of this word in pathology), and the predominance of 'basal' cells, are constant. The cell masses may be large and uniform, or narrow and ribbon-like. Small patches of squamous differentiation or even ker-atinisation may cause confusion with squamous carcinoma if one is not aware of their frequency in basal-cell carcinomas. Small cystic spaces form at times, some genuine, some the result of stromal degeneration. Inclusion of a few melanocytes from the original epidermis is common, and occasionally the tumour is sufficiently heavily pigmented to cause clinical confusion with melanoma. Little attention should be paid to the number of mitoses, which can be surprisingly numerous for such slowly-growing tumours. One variety meriting special mention is the sclerotic type, in which the stromal reaction to the tumour is unusually marked and small thin strands of epithelium are buried in dense fibrous tissue: this results in the edge being ill-defined and may lead to inadequate excision with consequent 'recurrence'.

Sites. Though they can be found anywhere on the skin (except the palms and soles) most basal-cell carcinomas occur in a relatively

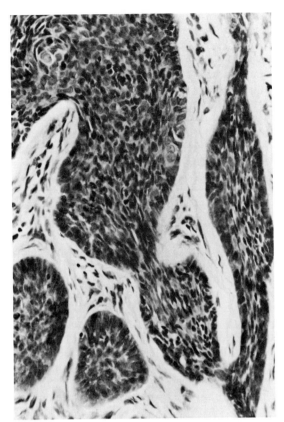

Fig. 27.35 Basal-cell carcinoma. The dermis is invaded by clumps of small, darkly-staining tumour cells resembling basal epidermal cells. The peripheral cells in places present a palisaded appearance. × 250.

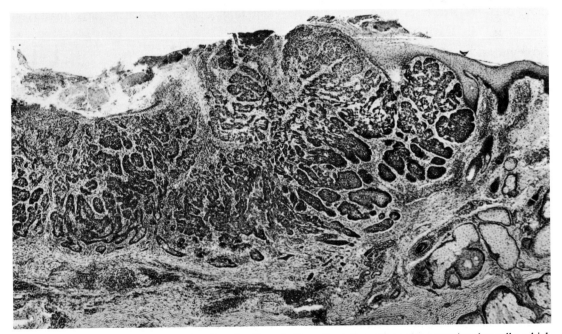

Fig. 27.36 Basal-cell carcinoma, showing the flat, shallow ulceration. Note the extension laterally which accounts for the 'rolled' border. × 33.

restricted area of the face, in front of the ears, above the mouth and below the supra-orbital ridges. In this area, sunlight produces far more basal-cell carcinomas than squamous carcinomas (in some parts of Australia it is the exception for a fair-skinned man to reach the age of 75 without having had at least one basal-cell carcinoma on the face). In other sites the reverse holds, and a radiation-induced basal-cell carcinoma of the trunk, for instance, or one arising in the margin of a varicose ulcer of the skin, is much less often seen than the corresponding squamous carcinoma.

Tumours of sweat glands (hidradenomas)

These form a distinct group of varied and often bizarre histological appearances but characteristically they exhibit a two-layered epithelium and show evidence of mucin secretion. Arising from the **eccrine sweat glands** are three main types: (1) from the intra-epidermal portion of the sweat duct, the *eccrine poroma*; (2) from the intradermal portion of the sweat duct, (*a*) the *nodular* and (*b*) the *tubular hidradenoma*. The nodular type (Fig. 27.37a) consists of solid masses and cords of cells containing an occasional duct-like structure containing mucin. The tubular type (Fig. 27.37b) consists of branching duct-like structures lined by a double

layer of epithelium and containing mucin embedded in a prominent fibrous stroma; (3) arising from the secretory coils, the *eccrine spiradenoma*. The majority of eccrine sweat gland tumours are benign although nodular hidradenomas may exhibit local invasion and recurrence after removal. True metastasising sweat gland tumours (hidradenocarcinomas) are rare. The **apocrine sweat glands** may also give rise to tumours, the commonest being the benign *hidradenoma papilliferum* of the vulva and the *cylindroma* or turban tumour of the scalp.

Tumours of pilo-sebaceous follicles

These are even less common than sweat gland tumours. True sebaceous adenomas are very rare. An uncommon tumour which probably arises in the hair matrix is the so-called '*benign calcifying epithelioma*' of Malherbe (pilomatricoma). This forms a slowly growing encapsulated rounded mass lying under the skin, arising anywhere on the body surface and at any age but most commonly in the first two decades. Calcification occurs in over 70 per cent and may be extensive and spectacular, sometimes with ossification. The tumour epithelial cells are small, darkly-staining and regular and form disproportionately large masses of

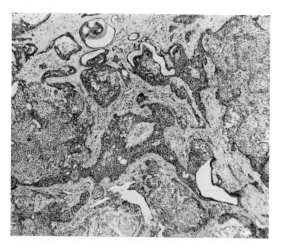 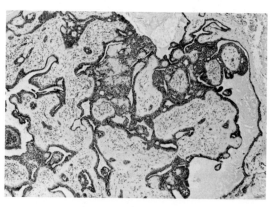

a   b

Fig. 27.37 Hidradenomas of intradermal sweat duct origin. **a.** Nodular hidradenoma, consisting of solid masses of pale-staining cells with occasional duct-like structures (which contain PAS-positive material). **b.** Tubular hidradenoma, showing the typical branching duct-like structures lined by two-layered epithelium and embedded in a hyaline stroma. × 30.

keratin in which ghosts of the cells that have formed it can often be seen. Rupture of the capsule may be followed by a foreign-body giant-cell reaction, which appears to predispose to the calcification, although direct calcification of ghost-cell areas of keratin in the intact tumour may also occur.

Molluscum sebaceum (kerato-acanthoma). This tumour-like but self-healing lesion is much commoner than any of the true hair follicle tumours. It occurs predominantly on the face of adults. A nodule in the skin appears and grows rapidly for about eight weeks, producing a rounded, slightly umbilicated mass of 10–20 mm diameter (Fig. 27.38). It stops growing, the central dimple enlarges and becomes dry and scaly, the central plug is discharged and the lesion heals: the whole process usually takes about six months.

Histologically, the resemblance to squamous carcinoma is very close during the active phase, so much so that it was only after 1950 that it won general recognition as a distinct lesion which did not require to be treated as a car-

cinoma. The appearances which mimic invasion are, however, the result of rapid irregular overgrowth of a group of hair follicles (Fig. 27.39).

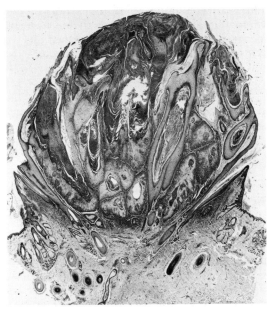

Fig. 27.39 Molluscum sebaceum. A lesion about the same age as Fig. 27.38. Note the resemblance to squamous carcinoma. × 12.

During the stationary phase, the epithelium so formed is progressively keratinised, and the resulting mass of keratin is finally discharged. Recognition of this lesion is obviously of great importance in treatment. An important diagnostic feature is the superficial nature of the lesion, well seen in Fig. 27.38: the apparently invasive deep surface lies at or above the level of the skin appendages. In the later stages, polymorphs migrate into the epithelial masses, a feature not usual in squamous carcinoma. It is important to examine histologically the edge of the lesion, which shows abrupt transition from normal to the hyperplastic epithelium. These features are of value in distinguishing the lesion from squamous carcinoma, although this is not always possible even when the clinical history is taken into account.

Self-healing squamous-cell carcinoma of the skin. This is a rare familial disorder, first described by Shaw Dunn and Ferguson Smith. It begins usually in early adult life, and is characterised by the appearance at intervals of tumours of the skin, mostly, but not exclusively, of

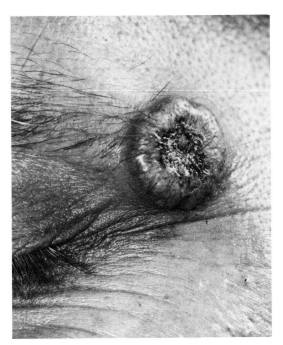

Fig. 27.38 Molluscum sebaceum. Clinical photograph of an eight-week-old lesion near the eye. A firm rounded nodule with epidermis stretched over the edge, and a central crater where the keratin core is exposed. × 1·5.

the exposed parts, which are indistinguishable histologically from squamous-cell carcinomas (Currie and Ferguson Smith, (1952). After some months of activity, each lesion in succession undergoes involution by keratinisation of the infiltrating columns of cells and discharge of the dead cells leaving shallow depressed pits. It is quite unrelated to molluscum sebaceum.

Melanocytic tumours

The following account attempts to give a clear if somewhat oversimplified explanation of a complex series of phenomena, interpretation of which is still controversial.

Early in fetal life specialised cells migrate from the neural crest and settle in the skin, the uveal tract of the eye and the leptomeninges, in which sites they are known as melanocytes. Melanocytic tumours arise from these cells. Those melanocytes which migrate to the skin come to lie among the basal cells of the epidermis in the ratio of 1 : 10 to 1 : 5, depending on the anatomical site. The number of melanocytes per unit area of skin is constant irrespective of race or skin coloration.

Occasionally some melanocytes fail to reach the epidermis, developing within the dermis to form a Mongolian spot or a more compact mass termed a blue naevus (p. 1083).

During infancy, the balance between the normal ratio of melanocytes to basal epidermal cells breaks down at a few or many sites: the melanocytes multiply too rapidly and become too numerous to be accommodated in their normal position. The lesions resulting from this proliferation of melanocytes are known as pigmented naevi. While precise details of the evolution of these lesions is not known, the probable course is shown in diagrammatic form in Fig. 27.40.

Initially the proliferating melanocytes replace the basal layer of the epidermis over a given area and at this stage the lesion is known as a *lentigo* (Fig. 27.40b). (This should not be confused with an ephilis or freckle, in which there is an increase in melanin pigmentation of the basal layer without an increase in the numbers of melanocytes). The next stage is more focal proliferation of the melanocytes and the formation of small nodules within the epidermis which bulge downwards into the dermis: this lesion is known as the *junctional naevus*

(Fig. 27.40c). Eventually the basement membrane is disrupted and some of the nodules or packets of melanocytes pass down into the dermis. At this stage, where there is a combination of junctional activity and nests of melanocytes in the dermis, the lesion is known as a *compound pigmented naevus* (Fig. 27.40d). The melanocytes which reach the dermis soon lose their melanin-synthesising enzymes, become smaller and lose the power to proliferate and are known as *naevus cells*. At or around puberty, in the majority of instances junctional activity ceases, the naevus cells in the dermis undergo further maturation and a certain amount of fibrosis occurs. At this stage the lesion is known as an *intradermal naevus* and may remain as such for life. (Fig. 27.40e).

While the above account is thought to represent the normal evolution of these lesions it should be emphasised that *maturation may be arrested at any of the stages described*. In addition, *similar stages of melanocytic proliferation may occur in adult life*, either after exposure to ultraviolet light or from as yet imperfectly understood hormonal changes.

The principal types of pigmented naevus are described below. They are extremely common lesions: few people have none at all and some have many: the mean number per person is said to be 18.

Lentigo. Clinically this presents as a flat blemish on any part of the skin surface, varying in colour from pale brown to deep black. *It is not possible to distinguish these lesions clinically with any certainty from junctional naevi*. Histologically one sees stretches of the basal layer of the epidermis replaced by melanocytes, which appear in fixed tissue sections as rounded cells with abundant clear cytoplasm. Many of the melanocytes contain varying amounts of fine granular brown melanin pigment. In the underlying dermis, macrophages containing coarser granules of darker melanin pigment are usually seen.

In older persons, on sun-exposed skin, a variant of the lentigo, the *lentigo maligna*, may be encountered (p. 1081).

Junctional pigmented naevus. As already stated, the clinical appearance of the junctional naevus is virtually indistinguishable from the lentigo. In older lesions, examined with a lens in a good light, small areas of darker speckled

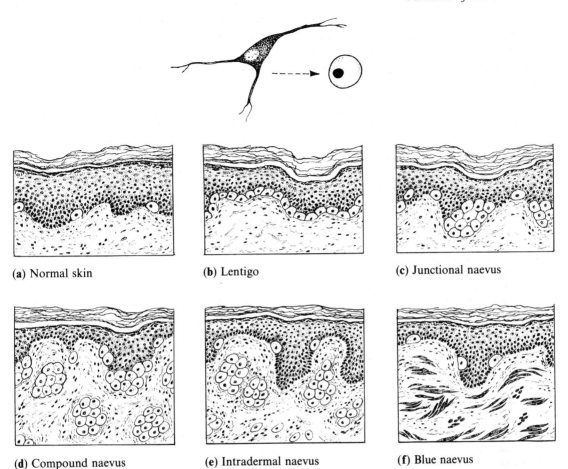

(a) Normal skin

(b) Lentigo

(c) Junctional naevus

(d) Compound naevus

(e) Intradermal naevus

(f) Blue naevus

Fig. 27.40 Diagram of the origin and evolution of pigmented naevi. At the top of the diagram the dendritic melanocyte, the cell of origin, is seen. Stained by the DOPA reaction, this has a triangular body with long branching processes (dendrites). In fixed tissue sections this cell appears rounded with clear cytoplasm. The distribution of melanocytes in normal skin is seen in (**a**). Replacement of the basal layer of the epidermis by melanocytes is the **lentigo** (**b**). Focal proliferation of melanocytes is the **junctional pigmented naevus** (**c**), and this proliferation at the dermo-epidermal junction is called **junctional change**. Some of these nodules descend into the dermis to become adult naevus cells and the combination of junctional change and intradermal naevus cells is the **compound pigmented naevus** (**d**). Junctional activity ceases and masses of mature naevus cells lie in the dermis, the **intradermal naevus** (**e**). Occasionally melanocytes en route from the neural crest may be arrested in the dermis where they form the **Mongolian spot or blue naevus** (**f**).

pigmentation, corresponding to the nests of junctional activity, can be detected.

Histologically the junctional naevus is composed of rounded aggregates (or packets) of melanocytes which, while occurring at any level of the epidermis, tend to be in the lower layers and to bulge down into the underlying dermis, giving the undersurface of the epidermis an irregular configuration (Fig. 27.41). It is this proliferation of melanocytes at the dermo-epidermal junction which gives the junctional naevus its name.

Compound pigmented naevus. This is the commonest type of pigmented naevus in late childhood. Clinically such lesions are usually raised above the surface: they may be papillomatous in appearance and vary in colour from pale brown to black. In some instances the hair follicles are increased in number and abnormally large, and various numbers of coarse dark hairs can be seen growing from the surface of the lesion. Rarely such hairy pigmented naevi may cover an extensive area of the skin surface (giant hairy naevus). Such cases may

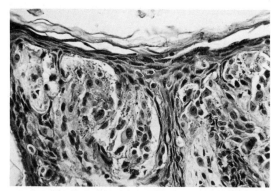

Fig. 27.41 Junctional pigmented naevus. Note the groups of melanocytes lying in the deeper part of the epidermis. × 200.

also be associated with diffuse meningeal melanomatosis and can undergo malignant transformation in childhood (see below).

Histologically compound naevi show junctional activity in the overlying epidermis. In the dermis are loose aggregates of rounded inactive-looking cells, some of which contain granules of melanin pigment. The deeper these cells lie in the dermis, the smaller they tend to be (Fig. 27.42). The cells are often called naevus cells but in order to avoid confusion with other naevi (e.g. angiomas) they should always be referred to as pigmented naevus cells. In the connective tissue of the dermis between the nests of pigmented naevus cells are found varying numbers of macrophages containing coarser granules of melanin pigment. The gross colour of pigmented naevi depends largely on the numbers and content of these macrophages.

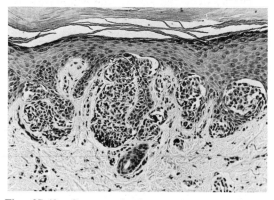

Fig. 27.42 Compound pigmented naevus. Some groups of proliferated melanocytes lie in the deeper part of the epidermis. Other groups have become separated from the epidermis and lie in the superficial dermis. × 100.

Juvenile melanoma. This variant of the benign compound pigmented naevus is important because it may easily be mistaken histologically for a malignant melanoma, especially if the age of the patient is not known. It is commonest in children although no age group is exempt. There is very extensive, active-looking junctional activity which may be of spindle cell type. This is associated with a more prominent intradermal component which may again contain many active-looking spindle cells. Associated histological features which are of considerable importance for diagnosis are pseudo-epitheliomatous hyperplasia and the presence of numerous large dilated vascular channels (Fig. 27.43). It is this latter feature which accounts for the reddish colour of these lesions to the naked eye.

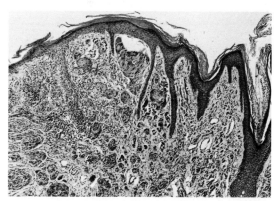

Fig. 27.43 Juvenile melanoma, showing junctional activity and extensive dermal infiltration. Note also the pseudo-epitheliomatous hyperplasia and dilated vascular channels. × 30.

Intradermal pigmented naevus. The vast majority of pigmented naevi in adults are of the intradermal type. Clinically these are similar in appearance to compound pigmented naevi, being sometimes raised and warty (Fig. 27.44), sometimes flat. Histologically there is no junctional activity in the epidermis although there may be an increase in the number of normal-looking melanocytes. The dermis is occupied by cells similar to those seen in the dermal component of the compound naevus (Fig. 27.45). In older lesions, particularly in the deeper parts, there is often considerable fibrosis and some of the nests of pigmented naevus cells merge imperceptibly into bundles of elongated cells which bear a close resemblance to neuri-

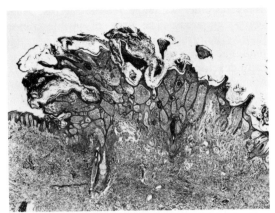

Fig. 27.44 Intradermal pigmented naevus of warty type. The dermal papillae are filled with naevus cells which extend widely in the underlying dermis. × 14.

lemmal cells or sensory nerve endings, both of which, like melanocytes, are of neural crest origin. Such appearances are of no practical significance.

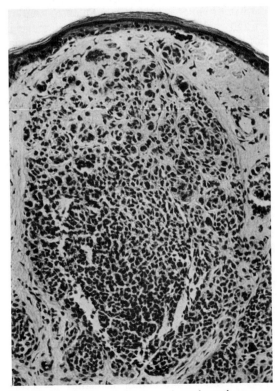

Fig. 27.45 Section through an intradermal naevus, showing collections of so-called 'naevus cells' underneath the epithelium. × 220.

Relationship of pigmented naevi to malignant melanoma

Malignant melanoma is exceedingly rare before puberty. The main exception to this is in the case of the giant hairy pigmented naevus, a significant number of cases of which have been reported where death resulted either from metastases from the skin or from diffuse meningeal melanomatosis.

After puberty any pigmented naevus with junctional activity has the potential to undergo malignant change, but the proportion of lesions which undergo such change must be extremely small as malignant melanoma is not a common tumour.

Histological assessment of a junctional naevous from an adult is often difficult, and multiple sections of a suspicious lesion should be examined. Features of the proliferated melanocytes which should raise the suspicion of malignancy include a high mitotic rate, a cell size appreciably larger than the adjacent keratinocytes and the presence of melanin pigment and aberrant melanocytes in the superficial part of the epidermis.

Prophylactic excision of all pigmented lesions in adults is clearly impractical and the clinical features which warrant complete excision and examination are given on p. 1083.

Malignant melanoma

This tumour, which arises from melanocytes, spreads locally and also by the lymphatics and blood to produce metastases. It arises in four main forms, described below.

Lentigo maligna or **Hutchinson's melanotic freckle** is a slowly growing, flat lesion of varying shades of brown, arising on the sun-exposed skin of the elderly. While this is essentially malignant melanoma *in situ*, it may be present for up to 20 years with different areas simultaneously developing and regressing. Over a period of observation the lesion may thus appear to move within the skin. Eventually invasive maligant melanoma may develop. Histologically the basal layer of the epidermis is replaced by dysplastic, pleomorphic melanocytes which have a high nuclear-cytoplasmic ratio, and which may aggregate to give collections of spindle-celled junctional activity (Fig. 27.46).

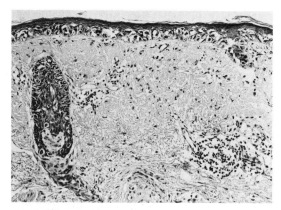

Fig. 27.46 Lentigo maligna. Melanocytes of variable appearance form a continuous deep layer in the epithelium and are seen also in the pilosebaceous unit. The dermis shows pronounced solar elastosis. × 30.

While there is little tendency to extend through the epidermis to the surface, the dysplastic melanocytes do extend into the skin appendages. Solar elastosis (degeneration and matting of the dermal elastic tissue) is always present. The areas of regression show various degrees of epidermal atrophy, upper dermal telangiectasia, fibroblastic reaction and melanin lying free or within macrophages. Invasive malignant melanoma arising on the basis of a lentigo maligna has a relatively good prognosis.

Superficial spreading melanoma. This is a slightly raised, variably coloured lesion which can occur anywhere on the skin. The colour varies from brown in actively melanogenic areas to blue, white or red in regressed and regressing areas. The area of visible abnormality is usually smaller than in lentigo maligna. Invasive malignant melanoma generally develops from superficial spreading melanoma *in situ* in 5 to 7 years. Histologically there is a population of dysplastic and pleomorphic melanocytes at the epidermal-dermal junction (Fig. 27.47): these cells spread through the epidermis rather like the carcinoma cells in Paget's disease (p. 983). The invasive tumour which results shows a variable histology but the cells often resemble epithelial cells. Diagnosis rests not on the invasive component but on the presence of abnormal melanocytes in the adjacent epidermis. Prognosis is worse than that for invasive melanoma arising in lentigo maligna, but somewhat better than that of nodular malignant melanoma.

Acral lentiginous and **mucosal melanomas.** These variants have recently been described as arising on the soles and palms and on mucosal surfaces respectively. They are characterised by melanocytic abnormality of the adjacent epidermis or mucosa which is similar to that of lentigo maligna except that actinic damage is not seen. The prognosis is similar to superficial spreading melanoma.

Nodular melanoma. The above three types of malignant melanoma are characterised by a clinically detectable phase of melanoma *in situ* ('horizontal growth phase') from which an invasive melanoma ('vertical growth phase') develops. In nodular malignant melanoma there

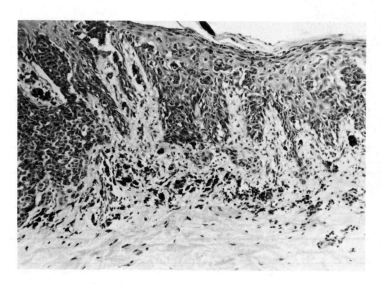

Fig. 27.47 Superficial spreading melanoma, showing proliferated dysplastic cells at the dermo-epidermal junction and in groups within the epidermis. On the left, invasion of the dermis has occurred. The black cells in the dermis are macrophages laden with melanin. × 80.

is neither clinical nor histological evidence of a horizontal growth phase. The invasive tumour apparently arises by transformation from a morphologically and numerically normal melanocyte population. The histology shows an epithelioid or spindle cell malignant melanoma (Fig. 27.48) with junctional activity confined to that area of epidermis immediately overlying the tumour. This variant carries the worst prognosis.

Other types of melanoma include the rare tumours which develop in congenital (bathing trunk) naevi and blue naevi. In some cases the patient presents with metastases and the primary tumour cannot be found.

The prognosis for patients with primary malignant melanoma is related to the depth of invasion of the tumour in the dermis, which may be assessed by comparison with the skin appendages (Clark, 1969) or by measuring the thickest part of the tumour (Breslow, 1970). The outlook is best when invasion is confined to the superficial dermis and worst when it has extended into the subcutaneous fat. Other morphological features which correlate with prognosis include the histogenetic types of melanoma (see above), the extent of ulceration, mitotic rate and local invasion of lymphatics.

Metastases occur commonly in the lymph nodes and also by blood spread, particularly to the liver, brain, lungs, bowel and bone marrow. Widespread metastases may also appear in the skin, where they differ from the primary tumour in the absence of junctional activity and of an inflammatory flare. Metastases from deeply pigmented primary melanoma sometimes produce little or no pigment.

Clinical features suggesting that a pigmented naevus or melanoma *in situ* has undergone aggressive change include alteration in colour, spreading of pigment to the adjacent skin, itching, bleeding, ulceration, increase in size and the development of satellite lesions. Such changes in character of a pigmented lesion in an adult warrant its excision and examination. Any new pigmented lesion developing after the age of 20 years should be regarded with suspicion and excised for histological assessment.

Blue naevus or 'melanophoroma'

In these lesions there are accumulations of deeply pigmented cells in the dermis (Fig. 27.40f). These are melanocytes in the sense that they produce melanin: they correspond to no normal human cell but have some homology with the frog melanophores—hence the alternative name. The lesions are blue in colour as a result of an optical effect due to their depth beneath the surface. Occasionally elements of blue naevi and ordinary pigmented naevi occur together in one tumour (the '**combined naevus**'), producing a very confusing histological picture. Malignancy in blue naevi is very rare.

Dermal tumours

With a few exceptions, these are less common and less important than the epithelial tumours. They are, however, too numerous in variety for any systematic treatment here and what follows consists only of notes on some of the more interesting kinds. Reference should be made to Chapter 13

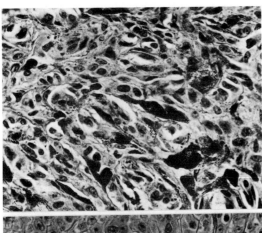

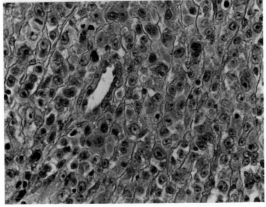

Fig. 27.48 Examples of nodular melanoma, illustrating the wide range of morphology. *Above*, a large spindle-celled tumour with abundant melanin production. *Below*, a tumour of epithelioid appearance with no obvious melanin production in this field. × 250.

for fibromas (p. 341), lipomas (p. 344) and angiomas (p. 348) and their variants, which include several important skin tumours. Neurofibromas will be found in Chapter 20 (p. 793). Lymphoid tumours and their precursors have been mentioned earlier in this Chapter (p. 1070).

The sclerosing angioma/dermatofibroma group

This group contains at least three seemingly distinct tumours (or apparent tumours) which often show transitions. However, it is likely, but not certain, that they are stages of a single process. The name *subepidermal nodular fibrosis* may be used for the whole group.

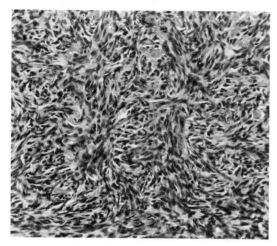

Fig. 27.49 Sclerosing angioma, showing the characteristic whorled pattern, with inconspicuous capillaries. × 154.

The process begins with a hypothetical *angioma*, perhaps too small to be clinically evident. This may undergo, as a result of trauma, a brief phase of haemorrhage and endothelial cell proliferation. The result is a brownish protruding mass, the so-called *sclerosing angioma*, which may reach 25 mm in diameter, though 10–15 mm is more usual, and which may readily be mistaken clinically for a malignant melanoma. Histologically, it shows dense masses of proliferating endothelial cells with numerous but inconspicuous angiomatoid vessels (Fig. 27.49) and numerous histiocytes and giant cells containing haemosiderin and lipid, both derived presumably from break down of erythrocytes.

Left alone, these lesions regress, most of the endothelial cells and the haemosiderin disappear and one is left with a collagenous nodule in the dermis containing numerous lipid-laden macrophages: this stage is called a *histiocytoma*.

Finally, the macrophages also disappear, and the result is a fibrous nodule, a *dermatofibroma*. Like its predecessors, this is a benign lesion, and commonest on the limbs. They can usually be readily distinguished from true fibromas: in the earlier stages by the persistence of some macrophages, in the later stages by very low cellularity and a general pattern suggesting rather a thickening or distortion of the dermis than new fibroblastic proliferation.

True fibroma of the dermis is very rare, but confusion is possible not only with dermatofibroma but with neurofibroma.

Dermatofibrosarcoma protuberans

Fibrosarcoma of the skin is represented by this lesion, which arises usually *de novo* from the skin of the trunk. It has the histology of any low-grade fibrosarcoma, and when small a characteristic hour-glass shape, with a base in the dermis and two nodules, one superficial pressing the epidermis outwards (hence 'protuberans') and one larger invading the deeper tissues. It is slow growing and rarely metastasises but recurs persistently after any but the most ruthless excision.

References

Breslow, A. (1970). Thickness, cross-sectional areas and depth of invasion in the prognosis of cutaneous melanoma. *Annals of Surgery* **172**, 902–8.

Clark, W. H. Jr., From, L., Bernadino, E. A. and Mihm, M. C. Jr. (1969). The histogenesis and biological behaviour of primary human malignant melanomas of the skin. *Cancer Research* **29**, 705–27.

Currie, A. R. and Ferguson Smith, J. (1952). Multiple primary spontaneously-healing squamous-cell carcinomata of the skin. *Journal of Pathology and Bacteriology*, **64**, 827–39.

McGovern, V. J., Mihm, M. C., Bailly, C., Booth, J. C., Clark, W. H., Cochran, A. J., Hardy, E. G., Hicks, J. D., Levene, A., Lewis, M. G., Little, J. H. and Milton, G. W. (1973). The classification of malignant melanoma and its histological reporting. *Cancer* **32**, 1446–57.

Further Reading

Ackerman, A. Bernard (1978). *Histologic Diagnosis of Inflammatory Skin Diseases*, pp. 863. Lea and Febiger, Philadelphia.

Lever, W. F. and Schaumburg-Lever, Gundula (1975). *Histopathology of the Skin*, 5th edn., pp. 793. Lippincott, Philadelphia.

Milne, J. A. (1972). *An Introduction to the Diagnostic Histopathology of the Skin*, pp. 362. Edward Arnold, London.

Montgomery, H. (1967). *Dermapathology* (2 vols.). Hoeber Medical Division, Harper and Row.

Pinkus, H. and Mehregan, A. H. (1976). *A Guide to Dermatohistopathology*, 2nd edn., pp. 724. Appleton–Century–Crofts, New York.

Index